Musculoskeletal Assessment
in Athletic Training and Therapy

Matthew R. Kutz, PhD, ATC, CSCS
Professor
School of Human Movement, Sport, and Leisure Studies
College of Education and Human Development
Bowling Green State University
Bowling Green, Ohio

Andrea E. Cripps, PhD, ATC
Associate Professor
School of Human Movement, Sport, and Leisure Studies
College of Education and Human Development
Bowling Green State University
Bowling Green, Ohio

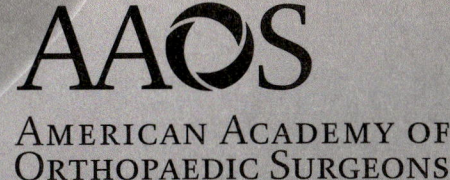

AAOS
AMERICAN ACADEMY OF ORTHOPAEDIC SURGEONS

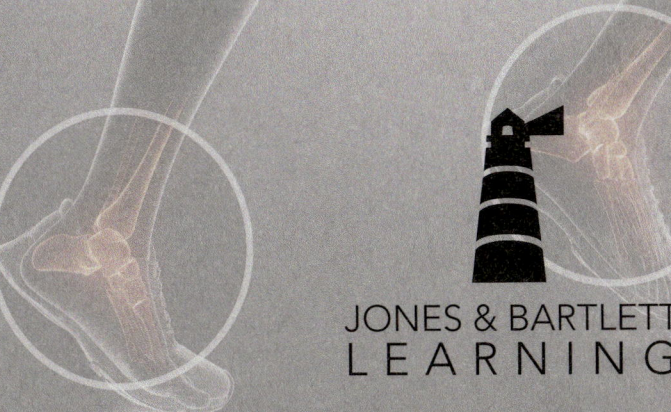

JONES & BARTLETT LEARNING

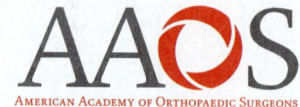

World Headquarters
Jones & Bartlett Learning
5 Wall Street
Burlington, MA 01803
978-443-5000
info@jblearning.com
www.jblearning.com

2020–2021 AAOS Board of Directors:
President: Joseph A. Bosco, III, MD, FAAOS
First Vice President: Daniel K. Guy, MD, FAAOS
Second Vice President: Felix H. Savoie, III, MD, FAAOS
Treasurer: Alan S. Hilibrand, MD, MBA, FAAOS
Past President: Kristy L. Weber, MD, FAAOS
Chair BOC: Thomas S. Muzzonigro, MD, FAAOS
Chair-Elect BOC: Wayne A. Johnson, MD, FAAOS
Secretary BOC: Claudette M. Lajam, MD, FAAOS
Chair BOS: C. Craig Satterlee, MD, FAAOS
Chair-Elect BOS: Kevin D. Plancher, MD, MPH, MS, FAAOS
Secretary BOS: Alexandra E. Page, MD, FAAOS

Lay Member: James J. Balaschak
Member at Large: Matthew P. Abdel, MD, FAAOS
Member at Large: James R. Ficke, MD, FAAOS
Member at Large: Rachel Y. Goldstein, MD, MPH, FAAOS
Member at Large: Alexander Vaccaro, MD, MBA, PhD, FAAOS
Ex-Officio: Thomas E. Arend, Jr., Esq., CAE

Editorial Credits:
Chief Education Strategist: Anna Salt Troise, MBA
Director, Publishing: Hans J. Koelsch, PhD
Senior Manager, Editorial: Lisa Claxton Moore
Senior Editor: Steven Kellert

Jones & Bartlett Learning books and products are available through most bookstores and online booksellers. To contact Jones & Bartlett Learning directly, call 800-832-0034, fax 978-443-8000, or visit our website, www.jblearning.com.

Substantial discounts on bulk quantities of Jones & Bartlett Learning publications are available to corporations, professional associations, and other qualified organizations. For details and specific discount information, contact the special sales department at Jones & Bartlett Learning via the above contact information or send an email to specialsales@jblearning.com.

Copyright © 2022 by The American Academy of Orthopaedic Surgeons

All rights reserved. No part of the material protected by this copyright may be reproduced or utilized in any form, electronic or mechanical, including photocopying, recording, or by any information storage and retrieval system, without written permission from the copyright owner.

The content, statements, views, and opinions herein are the sole expression of the respective authors and not that of Jones & Bartlett Learning, LLC. Reference herein to any specific commercial product, process, or service by trade name, trademark, manufacturer, or otherwise does not constitute or imply its endorsement or recommendation by Jones & Bartlett Learning, LLC and such reference shall not be used for advertising or product endorsement purposes. All trademarks displayed are the trademarks of the parties noted herein. *Musculoskeletal Assessment in Athletic Training and Therapy* is an independent publication and has not been authorized, sponsored, or otherwise approved by the owners of the trademarks or service marks referenced in this product.

There may be images in this book that feature models; these models do not necessarily endorse, represent, or participate in the activities represented in the images. Any screenshots in this product are for educational and instructive purposes only. Any individuals and scenarios featured in the case studies throughout this product may be real or fictitious, but are used for instructional purposes only.

The procedures and protocols in this book are based on the most current recommendations of responsible medical sources available at the time of publication. The American Academy of Orthopaedic Surgeons and the publisher, however, make no guarantee as to, and assume no responsibility for, the correctness, sufficiency, or completeness of such information or recommendations. Other or additional safety measures may be required under particular circumstances. Clinicians should use their own, independent medical judgment, in addition to open discussion with the patient, when developing patient care recommendations and treatment plans.

This textbook is intended solely as a guide to the appropriate procedures to be employed when rendering emergency care to the sick and injured. It is not intended as a statement of the standards of care required in any particular situation, because circumstances and the patient's physical condition can vary widely from one emergency to another. Nor is it intended that this textbook shall in any way advise emergency personnel concerning legal authority to perform the activities or procedures discussed. Such local determination should be made only with the aid of legal counsel.

15227-2

Production Credits
VP, Product Management: Amanda Martin
Director of Product Management: Cathy L. Esperti
Product Manager: Sean Fabery
Content Strategist: Andrew Labelle
Content Strategist: Carol Guerrero
Content Coordinator: Elena Sorrentino
Manager, Project Management: Lori Mortimer
Project Specialist: Kathryn Leeber
Director of Marketing: Andrea DeFronzo

VP, Manufacturing and Inventory Control: Therese Connell
Composition: Exela Technologies
Cover and Text Design: Michael O'Donnell
Senior Media Development Editor: Troy Liston
Rights Specialist: Rebecca Damon
Cover Image: (Main Image and Title Page) © CLIPAREA l Custom media/Shutterstock; (Background Image and Chapter Opener) © Sbayram/E+/Getty Images
Printing and Binding: LSC Communications

Library of Congress Cataloging-in-Publication Data
Names: Kutz, Matthew R., author. | Cripps, Andrea, author. | American Academy of Orthopaedic Surgeons, issuing body.
Title: Musculoskeletal assessment in athletic training and therapy / Matthew R. Kutz, Andrea Cripps.
Description: First edition. | Burlington, MA : Jones & Bartlett Learning, [2022] | Includes bibliographical references and index.
Identifiers: LCCN 2019050630 | ISBN 9781284151923 (paperback)
Subjects: MESH: Musculoskeletal System–injuries | Athletic Injuries–diagnosis | Physical Examination–methods
Classification: LCC RD97 | NLM WE 141 | DDC 617.1/027–dc23
LC record available at https://lccn.loc.gov/2019050630

6048

Printed in the United States of America
24 23 22 21 20   10 9 8 7 6 5 4 3 2 1

Brief Contents

Preface	viii
Acknowledgments	xi
About the Authors	xii
Contributors	xiii
Reviewers	xiv

UNIT I — Foundations — 1

- **CHAPTER 1** Taxonomy of Injury Pathology and Classifications 3
- **CHAPTER 2** The Examination Process 17
- **CHAPTER 3** Evidence-Based Injury Evaluation 29
- **CHAPTER 4** Diagnostic Imaging for Musculoskeletal Injuries 41

UNIT II — Lower Extremity Evaluation — 55

- **CHAPTER 5** Foot and Ankle 57
- **CHAPTER 6** Knee Joint 127
- **CHAPTER 7** Hip and Thigh 163

UNIT III — Upper Extremity Evaluation — 213

- **CHAPTER 8** Wrist and Hand 215
- **CHAPTER 9** Elbow 273
- **CHAPTER 10** Shoulder 337
- **CHAPTER 11** Abdomen and Thorax 413

Brief Contents

| CHAPTER 12 | **Spine** | 503 |
| CHAPTER 13 | **Head and Face** | 579 |

Index   **621**

Contents

Preface viii
Acknowledgments xi
About the Authors xii
Contributors xiii
Reviewers xiv

UNIT I Foundations 1

CHAPTER 1 Taxonomy of Injury Pathology and Classifications 3
Matthew R. Kutz, PhD, ATC, CSCS

Introduction 3
Introduction to Medical Terminology 4
Anatomic Reference Points 4
The Role of Disablement Models in the Evaluation Process 5
Categorizations of Physical Maturity 9
Categorizations of Injury 10
Common MOIs 10
Determining the Severity of Injuries 11
Summary 14
Critical Thinking Questions 14
Pearls and Pitfalls 15
References 15

CHAPTER 2 The Examination Process 17
Matthew R. Kutz, PhD, ATC, CSCS

Introduction 17
History 18
Inspection 19
Palpation 20
Special Tests 20
Record-Keeping Format (SOAP Notes) 26
On-Field and Emergency Evaluations 26
Summary 28

Critical Thinking Questions 28
Pearls and Pitfalls 28
Reference 28

CHAPTER 3 Evidence-Based Injury Evaluation 29
Jenny L. Toonstra, PhD, ATC, LAT

Introduction 29
Diagnostic Accuracy in the Evaluation Process 31
Summary 38
Critical Thinking Questions 39
Pearls and Pitfalls 39
References 39

CHAPTER 4 Diagnostic Imaging for Musculoskeletal Injuries 41
Andrea E. Cripps, PhD, ATC

Introduction 41
Diagnostic Imaging 41
Summary 53
Critical Thinking Questions 54
Pearls and Pitfalls 54
References 54

UNIT II Lower Extremity Evaluation 55

CHAPTER 5 Foot and Ankle 57
Christine Waters-Banker, PhD, ATC
Nicole Lounsberry Yates, MS, ATC, LAT

Introduction 57
Clinical Anatomy 58
Overview of Radiology and Imaging 84
Evaluation of the Foot and Ankle Joint ... 86
Pathologies of the Foot and Ankle 100

v

Critical Thinking Questions 124
Pearls and Pitfalls 124
References 124

CHAPTER 6 Knee Joint 127
Kaitlyn Shank, MEd, ATC, CCRP
Joseph M. Hart, PhD, ATC, FACSM, FNATA

Introduction 127
Clinical Anatomy 128
Overview of Radiology and Imaging 136
Evaluation of the Knee 138
Pathologies of the Knee 141
Summary 156
Critical Thinking Questions 160
Pearls and Pitfalls 160
References 161

CHAPTER 7 Hip and Thigh 163
Maureen K. Dwyer, PhD, ATC

Introduction 163
Clinical Anatomy 163
Overview of Radiology and Imaging 183
Evaluation of the Hip 184
Common Hip Pathologies 191
Muscle Injuries 199
Intra-articular Pathology 200
Snapping Hip Syndrome 201
Piriformis Syndrome 202
Hip Pointer 203
Stress Fractures 204
Pediatric Hip Diseases 204
SI Joint Pathology 205
Quick Tips for Evaluations for Pathology . . . 206
Critical Thinking Questions 208
Pearls and Pitfalls 208
References 208

UNIT III Upper Extremity Evaluation 213

CHAPTER 8 Wrist and Hand 215
Sara D. Rynders, MPAS, PA-C

Introduction 215
Clinical Anatomy 215
Overview of Radiology and Imaging 219
Evaluation of the Hand and Wrist 224
Conditions Causing Radial-Side Wrist Pain . . . 227
Conditions Causing Ulnar-Side Wrist Pain 240
Conditions of the Hand and Fingers 251
Finger PIP Joint Injuries 257
Finger Tendon Injuries: Jersey Finger
  and Mallet Finger 262
Critical Thinking Questions 270
Pearls and Pitfalls 270
References 271

CHAPTER 9 Elbow 273
Natalie L. Myers, PhD, ATC, PES
Aaron D. Sciascia, PhD, ATC, PES, SMTC

Introduction 273
Clinical Anatomy 274
Overview of Radiology and Imaging 288
Evaluation of the Elbow 289
Pathologies of the Elbow 294
Special Tests 309
Orthopaedic Special Tests 316
Summary 329
Critical Thinking Questions 331
Pearls and Pitfalls 331
References 331

CHAPTER 10 Shoulder 337
Mark R. Lafave, PhD, CAT(C)
Breda H.F. Eubank, PhD, CAT(C)

Introduction 337
Clinical Anatomy 338
Overview of Radiology and Imaging 355
Evaluation of the Shoulder 356
Common Shoulder Pathologies 360
Large Muscle Strains and Tears 390
Quick Tips for Evaluations for Pathology . . . 392
Critical Thinking Questions 408
Pearls and Pitfalls 408
References 408

CHAPTER 11 Abdomen and Thorax 413
Mikaela Boham, EdD, LAT, ATC

Introduction 413
Unique/Special History Questions 414

Observation 417	Pearls and Pitfalls 566
Palpation. 419	References 566
Muscles Used for Breathing 440	Appendix 12.A: Oswestry Low Back Pain Disability Questionnaire 572
Injury Conditions to the Thorax and Abdomen 441	Appendix 12.B: Neck Disability Index 574
Physical Activity Readiness Questionnaire (PAR-Q) 477	Appendix 12.C: Patient-Specific Functional Scale 576
Special Tests 477	Appendix 12.D: The Roland-Morris Disability Questionnaire 577
Orthopaedic Special Tests. 487	
Summary 497	
Critical Thinking Questions 498	
Pearls and Pitfalls 499	
References 499	

CHAPTER 12 Spine 503

Thomas G. Palmer, PhD, ATC, CSCS*D, TSAC
Andrea E. Cripps, PhD, ATC
Sara Stiltner, EdD, ATC

Introduction 503	
Clinical Anatomy 504	
Overview of Radiology and Imaging 521	
Evaluation of the Spine 521	
Common Spine Pathologies 537	
Summary 564	
Critical Thinking Questions 565	

CHAPTER 13 Head and Face 579

Johna K. Register-Mihalik, PhD, LAT, ATC, FACSM

Introduction 579	
Clinical Anatomy 579	
Overview of Radiology and Imaging 588	
Evaluation of the Head and Face 589	
Common Pathologies of the Head and Face 596	
Critical Thinking Questions 611	
Pearls and Pitfalls 611	
References 611	
Appendix 13.A: Sport Concussion Assessment Tool-5 613	

Index 621

Preface

Welcome to *Musculoskeletal Assessment in Athletic Training and Therapy*. As the title states, this text was written for students in professional athletic training and therapy programs as well as practicing clinicians. Musculoskeletal assessment is a foundation to sound clinical practice and an essential skill of a clinician. As the scope of practice for athletic trainers and therapists expands, being able to apply different musculoskeletal assessment techniques that inform an accurate clinical diagnosis becomes critical. With that goal in mind, this book attempts to address Domain 2 of the Board of Certification (BOC) *Practice Analysis, Seventh Edition*. Domain 2: Examination, Assessment, and Diagnosis, requires implementing systematic and evidence-based assessments that help to formulate a clinical diagnosis and an appropriate plan of care. Ultimately, developing the skills required to make a clinical diagnosis is needed to work interprofessionally and is central to offering the best plan of care for our patients regardless of practice setting.

Structure of the Text

As one might expect, this text includes instruction and examples on performing many common assessment techniques, such as goniometry for range of motion, manual muscle testing, neurovascular screens, and diagnostic imaging. To help with this, easy-to-use and -reference graphs, tables, pictures, images, and detailed descriptions are included. The chapters in this text are organized in a logical sequence and follow the HIPS (history, inspection, palpation, and special tests) systemic process of evaluation and assessment.

Although this text has many of the traditional and requisite aspects, it also includes a decidedly unique approach in that much of the content is formatted into tables. For example, there are narrative descriptions of many common joint laxity tests and other evaluation procedures, but much of the detail is presented in tabular format to allow the reader to quickly and easily reference key information.

Another unique and fun feature of this text is the personality that each expert author brings to his or her respective chapter. Although each chapter follows a general and obvious sequence, the way in which the content in each chapter is presented is unique. This was intentionally allowed to ensure that the authors were comfortable with his or her content and how he or she believes it should be presented and taught in the classroom. It is also a bold attempt to help the student understand the interprofessional aspect of clinical practice and specifically musculoskeletal assessment.

Approach

The authors of this text come from various places within the United States and Canada and, consequently, have differing scopes of practice, some with entirely different philosophies on the processes of examination. Furthermore, most authors are athletic trainers, but some are athletic therapists. Still others are physician assistants. This means different clinical experiences, different education, different scopes of practice, and different credentialing processes. With such a rich diversity of authors and varied backgrounds, it would be contrived and disingenuous to create a cookie-cutter outline to each chapter. After many conversations with editors, authors, and publishing partners (Jones & Bartlett Learning and the American Academy of Orthopaedic Surgeons), we are excited to let each author present the material in his or her own style and sequence. This allows you, the reader (student, clinician, and faculty), to assimilate multiple perspectives. For example, some authors are more formal, some are less formal, some prefer tables over narrative descriptions, and still others prefer narrative text for joint laxity tests with a summary table of all special tests at the end. All are thorough, detailed, and meaningful and present an accurate and viable approach to musculoskeletal assessment that the professional master's students can appreciate. It is our strong conviction that professional athletic training and therapy need to include this type of approach and this level of author diversity to cultivate expert clinicians who can accurately evaluate musculoskeletal pathology and integrate multiple perspectives on how that can be done.

Visual Walk-Through of This Text

Each chapter begins with an overview, learning objectives, and fun facts about the specific topic.

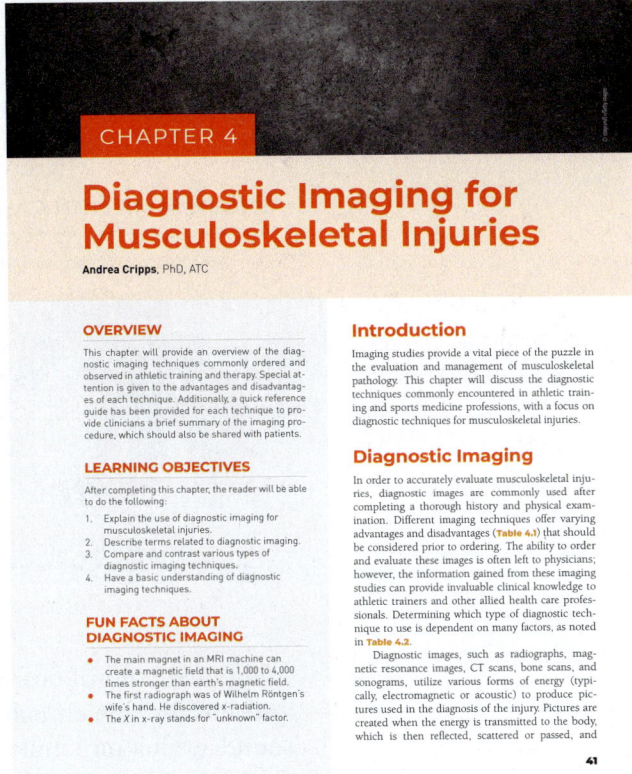

After the introductory content, there is a review of relevant clinical anatomy followed by evaluation techniques, common pathologies specific for each topic, and **Quick Tips for Evaluation** tables in several chapters.

Table 10.15 Humeral Fracture Quick Tips

Pathology	Description	Presentation (HIPS)	Special Tests/Imaging	Differential Diagnosis	5-Min Sideline Assessment Tips
Humeral fracture	This injury occurs as a result of significant upper body force or trauma.	A significant force is required to break this bone, so the sport or activity is important to note. Angulated fractures are relatively easy to discern, but stress fractures are less obvious. Aching and throbbing in the upper arm.	A percussion test at the distal end of the humerus may be useful clinically. Radiographs are confirmatory.	Glenohumeral impingement, rotator cuff pathology, long head of biceps brachii pathology, or triceps strain.	Feeling the continuity of the bony shaft compared to the opposite side can be useful.

HIPS, history, inspection, palpation, special tests.

Preface

Each chapter then concludes with a wrap-up that offers practical **Case Studies** with key questions and a **One-in-a-Million Case Study** that offers a look into a rare or unusual pathology.

CASE STUDY

This is a case presented by Butterwick et al.[91] related to a latissimus dorsi rupture. During the steer wrestling event at a rodeo performance, a professional steer wrestler reported to a member of the Canadian Professional Rodeo Sports Medicine Team with an injury to his right arm. In steer wrestling, the cowboy chases a steer while mounted on a horse, reaches down to grab its horns, drops down to the steer, and twists the steer to the ground. The mechanism of injury is similar to pectoralis major muscle strain in which the right shoulder was forced into abduction, external rotation, and horizontal abduction. During the twisting phase, the cowboy reported feeling a pop. He reported experiencing a burning sensation occurring at the superior aspect of the upper arm (ie, triceps brachii). Upon observation, the athletic therapist notices discoloration and swelling appearing over the back of the upper arm. An asymmetry was also noted over the posterolateral thorax. Active range of motion was full, but isometric testing was slightly limited in adduction and internal rotation. MRI was used to confirm the site and size of tear. The patient was successfully treated without surgery.

1. Are large muscles or muscle groups more or less susceptible to muscle tears?
2. What kinds of sports or activities have a large enough force to rupture large muscle groups?
3. What is a key history question the examiner should ask when he or she suspect a muscle rupture?
4. What does a defect in a muscle or tendon feel like and how would the examiner ensure he or she can find it?
5. Does a complete muscle rupture always have extreme pain associated with it?

ONE-IN-A-MILLION CASE STUDY

This is a case study presented by Lafave et al.[92] related to an AC joint sprain and concomitant first rib subluxation. The mechanism of injury is related to a cowboy falling off his horse and landing on the tip of his shoulder **(Figure 10.66)**. This is the same mechanism of injury as an AC joint sprain, and, in fact, the patient suffered a definitive AC joint sprain, based on his pain location. However, the unique aspect of this case had to do with the change in sensation or transient neurologic symptoms the patient complained about immediately. In addition to pain in the tip of his shoulder (ie, AC joint), he also complained of a jolt into his "pinky." Due to the fall from a height and the presence of neurologic symptoms, neck evaluation was important to rule out other conditions. Neck motion resulted in somewhat stiff range of motion around the first rib, particularly with side-bending and rotation. Two special tests were completed. The first was rib cephalad to caudad springing. It was hypomobile and sitting more cephalad than the unaffected side. The cervical lateral flexion and rotation test was completed and was also positive. The patient was sent to a physician for follow-up radiographs to confirm the AC joint sprain. He also had a first rib sprain that was in an elevated position. Traditional AC joint sprain treatment was implemented as well as first rib mobilization. The first rib mobilization resulted in almost immediate relief for the patient, taking pressure off the AC joint because it had been pushing upward on the clavicle.

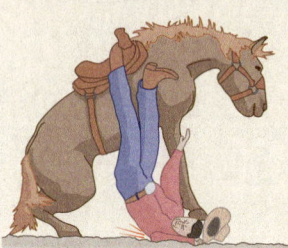

Figure 10.66 The mechanism of injury related to a rider falling off his horse and landing on the tip of his shoulder.

© Jones & Bartlett Learning.

Additional end-of-chapter features include **Pearls and Pitfalls**, which help students remember keys to sound evaluation strategies, and **Critical Thinking Questions** to bring all the content together for the student.

Navigate

Included with the purchase of each new print copy of *Musculoskeletal Assessment in Athletic Training and Therapy* is Navigate Advantage Access. Content offerings include:

- eBook
- Videos
- Instructor resources

Unlock a wealth of resources to promote comprehension through practical learning activities and study tools.

WRAP-UP

Critical Thinking Questions

1. What are the strengths and weaknesses in the design of the medial longitudinal arch? In what ways might changes in the shape of the arch affect structures farther up the kinetic chain?
2. What role could the windlass mechanism play in rehabilitation? How could it be manipulated to target specific tissues and structures?
3. Given the location of the retrocalcaneal bursa, how might it affect your assessment of Achilles tendon injury in both acute and chronic conditions?

Pearls and Pitfalls

- **Trust your physical examination.**
  - Diagnostic imaging is a useful tool, but it can be expensive and time consuming. In many cases, a sound and thorough physical examination is sufficient when evaluating soft-tissue injury to the foot and ankle, as demonstrated previously in this chapter. Remember to use the Ottawa Ankle Rules when trying to determine whether imaging of the foot and/or ankle is truly necessary.
- **Special tests are the last step in HIPS for a reason.**
  - Special tests are useful diagnostic tools that too often become a crutch to young clinicians. In the HIPS evaluation method, special tests are performed after the history, inspection, and palpation have all occurred. By the time special tests are performed, you should already have a differential diagnosis in mind, and special tests can help confirm or refute your assessments. Always take into consideration the diagnostic accuracy of the test and what that means for your evaluation. Not all foot and ankle special tests are created equal.
- **Reassess lingering injuries.**
  - An often-overlooked pathology is anterior impingement in the ankle. When a patient sustains a lateral or syndesmotic ankle sprain, changes in the joint can lead to lingering symptoms, such as pain and pinching in the anterior ankle. Rather than continuing to treat the same injury to no avail, reassess the problem. Are there biomechanical changes or differences in arthrokinematics compared to the healthy limb? A proper assessment is the foundation of a treatment plan, and it is important to remember that injuries can evolve over time.

References

1. Nwawka OK, Hayashi D, Diaz LE, et al: Sesamoids and accessory ossicles of the foot: anatomical variability and related pathology. *Insights Imaging* 2013;4(5):581-593.
2. Dedmond BT, Cory JW, McBryde A, Jr.: The hallucal sesamoid complex. *J Am Acad Orthop Surg* 2006;14(13):745-753.
3. Maceira E, Monteagudo M: Subtalar anatomy and mechanics. *Foot Ankle Clin* 2015;20:195-221.
4. Irwin TA, Lien J, Kadakia AR: Posterior malleolus fracture. *J Am Acad Orthop Surg* 2013;21(1):32-40.
5. Welck MJ, Zinchenko R, Rudge B: Lisfranc injuries. *Injury* 2015;46(4):536-541.
6. Panchani PN, Chappell TM, Moore GD, et al: Anatomic study of the deltoid ligament of the ankle. *Foot Ankle Int* 2014;35:916-921.

Acknowledgments

Any book, especially a textbook like this, undoubtedly requires a huge effort and tons of time. Draft revision after draft revision and on and on, a seemingly endless cycle and for some more repetitive than others. As such, there are many people to thank! Andrea and I (Matt) would first like to thank our families for their encouragement and support, without which nothing productive would ever happen. We also would like to recognize the authors who contributed to this manuscript. Your thoughtful contributions and seemingly endless revisions are greatly appreciated. As such, we shout out a hearty, "Thank you!" to all our authors! We would also like to thank all our colleagues, especially Chris Schommer, Nate Peters, Jess Kiss, Jenny Toonstra, and our school director, Ray Schneider, all of whom had to put up with our requests to reschedule meetings extend projects, and sometimes just endure our whining as we worked on this enormous project. Of course, there were several graduate assistants who helped us organize data and records for this project, and performed editing duties. Without your help early on, this task would have been overwhelming, so thanks to Beth McNutt, Gabrielle Caruso, and Kenny Hurley; we are so very appreciative for your help. Special thanks to Sean Fabery, Kathryn Leeber, Andrew LaBelle, and the rest of our project team at Jones & Bartlett Learning, who were so accommodating and patient as we learned to navigate your publishing and editing process. The publications team of the American Academy of Orthopaedic Surgeons also contributed significant insight into the content development and editorial process—thank you! Finally, we thank you, the reader. Without you, there is no book at all!

Matthew R. Kutz, PhD, ATC, CSCS
Andrea E. Cripps, PhD, ATC

About the Authors

Matthew R. Kutz, PhD, ATC, CSCS, is a professor at Bowling Green State University, an award-winning author, and an international athletic training scholar. He has lived and taught in Rwanda (Fulbright Scholar, University of Rwanda, College of Medicine and Health Science) and Australia (Visiting Research Fellow, Gold Coast University Hospital, and Griffith University). Matt is a member of the Commission on Accreditation of Athletic Training Education Ethics and Professional Standards Committee, the National Athletic Trainers Association International Committee, and the Educational Journal Committee. He serves as senior associate editor for the *Athletic Training Education Journal* and editor-in-chief of the *Journal of Sports Medicine and Allied Health Sciences*. He has been an athletic trainer for 26 years.

Andrea E. Cripps, PhD, ATC, is an associate professor and the program director of the athletic training graduate program at Bowling Green State University (BGSU). Prior to joining BGSU, she served as program director of the athletic training program at New Mexico State University. Dr. Cripps has degrees from Lake Superior State University and Central Michigan University and earned her PhD in Rehabilitation Science from the University of Kentucky. She currently serves as the web team coordinator for the Great Lakes Athletic Trainers Association. Dr. Cripps has been a certified athletic trainer for 13 years. Her research focuses on sensory deficits and long-term cognitive outcomes of patients with traumatic brain injury.

Contributors

Mikaela Boham, EdD, LAT, ATC
Texas A&M University - Corpus Christi
Corpus Christi, Texas

Andrea E. Cripps, PhD, ATC
Bowling Green State University
Bowling Green, Ohio

Maureen K. Dwyer, PhD, ATC
Newton-Wellesley Hospital
Newton, Massachusetts

Breda H.F. Eubank, PhD, CAT(C)
Mount Royal University
Calgary, Alberta, Canada

Joseph M. Hart, PhD, ATC, FACSM, FNATA
University of Virginia
Charlottesville, Virginia

Matthew R. Kutz, PhD, ATC, CSCS
Bowling Green State University
Bowling Green, Ohio

Mark R. Lafave, PhD, CAT(C)
Mount Royal University
Calgary, Alberta, Canada

Natalie L. Myers, PhD, ATC, PES
Texas State University
San Marcos, Texas

Thomas G. Palmer, PhD, ATC, CSCS*D, TSAC
Sport Science Initiatives; TPB, Inc.
Union, Kentucky

Johna K. Register-Mihalik, PhD, LAT, ATC, FACSM
University of North Carolina at Chapel Hill
Chapel Hill, North Carolina

Sara D. Rynders, MPAS, PA-C
University of Virginia
Charlottesville, Virginia

Aaron D. Sciascia, PhD, ATC, PES, SMTC
Eastern Kentucky University
Richmond, Kentucky

Kaitlyn Shank, MEd, ATC, CCRP
University of Virginia
Charlottesville, Virginia

Sara Stiltner, EdD, ATC
Texas A&M University - Corpus Christi
Corpus Christi, Texas

Jenny L. Toonstra, PhD, ATC, LAT
Bowling Green State University
Bowling Green, Ohio

Christine Waters-Banker, PhD, ATC
University of Hawai'i at Hilo
Hilo, Hawaii

Nicole Lounsberry Yates, MS, ATC, LAT
University of Delaware
Newark, Delaware

Reviewers

Melissa Davis, MA, ATC-L
Head Athletic Trainer
Athletic Training Services
Emory & Henry College
Emory, Virginia

R.T. Floyd, EdD, ATC, CSCS
Director of Athletic Training and Sports Medicine
and
Distinguished Professor
Department of Physical Education and Athletic Training
and
Chair, School of Health Sciences and Human Performance
College of Natural Science and Mathematics
University of West Alabama
Livingston, Alabama

William Gear, PhD, LAT, ATC
Assistant Professor, Program Director
Master of Athletic Training Program
University of Wisconsin – Green Bay
Green Bay, Wisconsin

Jason Graham, MS, LAT, ATC
Instructor, ATP Clinical Education Coordinator
Department of Health and Human Performance
College of Health and Behavioral Sciences
Fort Hays State University
Hays, Kansas

KyungMo Han, PhD, ATC, CSCS
Program Director and Associate Professor
Athletic Training Program
Department of Kinesiology
College of Health and Human Sciences
San José State University
San José, California

Jessica Hurlbut, MS, ATC, EMT
Assistant Athletic Director
Senior Woman Administrator
Athletic Department
College of Liberal Arts and Sciences
Alfred University
Alfred, New York

Joanne Klossner, PhD, ATC
Senior Lecturer
Department of Kinesiology
School of Public Health
University of Maryland
College Park, Maryland

Randy Meador, MS, ATC
Coordinator of Athletic Training Services
Head Men's Basketball Athletic Trainer
Clinical Preceptor
College of Physical Activity and Sport Sciences
West Virginia University
Morgantown, West Virginia

Angela Mickle, PhD, ATC
Director, Athletic Training
Department of Health and Human Performance
College of Education and Human Development
Radford University
Radford, Virginia

Karen E. Pfeifer, MS, ATC, LAT
Assistant Professor, Clinical Education Coordinator
Master of Athletic Training (MAT) Program
Sport Health Science Department
Life University
Marietta, Georgia

Scot Raab, PhD, ATC, LAT
Associate Professor
Department of Athletic Training
College of Health and Human Services
Northern Arizona University
Flagstaff, Arizona

Eric Scibek, MS, ATC, CSCS
Clinical Associate Professor
Department of Exercise Science
College of Health Professions
Sacred Heart University
Fairfield, Connecticut

Carrie Truebenbach, MS, MSPT, OCS
Clinical Associate Professor
Physical Therapy Program
College of Health Sciences
University of Wisconsin – Milwaukee
Milwaukee, Wisconsin

UNIT I

Foundations

CHAPTER 1	Taxonomy of Injury Pathology and Classifications	3
CHAPTER 2	The Examination Process	17
CHAPTER 3	Evidence-Based Injury Evaluation	29
CHAPTER 4	Diagnostic Imaging for Musculoskeletal Injuries	41

CHAPTER 1

Taxonomy of Injury Pathology and Classifications

Matthew R. Kutz, PhD, ATC, CSCS

OVERVIEW

This chapter is a basic overview of common vocabulary and terminology used in evaluating injuries and communicating findings. As an introductory chapter, this is a primer and should not be used as a substitute for a rigorous medical terminology course.

A taxonomy is a way of classifying and organizing information. In this chapter, the means to classify, define, and organize different injuries, including how disablement models contribute to the evaluation process, will be presented. Key anatomic positions and terms will be identified and discussed. Classification of the type and severity of ligamentous injuries, musculoskeletal injuries, and neurologic injuries also will be discussed. In addition, several key terms that are important for communicating clearly with other health care professionals will be defined.

LEARNING OBJECTIVES

After completing this chapter, the reader will be able to do the following:

1. Describe anatomically correct reference points and positions.
2. Use appropriate terminology to describe injury location relative to anatomic terms and reference points.
3. Describe various classifications of soft-tissue injury and levels of severity.
4. Use and describe correct nomenclature relative to injury classification.

FUN FACTS ABOUT TAXONOMY AND PATHOLOGY

- Taxonomy is a branch of science about the laws and principles of classifying things.
- In medieval Europe, doctors confirmed diagnosis of conditions by observing the smell, consistency, and even the taste of a patient's urine. Urine analysis was pioneered by Thomas Willis in the 1600s; he was the first to notice the characteristic sweet taste of urine from patients with diabetes.[1]
- The average human body carries 10 times more bacterial cells than human cells. Frighteningly, the strongest organisms on Earth are gonorrhea bacteria—they can pull 100,000 times their own body weight.[1]

Introduction

One of the fundamental aspects of successful assessment and diagnosis of orthopaedic and musculoskeletal injuries is being able to communicate accurately and concisely with patients and other health care providers. Failing to communicate clearly can hinder the clinician's effectiveness. Using proper anatomic references and injury terminology is essential to successful clinical practice. This chapter will provide a brief overview that can serve as a basis and reference point for clearly articulating, to all relevant stakeholders, the findings of a clinical examination.

Language naturally evolves over time as new discoveries are made and culture and society progress. An example of that within health care is a difference between the terms *tendinitis* and *tendinosis*.[2] Until recently, the term tendinitis was used to describe most tendon pathology; however, because the suffix *-itis* implies inflammation, it does not accurately describe many tendon pathologies.[2] Many tendon pathologies are degenerative in nature and, if because of the incorrect terminology the assumption is made that inflammation is the culprit, the condition may be managed inappropriately.[2] Therefore, it is important that correct terminology be used because of its direct contribution to decisions about intervention and treatment.

It is important to begin by explaining the differences between the terms pathology, etiology, epidemiology, diagnosis, and prognosis. Pathology is the study of the origin, nature, and course a disease takes and includes the conditions and processes of injury or disease. A pathologist is someone who studies the causes and effects of diseases. Etiology is a term that describes the cause or contributing factors to an injury or disease condition. Epidemiology is a particular branch of medicine that studies and explores the incidence, distribution, and possible control of diseases and injuries that affect health and quality of life. An epidemiologist is a person who is an expert in studying how diseases spread and how to control them. Diagnosis is the process of identifying the nature and characteristics of an illness or injury by exploring the signs and symptoms associated with the patient's particular complaint. A diagnosis is usually an outcome of a clinical or medical examination. A differential diagnosis is a process of diagnosis that requires identifying several possible conditions with similar signs or symptoms. The goal is to eventually narrow down those possibilities to a single diagnosis using deductive reasoning. Prognosis is the likely or predictable course that a disease or injury will take. For example, patients often ask after an injury or condition has been diagnosed, "What happens next?," "How long will the recovery take?," or something similar. The answer the clinician provides is usually in the form of a prognosis.

Introduction to Medical Terminology

A working knowledge of the key terms and how those terms are formed can help facilitate good communication and a clear understanding among health care professionals. Having a solid vocabulary base also helps to promote a sense of competence among the health care community.

A prefix is a letter or letters added to the beginning of a word, and a suffix is a letter or letters added to the end of a word. Most of the words used in medical terminology have their origins in either Latin or Greek. For example, *anti-* is of Greek origin and means against, used as a prefix in the term *antibody*. An example of a Latin suffix is *-ible*, which means capable or worthy of and is used in the term *flexible*. **Table 1.1** is a short list of common medical prefixes and suffixes that can help form the basis of good medical vocabulary.

Anatomic Reference Points

The anatomic position is the standard position the body is in when referencing specific locations or anatomic landmarks. It is an erect or supine posture with the body facing forward or anteriorly, the arms

Table 1.1 Common Orthopaedic Prefixes and Suffixes

Prefix	Meaning	Suffix	Meaning
Arter/io-	Artery	-algia	Pain
Arthro-	Joint	-cyte	Cell
Bio-	Life	-ectomy	Surgical removal
Chondro-	Cartilage	-emia	Blood or in the blood
Derm-	Skin	-ic/al	Pertaining to or relating to
Hemo-	Blood	-itis	Inflammation
Histo-	Tissue	-logy	Study of
Hyper-	Excessive or above	-ostomy	Surgical opening

Prefix	Meaning	Suffix	Meaning
Hypo-	Less or below	-otomy	Surgical incision
Myo-	Muscle	-penia	Deficiency or decrease from normal
Neuro-	Nerve	-plasia	Growth or cellular proliferation
Ortho-	Straight, correct, or erect	-sis	State of
Osteo-	Bone	-tomy	Incise or process of cutting into
Path-	Disease	-trophic	Nourishment
Thromb/o-	Clotting		

positioned at the patient's side with the palms of the hands facing forward, the lower limbs are straight and feet together pointing anteriorly or forward. Whenever a body region or anatomic structure is referred to, it is important to always describe it relative to the anatomic position. Failure to do so may lead to confusion and misunderstanding. **Figure 1.1** is a depiction of anatomic position.

From the anatomic position, three cardinal planes, which are imaginary lines that separate the body into segments, can be described. The imaginary line that separates the body into left and right segments is the sagittal plane. Within the sagittal plane, typical motions that occur are flexion, extension, dorsiflexion, and plantar flexion. Flexion movements are generally described as any decrease in joint angle, and extension is any increase in joint angle.

The imaginary line that separates the body into anterior and posterior segments (or front and back) is the frontal plane (also called the coronal plane). Within the frontal plane, typical motions that occur are abduction, adduction, and radial and ulnar deviation. Abduction is generally any movement away from the midline, and adduction is any movement toward the midline. Other motions that occur in the frontal plane include elevation, depression, inversion, and eversion.

The imaginary line that divides the body into superior and inferior sections (or top and bottom) is called the horizontal or transverse plane. Within the transverse plane, motions that occur are internal and external rotation, pronation, supination, and horizontal adduction and abduction. External rotation is the outward turning of a bone on a vertical axis, and internal rotation is an inward turning around a vertical axis. **Table 1.2** lists the terms (and synonyms, when available) that describe different parts and positions of the body. **Table 1.3** is a list with corresponding descriptions of common anatomic movements. **Figure 1.2** is a depiction of the cardinal planes of motion.

The Role of Disablement Models in the Evaluation Process

Many tissues in the body react to stress or injury in a predictable manner. Stress can take the form of physical, social, emotional, or psychological factors, each of which has an expected effect on the body and its systems. It is important to understand that these stresses can be compounded. For example, emotional stress is likely to influence the patient's reaction to the injury as well as his or her perception of pain.[3] Therefore, it is important that all health care professionals understand the complex nature of the injury process and how it contributes to disablement.

The examination process is a critical component to understanding this complex integration. During an orthopaedic examination, it is necessary to isolate the segment being examined. However, it is important to realize that other segments may contribute to the complaint and that the complaint may have an effect beyond the findings of clinical examination. For example, an athlete may experience a loss of range of motion (ROM), and that decreased ROM may affect more than his or her ability to compete—it may also have a negative effect on a different aspect of his or her life that falls outside the scope of competition.

Disablement models are a way to understand and organize the overall effect to multiple aspects of a patient's life and ability as a result of injury or illness. Disablement models are very useful to the clinician

6 **Chapter 1** Taxonomy of Injury Pathology and Classifications

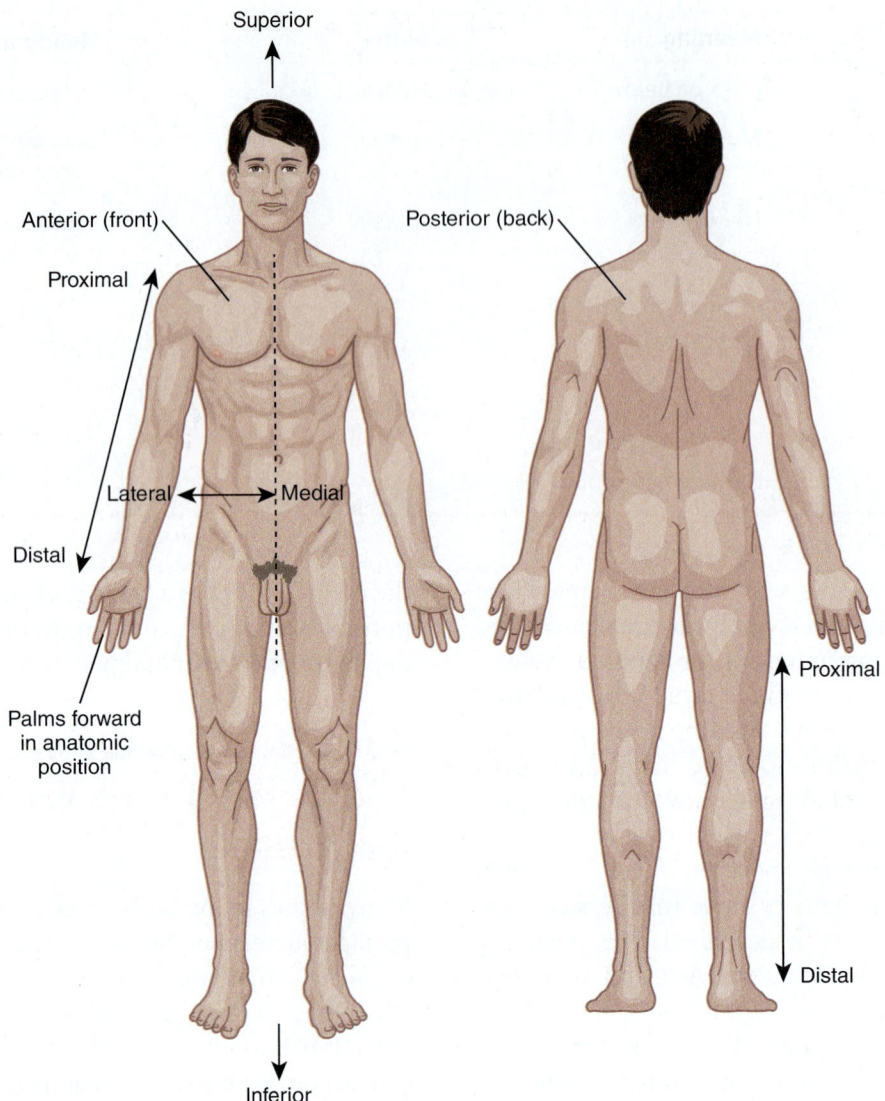

Figure 1.1 Drawings showing anatomic position, anterior and posterior.
© Jones & Bartlett Learning

Table 1.2 Common Anatomic Terms

Term	Possible Synonym	Definition
Abdominal		The region between the thorax and the pelvis
Anterior	Ventral/palmar	Toward the front
Appendicular		Includes the limbs or extremities (arms and legs)
Axial		Includes the head, neck, and trunk
Axillary		The armpit
Brachial		The upper arm
Celiac		The abdomen
Central		Near or close to the center
Cervical		The neck
Contralateral		On the opposite side

Term	Possible Synonym	Definition
Coronal		On top or top of the head
Costal		The ribs
Cubital		The elbow
Deep		Farther or farthest from the surface of the skin
Distal		Farther away from the reference point
Femoral		The thigh
Frontal	Coronal	Imaginary line that divides the body into anterior and posterior (front and back) sections
Gluteal		The buttock
Inferior	Caudal	Beneath or below; moving away from the head
Ipsilateral		On the same side
Lateral		Away from or outside of the midline of the body
Lumbar		The lower back
Medial		Near or toward the midline of the body
Parietal		The external wall of a body cavity
Peripheral		Farther away from the body center
Posterior	Dorsal/dorsum	Behind or back of the body
Prone		Lying face down on the stomach
Proximal		Closer to the point of reference
Sagittal		Imaginary line that divides the body into right and left sections
Superficial		Near the surface of the skin
Superior	Cranial/cephalic	Toward the head
Supine		Lying on the back
Transverse	Horizontal	Imaginary line that divides the body into superior and inferior (top and bottom) sections
Visceral		The covering of an internal organ

Table 1.3 Common Anatomic Terms Describing Joint Motion

Motion	Description
Flexion	Decreasing the joint angle between two bones
Extension	Increasing the joint angle between two bones
Circumduction	Moving a limb (arm or leg) around its proximal attachment such that the distal end rotates in a circle
Rotation	Inward or internal rotation is turning a bone (typically, the humerus, femur, or tibia) around the vertical axis toward the midline. Outward or external rotation is turning a bone around the vertical axis away from the midline
Dorsiflexion	Pulling the foot upward—raising the toes

(continues)

Table 1.3 Common Anatomic Terms Describing Joint Motion (continued)

Motion	Description
Plantar flexion	Moving the bottom of the foot downward—pointing the toes
Ulnar deviation	Bending the wrist/hand toward the fifth finger (little finger)
Radial deviation	Bending the hand or wrist toward the thumb
Supination	Rotating the forearm so that the palmar side of the hand faces upward
Pronation	Rotating the forearm so that the palmar side of the hand faces downward
Abduction	Moving the arms or legs away from the midline
Adduction	Moving the arms or legs toward the midline
Inversion	Moving the medial aspect of the foot toward the midline upward
Eversion	Moving the lateral aspect of the foot away from the midline upward

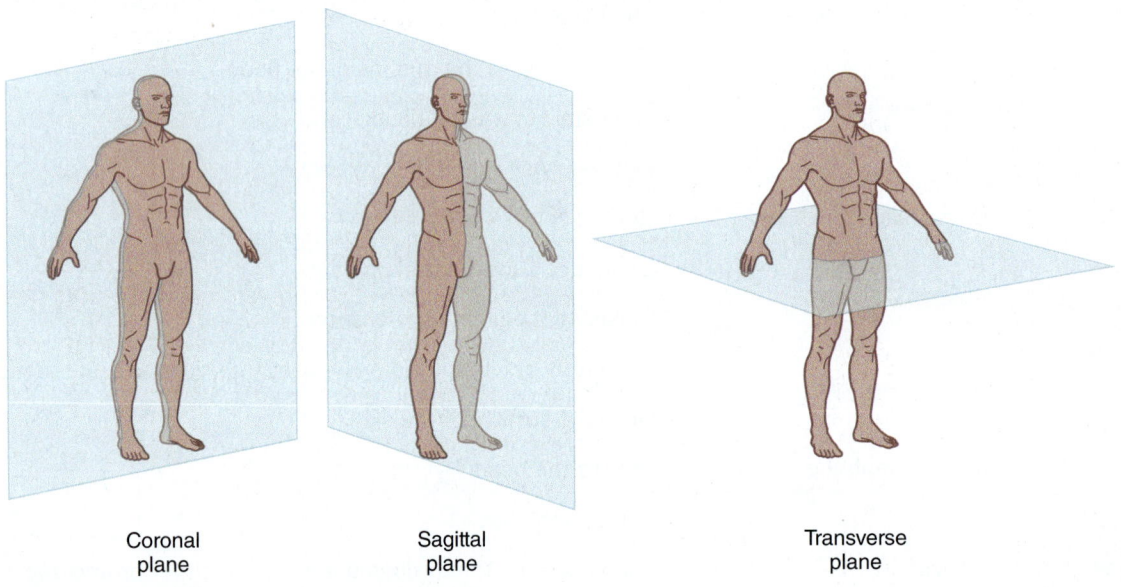

Figure 1.2 Drawings showing the anatomic planes.
© Jones & Bartlett Learning

and can help describe the parameters of a given injury by classifying it as an impairment, functional limitation, or disability, which in turn helps to determine personal and contextual outcomes of the injury.[4] There are several disablement models, but one of the more commonly used versions was developed by the World Health Organization and is often referred to as the International Classification of Functioning, Disability and Health, or ICF, model. **Figure 1.3** shows the disablement model framework.

To use a disablement model, the diagnosis should be first, followed by determining how that diagnosis contributes to any physical impairment. After the physical impairment is determined, it can then be used to help identify how the impairment(s) affect(s) activity (ie, functional limitation). After the patient's activity has been determined, the disablement model is useful in classifying the current level of participation or overall disability. Finally, that level of participation or disability can be used to determine overall outcomes of the diagnosis. In other words, the profound effect of understanding disablement models means that clinicians need to pay attention to more than just a loss of function. For example, a compromised anterior cruciate ligament may have a much more dramatic effect on a patient than simply the loss of ROM or stability. Disablement models aid clinicians by reiterating all the

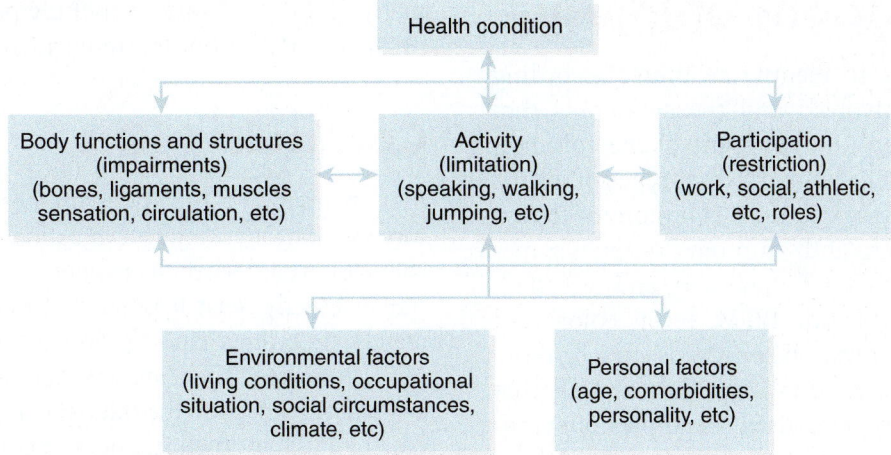

Figure 1.3 Disablement model framework.

Adapted from the National Athletic Trainers' Association, 2016. https://www.nata.org/icf-disablement-model

possible negative outcomes of the injury, including social and environmental risks.

As a case example, consider how multidirectional instability (MDI) of the shoulder—as a *diagnosed condition*—can affect an athlete. MDI may lead to a *physical impairment,* such as muscle weakness. That physical impairment contributes to the *functional limitation* of feeling weak or unstable when the shoulder is flexed and externally rotated. That functional limitation then means the athlete cannot *participate* in his or her chosen sport, or that participation is compromised or limited. Not being able to participate may have other consequences, such as losing a scholarship, a place on a team, or identity as an athlete, which are personal factors. It may also affect environmental or contextual factors, such as absence from team meetings and team activities because of an increased demand of treatment with the athletic trainer or more time in the athletic training clinic. Appropriately using disablement models helps the clinician see the bigger picture and helps the clinician to not become overly focused on treating the shoulder; instead, these models encourage the clinician to treat the entire patient and all of the associated outcomes of the injury from the emotional, physical, and psychosocial aspects.

Categorizations of Physical Maturity

During an evaluation, it is important to determine both the biologic and chronologic age of the patient. Chronologic age refers to how old the patient is in terms of years alive, whereas biologic age refers to the patient's physical maturity and related characteristics. Understanding these differences means that it is entirely possible to have two patients of the same chronologic age, but different biologic ages. For example, two 15-year-olds would be considered to be of different biologic ages if one has not yet experienced puberty, and therefore has not achieved skeletal maturity, and one has. Physical maturity is often categorized accordingly:[3]

- Infancy (pediatric) – 0 to 12 months of age
- Childhood (pediatric) – 12 months to 11 years of age
- Adolescence (pediatric) – approximately 11 through 18 years of age
- Adulthood – ages 18 to approximately 40 years of age
- Middle adulthood – approximately 40 to 60 years of age
- Older adulthood (geriatric) – approximately 60 years of age and older

Each of these categorizations has certain risk factors or special considerations that should be examined during the evaluation process. For example, during childhood, epiphyseal plates should be a consideration when evaluating bones. A second example would be during middle adulthood, when there is typically a slow decline in muscular strength, which should be accounted for during injury evaluation. This is pertinent when taking a history, as biologic and chronologic ages may affect several different physiologic and anatomic differences.

Categorizations of Injury

Often, it is possible to identify an injury according to the structures involved and the symptoms that present. This section outlines some of the common language used in identifying different types of injury. During the evaluation process, it is important to distinguish between signs and symptoms. A sign is something that can be observed, measured, and recorded. Examples of signs include ROM, fever, color, and heart rate. A symptom, however, is much more subjective and includes things the patient feels that cannot necessarily be measured. Examples of symptoms include dizziness, nausea, and pain. One of the objectives of a thorough and accurate evaluation is to determine the signs and symptoms of a particular patient's injury and distinguish between them.

Injuries can also be classified as acute or chronic. Acute injuries are typically considered to have a traumatic or sudden onset—in other words, a direct cause that the patient typically remembers and can recount when describing the mechanism of injury (MOI). Chronic injuries usually are insidious in nature, which means a gradual or unknown cause. Unlike acute injuries, chronic injuries typically result from an accumulation of submaximal or even minor and repetitive stresses. In many situations, chronic injuries are a result of inflammation and classified as inflammatory injuries. Common examples include bursitis, which is inflammation of the bursa; myositis, which is inflammation of the muscle or other connective tissue; neuritis, which is the inflammation of the nerve or nerve sheath; and tendinitis, which is inflammation of the tendon. Signs and symptoms of many of these conditions include pain, point tenderness, loss of motion or strength, and swelling.

Common MOIs

Identifying the MOI is the main focal point of the history portion of an injury evaluation. The MOI is typically discovered when the patient explains to the athletic trainer exactly what happened at the moments immediately preceding, during, and immediately after the injury occurred. There are several forces that could have a significant effect on the trauma being described by the patient. It is the athletic trainer's responsibility to attempt to determine which force or forces were involved in the MOI. Common forces that can cause damage to tissue include tensile force, compressive force, rotational force (or torsion), shear force, and direct force. **Figure 1.4** is a depiction of the different forces.

- Tensile force is a longitudinal stress pulling a structure in opposite directions that results in a "tearing" sensation.
- Compressive force is a force that presses two ends of a structure together that results in a "crushing" or "smashing" sensation.
- Rotational force (also known as torsion) is a rotating or spinning force that results in a "twisting" sensation.
- Shear force is a perpendicular force across the long axis of the structure that results in a "sliding" or "slipping" sensation.
- Direct force is a force that occurs from a direct blow to a particular structure and typically causes contusions, dislocations, and fractures.

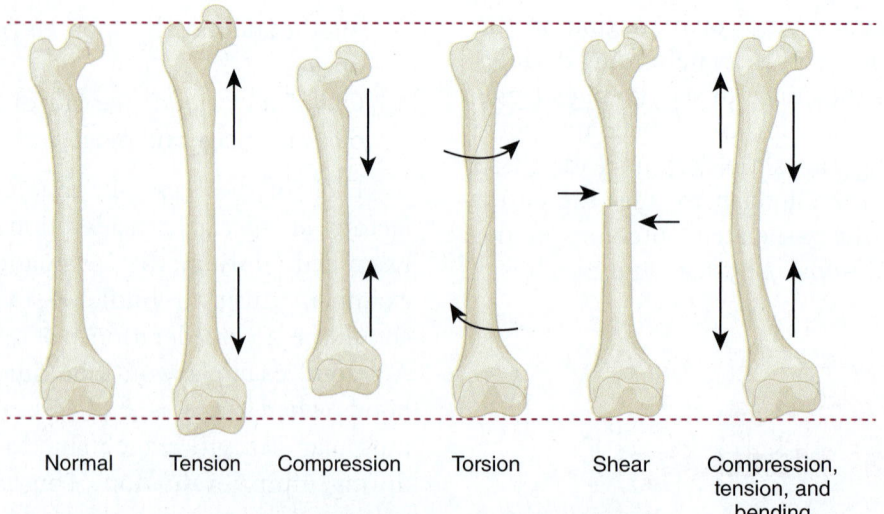

Figure 1.4 Drawing showing the forces affecting bone.
© Jones & Bartlett Learning

Determining the Severity of Injuries

Many injuries are classified according to the degree of severity or the extent of the damage to particular tissue. Often, these are identified by level or degree (eg, first degree, second degree, third degree). In the following section, different types of injury are identified and how they are graded by degree is described.

Ligament and Capsular Sprains

A sprain is an injury to a ligament or joint capsule and is a common type of joint injury. Ligaments hold bones together at their articulations and are integral to the joint. When one or more of these ligaments are injured, they are classified as a sprain. Sprains are described as either first-, second-, or third-degree injuries.

- First-degree sprain is generally a mild overstretch of the ligament and typically does not involve any tearing or disruption of the tissue. There usually is little disability associated with first-degree sprains except at the extreme ends of ROM.
- Second-degree sprain is generally an overstretch that has minor or partial disruption or tearing of the ligament. There is often some level of disability associated with second-degree sprains, and the signs and symptoms can vary considerably.
- Third-degree sprain is the most severe and is a complete disruption of the ligament. This means the ligament has torn in half, which is classified as a rupture. Often, the athlete will feel or hear a "pop" or "snap" at the time of the injury. There is usually a much more significant loss of function associated with this level of ligamentous injury. It is noteworthy that third-degree sprains are typically less painful than second-degree sprains; the reason for this is the absence of tensile force due to the complete rupture of the ligament.

Muscle and Tendon Strains

A strain is an injury to a muscle or tendon. Normally, ligaments will give way before a muscle or tendon; therefore, strains are often more traumatic or violent in nature. Like sprains, strains are also classified as first-, second-, or third-degree injuries.

- First-degree strain is characterized by a mild overstretching of a muscle or tendon. In a normal situation of first-degree strain, the fibers of the tissue remain intact, and pain is usually felt only when there is tension or load put on the injured tissue.
- Second-degree strain involves some minor tearing or more severe overstretch to the fibers of the muscle or tendon. Second-degree strains often have pain that is more acute and result in instant disability. They are also likely to lead to discoloration (ecchymosis), loss of motion, and decreased strength.
- Third-degree strain is when a muscle or tendon completely ruptures (tears in half). There is often instant disability and an audible pop associated with the injury. Third-degree strains typically will have a visible and palpable defect.

Severity and Classification of Nerve Injury

Nerve injuries are classified differently than sprains and strains. Similar to other classification models, each level of nerve injury increases in severity. Nerves are very sensitive to compression and ischemia, which is a loss or decrease of blood flow that is often associated with a secondary injury, such as compression from swelling or a laceration due to a fracture or dislocation. When assessing nerves, it is important to consider muscle function (eg, myotomes). Paralysis is the complete loss of muscle function, but there may be partial or no loss of function. Furthermore, there are varying degrees of sensation that can be associated with nerve injury: anesthesia, which is an absence of sensation; paresthesia, which is often described as numbness, tingling, and burning; and hyperesthesia, which is excessive or hypersensitivity. The three classes of nerve injury are neurapraxia (class I), axonotmesis (class II), and neurotmesis (class III). **Figure 1.5** is a depiction of nerve injuries.

- Neurapraxia (class I) is described as a temporary disruption of nerve conduction due to compression without any loss of axonal continuity. This is the mildest type of peripheral nerve injury. Generally, a full recovery is expected within a few days to weeks.
- Axonotmesis (class II) is demyelination combined with damage to the axon. Whereas neurapraxia is a compression injury, axonotmesis is when the axon is severed. However, the endoneurium (protective sheath of the nerve) is intact.
- Neurotmesis (class III) is when the entire nerve is completely disrupted.

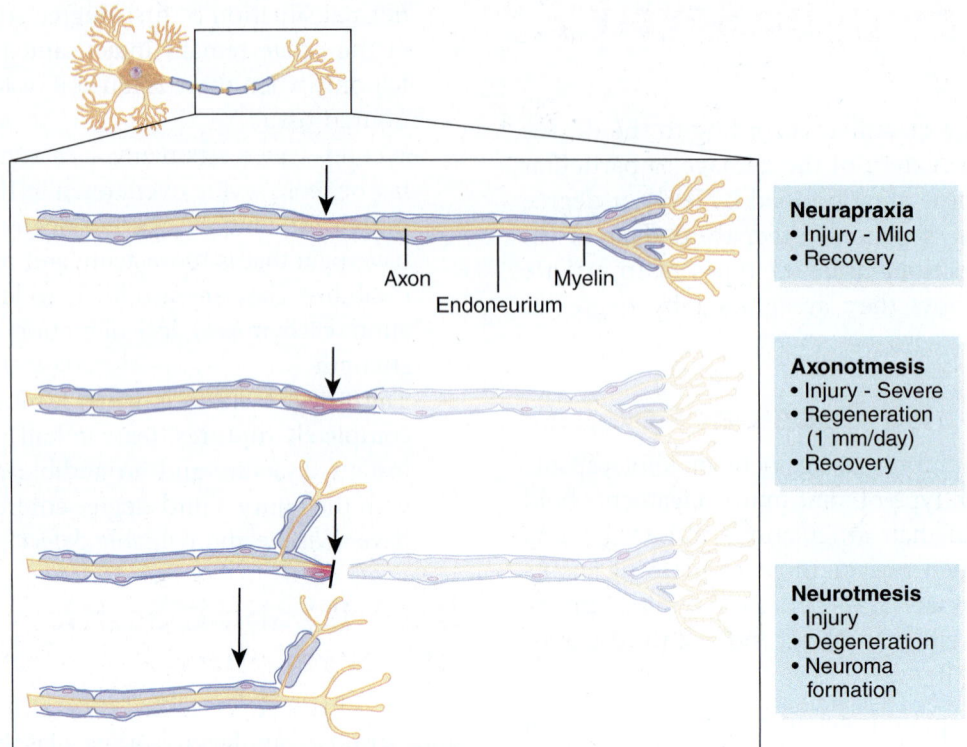

Figure 1.5 Seddon classification of nerve injury.
© Jones & Bartlett Learning

Types of Bone Injuries

Injuries to bone are classified as fractures, dislocations, or subluxations. A closed fracture generally describes a disruption to the bone without disruption to the surface of the skin. Fractures usually are caused by direct impact or indirect forces that exceed the strength of the bone. Depending on the type of force applied to the bone, there may be one of several different types of fracture. The common types of bone fracture consist of transverse, oblique, spiral, comminuted, linear, greenstick, compression, avulsion, and osteochondral. Some of these fracture types are shown in **Figure 1.6**. Minor or submaximal repetitive stresses may cause a stress fracture. There are also injuries to bone that can occur before the epiphyseal line (growth plate) has closed; injuries to epiphyseal plates are described according to the Salter-Harris classification, which is detailed in **Table 1.4** and depicted in **Figure 1.7**.

Other bone injuries include dislocations and subluxations. A dislocation occurs when the articulating surfaces of two bones completely disassociate.

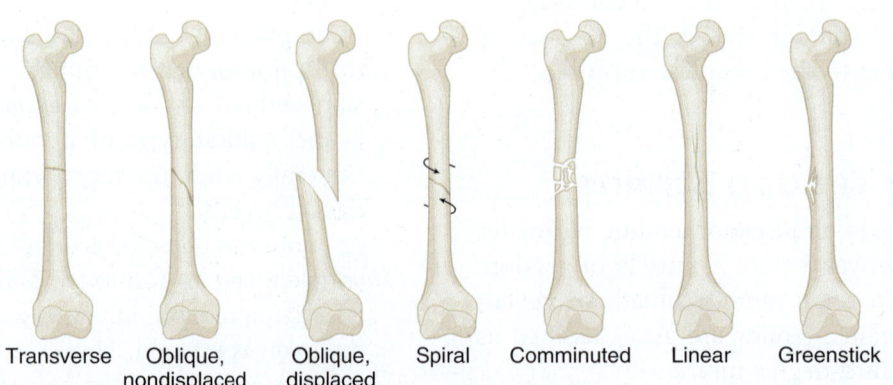

Figure 1.6 Drawings showing the types of bone fractures.
© Jones & Bartlett Learning

Table 1.4 Salter-Harris Classification of Epiphyseal Injuries

Type	Characteristics
I	Separation through the physis, usually through areas of hypertrophic and degenerating cartilage cell columns
II	Fracture through a portion of the physis that extends through the metaphyses
III	Fracture through a portion of the physis that extends through the epiphysis and into the joint
IV	Fracture across the metaphysis, physis, and epiphysis
V	Crush injury to the physis

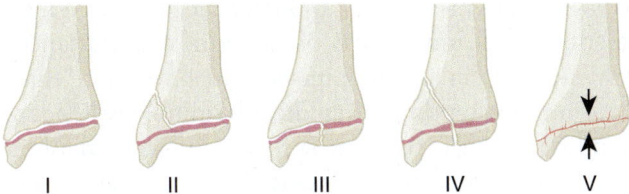

Figure 1.7 Salter-Harris classification of epiphyseal injuries. For complete definitions, see Table 1.4.
© Jones & Bartlett Learning

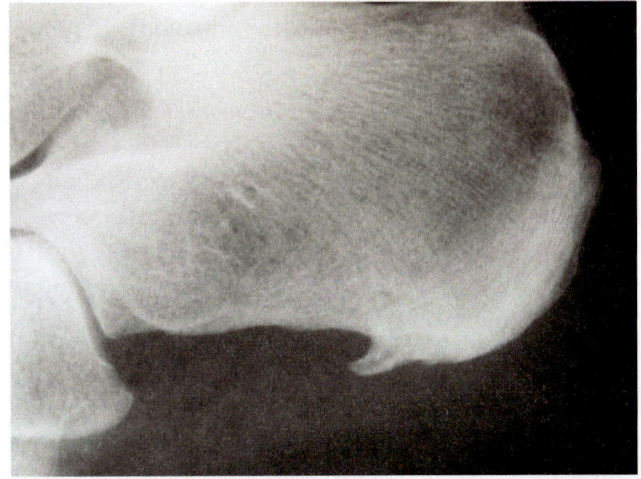

Figure 1.8 Radiograph showing a bone spur.
© Ralf Liebhold/Shutterstock

Sometimes, that disassociation may spontaneously reduce (go back into place without external intervention), but that is no less of a dislocation. Dislocations usually include a third-degree sprain of ligaments and joint capsules and possible strains or impingement to nearby muscles and tendons. A subluxation is an incomplete or partial disassociation of two articulating bones. Signs and symptoms of subluxations vary greatly depending on any associated injury to local soft tissue. An avulsion fracture is a type of fracture that involves tendons or ligaments. Sometimes, the bone fails before the ligament or tendon does; an avulsion fracture is when the tendon or ligament remains intact but pulls a piece of the bone off at the attachment.

Other injuries can also occur in bones from abnormal growth. For example, bone, when it heals, will respond to the stress placed on it (Wolff law); consequently, growth of extra or unwanted bone can occur if a regular force is placed on that bone during healing or growth. That additional bone growth is called an exostosis, or spur. A second type of injury is apophysitis, which is an inflammatory condition at the growth plate that typically occurs in younger athletes. This is sometimes referred to as "growing pains." **Figure 1.8** shows a bone spur.

Classification of Wounds

Wounds are injuries that break or damage the surface of the skin. There are several types of wounds, which are classified as abrasions, blisters, incisions, lacerations, punctures, avulsions, amputations, contusions, and hematomas. Contusions and hematomas are generally classified as closed wounds, whereas the others are considered open wounds. Open wounds penetrate or disrupt the surface of the skin.

- Abrasions, also known as "road rash" or a "strawberry," are the rubbing or scraping of the skin against an abrasive surface. Abrasions typically do not produce a lot of bleeding, but they do have a higher risk of infection.
- Blisters, usually caused by friction or shearing of the skin (also known to be caused by burns, extreme cold, or infections), are fluid-filled sacs under the epidermis.
- Incisions are slice wounds caused by a sharp object (eg, glass, razor, knife). Incisions can be very deep and consequently at high risk for infection and profuse bleeding.
- Lacerations are similar to incisions, but can be linear or an irregular-shaped tear of the skin.
- Punctures are holes that penetrate the skin (epidermis and usually the dermis). They can be deep or shallow.

- Avulsions are a violent tearing away of the skin (epidermis and dermis). They can range from minor to severe and typically bleed profusely.
- Amputations can be surgical or traumatic in nature and involve the complete removal or severing of body tissue (typically an extremity).
- Contusions are closed wounds (type of hematoma) resulting from a direct blow or crushing injury. Typically, blood accumulates under the skin and can become discolored (ecchymosis) and tender to touch.
- Hematomas are localized collections of blood outside of the blood vessels (pooling) from seeping of damaged capillaries. Like contusions, they are closed wounds.

Closed wounds, such as contusions and hematomas, although generally easily treatable, may lead to other complications if not cared for properly. One of those complications is heterotopic ossification. Heterotopic ossification (formerly known as myositis ossificans) is the formation of bone within the muscle's belly and fascia. The word heterotopic is used because it means occurring in an abnormal anatomic location. This form of injury typically occurs within larger muscle groups.

Summary

Good communication is more than just verbal and nonverbal communication: It begins with using proper terminology. Using correct vocabulary is a fundamental professional behavior and is critical for collegial collaboration and contributing to better patient outcomes. As health care becomes more collaborative and moves away from a disease-oriented approach toward a patient-oriented approach, accurate and representative terminology is of the utmost importance. Athletic trainers and therapists must have more than a base understanding of medical terminology. Understanding the basic prefixes, suffixes, and abbreviations is only the beginning. Knowing the correct terms and nomenclature associated with orthopaedic and musculoskeletal conditions as well as a variety of diseases facilitates communication between health care providers and helps to build rapport, which ultimately contributes to better patient outcomes.

WRAP-UP

Critical Thinking Questions

1. What are some common complaints you might expect from a patient who has shoulder pain that could be described as signs? What are some additional complaints that could be described as symptoms?
2. A patient comes to you complaining of pain on the lateral aspect of the ankle. Considering the anatomic structures in this area, what types of conditions might you suspect? Based on the signs and symptoms, how would you differentiate among the suspected structures?
3. Your team physician has just texted you to ask about one of the injuries that you evaluated. What are some of the key terms you would use to classify the type and severity of the injury to provide the team physician with the best information?
4. What are the anatomic reference points you would use to describe the following anatomic locations:
   a. The back side of the hand
   b. The top of the shoulder
   c. The outside of the thigh
   d. The sole of the foot when directed toward the opposite foot
   e. The left kidney relative to the heart
   f. The heart relative to the thoracic spine

Pearls and Pitfalls
- Always use anatomically correct terms (avoid using colloquialisms or common names of anatomy).
- Always try to distinguish between type and severity of injury.
- Strains occur to muscles and tendons, and severity is graded as first, second, and third degree.
- Sprains occur to ligaments, and severity is graded as first, second, and third degree.
- The three classes of nerve injury are called neurapraxia (class I), axonotmesis (class II), and neurotmesis (class III).

References
1. Biais N, Ladoux B, Higashi D, So M, Sheetz M: (2008) Cooperative retraction of bundled type IV pili enables nanonewton force generation. *PLoS Biol*;6(4):e87. https://doi.org/10.1371/journal.pbio.0060087.
2. Starkey C, Brown S: *Examination of Orthopedic & Athletic Injuries*, ed 4. Philadelphia, PA, FA Davis, 2015.
3. Shultz S, Houglum P, Perrin D: *Examination of Musculoskeletal Injuries*, ed 4. Champaign, IL, Human Kinetics, 2016.
4. Snyder AR, Parsons JT, Valovich McLeod TC, Curtis Bay R, Michener LA, Sauers EL: Using disablement models and clinical outcomes assessment to enable evidence-based athletic training practice, part I: disablement models. *J Athl Train* 2008;43(4):428-436.

CHAPTER 2

The Examination Process

Matthew R. Kutz, PhD, ATC, CSCS

OVERVIEW

This chapter focuses on the injury evaluation process and how a proper evaluation contributes to the clinical diagnosis and patient's plan of care. Many nuances to the injury evaluation process contribute to the identification and classification of an injury. These nuances also affect which body parts are evaluated relative to the primary injury, the treatment options, and the overall plan of care. It is impossible to identify and discuss every possible nuance during an evaluation in a text such as this. Therefore, the skilled clinician is required to integrate and assess a very complex "web" of information supplied by the patient, the clinician's observation of the injury (if he or she was there), the patient's presentation, the clinician's experience, valid and reliable research evidence, and the experience and input from reliable stakeholders (eg, other health care providers and observations from witnesses). Sometimes, the information gathered from all of these different sources may be contradictory, and so it must be carefully and thoroughly scrutinized.

In this chapter, a common framework for gathering relevant information about a patient's injury and associated signs and symptoms, history, inspection/observation, palpation, and special tests (known as HIPS, or HOPS by other clinicians), will be introduced. These are the four elements minimally required to gather enough information to form a clinical diagnosis. The ways in which that information is documented and recorded in a SOAP (subjective, objective, assessment, and plan) note will be discussed; these four sections are necessary to provide enough information in the medical record to ensure ongoing and adequate patient care.

LEARNING OBJECTIVES

After completing this chapter, the reader will be able to do the following:

1. Describe the injury evaluation process.
2. Understand the necessity of a systematic and organized approach to injury evaluation.
3. Articulate key questions to ask when taking a history.
4. Understand the importance and necessity of inspections, palpations, and special tests.
5. Understand the difference between the HIPS injury assessment and the SOAP note-taking format.
6. Understand the difference between primary and secondary evaluations.

FUN FACTS ABOUT INJURY EVALUATION

- Although all injury evaluations should be structured and organized, they do not necessarily have to follow a prescribed sequence.
- Injury evaluations should be divided into primary and secondary assessments. Primary assessments deal with life-threatening conditions and secondary assessments deal with non–life-threatening conditions.

Introduction

One of the key domains within athletic training is for the athletic trainer to be proficient at examination, assessment, and diagnosis. The examination process should be systematic and organized, and it should contribute to a valid clinical diagnosis and the patient's plan of care. However, the evaluation need not always follow a prescribed sequence. For example, there are differences between a formal clinical evaluation (in a controlled environment) and an on-field evaluation (during competition or practice, usually in front of spectators). In certain situations, the clinician may decide to abbreviate or reorder one aspect of the evaluation to expedite the process or to accommodate a more emergent situation. There are also distinctions to be made between primary and secondary evaluations. A primary evaluation assesses life-threatening conditions, whereas a secondary evaluation assesses non–life-threatening conditions.

All injury evaluations, regardless of type, should be structured and organized. The examination process is generally structured according to history, inspection (or observation), palpations, and special tests. The acronym HIPS (or HOPS) is commonly used to delineate this evaluation format. In the next sections, the HIPS framework and each of these aspects will be discussed.

History

Taking and recording a patient's history is considered by many clinicians to be the most revealing portion of the evaluation process. An accurate history is very important for determining a differential diagnosis, which is a list of the possible diagnoses associated with a patient's complaint. The process of a differential diagnosis requires that the clinician begin to differentiate between two or more conditions that share common signs or symptoms. Although signs and symptoms are sometimes used interchangeably, they have important differences: symptoms are generally subjective, whereas a sign is more objective. More specifically, a sign is something that can be observed, measured, and recorded by a health care professional, and a symptom is something that the patient feels and may or may not be able to explain or measure. For example, a patient with a fever may show a *sign* of a certain temperature, say 102°F, and the *symptom*s of headache and fatigue. Using the HIPS framework of injury evaluation, the clinician is better able to form a differential diagnosis and determine between signs and symptoms. **Table 2.1** is a breakdown of the HIPS framework used in a clinical examination.

An accurate history can be extremely revealing for the clinician and can help uncover many salient issues. One of the most significant aspects that a good history contributes to is uncovering the mechanism of injury (MOI). Identifying the MOI often reveals the specific cause of or at least identifies the event that immediately preceded the injury as well as informs the clinician of any underlying medical conditions that may contribute to or influence the current condition and quality of life. Discovering the MOI is critical to determining the forces that have been applied to the injured body structures.

The history-taking process requires active listening, thorough note taking, and skills at framing open-ended questions. Although a history usually occurs at

Table 2.1 HIPS Framework

Framework Elements	Description
Subjective Component	
History	The clinician asks the patient about the onset and mechanism of the injury and associated signs and symptoms.
Objective Components	
Inspection/Observation	The clinician observes how the patient presents with the injury (gait, posture, etc) as well as any measurable factors, such as edema, ecchymosis, atrophy, range of motion, signs of infection, and other observable characteristics of the injury.
Palpation	The clinician begins to "feel and touch" the injured area to identify areas of point tenderness, swelling, pain, or discomfort and may also use it in conjunction with assessing range of motion in determining end feel.
Special tests	The clinician intentionally stresses the joint or injured body part to assess the integrity of the structures and soft tissue near and around the injury, which helps to determine extent and involvement of the injury. Other special tests include neurologic screening and muscle function tests (eg, break tests or manual muscle tests).

the beginning of the evaluation, it is often necessary to revisit it throughout the entire evaluation process. A thorough history provides information about the activity that was being performed when the injury occurred, the extent of the injury, the anatomic structures involved in the injury, and any limitations in participation or desired activities that resulted from the injury.

Taking a history typically involves asking about past medical history as well as history of the current condition. Past medical history helps the clinician to establish any previous history that is relevant to the current condition (eg, any previous surgeries, previous injuries, residual complaints, general health status, or current medications). It is also important to identify any comorbidities. Comorbidity, or when a patient has one or more distinct conditions, is associated with worse health outcomes, more complex clinical management, and increased cost of care.[1] A thorough history includes asking questions about other medical conditions, including comorbidities. The history of the current condition is to identify the cause of the current complaint. It is necessary, at this point, to determine current level of function, which is to determine any restrictions to current activity and any limitations the patient may be experiencing in any aspect of life. These limitations transcend sports participation and include activities of daily living. A thorough history can also help determine any changes in activity that have occurred and, if activity is still possible, helps to identify if there any changes to activity patterns.

Gathering Information During a History

When taking a history, it is necessary to help the patient focus on his or her primary complaint. The primary complaint is the patient's perception of the current injury. It may be necessary to gather information relative to past medical history, but the clinician should help the patient focus on the primary complaint first. It is also extremely important that the clinician learn to ask open-ended questions. Asking questions that require only yes or no responses, known as closed-ended questions, may not provide enough information to make an accurate assessment. Open-ended questions require the patient to go into more detail and provide more information. Open-ended questions about the primary complaint and the mechanism of injury include questions such as the following:

1. What is the problem?
2. What hurts?
3. When did the injury occur?
4. What activities cause pain?
5. What activities reduce pain?
6. Describe the type/sensation of pain (stabbing, aching, throbbing, radicular, radiating, etc).
7. How did the injury occur/how did you do it?
8. If you landed awkwardly, how did you land?
9. What position was the joint in when you got hurt?
10. How long ago was the injury?
11. Do you remember anything specific that happened immediately before or after the injury?
12. Did you hear any noises (eg, click, pop, snap, or crack) when the injury occurred?

It may also be beneficial to use a mnemonic to help remember what questions should be asked. One such mnemonic that aids in the collection of a relevant history is OPQRST:

1. O = Onset of the injury—What happened?
2. P = Provocation—What makes this problem feel better or worse?
3. Q = Quality of the pain—How would you describe the pain?
4. R = Region or radiation—Where is the pain?
5. S = Severity—How bad is the pain?
6. T = Timing—How long has it been hurting? Did the symptoms change?

Asking questions such as these will help the clinician make an informed and accurate clinical diagnosis. The more specific the questions can be without badgering the patient, the more likely that meaningful and accurate information will be obtained.

Finally, it is also important that the clinician be aware of the patient's level of frustration and anxiety during the history, especially if it is a relatively acute injury. Being aware of the patient's demeanor during this portion of the examination is an important segue to observation.

Inspection

Inspection (others may refer to this portion as observation) is the next aspect within the HIPS framework and includes observing how the patient presents his or her *signs* and *symptoms*. In an ideal situation, the clinician observes the injury in real time. However, that is not always the case; most of the time, the patient presents to the clinician after the injury has occurred. Inspection includes obtaining a general overview of the appearance of the injury and the patient, including the symmetry of the patient's body; the patient's posture, gait, and level of consciousness; and an observation of general motor function. Additionally, it is important to note any deformity, swelling, discoloration, scars, cuts or abrasions, redness, ecchymosis, and any other skin abnormalities.

Additionally, it may be important to note general inspections, especially if the patient is unknown to the clinician, of the patient's well-being, willingness and ability to move, age, physical condition, and personal hygiene. Questions for the clinician to consider during inspection of the patient include the following:

1. What is the patient's level of consciousness/is the patient oriented to his or her surroundings?
2. What is the patient's level of irritability?
3. Does the patient appear to be relatively healthy and practice good hygiene?
4. Does the patient make good eye contact, and is he or she able to articulate?
5. What are the general speech patterns of the patient (slurred, hoarse, fast, etc)?

When visually scanning appearance, it is important to note symmetry of the patient's body. For example, are the shoulder heights relatively equal; posture upright; spinal curves normal; and feet, knees, and elbows "normal"? When observing, make note of pes planus, pes cavus, genu recurvatum, genu valgus, genu varus, and elbow carrying angle.

Further inspection of the injury site may include a general or quick assessment of motor function. For example, is the patient able to bend over (flex); bend to the side; rotate the head, neck, and spine; walk on the heels and toes; and flex and extend the shoulders over and above the head? While the patient is performing these general motor tasks, it is important to observe the ease or difficulty with which he or she performs these tasks, making note of any intense pain or discomfort. If any inflammation or other changes in the appearance of the joint are noted, the clinician must be able to determine whether these changes are edema or effusion. Edema, also known as swelling, is typically extra-articular (outside of the joint capsule), whereas effusion is usually intra-articular (inside the joint capsule). It may be necessary for the clinician to perform special tests, such as a sweep test, to identify effusion. When inflammation is suspected, but not readily obvious, it may be necessary for the clinician to record girth measurements. Girth measurements generally require measuring the circumference of a body part where swelling is suspected. It is important to note nearby anatomic landmarks so that measurements are more reliable.

Palpation

Palpation is the part of the examination where the clinician "touches and feels" the patient's injury. It is important to obtain consent from any patient during a physical examination, but it is especially important, and should be done formally, when the patient is a minor. Ask the patient whether he or she has a preference regarding the sex of the clinician. If it is possible, this preference should be accommodated. However, if it is not possible and the evaluation needs to continue, there should be a third party observing; it is best that the third party be another clinician or the patient's parent or guardian (if a minor).

General rules of palpation include bilateral comparison and feeling the temperature of the skin, feeling for any swelling, noting any areas of point tenderness, identifying crepitus, feeling for deformity, noting end feel with passive range of motion (ROM), noting any muscle spasms, determining sensations on the skin, and assessing pulse and capillary refill. Bilateral comparison means that it is necessary to palpate paired anatomic structures. For example, when assessing an injured right forearm, it is important to assess the left forearm to establish a baseline. In addition to bilateral comparison, palpation should begin with gentle pressure that gradually increases. Palpation should always be initiated on structures away from (distal) the most sensitive area and move toward the injured area. Palpating the unaffected side first and waiting to palpate the most painful area until last helps to build rapport with the patient and reduces residual pain for subsequent palpitations.

As a precaution, it may be necessary that the clinician wears protective gloves, and the clinician should always have clean, warm hands. To maximize palpation, the clinician must have an accurate and proficient knowledge of clinical anatomy. Knowledge of surface anatomy, such as the bones, bony landmarks, origins and insertions of muscles, circulatory system, and location of bursa, is necessary; without such knowledge, it may be difficult to form an accurate clinical diagnosis.

Special Tests

After the history, inspection, and palpation have been completed, it is important to perform special tests, which are necessary to assess the integrity of the body's tissues (eg, ligaments, tendons, muscles, cartilage, bones). In most situations, special tests are performed last; however, it is not uncommon, especially in emergent, on-field, or follow-up situations, for these tests to come earlier in the assessment process. Regardless of the situation, special tests should not be

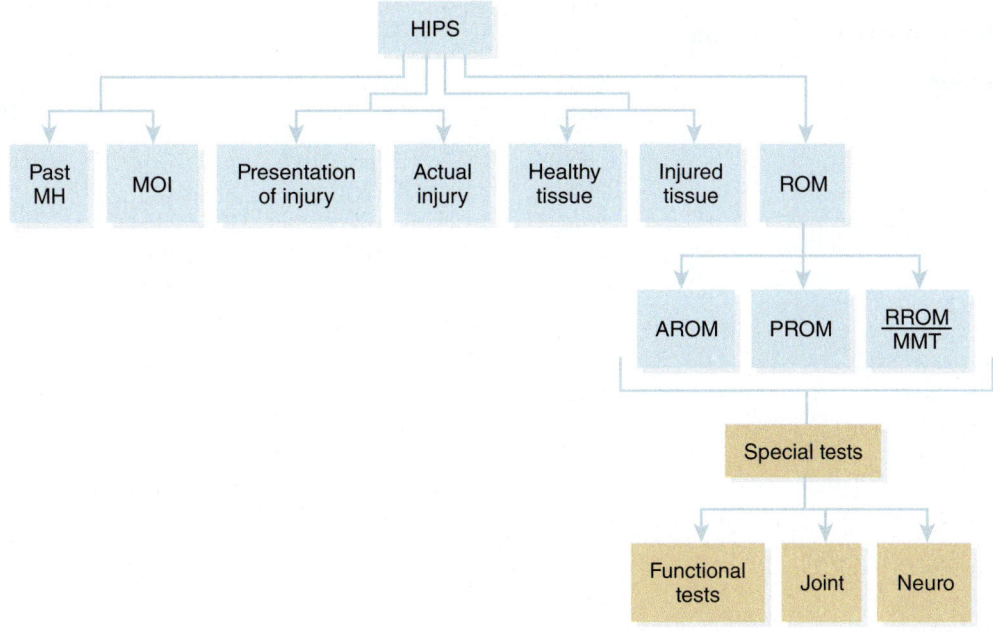

Figure 2.1 Concept map of HIPS framework.
AROM, active range of motion; HIPS, history, inspection, palpation, special tests; MH, medical history; MMT, manual muscle testing; MOI, mechanism of injury; PMH, past medical history; PROM, passive range of motion; ROM, range of motion; RROM, resisted range of motion.
© Jones & Bartlett Learning

completed until fractures, dislocations, and musculotendinous ruptures have been ruled out. **Figure 2.1** is a concept map of the overall HIPS framework.

Special tests include a variety of interventions:

1. Functional tests (basic and sport specific)
2. ROM and end feel (Note: Some clinicians may include ROM testing during the inspection portion of the assessment.)
3. Ligamentous stress test
4. Neurologic tests

Each of these special tests, the *S* of HIPS, is briefly described in the next paragraphs. Specific special tests and related components are described in more detail in later chapters.

Functional Tests

Functional testing takes two forms during the examination process. The first is basic functional testing, which includes tasks such as walking, standing up from a chair, sitting down, opening a door, lifting, reaching, pushing, pulling, ascending and descending stairs, or other rudimentary functional activities (sometimes referred to as activities of daily living). Functional tests can be as simple as weight bearing or balancing in an upright position. Obviously, these basic functional tests come early in the examination and are used to determine a patient's limitations and disability as well as the overall extent of the injury.

Later in the examination process, as the clinician reassesses the patient to determine how much progress has been made, when to progress, or even to determine return to play, it is likely that sport-specific functional tests will be used. Sport-specific functional testing includes running, jumping, diagonal movements, changes of direction, balancing on unstable surfaces, kicking or throwing, and any other movements that the sport requires. In both the basic and sport-specific versions, functional tests are used to determine the extent of the patient's balance, coordination, agility, strength, endurance, and power, all of which are essential to performing a thorough evaluation.

ROM and End Feel

Typically, ROM occurs during the special tests portion of the evaluation. However, some clinicians may prefer to perform ROM testing earlier in the examination. Regardless of when it occurs, ROM is a must for a complete evaluation. It can be measured objectively with a goniometer (**Figure 2.2**), and typical ranges for selected joints are listed in **Table 2.2**.

Typically, ROM assessment occurs in the following order: active range of motion (AROM), passive range of motion (PROM), and resisted range of motion (RROM). If the patient is able to perform satisfactory AROM, then PROM and RROM can be assessed. However, if the patient is unable to perform AROM, then RROM is either not necessary or

Table 2.2 Normal Ranges of Motion

Joint	Motion	Range of Motion	Joint	Motion	Range of Motion

Cervical	Flexion
	Extension
	Lateral flexion
	Rotation
		0°–80°
		0°–70°
		0°–45°
		0°–80°
			Digits 2 to 5
			  MCP
			  PIP
			  DIP
				
				Flexion
				Extension
				Abduction
				Flexion
				Flexion
					
					0°–90°
					0°–45°
					0°–20°
					0°–100°
					0°–90°

Lumbar	Forward flexion Extension Lateral flexion Rotation	0°–60° 0°–35° 0°–20° 0°–50°	Hip	Flexion Extension Abduction Adduction Internal rotation External rotation	0°–120° 0°–30° 0°–40° 0°–30° 0°–40° 0°–50°
Shoulder	Flexion Extension Abduction Internal rotation External rotation Horizontal abduction/adduction	0°–180° 0°–60° 0°–180° 0°–70° 0°–90° 0°–130°	Knee	Flexion Extension Medial rotation with knee flexed Lateral rotation with knee flexed	0°–135° 0°–15° 0°–25° 0°–35°
Elbow	Flexion Extension	0°–150° 0°–10°	Ankle	Dorsiflexion Plantar flexion Pronation Supination	0°–20° 0°–50° 0°–30° 0°–50°
Forearm	Pronation Supination	0°–80° 0°–80°	Subtalar	Inversion Eversion	0°–5° 0°–5°

Wrist	Flexion
	Extension
	Ulnar deviation
	Radial deviation
		0°–80°
		0°–70°
		0°–30°
		0°–20°
			Hallux
			  1st MTP
			
			  1st IP
				
				Flexion
				Extension
				Flexion
					
					0°–45°
					0°–75°
					0°–90°

Thumb
  CMC
 	
  MCP
  IP
	
	Abduction
	Flexion
	Extension
	Opposition
	Flexion
	Flexion
		
		0°–70°
		0°–15°
		0°–20°
		Tip of thumb to tip of fifth finger
		0°–50°
		0°–80°
			Toes 2 to 5
			  MTP
			
			  PIP
			  DIP
				
				Flexion
				Extension
				Flexion
				Flexion
				Extension
					
					0°–40°
					0°–40°
					0°–35°
					0°–30°
					0°–60°

CMC, carpometacarpal; DIP, distal interphalangeal; IP, interphalangeal; MCP, metacarpophalangeal; MTP, metatarsophalangeal; PIP, posterior interphalangeal.

contraindicated (PROM can still be assessed in the absence of AROM). **Figure 2.3** shows the use of a goniometer.

AROM is a joint motion performed voluntarily by the patient via muscular contraction. Unless contraindicated, AROM should be performed before PROM. AROM is an indication that the patient is willing and able to move the injured joint and contract the associated muscles. When the patient is not able to perform AROM, it is typically an indication of a neuromuscular injury. An accurate AROM assessment includes determining specific ranges (Table 2.2) as well as noting the patient's willingness to move and the ease of that movement. During an AROM assessment, the clinician must note the point during the range where pain begins, the painful arc (the presence of pain at specific joint angles), and the type of pain associated with the complaint. If the patient suspects that a particular movement will be painful and exhibits apprehension, it should be performed last or terminated if apprehension is noticed.

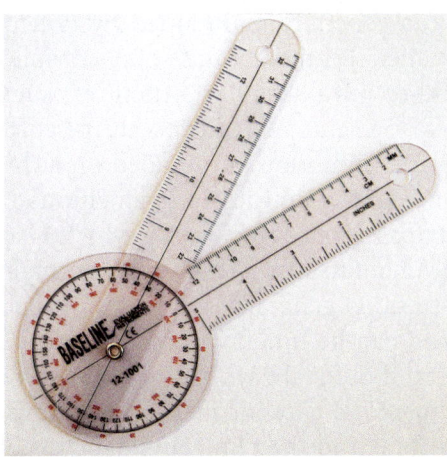

Figure 2.2 An example of a goniometer.
© Jones & Bartlett Learning

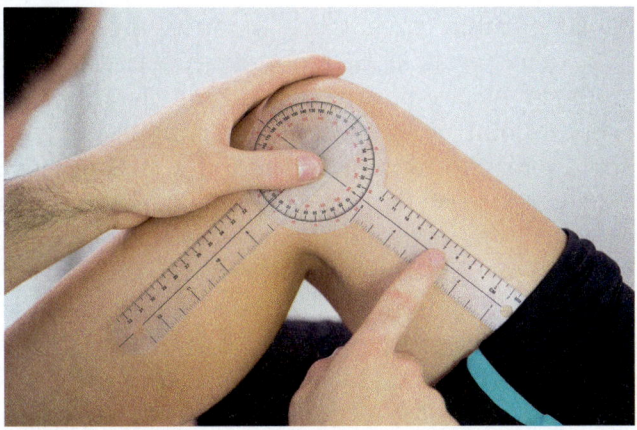

Figure 2.3 Example of a goniometric measurement.
© ESB Professional/Shutterstock

PROM is motion where the clinician "moves" the patient's injured body part without any assistance from the patient. Positioning the patient for PROM is important. The patient should be relaxed and in a non–weight-bearing position. The rationale to performing PROM is that it distinguishes between contractile and noncontractile tissue. Typically, if there is pain with PROM, it is an indication that the injury is to noncontractile tissue; if there is no pain with PROM, but pain is present with AROM, it is an indication of injury to contractile tissue. Another important component of PROM is gentle overpressure. Typically, PROM will show greater ranges than AROM because the clinician will apply gentle overpressure to determine end feel.

Normal end feels include soft, firm, and hard. Soft end feels result from tissue approximation, which is when two body parts touch. An example of a soft end feel as a result of tissue approximation is elbow flexion when the forearm and bicep touch. A firm end feel results from soft-tissue stretch (eg, muscular, capsular, ligamentous). An example of a firm end feel is when the end range of a muscle begins to feel tight during flexibility testing. A hard end feel results from bone-to-bone contact. An example would be elbow extension during which the olecranon process fits into the olecranon fossa.

Abnormal end feels occur when any of the normal end feels occur out of place (eg, if the clinician recognizes a hard end feel when there should be a soft end feel, or a firm end feel when there should be a hard end feel). In addition to these three abnormal end feels, there is an empty end feel, which is the absence of any sensation at all. This is when, at the end range, the clinician does not notice any tissue resistance and the patient does not have any pain.

RROM is motion during which the clinician resists the patient's voluntary movement. Some clinicians refer to this as manual muscle testing or break testing. RROM/manual muscle testing is a way to evaluate voluntary muscle contraction by asking the patient to perform movements of the joint against gravity or manual resistance. It can also be described as gentle to moderate resistance applied by the clinician throughout the patient's available ROM. **Figure 2.4** shows examples of selected manual muscle tests. Break tests are when overload is applied to a patient when holding a static (isometric) position. The intent is for the patient to hold a static position (isometric contraction), for example, elbow flexion at 90°, while the clinician tries to gently, but forcefully, move the forearm and consequently the elbow back to neutral or into extension. **Table 2.3** is the typical scale used to grade manual muscle tests.

During RROM testing, muscle strength is graded on a six-point numeric scale. Some clinicians use plusses and minuses within this scale. For example, if the clinician estimates that a patient's strength is approximately 90%, the rating would be 4+ (falling between 4 and 5). A plus and minus system can be added for any number between 1 and 4 on the strength scale to add further specificity and detail to the medical record.

RROM is necessary because it will help detect neuromuscular involvement in any injury. The presence of pain during RROM testing should be noted, and the test may need to be repeated before pain or weakness is noted.

Ligamentous Stress Test

After ROM testing is complete, it is necessary to perform a series of tests that assess the integrity of the joint and its associated structures. Joint

Chapter 2 The Examination Process

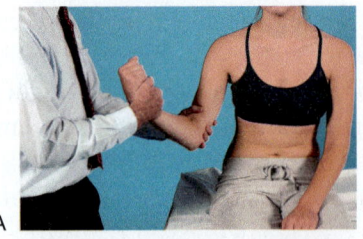
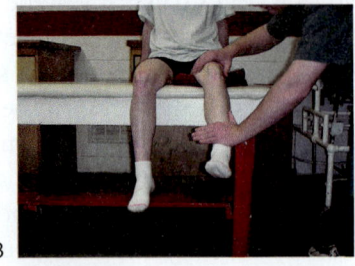
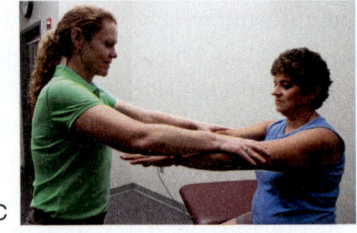

Figure 2.4 Examples of manual muscle testing. **A.** The elbow. **B.** The knee. **C.** The shoulder.

A. © Jones & Bartlett Learning; B. Used with permission from http://at.uwa.edu/mmt/knee.htm; C. © Jones & Bartlett Learning

Table 2.3 Manual Muscle Testing Scale

Numeric Value	Grade Name	Percentage	Clinical Description
0	Zero	0%	No muscle contraction
1	Trace	5%	Evidence of muscular contraction, no joint movement
2	Poor	20%	Complete range of motion with some assistance or gravity eliminated
3	Fair	50%	Complete range of motion against gravity
4	Good	80%	Complete range of motion against gravity and some resistance
5	Normal	100%	Complete range of motion against gravity with negative break test

integrity is generally maintained by noncontractile tissues called ligaments and joint capsules; sometimes, other intra-articular structures, such as cartilage, are present. Stress tests are performed in a single plane of motion and graded on a three-point scale for severity. Injuries to ligamentous tissue are referred to as sprains. Instability, which is the failure of the ligament to sustain the joint's normal function under stress, is generally the result of ligamentous injury and can be functional or dynamic. Ligamentous tests should always be performed bilaterally and compared to baseline metrics. Positioning of the patient's joint and the clinician's hands is of utmost importance to ensure proper angle during ligamentous testing. Generally, when examining for joint laxity and ligamentous injury, the proximal segment of the joint is stabilized, and the distal segment is moved. Failure to properly position the patient's joint may result in false-positive or false-negative findings. A false-positive ligamentous test result is when a joint or ligament is not injured, but testing appears to indicate an injury; a false-negative ligamentous test result is when a joint or ligament is actually injured, but testing does not reveal the injury. Typically, false-negative test results are a consequence of muscle guarding or faulty joint positioning during testing.

The three-point scale for ligamentous sprains is as follows:

- Grade 1 has a normal ligamentous end feel and is described as a minor stretching of the ligament with little or no tearing of the fibers. Pain is present, but stability is comparable upon bilateral comparison.
- Grade 2 has a soft or abnormal end feel and is described as partial tearing of the fiber. There is moderate instability when compared bilaterally.
- Grade 3 has an empty end feel and is described as a complete tearing of the ligament.

In addition to ligamentous stress tests, there are other tests that have been developed by clinicians that target specific body parts (eg, bones, muscle, or tendon). Generally speaking, these tests are more detailed than ligamentous tests; they often occur across multiple planes of motion and are not generally graded on severity (except for strains, which are injuries to muscles and tendons that are also graded on a three-point scale). In many cases, special tests are reported as positive or negative. An example of a special test would be the Yergason test, which is a technique used to assess pathology to the bicipital tendon at the bicipital groove.

Neurologic Tests

Neurologic testing is very complex, so it will be discussed only briefly here. Basic neurologic testing includes dermatomes, myotomes, and reflexes.

The sensory component of a neurologic test requires assessing dermatomes. **Figure 2.5** identifies the possible dermatomes that should be assessed during injury evaluation. Dermatomes can be assessed by using different pressures and sensations on the surface of the skin. For example, a patient should be able to distinguish between a cotton ball, pinprick, and feather, and between light pressure versus deep pressure. When performing a dermatome assessment, the clinician should ask the patient about the sensations and whether or not the sensations are similar when compared bilaterally.

The motor component of neurologic testing requires assessing myotomes. Myotomes are the nerve roots that innervate specific muscles or muscle groups. **Table 2.4** identifies the myotomes and their associated neuromuscular motions. When performing a myotome assessment, the clinician instructs the patient to demonstrate specific movements or motions, which the clinician evaluates for the quality and strength of a given muscular contraction and the coordination of associated muscular contractions. Weakness in a myotome may indicate possible injury to the nerve or nerve root.

Reflexes should also be assessed during neurologic testing. Assessing reflexes can indicate damage to the central nervous system; reflexes, and specifically deep tendon reflexes, may be diminished or even absent if the nerve root is injured. Abnormal reflexes should be considered relevant only in conjunction with sensory or

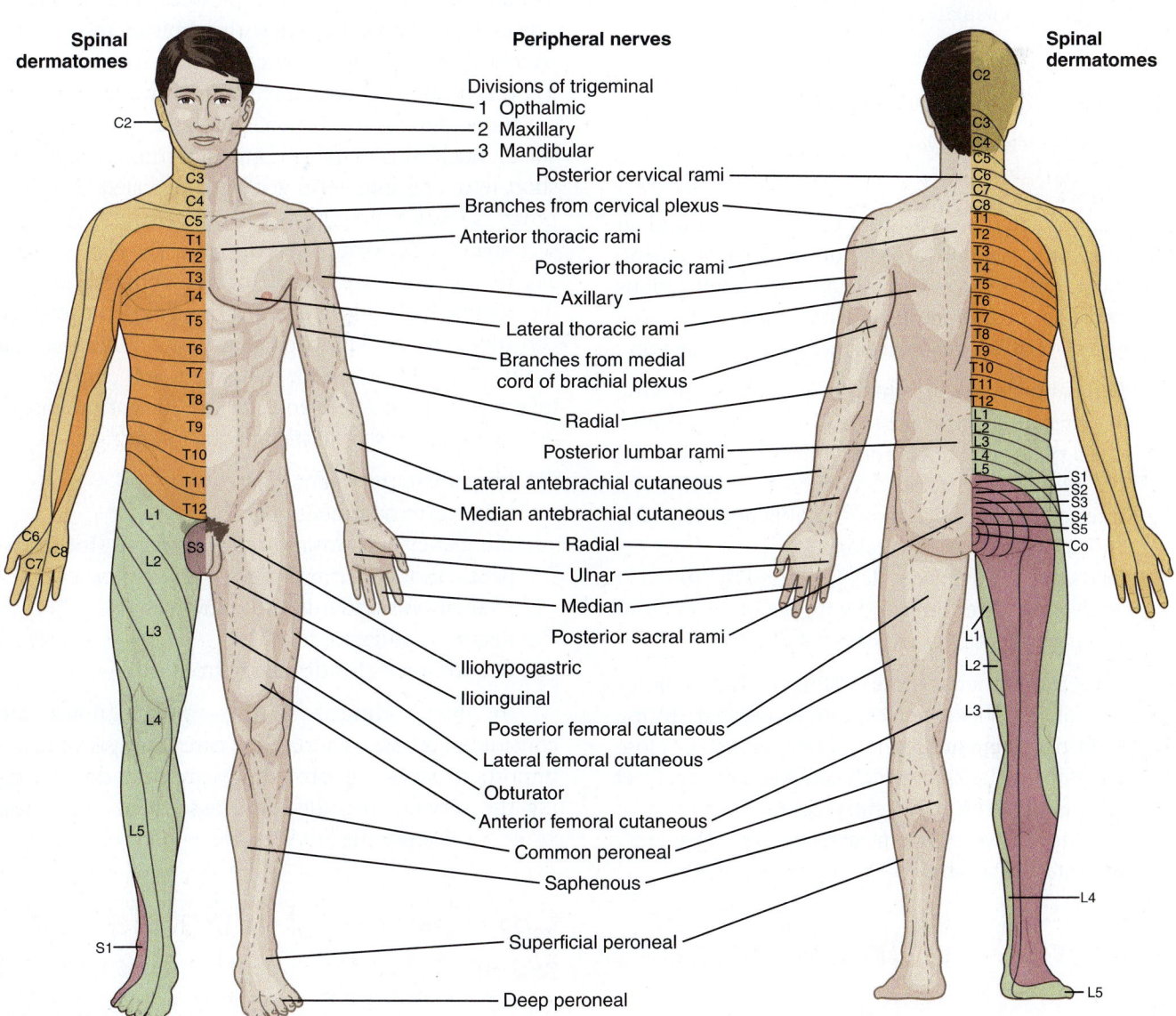

Figure 2.5 Anatomic drawing identifying the dermatomes.

© Jones & Bartlett Learning

Table 2.4 Common Myotomes

Nerve Root	Motion
C1, C2	Cervical flexion
C3	Cervical side flexion
C4	Scapula elevation
C5	Shoulder abduction
C6	Elbow flexion and wrist extension
C7	Elbow extension and wrist flexion
C8	Thumb extension
T1	Finger abduction
L1, L2	Hip flexion
L3	Knee extension
L4	Ankle dorsiflexion
L5	Big toe extension
S1	Ankle plantar flexion
S2	Knee flexion

motor abnormalities, as it is not uncommon to find an abnormal reflex without sensory or motor involvement. Pathologic reflexes can indicate motor neural lesions and serve as an indication of a pathologic condition. Examples of pathologic reflexes include the following:

- The Babinski reflex, which is elicited by stroking the lateral aspect of the sole of the foot, can indicate a pyramidal tract lesion if the big toe extends.
- The Oppenheim reflex is elicited by stroking the anterior medial portion of the tibia and may also indicate pyramid tract lesion.
- A positive Brudzinski reflex is elicited by passively flexing the lower limb and with the opposite limb also moving; it may indicate meningitis.

Finally, peripheral nerve testing includes motor function of peripheral nerves and is assessed during ROM testing. There are several peripheral nerves close to the surface of the skin, which can be tested via Tinel sign; this is performed by light pressure or tapping of the skin directly over a superficial nerve. A positive Tinel sign indicates irritation or compression of the nerve.

Record-Keeping Format (SOAP Notes)

Another critical component to a thorough evaluation is accurate records. After documenting the initial injury, it is important to keep up-to-date and accurate progress notes. These progress notes are essential to ensuring and maintaining proper patient care. The standard format for notes documenting the patient's progress is referred to as SOAP notes. Health care professionals in a variety of disciplines use this SOAP format.

The *subjective* aspect of the report refers to the current feelings of the patient. These feelings cannot be validated via objective measurements; they are simply how the patient reports feeling that day and are an indicator of the ongoing status of the patient's recovery. The *objective* aspect of the report refers to any objective measures that can be reported; these may include follow-up special tests, ROM, strength measurements, girth measurements, or other measurable outcomes. It is not necessary to repeat the entire initial evaluation when recording objective notes, but they should be thorough and address any changes from previous measurements. The *assessment* aspect is where the clinician assesses the patient's prognosis and may confirm or reiterate a clinical diagnosis. The assessment primarily addresses two questions: how is the patient progressing and is he or she on track? It is in the assessment portion where both short-term and long-term goals are indicated as well as progress toward those goals and any setbacks. The final section of the SOAP record is the plan. The *plan* is where any interventions are noted. Interventions can include therapeutic modalities, remedial or advanced exercises, consultations, and functional activities. These are all outlined in this section for the patient and clinicians to follow and use as a reference for the current prognosis. A thorough plan should include the following:

1. Immediate treatment goals
2. Long-term treatment goals
3. Frequency and duration of treatments (for therapeutic modalities and therapeutic exercises)
4. Evaluation standards and outcomes
5. Required patient education
6. Requirements for discharge from care

In many clinical settings, SOAP notes are considered a basic standard of care; they serve as an important aspect of providing care and documenting the services provided and associated outcomes. Table 2.5 is a sample SOAP note.

On-Field and Emergency Evaluations

When assessing an injury in an emergency, and after ruling out life-threatening conditions, the typical HIPS framework still applies, but can be implemented with greater flexibility. However, regardless

Table 2.5 Sample SOAP Note

Section	Sample
Subjective	Patient reports feeling "better" today. Reported sleeping well last night despite some "minor throbbing" in the left ankle. Patient reported walking yesterday with virtually no pain.
Objective	Yesterday's radiograph ruled out fracture. Patient reports pain is 2/10. Ranges of motion for dorsiflexion, plantar flexion, inversion, and eversion are within normal limits; manual muscle tests for both dorsiflexion and plantar flexion are 4/5. Negative talar tilt test; negative anterior drawer test; patient indicates a small amount of pain with Kleiger test.
Assessment	Patient continues to present with symptoms indicating grade 1 syndesmosis sprain of left ankle. Patient should be able to increase tolerance of current exercise program. Continue weight-bearing exercises and add 10 lb to stationary calf press.
Plan	All exercises should be completed with brace or tape. Continue current exercise regimen and add 3 × 10 bodyweight lunge walks and 3 × 10 lateral skipping.

of the level of urgency, the clinician should at least take a modified history and determine the location of the pain, presence of any neurologic signs and symptoms, the mechanism of injury, and associated sounds (crack or pop associated with the injury). Occasionally, multiple patients are injured at the same time, in which case the clinician should perform triage. Triage is the rapid assessment of all injured parties to determine who has the most serious injuries.

After a modified history has been performed, on-field or emergent inspection/observation would include checking the surrounding environment for additional dangerous conditions or clues about the MOI. The clinician should note body position of the patient (eg, supine, prone, or sideline) and note any gross deformity or posture. For example, is the patient found in extension of all four extremities (eg, decerebrate rigidity), or extension of the legs and flexion of the upper extremities, including wrists and fingers (eg, decorticate rigidity)? **Figure 2.6** is an example of the types of rigidity. Additional observation would include how the patient presents the injury—is he or she protecting a limb or limping? Note the patient's level of responsiveness and any associated signs of head trauma.

On-site and emergent palpation should include bony palpitations for possible fractures as well as for gross deformity, specific deformity, skin temperature, and any swelling. On-site and emergency special testing can include quick assessments of ROM and weight bearing as well as any specialized joint integrity tests. On-site neurologic testing can include cutaneous sensation (dermatomes) and gross motor function. Finally, the clinician should inspect any damaged equipment and use safe and appropriate techniques to remove any equipment that hinders the patient's

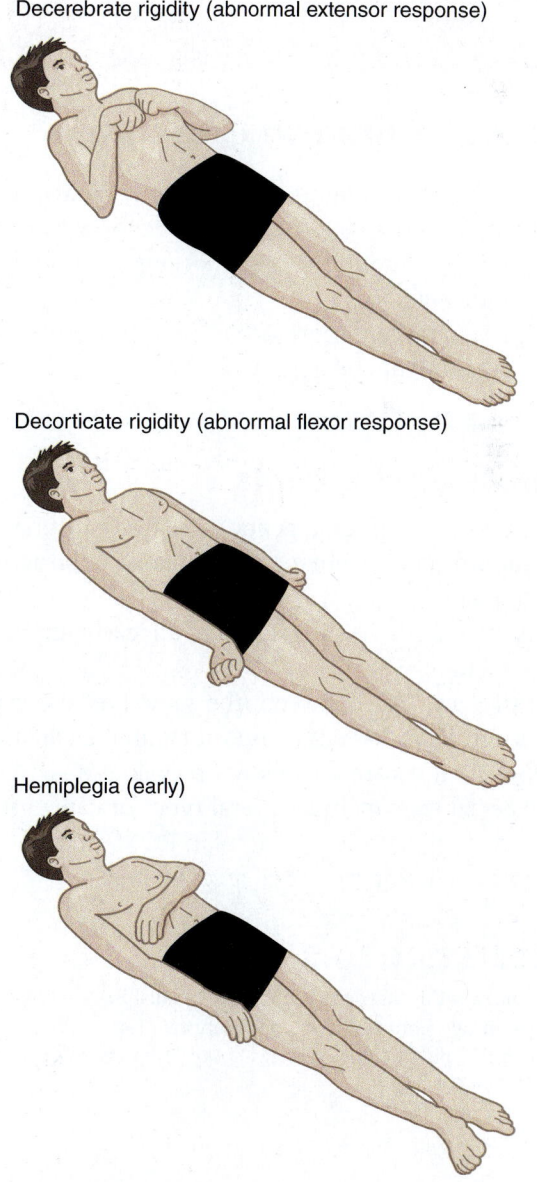

Figure 2.6 Abdominal postures showing rigidity in comatose patients.

© Jones & Bartlett Learning

immediate well-being. The injured patient should be moved only when deemed safe to do so. Under no circumstances should coaches, players, officials, or other bystanders prematurely move the patient, nor should the clinician allow any bystanders to pressure or expedite moving a patient before it is deemed safe.

Summary

Performing a thorough evaluation of an injured patient should be structured and organized. That structure typically follows the HIPS framework. Evaluating an injured patient can be extremely complex and require integrating and assimilating information from multiple sources, including the history, inspection, palpation, and special tests. The clinician should take care to thoughtfully and thoroughly report initial findings as well as follow-up findings in a SOAP format. Using the HIPS framework and the SOAP format increases the likelihood of an accurate clinical diagnosis and allows the clinician to develop a well-informed plan of care.

WRAP-UP

Critical Thinking Questions

1. When assessing range of motion (ROM), what might differences between deficits in passive range of motion and active range of motion indicate?
2. Discuss the importance of performing all assessments bilaterally.
3. How is an on-site or emergent assessment/evaluation different from a clinical evaluation?
4. Describe the difference between a false-positive and a false-negative test result.
5. What is the value of end feel during a clinical musculoskeletal/orthopedic evaluation and helping to reach a clinical diagnosis?

Pearls and Pitfalls

- Unless in an emergency situation, evaluations should be systematic and follow a structured sequence.
- Active ROM testing can be an early myotome screen.
- HIPS and SOAP are not the same types of evaluation. HIPS format is used for initial evaluations; SOAP notes are for follow-up evaluations.
- Special tests include several types or categories of tests (eg, neurologic, vascular, ROM) and not *only* joint laxity or structural assessments.
- Clinician positioning is just as important as patient positioning in order to perform special tests correctly.
- Functional tests are both general and specific. Used early in an evaluation, they can indicate basic activities of daily living—for example, standing, bending, walking, and sitting—and, later in the evaluation, they can be sport-specific activities (eg, running, jumping, and cutting).

Reference

1. Valderas JM, Starfield B, Sibbald B, Salisbury C, Roland M: Defining comorbidity: implications for understanding health and health services. *Ann Fam Med* 2009;7(4): 357-363.

CHAPTER 3

Evidence-Based Injury Evaluation

Jenny L. Toonstra, PhD, ATC, LAT

OVERVIEW

This chapter provides an overview of evidence-based practice (EBP) as it relates to clinical evaluation and diagnosis. Concepts such as reliability, validity, sensitivity, specificity, and receiver operating characteristic (ROC) curves will be explained in the context of clinical decision making. Understanding the interpretation of these values will assist students in applying the concepts of EBP to make informed decisions regarding the clinical usefulness of commonly used diagnostic tests.

LEARNING OBJECTIVES

After completing this chapter, the reader will be able to do the following:

1. Describe the role of EBP in the evaluation and diagnosis process.
2. Define the diagnostic properties of clinical tests and describe how these concepts can be used to inform clinical decision making.
3. Interpret sensitivity, specificity, and ROC curve values to determine the clinical usefulness of commonly used diagnostic tests.

FUN FACTS ABOUT EVIDENCE-BASED PRACTICE

- EBP helps clinicians stay current on standardized practices.
- EBP improves the transparency and accountability of the clinician.
- EBP improves quality of care.

Introduction

Evidence-based practice (EBP) provides the groundwork for clinical decision making and high-quality, patient-centered care. Evidence-based medicine has been defined as the "conscientious and judicious use of current best evidence in making decisions about the care of individual patients."[1] Inherent in this definition is the merging of relevant scientific evidence, patient values and expectations, and clinical judgment and expertise. EBP is not a new concept in athletic training. It is included as a core competency in the Commission on Accreditation of Athletic Training Education's *2020 Standards for Accreditation of Professional Athletic Training Programs*.[2] It has been shown that EBP improves patient care, promotes critical thinking, demonstrates effectiveness of athletic training interventions, encourages third-party reimbursement, and enhances the reputation of athletic training within the health care industry.[3] Although athletic trainers perceive EBP as valuable, barriers to implementing EBP into clinical practice still exist. These barriers include limited access to scientific research, lack of time, and lack of relevance and applicability to clinical practice.[4] The goal of this chapter is to remove some of those barriers by assisting clinicians in the understanding, interpretation, and relevance of EBP in diagnostic research.

Clinical evaluation of injuries and illnesses is a systematic process that involves decision making at many levels. Determining which tests are most appropriate for ruling in or ruling out a specific pathology can be a daunting process. For example, there are multiple tests to assess for superior labrum anterior to posterior (SLAP) lesions. Should the clinician perform every test on every patient with a suspected SLAP lesion? If not, which test(s) should he or she use to rule in or rule out the presence of a SLAP lesion? Applying EBP throughout the evaluation process assists the clinician in selecting the most accurate and reliable clinical tests. This, in turn, expedites the examination process, produces more accurate diagnoses, and ultimately aids the clinician in developing effective management strategies. Therefore, it is vital that clinicians understand and appreciate evidence-based medicine in the context of injury evaluation. First, however, clinicians must understand the role that each component of EBP plays with respect to injury evaluation and diagnosis.

The body of scientific evidence related to athletic training interventions, prognoses, and diagnoses continues to grow. As this evidence base grows, it is imperative for clinicians to be able to critically evaluate the evidence and determine what diagnostic tools they will incorporate into their clinical practice. This process of critical appraisal includes an assessment of the methodologic quality of the study and its relevance to clinical practice. Although an assessment of methodologic quality is beyond the scope of this chapter, it may be helpful to note that the Quality Assessment of Diagnostic Accuracy Studies, or QUADAS-2, is a tool developed to assess the quality of diagnostic accuracy studies,[5] and may be a useful resource for clinicians when evaluating studies. This chapter, rather, will focus on the interpretation of diagnostic studies and determine their relevance and applicability to clinical practice. The first question a clinician should ask when assessing a diagnostic study is, "Are the patients in this study representative of the patients in my clinical practice?" If the answer is no, the clinician should interpret the results of the study with caution. For example, a study evaluating the accuracy of the Thessaly test in diagnosing meniscal tears in adolescents may not be applicable to a clinician who primarily treats elderly patients. Without evidence demonstrating the accuracy of the Thessaly test in elderly patients, the clinician must rely on his or her clinical judgment and expertise as well as the unique clinical presentation of the patient to determine if utilizing the Thessaly test is warranted.

Relevant scientific research is not a be-all and end-all. Clinical judgment and expertise also factor into whether a clinician decides to incorporate a specific diagnostic test into clinical practice. Although a test may demonstrate high degrees of diagnostic accuracy, this evidence is futile if the clinician is unfamiliar with that test or has little experience performing the test. For example, the Thessaly test has demonstrated high diagnostic accuracy values for meniscal pathology.[6] However, the Thessaly test is a relatively new test and may be unfamiliar to some clinicians. As such, their clinical results may not demonstrate similar degrees of accuracy as the evidence indicates. As scientific research continues to evolve and grow within the profession of athletic training, it becomes the responsibility of clinicians to remain current with new diagnostic tests, especially if they improve clinical decision making.

Patient-centered care is at the core of evidence-based medicine. Without considering patient values, preferences, goals, and unique circumstances, scientific research and clinical experience are meaningless. Weighing the evidence of diagnostic studies must always be considered relative to the unique characteristics of the patient. For example, a clinician may elect to use the Thessaly test in a patient with a suspected meniscus tear because the test has a high degree of diagnostic accuracy. Furthermore, the clinician may also be very comfortable performing this test on patients with suspected meniscal pathology. However, careful consideration should be given to a patient who presents with weight-bearing limitations due to pain, swelling, and/or feelings of instability. Although the evidence clearly demonstrates that the Thessaly test is superior for diagnosing meniscal lesions and it may be the preferred test based on clinical experience and preference, it would not be appropriate to utilize in this scenario given the patient's circumstances. The clinician may then consider performing the McMurray test and/or the Apley compression and distraction test as a substitute because these tests do not require weight bearing.

Integrating the best evidence into injury evaluation requires the clinician to evaluate the strength and clinical usefulness of the evidence relative to diagnostic accuracy; consider the evidence relative to the unique characteristics of the patient; and, finally, consider the evidence relative to his or her clinical expertise. The result is increased confidence in injury evaluation and diagnosis, improved decision making regarding appropriate management, and quality patient-centered care. **Figure 3.1** demonstrates the physical examination process and the relationship among relevant scientific research, clinical expertise, and patient values.

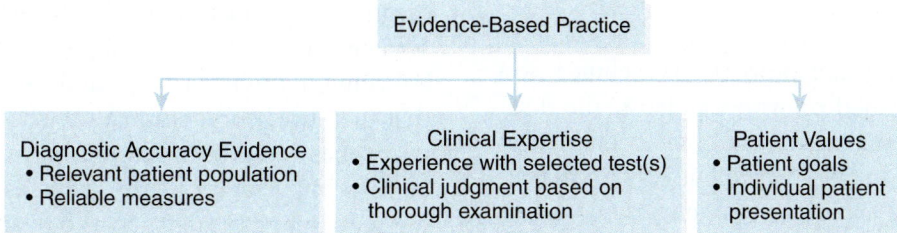

Figure 3.1 Flow chart outlining evidence-based practice in injury evaluation.
© Jones & Bartlett Learning

Diagnostic Accuracy in the Evaluation Process

During the evaluation process, information and clinical outcomes are gathered from the patient through a systematic and thorough examination. A variety of clinical assessment tools are available during this process to determine a patient's degree of dysfunction and impairment and to determine the appropriate course of treatment. These tools also aid the clinician in ruling in or ruling out a specific pathology. Examples of clinical assessment tools include goniometric and girth measurements, special tests, and patient-reported outcome measures. These tools provide the clinician with valuable information regarding the degree of impairment and progress with rehabilitation interventions. However, for these tools to be useful in the diagnosis and management of injuries, they need to demonstrate reliability, validity, and diagnostic accuracy. Clinicians should, at a minimum, be able to interpret diagnostic accuracy studies to determine relevance and clinical usefulness of assessment tools. The usefulness of these clinical tests is usually described in terms of reliability, validity, sensitivity, specificity, and likelihood ratios. The next section provides a description and interpretation of each term, along with a clinical example, using the following hypothetical scenario.

CASE STUDY

Jim was recently hired as an athletic trainer for a busy orthopaedic practice that specializes in shoulder injuries. During his first week, he notices one of the physicians, Dr. Potts, perform a test on a patient with a suspected superior labrum anterior to posterior (SLAP) lesion. He does not recall learning this test while in school, so he approaches the physician after clinic to inquire about this new test. Dr. Potts tells Jim that she developed the test (which she refers to as the Potts maneuver) 2 years earlier and thinks that it is more accurate than other tests for diagnosing SLAP lesions. Jim decides to conduct a study to assess the diagnostic accuracy of the Potts maneuver in diagnosing SLAP lesions. For the next 24 months, he collects data on 100 patients who report to his clinic with a suspected SLAP lesion. Data collected include the results of the Potts maneuver (positive or negative) and the patient's MRI study (SLAP lesion or no SLAP lesion). **Table 3.1** summarizes the results of Jim's 2-year study.

Table 3.1 Results of the Potts Maneuver

	MRI Results	
	SLAP Lesion	**No SLAP Lesion**
Test (+) **Potts Maneuver**	Potts Maneuver (+) SLAP Tear (38 Patients)	Potts Maneuver (+) No SLAP Tear (7 Patients)
Test (−) **Potts Maneuver**	Potts Maneuver (−) SLAP Tear (2 Patients)	Potts Maneuver (−) No SLAP Tear (53 Patients)

SLAP, superior labrum anterior to posterior.

Reliability

Reliability is an important property of a clinical test that must be established prior to evaluating the diagnostic accuracy of that test. Reliability is defined as the consistency of a test or instrument.[7,8] Clinical tests used during injury evaluations should demonstrate consistency of results when performed under similar conditions, in the absence of a change in signs and symptoms, and between clinicians. For example, if a clinician suspects an anterior cruciate ligament (ACL) rupture, he or she might perform a Lachman test. If the Lachman test result is positive in a patient with an ACL rupture, then it would be reasonable to expect that the Lachman test result would also be positive if performed by a different clinician and when performed the following day, assuming the patient had not undergone reconstructive surgery. If the Lachman test does not produce consistent results across these conditions, then it cannot demonstrate accuracy in ruling in or ruling out the presence of an ACL rupture.

Reliability has often been defined in terms of intrarater and interrater reliability. In the context of the injury evaluation process, intrarater reliability indicates the degree of consistency in a clinical test when performed by the same clinician on multiple occasions.[7] Using the hypothetical clinical scenario, the Potts maneuver would demonstrate intrarater reliability if the same clinician performed the test on the same patient, on consecutive days, with the same result. Stated differently, if a patient reported to the clinic with a suspected SLAP lesion and the Potts maneuver had a positive result, it is reasonable to assume that the result would be positive the following day, assuming the patient had not undergone treatment. Interrater reliability, however, reflects the degree of consistency of a clinical test when performed on the same patient, under the same conditions, by different examiners.[7] If the Potts maneuver were to be performed in the same manner by two different clinicians on a patient with a SLAP lesion, it is reasonable to expect that both examiners would attain a positive test result. The interrater reliability of diagnostic tests is more difficult to establish given that clinicians often perform clinical tests using different hand placements and varying levels of force.

Validity

Validity is an important characteristic of clinical tests. Although reproducibility of clinical test results must be established to ensure diagnostic accuracy, the validity of the test itself needs to be considered prior to clinical application. Validity, in the context of the physical examination process, is the degree to which a diagnostic test measures what it intends to measure.[7] If there is interest in assessing the core temperature of an individual with a suspected heat illness, a device that measures core temperature should be used. Rectal probes have been shown to be a valid measure of core body temperature, whereas other devices to measure temperature, such as oral and tympanic thermometers, have been shown to underestimate core temperature.[9] Furthermore, when using special tests for diagnosing ACL sprains of the knee, clinicians should select tests that have been shown to effectively evaluate the integrity of the ACL. Correct diagnoses rely on the ability of a test to indicate whether pathology is present. The diagnostic validity of a clinical test is established by comparing the results of the test to a diagnostic gold standard and by utilizing statistics, such as sensitivity and specificity. These concepts will be explained further in the following sections.

Diagnostic Gold Standard

Before diagnostic accuracy of a clinical test can be determined, the results of the test are compared to a gold standard, sometimes referred to as a reference criterion. A diagnostic gold standard test will confirm the presence or absence of a specific pathology and will thus determine whether the clinical test was accurate in ruling in or ruling out an injury. Gold standard tests are usually more invasive, time consuming, and expensive. Examples of gold standard tests include arthroscopy, MRI, and ultrasonography. **Table 3.2** provides examples of gold standard references for several common orthopaedic special tests.[10-16]

There are two things to think about regarding diagnostic gold standard tests. First, diagnostic gold standards must also demonstrate reliability and validity in identifying the presence or absence of pathologic findings. The clinical scenario comparing the results of the Potts maneuver to the gold standard MRI in confirming the presence or absence of a SLAP lesion can be considered here. If an accurate diagnosis of SLAP lesions is not made by either the radiologist or the imaging study itself, then utilizing MRI as the gold standard test as a comparison for the Potts maneuver is meaningless. Second, it is assumed that not all patients evaluated in a clinical setting will undergo additional diagnostic tests to confirm the presence or absence of pathology. Rather, clinicians use clinical judgment based on a thorough examination to determine the most appropriate management. Additional diagnostic testing is usually reserved for patients who may require surgical intervention or for patients whose condition is not improving with

Table 3.2 Examples of Gold Standard References for Common Orthopaedic Tests

Joint	Special Tests	Pathology	Gold Standard
Shoulder	Hawkins-Kennedy	Subacromial impingement	Arthroscopy and ultrasonography
	Drop arm	Rotator cuff pathology	Ultrasonography
	Yergason	Biceps tendon pathology	Arthroscopy
	Speed	Biceps tendon pathology	Arthroscopy
	O'Brien	Labral pathology/SLAP lesion	Arthroscopy
Hip	FADDIR	FAI	MRA
	FABER	FAI	Intra-articular injection and MRA
	Scour	Labral pathology	Intra-articular injection and MRA
	Compression	Labral pathology	
Knee	Thessaly	Meniscal pathology	Arthroscopy
	McMurray	Meniscal pathology	Arthroscopy
	Anterior drawer	ACL sprain	Arthroscopy
	Lachman	ACL sprain	Arthroscopy
	Pivot shift	ACL sprain	Arthroscopy
Foot and Ankle	Anterior drawer	Talocrural joint laxity	Stress fluoroscopy
	Medial talar tilt	Talocrural joint laxity	Stress fluoroscopy
	External rotation	Syndesmosis joint laxity	MRI
	Thompson	Achilles tendon rupture	MRI and ultrasonography

ACL, anterior cruciate ligament; FABER, flexion, abduction, external rotation; FADDIR, flexion, adduction, internal rotation; FAI, femoroacetabular impingement; MRA, magnetic resonance angiography; SLAP, superior labrum anterior to posterior.

Data from Hegedus EJ, Goode AP, Cook CE, et al.: Which physical examination tests provide clinicians with the most value when examining the shoulder? Update of a systematic review with meta-analysis of individual tests. Br J Sports Med 2012;46(14):964-978.

nonsurgical treatment. Diagnostic gold standard tests are used in research studies as a comparison to clinical examination tests to determine the accuracy and clinical usefulness of the test.

When performing a clinical test during an injury evaluation, there are four possible outcomes:

- *True Positive*: the clinical test is positive and the diagnostic gold standard confirms the presence of pathology. In other words, both tests are positive. Using the hypothetical Potts maneuver as an example, a true-positive outcome would occur when the Potts maneuver was positive and the MRI study was also positive for a SLAP lesion. As can be seen in Table 3.1, there were a total of 38 true-positive outcomes.
- *False Positive*: the clinical test is positive, but the diagnostic gold standard confirms the absence of pathology. Stated differently, the clinical test incorrectly identified the presence of pathology when there were no pathologic findings present. Using the hypothetical scenario, a false-positive outcome would occur when the Potts maneuver was positive, indicating a possible SLAP lesion, but the MRI study was negative for labral pathology. As can be seen in Table 3.1, there were a total of seven false-positive outcomes.
- *True Negative*: the clinical test is negative and the diagnostic gold standard confirms the absence of pathologic findings. In other words, both tests are negative. In the hypothetical scenario, a true-negative outcome would occur when the Potts maneuver was negative and the MRI study confirmed that the patient did not have a SLAP lesion. As shown in Table 3.1, there were a total of 53 true-negative outcomes.
- *False Negative*: the clinical test is negative, but the diagnostic gold standard confirms the presence of pathologic findings. Stated differently, the clinical test incorrectly identified a pathology as not being present when the pathology was present. Using the hypothetical scenario, a false-negative outcome would occur when the Potts maneuver was negative, but the MRI study revealed a SLAP lesion. As shown in Table 3.1, there were a total of two false-negative outcomes.

Documenting the outcomes of a clinical test and comparing those results to a reliable and valid diagnostic gold standard will provide a measure of diagnostic accuracy. Ideally, clinical tests will have high rates of true-positive and true-negative outcomes. These tests would be classified as having a high degree of diagnostic accuracy when ruling in or ruling out pathologic findings. However, this is not always the case. In fact, some tests commonly used during injury evaluations have demonstrated false-positive or false-negative outcomes. A common example is the Finkelstein test, used to assess for the presence or absence of de Quervain tenosynovitis. This test often produces false-positive results, as indicated when pain is present in the absence of pathology.

Sensitivity and Specificity

During an injury evaluation, clinicians perform various special tests that are generally categorized as positive or negative. Positive tests may be indicated by pain, laxity, apprehension, or a catching sensation. Sometimes, positive tests indicate that pathology is present, whereas negative tests indicate that pathology is not present. Clinicians use the results of these tests in conjunction with a history and physical examination to determine a final working diagnosis and develop a treatment plan. Sensitivity and specificity are two common measures of diagnostic accuracy that identify the number of true-positive and true-negative outcomes.

Sensitivity is defined as the proportion of patients **with the suspected pathology** (as confirmed with a gold standard test) who will have a **positive clinical test**.[17] Sensitivity refers to only patients with pathologic findings. Therefore, sensitivity is sometimes referred to as the true-positive rate. According to the results of the hypothetical scenario in Table 3.1, the diagnosis of a SLAP lesion was made in a total of 40 patients (of the original 100), as indicated on MRI. Of these 40 patients, the Potts maneuver had a positive result in 38 (true-positive outcome) and a negative result in 2 (false-negative outcome). Therefore, to determine the accuracy of the Potts maneuver in correctly identifying patients with a SLAP lesion, the following calculation for sensitivity can be used:

$$\frac{\textit{True-Positive Rate of the Potts Maneuver (38 patients)}}{\textit{Total Number of Patients With SLAP Lesions (40 patients)}} = 0.95$$

This can be interpreted in the following way: the Potts maneuver correctly identified (positive test result) 95% of those patients who had a SLAP lesion. Only 5% of patients had a false-negative test result (ie, the Potts maneuver test result was negative, but the patient had a SLAP lesion). The Potts maneuver, therefore, is a highly sensitive test. This can be interpreted in another way as well. Because only 5% of patients had a false-negative result with the Potts maneuver, a highly sensitive test is one in which a **negative clinical test** accurately **rules out** pathology. Because there were very few false-negative results, clinicians can therefore be confident that, when the Potts maneuver test result is negative, the patient does not have the suspected pathology.

Specificity is defined as the proportion of patients **without the suspected pathology** (as confirmed with a gold standard test) who will have a **negative clinical test**.[17] Specificity refers to only patients without pathologic findings. Therefore, specificity is sometimes referred to as the true-negative rate. Referring once again to the hypothetical scenario in Table 3.1, a total of 60 patients (of the original 100) had a normal MRI study (no evidence of a SLAP lesion). Of these 60 patients, the Potts maneuver had a negative result in 53 (true-negative outcome) and a positive result in 7 (false-positive outcome). Therefore, to determine the accuracy of the Potts maneuver in correctly identifying patients **without a SLAP lesion**, the following calculation for specificity can be used:

$$\frac{\textit{True-Negative Rate of the Potts Maneuver (53 patients)}}{\textit{Total Number of Patients Without SLAP Lesions (60 patients)}} = 0.88$$

This can be interpreted in the following way: the Potts maneuver correctly identified (negative test) 88% of patients who did not have a SLAP lesion; only 12% of patients had a false-positive test result (ie, the Potts maneuver test result was positive, but the patient did not have a SLAP lesion). The Potts maneuver, therefore, is a highly specific test. Again, this can also be interpreted to indicate that, because only 12% of patients had a false-positive Potts maneuver test result, a highly specific test is one in which a **positive clinical test** accurately **rules in** pathology. Because there were very few false-positive test results in this scenario, clinicians can therefore be confident that, when the Potts maneuver test result is positive, the patient does have a SLAP lesion. A common mnemonic (SpPin and SnNout) can help clinicians differentiate between sensitivity and specificity. These helpful hints are presented in **Table 3.3**.

Interpreting Sensitivity and Specificity Values

Although the hypothetical situation previously described required calculation to determine sensitivity and specificity, statistics is not the focus of this chapter. Rather, the goal of this chapter is to assist clinicians in

Table 3.3	Sensitivity and Specificity Helpful Hints
Mnemonic	Meaning
SnNout	• High **Se**nsitivity, **N**egative test, rule **out** • A highly sensitive test will have very few false-negative results. Thus, clinicians can be confident that, when the test is negative, the patient does **not** have the pathology.
SpPin	• High **Sp**ecificity, **P**ositive test, rule **in** • A highly specific test will have very few false-positive results. Thus, clinicians can be confident that when the clinical test is positive, the patient **has** the pathology.

interpreting sensitivity and specificity values reported in the literature. In an ideal clinical setting, clinical tests would demonstrate sensitivity and specificity values near 100%. However, this is not usually the case with most clinical tests. What, therefore, is considered good sensitivity? What is considered good specificity? Is it more important to have higher values of sensitivity or higher values of specificity? Unfortunately, there are no clearly established guidelines that provide acceptable values of sensitivity and specificity. As a rule of thumb, clinicians should use their clinical judgment and expertise for clinical tests with a sensitivity or specificity value below 0.80. In clinical tests with values below 0.50, clinicians can conclude that the test is no more accurate than the flip of a coin.

To interpret the clinical usefulness of sensitivity and specificity values, clinicians should consider how the test is being used and whether a high degree of false-positive or false-negative results are acceptable. For example, the Homan sign is a clinical test that is used to assess for the presence of a deep vein thrombosis (DVT). When compared to the gold standard, venography, the Homan sign has reported sensitivity values as low as 0.10 and specificity values greater than 0.80.[18] A specificity value of 0.80 indicates that 20% of patients without a DVT had a positive Homan sign. In this situation, the worse-case scenario would be an unnecessary venography. When the sensitivity of the Homan sign is interpreted, a value of 0.10 indicates that in 90% of patients with a DVT, the Homan sign was negative (false-negative result). Using this information, clinicians cannot be confident that a patient does not have a DVT when the Homan sign is negative because it is missed 90% of the time. If clinicians relied solely on the results of the Homan sign for the diagnosis of DVT, the results could be catastrophic. In this case, it would be preferable for the Homan sign to have a higher degree of sensitivity than specificity. Again, clinical judgment and expertise are important considerations in this scenario. In addition to the results of the Homan sign, clinicians should also consider the patient's signs and symptoms, including leg tenderness, difference in calf circumference, and warmth to determine the appropriate management.

Likelihood Ratios

Although sensitivity and specificity values provide clinicians with valuable information regarding a diagnostic test, these values cannot be used to definitively make a diagnosis. A Lachman test may be positive, but what does that indicate about the likelihood that the patient has an ACL sprain? A more clinically useful value would determine the probability that a patient has or does not have pathologic findings based on the results of the diagnostic test. Sensitivity and specificity cannot predict the probability of a pathology based on clinical tests. Rather, they describe the accuracy of the clinical test compared to the diagnostic gold standard. Sensitivity and specificity, however, can be combined into one measure called a likelihood ratio. Likelihood ratios provide a summary of how many times more (positive) or less (negative) likely patients are to have pathologic findings based on the results of the clinical examination. Thus, they allow clinicians to best apply the results of diagnostic tests to the individual patient. Because likelihood ratios combine sensitivity and specificity values, a diagnostic gold standard is still required as a comparison.

A positive likelihood ratio applies to clinical scenarios where a clinical test is positive. It is defined as the probability of a patient with a pathology having a positive clinical test divided by the probability of a patient without that same pathology having a positive test.[19] Therefore, a positive likelihood ratio calculates the probability of having pathologic findings based on the outcome of a clinical test. Mathematically speaking, a positive likelihood ratio can be calculated as follows:

$$Sensitivity \div (1 - Specificity)$$

A large positive likelihood ratio indicates that a patient with a positive clinical test is **likely** to have the associated pathology. Conversely, a small positive likelihood ratio does not provide much diagnostic certainty regarding the results of a clinical test. Considering the hypothetical scenario using the Potts maneuver, the positive likelihood ratio can be calculated as 0.95 ÷ (1 − 0.65) = 2.7. This can be interpreted to mean that a patient with a SLAP lesion is 2.7 times more likely to have a positive Potts maneuver test result than a patient without a SLAP lesion.

A negative likelihood ratio applies to clinical scenarios where a clinical test is negative. It is defined as the probability of a patient with pathologic findings having a negative clinical test result divided by the probability of a patient without the same pathologic findings having a negative clinical test result.[19] A negative likelihood ratio considers the true-negative and false-negative rates of clinical test results and calculates the probability that pathologic findings are present in the presence of a negative clinical test result. Negative likelihood ratios can be calculated using the following formula:

$$(1 - Sensitivity) \div Specificity$$

A small negative likelihood ratio indicates that a patient with a negative clinical test is **not likely** to have the associated pathology. Larger negative likelihood ratios, however, indicate that the results of the clinical test do not provide much diagnostic certainty. Using the hypothetical scenario, the negative likelihood ratio of the Potts maneuver can be calculated as (1 − 0.95) ÷ 0.65 = 0.08. This can be interpreted to mean that the probability of having a negative Potts maneuver test result for patients with SLAP lesions is 0.08 times that of those without a SLAP lesion. It can also be interpreted to mean that patients without SLAP lesions are 12 times more likely to have a negative Potts maneuver test result than patients with a SLAP lesion.

Interpreting the Magnitude of Likelihood Ratios

Likelihood ratios provide meaningful information regarding the probability of pathologic findings based on the results of a clinical test. However, application of likelihood ratio values into clinical practice requires interpretation of their magnitude. As stated previously, larger positive likelihood ratios (>10) indicate a greater probability of pathologic findings when a clinical test is positive, whereas a smaller negative likelihood ratio (<0.1) indicates that a negative clinical test result is less likely to occur in patients with the associated pathology. As likelihood ratios near 1, they provide very minimal clinical significance regarding the probability of pathologic findings based on the results of a clinical test.[20] **Table 3.4** provides a description of the magnitude of likelihood ratios for clinical practice. **Table 3.5** provides diagnostic accuracy values (sensitivity, specificity, positive likelihood ratios, and negative likelihood ratios) for common orthopaedic special tests.[10-14, 16]

Table 3.4 Clinical Interpretation of Likelihood Ratio Magnitudes

Positive Likelihood Ratio	Negative Likelihood Ratio	Clinical Interpretation
>10	<0.1	Large magnitude, clinically meaningful
5–10	0.1–0.2	Moderate magnitude, usually clinically meaningful
2–5	0.2–0.5	Small magnitude, sometimes clinically meaningful
1–2	0.5–1	Very small magnitude, clinically unimportant

Data from Jaeschke R, Guyatt GH, Sackett DL, et al: Users' guides to the medical literature. III. How to use an article about a diagnostic test. B. What are the results and will they help me in caring for my patients? The Evidence-Based Medicine Working Group. *JAMA* 1994;271(9):703-707.

Receiver Operating Characteristic Curves

This chapter has discussed concepts of diagnostic accuracy for clinical tests that have a dichotomous outcome, meaning the test has two possible outcomes: positive or negative. Positive special test results are considered abnormal and are often associated with a specific pathology. However, not all clinical tests have dichotomous outcomes. Clinical tests with continuous variable outcomes, such as blood glucose, blood pressure, and temperature, are commonly used to assist in making clinical diagnoses. Rather than a positive clinical test result determining the presence of pathology, clinicians must be able to identify a cutoff point for what constitutes a normal versus abnormal test. A patient with a suspected heat illness in whom core temperature is assessed using a rectal probe can be used as an example. It has been established that patients with a core temperature lower than 105°F are likely experiencing heat exhaustion, whereas patients with a core temperature higher than 105°F are likely experiencing heatstroke.[21] This distinction in core temperature is critical because the management is vastly different and may have serious consequences if treatment is mismanaged or delayed. The receiver operating characteristic (ROC) curve is a common method for selecting an optimal cutoff point for a diagnostic test. These curves are also useful for comparing the diagnostic accuracy of two or more clinical tests.

Table 3.5 Diagnostic Accuracy Values of Common Orthopaedic Special Tests

Special Test	Sensitivity	Specificity	Positive Likelihood Ratio	Negative Likelihood Ratio
Hawkins-Kennedy	0.80	0.56	1.84	0.35
Speed	0.20	0.78	0.90	1.03
FADDIR	0.94	0.09	1.02	0.45
Lachman	0.85	0.94	10.2	0.2
Anterior drawer, knee	0.55	0.92	7.3	0.5
McMurray	0.61	0.84	3.2	0.52
Thessaly	0.75	0.87	5.6	0.28
Anterior drawer, ankle	0.74	0.38	1.2	0.66
Thompson	0.96	0.93	13.47	0.04

FADDIR, flexion, adduction, internal rotation.
Data from Hegedus EJ, Goode AP, Cook CE, et al.: Which physical examination tests provide clinicians with the most value when examining the shoulder? Update of a systematic review with meta-analysis of individual tests. Br J Sports Med 2012;46(14):964-978.

ROC curves provide a visual representation of the accuracy of a diagnostic test in its ability to discriminate between patients with or without pathologic findings.[22] The curve is created by calculating the sensitivity and specificity of a diagnostic test at every possible cutoff point and then plotting the sensitivity (true-positive rate) on the y-axis against 1 minus specificity (false-positive rate) on the x-axis. As mentioned previously, it is preferable for tests to have high degrees of both sensitivity and specificity. This is not always the case, however. Using a ROC curve provides a cutoff value in which the optimal sensitivity and specificity of a diagnostic test are achieved. This is the point at which the test is most useful for making clinical decisions. When viewing a ROC curve, a diagonal line that runs from the lower left-hand corner to the upper right-hand corner can be seen. This is provided as a reference line. When cutoff scores lie on this reference line, the clinical test is unable to discriminate between those with pathologic findings and those without. In other words, this line represents a test with a high number of false-positive and false-negative results. A clinical test that is both highly sensitive and specific will present graphically as a "curve" to the left side of the reference line. The closer the ROC curve is to the upper left-hand corner (or the further away the ROC curve is from the reference line), the better the clinical test at discriminating between patients with pathologic findings and those without. This is also known as the area under the curve (AUC). The greater the AUC, the better the test discriminates between patients with and without pathologic findings. When using a ROC curve to compare the diagnostic accuracy of two clinical tests, the test that is further from the reference line is the more accurate test. Research studies that use ROC curves to report on the diagnostic accuracy of a test will include the AUC value. When the AUC is closer to 1, the more accurate the test; when the AUC is closer to 0.5 (reference line), the less accurate the test.[23] Table 3.6 provides a description of the interpretation of AUC values for clinical practice. It is important to note that the AUC values may change if the test is performed on a different patient population and/or under different testing conditions. Therefore, clinicians should be mindful of the patient population reported in a research study. If the patient population on which the study is conducted is vastly different from the clinician's typical patients

Table 3.6 Area Under the Curve Interpretation

AUC Value	Clinical Interpretation
>0.9	High degree of accuracy
0.7–0.9	Moderate degree of accuracy
0.5–0.7	Low degree of accuracy
0.5	Poor degree of accuracy

AUC, area under the curve.
Data from Fischer JE, Bachmann LM, Jaeschke RA: A readers' guide to the interpretation of diagnostic test properties: clinical example of sepsis. Intensive Care Med 2003;29(7):1043-1051.

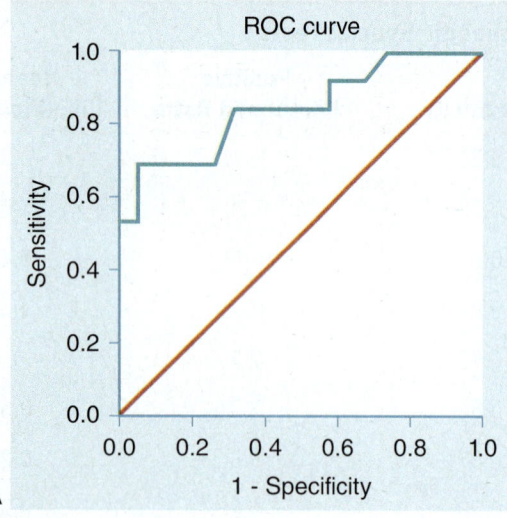 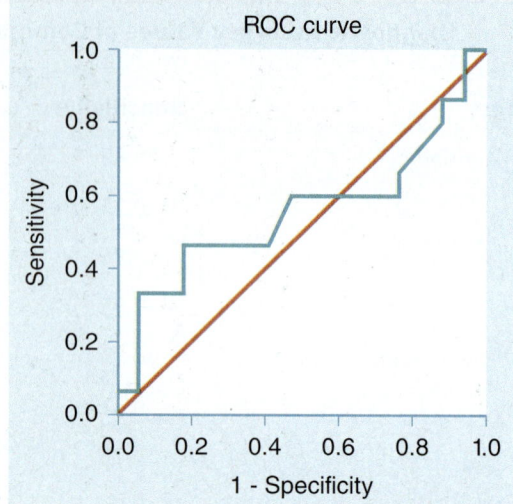

Figure 3.2 Receiver operating characteristic (ROC) curves. **A.** Example of a good diagnostic test. **B.** Example of a poor diagnostic test.

© Jones & Bartlett Learning

(eg, age, sex, activity level), then the clinician should interpret the results of the test with caution.

What follows are two examples of ROC curves, using fictitious data. **Figure 3.2A** represents a diagnostic test with a high degree of accuracy in identifying patients with and without pathologic findings. The red line represents the reference line, whereas the blue line represents the diagnostic accuracy of the clinical test. The farther (distance) the blue line is from the red line, the more accurate the test. As seen on the right of the graph, the AUC has been calculated as 0.848, which indicates that this fictitious test has a moderate degree of accuracy. **Figure 3.2B** represents a clinical test with a low degree of accuracy. In this figure, the blue line is much closer to the reference line, indicating that the clinical test has poor accuracy when identifying patients with and without pathologic findings.

In addition to using ROC curves as a graphic representation of the diagnostic accuracy of a clinical test, they can also be used to establish a cutoff point for clinical tests that use continuous variables as outcomes. An ideal clinical test has 100% sensitivity and specificity and thus accurately identifies all patients with a specific pathology and all patients without a specific pathology. However, because not all clinical tests are perfect, it would be helpful to determine a score or outcome that best differentiates between patients with pathologic findings and those without. This score is known as a cutoff point. On a ROC curve, the cutoff point is calculated as the point on the curve that is closest to the upper left-hand corner of the graph. This point corresponds to the value that has the highest degree of sensitivity and specificity.[24]

The Functional Movement Screen (FMS) is an example in the athletic training literature that uses a cutoff point to differentiate patients at risk for injury. In one study,[25] collegiate athletes completed an FMS prior to the start of their season. The FMS includes seven tests that assess flexibility and stability in various planes of movement to determine if movement asymmetries exist. Players received a composite FMS score, ranging from 0 to 21, where higher scores indicated fewer asymmetries. Following completion of FMS testing, players were followed over the course of a season and all injuries were recorded. Results from the ROC analysis established a cutoff score of 14, which indicated that players with a score of 14 or less on the FMS were at greater risk of injury during the season than players with a score greater than 14. This study provides an example of using a ROC curve to establish a cutoff score for differentiating between patients with pathologic findings and those without.

Summary

Diagnostic tests are used as supplements to clinical evaluations. Results of clinical tests are used in conjunction with history, palpation, range of motion, strength testing, neurologic testing, and functional tests to provide a complete picture of the pathology and determine the appropriate management. Which diagnostic tests to use as supplements to the clinical evaluation process is determined by the clinician's expertise, the patient's values and goals, and the most relevant scientific evidence. Evidence, such as the validity, reliability, and diagnostic accuracy of clinical tests, should drive clinical decision making. It is essential for clinicians to have the skill set necessary for performing clinical tests properly, but also to interpret the results of research studies that report the diagnostic accuracy of tests. This will allow for the selection of the most appropriate clinical tests, which leads to more accurate clinical decision making, diagnoses, and management of injuries and illnesses.

WRAP-UP

Critical Thinking Questions

1. What role does evidence-based medicine play in the injury evaluation process?
2. How is the validity of a clinical test established?
3. Differentiate between sensitivity and specificity. How can clinicians use these values to make decisions about the clinical usefulness of a test?
4. A new clinical test has a positive likelihood ratio of 4.3 and a negative likelihood ratio of 0.01. How are these values interpreted? Would you use this new clinical test? If so, why?
5. How can receiver operating characteristic curves be used to make clinical decisions?

Pearls and Pitfalls

- Evidence-based medicine is the integration of relevant evidence, clinical expertise, and patient values. Each of these components must be considered in the context of injury evaluation to determine which clinical tests are most useful when diagnosing pathologies.
- Clinical tests must demonstrate reliability (reproducibility and consistency of results) and validity (degree to which a clinical test measures what it intends to measure) to be considered useful in injury evaluation and diagnosis.
- Sensitivity is a measure of diagnostic accuracy in patients with pathologic findings. A highly sensitive test has few false-negative results, and therefore is accurate in ruling out pathology.
- Specificity is a measure of diagnostic accuracy in patients without a pathology. A highly specific test has few false-positive results, and therefore is accurate in ruling in a pathology.
- Positive and negative likelihood ratios provide clinicians with the probability that a patient has a pathology based on the results of clinical tests. Clinical tests with a high likelihood value (>10) indicate a greater probability that a patient has pathologic findings when a clinical test is positive. Conversely, clinical tests with a low negative likelihood value (<0.01) indicate that a negative clinical test is less likely to occur in a patient with pathologic findings.
- Receiver operating characteristic curves provide information regarding the diagnostic accuracy of clinical tests with continuous variables by establishing cutoff points, which aid in distinguishing between those patients with pathologic findings and those without pathologic findings.

References

1. Sackett DL, Rosenberg WM, Gray JA, Haynes RB, Richardson WS: Evidence based medicine: what it is and what it isn't. *BMJ* 1996;312(7023):71-72.
2. Commission on Accreditation of Athletic Training Education: 2020 Standards for Accreditation of Professional Athletic Training Programs. https://caate.net/wp-content/uploads/2019/02/2020-Standards-Final-2-20-2019.pdf. Accessed March 18, 2019.
3. Steves R, Hootman JM: Evidence-based medicine: what is it and how does it apply to athletic training? *J Athl Train* 2004;39(1):83-87.
4. McCarty CW, Hankemeier DA, Walter JM, Newton EJ, Van Lunen BL: Use of evidence-based practice among athletic training educators, clinicians, and students, Part 2: Attitudes, beliefs, accessibility, and barriers. *J Athl Train* 2013;48(3):405-415.
5. Whiting PF, Rutjes AW, Westwood ME, et al: QUADAS-2: a revised tool for the quality assessment of diagnostic accuracy studies. *Ann Intern Med* 2011;155(8):529-536.
6. Karachalios T, Hantes M, Zibis AH, Zachos V, Karantanas AH, Malizos KN: Diagnostic accuracy of a new clinical test (the Thessaly test) for early detection of meniscal tears. *J Bone Joint Surg Am* 2005;87(5):955-962.

7. Rubin AB: *Practitioner's Guide to Using Research for Evidence-Based Practice.* Hoboken, NJ, John Wiley & Sons, 2012.
8. Hopkins WG: Measures of reliability in sports medicine and science. *Sports Med* 2000;30(1):1-15.
9. Casa DJ, Becker SM, Ganio MS, et al: Validity of devices that assess body temperature during outdoor exercise in the heat. *J Athl Train* 2007;42(3):333-342.
10. Hegedus EJ, Goode AP, Cook CE, et al: Which physical examination tests provide clinicians with the most value when examining the shoulder? Update of a systematic review with meta-analysis of individual tests. *Br J Sports Med* 2012;46(14):964-978.
11. Reiman MP, Goode AP, Cook CE, Holmich P, Thorborg K: Diagnostic accuracy of clinical tests for the diagnosis of hip femoroacetabular impingement/labral tear: a systematic review with meta-analysis. *Br J Sports Med* 2015;49(12):811.
12. Smith BE, Thacker D, Crewesmith A, Hall M: Special tests for assessing meniscal tears within the knee: a systematic review and meta-analysis. *Evid Based Med* 2015;20(3):88-97.
13. Benjaminse A, Gokeler A, van der Schans CP: Clinical diagnosis of an anterior cruciate ligament rupture: a meta-analysis. *J Orthop Sports Phys Ther* 2006;36(5):267-288.
14. Croy T, Koppenhaver S, Saliba S, Hertel J. Anterior talucrural joint laxity: diagnostic accuracy of the anterior drawer test of the ankle. *J Orthop Sports Phys Ther.* 2013;43(12):911-919.
15. de Cesar P, Avila E, de Abreu M: Comparison of magnetic resonance imaging to physical examination for syndesmotic injury after lateral ankle sprain. *Foot Ankle Int* 2011;32(12):189-192.
16. Maffulli N: The clinical diagnosis of subcutaneous tear of the Achilles tendon: a prospective study in 174 patients. *Am J Sports Med* 1998;26(2):266-270.
17. Akobeng AK: Understanding diagnostic tests 1: sensitivity, specificity and predictive values. *Acta Paediatr* 2007;96(3):338-341.
18. Richards KL, Armstrong JJK, Tikoff G, et al: Non-invasive diagnosis of deep vein thrombosis. *Arch Intern Med* 1976;136:1091-1096.
19. Akobeng AK: Understanding diagnostic tests 2: likelihood ratios, pre- and post-test probabilities and their use in clinical practice. *Acta Paediatr* 2007;96(4):487-491.
20. Jaeschke R, Guyatt GH, Sackett DL: Users' guides to the medical literature. III. How to use an article about a diagnostic test. B. What are the results and will they help me in caring for my patients? The Evidence-Based Medicine Working Group. *JAMA* 1994;271(9):703-707.
21. Casa DJ, DeMartini JK, Bergeron MF, et al: National Athletic Trainers' Association position statement: exertional heat illnesses. *J Athl Train* 2015;50(9):986-1000.
22. Akobeng AK: Understanding diagnostic tests 3: receiver operating characteristic curves. *Acta Paediatr* 2007;96(5):644-647.
23. Fischer JE, Bachmann LM, Jaeschke R: A readers' guide to the interpretation of diagnostic test properties: clinical example of sepsis. *Intensive Care Med* 2003;29(7):1043-1051.
24. Fan J, Upadhye S, Worster A: Understanding receiver operating characteristic (ROC) curves. *CJEM* 2006;8(1):19-20.
25. Garrison M, Westrick R, Johnson MR, Benenson J: Association between the functional movement screen and injury development in college athletes. *Int J Sports Phys Ther* 2015;10(1):21-28.

CHAPTER 4

Diagnostic Imaging for Musculoskeletal Injuries

Andrea E. Cripps, PhD, ATC

OVERVIEW

This chapter will provide an overview of the diagnostic imaging techniques commonly ordered and observed in athletic training and therapy. Special attention is given to the advantages and disadvantages of each technique. Additionally, a quick reference guide has been provided for each technique to provide clinicians a brief summary of the imaging procedure, which should also be shared with patients.

LEARNING OBJECTIVES

After completing this chapter, the reader will be able to do the following:

1. Explain the use of diagnostic imaging for musculoskeletal injuries.
2. Describe terms related to diagnostic imaging.
3. Compare and contrast various types of diagnostic imaging techniques.
4. Have a basic understanding of diagnostic imaging techniques.

FUN FACTS ABOUT DIAGNOSTIC IMAGING

- The main magnet in an MRI machine can create a magnetic field that is 1,000 to 4,000 times stronger than earth's magnetic field.
- The first radiograph was of Wilhelm Röntgen's wife's hand. He discovered x-radiation.
- The *X* in x-ray stands for "unknown" factor.

Introduction

Imaging studies provide a vital piece of the puzzle in the evaluation and management of musculoskeletal pathology. This chapter will discuss the diagnostic techniques commonly encountered in athletic training and sports medicine professions, with a focus on diagnostic techniques for musculoskeletal injuries.

Diagnostic Imaging

In order to accurately evaluate musculoskeletal injuries, diagnostic images are commonly used after completing a thorough history and physical examination. Different imaging techniques offer varying advantages and disadvantages (**Table 4.1**) that should be considered prior to ordering. The ability to order and evaluate these images is often left to physicians; however, the information gained from these imaging studies can provide invaluable clinical knowledge to athletic trainers and other allied health care professionals. Determining which type of diagnostic technique to use is dependent on many factors, as noted in **Table 4.2**.

Diagnostic images, such as radiographs, magnetic resonance images, CT scans, bone scans, and sonograms, utilize various forms of energy (typically, electromagnetic or acoustic) to produce pictures used in the diagnosis of the injury. Pictures are created when the energy is transmitted to the body, which is then reflected, scattered or passed, and

Table 4.1 Imaging Modalities

Modality	Advantages	Disadvantages
Radiography	• Readily available • Inexpensive • Easily interpreted • Accurate[a]	• Radiation exposure • Poor tissue contrast • High reliance on technician experience • Two dimensional
CT	• Three dimensional • Axial imaging • High-quality images • Rapid	• Highest amount of radiation • Patient must be completely still • High metal artifact • Poor soft-tissue contrast
MRI	• Highest contrast resolution	• Costly • Patient must be completely still • High metal artifact • Time consuming
Bone scan	• Very sensitive	• Not specific
Ultrasonography	• Very safe • Inexpensive	• Small field of view • Experience needed to interpret results accurately • High amount of artifact
Nerve conduction studies/electromyography	• Sensitive • Safe	• Invasive (electromyography) • Experience needed to interpret results accurately

[a]Accuracy depends on the technician performing the imaging, the physician interpreting the image, and the type of injury (ie, acute stress fractures are often difficult to see on standard radiographs).

collected. From this collected energy, a two- or three-dimensional image is created. The angle at which the energy is presented to the body is essential in achieving the clearest image; therefore, patient positioning is essential when ordering any diagnostic images (Figure 4.1). Anteroposterior (AP) refers to energy passing from anterior to posterior, whereas posteroanterior (PA) refers to energy passing from posterior

Table 4.2 Factors to Consider When Choosing a Diagnostic Technique

Cost	• Insurance restrictions. Often, a standard radiograph needs to be ordered and interpreted prior to advanced diagnostic techniques being approved. • Costs vary greatly among techniques. Evaluating the appropriateness of the technique ordered will help to limit the overall cost.
Availability	• Identification of the equipment in the area or surrounding area. There is no point in ordering an advanced imaging technique if it is not feasible for the patient to get to the location. • Can the patient be seen immediately, or does he or she need to schedule an appointment? Often, standard radiographs can be done the same day, whereas MRI or other advanced imaging methods need to be scheduled (unless in emergency situations).
Risks to the patient	• The use of many of these techniques is contraindicated in pregnancy. • Metal within the body can cause additional harm to the patient. • Radiation exposure increases with each image ordered.
Patient values	• Time requirements vary greatly among techniques. Standard radiographs can often be completed within minutes, but functional MRI can take hours to complete. • Concerns. Patients may experience claustrophobia during some of the procedures, and this should be considered a limiting factor in decision making. • Pain. To obtain certain images, positioning may cause pain to the patient.

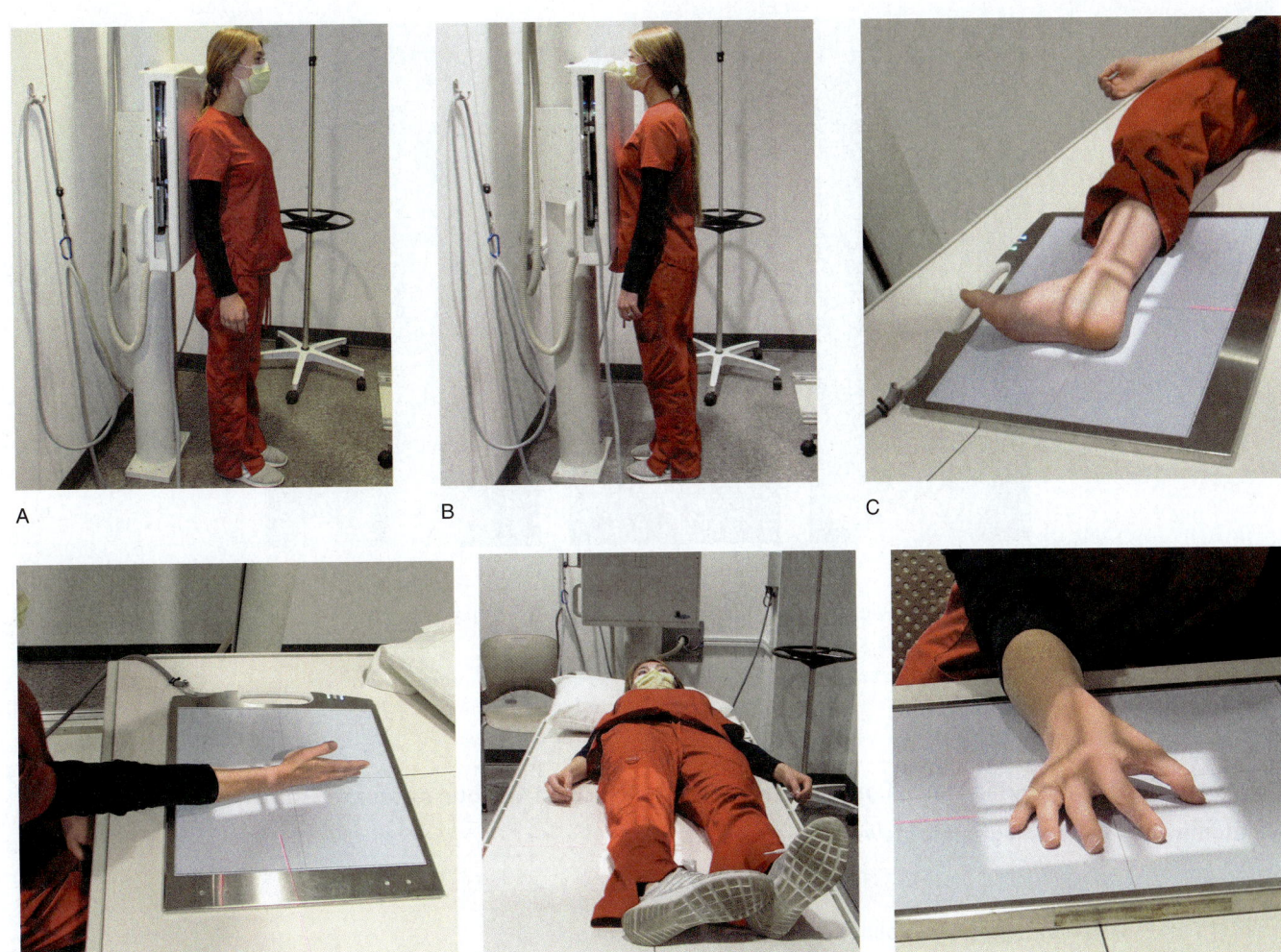

Figure 4.1 Photographs of patient positioning while taking diagnostic images. **A.** AP projection. **B.** PA projection. **C.** Mediolateral projection (ankle). **D.** Lateromedial projection (wrist). **E.** AP oblique projection–medial rotation (from AP). **F.** PA oblique projection–lateral rotation (from PA).

Courtesy of Andrea Cripps.

to anterior. Left- or right-lateral projections refers to energy passing from the right or left side, and oblique views refer to energy passing through the body at an angle.

Radiography

Most commonly referred to as x-ray, radiography uses a form of electromagnetic energy to pass through the body. When that energy is decreased on the other side (as bone absorbs or disperses more energy than soft tissue) a bright (or white) image is produced on the film (**Figure 4.2**).

Radiographs are typically ordered prior to more complex imaging studies (MRI, CT) because of their relatively low expense, low radiation exposure, and easy accessibility. However, radiographs are used mainly to diagnose fractures, and they may not be sensitive enough to diagnose stress fractures or other small fractures, such as in the carpal bone.[1,2] When ordering a radiograph, a minimum of two views should be ordered in perpendicular planes (AP and lateral).[3] Additionally, when ordering radiographs to diagnose a fracture, the joints above and below a suspected injury site are often evaluated for joint dislocations or additional fractures. Complex joints (wrist, elbow, pelvis, or ankle) often require specialized views (**Table 4.3**), and bilateral images should be ordered in pediatric patients when a physical injury is suspected.

The patient should be informed to wear loose clothing that can be easily manipulated or removed to expose the area to be imaged. A lead shield will be placed over reproductive organs to protect them from radiation exposure. If stress radiographs are ordered to determine the effect that stress has on a

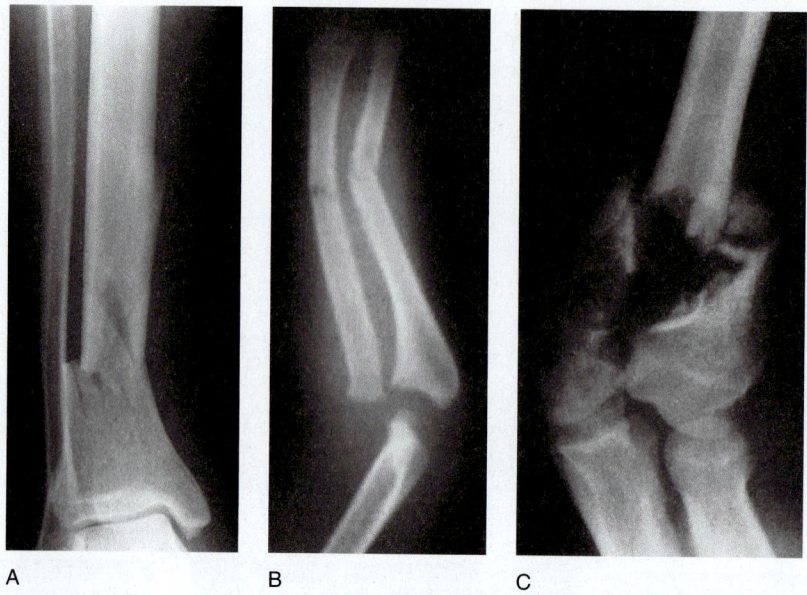

Figure 4.2 Radiographs of skeletal fractures. **A.** Distal tibia fracture. **B.** Radial and ulnar fracture. **C.** Distal humeral fracture.

Reproduced from Bedi A, Le TT, Karunakar MA: Surgical treatment of nonarticular distal tibia fracture. *J Am Acad Orthop Surg* 1998;6(4):215-224. Panel C reproduced with permission from Mayo Foundation for Medical Education and Research.

Table 4.3 Radiographic Views Commonly Ordered to Evaluate Various Anatomic Regions

Anatomic Region	Radiographic Views
Upper Extremity	
Fingers	PA, lateral, and oblique with fingers separated
Hand	PA, lateral (oblique)
Wrist	PA, lateral with wrist in neutral position (consider scaphoid views for anatomic snuffbox tenderness)
Forearm	AP, lateral
Elbow	AP, in supination, lateral in 90° of flexion (consider radial head views for direct tenderness over radial head)
Humerus	AP, lateral
Shoulder	AP in internal and external rotation, scapular-Y lateral, axillary lateral view (for all trauma/suspected dislocations); consider Zanca view for acromioclavicular joint pathology
Lower Extremity	
Hip	AP in internal rotation, frog-lateral, or cross-table lateral if necessary
Femur	AP, lateral
Knee	AP, lateral, and tunnel views; oblique view to see fibular head; add AP weight bearing view for arthritis evaluation
Tibia/fibula	AP, lateral
Ankle	AP, lateral, mortise
Foot	AP, lateral, internal oblique (weight-bearing views for Lisfranc injury, alignment abnormalities)
Calcaneus	AP, lateral, Harris axial view
Toes	AP, lateral, oblique

Axial Skeleton	
Cervical spine	AP, lateral (trauma series also should include odontoid view and C7 swimmer's view; consider lateral flexion/extension views for patients with rheumatoid arthritis and suspected instability)
Thoracic spine	AP, lateral
Lumbar spine	AP, lateral
Pelvis	AP (consider Judet views for acetabular fractures, inlet/outlet views for pelvic ring injuries)

joint (or to check integrity of ligamentous structures [**Figure 4.3**]), specialized positioning and weights or manual traction is applied by the technician.

If an arthrogram is ordered to evaluate articular cartilage or capsular tissue, the patient should inform the technician of any allergies because a local anesthetic is used prior to the injection of a contrast medium into the joint space. Patients undergoing arthrography should be informed that joint discomfort is common for 24 to 48 hours after the procedure. Last, other forms of radiographic images include angiograms and myelograms, which both involve the absorption of various dyes to check the integrity of soft-tissue structures; however, these methods are increasingly less common because of the advancement of MRI technologies.

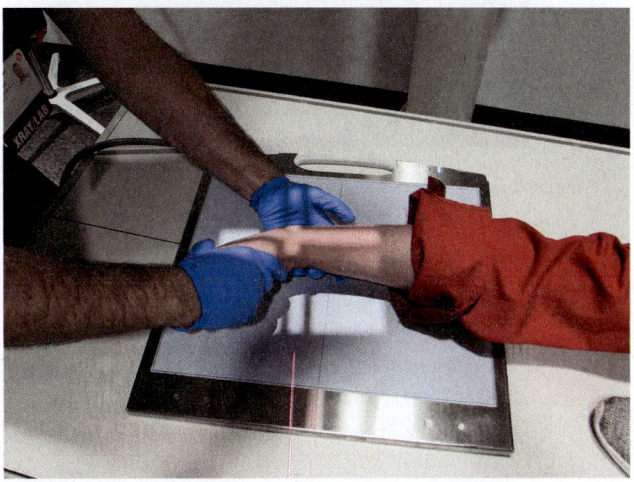

Figure 4.3 Patient stabilization for stress radiograph.
Courtesy of Andrea Cripps.

Radiography Quick Reference Guide

Indications
- Bone and joint deformities
- Pain or decreased joint motion
- Localized tenderness
- Abnormal asymmetry or mass
- Suspected foreign body

Best Uses
- Bone abnormalities, including fractures, joint surfaces, and joint spaces
- Pathologies of the articular cartilage and capsular tissues (arthrogram)
- Blood vessel diagnosis (angiogram)
- Spinal cord pathologies (myelogram)

Length of Procedure
- Standard radiographs: 5 to 10 minutes
- Arthrogram: 45 to 60 minutes

Comments
- Interpretation is best done via ABCs method:[4]
  - Alignment: Observe the relationship of bones around joints and the continuity of the bones for proper alignment and spacing (**Figure 4.4**).

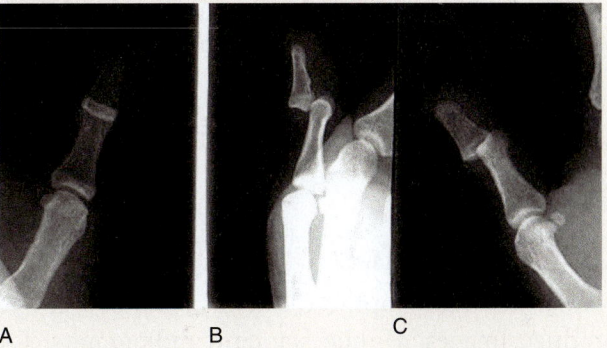

Figure 4.4 A. PA view of overlapping phalangeal joint margins. **B.** AP view demonstrating a lateral talar shift. **C.** Lateral view showing no overlap or edges.

- Bones: Each bone should be observed independently and then as a whole. Evaluate the margins of each bone, observing for abnormalities in shape, color, and consistency. Note: Cortical bone should be the brightest, and cancellous bone is darker. Decreases in bone density appear as darkened areas (**Figure 4.5**).

(continues)

Radiography Quick Reference Guide

(continued)

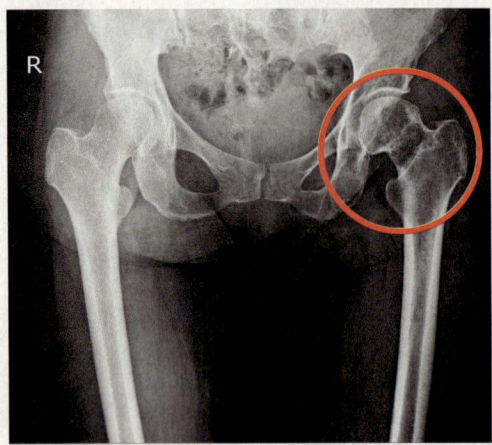

Figure 4.5 Radiolucent appearance of fracture.
© Richman Photo/Shutterstock

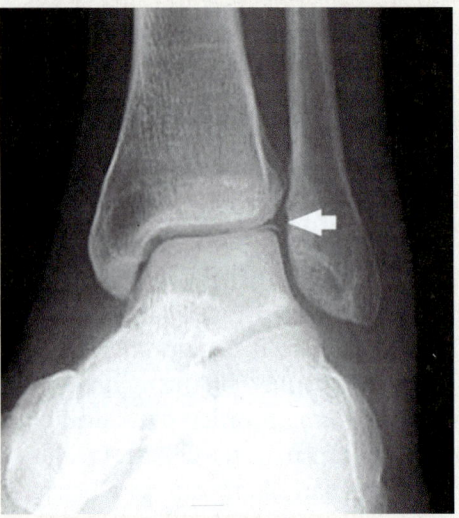

Figure 4.6 Talar dome avulsion fracture (arrow).

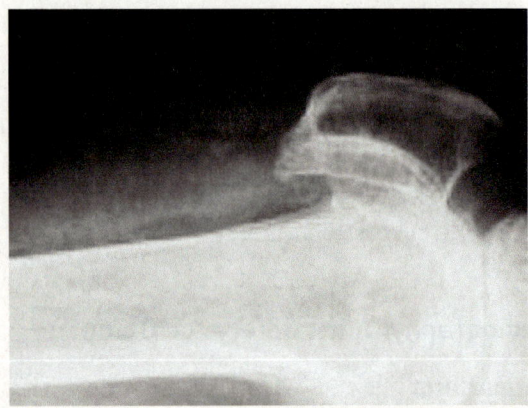

Figure 4.7 Knee effusion.

- Cartilage and joints: Although cartilage cannot be seen on radiographs, the soft tissue that makes up the cartilage and ligaments is evaluated for what is not seen, rather than what is. Each joint space and articular surface should be checked independently, observing for congruity and separation of the margins, any overlap in bone, uniform joint space, and articular fractures (**Figure 4.6**).
- Soft tissue: Although soft tissue cannot be imaged with a radiograph, swelling within the confines of the tissue can be determined. Additionally, fat pad locations can indicate a suspected fracture or dislocation (**Figure 4.7**).
- Female patients of childbearing age should inform the technician if they are or suspect they may be pregnant.

Figures 4.4, 4.6, and 4.7 courtesy of the editor of the South African Radiographer. Williams IJ: Appendicular skeleton: ABCs image interpretation search strategy. *S African Radiographer* 2013;51:2:9-14.

Computed Tomography

Similar to radiography, CT uses x-ray sources to produce images. Unlike standard radiographs, CT rotates around the body (**Figure 4.8**) to produce detailed images. During this rotation, the x-ray source and detectors are sending and receiving absorption data. The data are then compiled by a computer and projected as an image. These images can be viewed as either a two-dimensional (slice) or a three-dimensional image.[5] CT is performed to diagnose a specific pathology and is the best modality for evaluating intra-articular and complex fractures, such as those in the scapula, spine, and pelvis. Intravenous or oral administration of various contrast dye can be used to evaluate the integrity of soft tissues, including arteries and veins (angiography) (**Figure 4.9**).

Patients should wear loose-fitting clothing without any zippers or other metal objects that may distort the image. Often, patients will be given a hospital gown to wear to ensure no distortion of the image and may be required to remove jewelry, hearing aids, dentures, or glasses. For patients undergoing angiography, they will need to refrain from consuming anything other than clear liquids for the preceding 12 to 24 hours. CT with injected contrast is contraindicated for patients with certain kidney diseases. Also, patients with claustrophobia or larger patients may not be suitable candidates for CT. Some patients may be allergic to the dye used for contrast imaging.

Diagnostic Imaging   47

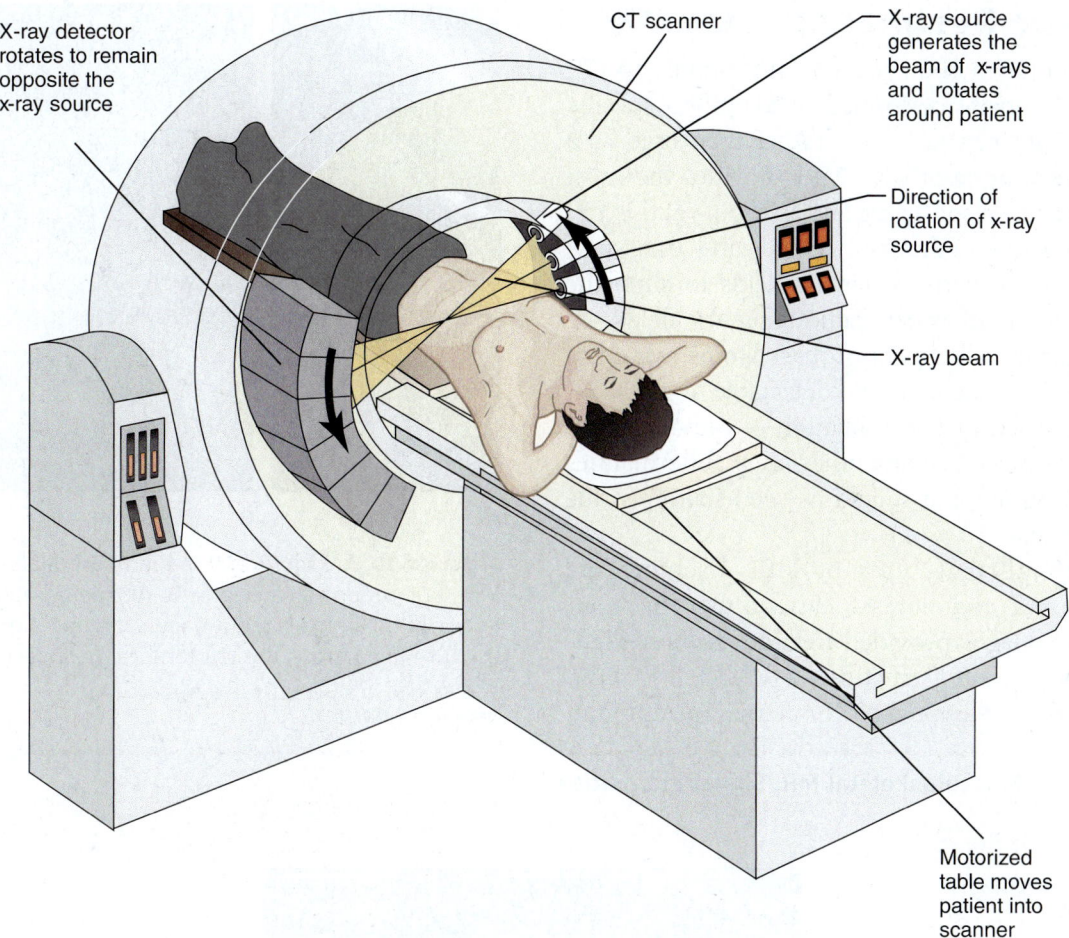

Figure 4.8 CT scanner.
© Jones & Bartlett Learning

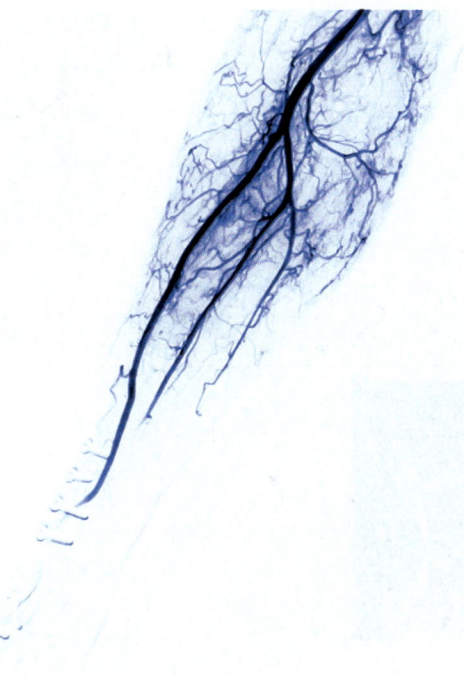

Figure 4.9 Angiography of the arm.
© samunella/shutterstock

CT Quick Reference Guide

Indications
- Intra-articular or advanced fracture evaluation
- Evaluation of bone fragment size and location for surgical planning
- Bone tumor evaluation

Best Uses
- Soft-tissue, bony, or articular cartilage lesions
- Identification of ligamentous or tendinous pathologies
- Artery and/or vein pathologies (angiography)

Length of Procedure
- 5 to 30 minutes; spiral CT requires less time

Comments
- Female patients of childbearing age should inform technician if they are or suspect they may be pregnant.
- Use extreme caution when ordering CT for children, as increased radiation exposure produces a slight increase in cancer risk.

Magnetic Resonance Imaging

Soft-tissue injuries often require MRI. Similar to CT, MRI is traditionally performed to identify a specific pathology (eg, meniscal tear), rather than used as a general screening approach. MRI provides the most detailed images of soft tissue and the spine and is referenced in terms of frontal, sagittal, and transverse planes. Using powerful magnetic fields to align the hydrogen atoms of water, radiofrequency fields are used to alter the alignment of these atoms, which in turn produces a magnetic field detectable by the scanner. MRI is used in the evaluation of tumors, stress fractures (**Figure 4.10**), and other bony abnormalities (eg, osteomyelitis), but should be used sparingly due to the high cost.

Several different types of MRI machines are available, and radiologists can adjust the contrast of the images provided in order to best identify the soft-tissue structures (**Table 4.4**), fluid accumulations (**Figure 4.11**), or nerve entrapment.

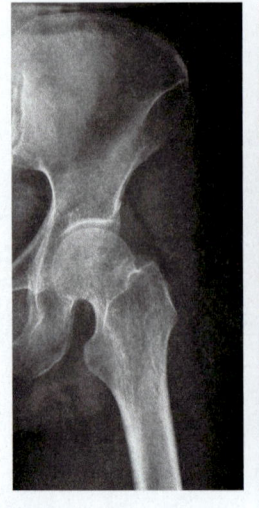
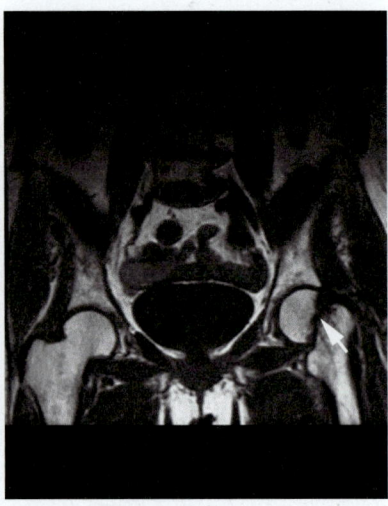

Figure 4.10 A. Fracture of the femoral neck seen on MRI, but not on radiography. **B.** AP radiograph of the left femur of the same patient shows the low-signal intensity fracture line across the left femoral neck (arrow).

Reproduced from Johnson TR, Steinbach LS, eds: *Essentials of Musculoskeletal Imaging*. Rosemont, IL, American Academy of Orthopaedic Surgeons, 2004, p 435.

Table 4.4 Musculoskeletal MRI Signal Intensities

Brain

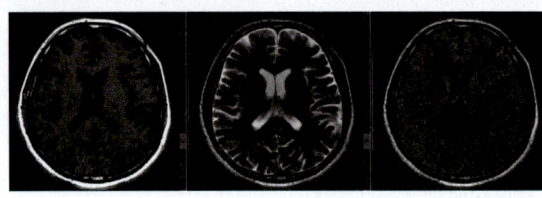

© springsky/Shutterstock

Tissue	T1-weighted	T2-weighted	FLAIR
CSF	Dark	Bright	Dark
White matter	Light	Dark gray	Dark gray
Gray matter	Gray	Gray	Gray
Cortex	Gray	Light gray	Light gray
Fat (within bone marrow)	Bright	Light	Light
Fluid (eg, edema, infarction)	Dark	Bright	Bright

Spine and Extremities

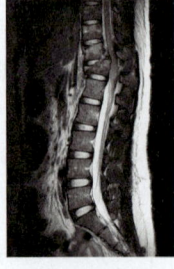
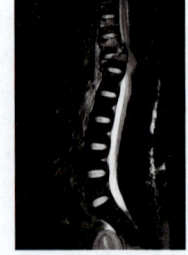

© Tossaporn Buttabut/Shutterstock

Tissue	T1-weighted	T2-weighted
CSF	Dark	Bright

Spine and Extremities		
Skeletal muscle	Gray	Dark gray
Spinal cord	Gray	Light gray
Adipose tissue and bone marrow	Bright	Light
Intervertebral discs	Gray	Bright
Air (eg, pharynx)	Very dark	Very dark
Fibrocartilage (eg, labrum, menisci, triangular fibrocartilage)	Dark	Dark
Fluid (eg, edema, tears, cysts)	Dark	Bright

Note: Longitudinal relaxation time (T1) is the time constant that determines the rate at that excited protons return to equilibrium. Transverse relaxation time (T2) is the time constant that determines the rate at which excited protons reach equilibrium or go out of phase with each other. Fluid-attenuated inversion recovery (FLAIR) is similar to T2 except abnormalities remain bright, but normal cerebrospinal fluid (CSF) is attenuated and made dark, which makes this sequence sensitive to pathologies and makes the differentiation between CSF and an abnormality much easier to see.
Data from Preston, D: Magnetic resonance imaging (MRI) of the brain and spine: basics. Casemed, 30 Nov 2006, https://casemed.case.edu/clerkships/neurology/Web%20Neurorad/MRI%20Basics.htm. Accessed 15 Sept. 2019.

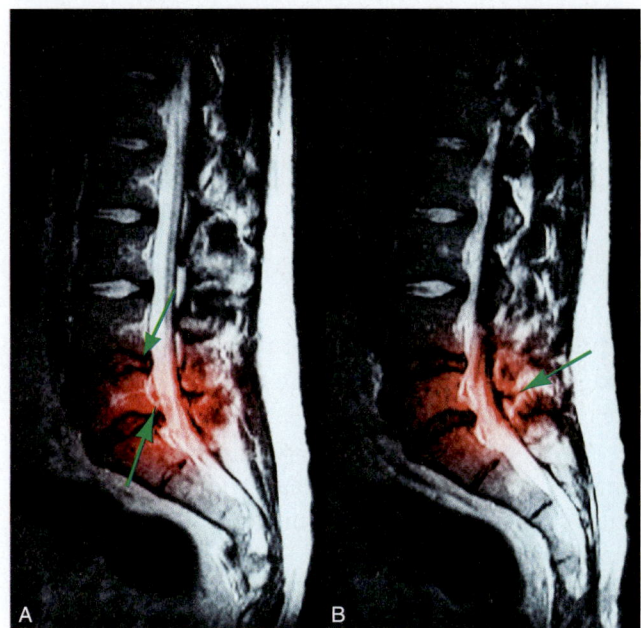

Figure 4.11 MRI of soft-tissue injury. **A.** Lumbosacral anterior herniated disk at L4-L5 (arrows). **B.** Lumbosacral posterior disk herniation at L3-L4.
© DeymosHR/Shutterstock

pacemaker), or cause image distortion (eg, braces, metal tooth fillings, tattoos [including permanent makeup]) during the imaging process. Health professionals should also take note of body size and presence of claustrophobia because standard MRI machines are quite small; larger patients and patients with claustrophobia would be better suited to using open MRI if available. Often, patients will be given a hospital gown to wear to ensure no metal objects enter the MRI suite, as even something as small as a metal button can get pulled into the scanner. Patients will be required to remove jewelry, hearing aids,

Additionally, various contrast agents can be injected into a joint or intravenously to provide further contrast detail. Magnetic resonance arthrography is a form of MRI in which a contrast material is injected into the bloodstream prior to obtaining the MRI study. The intent is to visualize the blood vessels (**Figure 4.12**). Last, functional MRI (fMRI) is used to detect metabolic changes in the brain. Often used to evaluate brain activity following a stroke or traumatic brain injury, fMRI can be used to visualize functional as well as structural changes in the brain.

Patients should be questioned about any implanted metal within the body that could heat up, dislodge (aneurysm clips), malfunction (cardiac

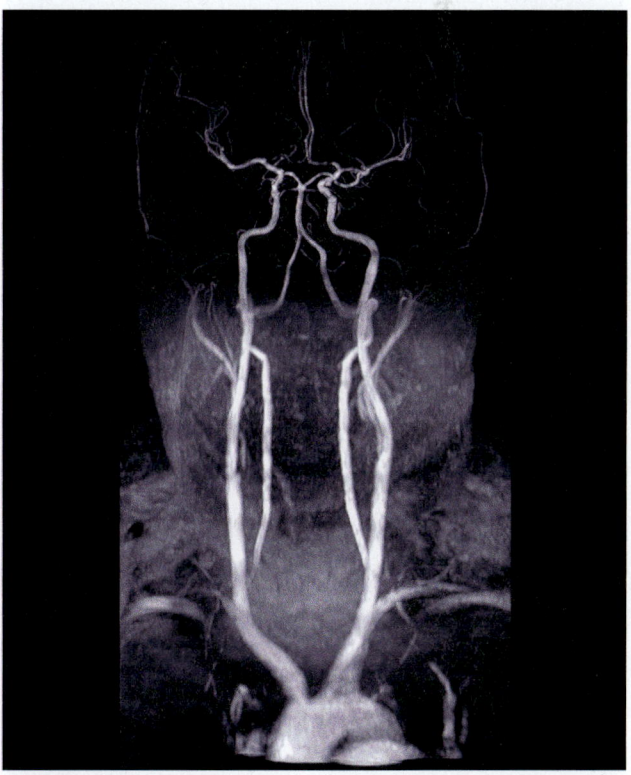

Figure 4.12 Magnetic resonance angiography.
© samunella/Shutterstock

MRI Quick Reference Guide

Indications
- Stress fractures
- Meniscal pathologies
- Spinal cord and disk pathologies
- Ligamentous or tendinous pathologies
- Tumor (soft tissue or bone) evaluation
- Osteonecrosis or osteomyelitis

Best Uses
- Ligamentous and meniscal injuries
- Blood vessel pathologies (magnetic resonance arthrography)
- Assessment of brain function (fMRI)

Length of Procedure
- 15 to 45 minutes

Comments
- Female patients of childbearing age should inform technician if they are or they suspect they may be pregnant.

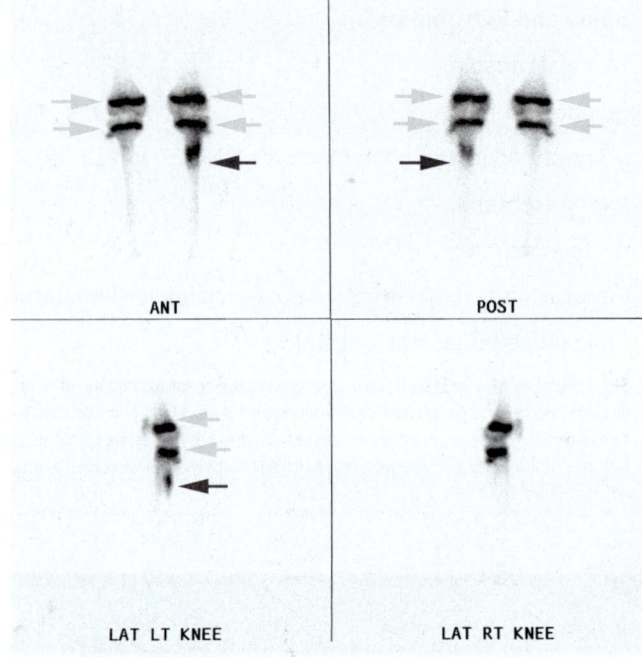

Figure 4.13 Bone scan of the lower extremity.

Reproduced from Johnson TR, Steinbach LS, eds: *Essentials of Musculoskeletal Imaging*. Rosemont, IL, American Academy of Orthopaedic Surgeons, 2004.

dentures, or glasses. Earplugs can be used during the testing to minimize the sound.

Scintigraphy (Bone Scan)

Bone scans are very useful in identifying common pathologies of the bone, including tumors, stress fractures, degenerative disease, and infections. As is usually done for all forms of nuclear medicine, after an injection (most commonly technetium-99m [Tc-99m]), the patient is asked to lie still while the scintillation camera processes the gamma radiation (emitted by Tc-99m) and forms a two-dimensional image. The radionuclide Tc-99m is localized to areas of metabolic bone activity, which appear as darkened spots (**Figure 4.13**) on the bone scan image. These darkened areas are then correlated with clinical signs and symptoms to confirm the diagnosis.

Diagnostic Ultrasonography

Diagnostic ultrasonography (sonograms) should not be confused with therapeutic ultrasonography. Using piezoelectric transducers, both ultrasonograms and ultrasound therapy depend on the transmission of sound waves through soft tissue. The difference between the two types of ultrasonography is in the sound wave frequency. Ultrasound therapy uses sound waves of 0.75-3 megahertz (MHz), whereas ultrasonograms use sound waves with frequencies between 1 and 15 MHz, depending on the depth and type of tissue being imaged, with deeper tissues requiring lower frequencies and superficial tissues normally requiring frequencies between 7 and 15 MHz.

To produce the image, the sound wave echoes are recorded after they have bounced off internal structures. Different tissues produce different echo

Bone Scan Quick Reference Guide

Indications
- Infections and inflammatory disorders
- Metastatic disease
- Tumors
- Metabolic bone disease

Best Uses
- Identification of increased metabolic activity (Note: Often yields a false-positive result in endurance athletes)

Length of Procedure
- 25 to 40 minutes

Comments
- Female patients of childbearing age should inform technician if they are or they suspect they may be pregnant.

Diagnostic Imaging

can often be identified using sonograms. Ultrasonographic imaging poses very little risk to the patient and is portable, inexpensive, and easy to obtain, which makes its use very popular. However, advanced skill is necessary to not only perform the procedure but also to interpret the image. Last, patients with excessive adipose tissue may have degraded results, as the ultrasound waves are scattered as a result of the dense tissue.

Nerve Conduction Study/Electromyography

Studies involving the pathologies of the peripheral nerves and the muscles they innervate are done using either a nerve conduction study (NCS) or electromyography. Both of these techniques identify the integrity of the nerves and determine the speed at which nerves are transmitting information.

The NCS is noninvasive and involves the stimulation of a motor peripheral nerve, using an electrical current. The signal is then recorded on a muscle that is innervated by the nerve (eg, tibialis anterior muscle activity recorded when the deep peroneal nerve is stimulated [**Figure 4.15**]). The latency (time it takes for the impulse to travel to the target muscle) and amplitude (the magnitude of the

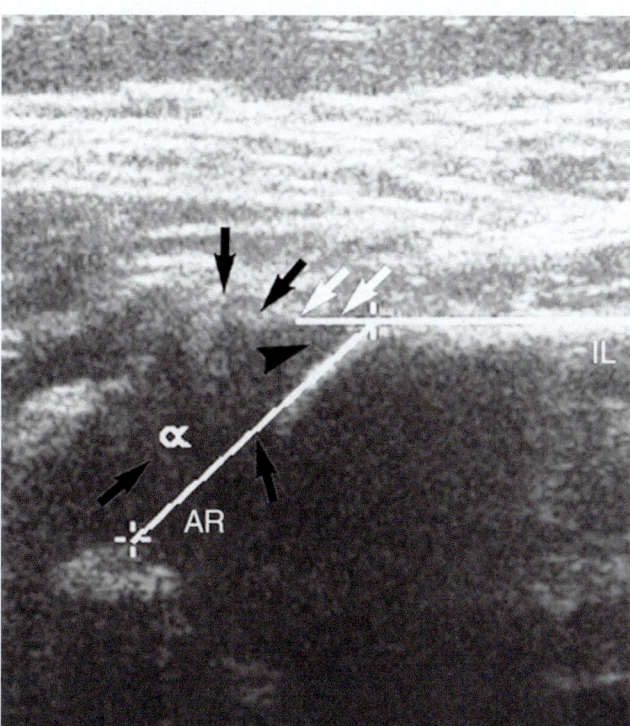

Figure 4.14 Coronal ultrasound of pediatric hip dysplasia demonstrates the cartilaginous femoral head (black arrows), labrum (white arrows), and (alpha symbol) angle (arrowhead).
AR, bony acetular roof; IL, iliac wing.

Reproduced from Armstrong AD, Hubbard MC. eds: *Essentials of Musculoskeletal Care*, ed 5. Burlington, MA, American Academy of Orthopaedic Surgeons, 2015.

patterns, which are then converted to an image. The image is presented as tissue cross sections (**Figure 4.14**), which can then be interpreted. Muscle pathology, tendinopathy, and ligamentous pathologies

Ultrasonography Quick Reference Guide

Indications
- Joint effusion
- Tendinopathy
- Ligament pathology
- Soft-tissue masses
- Infantile hip dysplasia

Best Uses
- Joint and soft-tissue pathology
- Injection guide

Length of Procedure
- 10 to 40 minutes

Comments
- Although generally considered safe, extra precaution should be taken when performing ultrasonography around any fluid-filled organ.

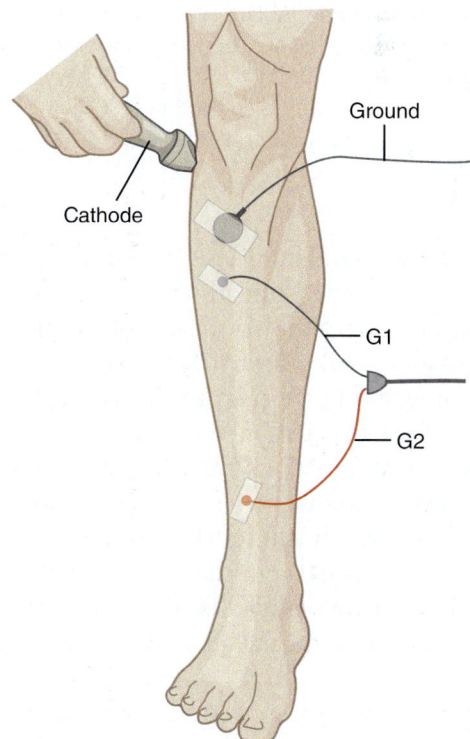

Figure 4.15 Tibialis anterior nerve conduction study.
© Jones & Bartlett Learning

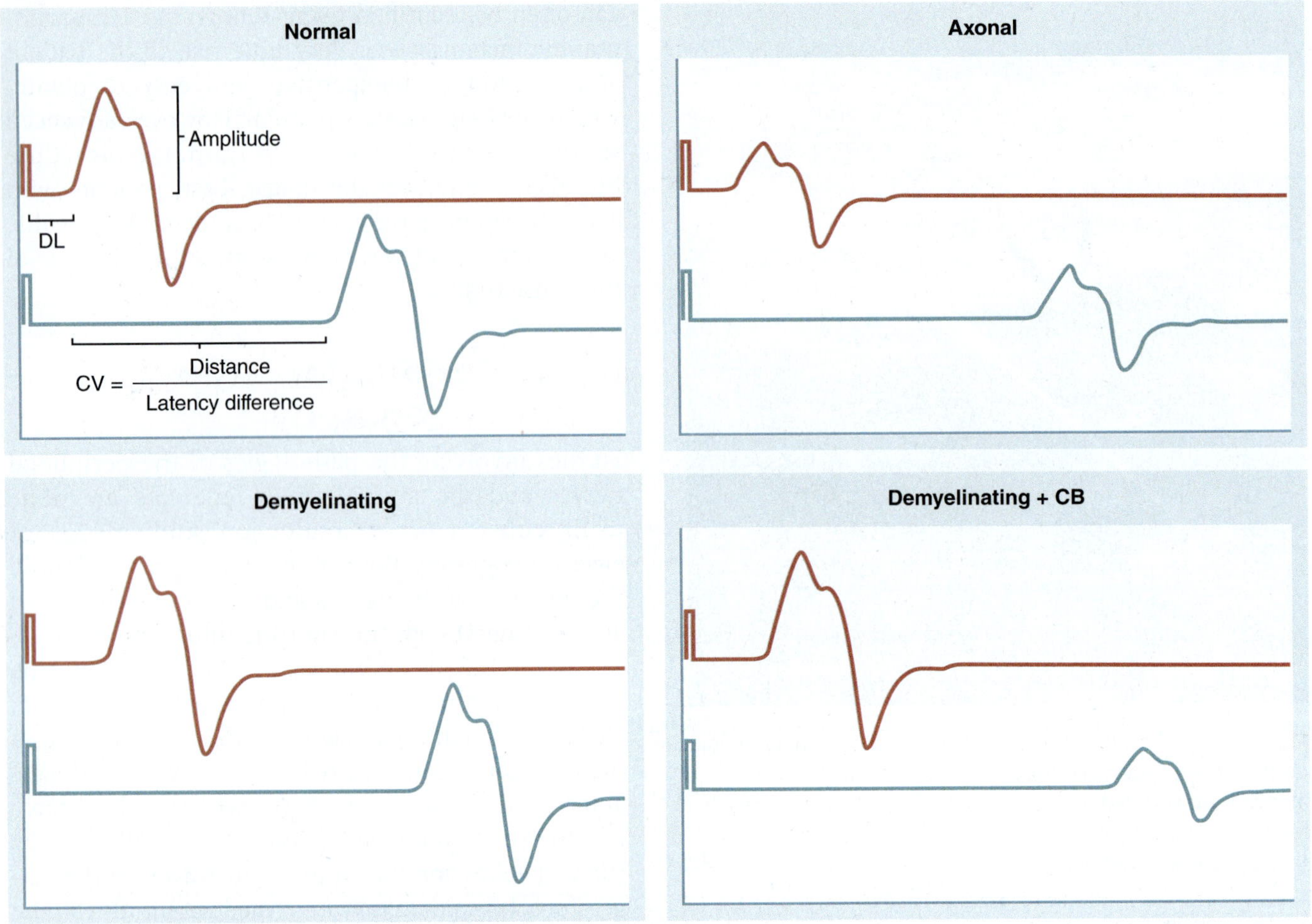

Figure 4.16 Normal versus abnormal nerve conduction study. The red lines show proximal stimulation and the blue lines show distal stimulation. **A.** Normal nerve conduction. **B.** Axonal Injury where the axons are no longer functioning. NCS shows lower amplitudes but relatively preserved DL and CV. **C.** Demyelinating nerves produce similar amplitues but slowed CV and prolonged DL. **D.** Demlinating + CB nerves produce slowed CV but with similar amplitude proximal. Distally, the nerve shows low amplitude and prolonged DL.
CB, conduction block; CV, conduction velocity; DL, distal latency.
© Jones & Bartlett Learning

response) are recorded. These values are compared to the original signal strength and can be compared bilaterally to determine the health of the peripheral nerve (**Figure 4.16**). The NCS is done at multiple points along the nerve path to determine the presence of pathology, most often an entrapment.

Electromyography is an invasive procedure and involves the use of a thin detecting needle (**Figure 4.17**), which is inserted into the muscle. The needle sends a signal into the muscle; that signal is recorded. Electrical activity is then compared to the resting muscle and during an active muscle contraction (**Figure 4.18**).

Patients undergoing electromyography should be informed of possible muscle soreness following the procedure; patients who are taking anticoagulants should be informed of increased risk of hematomas and increased bleeding time. The NCS poses very little risk to patients and can be completed very quickly; however, patients may experience a slight shock when electrical current is applied. Advanced skill is required to perform and interpret results.

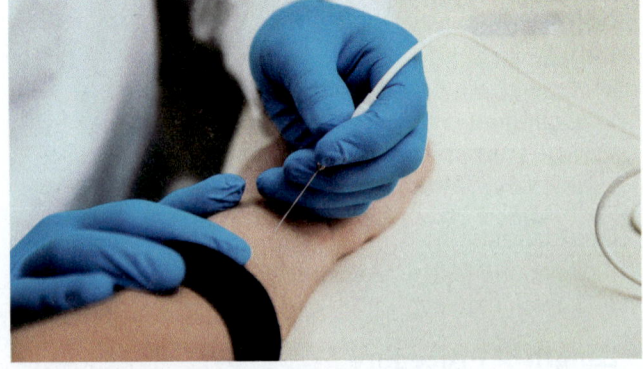

Figure 4.17 Electromyography.
© Roman Zaiets/Shutterstock

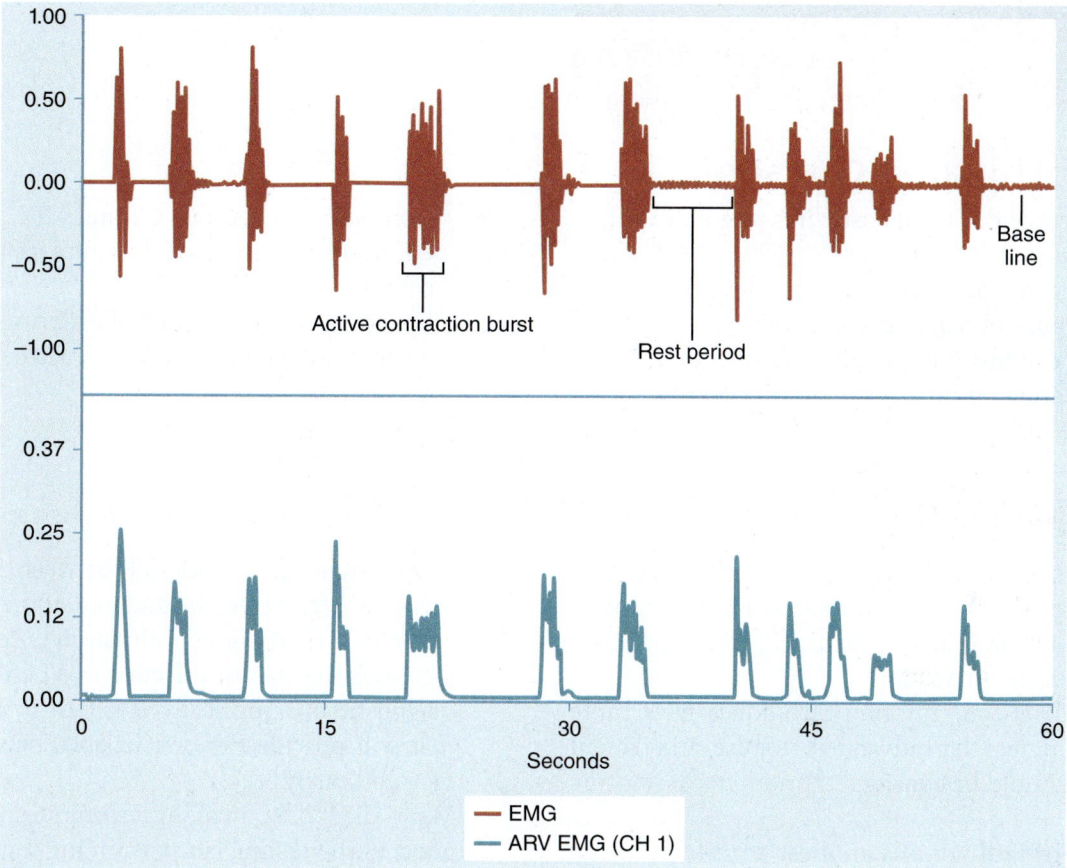

Figure 4.18 Sample electromyography (EMG) results. The top graph represents a traditional raw recording from a voluntary neuromuscular activation. Note the active contraction burst (the start to end of one contraction), the raw baseline noise value (the value when the muscle is relaxed), and the rest period (the time from the end of one contraction to the beginning of the next). The bottom graph shows the rectified EMG recording where all the negative amplitudes have been converted to positive amplitudes. This is so the amplitude parameters (mean, peak/max value) can be calculated (raw EMG has a mean value of zero).
ARV, average rectified value EMG; CH, Channel

© Jones & Bartlett Learning

Nerve Conduction Study/Electromyography Quick Reference Guide

Indications
- Carpal tunnel syndrome
- Nerve root injuries
- Idiopathic foot drop

Best Uses
- Nerve pathologies

Length of Procedure
- 30 minutes to 2 hours

Comments
- Patients with nerve injury should wait 3 to 4 weeks before undergoing an EMG test.
- Obese and edematous limbs will reduce the accuracy of nerve conduction studies.

Summary

Diagnostic imaging is a cornerstone of the evaluation and subsequent management of musculoskeletal pathologies, in that many pathologies have a way of being accurately diagnosed without the use of diagnostic imaging. Deciding which imaging studies to order is often dependent on a number of factors, including but not limited to cost, patient values, and suspected pathology; each of these factors is just as important as the next, and each one needs to be considered and discussed with the patient prior to ordering. It is essential for clinicians to understand the advantages and disadvantages of each of the diagnostic images and to also realize that not every diagnostic imaging technique is appropriate in every situation. Last, clinicians should understand and appreciate the expertise required to perform and interpret many of the diagnostic imaging techniques.

WRAP-UP

Critical Thinking Questions

1. What role does diagnostic imaging play in the injury evaluation process?
2. How can a patient's values dictate the outcomes of diagnostic imaging?
3. How can insurance companies direct the evaluation and management process of a soft-tissue injury?
4. Compare and contrast CT and MRI. How can clinicians use one modality in place of the other?
5. Describe the importance of ordering the correct radiologic view for a fracture or dislocation.

Pearls and Pitfalls

- Diagnostic imaging plays a critical role in the evaluation process. Many injuries cannot be properly diagnosed, and thereby managed, without the use of diagnostic imaging.
- Many diagnostic imaging techniques have more disadvantages than advantages for use, and patient values should be considered prior to ordering any image.
- Standard radiographs are best used for skeletal pathologies, whereas MRI, CT, and ultrasonography are used to evaluate the integrity of the soft tissue.
- Often, there is a trade-off between safety and accuracy (eg, nerve conduction studies are more accurate when done invasively; however, it increases the risk of infection). When ordering a diagnostic imaging study, it is best to order a test that will provide the best balance between accuracy and safety.
- Many diagnostic imaging techniques are only as good as the technician performing the test or the radiologist interpreting the tests. Therefore, when you find good technicians or radiologists, hold on to them!

References

1. Chakravarty D, Sloan J, Brenchley J: Risk reduction through skeletal scintigraphy as a screening tool in suspected scaphoid fracture: a literature review. *Emerg Med J* 2002;19:507.
2. Gaeta M, Mintoli F, Scribano E, et al: CT and MR imaging findings in athletes with early tibial stress injuries: comparison with bone scintigraphy findings and emphasis on cortical abnormalities. *Radiology* 2015;235:553-561.
3. Chan O: *ABC of Emergency Radiology*, ed 3. West Sussex, England, UK, Wiley-Blackwell Publishing, 2013.
4. Williams IJ: Appendicular skeleton: ABCs image interpretation search strategy. *S African Radiographer* 2013;51:2.
5. D'Orsi CJ: Radiology and magnetic resonance imaging, in Greene HL, Glassock RJ, Kelley MA, eds: *Introduction to Clinical Medicine*. Philadelphia, PA, BC Decker, 1991, p 91.
6. Kimura J: *Principles of Nerve Conduction Studies*. Oxford, England, UK: Oxford University Press, 2013.

UNIT II

Lower Extremity Evaluation

CHAPTER 5	Foot and Ankle	57
CHAPTER 6	Knee Joint	127
CHAPTER 7	Hip and Thigh	163

CHAPTER 5

Foot and Ankle

Christine Waters-Banker, PhD, ATC
Nicole Lounsberry Yates, MS, ATC, LAT

OVERVIEW

This chapter provides an in-depth overview of the structures, functions, assessments, and pathologies of the foot and ankle. Emphasis will be placed on evaluation techniques and injuries commonly encountered within the field of athletic training and therapy.

LEARNING OBJECTIVES

After completing this chapter, the reader will be able to do the following:

1. Describe the anatomy of the foot and ankle, including bone, muscle, and ligaments.
2. Explain the various articulations of the foot and ankle and their associated supporting structures.
3. Identify common imaging techniques and their usefulness in the diagnosis of foot and ankle injuries.
4. Describe different fractures of the foot and ankle.
5. Differentiate between common foot and ankle pathologies, based on history, inspection, palpation, and special tests.
6. Discuss the diagnostic accuracy of special tests for the foot and ankle and how that relates to clinical evaluation.

FUN FACTS ABOUT THE FOOT AND ANKLE

- The navicular bone is sometimes referred to as the scaphoid bone. Navicular is generally used to avoid confusion with the scaphoid bone in the wrist.
- The Achilles tendon is the largest and strongest tendon in the entire human body.
- Shoe sizes were once measured in barleycorns. It became standard in the 14th century when King Edward of England signed a royal decree that barleycorn be used as a unit of measurement for shoe sizes. The decree also included a proclamation that three lengths of barleycorn were equivalent to 1 inch.
- The world's oldest leather shoe was found in Armenia in 2010 and dates back to about 3500 BC.

Introduction

The foot and ankle act as a unit and form the base of the kinetic chain. Together, they absorb and transfer force quickly over a diverse range of activities. As they make contact with the ground, the foot and ankle adapt to a variety of terrains, making them vulnerable to myriads of injuries. The complexity of the foot and ankle allows for specialized movements; however, it often complicates evaluation and proper diagnosis. As weight-bearing structures, the foot and ankle introduce numerous challenges in the maintenance and rehabilitation phases of injury management. It is important for clinicians to have a thorough understanding of the extensive and unique anatomy of the foot and ankle to better realize not only acute mechanisms of injury but also the chronic pathologies associated with instability.

Clinical Anatomy

Bones of the Foot and Ankle

The foot is composed primarily of 26 bones, excluding the sesamoid bones (**Figure 5.1**). The bones of the foot include the following (listed distal to proximal): 14 phalanges, 5 metatarsals, and 7 tarsal bones (navicular; the medial, intermediate, and lateral cuneiforms; cuboid; calcaneus; and talus). The foot and the lower leg connect to form the ankle, or mortise joint, which includes the talus of the foot and the tibia and fibula bones of the lower leg.

Phalanges and Metatarsals

Phalanges and metatarsal bones comprise the long bones of the foot. They are cylindrical bones that make up the forefoot region of each foot. The individual toes, not including the first toe (or hallux), are constructed by three phalanges: distal, intermediate, and proximal; the hallux consists of distal and proximal phalanges only. The phalanges provide a wide base to the foot to distribute weight and improve balance. The metatarsals form articulations with the proximal phalanges and the tarsal bones of the foot, serving to transmit force between the forefoot and the midfoot tarsal bones. Two sesamoid bones are located on the plantar aspect of the first metatarsophalangeal (MTP) joint and are described in the following section.

Sesamoids

Sesamoid bones are small ovoid or nodular-shaped bones that are either partially or fully embedded within a tendon and may be bipartite or multipartite in nature[1] (**Figure 5.2**). Named for their sesame seed–like appearance, sesamoid bones can vary greatly in prevalence.[2] However, the hallucal sesamoids are always present on the plantar aspect of the distal head (or sometimes simply referred to as the head) of the first metatarsal of the human foot. The medial (tibial) and lateral (fibular) hallucal sesamoids are embedded within the medial and lateral flexor hallucis brevis tendons, respectively, as the tendons insert onto the first metatarsal head. The larger medial sesamoid is commonly associated with a bipartite variation that can often be misdiagnosed as a fracture.[1] Receiving additional tendinous attachments from the adductor and abductor hallucis muscles, the sesamoids are further stabilized via ligamentous attachments.[2] Hallucal sesamoids play a very important role in regard to foot function. Hallucal sesamoids can transmit approximately 50% of body weight and loads greater than 300% during the push-off phase.[2] They serve to disperse load, thereby protecting the first metatarsal and flexor tendons. Like other sesamoid bones throughout the body, the hallucal sesamoids provide a powerful

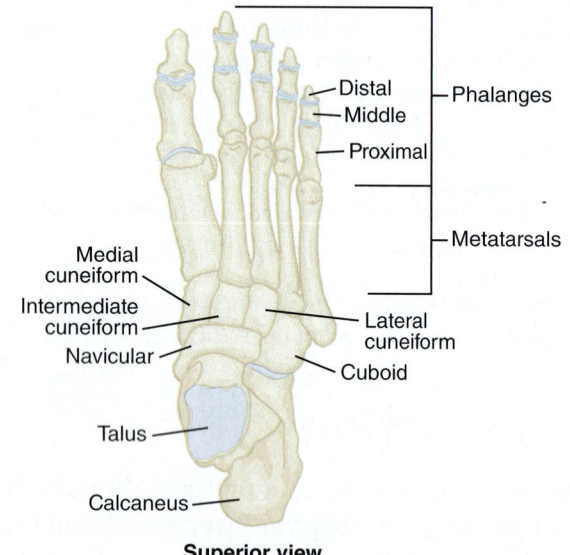
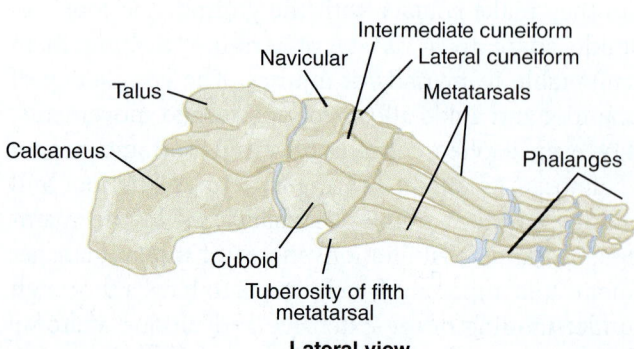

Figure 5.1 Drawings showing skeletal anatomy of the foot and ankle.
© Jones & Bartlett Learning

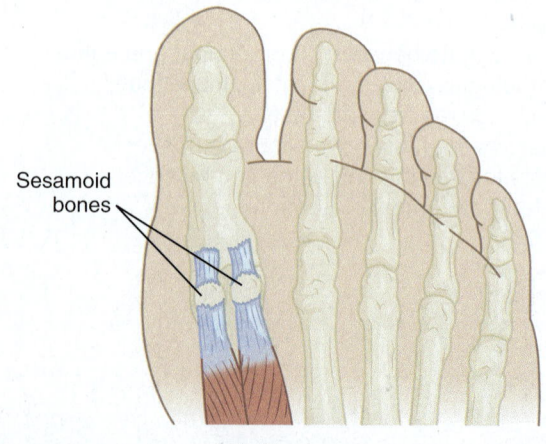

Figure 5.2 Drawing showing sesamoid bones of the foot.
© Jones & Bartlett Learning

biomechanical advantage to the tendon by increasing the moment arm of the flexor hallucis tendon.[2]

Tarsals

Seven tarsal bones comprise the midfoot and rearfoot regions of the foot. The Greek root of the word *tarsals* is *tarsos*, meaning flat surface, or translated to sole of the foot, which can be applied to both the tarsals of the midfoot and the metatarsals of the forefoot. The medial cuneiform, intermediate cuneiform, lateral cuneiform, and cuboid are shorter, cubelike bones that articulate with the metatarsal bones. The navicular bone is a longer rectangular bone with a slight concavity resembling a boat or canoe; the Latin root *nav* or *navicula* means ship or boat, hence, the name. The navicular is the keystone of the medial arch of the foot, and, in addition to articulating with the cuboid, it forms articulations with the talus and calcaneus bones (described in the following paragraphs).

Talus. The talus has a uniquely complex geometric shape that includes a distinct dome. Approximately 60% of the talar surface is covered in articular cartilage, and it is completely absent of muscular attachment.[3] Therefore, movement of the talus is initiated and carried out through the surrounding structures. The talus is positioned superior to the calcaneus over the bony projection known as the sustentaculum tali. The base of the talus is described as the body, whereas the dome is described as the head, with a neck between the two. The head consists of a groove referred to as the trochlea (from the Latin *trochlea,* meaning pulley), so named, as it resembles the groove found in a pulley system. The trochlea articulates with the tibia and fibula long bones to form the mortise joint (**Figure 5.3**). The anterior aspect of the talus is wider than the posterior aspect, therefore, promoting a greater range of motion in plantar flexion than dorsiflexion of the ankle.

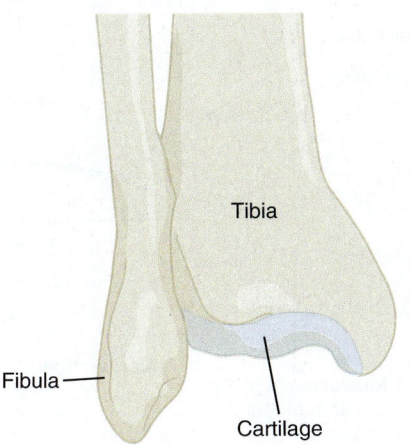

Figure 5.3 Drawing showing the ankle mortise.
© Jones & Bartlett Learning

Calcaneus. Largest of the tarsal bones, the calcaneus forms the rounded heel of the foot, which makes initial contact with the ground during the heel-strike phase of gait. The calcaneus has several important bony anatomic landmarks. The tuberosity of the calcaneus serves as an attachment site for the Achilles tendon, the medial plantar aspect of the calcaneus serves as an attachment for connective tissue structures (ie, plantar fascia), and the peroneal tubercle serves as a point of stability and divergence of the peroneal tendons on the lateral aspect. Furthermore, the calcaneus gives rise to the shelflike sustentaculum tali, which provides support to the talus in addition to providing a sliding surface for several tendons of the medial aspect of the foot and an attachment site for the calcaneonavicular ligament (or spring ligament).

Tibia and Fibula

The tibia and fibula are long bones of the lower leg and are often referred to as the shank. The fibula is a slender long bone located on the lateral aspect of the lower leg, primarily serving as an attachment site for lateral musculature. The distal end of the fibula forms the smaller and slightly posterior lateral malleolus.

The tibia is second to the femur as the longest bone in the body and is the primary weight-bearing bone of the leg. The tibia is triangular in shape and therefore has posterior, medial, and lateral surfaces that serve as the attachment sites for numerous muscles. The medial aspect lies just below the subcutaneous layer of the skin, leaving the periosteal surface of the bone vulnerable to injury. The inferior third of the tibial shaft has the highest prevalence for lower leg fractures; this is often attributed to the change in shape from a more triangular to a columnar configuration, presenting an anatomic weakness. The distal portion of the tibia forms the larger and slightly more anterior medial malleolus. The distal articular surface, referred to as the tibial plafond (French origin: *plat,* meaning flat, and *fond,* meaning bottom), extends posteriorly as well, comprising the posterior malleolus.[4]

Articulations and Ligamentous Support of the Foot and Ankle

There are numerous articulations that accompany the great number of bones in the foot and ankle that allow for movement and stability. The foot and ankle complex comprises both long bones (phalanges, metatarsals, tibia, fibula) and short bones (tarsals). The foot can be divided into three major regions: the forefoot, midfoot, and hindfoot, with the distal portion of the shank forming the talocrural (ankle), also referred to as a mortise joint (**Figure 5.4**). These articulations are categorized as they relate to each region from distal to proximal.

Forefoot

The forefoot is the most distal aspect of the foot and can be further subdivided into first ray and lateral forefoot portions.

First Ray and Hallux. Also referred to as the medial forefoot, the first ray is composed of the first metatarsal and the medial cuneiform bones and is arguably one of the most important mechanical structures of the forefoot. The first ray functions to provide transmission of force during weight bearing and arch stability throughout the midstance and propulsion phases of gait. As the foot moves from heel strike to midstance, the triceps surae muscles contract, tightening the plantar fascia and moving the foot into plantar flexion. As the foot begins to plantarflex, the toes dorsiflex, drawing the plantar fascia taut and raising and stabilizing the longitudinal arches, particularly the medial arch, in preparation for push-off. Weight is transferred to the first MTP joint, and push-off occurs through the proximal and distal phalanges of the hallux. This mechanism is referred to as the windlass mechanism and can be easily achieved by dorsiflexing the toes during a static stance (medial arch will rise). Because proper transfer of force is required for propulsion, any disruption of first ray stability, either through hypomobility or hypermobility, can limit the functional performance of the foot.

Lateral Forefoot. The lateral forefoot is composed of the remaining metatarsals and the associated phalanges. The forefoot stabilization is provided via numerous collateral ligaments at each of the proximal and distal phalanges and by the transverse and plantar metatarsal ligaments at the MTP joints.

Tarsometatarsal, or Lisfranc, Joint

The tarsometatarsal (TMT) joint, also referred to as the Lisfranc joint, is named for the French surgeon, Jacques Lisfranc de St. Martin, who first described the displacement of the metatarsals from the tarsus in 1815, is now referred to as a Lisfranc injury.[5] The TMT joint is composed of the articulations that join

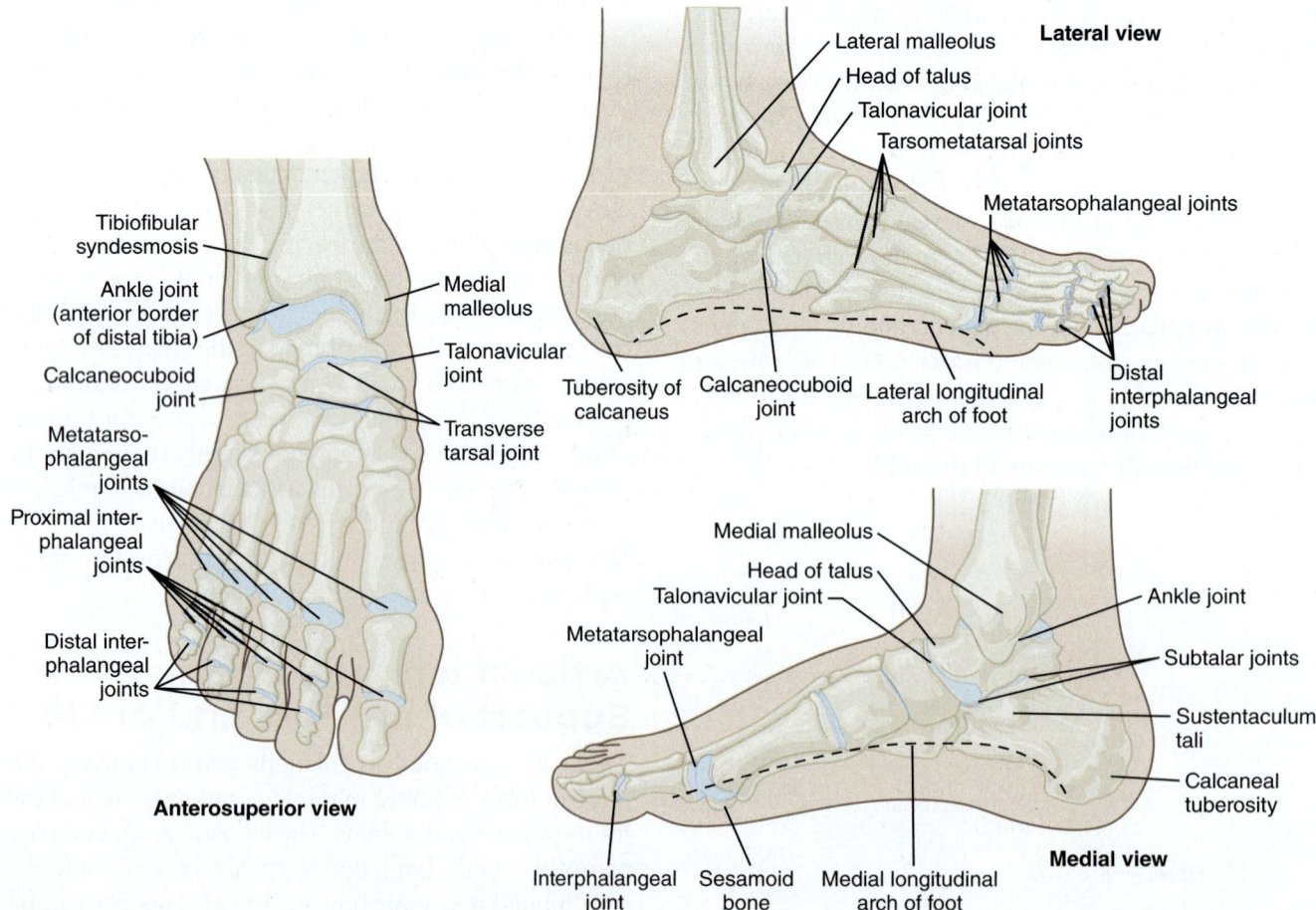

Figure 5.4 Drawings showing the articulations of the foot based on anatomic zones.
© Jones & Bartlett Learning

the midfoot and forefoot. Often divided into medial and lateral aspects, the medial aspect of the TMT joint consists of the medial, intermediate, and lateral cuneiforms and their articulations with the first, second, and third metatarsals.[5] The lateral aspect of the TMT joint consists of the remaining cuboid tarsal bone and its articulations with the fourth and fifth metatarsals.[5] The TMT joint forms a stable bony arch, referred to as a Roman arch because of its resemblance to traditional Roman stone arches with a keystone configuration. The keystone of the TMT arch is the base of the second metatarsal, and, as such, the second metatarsal plays a large role in the bony stability of the TMT joint. Therefore, a shallow alignment of the second TMT joint is a risk factor for a Lisfranc injury.[5] The Lisfranc ligament strengthens the TMT articulation and helps to maintain the midfoot arch, extending from the base of the second metatarsal to the plantar aspect of the medial cuneiform.[5] Additionally, interosseous ligaments span the joint, from the plantar aspect of the distal second metatarsal head through to the fifth metatarsal head, and, together, these ligaments further bolster the stability of the keystone and TMT joint, respectively.

Midfoot

The midfoot consists of the tarsal bones (navicular, cuneiforms, and cuboid). Supported by connective tissue, ligaments, and muscles, the tarsal bones form a half dome with the combination of the medial, lateral, and transverse arches (**Figure 5.5** and **Figure 5.6**). This dome is key for the transmission and attenuation of forces as the foot meets the ground, providing

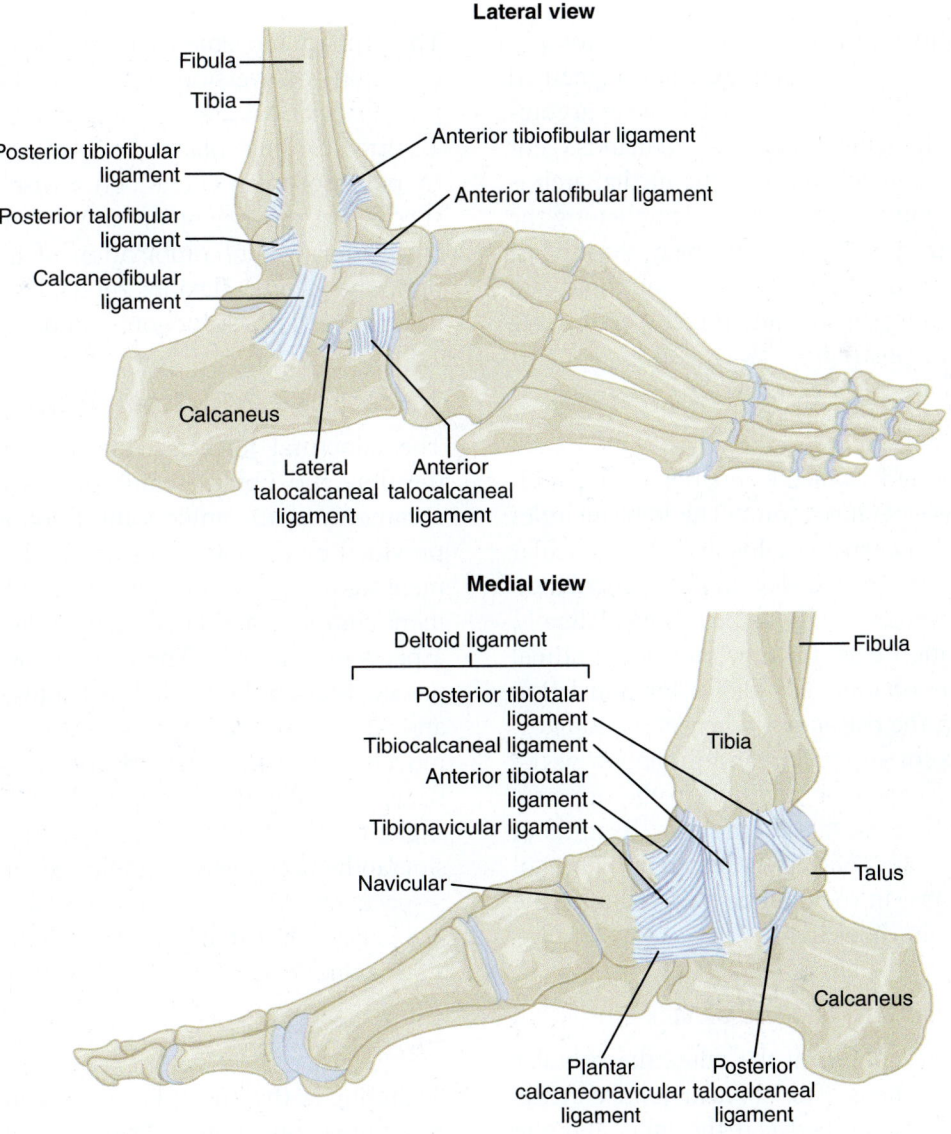

Figure 5.5 Drawings showing ligamentous support of the foot (medial and lateral).

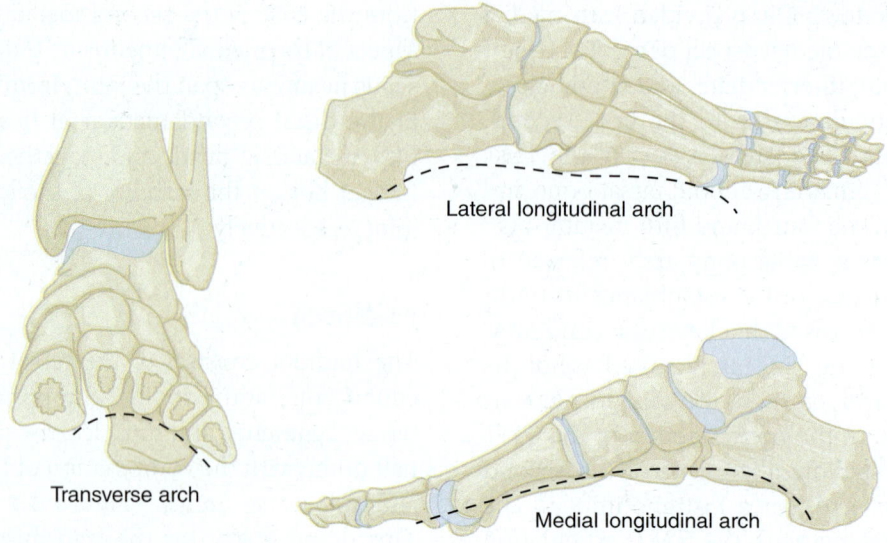

Figure 5.6 Drawings showing arches of the foot.
© Jones & Bartlett Learning

both static stability and dynamic adaptability for various surfaces. The foot is a complex, multisegmented system, and the midfoot plays a crucial role in accommodating ever-changing functional demands. For example, during slow locomotion, the medial arch is more compliant and flattens, thereby lengthening the foot and maximizing balance. Conversely, during fast locomotion, the medial arch becomes more rigid and inflexible, shortening the foot and thereby optimizing propulsion during push-off.

Transverse Tarsal, or Chopart, Joint

Motion is transferred from the forefoot to the midfoot via the transverse tarsal joint. The joint includes the articulation between the talus and the navicular on the medial aspect of the foot and the articulation between the calcaneus and the cuboid bone, laterally. Two axes of rotation exist for this joint: longitudinal and oblique. The oblique axis allows for translation of the cuboid on the calcaneus, whereas the longitudinal axis allows for supination and pronation of the cuboid on the calcaneus in addition to the opposite rotation of the transverse tarsal joint from the midfoot in the transverse plane. Furthermore, manipulation of the transverse tarsal in the oblique axis will alter the height of the longitudinal arches.

Hindfoot and Subtalar Joint

The hindfoot is composed of the talus, the subtalar joint, and the calcaneus. The subtalar joint consists of multiple articulations between the talus and the calcaneus (talocalcaneal), in addition to the talus, calcaneus, and navicular bones (talocalcaneonavicular).

The primary movements at this joint are described as inversion and eversion of the foot. However, the complex articulations create an axis of rotation that crosses all three cardinal planes from anterior-superomedial to posterior-inferolateral, otherwise described as a specialized movement of supination and pronation. Supination is the combination of inversion, adduction, and plantar flexion; pronation is the combination of eversion, abduction, and dorsiflexion.

Talocrural (Mortise) Joint

The talocrural joint is composed of the talus and the tibia and fibula (shank) and is referred to most commonly as the ankle joint. Support of the joint is provided by the joint capsule in addition to the ligamentous structures on both the medial (deltoid ligament complex) and lateral (lateral ligament complex) aspects of the joint. The axis of the talocrural joint passes through the medial malleolus, the talar dome, and the lateral malleolus. Although the primary movements of the joint are dorsiflexion and plantar flexion, the slightly oblique angle of the axis allows for slight movements of eversion/adduction and inversion/abduction during dorsiflexion or plantar flexion, respectively. As its namesake would suggest, the mortise joint is most stable when the joint is positioned at a 90° angle.

Shank

Beginning at the knee, the shank consists of the tibia and fibula long bones. Proximally, the tibia articulates with the distal femur, and the fibula articulates with the lateral condyle of the tibia. As mentioned previously, the distal portions of the tibia and fibula form the medial and lateral malleoli, respectively. The shank is stabilized by the interosseous ligament, which runs the length of the diaphyses, in addition to the superior/inferior anterior and posterior tibiofibular ligaments. Although the fibula does not articulate with the knee directly, it bears approximately 10% to 30% of the axial load. During ankle motion, the tibia internally rotates with rearfoot pronation, and the fibula translates and/or rotates during dorsiflexion and plantar flexion across all cardinal planes.

Soft-Tissue Anatomy of the Foot and Ankle

Ligamentous Anatomy

The bones and ligaments provide passive support to the skeletal system. Ligaments bridge the bones and provide stability to the articulations, or joints, which two or more bones create. Ligaments provide this stability by resisting excessive motion at the joint, which would otherwise separate the bony ends. If ligamentous structures become lax or damaged when subjected to excessive tension, joint instability occurs.

To better conceptualize joint function, it is important to consider structure, organization, and purpose. The human body is generally designed in repeating fashion. Each joint exists in a pair, with similar joint configurations appearing in the upper and lower extremities, with slight functional differences. For example, the first ray of the hand, which consists of the thumb phalanges and first metacarpal, requires great mobility to oppose the other fingers of the hand, allowing the fingers to grip and hold objects. However, the first ray of the foot, which displays an anatomic structure similar to the hand (composed of the first toe phalanges, first metatarsal, and medial cuneiform), does not oppose the other toes and instead is designed to have rather fixed motion. As discussed previously, this design plays an important role in propulsion during toe-off and provides stability during weight bearing.

A hypermobile first ray of the foot would be detrimental to function, whereas hypermobility is greatly appreciated in the hand. When examining the passive support structures that make this possible, it is clear that slight bony modifications, such as the concavity and shape of the specialized saddle joint provided by the trapezium and the first metacarpal and the minimal ligamentous support, allow for great movement of the thumb. Evaluation of the foot reveals arthrodial joints at the tarsometatarsal level, surrounded by thick, strong, ligamentous structures, that allow for very little movement, thereby promoting great stability (Figure 5.5).

When trying to understand and/or visualize the stability provided by a particular ligament, its name provides a description. As an example, the role of the anterior talofibular ligament (ATFL), the most commonly injured lateral ankle ligament, can be studied. Its name describes its exact placement in the body, as it connects the talus and the fibula bones on the anterolateral aspect of the ankle.

To understand how the ATFL provides anterolateral support, recall that the talus has a domed component with a trochlear groove that articulates with the tibia and the fibula as a part of the mortise joint. This dome allows the talus the freedom to roll anteriorly and posteriorly, creating plantar flexion and dorsiflexion movements. When the foot is in a plantarflexed position, the dome rotates anteriorly, and the collateral stability that is provided by the tibia and fibula on either aspect of the talar dome is reduced; this makes plantar flexion the most unstable position as the talus begins to translate anteriorly. Without support, the talus could completely dislodge (dislocate) from the mortise joint. As mentioned previously, the ATFL connects the talus to the fibula at the lateral malleolus. This placement allows for the talus to be stabilized—or, rather, anchored—to the fibula, preventing its anterior translation. Therefore, the ATFL is said to resist anterior translation of the ankle. When the talus is forcibly translated anteriorly, it produces tension of the ATFL as the ligament is pulled away from the fibula. If the force exceeds the tensile properties of the ligament, the ligament will fail, causing injury.

Understanding the role ligaments play provides great insight into mechanisms of injury (MOIs). Gathering a thorough history that describes an MOI directs the clinician to the site of injury and allows for a thorough and precise orthopaedic examination. For example, if an individual describes pain over the anterolateral aspect of the ankle and an incident in which his or her foot was plantarflexed while rolling laterally (inversion), it is highly probable that the ATFL may have been damaged. To rule in or rule out this diagnosis, a clinician would assess anterior drawer movement (special test) via anterior translation of the talus and determine whether pain and/or excessive laxity exists.

Many ligaments are required to provide both stability and flexibility to the multitude of bones and joints that comprise the foot and ankle. The major ligamentous structures of the foot and ankle are grouped by the joint in which stability is provided and listed from distal to proximal.

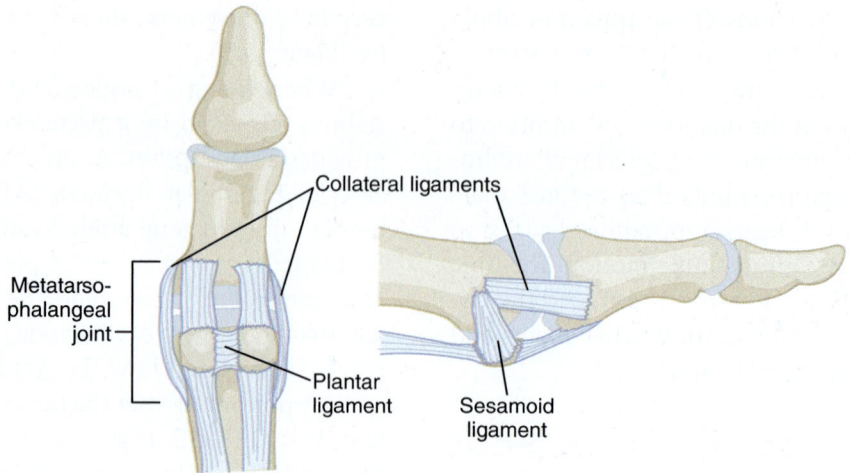

Figure 5.7 Inferior view (left) and lateral view (right) drawings showing collateral ligaments of the metatarsophalangeal joint.

© Jones & Bartlett Learning

Phalangeal and MTP Joint Stabilization.

The MTP joints and interphalangeal joints are surrounded by a synovial joint capsule that is supported by collateral ligaments (**Figure 5.7**). The capsule and ligaments provide support for these joints and can be evaluated using valgus and varus stress tests. In addition to the joint capsule and collateral ligaments, the dorsal aspect of the MTP joint capsule is further supported by the plantar fascia and the deep transverse metatarsal ligaments. On the dorsal aspect of the distal interphalangeal joints two through five, a connective tissue structure, referred to as the extensor hood/expansion, extends from the extensor tendons, providing additional dorsal support to the joints (**Figure 5.8**).

Forefoot and Midfoot Stabilization.

The Lisfranc joint is the junction between the forefoot and the midfoot at the TMT joint junction. The midfoot is further composed of the talocalcaneonavicular and calcaneocuboid joints. These regions are supported by plantar, dorsal, and interosseous ligaments. The proper Lisfranc ligament provides stability at the TMT joint articulation, originating from the base of the second metatarsal and extending to the plantar aspect of the medial cuneiform (**Figure 5.9**). For the talocalcaneonavicular joint, the plantar calcaneonavicular ligament (or spring ligament) originates on the sustentaculum tali of the calcaneus and inserts on the inferior-posterior aspect of the navicular tubercle. The calcaneocuboid joints are stabilized by dorsal and plantar calcaneocuboid ligaments, the long plantar ligament, and the plantar fascia.

Subtalar Joint Stabilization.

The talus is stabilized by the posterior talocalcaneal ligament, the anterior (interosseous) talocalcaneal ligament, and the lateral talocalcaneal ligament (**Figure 5.10**). The posterior talocalcaneal ligament originates from the posterior-inferior aspect of the talus and extends

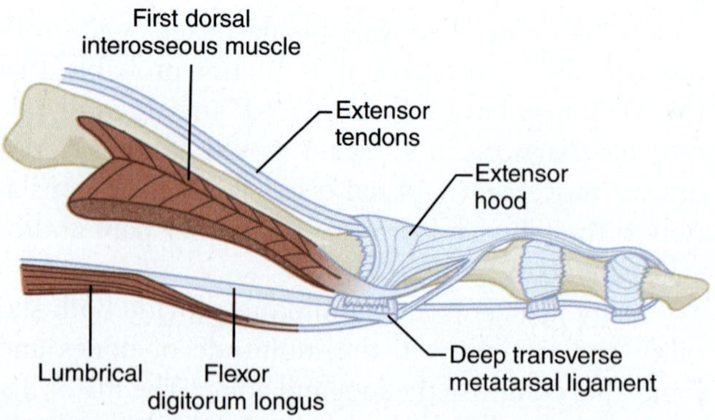

Figure 5.8 Drawing showing distal interphalangeal joint extensor hood/expansion.

© Jones & Bartlett Learning

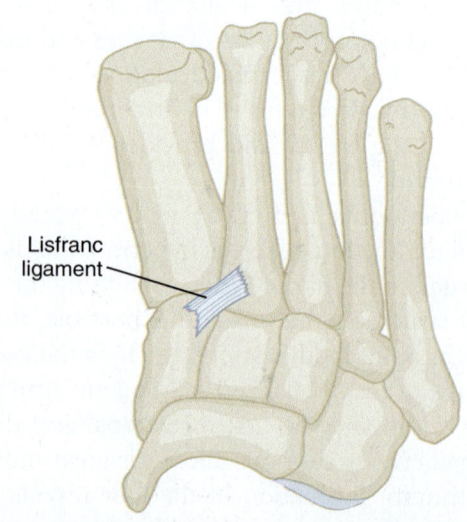

Figure 5.9 Drawing showing the Lisfranc ligament.

© Jones & Bartlett Learning

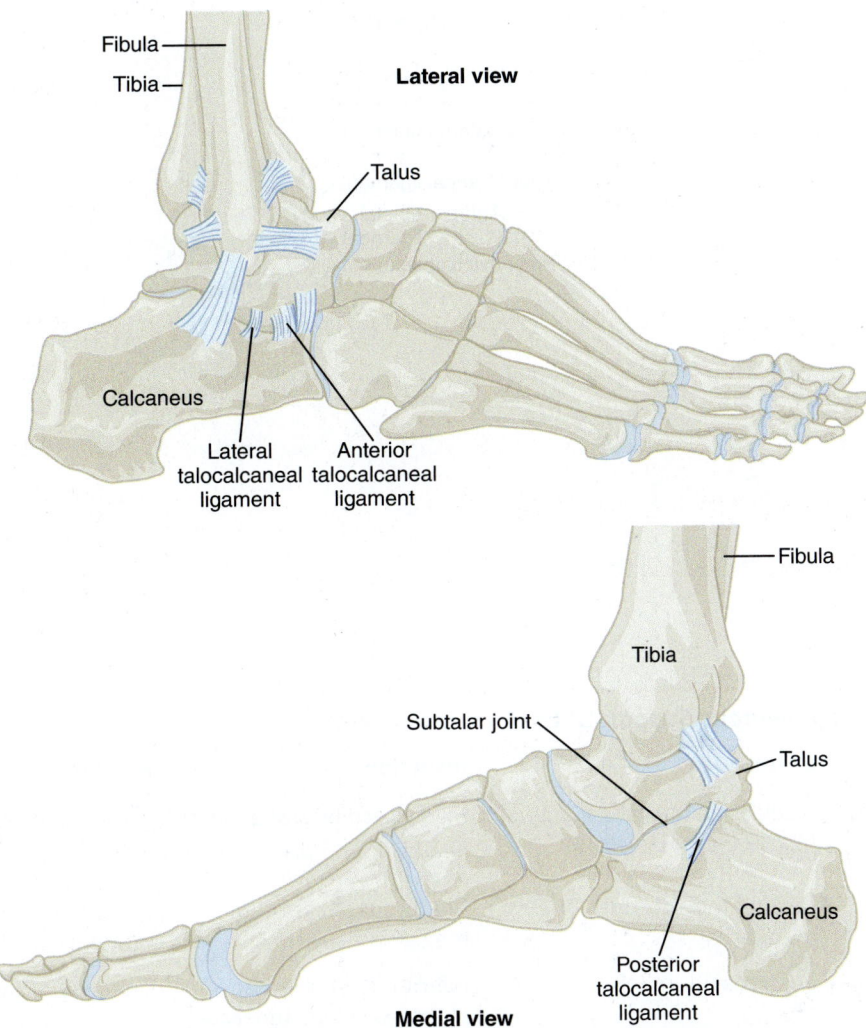

Figure 5.10 Drawings showing the talocalcaneal ligaments (posterior, anterior, and lateral).
© Jones & Bartlett Learning

to the superior aspect of the calcaneus, whereas the anterior talocalcaneal ligament originates on the anterolateral aspect of the talus and extends inferiorly to the superior-anterior aspect of the calcaneus within the sinus tarsi. Last, the lateral talocalcaneal ligament originates on the lateral aspect of the talus, posterior to the anterior talocalcaneal ligament and inferior to the anterior aspect of the lateral malleolus, extending inferiorly and posteriorly to insert on the lateral aspect of the calcaneus superior to the peroneal trochlea.

Medial Ankle Stabilization. Medial stabilization of the ankle joint is mostly provided by a large, triangular ligamentous fan, referred to as the deltoid ligament complex (**Figure 5.11**). The complex is composed of multiple ligaments, including the posterior tibiotalar ligament (superficial and deep); the tibiocalcaneal ligament (superficial and deep); the anterior tibiotalar ligament; the tibionavicular ligament; and, in some cases, fibers to the spring ligament.

In general, the deltoid ligament originates from the medial malleolus and extends to the talus, calcaneus, and navicular bones to resist eversion and the lateral subluxation of the talus in severe ankle fractures.[6] The origin and insertion points for each individual medial ankle ligament are presented in **Table 5.1**.

Lateral Ankle Stabilization. Lateral ankle stabilization is provided by three major lateral ankle ligaments: the anterior talofibular ligament; the calcaneofibular ligament; and the strongest of the three ligaments, the posterior talofibular ligament (**Figure 5.12**). These three ligaments extend to stabilize the lateral aspect of the talocalcaneal unit of the mortise joint, resisting inversion. The origin and insertion points for the individual lateral ankle ligaments are presented in Table 5.1.

Distal Tibiofibular Stabilization. Stability of the distal tibiofibular articulation, referred to as the syndesmosis/syndesmotic joint, is provided by the distal interosseous tibiofibular ligament and the

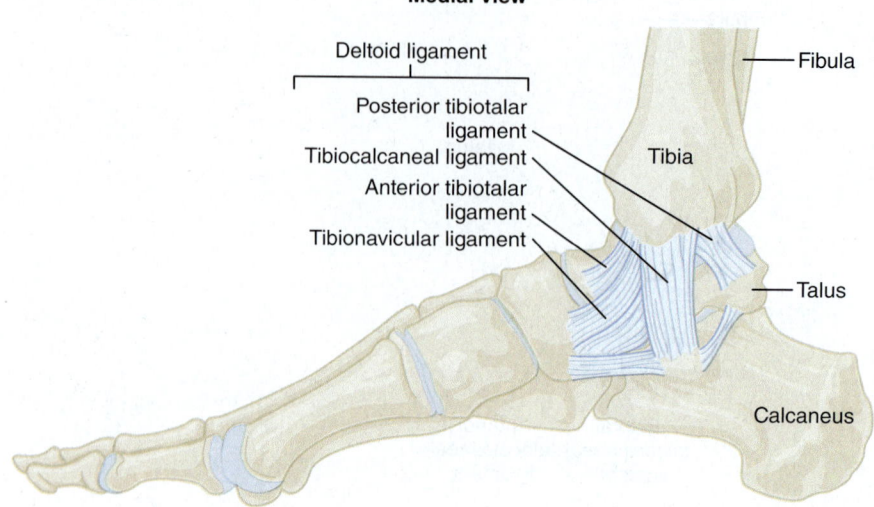

Figure 5.11 Drawing showing the deltoid ligaments.
© Jones & Bartlett Learning

Table 5.1 Major Ligamentous Support of the Foot and Ankle

Ligament	Origin	Insertion	Resists
Collateral ligaments	Medial and lateral aspects of all DIP and MTP joints	Medial and lateral aspects of all DIP and MTP joints	Valgus and varus forces at the joint
Lisfranc ligament	Base of the second metatarsal	Plantar aspect of the medial cuneiform	Dorsal displacement of metatarsal bases
Spring ligament	Sustentaculum tali	Inferior-posterior aspect of the navicular tubercle	Collapse of the medial arch
Medial (Deltoid) Ligament Complex			
Posterior tibiotalar ligament	Posterior medial aspect of the medial malleolus	Superoposterior aspect of the talus	Eversion of the ankle; deep portion resists axial rotation of the talus
Tibiocalcaneal ligament	Medial aspect of the medial malleolus	Superior aspect of the sustentaculum tali	Eversion of the ankle
Anterior tibiotalar ligament	Anteromedial aspect of the medial malleolus	Superoanterior aspect of the talus	Eversion of the ankle; deep portion resists axial rotation of the talus
Tibionavicular ligament	Anterior aspect of the medial malleolus	Dorsomedial aspect of the navicular	Eversion of the ankle
Lateral Ankle Ligament Complex			
Anterior talofibular ligament	Anterior margin of the lateral malleolus	Talar body immediately anterior to the lateral malleolus	Inversion of the ankle in dorsiflexion and the anterior translation of the talus on the tibia
Calcaneofibular ligament	Inferior-anterior margin of the lateral malleolus; inferior to the anterior talofibular ligament	Posterior region of the lateral calcaneal surface	Inversion of the ankle
Posterior talofibular ligament	Malleolar fossa on the medial surface of the lateral malleolus	Posterolateral talus	Limits posterior displacement of the talus of the tibia in dorsiflexion and extreme inversion

Ligament	Origin	Insertion	Resists
Syndesmotic Ankle Ligament Complex			
Anterior inferior tibiofibular ligament	Longitudinal tubercle on the anterior aspect of the lateral malleolus	Anterolateral tubercle of the tibia	Lateral displacement of the fibula
Posterior inferior tibiofibular ligament	Posterior malleolus (posterior tubercle of the tibia)	Posterior lateral malleolus	Lateral displacement of the fibula
Interosseous ligament	Anteroinferior triangular segment of the medial aspect of the distal fibular shaft	Lateral surface of the distal tibia	Lateral displacement of the fibula

DIP, distal interphalangeal; MTP, metatarsophalangeal.

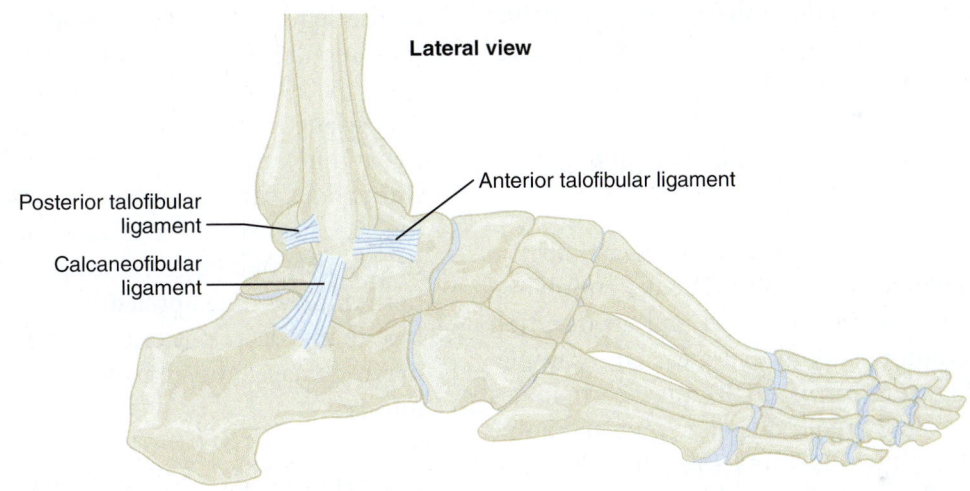

Figure 5.12 Drawing showing the lateral ankle ligaments: anterior talofibular ligament, calcaneofibular ligament, and posterior talofibular ligament.

© Jones & Bartlett Learning

anterior tibiofibular and posterior tibiofibular ligaments (**Figure 5.13**). The interosseous membrane is a thick connective tissue sheet that attaches the tibia and fibula, runs almost the entire length of the bones, and distally forms the interosseous tibiofibular ligament.[7]

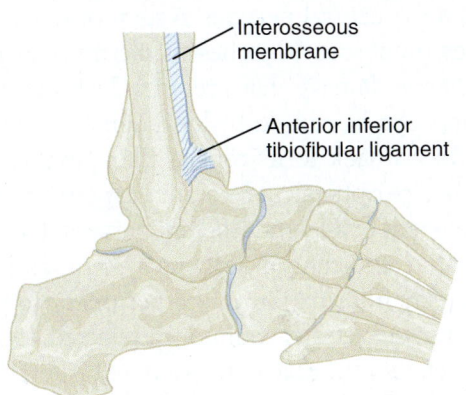

Figure 5.13 Drawing showing the tibiofibular ligament and interosseous membrane.

© Jones & Bartlett Learning

The combination of these structures allows for the tibia and fibula to adapt to the changing width of the talus. The fibula slightly ascends and rotates medially during dorsiflexion to provide maximum width and slightly descends and rotates laterally during plantar flexion (minimum width).[8] Together, these structures resist axial, rotational, and translational forces that would separate the tibia and fibula.[8] Origin and insertion points of the anterior and posterior tibiofibular ligaments are detailed in Table 5.1.

Musculotendinous Anatomy

Unlike the bones and ligaments that provide passive support, the muscles of the body provide what is called active support. Skeletal muscle is the only tissue in the body that can be voluntarily contracted. These muscular contractions are used daily to perform a variety of fine and gross motor tasks, from typing on a keyboard to running a mountain trail.

Knowing the origin and insertion of a muscle is crucial to understanding its action. Think of the origin as the anchor of the muscle. As a muscle contracts, the insertion is drawn toward the origin, or anchor. For example, the tibialis anterior (TA) muscle originates on the lateral condyle and proximal half of the tibia; its long tendon inserts on the medial cuneiform and the base of the first metatarsal. When the TA contracts, it pulls from the medial aspect of the first metatarsal base, toward the lateral condyle of the tibia, thereby bringing the foot/ankle into a dorsiflexed position. Therefore, the major action of the TA is dorsiflexion. Additionally, because of the orientation of the muscle and its line of action (pulling medially to laterally), the TA provides slight inversion and adduction of the foot. Last, because the TA tendon travels along the medial and plantar aspects of the foot, it provides some support to the medial arch as well.

Intrinsic Versus Extrinsic Muscles of the Foot

Muscles can be described or categorized as intrinsic or extrinsic relative to the joint they are supplying. An intrinsic muscle has an origin and an insertion point that pertain strictly to that area. For example, the flexor digitorum brevis (FDB) muscle originates and inserts in the foot and does not cross the ankle joint. Therefore, the FDB acts solely on the foot. However, the flexor digitorum longus (FDL) originates on the middle posterior aspect of the tibial shaft, far from its insertion on the plantar aspect of the distal phalanges of the second through fifth toes. The tendon of the FDL crosses the ankle mortise joint in addition to the toes and therefore has actions on both. Although its primary action is the flexion of the second through fifth toes, it also plays a small role in both plantar flexion and inversion of the ankle mortise joint. Understanding the intrinsic or extrinsic nature of a muscle is yet another illustration that underscores the importance of knowing the origins and insertions of muscles. The organization of the intrinsic and extrinsic muscles of the foot is outlined in **Tables 5.2** and **5.3**.

Both of the flexor digitorum muscles perform flexion of the toes; however, each muscle performs this action over a very different range. The architectural differences of these two muscles (eg, cross-sectional areas of the muscle bellies, the length of the tendons) play a critical role in the ability to flex the toes. Toe flexion is required throughout varying degrees of ankle plantar flexion and dorsiflexion, not just the range of motion (ROM) supplied by the MTP joints and the proximal and distal interphalangeal joints. Therefore, these muscles work synergistically to provide a biomechanical advantage necessary for function. This information can be useful when performing an evaluation. Knowing the actions, origins, and insertions allows clinicians to isolate muscles of interest for manual muscle testing with proper positioning of a limb. This understanding can also explain muscle behavior during an injury.

The muscles of the leg are separated by fibrous septae and categorized as compartments. The lower leg is composed of four unique compartments (**Table 5.4**). Consider a scenario in which there is a significant traumatic blow to the lower leg, resulting in the swelling of the deep posterior compartment of the leg (compartment syndrome). When testing toe function, toe extension would be normal; however, toe flexion would likely be considered weak. The strength of toe flexion, in addition to dorsiflexion and inversion, may change as the ankle is moved throughout various degrees of flexion and dorsiflexion. Because the FDB is not damaged directly, toe flexion may not entirely disappear. However, because both muscles are supplied by the tibial nerve, swelling in the deep posterior compartment may cause nerve damage, thereby affecting the action of both muscles.

Neurologic Anatomy

The tibial and peroneal nerves are the main branches from the sciatic nerve that supply the lower leg, ankle, and foot. The tibial nerve branches into the medial and lateral plantar nerves that supply the foot (**Figure 5.14** and **Figure 5.15**).

The importance of understanding muscle innervation was briefly highlighted in the aforementioned injury scenario (compartment syndrome). The peripheral nervous system is a network of nerves extending from the central nervous system of the spine that supplies numerous branches to the muscles it innervates. Nerve damage that presents dysfunction in the periphery can be caused by local damage to the nerve or be traced back to its root at the spinal cord. Furthermore, peripheral nerves are categorized as being either efferent or afferent: Afferent nerves relay information back to the central nervous system, and efferent nerves relay information to the periphery to promote a response or action, commonly referred to as afferent and efferent feedback, respectively. Afferent nerves provide feedback of numerous variables associated with motor control (eg, length, rate, and power of a muscular contraction) and sensation or proprioception

Clinical Anatomy

Table 5.2 Intrinsic Muscles of the Foot Organized by Layer From Superficial to Deep

Muscle	Origin	Insertion	Action	Innervation (Nerve Root)	Palpation	Manual Muscle Test
Plantar Muscles of the Foot						
First Layer (Most Superficial, Palpable Layer)						
Central: Flexor digitorum brevis **Flexor digitorum brevis manual muscle test.** Patient long-sitting. Stabilize the foot. Instruct the patient to flex IP joints of the second through fifth toes. Try to move the patient's toes into extension.	Medial calcaneal tuberosity and plantar aponeurosis	Two tendon slips from each of the four tendons insert on the medial and lateral aspects of the intermediate (middle) phalanx for the second through fifth toes	Flexion of the intermediate phalanges of second through fifth toes	Medial plantar (L1, L5, S1)	**Muscle belly:** Can be palpated near the origin at the medial calcaneal tuberosity and along the length of the arch. **Tendons:** Palpate along the length of the muscle belly toward the second through fifth toes; the muscle will split into four tendon slips to insert on the DIP joints. *Note:* Instruct the patient to flex his or her toe to help with palpation of the muscle.	Stabilize the foot and instruct the patient to flex the toes with and without manual resistance of the second through fifth toes.
Medial: Abductor hallucis **Abductor hallucis manual muscle test.** Patient long-sitting. Stabilize the foot. Instruct patient to move first phalange into abduction. Try to move the patient's toe into neutral/adduction.	Medial calcaneal tuberosity and plantar aponeurosis	Medial plantar surface of the first proximal phalanx and medial sesamoid bone	Abducts the first toe and assists in first toe flexion at the MTP joint	Medial plantar (L4, L5, S1)	**Muscle belly:** Can be palpated on the posterior medial plantar aspect of the foot. **Tendon:** The belly will give rise to a long tendon that runs along the medial aspect of the first metatarsal.	Stabilize the foot and apply resistance to the medial aspect of the first toe while asking the patient to push against your finger. *Note:* It may be easier for the patient to collectively spread the toes against your resistance of holding them together.

(continues)

Table 5.2 Intrinsic Muscles of the Foot Organized by Layer From Superficial to Deep (continued)

Muscle	Origin	Insertion	Action	Innervation (Nerve Root)	Palpation	Manual Muscle Test
Lateral: Abductor digiti minimi **Abductor digiti minimi manual muscle test.** Patient long-sitting. Stabilize the foot. Instruct patient to abduct the fifth phalange. Try to move the patient's toe into neutral/adduction.	Lateral process of the calcaneus and plantar aponeurosis	Lateral aspect of the proximal phalanx of the fifth toe	Flexion of the fifth MTP joint and assists in abduction of the MTP joint	Lateral plantar (S1, S2)	**Muscle belly:** Can be palpated at the lateral plantar aspect of the calcaneus. **Tendon:** The belly of the muscle runs obliquely toward the lateral aspect of the foot along the dorsal and lateral aspect of the fifth metatarsal.	Stabilize the foot and apply resistance to the lateral aspect of the fifth toe while asking the patient to push against your finger. ***Note:** It may be easier for the patient to collectively spread his or her toes against your resistance of holding them together.
Second Layer						
Quadratus plantae	Medial and lateral heads insert on the medial and lateral aspects of the plantar surface of the calcaneus	Posterior and lateral aspects of the flexor digitorum longus tendon	Assists the flexor digitorum longus in flexion of the second through fifth toes (modifies the angle of pull)	Lateral plantar (S1, S2)	Not readily palpable.	Stabilize the foot and instruct the patient to flex toes with and without manual resistance of the second through fifth toes.
Lumbrical muscles of the foot **Lumbrical muscles of the foot manual muscle test (flexion).** Patient long-sitting. Stabilize the foot. Instruct patient to flex MTP joints of the second through fifth toes without flexion of the IP joints. Try to move the toes at the MTP joints into extension.	Tendons of the flexor digitorum longus	Bases of the proximal phalanges of the second through fifth toes via the extensor digitorum tendons (plantar aspect)	Flexes the proximal phalanges at the MTP joint of the second through fifth toes and assists in extension of the middle and distal phalanges of the second through fifth toes at the interphalangeal joints	Medial and lateral plantar (L4, L5, S1, S2)	Not readily palpable.	**Flexion:** Stabilize the foot and instruct the patient to flex toes with or without resistance applied at the MTP joints of the second through fifth toes. **Extension:** Stabilize the foot and instruct the patient to extend the toes with or without resistance applied to the middle and distal phalanges of the second through fifth toes at the interphalangeal joints.

Clinical Anatomy | 71

Lumbrical muscles of the foot manual muscle test (extension). Patient long-sitting. Stabilize the foot. Instruct patient to extend MTP joints of the second through fifth toes without extending IP joints. Try to move the toes at the MCP joints into flexion.

Third Layer

Flexor hallucis brevis	Medial plantar surface of the cuboid and lateral cuneiform	Two tendons insert on the medial and lateral plantar aspect of the proximal phalanx of the first toe	Flexion of the first MTP joint	Medial plantar (L4, L5, S1)	Not readily palpable.	Stabilize the foot and instruct the patient to flex the first toe with or without resistance applied to the plantar aspect of the toe.

Flexor hallucis brevis manual muscle test. Patient long-sitting. Stabilize the foot. Instruct patient to flex first MTP joint. Try to move the patient's toe into extension.

(continues)

Table 5.2 Intrinsic Muscles of the Foot Organized by Layer From Superficial to Deep (continued)

Muscle	Origin	Insertion	Action	Innervation (Nerve Root)	Palpation	Manual Muscle Test
Adductor hallucis	**Oblique head:** Bases of the second through fourth metatarsals and tendon sheath of the peroneus longus **Transverse head:** Plantar ligament of the third through fifth MTP joints	Lateral surface of the base of the proximal phalanx of the first toe	Adducts the first MTP joint and assists in flexing the MTP joint	Lateral plantar (S1, S2)	Not readily palpable.	Stabilize the foot and place a finger between the first and second toes. Instruct the patient to resist against resistance applied to the lateral aspect of the first toe.
Flexor digiti minimi brevis	Plantar aspects of the cuboid and base of the fifth metatarsal	Plantar aspect of the proximal phalanx of the fifth toe	Flexes the fifth toe at the MTP joint	Lateral plantar (S1, S2)	Not readily palpable.	Stabilize the foot and instruct the patient to flex the toes with or without resistance applied to the plantar aspect of the fifth toe.
Fourth Layer (Deepest Layer)						
Plantar interossei	Medial aspect of the third through fifth metatarsals	Medial aspect of the proximal phalanges of the third through fifth toes	Adducts the third through fifth toes at the MTP joints, assists in flexing the third through fifth toes at the MTP joints, and can assist in extension of the third through fifth toes at the IP joints	Lateral plantar (S1, S2)	Not readily palpable.	Stabilize the foot and place your fingers between the patient's third through fifth toes. Instruct the patient to squeeze against the resistance of your fingers.

Plantar interossei manual muscle test. Patient long-sitting. Stabilize the foot. Place your fingers between the patient's third through fifth toes and instruct him or her to squeeze against your fingers.

Muscle	Attachment 1	Attachment 2	Action	Innervation	Palpation	Manual Muscle Test
Dorsal interossei	The inner surface of all metatarsal bones	**First:** Medial surface of proximal phalanx of the second toe **Second through fifth:** Lateral surface of proximal phalanges of the second through fourth toes	Abducts second through fourth toes at the MTP joints and flexes second through fourth toes at the MTP joints	Lateral plantar (S1, S2)	Not readily palpable.	Stabilize the foot and grasp the patient's second through fourth toes. Instruct the patient to spread the toes against your grip. **Dorsal interossei manual muscle test.** Patient long-sitting. Stabilize the foot. Grasp the patient's toes on the medial and lateral sides of the second through fourth toes, and instruct patient to try to spread toes.

Dorsal Surface

Muscle	Attachment 1	Attachment 2	Action	Innervation	Palpation	Manual Muscle Test
Extensor digitorum brevis	Lateral superior (dorsal) aspect of the calcaneus	Second through fourth toes via the extensor digitorum longus tendons	Extends the second through fourth toes at the MTP joints and the IP joints	Deep peroneal (L5, S1)	**Muscle belly:** Can be palpated through the sinus tarsi. Place your finger within the sinus, and instruct the patient to extend the toes.	Stabilize the foot and instruct the patient to extend the toes with or without resistance applied to the dorsal aspect of the second through fourth toes. **Extensor digitorum brevis manual muscle test.** Patient long-sitting. Stabilize plantar surface of foot. Instruct patient to extend all joints of second through fifth toes. Try to move patient's toes into flexion.

DIP, distal interphalangeal; IP, interphalangeal; MTP, metatarsophalangeal. All figures in table © Jones & Bartlett Learning.

Table 5.3 Muscles of the Lower Leg and Ankle (Extrinsic to the Foot) Organized by Compartment

Muscle	Origin	Insertion	Action	Innervation (Nerve Root)	Palpation	Manual Muscle Test
Anterior Compartment						
Anterior: Tibialis anterior	Lateral condyle of the tibia, the proximal and lateral surface of the tibial shaft, and interosseous membrane	Medial and plantar surfaces of the medial cuneiform and the base of the first metatarsal	Inverts the foot and dorsiflexes the ankle (talocrural joint)	Deep peroneal (L4, L5, S1)	**Muscle belly:** Can be palpated on the anterior surface of the tibia. **Tendon:** Can be palpated on the central dorsal aspect of the foot. Tendon can be seen with dorsiflexion.	Stabilize the lower leg and instruct the patient to dorsiflex the foot with or without resistance applied to the dorsal aspect of the midfoot.
Tibialis anterior manual muscle test. Patient long-sitting. Stabilize the lower leg. Instruct patient to dorsiflex and invert ankle. Try to move the patient's ankle into plantar flexion and eversion.						
Lateral: Extensor digitorum longus	Lateral condyle of the tibia, anterior proximal shaft of the fibula, and interosseous membrane	Middle and distal phalanges of the second through fifth toes	Extends the second through fifth toes and assists in foot eversion and ankle dorsiflexion (talocrural joint)	Deep peroneal (L4, L5, S1)	**Muscle belly:** Can be palpated on the mid to distal third of the lateral tibia shaft, lateral to the tibialis anterior muscle. Can be felt with active toe extension. **Tendon:** Four tendon slips can be palpated on the dorsal aspect of the foot to the second through fifth toes during toe extension.	Stabilize the foot and instruct the patient to extend the toes with or without resistance applied to the second through fifth toes.
Extensor digitorum longus manual muscle test. Patient long-sitting. Stabilize the plantar surface of the foot. Instruct patient to extend all joints of the second through fifth toes. Try to move the patient's toes into flexion.						

Lateral: Peroneus tertius	Distal anterior surface of the fibular shaft and interosseous membrane	Dorsal surface of the styloid process of the fifth metatarsal	Everts the foot and assists in dorsiflexion of the ankle (talocrural joint)	Deep peroneal (L4, L5, S1)	Difficult to distinguish. **Muscle belly:** May be felt on the distal anterolateral surface of the tibia during active eversion.	Stabilize the lower leg and instruct the patient to evert the ankle with or without resistance applied to the lateral aspect of the foot. *****Note:** This muscle largely serves as a synergist muscle to the peroneal, TA, and EDL muscles and is not the chief evertor or dorsiflexor of the foot.
Peroneus tertius manual muscle test. Patient long-sitting. Stabilize the lower leg. Instruct patient to evert and dorsiflex the ankle. Try to move the patient's ankle into inversion and plantar flexion.						
Deep: Extensor hallucis longus	Anterior middle surface of the fibular shaft and interosseous membrane	Base of the distal phalanx of the first toe	Extends the first MTP joint and assists in dorsiflexion of the ankle (talocrural joint) and inversion of the foot	Deep peroneal (L4, L5, S1)	**Muscle belly:** Difficult to palpate, as it lies deep to the TA and EDL muscles. **Tendon:** Can be palpated on the dorsal medial aspect of the foot to the first toe and is visually prominent during first toe extension.	Stabilize the foot/lower leg and instruct the patient to extend the first toe with or without resistance applied to the dorsal aspect of the first toe.
Extensor hallucis longus manual muscle test. Patient long-sitting. Stabilize the foot. Instruct patient to extend the MTP and IP joints of the first toe. Try to move the patient's toe into flexion.						

(continues)

Table 5.3 Muscles of the Lower Leg and Ankle (Extrinsic to the Foot) Organized by Compartment (continued)

Muscle	Origin	Insertion	Action	Innervation (Nerve Root)	Palpation	Manual Muscle Test
Lateral Compartment						
Superficial: Peroneus longus **Peroneus longus manual muscle test.** Patient long-sitting. Stabilize the lower leg. Instruct patient to evert and plantarflex the ankle. Try to move the patient's ankle into inversion and dorsiflexion.	Head of the fibula and the proximal two-thirds of the lateral fibular shaft	Dorsal base of the first metatarsal and medial cuneiform	Everts the foot and assists in plantar flexion of the ankle (talocrural joint)	Superficial peroneal (L4, L5, S1)	**Muscle belly:** Can be palpated at the proximal lateral aspect of the fibula during active eversion. **Tendon:** Can be palpated and is visually prominent just superior, posterior, and inferior to the lateral malleolus as it travels to the styloid process of the fifth metatarsal.	Stabilize the lower leg and instruct the patient to evert the ankle with or without resistance applied to the lateral aspect of the foot.
Deep: Peroneus brevis **Peroneus brevis manual muscle test.** Patient long-sitting. Stabilize the lower leg. Instruct patient to evert the ankle. Try to move patient's ankle into inversion.	Distal two-thirds of the lateral fibular shaft	Styloid process of the fifth metatarsal	Everts the foot and assists in plantar flexion of the ankle (talocrural joint)	Superficial peroneal (L4, L5, S1)	**Muscle belly:** Difficult to palpate, as it lies deep to the peroneus longus muscle. **Tendon:** Can be palpated and is visually prominent just superior, posterior, and inferior to the lateral malleolus as it inserts on the styloid process of the fifth metatarsal.	Stabilize the lower leg and instruct the patient to evert the ankle with or without resistance applied to the lateral aspect of the foot.

Clinical Anatomy

Superficial Posterior Compartment

Superficial: Gastrocnemius	Posterior surfaces of the medial and lateral femoral condyles	Calcaneus via the Achilles tendon	Plantarflexes the ankle (talocrural joint) and flexes the knee	Tibial (S1, S2)	**Muscle bellies:** The medial and lateral bellies of the gastrocnemius can be palpated in the upper one-third of the posterior aspect of the lower leg. They can be traced to their origin on the femoral condyles through the popliteal fossa (posterior aspect of the knee). **Tendon:** Continue to trace the bellies distally until they blend into the Achilles tendon that inserts on the posterior aspect of the calcaneus.	Instruct the patient, with knees extended, to plantarflex the foot with or without resistance applied to the plantar aspect of the foot. You can apply resistance while the patient is positioned on an examination table or use the resistance from the ground while the patient is weight bearing. ***Note:** The gastrocnemius is an active dorsiflexor when the knee is in extension.

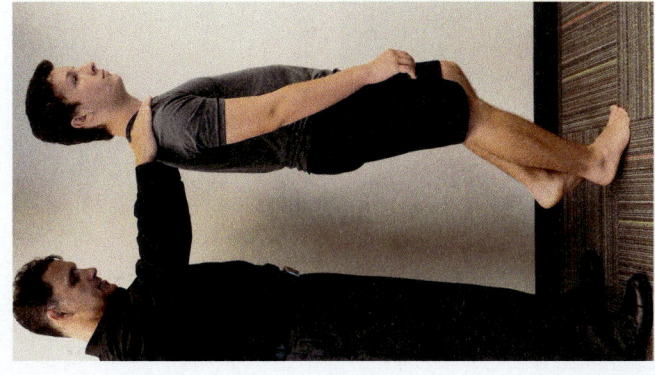

Gastrocnemius manual muscle test. Patient standing (can be holding onto chair or end of examination table for stability). Instruct patient to rise up on toes, pushing body weight directly upward. Push down on the patient's shoulders.

(continues)

Table 5.3 Muscles of the Lower Leg and Ankle (Extrinsic to the Foot) Organized by Compartment *(continued)*

Muscle	Origin	Insertion	Action	Innervation (Nerve Root)	Palpation	Manual Muscle Test
Deep: Soleus	Soleal line on the proximal posterior surface of the tibia, middle third of the medial tibial border, and the posterior aspect of the fibular head	Calcaneus via the Achilles tendon	Plantarflexes the ankle (talocrural joint)	Tibial (L5, S1, S2)	**Muscle belly:** The soleus lies deep to the gastrocnemius, but medial and lateral aspects of the belly can be palpated distal to the medial and lateral gastrocnemius heads as they blend into the Achilles tendon. **Tendon:** The soleus also comprises the Achilles tendon.	To isolate the soleus from the Achilles tendon, the patient will need to lie prone. Bend the knee to 90°, and instruct the patient to plantarflex the foot with or without resistance applied to the plantar side of the foot. ***Note:** The gastrocnemius is disengaged when the knee is flexed, allowing for the isolation of the soleus muscle.

Soleus manual muscle test #1. Patient lying prone with knee flexed to 90°. Stabilize lower leg. Instruct patient to plantarflex the ankle. Try to move the patient's ankle into dorsiflexion.

Soleus manual muscle test #2. Patient lying prone with foot hanging off table. No stabilization necessary. Instruct patient to plantarflex foot. Distract the patient's calcaneus while also moving the patient's ankle into dorsiflexion.

Clinical Anatomy

Deep: Plantaris	Distal portion of the lateral supracondylar line of the femur	Calcaneus via the Achilles tendon	Weak plantar flexion of the ankle and flexion of the knee	Tibial (L4, L5, S1, S2)	**Muscle belly:** The belly of the plantaris can be palpated between the proximal aspect of the medial and lateral gastrocnemius heads at the popliteal fossa (posterior aspect of the knee). The belly is approximately 1 inch wide. **Tendon:** The plantaris has the longest tendon in the body, which runs deep to the gastrocnemius muscle and is not palpable; however, the tendon blends into the Achilles tendon.	As a weak plantar flexor of the ankle and flexor of the knee, the plantaris is difficult to isolate. Its contributions as a synergist are tested with the actions of the gastrocnemius and soleus muscles.

Plantaris manual muscle test. Tested with gastrocnemius.

(continues)

Table 5.3 Muscles of the Lower Leg and Ankle (Extrinsic to the Foot) Organized by Compartment

(continued)

Muscle	Origin	Insertion	Action	Innervation (Nerve Root)	Palpation	Manual Muscle Test
Deep Posterior Compartment						
Deep: Flexor hallucis longus	Middle half of the posterior fibular shaft	Plantar surface of the distal phalanx of the first toe	Flexes the first toe at the MTP and interphalangeal joints; weak plantar flexor of the ankle; assists with inversion	Tibial (L5, S1, S2)	**Muscle belly:** Lies deep to the soleus muscle and is difficult to palpate but may be felt on the distal and medial aspect of the lower leg during first toe flexion. **Tendon:** Can be palpated as the third tendon posterior to the medial malleolus.	Stabilize the lower leg and instruct the patient to flex his or her first toe with or without resistance applied to the plantar aspect of the first toe.
Flexor hallucis longus manual muscle test. Patient long-sitting. Stabilize the foot. Instruct patient to flex the first IP joint. Try to move the patient's toe into extension.						
Deep: Flexor digitorum longus	Middle posterior surface of the tibial shaft	Plantar aspect of the distal phalanges of the second through fifth toes	Flexes the second through fifth toes at the MTP and interphalangeal joints; weak plantar flexion of the ankle (talocrural joint); assists in inversion of the foot	Tibial (L5, S1, S2)	**Muscle belly:** Difficult to palpate but may be felt during flexion of the second through fifth toes on the distal and medial aspect of the lower leg. **Tendon:** Can be palpated; the tendon is the second tendon located posterior to the medial malleolus (posterior to the tibialis posterior).	Stabilize the lower leg and instruct the patient to flex the toes with or without resistance applied to the plantar aspect of the second through fifth toes.
Flexor digitorum longus manual muscle test. Patient long-sitting. Stabilize the foot. Instruct patient to flex the DIP joints of the second through fifth toes. Try to extend the patient's toes.						

Clinical Anatomy

Muscle	Origin	Insertion	Action	Innervation	Palpation	Manual muscle test
Deep: Tibialis posterior	Proximal posterior aspects of tibial and fibular shafts, and interosseous membrane	Navicular tubercle; sustentaculum tali; and plantar aspect of cuneiforms, cuboid, and second through fourth distal metatarsal heads	Inverts the foot and assists in plantar flexion at the ankle (talocrural joint)	Tibial (L5, S1, S2)	**Muscle belly:** Difficult to palpate but may be felt during inversion and plantar flexion of the foot on the distal and medial aspect of the lower leg. **Tendon:** Can be palpated; the tibialis posterior tendon is positioned immediately posterior to the medial malleolus.	Stabilize the lower leg and instruct the patient to invert the foot with or without resistance applied to the medial aspect of the foot. The tibialis posterior can also be tested by palpating the distal and medial aspect of the lower leg while asking the patient to dorsiflex the foot with or without resistance applied to the plantar aspect of the foot.

Tibialis posterior manual muscle test. Patient long-sitting. Stabilize the lower leg. Instruct patient to invert and plantarflex the ankle. Try to move the patient's ankle into eversion and dorsiflexion.

EDL, extensor digitorum longus; IP, interphalangeal; MTP, metatarsophalangeal; TA, tibialis anterior.
All figures in table © Jones & Bartlett Learning.

Table 5.4 Lower Leg Compartments

Name of Compartment		Anterior Compartment	Lateral Compartment	Deep Posterior Compartment	Superficial Compartment
Soft-tissue structures	Muscles	• Tibialis anterior • Extensor hallucis longus • Extensor digitorum longus • Peroneus tertius	• Peroneus longus • Peroneus brevis	• Tibialis posterior • Flexor digitorum longus • Flexor hallucis longus	• Gastrocnemius • Soleus • Plantaris
	Soft tissue	• Deep peroneal nerve • Anterior tibial artery	• Superficial peroneal nerve • Peroneal artery	• Peroneal vessels • Tibial nerve • Posterior tibial vessels	

(eg, pressure, temperature, pain, and location). Efferent nerves innervate muscles and are responsible for muscular contraction (motor control) and reflexes.

Neurologic symptoms are related to the location (ie, level) at which the damage exists. In the compartment syndrome example, the tibial nerve is located in the deep posterior compartment and may be compressed/damaged if the deep posterior compartment swells. Damage at this level of the tibial nerve would affect not only the local muscular innervations but

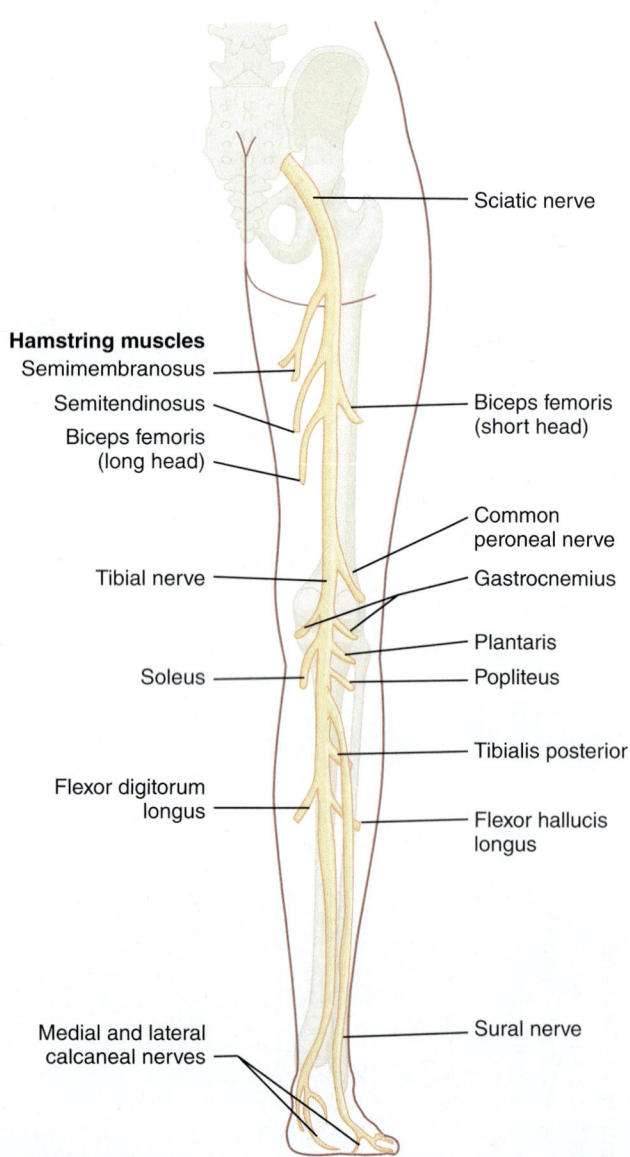

Figure 5.14 Drawing showing lower leg neural anatomy branching from the sciatic nerve.

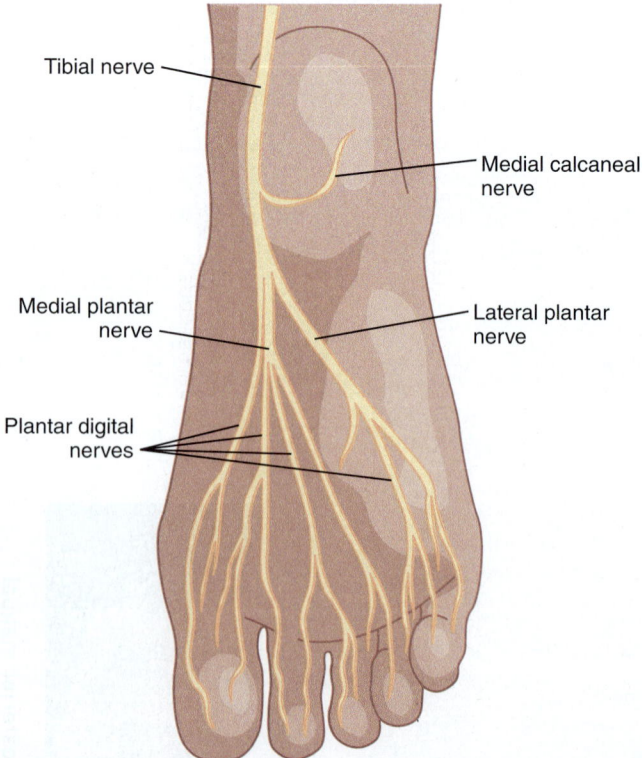

Figure 5.15 Drawing showing plantar nerve branches of the foot.

all distal branches (ie, the medial and lateral plantar nerves) as well. Although the tibial nerve is a continuation of the larger sciatic nerve, damage at the level of the lower leg would not affect any muscular function above the level of the injury. Information regarding the innervations for each muscle is listed in Tables 5.2 and 5.3.

Damage that takes place at the spinal cord at the level of the nerve root typically results in diminished motor and sensory functions for the muscles and cutaneous areas it supplies. Nerve root testing can be performed via myotome, dermatome, and reflex testing. The nerve roots associated with their respective muscles are listed in Tables 5.2 and 5.3. A body map of dermatomes is shown in **Figure 5.16**, and myotome and reflex testing for the ankle and foot is outlined in **Table 5.5**.

Vascular Anatomy

Similar to the nervous system, the cardiovascular system constitutes a vast network of vessels that supply blood to the lower limbs. The anterior and posterior tibial arteries are the main sources of oxygenated blood supply to the lower leg, ankle, and foot (**Figure 5.17**). The anterior tibial artery branches into the dorsal pedal and the dorsal metatarsal arteries, which supply blood to the dorsal aspect of the foot. The posterior tibial artery branches into the lateral plantar, medial plantar, and plantar arterial arch, which supply blood to the plantar aspect of the foot. Location and palpation instructions for the dorsal pedal artery (branch of the anterior tibial artery) and the posterior tibial artery are discussed later in this chapter. It is important to assess the vascular status of the distal limb with severe injury, especially if there is concern that a compromise of the blood supply has occurred (eg, fracture, dislocation, or hemorrhage). A diminished or absent distal pulse constitutes a medical emergency, as prolonged loss of oxygen to the tissue will result in tissue death and lead to possible amputation.

Deoxygenated blood is taken from the lower leg, ankle, and foot via veins. The medial and lateral plantar veins drain blood from the plantar aspect of the foot to the posterior tibial vein. The dorsal venous arch and the dorsal pedal veins drain blood from the dorsal aspect of the foot to the anterior tibial vein. In the lower leg, blood is drained via the posterior tibial, anterior tibial, and peroneal veins. Figure 5.17 provides a visual overview of the vascular anatomy of the lower leg, ankle, and foot. **Figure 5.18** provides a visual overview of the muscular anatomy of the lower leg, ankle, and foot.

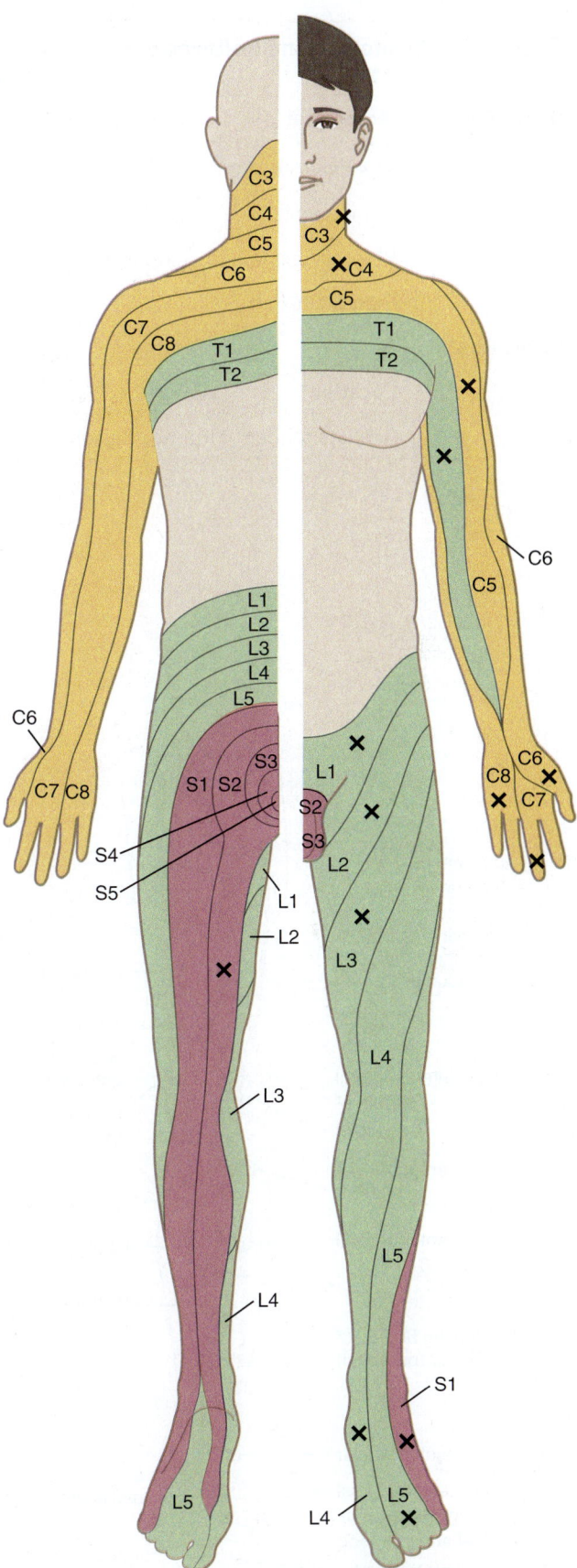

Figure 5.16 Body map of dermatomes (specific skin regions to test within each dermatome indicated with an X).

© Jones & Bartlett Learning

Table 5.5 Myotomes and Reflexes of the Ankle and Foot

Nerve Root	Motor Test
L4	Ankle dorsiflexion
L5	Toe extension
S1	Plantar flexion and ankle eversion
S2	Plantar flexion

Nerve Root	Reflex Testing	
	Location	Action
S1	Achilles tendon	Plantar flexion

Overview of Radiology and Imaging

Common Radiographic Views

A standard foot radiograph series includes dorsal to plantar, lateral, and medial oblique views.[9,10] The medial oblique view involves positioning the patient for a dorsal to plantar view and angling the foot 30° to 40° medially. The dorsal to plantar view is best for assessing the metatarsals in anatomic position, whereas the medial oblique view is useful for evaluating the tarsal bones.[11] When there is concern for a possible Lisfranc injury (instability of the Lisfranc

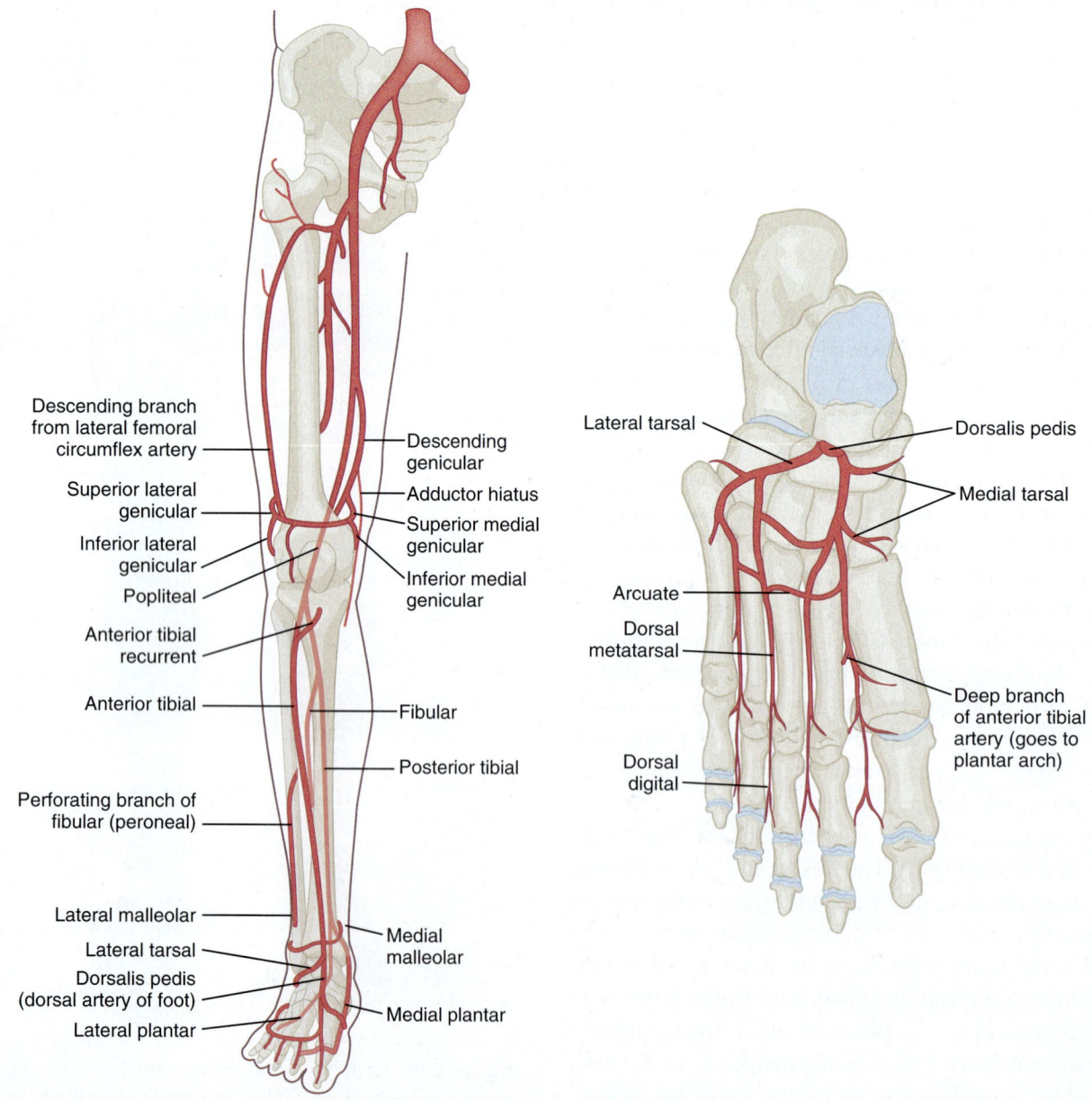

Figure 5.17 Drawings showing vascular anatomy of the lower leg, ankle, and foot.

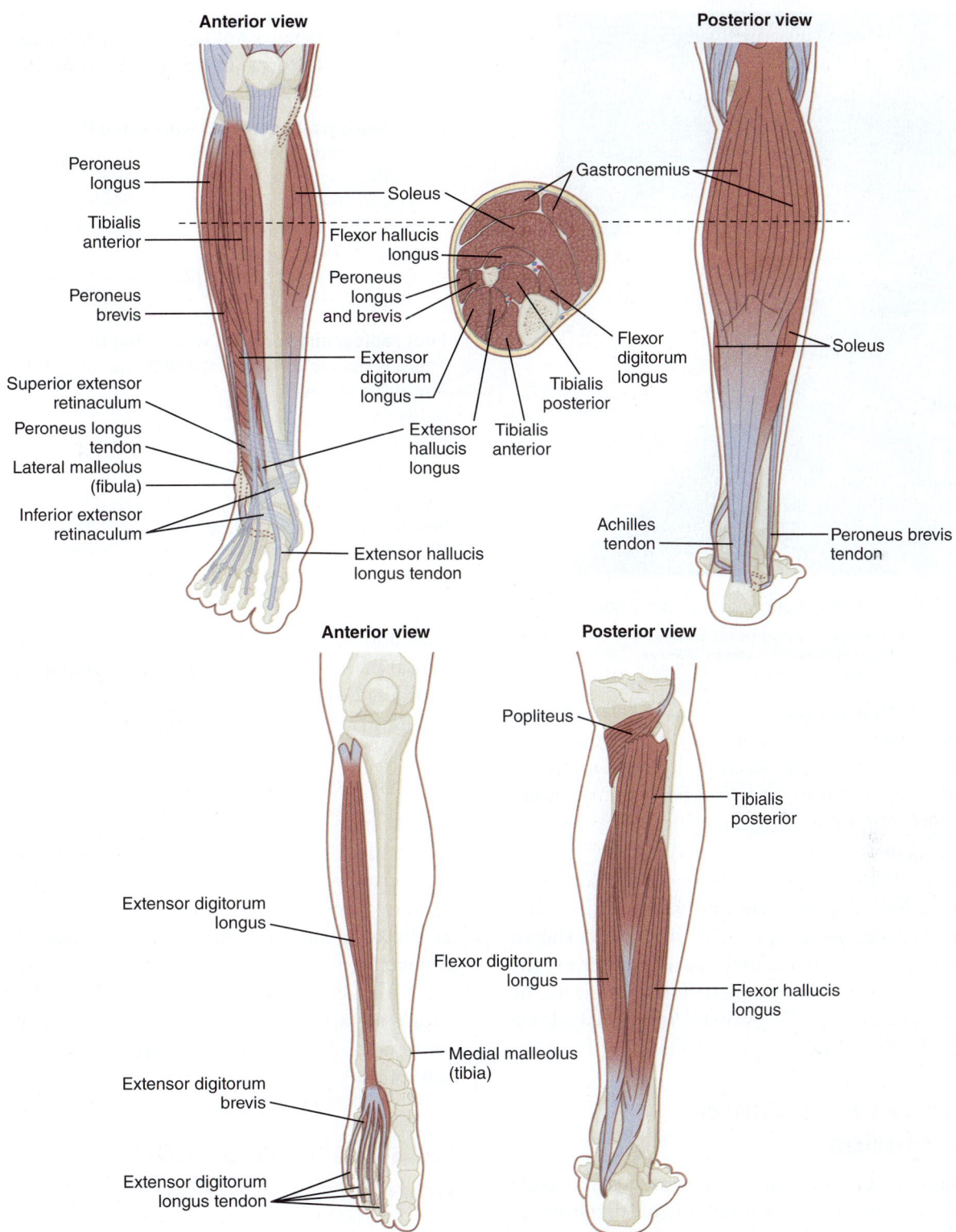

Figure 5.18 Drawings showing muscular anatomy of the lower leg, ankle, and foot.
© Jones & Bartlett Learning

joint due to ligamentous sprain or midfoot fracture), a weight-bearing view or a stress view in which the forefoot is abducted may be indicated[11] (**Figure 5.19**).

Standard radiographic views for the ankle consist of a series of three images, which include anterior to posterior (AP), lateral, and mortise views.[10,12] The mortise view involves positioning the patient for an AP view and then internally rotating the tibia approximately 15° to 30°. In some cases, an oblique view may be ordered, which is similar to the mortise view, except the leg is rotated medially to 45°. Mortise and oblique views are preferred when evaluating for syndesmotic

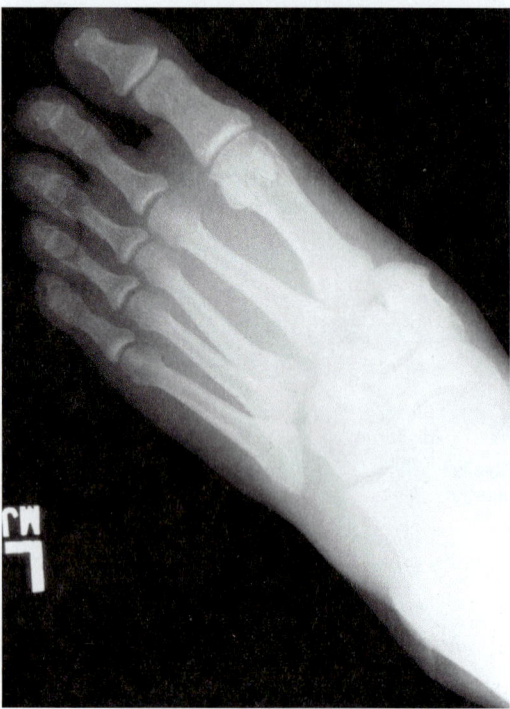

Figure 5.19 Radiograph showing Lisfranc injury.

Benejam CE, Potaczek SG. Unusual presentation of Lisfranc fracture dislocation associated with high-velocity sledding injury: a case report and review of the literature. J Med Case Rep. 2008;2:266. Published 2008 Aug 11. doi:10.1186/1752-1947-2-266

Table 5.6 Ottawa Ankle Rules for Radiograph Referral in Acute Lateral Ankle Sprains

Ankle radiograph series is warranted if:
Pain near either malleoli (distal 6 cm of the fibula or tibia) **AND** one or more of the following: <ul><li>Age 55 years or older, **OR**</li><li>Unable to bear weight or walk four consecutive steps, **OR**</li><li>Bone tenderness at the posterior edge of either malleoli</li></ul>
Foot radiograph series is warranted if:
There is pain in the midfoot **AND** bone tenderness at any of the following: <ul><li>Navicular</li><li>Cuboid</li><li>Base of the fifth metatarsal</li></ul>

Ankle rules: Sensitivity, 97.9% to 99.8%; specificity, 28.8% to 42.3%*
Midfoot rules: Sensitivity, 97.2% to 99.8%; specificity, 28.8% to 57.1%*
*Sensitivity and specificity values are largely based on the adult population

injury. Although sometimes still used, talar tilt and anterior drawer stress views have not been shown to be valid means of assessment for ankle ligament injury.[13,14]

Although useful in detecting bony injury, radiographs are not ideal for examining injury to supporting ligaments of the ankle. A quality clinical examination has been shown to be more effective in evaluating for ankle ligament injury than plain radiographs. The Ottawa Ankle Rules have been shown to be a very useful clinical tool when determining the need for radiologic examination for fracture in the ankle[15,16] (**Table 5.6**). To evaluate severe soft-tissue injury, MRI should be used.

Common MRI Views and Injuries

MRI is the preferred modality for assessing soft-tissue injury.[17] Superior to other forms of soft-tissue imaging, MRI has very high sensitivity and specificity values for multiple tendinous and ligamentous injuries.[18] When examining the foot, a series of views including oblique axial, oblique coronal, and oblique sagittal planes are used.[19] The oblique axial scan runs parallel to the metatarsal bones, whereas the oblique coronal scan runs perpendicular to the metatarsals; the oblique sagittal scan provides sagittal images of each ray in the forefoot and extends posteriorly through the hindfoot. Most MRI studies for the ankle consist of a standard series of views in the axial, coronal, and sagittal planes.[19] In some cases, an oblique scan may be ordered to examine for subtle injuries to the peroneal longus and brevis and tibialis posterior tendons.

Other Imaging Options

Other common types of diagnostic imaging modalities include CT and diagnostic ultrasonography. CT is preferred when examining for smaller or more subtle bony abnormalities.[9] Diagnostic ultrasonography has become more common in recent years because of increased accessibility of equipment and training. Although still not as precise as MRI, diagnostic ultrasonography has been shown to be useful in the assessment of lateral ankle ligament injury and tendon injury.[20-22]

Evaluation of the Foot and Ankle Joint

Chronic injuries rarely, if ever, occur in isolation, and acute injuries rarely, if ever, remain isolated to a single joint. The concept of a kinetic chain is critically important for a thorough full-body evaluation, and, because of the bipedal nature of humans, a great place to begin for any injury is at the foot and ankle. The toes, foot, and ankle function as a unit or system and should be evaluated as such. A detailed evaluation of foot position, arches, and gait can provide great insight into a patient's biomechanics and functional movement patterns that are either causing or lending to pathology. The following paragraphs provide an overview of the elements that comprise a thorough evaluation of the foot and ankle, often referred to as the HIPS/HOPS (History, Inspection/Observation, Palpation, Special Tests) evaluation procedure.

History

Just as with any injury, a thorough history often provides rich information to reach the proper diagnosis of a foot and/or ankle injury. Armed with a sound understanding of anatomy and musculoskeletal evaluation tools, skilled clinicians display mastery in the art of history taking. History questions should be open ended and avoid any type of suggestive answers. When required, examples to answers can be given; however, a variety of answers should be provided to avoid influencing a patient's response. When collecting history, clinicians will want to record important information regarding the onset of injury, MOI, type of injury, symptoms, duration of symptoms, and previous history of injuries to the area in question. Patient responses to the following questions regarding history build the foundation for additional related inquiry and serve as a guide for the remainder of the examination.

Location of Pain and Type of Pain

Clinicians should ask the patient to indicate the area of greatest pain. It is common for patients to indicate pain over a rather general area; however, the patient should be asked to identify any specific locations. Additionally, because pain can be referred to distal locations (eg, compartment syndrome), the type of pain can be especially helpful to determine whether damage to nervous structures is the source of pain. Common descriptions for neurologic pain include sharp/stabbing pain, tingling pain, shooting pain, and hypersensation or hyposensation. Muscular pain, however, is usually described as being dull and/or achy. Ligamentous pain is rather localized, and pain following a bone fracture is typically severe in the acute phase and can be exacerbated with muscular contraction.

Onset and Duration of Pain

The onset of pain can serve different purposes. A clinician should capture both the initial occurrence of pain (which also helps to establish duration) and whether there are particular circumstances in which pain is triggered. For example, neurologic pain can be constant, can travel or radiate, or may appear during certain times of the day or after certain types of activities (eg, moving around after sitting for an extended period of time). Muscular pain can be related to specific movements or perhaps the repetition of movements. Ligamentous pain is often experienced during instances of joint instability. Furthermore, establishing the duration of pain becomes an important part of identifying the injury as acute, chronic, or idiopathic.

Mechanism of Injury

Particularly for acute injuries, the MOI is often one of the most important aspects of an evaluation, as it alone can serve as a foundation to formulate a differential diagnosis. Clinicians should ask the patient to describe, in detail, the events leading up to, during, and following the injury. If possible, patients can also be encouraged to demonstrate the MOI on the uninjured limb. Depending on the duration of the injury, the mechanism of chronic—and especially idiopathic—injuries can sometimes be harder to establish, has been forgotten, or is unknown.

Changes in Activity or Training

Changes from one activity to another with little to no training or a sudden increase in training volume can result in both acute and chronic injuries in any circumstance. Identification of perhaps more obviously chronic injuries may be tied to an athlete's sport of interest. For example, shoulder instability is not uncommon with overhead athletes, and medial tibial stress syndrome is common with track athletes. However, chronic injuries to the foot and/or ankle can be seen across all sports, regardless of the specific sporting activity. For this reason, it is important to ask questions regarding changes in activity, changes in footwear (ie, new shoes), use of old footwear, training on a different ground surface, or training on a sloped ground surface. These questions sometimes can provide helpful clues to less obvious foot and/or ankle injuries. It may be helpful for athletic trainers to request training logs from athletes (particularly of endurance athletes) to keep track of the volume, intensity, and mileage of shoes.

Previous History of Injury

The greatest predictor of injury is previous injury. Previous injury to the foot and/or ankle complex puts athletes at a far greater risk for a repeat injury to the same structure. If an athlete reports previous history of injury, the athletic trainer can ask the athlete to compare the injuries in mechanism, severity, and location of pain. Repeat injuries should be a red flag for a more thorough evaluation of chronic instability, and rehabilitation protocols should be structured to address these issues. Particularly regarding the foot and ankle, chronic instability can result in diminished proprioception and may be a source of injury to other areas of the body.

Additional Pertinent Medical History

The foot can often be a source of disease manifestation, so it is important to collect any additional information regarding various disease conditions. The foot can be subject to arthritis, and skin ulcerations associated with diabetes may also develop along with circulatory issues (given the distance from the heart), neuropathies, and cutaneous melanomas. When skin abnormalities or neuropathies are present, it is important to remember to keep these disease conditions as potential differential diagnoses until they can be ruled out appropriately.

Inspection

Athletic trainers are in a unique position to witness many of the injuries they evaluate. This is very uncommon in any other area of health care and provides a very helpful understanding of the MOI before the formal evaluation begins. However, as with any clinician, informal observation should begin from the moment a patient presents with a request for examination.

Posturing and/or Weight-Bearing Status

As the patient moves, observe how he or she is posturing (eg, self-splinting with shoulder/elbow injury). Regarding the foot and ankle, observe whether the patient can distribute his or her weight evenly or if there is a noticeable disruption in gait (limp or antalgic gait). These findings often provide clues as to the location and sometimes type of injury. For example, if an individual is unable to bear weight or walk, the possibility of a fracture of the midfoot or ankle should comprise a part of the differential diagnosis until ruled out.

Presence of Deformities

Observe whether there are any obvious gross (eg, dislocations, fractures) or anatomic (eg, pes planus, hallux valgus) deformities present. Depending on the situation, these deformities can be either directly or indirectly related to the injury in question.

Foot Type

At the beginning of a more formal foot and ankle evaluation, a clinician should take note of the type of foot alignment an individual has. Alignments typically fall into three general categories: neutral, pronated, or supinated (**Figure 5.20**).

Pronation. Individuals with a pronated foot are often described having a flat medial arch and walking on the inside sole of their foot. A quick evaluation of the sole of the shoes likely shows a wear pattern on the medial aspect of the shoe (**Figure 5.21**).

Supination. The supinated foot is the opposite of the pronated foot. A person with a supinated foot often is described as having a high, rigid medial arch and walking on the lateral border of the foot, applying excessive stress to the fifth metatarsal. An evaluation of the sole of a shoe of a person with a supinated foot typically shows a wear pattern on the lateral aspect of the sole. **Table 5.7** outlines the criteria for pronated and supinated classifications.[23]

Neutral. Feet not meeting the criteria for pronation and supination should be classified as neutral. For what is referred to as an "ideal foot," subtalar neutral would be expected to be present during static stance.[24] However, there is limited population-level evidence to support a definition for an ideal or neutral foot. In a study evaluating 121 men and women with no previous history of foot issues, the majority were found to have a subtalar neutral alignment with slight valgus (mean of 2°). Interestingly, none of the individuals participating in the study was considered to have an ideal foot, as the mean values for forefoot varus and calcaneal valgus were 6° and 7°.[24] The study also showed that women had greater ankle and subtalar joint ROM compared to men. The investigators concluded that the parameters for a neutral foot should be established from normative data obtained through large population-based studies of healthy individuals, rather than based on theoretical concepts, in order to provide an appropriate range of "normal" or "ideal."

Skin Abnormalities

Initial inspection should quickly note any skin abnormalities, such as calluses, blisters, corns, bunions, plantar warts, open wounds/ulcerations, or infections present on the foot. The presence of calluses, blisters, and bunions may be an indicator of

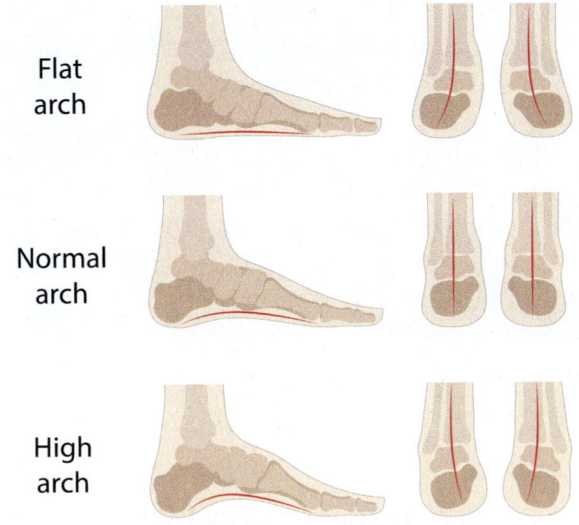

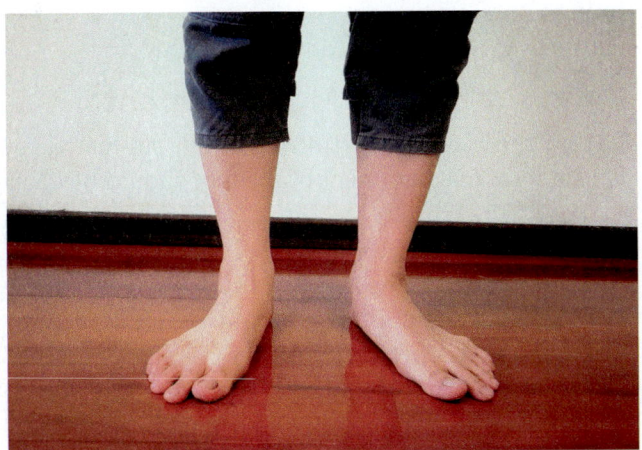

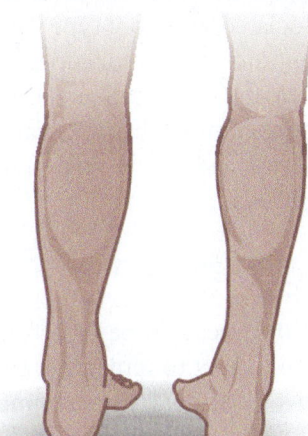

Figure 5.20 **A.** A drawing of foot arches. **B.** Photograph showing pronated foot type. **C.** Drawing showing supinated foot type.

A. © Olga Bolbot/Shutterstock; **B.** © Piyada Jaiaree/Shutterstock; **C.** © Jones & Bartlett Learning

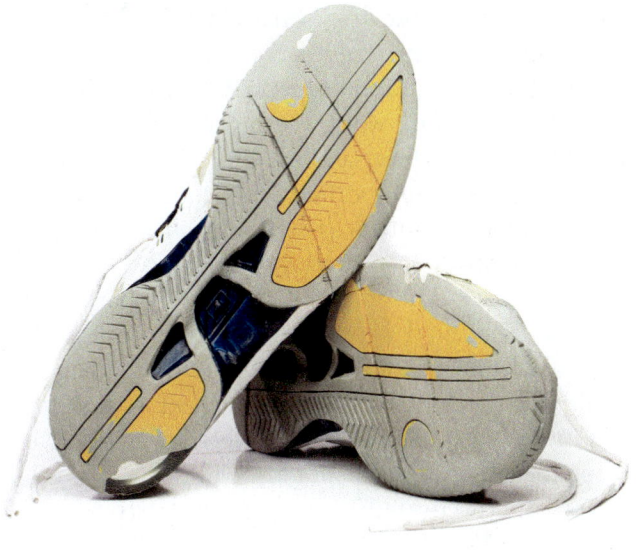

Figure 5.21 Shoe wear patterns.

© Bill Oxford/E+/Getty Images

poorly fitting shoes causing undue pressure and/or friction or can be related to poor biomechanics. Blisters can also be associated with fungal infections, such as athlete's foot (tinea pedis), which can cause peeling and cracking of the skin. Bunion formation (inflamed bursa) can be found on the first MTP joint or as a bunionette deformity on the fifth MTP joint. Corns (thickening of the stratum corneum of the skin) typically appear in areas of pressure that are not weight bearing in nature. Hard corns are often found on the dorsal aspect of the proximal interphalangeal joints, and soft corns typically form in the webbing of the toes. Ingrown toenails are a growth of the nail

Table 5.7 Evaluating Foot Type[a]

	Pronated	Supinated
Calcaneus	Must be everted greater than 3° as measured perpendicularly to the ground	Must be inverted greater than 3° as measured perpendicularly to the ground
Medial bulge at the talonavicular joint	Must be present due to the excessive rotation (adduction) of the talar head	Must *not* be present
Medial arch[b]	Low to the ground	Arch is high

[a] Any foot not meeting either criteria should be classified as a neutral foot.
[b] This can be assessed by measuring navicular displacement with various evaluation tools, such as Feiss line, navicular drop test, or supple pes planus test.

(most commonly the first toenail) into the skin, which often results in a painful infection of the surrounding nail bed. On the plantar aspect of the foot, it is common to find plantar warts; these warts are usually flat and rounded in shape and are caused by the *Verruca vulgaris* virus. Unlike calluses, they are point tender and may be described as stepping on a pebble. As discussed previously, ulcerations may be attributed to diabetes, and abnormal or unusually dark moles may be associated with cutaneous melanomas. Any skin abnormality can affect the biomechanics and health of the foot by altering the gait and providing increased opportunity for infection, respectively. Therefore, these issues should be addressed as soon as they are discovered.

Hematomas

Hematomas can be found under the beds of the toenails, referred to as a subungual hematoma (**Figure 5.22**). Hematomas are usually the result of macrotrauma, such as a direct blow to the foot (eg, dropping something on a toe) or from chronic microtrauma, such as running in ill-fitting shoes. Blood collects under the nail, causing painful pressure. This pressure can be relieved through drilling or melting a hole in the nail with an electrocautery tool (**Figure 5.23**). It is important to note that hematomas that develop from acute compressive trauma may be secondary to a fracture.

Toe Deformities

During foot inspection, clinicians should take note of important toe alignments that may contribute to a variety of foot injuries and/or biomechanical issues.

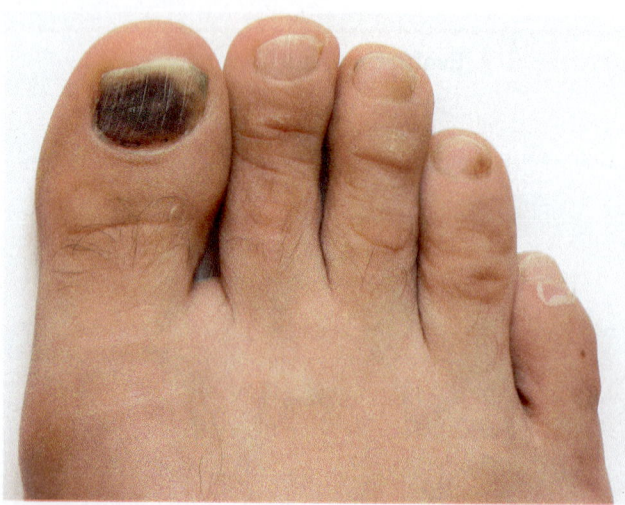

Figure 5.22 Photograph showing subungual hematoma of the toe.
© Jones & Bartlett Learning

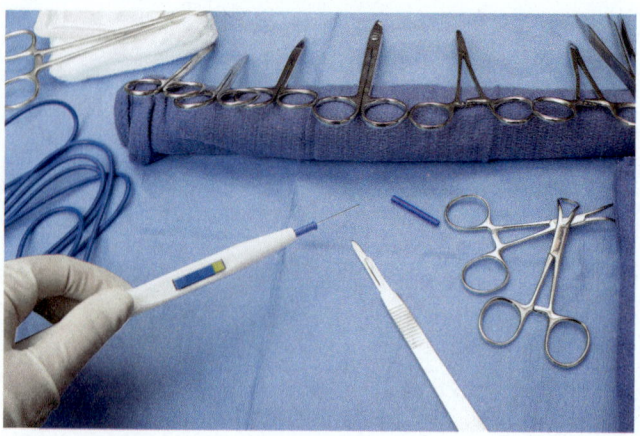

Figure 5.23 An electrocautery tool.
© Sherry Yates Young/Shutterstock

Table 5.8 lists the different types of toe deformities and their defining characteristics (**Figures 5.24** through **5.27**).

Presence of Foot Malalignment

Beyond the classification of pronated, supinated, or neutral foot, malalignment of the foot should be characterized when present. These alignments include valgus and varus deviations of the rearfoot and forefoot. Generally, valgus deformities refer to a lateral deviation, or abduction, from the neutral position. Varus deformities refer to a medial deviation, or adduction, from the neutral position. To evaluate these deviations, clinicians will need to view the rearfoot (posterior aspect) from the heel and the forefoot (anterior aspect) from the toes. These malalignments are often associated with foot types of either pronation or supination and arch deformities, such as pes planus and pes cavus (discussed later). **Table 5.9** outlines the characteristics of valgus and varus alignments of the rearfoot and forefoot.[23] **Figure 5.28** shows both types of alignments.

Arch Deformities

Although deformities can be structural (anatomic) in nature, it is important to remember that they may also be caused by functional muscle imbalances. When evaluating the overall posture of the foot, it is important to not only observe the deformities that are present but also to evaluate the potential contribution of bony structures (eg, navicular bone) and associated muscles to the pathology. Proper evaluation can help in the diagnosis of a structural versus a functional problem, which will greatly aid in the development of therapeutic exercise strategies or better inform the need for

Table 5.8 Characteristics of Toe Deformities

	Figure 5.24 Photograph showing hallux valgus. © Jones & Bartlett Learning	**Figure 5.25** Photograph showing Claw toe. © Andrea De Meo/Shutterstock	**Figure 5.26** Drawings showing Morton toe. © Aksanaku/Shutterstock	**Figure 5.27** Photograph showing hammer toe. © paulaah293/Shutterstock
Observable deviation	The first toe deviates laterally (abduction) at the first MTP joint and, in extreme cases, crosses under the second toe. A bunion develops on the medial aspect of the first MTP joint.	Toes appear to completely curl and are held in a constantly flexed state.	The second toe is longer than the first toe, causing excessive pressure on the second toe.	Toes appear to be partially curled or flexed at the PIP joint, but the distal phalanges remain extended.
Anatomic reasoning	Progressive subluxation of the first MTP join accompanied by bunion formation. Results in 20° deviation from neutral.	Contracture of the interosseous muscles, the lumbrical muscles, or both results in the hyperextension of the MTP joints and flexion at both the PIP and DIP joints of toes two through five.	First metatarsal is anatomically shorter than the second metatarsal.	Contractures of both the toe flexors and extensors result in the hyperextension of the MTP joints, flexion of the PIP joints, and extension of the DIP joints in toes two through five.

DIP, distal interphalangeal; MTP, metatarsophalangeal; PIP, proximal interphalangeal.

Table 5.9 Characteristics of Valgus and Varus Alignments of the Foot

	Rearfoot Valgus	Rearfoot Varus	Forefoot Valgus	Forefoot Varus
Observable deviation	The calcaneus is everted in relation to the long axis of the tibia	The calcaneus is inverted in relation to the long axis of the tibia	With rearfoot in a neutral position: The fifth metatarsal is elevated in relation to the first metatarsal	With rearfoot in a neutral position: The first metatarsal is elevated in relation to the fifth metatarsal
Biomechanical alterations	Hypermobility of the rearfoot leads to increased pronation	Rigid rearfoot leads to increased supination during weight bearing and prolonged moments of supination and pronation during gait	The first metatarsal contacts the ground earlier in the gait cycle, resulting in eversion followed by supination of the forefoot	Pronation is increased during gait, as the first metatarsal must travel farther to make contact with the ground

orthotic devices. The medial arch should be assessed in both a weight-bearing and non–weight-bearing position to evaluate alterations, adaptations, or compensations that may arise when changing positions. Because the navicular bone is the keystone of the medial longitudinal arch, a rise or drop in its position can influence the alignment of the foot. Using tests to assess navicular displacement will be helpful in determining foot behavior.

Pes Planus. From Latin roots, *pes* is the word for foot, and *planus* means flat. Pes planus, or flatfoot, (**Figure 5.29**) is also referred to as a fallen arch. The navicular bone is displaced inferiorly in a flat foot,

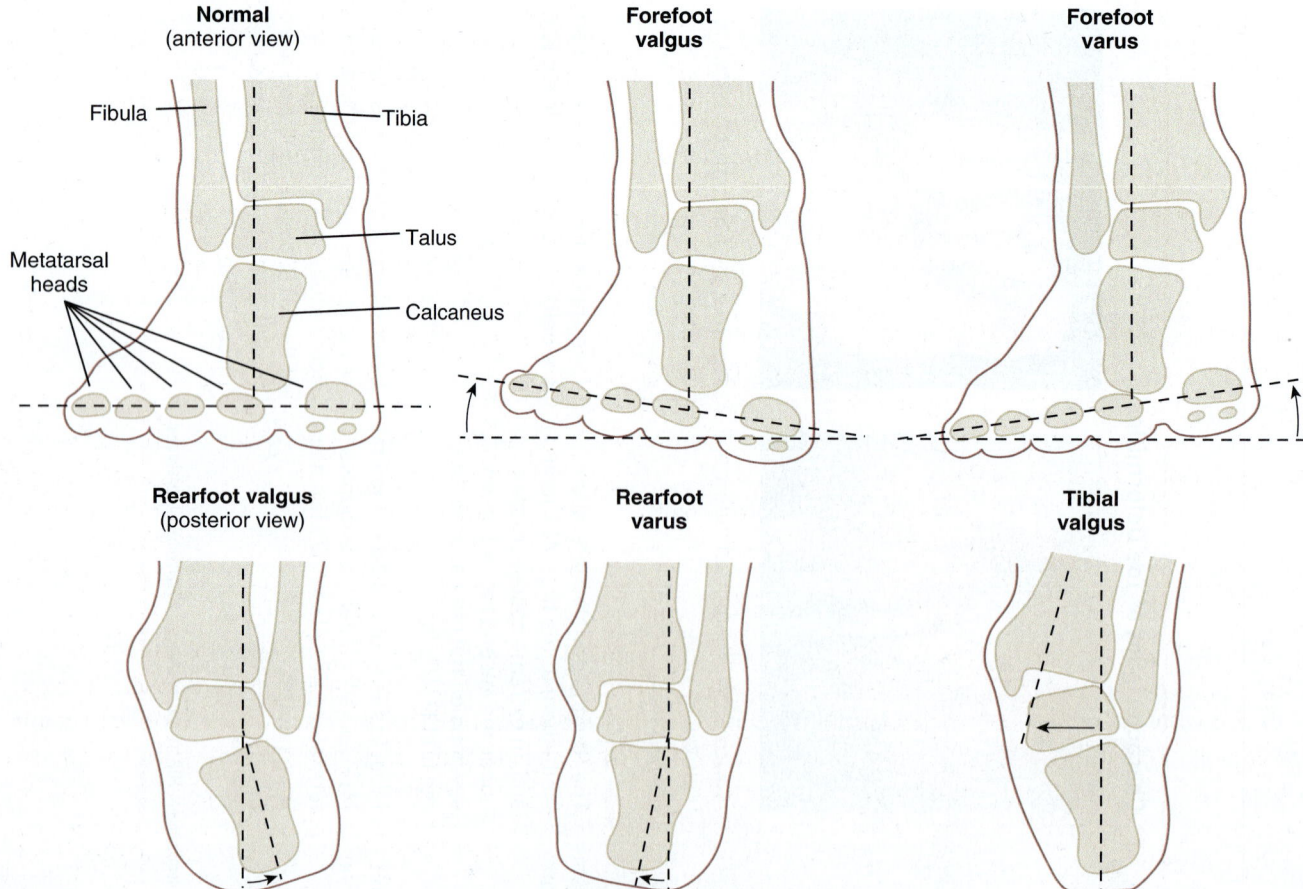

Figure 5.28 Drawings showing valgus and varus alignments of the foot.

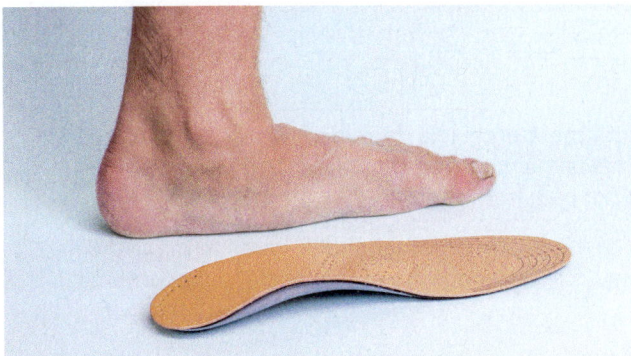

Figure 5.29 Photograph of a foot with pes planus and an orthotic device showing a normal arch.
© VLADIMIR VK/Shutterstock

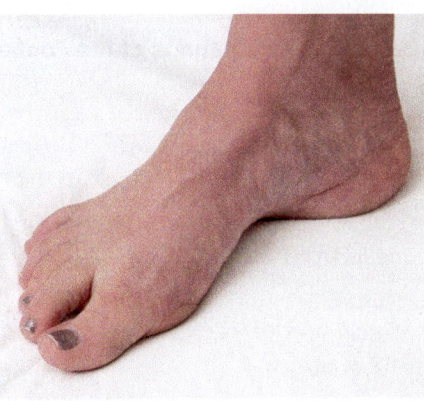

Figure 5.30 Photograph of a foot with pes cavus.
© Jones & Bartlett Learning

which allows the talar head to rotate medially. The talus becomes more prominent, creating a noticeable bulge along the medial longitudinal arch. Individuals with a flat foot may complain of soreness in this area of the foot, from the pressure applied by their shoe. Trauma to structures that support the medial arch, such as the spring ligament, plantar fascia, and anterior and posterior tibialis muscles, or fracture to the navicular bone/accessory navicular may result in pes planus.

Individuals with pes planus can be subcategorized into having either rigid pes planus (structural) or supple pes planus. With supple pes planus, the medial longitudinal arch appears when the person is in a non–weight-bearing position; however, once the person is bearing weight, the arch flattens, or disappears. Supple pes planus may be more functional in nature and may be helped with the use of orthotic devices.

Pes planus is often congenital, and, depending on a person's biomechanics, individuals with flat feet may never experience issues. However, individuals with pes planus typically put additional stress on the medial structures of the foot and spend prolonged periods of time in pronation. This can result in a hypermobile first ray, development of stress fractures, and a higher risk for other musculoskeletal injuries, both acute and chronic in nature.

Pes Cavus. *Cavus* is Latin, meaning hollow or vaulted; therefore, pes cavus (**Figure 5.30**) is the opposite of pes planus and is translated to mean high-arched foot. Pes cavus has been associated with the muscle imbalance highlighted earlier, but it is also common with neurologic diseases, such as cerebral palsy.

Pes cavus is congenital in nature and may not lead to symptoms. However, individuals with pes cavus put additional stress on lateral and forefoot structures and may spend prolonged periods in supination. Like pes planus, pes cavus can also lead to an increased likelihood of both acute and chronic injuries.

Bilateral Comparison

If possible, compare the injured with the uninjured limb and note obvious differences. With many injuries, this would include the presence and absence of swelling, redness, discoloration, or heat in the injured and uninjured limb, respectively. Additionally, defined anatomic landmarks should be relatively similar between limbs, as should limb length. If the length of the limbs and/or landmarks are altered, this could provide useful information for diagnosis.

Palpation

When performed properly, palpation can provide great insight into the location and condition of a structure. When performed poorly, palpation can worsen the severity of an injury and/or cause guarding, thereby hindering the ability to perform special tests accurately. Clinicians should initially place their hands and fingers away from the site of injury and assess anatomic landmarks not expected to be painful, orient themselves to the patient's local anatomy, and then slowly and gently move toward the site of injury. Skilled clinicians are very adept at finding and recognizing subtle differences in bony and soft-tissue structures. It is highly recommended that clinicians practice their palpation skills often, with a wide variety of both inanimate objects and body types to familiarize themselves with various presentations of "normal" conditions. Quick palpation guides were presented previously in Tables 5.2 and 5.3. **Tables 5.10** and **5.11** provide detailed instructions for a systematic approach to the palpation of the important bony and soft-tissue landmarks of the foot and ankle, organized by region and tissue type.

Table 5.10 Bony Palpations of the Foot and Ankle

Medial Aspect

Head of the first metatarsal and MTP joint	The distal head of the first metatarsal is a prominent landmark palpated at the ball of the foot. This is the most common area for gout and bunion formation and is the site of pain from turf toe.
Medial cuneiform	Palpate along the shaft of the first metatarsal until it flares to make the first metatarsocuneiform joint. The distal portion of the medial cuneiform can be felt here.
Navicular tubercle	The medial cuneiform articulates with the navicular bone. Continue to move proximally until the next bony prominence is reached. This is the navicular tubercle. The navicular bone articulates with the talus, all three cuneiforms, and the cuboid and is therefore very important to the support of the midfoot. If the navicular tubercle is overly prominent, it may rub against the medial aspect of the shoe, causing pain.
Head of the talus	Moving slightly superior (proximally) from the navicular tubercle and just posterior to the medial malleolus, the talar head can be palpated here. In a neutral position it is slightly recessed; however, moving the foot into an everted position will rotate the talar head medially, and it will become palpable. The head of the talus will be rotated medially in individuals with a pes planus foot.
Medial malleolus	Superior (proximal) to the head of the talus is the prominent medial malleolus, the distal end of the tibia.
Sustentaculum tali	From the medial malleolus, move toward the plantar aspect of the foot until a small shelflike prominence is reached. This landmark can be difficult to palpate. It serves as support for the talus and an attachment site of the spring ligament. Because of this attachment, it may feel more like a soft-tissue landmark and be tender to the touch, even when no injury is present.
Medial tubercle of the talus	The medial tubercle of the talus is barely palpable and lies just posterior and slightly inferior to the medial malleolus (slightly proximal to the sustentaculum tali). This serves as an attachment site for the posterior aspect of the deltoid ligament and can be better realized when everting and inverting the foot.

Lateral Aspect

Fifth MTP joint	The head of the fifth metatarsal/MTP joint is the lateral ball of the foot.
Base of the fifth metatarsal (styloid process)	Palpate proximally along the shaft of the fifth metatarsal until it flares laterally to a point. This is the base of the fifth metatarsal, which is also referred to as the styloid process. This is one of the more prominent landmarks of the lateral aspect of the foot and is a good source of orientation. This is also the site where the peroneus brevis attaches to the foot. The peroneus longus tendon lies directly behind the flare of the styloid process where it dives to the plantar aspect and across to the first MTP joint.
Cuboid	Posterior (proximal) to the flare of the styloid process is the cuboid bone.
Calcaneus	Continue proximally along the lateral aspect of the foot to identify the lateral arch of the foot, which is much smaller and less noticeable than the medial longitudinal arch, due to the structural anatomy and the fat pad located in this region. The calcaneus is subcutaneous in this area and easily palpable.
Peroneal tubercle	The peroneal tubercle is a prominent bony landmark on the lateral aspect of the calcaneus just inferior to the lateral malleolus. Fairly long at approximately 0.25 inch in length, the peroneal tubercle separates the peroneus longus and brevis tendons as they pass around the lateral aspect of the calcaneus.

Lateral Aspect	
Lateral malleolus	The lateral malleolus is just superior to the peroneal tubercle and is one of the more prominent bony landmarks of the ankle. The lateral malleolus is the distal end of the fibula; it extends farther distally and is located more posteriorly than the medial malleolus.
Sinus tarsi	Stabilize the patient's foot at the calcaneus, and then palpate the anterior aspect of the lateral malleolus. In this area, there is a soft-tissue depression, referred to as the sinus tarsi. Invert the foot slightly in order to possibly feel the talar neck. The ATFL also lies beneath this landmark, and swelling is often seen in the sinus tarsi soon after ATFL injury.
Dome of the talus	With the thumb positioned in the sinus tarsi, invert and dorsiflex the foot. A portion of the dome of the talus will become palpable as it rotates out of the mortise joint.
Inferior tibiofibular joint	Immediately superior (proximal) to the sinus tarsi and the talus is the inferior tibiofibular joint. The AITFL overlies this joint, making it difficult to palpate. However, in the event of a high ankle sprain, these bones may separate with injury to the AITFL.
Hindfoot	
Dome of the calcaneus	The dome of the calcaneus is what is referred to as the heel of the foot. If the posterior aspect of the foot is moved, the dome of the calcaneus can be palpated rather easily.
Medial tubercle	The medial tubercle of the calcaneus can be palpated on both the posterior medial aspect of the foot and the plantar surface of the foot. Move the thumb along the medial aspect of the heel until the tubercle on the medial plantar aspect is reached and then continue to the plantar aspect, where it is hardly palpable due to numerous soft-tissue attachments at this site (abductor hallucis, flexor digitorum brevis, and plantar fascia). This can be a place of bone spur development and, as such, can be quite tender to the touch.
Plantar Surface	
Sesamoid bones	From the medial tubercle of the calcaneus, palpate along the medial border of the foot until the first metatarsal head is reached. If pressed firmly, the two sesamoid bones embedded within the flexor hallucis tendon can be distinguished. Inflammation of the sesamoids (sesamoiditis) will result in pain/tenderness in this area.
Metatarsal heads	Move laterally from the first metatarsal head to palpate each of the remaining metatarsal heads. They can be better realized with the thumb being placed on the plantar aspect and the index finger, on the dorsal aspect. Grasp each head between the thumb and finger, and check to see whether any of the heads appear more prominent than the others. If so, this metatarsal will bear more weight than it should and therefore may be subject to injury.

AITFL, anterior inferior tibiofibular ligament; ATFL, anterior talofibular ligament; MTP, metatarsophalangeal.

Special Tests

Using information collected during the history, inspection, and palpation portions of the evaluation, a differential diagnosis is formulated to inform the use of special tests designed to orthopaedically assess the injured structure(s). Reported as a positive or negative result, special tests are intended to either rule in (positive test or lack of conclusive negative test) or rule out (negative test) potential injuries by recreating the MOI. In some cases, unexpected or inconclusive results of special tests may lead to additional potential diagnoses, requiring further examination. However, with a thorough understanding of anatomy, basic biomechanical principles, MOIs, open- and closed-chain kinematics, and mechanical tissue properties, many special

Table 5.11 Soft-Tissue Palpations of the Foot and Ankle

Medial Aspect	
Bursa at the first MTP joint	Normally, healthy bursae are not palpable. However, when they become inflamed (bursitis), they swell and become more obvious to observe and palpate. An inflamed bursa may be palpable at the first MTP joint.
Spring ligament	Helps to support the talus, which lacks bony and muscular attachment support. The spring ligament extends from the sustentaculum tali to the navicular tubercle, providing support to the medial arch, and can be palpated between these two structures. In the presence of pes planus, the talar head rotates medially, applying pressure to the spring ligament, stretching both it and the tibialis posterior tendon, which also provides medial support to the talus and attaches to the navicular tubercle.
Deltoid ligament complex	The deltoid ligament can be palpated just inferior to the medial malleolus. It is a very broad and strong ligament complex composed of four segments. Because of its broad attachment, it is difficult to determine distinct borders of the ligament through palpation. However, upon injury to the deltoid, pain and laxity in eversion will be located in this region.
Tibialis posterior tendon	From the medial malleolus, palpation moves posteriorly into the soft-tissue depression between the malleolus and the Achilles tendon. Within this depression lie several important structures. From anterior to posterior, they follow the mnemonic Tom, Dick, ANd Harry (Tibialis posterior, flexor Digitorum longus, posterior tibial Artery, tibial Nerve, and flexor Hallucis longus tendon). The most anterior is the tibialis posterior tendon. It passes immediately behind the medial malleolus and can be made more prominent by asking the patient to invert and dorsiflex the foot.
Flexor digitorum longus tendon	Posterior to the tibialis posterior tendon is the flexor digitorum longus tendon. To make this tendon more prominent, simply ask the patient to flex the toes.
Posterior tibial artery and tibial nerve	Posterior to the flexor digitorum is the posterior tibial artery and the tibial nerve. The nerve may be indistinguishable, but this is the area in which the posterior tibial pulse can be taken by lightly pressing the artery against the medial malleolus. The posterior tibial artery is the main blood supply of the foot and therefore is important when assessing distal pulses following severe injury.
Flexor hallucis longus tendon	Just posterior to the posterior tibial artery and tibial nerve is the flexor hallucis tendon. To make this tendon more prominent, ask the patient to flex his or her first toe.
Dorsal Aspect	
Tibialis anterior tendon	Between the malleoli, the TA tendon is the most medial and prominent of the three tendons on the dorsal aspect of the foot. It inserts on the dorsal medial aspect of the medial cuneiform and the base of the first metatarsal head. As the primary dorsiflexor, injury to the TA can result in foot drop. To palpate, instruct the patient to dorsiflex the foot.
Extensor hallucis longus tendon	Lateral to the TA is the extensor hallucis longus tendon. Instruct the patient to extend his or her first toe, and the tendon will become most prominent lateral to the TA at the ankle joint, where it can then be traced to its insertion on the dorsal aspect of the first toe.
Extensor digitorum longus tendon(s)	Just lateral to the extensor hallucis longus tendon is the extensor digitorum longus tendon. After passing the mortise joint, the tendon separates into four slips that insert on the dorsal aspect of toes two through five. To better realize this tendon and the individual slips, ask the patient to extend the toes with or without resistance.
Dorsal pedal artery	The dorsal pedal artery lies between the extensor hallucis longus tendon and the extensor digitorum longus tendon; however, it is not always present in every person. The artery is subcutaneous and can be used to assess a distal pulse of the foot. It is a secondary supply to the posterior tibial artery.

Lateral Aspect	
Anterior talofibular ligament	The ATFL runs from the anterior aspect of the lateral malleolus to the lateral aspect of the talar neck, the area that lies just beneath the sinus tarsi. The ATFL is the most commonly injured ligament in an ankle injury. Therefore, the area of the sinus tarsi is the best area to detect injury to the ligament, based on tenderness and swelling, and will allow for great translation with an anterior drawer test.
Calcaneofibular ligament	The CFL extends from the inferior aspect of the distal fibular head (lateral malleolus) to the lateral wall of the calcaneus on a small tubercle slightly posterior to the peroneal tubercle. The CFL is typically injured in severe ankle injuries, as it is the second ligament to tear following injury to the ATFL. Pain will be detected in this area and greater inversion range of motion allowed with this type of injury.
Posterior talofibular ligament	Originating from the posterior edge of the lateral malleolus, the posterior talofibular ligament inserts on a small lateral tubercle on the posterior aspect of the talus. It is a strong ligament that is rarely injured, as its main job is to resist anterior translation of the fibula (typically takes place with ankle dislocations). This ligament is not palpable; when injured, pain and swelling will be present in this location with a positive posterior drawer test.
Peroneal longus and brevis tendons	Both tendons pass immediately posterior to the lateral malleolus and can be better observed when the patient is asked to evert the foot. Because of their subcutaneous position, they can often be seen splitting at the peroneal tubercle and can be traced to their respective insertion sites. The retinaculum holds the peroneal tendons to the tubercle, and the tendons are contained within synovial sheaths. As a result, they are subject to tenosynovitis and snapping syndrome if there is injury to the tendons or the retinaculum, respectively.
Extensor digitorum brevis muscle	The belly of the extensor digitorum brevis muscle lies just below the sinus tarsi. Therefore, when palpating the sinus tarsi, instruct the patient to extend the toes, and the belly of the muscle can be felt contracting.
Posterior Aspect	
Achilles tendon	One of the most prominent features on the posterior aspect of the foot and ankle is the Achilles tendon. The Achilles tendon is the thick, cordlike tendon that extends from the calf and inserts on the calcaneus. A tear in the Achilles tendon can result in the complete loss of the natural contour created by the tendon, leaving a notable concavity.
Retrocalcaneal bursa	In a noninflamed state, the retrocalcaneal bursa cannot be palpated; even inflamed, it may be difficult to distinctively palpate, as it lies between the anterior surface of the Achilles tendon and the posterior superior angle of the calcaneus.
Calcaneal bursa	This bursa is not palpable in a noninflamed state. However, when irritated, it may be observed, as it lies subcutaneously on the posterior aspect of the Achilles tendon at the insertion on the calcaneus.
Plantar Aspect	
Plantar aponeurosis (plantar fascia)	Can be palpated along the length of the foot. However, it may be found most tender at its insertion on the medial tubercle of the calcaneus, where bone spurs often form, causing considerable pain with heel strike and palpation.

ATFL, anterior talofibular ligament; CFL, calcaneofibular ligament; MTP, metatarsophalangeal; TA, tibialis anterior.

tests can be easily understood and re-created, even if the clinician is unfamiliar with a particular injury or specific special test; the basic principles of testing structural integrity related to the MOI remain the same.

Special tests pertaining to specific foot and ankle pathologies will be discussed later, complete with sensitivity, specificity, and likelihood values when available. Detailed information regarding individual pathologies is presented later in this chapter.

Open- and Closed-Chain Kinematics

An understanding of open- and closed-chain kinematics is required before attempting to conduct special tests. Open-chain kinematics describes motion in which the distal end of a limb is free to move, whereas closed-chain kinematics describes motion in which the distal end of the limb is fixed. These concepts are important because they inform the clinician which part of the limb will be acting on the surrounding structures. In the foot and ankle, for example, any time the foot is in contact with a surface, the leg is operating as a closed-chain system. This means the talus is fixed in the mortise joint and the shank (tibia and fibula) is moving or acting on the talus. However, in relation to the knee joint, the tibia is fixed, and the femur is acting on the tibia. Conversely, if the foot is not in contact with a surface, the leg is operating as an open-chain system, meaning that, because the distal portion is free to move, the talus is now operating on a fixed shank and, at the knee, the tibia is now moving on a fixed femur. Therefore, it is important to recognize whether a special test, MOI, or even therapeutic exercise would be defined as being open- or closed-chain, as these definitions determine which aspect of the limb can be manipulated in respect to the joint and/or structure of interest.

Normal Gait

Gait is a cyclical movement that can be categorized into two major phases related to either closed- or open-chain movement. The stance phase constitutes approximately 60% of one complete step cycle from the point of heel strike through to push-off, making it a closed-chain event. The remaining 40% of the step cycle is open chain in nature and is referred to as the swing phase. During the stance phase, the heel strikes the ground, absorbing the impact as the foot supinates (loading response). From supination, the foot transfers the weight of the body medially, which is absorbed by the medial longitudinal arch (midstance). The foot continues to move into pronation as the weight of the body is transferred forward (terminal stance) and onto the first MTP joint for push-off. As the swing phase begins (initial swing), the foot is in a plantarflexed position following push-off. As the knee flexes to bring the foot forward (midswing), the ankle dorsiflexes and supinates to prepare for heel strike (terminal swing). **Figure 5.31** shows the different phases of gait through a single step cycle.

As the foot contacts the ground, it moves from a supinated to a pronated position. However, anyone spending abnormal periods of time in any area of a gait cycle may display a pathologic gait pattern. Pathologic gait patterns can be highly influenced by the type of foot/arch a person may have. For example, individuals with pronated feet often spend little, if any, time in the supination phases of gait. This results in added stress to the medial structures of the foot. These individuals typically have a flat medial longitudinal arch and a *hyper*mobile first ray. Conversely, individuals with a supinated foot spend far less time in pronation. They often stress the lateral structures of their feet; distribute their weight across the second through fifth toes, which are not built to support a large share of the body weight; and have a high and rigid medial longitudinal arch and a *hypo*mobile first ray.

When a clinician is familiar with neutral gait patterns, abnormal gait patterns can be relatively easy to spot. Evaluating the wear pattern on the sole of a shoe may be another tool a clinician can use to learn more about a person's gait. With a neutral gait, the wear pattern on the bottom of the shoe travels from the heel along the posterior lateral aspect of the shoe, diagonally across to the first MTP joint and the first toe.

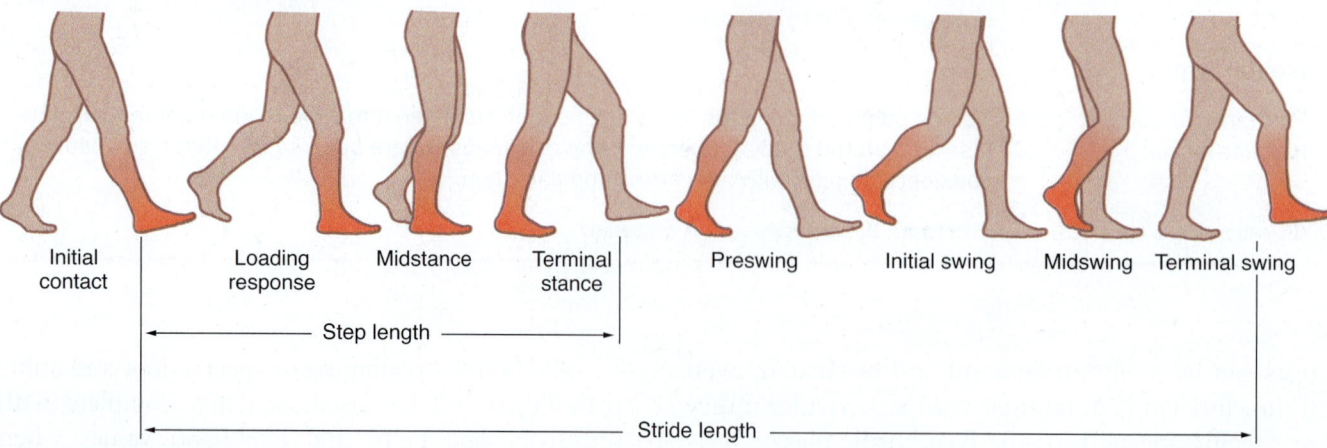

Figure 5.31 Phases of gait.

© Jones & Bartlett Learning

However, with a pronation gait pattern the wear pattern will mostly be evident on the medial aspect of the sole and, for a supination gait pattern, the lateral aspect of the sole (Figure 5.21).

Pathomechanics, such as abnormal gait patterns, can be related to either functional (eg, muscular imbalance, poor activation patterns, abnormal joint ROM) or structural (anatomic) issues and possibly a combination of both. Functional pathomechanics can and should be addressed with therapeutic exercises focused on correcting muscular imbalances and/or muscular activation patterns and joint mobility. The treatment of structural issues is determined by the degree or severity of the dysfunction. Less severe structural issues that result in an abnormal gait pattern may be addressed by customized orthotic devices. However, more debilitating structural issues may need to be addressed surgically.

Range of Motion

Evaluating the ROM of a limb, or, more specifically, a joint, can be extremely useful in determining both the severity of the injury and the tissue involved. There are three stages of ROM to be evaluated, and it is recommended that ROM be evaluated prior to performing any special tests. The three types of ROM—active ROM (AROM), passive ROM (PROM), and resistive ROM (RROM)—are presented in **Table 5.12**. Instructions for performing ROM in relation to

Table 5.12 Types of Range of Motion

	AROM	PROM	RROM
Performed by	The patient under his or her own will; patients actively contract their muscles and attempt to move the injured limb through the appropriate full ROM for any particular joint.	The clinician; after the patient has relaxed the limb, the clinician attempts to move the injured limb through the appropriate full ROM for any particular joint.	The patient; with manual resistance applied by the clinician or, in some cases, a surface (eg, ground) or object.
Indicated	For any injury; ask the patient whether he or she can or is willing to move the limb.	If a patient cannot achieve full AROM for that limb at any particular joint, the clinician properly isolates the joint of interest and attempts to move the limb passively to assess the quality of movement and end points.	If the patient is able to perform full or partial ROM, the clinician may apply resistance to assess the strength, quality, and endurance of the movement.
Contraindicated	Avoid if a fracture or dislocation is suspected.	Caution should be used if a fracture or dislocation is suspected.	Should not be performed if the patient cannot perform AROM or there is a suspected fracture/dislocation.
Primary structure being assessed	Tests the integrity of active structures and the patient's ability to contract and use his or her musculature. Inability or unwillingness to perform movement may be related to fracture, dislocation, or complete rupture of the tendon from the bone. Inability to perform full AROM at any particular joint can be directly related to muscular strain injury or obstruction of the joint (eg, meniscal tears, loose bodies).	Tests the integrity of passive structures: bone and ligament. Excessive joint ROM can be related to ligament damage resulting in joint instability (soft or lack of end point). Inability to passively reach full ROM may be due to bony disturbances (eg, loose bodies), osteochondral defects (hard end points), or muscular contractures (firm end points).	Tests the quality or strength of muscular contraction. If a patient can perform AROM but pain/discomfort is reported with the movement, resistance is applied to test the level of strength and endurance of contraction (to be compared bilaterally).

AROM, active range of motion; PROM, passive range of motion; ROM, range of motion; RROM, resistive range of motion.

injury evaluation are presented later in this chapter, in which the evaluation of common pathologies is presented.

Pathologies of the Foot and Ankle

Common Pathologies

Musculoskeletal injuries to the foot and ankle are common across all sports. Over a 2-year period at a large Division I athletics program, foot and ankle injuries comprised 27% of all musculoskeletal injuries.[25] It was determined that 21% of these injuries resulted in lost playing time.[25] Some sports and populations have a higher risk for sustaining foot and ankle injuries; however, the mechanisms of injury are consistent throughout. In the aforementioned study, it was determined that athletes at the highest risk for foot and ankle injury were those who participated in women's gymnastics, cross-country, and soccer, and men's cross-country.[25] Although not an exhaustive list, the more common injuries to the toes, foot, ankle, and lower leg are presented in the following paragraphs. **Table 5.13** presents a quick sideline assessment of foot and ankle motor function and ROM. Additional details about individual pathologies are presented in the next section. A quick reference guide for special test of the foot and ankle is presented later in this chapter in Table 5.32.

Metatarsalgia

Metatarsalgia, or metatarsal pain, is defined as pain in the forefoot typically present under one or more metatarsal heads.[26] Metatarsalgia is classified into three categories: primary, secondary, and iatrogenic.[26] Primary metatarsalgia is considered to be related to inherent anatomic characteristics that disrupt the distribution of force, such as when the second metatarsal absorbs more force with a congenital shorter first metatarsal. Secondary metatarsalgia develops after another issue, such as a disease or neurologic disorder. Finally, iatrogenic metatarsalgia describes a condition that develops following forefoot surgery.

Evaluation for metatarsalgia should include a thorough evaluation of foot type and gait. Additional radiographic imaging may be helpful in determining potential anatomic issues contributing to the condition. Referral to a podiatrist may be warranted.

Neuromas

A potential cause of metatarsalgia may be the presence of an interdigital neuroma (**Figure 5.32**). A neuroma is a benign growth of nervous tissue that elicits a painful burning on the plantar aspect of the foot.[27] Morton neuroma is the most common reason for the diagnosis of metatarsalgia and is typically located in the interdigital space between the third and fourth toes.[27] A bulge between the toes may be noticeable, and the pain is exacerbated with compression, such as with tight-fitting shoes or direct palpation.

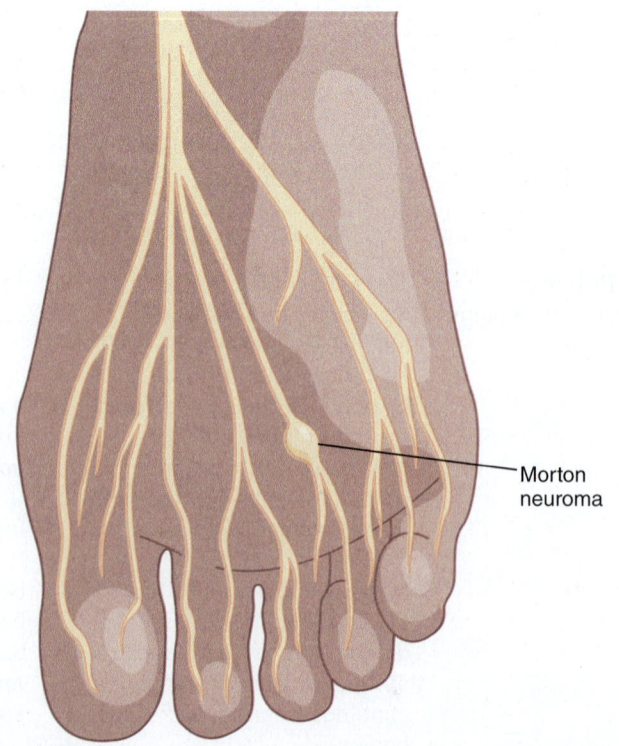

Figure 5.32 Drawing of the foot showing an interdigital neuroma.

© Jones & Bartlett Learning

Table 5.13 Motor Function of the Foot and Ankle (Quick Myotome and Range of Motion Test)

Action/Instruction	Associated Myotome
Walk on toes	Walking on the toes tests plantar flexion and the muscles associated with S1/S2 nerve roots.
Walk on heels with toes extended	Walking on the heels tests dorsiflexion/toe extension and the muscles associated with L4/L5.
Walk on the lateral edge of the feet	Walking on the lateral border of the foot tests inversion and the peroneal muscles associated with L4/L5/S1.
Walk on the medial edge of the foot	Walking on the medial border of the foot tests eversion and the muscles associated with S1.

Nonsurgical treatment focuses on the use of orthotic devices to ease loading of the metatarsals.[27] Additionally, steroid injection can be used to minimize pain. Prolonged issues with Morton neuroma may require radiographic imaging to evaluate any potential anatomic causes regarding development.[27] Surgical excision may be require if nonsurgical approaches fail. As with metatarsalgia, a sound evaluation of foot type and gait should be performed; referral to a podiatrist may be warranted.

Turf Toe

Turf toe is a hyperextension of the first MTP joint and therefore may take place during a multitude of activities; however, it is most commonly experienced in sports that take place on artificial turf.[28] The hyperextension of the first MTP joint results in a sprain of the joint capsule and a strain of the flexor hallucis longus tendon. Following a turf toe injury, individuals typically complain of pain during push-off and, depending on the severity, may completely avoid push-off, thereby noticeably altering their gait. Taping techniques that promote flexion while limiting toe extension can be used and may provide some relief.[28] Additionally, reinforcing the individual's shoe to make the toe plate more rigid (adding a plate or rigid orthotic device) may also limit extension and allow the individual to return to activity. As with any sprain, turf toe responds best to adequate rest for healing. If not treated appropriately, turf toe can become a chronic injury and result in complete removal from activity. Details of the sideline evaluation of turf toe are presented in **Table 5.14**, and further evaluation details are presented in **Table 5.15**.

Plantar Fasciitis

The plantar fascia is a thick connective tissue band (**Figure 5.33**) that supports the arch of the foot and acts as a shock absorber during weight-bearing activities.

Table 5.15 Evaluation of Turf Toe

History	
Classification	Acute
MOI	Hyperextension of the first MTP joint; mechanism may be described as the foot slipping during push-off
S/S	Pain at the first MTP joint; described with push-off phase of gait
Observation	
Swelling	Swelling may be present at the first MTP joint
Discoloration	Ecchymosis may be present at the first MTP joint
Palpation	
Pain	Pain when the first MTP joint is palpated
Special Tests	
AROM and PROM	Pain with active flexion of the first toe due to the strain of the flexor hallucis tendon Pain with passive extension of the first toe as it stretches the flexor hallucis tendon
RROM	Decreased toe flexion strength
Special Test	N/A

AROM, active range of motion; MOI, mechanism of injury; MTP, metatarsophalangeal; N/A, not applicable; PROM, passive range of motion; RROM, resistive range of motion; S/S, signs and symptoms.

Plantar fasciitis is one of the most common causes of heel pain.[29,30] The cause of plantar fasciitis is thought to be related to biomechanical overuse issues that lead to the development of microtears and subsequent inflammation at the origin of the medial calcaneal tubercle.[29]

Table 5.14 Turf Toe Quick Tips

Pathology	Description	Presentation (HIPS)	Special Tests/Imaging	Differential Diagnosis	5-Min Sideline Assessment Tips
Turf toe	Sprain (stretching or tearing) of the fibrocartilaginous plate of the first MTP joint capsule	Acute onset with the hyperextension of the first MTP joint MOI. Pain and swelling on the plantar aspect of the first MTP joint.	N/A	• Metatarsal or phalangeal fracture • MTP joint dislocation • Sesamoid fracture or stress fracture (rule out multipartite sesamoid)	Pain is present upon palpation of the plantar aspect of the first MTP joint. Increased pain is experienced upon passive hyperextension of the first toe at the MTP joint.

HIPS, history, inspection, palpation, special tests; MOI, mechanism of injury; MTP, metatarsophalangeal; N/A, not applicable.

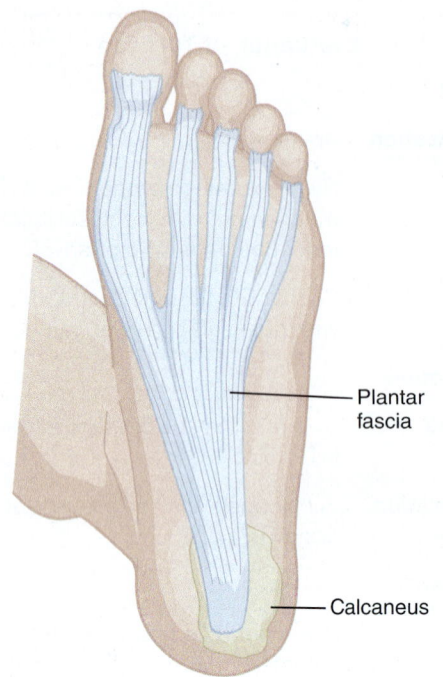

Figure 5.33 Drawing of the foot showing the plantar fascia.

© Jones & Bartlett Learning

However, histologic examinations have demonstrated a lack of acute inflammation, suggesting a degenerative disorder, more aptly referred to as plantar fasciosis.[29,30]

Patients typically present with pain that occurs first thing in the morning as the tissue is stretched when getting out of bed. The pain reportedly improves with movement; however, it worsens over the course of the day.[30] Upon evaluation, pain is elicited with the palpation of the medial calcaneal tubercle.[29,30] The patient will also experience pain with active and passive dorsiflexion of the foot as the fascia is stretched.

Differential diagnosis should include development of a bone spur on the calcaneus, and therefore radiographic imaging may be required.[29,30] Nonsurgical management may include the use of orthotic devices to correct possible foot types, such as pes cavus or pes planus. Use of a night splint to hold the foot in dorsiflexion during sleep or change of shoes may help relieve some of the painful symptoms.[30] Anti-inflammatory agents may provide relief, depending on whether active inflammation is present. Surgical management to release the fascia may be necessary if nonsurgical treatment fails.[29,30] Quick tips for the sideline evaluation of plantar fasciitis are presented in **Table 5.16**, and details regarding the evaluation of plantar fasciitis are presented in **Table 5.17**.

Ankle Sprains

Lateral Ankle Sprains. The lateral ankle sprain (**Figure 5.34**) is the most common lower extremity musculoskeletal injury experienced in both the

Table 5.16 Plantar Fasciitis Quick Tips

Pathology	Description	Presentation (HIPS)	Special Tests/ Imaging	Differential Diagnosis	5-Min Sideline Assessment Tips
Plantar fasciitis	Inflammation of the plantar fascia; possible pulling away of the fascia from the calcaneal tubercle.	Insidious onset, unresolved acute injury. Pain on the plantar aspect of the foot, most notably at the medial calcaneal tubercle, which worsens with weight bearing.	N/A	Tarsal tunnel (posterior tibial nerve entrapment).	Pain is sharp upon weight bearing and palpation of the medial calcaneal tubercle. Greatest pain is experienced in the morning upon getting out of bed and after being non–weight bearing for extended periods of time. Pes planus and pes cavus may be predisposing factors. Rule out tarsal tunnel with Tinel sign (tapping on the posterior tibial nerve at the posterior aspect of the medial malleolus).

HIPS, history, inspection, palpation, special tests; N/A, not applicable.

Table 5.17 Evaluation of Plantar Fasciitis

History	
Classification	Typically chronic/idiopathic Acute (strain)
MOI	Chronic: Indications of overuse (eg, sudden increase in volume), poor footwear, arch disfunction Idiopathic: May not have an obvious injury incident Acute: Forced dorsiflexion
S/S	Pain at the medial calcaneal tubercle on the plantar aspect of the foot Pain along the length of the plantar fascia (throughout the arch) Pain with weight bearing Pain is usually intense first thing in the morning when getting out of bed May be described as a stabbing or tearing pain
Observation	
Swelling	Swelling may be noticeable at the medial calcaneal tubercle
Foot type	Pes planus or pes cavus
Palpation	
Pain	Pain is elicited with palpation of the medial calcaneal tubercle and along the arch of the foot
Special Tests	
AROM and PROM	Decreased dorsiflexion Pain with dorsiflexion (both active and passive)
RROM	Decreased strength in plantar flexion, particularly during weight bearing
Special Test	N/A; Tinel sign to rule out posterior tibial nerve entrapment

AROM, active range of motion; HIPS, history, inspection, palpation, special tests; MOI, mechanism of injury; N/A, not applicable; PROM, passive range of motion; RROM, resistive range of motion; S/S, signs and symptoms.

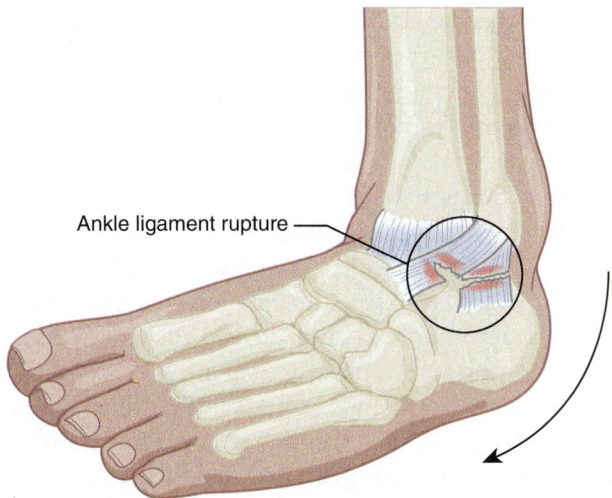

Figure 5.34 A drawing of a lateral ankle sprain.

© Jones & Bartlett Learning

have a twofold risk of recurrence within 1 year of the initial injury.[32] The mechanical and sensorimotor impairments that can develop following an acute ankle injury can lead to the development of chronic ankle instability issues.[32] The foot and ankle comprise a system that works together to absorb and transfer the ground-reaction forces experienced as the foot makes contact with the ground and adjusts throughout the course of gait. Instability can largely affect biomechanics throughout the body and further promote the development of musculoskeletal pathologies and/or pathomechanical movements that increase risk for additional injury. Furthermore, chronic ankle instability can have a negative effect on activity over a patient's life span and contribute to the development of anterior ankle impingement and/or posttraumatic osteoarthritis.[31]

Emergency department data suggest that a substantial number of individuals seek emergency medical treatment for lateral ankle sprains.[31,33] A fracture is diagnosed in approximately 15% of people presenting to the emergency room with an ankle injury, with an ankle sprain diagnosed in most of these people. These ligamentous injuries can be correctly diagnosed without the use of costly and unnecessary diagnostic imaging. The Ottawa Ankle Rules is one such way to determine whether an individual should be referred for radiography. When used appropriately, the Ottawa Ankle Rules have almost 100% sensitivity and decrease the ordering of ankle films by more than 30%.[33] A detailed overview of the Ottawa Ankle Rules is presented in Table 5.6.

Considering the high rate of injury and reinjury, it is important that clinicians not only perform a sound clinical diagnostic assessment but also evaluate and

athletic and the general population. Lateral ankle sprains have a slightly higher occurrence in women (57%) than in men (43%) and are most common in individuals age 18 to 25 years.[31] It is reported that approximately 70% of the general population will experience an ankle injury in their lifetime.[32] In the United States, the incidence of lateral ankle sprains is reported at 3.02 per 1,000 persons, as captured in the Nationwide Emergency Department Sample dataset.[31] This finding is significant because ankle injuries monitor mechanical and sensorimotor impairments throughout the treatment and rehabilitation process following a lateral ankle sprain.[32] Important mechanical and sensorimotor issues to consider include regular evaluation of pain, swelling, ROM, gait, static and dynamic postural balance, and muscular strength.[32] Impairments in each of these areas are often identified in individuals with chronic ankle instability.[32] A detailed overview of recommendations for acute lateral ankle sprain injuries is presented in the International Ankle Consortium Consensus Statement.[32]

The lateral malleolus extends farther distally than the medial malleolus, creating an anatomic configuration that allows for greater inversion than eversion motion at the ankle joint.[7] Although injuries are multifactorial in nature, bony anatomy is a primary reason lateral (inversion) ankle sprains occur more commonly than medial (eversion) and syndesmotic (often referred to as high ankle) sprains.[7,31] Lateral ankle stability is largely provided by the three main ligaments of the lateral complex. The most commonly damaged lateral ligament is the ATFL, followed by the CFL and, rarely, the PTFL. Detailed anatomic descriptions of the individual lateral ankle ligaments are presented in Table 5.1. Quick tips for the sideline evaluation of lateral ankle sprains are presented in **Table 5.18**. The collective application of anatomy, MOI, and components of orthopaedic evaluation for the lateral ankle sprain is summarized in **Table 5.19**, and special tests are described in Table 5.32.

Medial Ankle Sprains. The deltoid ligament is the strongest of the ankle ligaments; it resists excessive eversion at the subtalar joint and external rotation of the talus and therefore provides support to the medial aspect of the ankle joint.[7] Isolated eversion injuries to the deltoid ligament are rare. Estimates range from less than 1% of all ankle injuries captured across the United States in the National Emergency Department Sample dataset over a 2-year period to approximately 10% to 15% of ankle injuries.[6,31] However, it is important to consider that nearly 80% of ankle fractures have a supination-external rotation MOI and approximately 40% of deltoid ligament injuries are associated with ankle fractures.[34] It is not uncommon for medial ankle injuries to also result in lateral malleolar fracture because of the bony restriction provided during eversion of the ankle. Therefore, careful attention to the lateral structures during a medial ankle injury is warranted.

Similar to lateral ankle injuries, injury to the deltoid ligament complex can result in medial ankle instability, which can transition into chronicity.[34] The talus may tilt or even displace laterally when medial support is compromised.[35] Patients who experience an acute eversion trauma typically experience significant pain, an inability to bear weight, and swelling of the joint. However, individuals in whom chronic instability develops will describe the joint as giving away, particularly when walking on uneven surfaces or up a hill.[35] The spring ligament may be involved as well, lending to a collapse of the medial longitudinal arch (pes planus). Because of the close association of the spring ligament and, in some cases, the blending of the spring ligament into the deltoid ligament complex, the damage to the spring ligament should be considered and assessed upon evaluation.[6] High rotational forces coupled with forced dorsiflexion experienced with an eversion mechanism commonly result in injury to the tibiofibular and syndesmotic ligaments, referred to as a high ankle sprain.[7] A thorough differential diagnosis should include evaluation for a syndesmotic ankle sprain.

Table 5.18 Lateral Ankle Sprain Quick Tips

Pathology	Description	Presentation (HIPS)	Special Tests/ Imaging	Differential Diagnosis	5-Min Sideline Assessment Tips
Lateral ankle sprain	Stretching or tearing of one or multiple lateral ankle ligaments: ATFL, CFL, and/or PTFL	Acute onset, with inversion/dorsiflexion MOI. Pain, swelling, and discoloration present on the lateral aspect of the ankle (sinus tarsi).	ATFL: Anterior drawer CFL: Talar tilt (inversion stress test) PTFL: Posterior drawer	Fracture of the medial malleolus Fracture of the fifth metatarsal Avulsion of the peroneal brevis tendon from the styloid process	Swelling and painful palpation in the sinus tarsi is indicative of ATFL sprain. See Ottawa Ankle Rules for decision to refer for imaging.

ATFL, anterior talofibular ligament; CFL, calcaneofibular ligament; HIPS, history, inspection, palpation, special tests; MOI, mechanism of injury; PTFL ligament; PTFL, posterior talofibular ligament.

Table 5.19 Evaluation of Lateral Ankle Sprain

History	
Classification	Acute injury
MOI	Inversion of the subtalar joint with or without plantar flexion
S/S	Sudden onset of pain on the lateral portion of the ankle immediately anterior and/or inferior to the lateral malleolus
Inspection	
Swelling	Within the sinus tarsi and around the lateral malleolus. With severe (grade II/III) and later stages of healing, swelling may be spread across the dorsum of the foot and toes
Discoloration	Ecchymosis (bruising) around the sinus tarsi and lateral malleolus that spreads and changes colors (black/blue to green/yellow) throughout healing
Palpation	
Pain	Sinus tarsi, inferior to the lateral malleolus, peroneal tendons. Pain localized to the malleolus and styloid process may be indicative of fracture.
Special Tests	
AROM and PROM	Pain/soreness is likely in all ROM. Inversion recreates MOI and causes pain to damaged structures (ATFL and CFL) Eversion will elicit pain with contraction of peroneal muscles if strained Plantar flexion may be included in MOI, and the anterior rotation of the talar head may irritate the ATFL and CFL Dorsiflexion may elicit pain via the peroneal muscles and at the posterior aspect of the ankle in the rare PTFL sprain
RROM	Decreased strength is likely to be found in all motions; extreme weakness with eversion may be indicative of peroneal brevis avulsion from the styloid process of the fifth metatarsal
ATFL	Anterior drawer
CFL	Inversion stress test (talar tilt test)
Fracture	Squeeze, bump, or tuning fork

AROM, active range of motion; ATFL, anterior talofibular ligament; CFL, calcaneofibular ligament; MOI, mechanism of injury; PROM, passive range of motion; PTFL, posterior talofibular ligament; RROM, resistive range of motion; S/S, signs and symptoms.

In addition to malleolar fractures, tibial plafond fractures, talar fractures, and osteochondral lesions can be associated with deltoid ligament injury.[35] Surgical intervention is often recommended, particularly for unstable fracture injuries.[35] Detailed anatomic descriptions of the individual ligaments comprising the deltoid ligament complex are presented in Table 5.1. Quick tips for the sideline evaluation of medial ankle sprains are presented in **Table 5.20**. The collective application of anatomy, MOI, and components of orthopaedic evaluation for the medial ankle sprain is summarized in **Table 5.21**, and special tests are described in Table 5.32.

Syndesmotic or High Ankle Sprains.

Syndesmosis injuries include sprains of the interosseous ligament and/or the anterior and posterior tibiofibular ligaments that stabilize the distal syndesmosis joint of the fibula and tibia.

Although several MOIs for syndesmosis injury have been reported, these injuries are quite rare, occurring less frequently than eversion ankle sprains with a reported incidence of 0.0062 per 1,000 person-years.[31] Higher occurrence is seen in the athletic population, comprising approximately 11% of all ankle injuries. Various MOIs include inversion, plantar flexion, pronation, and internal rotation; however, the two most commonly recognized MOIs are external rotation and hyperdorsiflexion.[7,36] The talus places upward and rotational pressure within the mortise joint during excessive external rotation and/or hyperdorsiflexion, laterally displacing the fibula and effectively spreading the syndesmosis joint.[7]

Table 5.20 Medial Ankle Sprain Quick Tips

Pathology	Description	Presentation (HIPS)	Special Tests/ Imaging	Differential Diagnosis	5-Min Sideline Assessment Tips
Medial ankle sprain	Stretching or tearing of the deltoid ligament complex	Acute onset, with eversion MOI. Pain, swelling, and discoloration on the medial aspect of the ankle	Talar tilt (eversion stress test) Kleiger test (external rotation/ dorsiflexion)	Fracture of the lateral malleolus Talar dome fracture High ankle/ syndesmosis sprain	Pain and swelling over the lateral malleolus are indicative of distal fibular fracture. Difficulty with weight bearing with pain at the anterior distal tibiofibular syndesmosis is indicative of a high ankle sprain.

HIPS, history, inspection, palpation, and special tests; MOI, mechanism of injury.

Table 5.21 Evaluation of Medial/High Ankle Sprain

History	
Classification	Acute injury
MOI	Eversion of the subtalar joint; typically accompanied by extreme dorsiflexion
S/S	Sudden onset of pain on the medial portion of the ankle immediately anterior and/or inferior to the lateral malleolus Pain may also be indicated superior to the medial malleolus at the inferior tibiofibular joint (high ankle sprain) and on the lateral malleolus (fracture)
Observation	
Swelling	Swelling on the medial aspect of the ankle at the deltoid ligament around the medial malleolus which may spread to the dorsum of the foot; swelling may also be found superior to the medial malleolus at the inferior tibiofibular joint at the AITFL and over the lateral malleolus
Discoloration	Ecchymosis around medial malleolus that spreads and changes colors (black/blue to green/yellow) throughout healing; ecchymosis may be present at AITFL and lateral malleolus
Palpation	
Pain	Pain over the deltoid ligament Pain at the inferior tibiofibular joint may be indicative of an AITFL/syndesmosis sprain Pain directly over the lateral malleolus may be indicative of a distal fibular fracture
Special Tests	
AROM and PROM	Pain/soreness is likely in all ROM Eversion with dorsiflexion re-creates MOI and causes pain to damaged structures (deltoid ligament and AITFL) Inversion will elicit pain with contraction of the tibialis posterior muscle if strained. Dorsiflexion may be included in MOI, and superior translation of the talar head into the mortise joint may cause considerable pain with a high ankle sprain (AITFL and syndesmosis). Plantar flexion may elicit pain as the talar head rotates anteriorly against the AITFL, and the tibialis posterior muscle contracts.
RROM	Decreased strength is likely to be found in all motions
Deltoid and AITF Ligaments	Eversion stress test (talar tilt); with dorsiflexion and external rotation (Kleiger test)
Fracture	Squeeze, bump, or tuning fork

AITFL, anterior inferior tibiofibular ligament; AROM, active range of motion; MOI, mechanism of injury; PROM, passive range of motion; ROM, range of motion; RROM, resistive range of motion; S/S, signs and symptoms.

Individuals experiencing a syndesmosis sprain will present with pain on the anterior aspect of the ankle that intensifies with dorsiflexion, making weight bearing difficult. Syndesmosis sprains typically require a longer healing time, immobilization, and reduced weight bearing.[36] Because of a similar MOI, syndesmosis sprains can often occur concurrently with deltoid ligament sprains and ankle fractures. Lateral displacement and rotational forces sustained by the fibula may result in a Maisonneuve fracture of the proximal tibia.[36] The full length of the fibula should be palpated when a syndesmotic sprain is suspected to assess the possibility of a proximal fibular fracture. Detailed anatomic descriptions of the individual ligaments of the syndesmosis joint complex are presented in Table 5.1. Quick tips for the sideline evaluation of high/syndesmotic ankle sprains are presented in Table 5.22. The collective application of anatomy, MOI, and components of orthopaedic evaluation for the syndesmotic ankle sprain is summarized in Table 5.21.

Achilles Tendon Injuries

Achilles Tendinosis. Formerly referred to as Achilles tendinitis, Achilles tendinosis is a chronic condition that is characterized by the degradation of the collagen and elastin components of the Achilles tendon.[37] This change in collagen and elastin content alters the mechanical properties that are crucial to the proper functioning of this powerful tendon. Because tendons are largely avascular, tendinosis is not characterized by the presence of inflammation.[37] In chronic tendinosis injuries, many of the changes to the tendon's collagen and elastin matrix persist without a significant increase in inflammatory cells.[37] The lack of inflammation and remodeling of the matrix tissue may prevent optimal healing from taking place.

Individuals with Achilles tendinosis typically complain of pain along the length of the Achilles tendon and at the insertion site on the posterior aspect of the heel that lasts for at least 3 weeks or longer. Pain is usually greatest in the morning when getting out of bed as the tendon is stretched upon weight bearing. Sometimes, the pain is so excruciating that individuals describe having to crawl until the pain subsides. This pain can also take place after sitting for extended periods of time and may be relieved with extended activity as the tendon becomes more elastic.

Although the tendon is largely avascular, the peritendinous sheath that surrounds the tendon does have a vascular supply and may be subject to acute bouts of inflammation. In these cases, standard acute care protocols may be beneficial. When treating a patient with Achilles tendinosis, it is important to remember that the tendon is composed of the muscles that make up what is called the triceps surae group: the medial and lateral heads of the gastrocnemius, the soleus, and the plantaris muscles. Rehabilitation of the Achilles tendon should focus on the strengthening of these muscles. In fact, Achilles tendinosis injuries have been shown to positively respond to eccentric muscle training.[38] For short-term relief, a heel wedge may be added to a shoe to relieve loading on the Achilles tendon, and a donut pad can also be used to reduce shoe irritation at the heel. Quick tips for the sideline evaluation of Achilles tendinosis are presented in Table 5.23. Details regarding the evaluation of Achilles tendinosis are summarized in Table 5.24, and special tests are described in Table 5.32.

Achilles Tendon Rupture. Achilles tendon rupture is a complete tear of the Achilles tendon, referred to as a grade III tear. Unlike tendinopathy, acute ruptures of the Achilles tendon are characterized by a large inflammatory response.[37] The tendon

Table 5.22 High Ankle/Syndesmosis Sprain Quick Tips

Pathology	Description	Presentation (HIPS)	Special Tests/ Imaging	Differential Diagnosis	5-Min Sideline Assessment Tips
High ankle/ syndesmosis sprain	Stretching or tearing of the distal tibiofibular syndesmosis and/or the anterior and posterior distal tibiofibular ligaments	Acute onset, with an eversion in combination with forceful dorsiflexion MOI.	Kleiger test (external rotation/ dorsiflexion)	Medial ankle sprain Distal fibular fracture Maisonneuve fracture (proximal third of the fibula)	ROM is typically restricted in all directions due to pain, most notable difficulty when performing external rotation and dorsiflexion. Perform squeeze test to rule out fracture.

HIPS, history, inspection, palpation, and special tests; MOI, mechanism of injury; ROM, range of motion.

Table 5.23 Achilles Tendinosis Quick Tips

Pathology	Description	Presentation (HIPS)	Special Tests/Imaging	Differential Diagnosis	5-Min Sideline Assessment Tips
Achilles tendinosis	Degradation and alteration of the elastin and collagen content of the tendon	Insidious onset. Presents as a chronic condition lasting several weeks to months; could be in response to overuse. Pain reported along the length of the tendon. Thickening of the tendon can be seen when compared bilaterally.	N/A	Partial tear of the Achilles tendon	Pain and crepitus can be present during PROM. Patient will often remark that the greatest pain is experienced early in the morning upon getting out of bed and after sitting for extended periods of time. Pain usually subsides with activity.

HIPS, history, inspection, palpation, and special tests; PROM, passive range of motion.

Table 5.24 Evaluation of Achilles Tendinosis

History	
Classification	Chronic/idiopathic injury
MOI	Chronic: Indications of overuse (eg, sudden increase in volume), poor footwear Idiopathic: May not have an obvious injury incident
S/S	Pain at the site of the Achilles tendon; usually hurts first thing in the morning when getting out of bed or after sitting for prolonged periods of time with the tendon in a shortened position
Observation	
Swelling	Swelling may be present in an acute flare-up, but more likely a thickening of the involved tendon will be noticeable
Discoloration	Skin often appears red around the area of the tendon
Palpation	
Pain	Pain along the length of the tendon and may be intense at the insertion on the calcaneus
Crepitus	May be present, depending on the duration of the condition
Special Tests	
AROM and PROM	Pain/soreness is likely with both plantar flexion and dorsiflexion of the ankle Plantar flexion pain will be from contraction of the Achilles tendon; however, in some cases, patient may explain that pain gets better with activity Dorsiflexion pain will be from the stretch of the Achilles tendon. Dorsiflexion ROM may be limited
RROM	Decreased strength with plantar flexion
Special Test	If partial tear is suspected, Thompson squeeze test is warranted

AROM, active range of motion; MOI, mechanism of injury; PROM, passive range of motion; ROM, range of motion; RROM, resistive range of motion; S/S, signs and symptoms.

is composed of the triceps surae muscle group, which includes the primary and powerful plantar flexors of the ankle. Individuals often describe hearing a pop and feeling a sensation of someone either kicking or shooting them in the back of the leg or stepping on their heel. Individuals will likely be unable to plantarflex the ankle and will need assistance walking with crutches or a boot. The tendon can be repaired surgically or nonsurgically through a series of castings that gradually alter the position

Table 5.25 Achilles Tendon Rupture Quick Tips

Pathology	Description	Presentation (HIPS)	Special Tests/ Imaging	Differential Diagnosis	5-Min Sideline Assessment Tips
Achilles tendon rupture	Compete tear of the Achilles tendon	Acute onset with forceful dorsiflexion MOI. Pain, swelling, discoloration, and gross deformity are present at the site of rupture. Active dorsiflexion is weak or nonexistent; unable to dorsiflex against body weight. Typically occurs in males older than 30 years.	Thompson test	Partial tear of the Achilles tendon	Injury is often described as being kicked or shot in the back of the leg. There may be an audible pop. Noticeable concavity where the tendon is no longer intact. Dorsal pedal pulse should be monitored.

HIPS, history, inspection, palpation, and special tests; MOI, mechanism of injury.

of the ankle joint. The muscles of the Achilles tendon are very powerful, which makes for a nonsurgical and lengthy rehabilitation to ensure full fusion of the tendinous ends and strength prior to return to activity. Quick tips for the sideline evaluation of an Achilles tendon rupture are presented in **Table 5.25**, and further details regarding evaluation of an Achilles tendon rupture are provided in **Table 5.26**, and special tests are described in Table 5.32.

Fractures

Fractures of the lower leg and ankle can be common across many sports. Contact sports (eg, football) and high-velocity sports (eg, alpine skiing) are at greater risk for acute fractures, and sports that mostly use the feet (eg, soccer, endurance running) are at greater risk for chronic stress fractures. Quick tips for the sideline evaluation of common ankle fractures are presented in **Table 5.27**. Additional common fractures and their signs and symptoms and radiograph presentations are discussed later.

Jones Fracture. A Jones fracture (**Figure 5.35**) is a transverse fracture of the fifth metatarsal of the foot at the metadiaphysis, between the base and shaft, of the fifth metatarsal. Common mechanisms of injury include an inversion mechanism, in which the lateral border of the foot rotates under the full body weight of the individual, and blunt trauma.[19] Swelling and ecchymosis typically appear throughout the midfoot region, and pain is usually localized at the fracture site on the fifth metatarsal. Crepitus may be felt upon palpation of the fifth metatarsal. Quick tips for the sideline evaluation of a Jones fracture are presented in **Table 5.28**.

Growth Plate Fractures. Growth plate fractures take place in the adolescent population during pubertal development, before their bones are completely calcified. Growth plates are cartilaginous ossification centers responsible for longitudinal bone growth. These areas are considerably weaker than the tendons and ligaments that often attach either directly to the growth plate (primary ossification center) or to an apophysis/tuberosity (secondary ossification center).[39] Therefore, if the internal or external forces applied to a joint are sufficient enough to cause injury, the bone will often fail before the corresponding ligamentous or muscular attachments fail.[39] As a result, the growth plate will fracture, or a portion of the bone will become detached (avulsed) from the bone by the force produced by a ligament or tendon (referred to as an avulsion fracture). It is important to be aware of the common growth plate fractures seen in the adolescent population for the foot and ankle.

Avulsion Fracture of the Distal Fibula. An avulsion of the lateral malleolus (**Figure 5.36**) involving the ATFL can take place during a lateral ankle sprain injury. Adolescent patients with a mechanism of an inversion ankle sprain injury with pain directly on the lateral malleolus or within 6 cm superior to the lateral malleolus should be referred to a physician to rule out an avulsion fracture.[15,16] A squeeze test or bump test may be positive for pain in

Table 5.26 Evaluation of Achilles Tendon Rupture

History	
Classification	Acute
MOI	Complete tear of the Achilles tendon following a forceful plantar flexion contraction
S/S	Pain at the site of the Achilles tendon that may subside shortly after rupture Often described as a feeling of getting shot or kicked in the back of the heel Inability to plantarflex the foot; cannot push off during gait Middle-aged individual (more males than females)
Observation	
Swelling	Swelling may be present in absence of the tendon
Discoloration	Ecchymosis at the posterior aspect of the lower leg
Gross Deformity	Loss of contour to the back of the lower leg
Palpation	
Pain	Pain along the tendon
Defect	Palpable defect: Missing tendon
Special Tests	
AROM and PROM	Patient may not be able to bear weight Unable to perform active plantar flexion due to the lack of the muscular connection; weak plantar flexion may be achieved through tibialis posterior, toe flexors, and peroneal muscles. Pain may be elicited with dorsiflexion
RROM	Extremely weak to absent plantar flexion
Special Test	Thompson squeeze test

AROM, active range of motion; MOI, mechanism of injury; PROM, passive range of motion; RROM, resistive range of motion; S/S, signs and symptoms.

Table 5.27 Ankle Fracture Quick Tips

Pathology	Description	Presentation (HIPS)	Special Tests/ Imaging	Differential Diagnosis	5-Min Sideline Assessment Tips
Lateral malleolus fracture	Fracture of the lateral malleolus or avulsion fracture via detachment of the ATFL	Acute onset following trauma or inversion MOI. Presents with pain, swelling, and discoloration over the lateral malleolus; gross deformity may or may not be present.	Radiograph Anterior drawer	Lateral ankle sprain	Pain directly on or within 6 cm of the lateral malleolus should be referred for radiograph. A suspected grade II/III tear of the ATFL could be indicative of an avulsion fracture and should be referred for radiograph (particularly in the adolescent population).

Pathologies of the Foot and Ankle

Pathology	Description	Presentation (HIPS)	Special Tests/ Imaging	Differential Diagnosis	5-Min Sideline Assessment Tips
Medial malleolus fracture	Fracture of the medial malleolus or avulsion fracture via detachment of the deltoid ligament complex	Acute onset following trauma or eversion MOI. Patient presents with pain, swelling, and discoloration over the medial malleolus; gross deformity may or may not be present	Radiograph Talar tilt (eversion stress test)	Medial ankle sprain High ankle/ syndesmosis sprain	Pain directly on or within 6 cm of the medial malleolus should be referred for a radiograph. A suspected grade II/III tear of the deltoid ligament could be indicative of an avulsion fracture and should be referred for radiograph (particularly in the adolescent population).
Bimalleolar/ trimalleolar fracture and/ or ankle dislocation	Fractures of two or all three malleoli (lateral, medial, and posterior) Dislocation of the mortise joint	Acute onset following trauma; excessive swelling and gross deformity are typically present	Radiograph CT scan may be recommended	Tibia/fibula fractures above the ankle joint	Gross deformity is typically present. Stabilize and prepare for transportation to hospital. Monitor dorsal pedal pulse.

ATFL, anterior tibiofibular ligament; HIPS, history, inspection, palpation, and special tests; MOI, mechanism of injury.

the area of the fracture. Additionally, because of the proximity of the lateral malleolus to the surface of the skin, the use of a tuning fork may elicit a positive response for pain or discomfort when compared to the noninjured foot.

Avulsion Fracture of the Fifth Metatarsal, Styloid Process. An avulsion fracture of the styloid process (**Figure 5.37**) is the most common fracture of the fifth metatarsal.[19] The peroneal brevis muscle inserts on the styloid process of the fifth metatarsal bone and is a common culprit of avulsion fracture during an inversion ankle sprain. It is quite normal for the styloid process to be painful during an inversion mechanism. Additionally, as the peroneal muscles are often strained, it is also not uncommon for active eversion to be weak, even without a peroneal brevis avulsion. However, if pain is specifically indicated over the styloid process and/or it remains painful without improvement over the acute stage of an inversion ankle injury, adolescents should be referred to rule out a peroneal brevis avulsion fracture. Although weak, the patient will be able to perform eversion, as the peroneus longus remains intact (insertion at base of the first metatarsal and medial cuneiform). A modified bump test of the fifth toe may be positive. Because the styloid process lies just beneath the surface of the skin with little subcutaneous tissue, the use of a tuning fork may elicit a positive response for pain or discomfort when compared to the noninjured foot. Quick tips for the sideline evaluation of an avulsion fracture of the fifth metatarsal are presented in **Table 5.29**. Although adolescents are at a higher risk for this type of avulsion fracture, a peroneal brevis avulsion fracture can occur in adults.

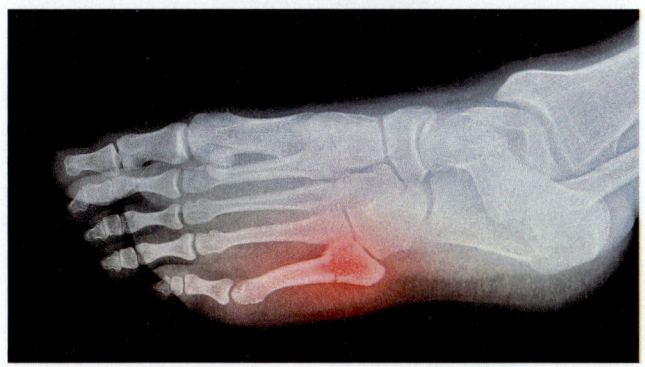

Figure 5.35 Radiograph showing a Jones fracture.
© Yinspire/Shutterstock

Table 5.28 Jones Fracture Quick Tips

Pathology	Description	Presentation (HIPS)	Special Tests/ Imaging	Differential Diagnosis	5-Min Sideline Assessment Tips
Jones fracture	Fracture of the fifth metatarsal approximately 1 cm distal to the styloid process	Acute onset after rolling or landing on the lateral side of the foot (supination). Presents with pain on the lateral aspect of the foot, with point tenderness just at/ below the base of the fifth metatarsal	Radiograph	Avulsion fracture of the styloid process Peroneal tendon strain Contusion and swelling associated with lateral ankle sprain	Pain elicited upon palpation of the proximal fifth metatarsal. May be diffuse if associated with lateral ankle sprain, but point tenderness will develop over the acute injury period (72 hours). Pain or discomfort may be experienced with the application of a tuning fork when compared bilaterally.

HIPS, history, inspection, palpation, special tests.

Calcaneal Apophysitis. Although not a fracture, calcaneal apophysitis, often referred to as Sever condition (previously known as Sever disease), is characterized by the inflammation of the apophysis on the posterior aspect of the calcaneus at the insertion of the Achilles tendon. Adolescents experience this injury when inflammation of the apophysis develops as a result of the repetitive tension to the secondary ossification center, applied by the Achilles tendon (triceps surae contraction).[40] Adolescents who participate in endurance sports or sports with repetitive jumping, such as basketball, are at the highest risk for the development of this condition.[40] Because the Achilles tendon pulls on the secondary ossification center, the osteophytes attempt to strengthen the apophysis with the addition of calcified bone.[40] This excessive calcification, over time, can lead to an exaggerated protrusion at the posterior aspect of the calcaneus. This protrusion can become a lifelong nuisance because it is often a source of irritation when wearing shoes. Apophysitis is usually

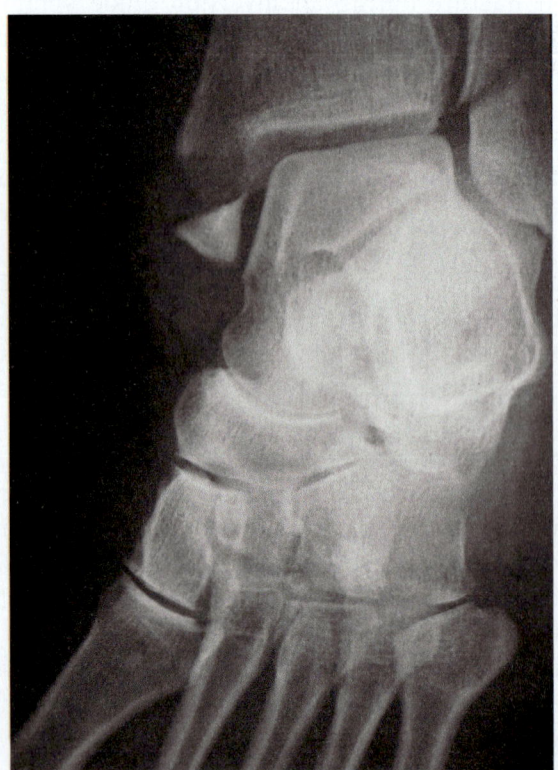

Figure 5.36 Radiograph showing avulsion of the lateral malleolus.

© kuehdi/Shutterstock

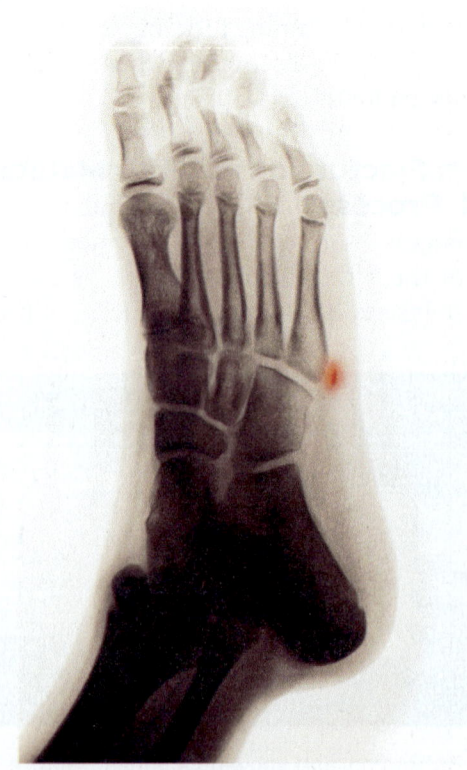

Figure 5.37 Radiograph showing avulsion fracture of the styloid process.

© Callista Images/Image Source/Getty Images

Table 5.29 Avulsion Fracture of the Fifth Metatarsal Quick Tips

Pathology	Description	Presentation (HIPS)	Special Tests/ Imaging	Differential Diagnosis	5-Min Sideline Assessment Tips
Avulsion fracture of the fifth metatarsal	Fracture of the styloid process of the fifth metatarsal via detachment of the peroneus brevis muscle	Acute onset after inversion MOI. Pain on the lateral aspect of the foot, with point tenderness just at the base of the fifth metatarsal. May present with crepitus	Radiograph	Jones fracture Peroneal tendon strain Contusion and swelling associated with lateral ankle sprain	AROM will be diminished or weak with eversion when compared bilaterally.

AROM, active range of motion; HIPS, history, inspection, palpation, and special tests; MOI, mechanism of injury.

rather painful, particularly when pressure from shoes or palpation is applied to the posterior aspect of the calcaneus. Donut pads can be used to help redistribute pressure away from the insertion site; however, the best treatment is to provide sufficient rest for the healing and strengthening of the apophysis without constant loading from the Achilles tendon. Quick tips for the sideline evaluation of calcaneal apophysitis are presented in **Table 5.30**.

Tibial and Fibular Ankle Fractures. Distal tibia and fibular ankle fractures can sometimes be hard to distinguish from ligamentous injury if gross deformity is not present. Nondisplaced fractures often present similarly to severe ligamentous injuries, with pain, swelling, and discoloration around the joint. The Ottawa Ankle Rules, presented in Table 5.6, should be used to determine whether referral for radiography is warranted.[15,16,41] Displaced fractures may also result in the dislocation of the joint. The limb should be stabilized for transport, and circulation should be monitored via the dorsal pedal pulse.

Stress Fractures. When bone is subjected to repeated submaximal stress over time, microscopic injuries can accumulate and result in a stress fracture, which may, if untreated, progress to a complete fracture.[42,43] Stress fractures result from an imbalance of osteoclastic over osteoblastic activity at a localized region of the bone.[43] This imbalance can be influenced by several factors, such as an increase in training volume, a change in terrain, and poor nutrition.[43] Among the most common locations, the metatarsals of the foot and the tibia rank as the two most common locations for stress fractures.[42,43] Metatarsals account for approximately 38% of all stress fractures in the lower limb, most commonly occurring in the second and third metatarsals.[42] Among tibial stress fractures, 58% occur in the distal third of the bone, followed by 30% in the middle third, and finally 13% in the proximal third. Although not as common, the calcaneus, navicular, talus, cuneiforms, and sesamoids may experience stress fractures as well.[42,43]

Stress fractures develop over time and therefore may appear to have more of an insidious onset. Patients

Table 5.30 Calcaneal Apophysitis Quick Tips

Pathology	Description	Presentation (HIPS)	Special Tests/ Imaging	Differential Diagnosis	5-Min Sideline Assessment Tips
Calcaneal apophysitis (formerly, Sever disease)	Apophysitis of the secondary ossification center at the insertion site of the Achilles tendon in the adolescent population	Insidious onset that presents as an overuse, chronic condition. Presents with pain, swelling, and redness on the posterior aspect of the calcaneus	N/A	Achilles tendinosis Retrocalcaneal bursitis	Adolescent injury typically seen with an increase in activity. Take a thorough history to establish duration of current and previous episodes as well as change in activity volume, terrain, and/or footwear. Donut pad may provide relief.

HIPS, history, inspection, palpation, special tests.

Table 5.31 Stress Fractures Quick Tips

Pathology	Description	Presentation (HIPS)	Special Tests/ Imaging	Differential Diagnosis	5-Min Sideline Assessment Tips
Stress fractures	Imbalance of bone resorption and bone remodeling; increase in osteoclastic (resorption) activity	Insidious onset due to overuse; typically experienced with cyclic activity (eg, endurance running)	Bump test Tuning fork Bone scan Radiograph CT scan	Dependent on suspected area	Patient will present with nonspecific but localized pain that may intensify after activity. Endurance athletes, particularly females with amenorrhea, are at high risk.

HIPS, history, inspection, palpation, special tests.

will typically present with a dull, achy/nonspecific pain that is rather localized. Data show that 21.5% of stress fractures are recurrent injuries and that approximately 20% are season ending.[43] Advanced stress fractures may present in a radiograph as a calcification on the bone surface; however, stress fractures often do not appear on a radiograph, and therefore a bone scan is required to identify a stress fracture.

Endurance athletes tend to be at the highest risk for the development of stress fractures. Additionally, women experience much higher rates of stress fractures compared to men (9.13 versus 4.44 per 100,000 athletic exposures).[43] High occurrence in women is often associated with a condition known as female athlete triad. Female athlete triad consists of three concurrent clinical entities: menstrual dysfunction, low energy availability due to a lack of appropriate caloric intake (with or without an eating disorder), and decreased bone mineral density.[44] Because of the complex multifactorial nature of stress fracture etiology, a thorough history can assist in determining factors that may contribute to the development of a stress fracture. Quick tips for the sideline evaluation of lower limb stress fractures are presented in **Table 5.31**. **Table 5.32** is a summary of the special tests related to the foot and ankle.[45-66]

Quick Tips for Evaluations

Foot and Ankle: The Ottawa Ankle Rules

The Ottawa Ankle Rules were developed as a quick orthopaedic evaluation tool to rule out fracture or the need for radiographic images following foot/ankle injury.[15] Approximately 15% of people presenting to the emergency room with an ankle injury leave with a fracture diagnosis; most of these people (85%) receive the far more common diagnosis of ankle sprain injury.[33] Approximately 23,000 people visit the emergency room daily in the United States seeking care for an injured ankle.[33] This translates to a large and unnecessary economic burden associated with emergency room costs, specifically radiographs. The Ottawa Ankle Rules can be used with a lateral (inversion) ankle sprain in both adults and adolescents, regardless of whether the foot was in a plantarflexed position. By using the Ottawa Ankle Rules, clinicians and other allied health care providers, such as athletic trainers and physical therapists, can detect almost 100% of fractures that would require radiographic evaluation.[16,33]

To reduce unnecessary radiographs and patient exposure to radiation, the Ottawa Ankle Rules were developed through the careful evaluation of the presenting characteristics of 750 patients in the emergency departments of the Ottawa Civic and Ottawa General hospitals.[15] From this study, the clinicians established that individuals who present with pain within the malleolar zone (distal 6 cm of the fibula or tibia) and/or the posterior edge of either malleoli *and* are (1) age 55 years or older or (2) unable to bear weight and complete at least four consecutive walking steps are at high risk for fracture, and a radiograph should be obtained (rules summarized in Table 5.6).[15,16,33] A radiograph may also be warranted if there is pain in the midfoot *and* bone tenderness is present at any of the following bones: navicular, cuboid, and base of the fifth metatarsal.[15,16,33]

Developed and established in 1992, the Ottawa Ankle Rules have remained a mainstay in orthopaedic diagnostic tools, as a more recent systematic review and meta-analysis of the Ottawa Ankle Rules literature shows 97.9% to 99.8% sensitivity and 28.8% to 42.3% specificity.[16] A higher sensitivity means the Ottawa Ankle Rules are better at ruling out the possibility of a fracture, rather than diagnosing a fracture. Therefore, clinicians can be rather confident that, if all the employed rules are found to be negative, there is a less than 2% chance that a fracture exists, otherwise referred to as a false negative. The Ottawa Ankle Rules have been found to be more sensitive in the adult population; however, the rules still have a high sensitivity in the adolescent population at 94.9% to 99.1%.[16] Variation of sensitivity between the adult and adolescent populations is likely due to the difference in bony development from adolescent to adult.

Pathologies of the Foot and Ankle

Table 5.32 Special Tests for the Orthopaedic Evaluation of the Foot and Ankle

Test	Patient Position	Procedure	Positive Test	Implication	Evidence
Navicular drop	**Beginning** Seated in a chair with foot on the ground in talar neutral **Ending** Standing with feet approximately 6 inches apart	Mark the location of the navicular tuberosity. While the patient is seated, place him or her in the talar neutral position, and mark a line on a piece of paper to denote the height of the tuberosity from the ground (A). Have the patient stand naturally, and mark the height again using the same paper (B).	Change in navicular height of 1 cm or greater	Overpronation; functional pes planus	Not reported or inconclusive
Feiss line	**Beginning** Seated on table with legs extended **Ending** Standing with feet approximately 6 inches apart	Mark the tip of the medial malleolus and the base of the first metatarsophalangeal joint; then draw a line between the points, and note the position of the navicular tuberosity (A). Once the patient is bearing weight, ensure the marks are still accurate, and note the position of the navicular tuberosity once again (B).	Navicular tuberosity located below the line in seated or standing position	Low navicular tuberosity seated; Congenital pes planus Navicular in line, which then drops below line when standing; Functional pes planus	Not reported or inconclusive

(continues)

Chapter 5 Foot and Ankle

Table 5.32 Special Tests for the Orthopaedic Evaluation of the Foot and Ankle *(continued)*

Test	Patient Position	Procedure	Positive Test	Implication	Evidence
Anterior drawer test (ankle)	Seated on the end of a table with the knee flexed	With one hand stabilizing the lower leg, use the other hand to grasp the calcaneus. Use the forearm to support the foot in a slightly plantarflexed position. Glide the calcaneus and talus anteriorly while stabilizing the lower leg.	Anterior translation of the talus on the mortise that is greater than the uninvolved side or production of pain	Sprain of the anterior talofibular ligament	**Sn:** 74% to 96% **Sp:** 67% to 100% **+ LR:** Small to moderate **− LR:** Small
Talar tilt test (inversion)	Seated on the end of a table with the knee flexed	With one hand stabilizing the lower leg, use the other hand to grasp the talus and calcaneus. Maintain the foot in a neutral or slightly dorsiflexed position while bringing the ankle into inversion. *Note:* The thumb or forefinger of the stabilizing hand can be placed just inferior to the lateral malleolus to feel for any gapping.	Excessive tilt or gapping when compared to the uninvolved side or production of pain	Sprain of the calcaneofibular ligament	**Sn:** 30% to 50% **Sp:** 88% to 95% **+ LR:** Small to moderate **− LR:** Small

Pathologies of the Foot and Ankle

Talar tilt test (eversion)	Seated on the end of a table with the knee flexed	With one hand stabilizing the lower leg, use the other hand to grasp the talus and calcaneus. Maintain the foot in a neutral or slightly dorsiflexed position while bringing the ankle into eversion. ***Note:** The thumb or forefinger of the stabilizing hand can be placed in the area of the deltoid ligament to feel for any gapping.	Excessive tilt or gapping when compared to the uninvolved side or production of pain	Sprain of the deltoid ligament	Not reported or inconclusive
Subtalar glides (medial and lateral) A (medial) B (lateral)	Medial glide: Side-lying on the limb being tested Lateral glide: Side-lying on the limb not being tested with a towel roll beneath the distal tibia	With one hand stabilizing the talus in the mortise, use the other hand to grasp the calcaneus. Apply a downward force to glide the calcaneus on the talus.	Increase or decrease in translation when compared to the uninvolved side	Medial glide: Decreased mobility may be associated with calcaneal eversion and decreased pronation. Excessive medial glide has also been associated with lateral ankle sprains Lateral glide: Decreased mobility may be associated with calcaneal inversion and decreased supination	Medial **Sn:** 58% **Sp:** 88% **+ LR:** Small **− LR:** Small Lateral Not reported or inconclusive

(continues)

Table 5.32 Special Tests for the Orthopaedic Evaluation of the Foot and Ankle (continued)

Test	Patient Position	Procedure	Positive Test	Implication	Evidence
Forced dorsiflexion test	Seated on the end of a table with the knee flexed	Use one hand to grasp the calcaneus and apply pressure to the anterolateral ankle (sinus tarsi region) using the thumb. Use the other hand to passively dorsiflex the ankle to end range.	Reproduction of pain or increase in pain reported from thumb pressure	Anterior ankle impingement	Sn: 95% Sp: 88% + LR: Moderate − LR: Large
Cotton test	Supine with foot off the table	With one hand stabilizing the mortise (do not compress the syndesmosis), use the other hand to grasp the calcaneus and talus. Apply force to move the talus laterally.	Increased translation of the talus when compared to the uninvolved side or pain in the area of the distal tibiofibular joint	Anterior inferior tibiofibular ligament sprain	Sn: 25% Other values not reported or inconclusive
Kleiger test	Seated on the end of a table with the knee flexed	With one hand stabilizing the mortise (do not compress the syndesmosis), use the other hand to grasp the medial aspect of the calcaneus and externally rotate the foot. To test the syndesmosis, dorsiflex the foot slightly. To test the deltoid ligament, keep the foot neutral or slightly plantarflexed.	Syndesmosis: Pain in the anterolateral ankle Deltoid ligament: Pain in the medial foot or translation away from the medial malleolus	Anterior inferior tibiofibular ligament sprain (anterior pain) or deltoid ligament sprain (medial pain)	Not reported or inconclusive

A (testing the syndesmosis)

B (testing the deltoid ligament)

Pathologies of the Foot and Ankle

Squeeze test	Supine in knee extension	Use both hands to compress the tibia and fibula together. Squeeze proximally to test the syndesmosis. Squeeze away from the site of pain, and move gradually closer if fracture is suspected.	<u>Syndesmosis</u> Pain at the distal tibiofibular joint <u>Fracture</u> Pain elicited at or near the compression site	Anterior inferior tibiofibular ligament sprain or fracture	<u>Syndesmosis</u> **Sn:** 30% **Sp:** 93% **+ LR:** Small **− LR:** Small <u>Fracture</u> Not reported or inconclusive
Dorsiflexion compression test	Standing	Have the patient dorsiflex by driving the knee forward over a planted foot until he or she reaches end range or produces pain (A). Apply compression around the malleoli to squeeze the syndesmosis together, and have the patient repeat the motion (B).	Decrease in pain when compression is applied or increased available motion when compression is applied.	Anterior inferior tibiofibular ligament sprain	Not reported or inconclusive

(continues)

Table 5.32 Special Tests for the Orthopaedic Evaluation of the Foot and Ankle (continued)

Test	Patient Position	Procedure	Positive Test	Implication	Evidence
Dorsiflexion eversion test	Side-lying on the limb being tested	Use one hand to bring the foot into maximal dorsiflexion and eversion while extending the toes. Hold this position for 5 to 10 seconds. Use the other hand to palpate the tibial nerve posterior to the medial malleolus.	Numbness, pain, or increased tenderness to palpation of the tibial nerve	Tarsal tunnel syndrome	Numbness Sn: 25% Sp: 95% to 100% + LR: Large - LR: Small Pain Sn: 57% Sp: 95% to 100% + LR: Large - LR: Small Tenderness Sn: 98% Sp: 95% to 100% + LR: Large - LR: Large
Tinel sign (ankle)	Seated or supine with the leg extended	Use one or two fingers to tap over the medial aspect of the ankle, posterior to the medial malleolus over the tibial nerve.	Pain or tingling along the path of the tibial nerve	Tarsal tunnel syndrome	Sn: 17% to 58% Sp: 80% + LR: Small - LR: Small
Thompson test	Prone with foot off the edge of the table	Use one hand to squeeze the muscle belly of calf.	Lack of plantar flexion upon squeezing the calf	Achilles tendon rupture	Sn: 96% Sp: 93% + LR: Large - LR: Large

Pathologies of the Foot and Ankle

Test	Position	Procedure	Positive Finding	Indicates	Statistics
Bump/percussion test	Seated or supine with the foot and ankle off the edge of the table	Use the nondominant hand to stabilize the foot in a neutral position. Use the other hand to firmly bump the heel using the palm of the hand.	Localized pain at the site of injury	Fracture	Not reported or inconclusive
Tuning fork test	Seated or supine with leg extended	Place an active tuning fork on a bony prominence distal to the site of injury/pain. Place a stethoscope head proximal to the site on the same bone (eg, if a fibular fracture is suspected, place the tuning fork on the lateral malleolus and the stethoscope on the fibular head).	Diminished sound or absence of sound in the involved limb compared to the uninvolved side. Patient report of pain with tuning fork application or difference in sensation when compared bilaterally	Fracture	**Sn:** 75% to 92% **Sp:** 67% to 80% **+ LR:** Small **− LR:** Small

LR, likelihood ratio; Sn, sensitivity; Sp, specificity.
All figures in table © Jones & Bartlett Learning.

CASE STUDY 1

During a volleyball match, a 16-year-old girl who plays center lands on her opponent's foot under the net after coming down from a blocked shot. The athletic trainer observes from courtside that the player's right foot inverted, rolling on to the lateral aspect of the foot and ankle, while in a plantarflexed position. Because the player is unable to bear weight, the athletic trainer and a fellow teammate help her to the bench. Upon observation, the athletic trainer notices there is already significant swelling of the dorsal lateral aspect of the ankle; however, no other gross deformities are present. During palpation, the athlete reports a significant amount of pain over the sinus tarsi. When asked to perform AROM movements of the foot and ankle, the athlete seems both unwilling and unable to perform full eversion due to pain and noticeable weakness. Dorsiflexion is equally as painful. The anterior drawer test is positive for both pain and laxity; talar tilt is positive for pain but negative for laxity. Because of the level of pain, the athletic trainer decides to apply an ice bag and give the athlete time to recover from the acute pain before evaluating further.

1. What is your differential diagnosis? List two or three potential injuries, based on the information provided in the case study.
2. Which lateral ankle ligament do you suspect is most likely involved in this injury?

Follow-up: After 15 minutes, the athletic trainer removes the ice bag and reexamines the ankle. Further palpation of important anatomic landmarks results in the detection of localized pain over the base of the fifth metatarsal (styloid process). When asked to stand, the athlete is able to apply only partial weight to the right foot. However, when asked whether she can walk, she is able to take only two steps.

1. What is your new differential diagnosis, following this updated information?
2. What is your major concern at this point, and what is your immediate course of action?
3. Considering the athlete's age, if localized pain had been present in the lateral malleolar zone, what additional injury would you need to have on your differential diagnosis?
4. Is there equal concern of avulsion fractures occurring in the adult population with lateral ankle sprains?

CASE STUDY 2

During practice, a 22-year-old woman who is a gymnast overrotates off the vault and lands on the medial aspect of her foot in an everted position. She reports extreme pain on the anteromedial aspect of the ankle just inferior to the medial malleolus. She is unable to bear weight and therefore cannot walk. The coach helps the athletic trainer carry the athlete off the mats and into the athletic training clinic for closer evaluation. Upon observation, the athletic trainer notices a considerable amount of swelling on both the anterior and lateral aspects of the ankle. During palpation, the athlete reports extreme pain over the area of the deltoid ligament and extreme point tenderness on the lateral malleolus as well. The athlete is unwilling to perform AROM movements.

1. What is your differential diagnosis? List two or three potential injuries based on the information provided.
2. Are PROM movements by the athletic trainer warranted at this time?
3. What is the potential concern with pain over the lateral malleolus?
4. What is your immediate course of action?

Follow-up: Radiographs are positive for a distal fibular head fracture associated with a medial ankle sprain to the deltoid ligament complex.

1. Describe how the lateral malleolus would fracture with an eversion mechanism.

CASE STUDY 3

A 45-year-old man reports to a clinic complaining of pain at the back of his right heel that has lasted for approximately 3 to 6 months. He enjoys golfing on the weekends and walking the course, but he has had considerable discomfort recently. He reports that his pain is at its worst in the morning. His pain tends to flare up throughout the day when he has been sitting for more than 30 minutes and after he plays a round of golf. He has no known MOI, and self-treatment with NSAIDs has provided little, if any, relief. He has not bought any new shoes recently; however, he remarks that the pressure from all of his shoes irritates the condition at times and he has been wearing the same golf shoes for the past 2 years.

Upon observation, the athletic trainer notes that the right Achilles tendon appears broader than the left tendon and the skin in that area is noticeably red. The tendon is tender/painful to the touch, particularly at the insertion on the posterior aspect of the heel. The patient has AROM within normal limits for plantar flexion and reports discomfort with dorsiflexion. PROM is slightly limited in dorsiflexion compared to the left foot, and the patient reports pain at end range. Thompson test is negative for Achilles tendon rupture or partial tear.

1. What is your diagnosis, based on the aforementioned findings?
2. Why do you believe this injury has responded poorly to NSAIDs?
3. What steps can be taken at this time to put less strain on the Achilles tendon during walking and provide pain relief for the patient?
4. Do you think radiographs would be recommended in this case?

Follow-up: After 6 weeks of treatment and a rest from golf, the patient's pain has started to subside, and he is becoming more functional. The patient and the athletic trainer have decided to start adding some golf activity back into the patient's routine.

1. Now that the patient's pain is starting to subside and his gait is returning to normal, what additional assessment would you suggest be performed in preparation for returning to activity?
2. What recommendations would you provide regarding the patient's footwear?

CASE STUDY 4

During a weekend wrestling tournament, a 20-year-old male wrestler reports to the athletic trainer complaining of pain in his right great toe. He describes that, during his match, he was positioned low to the ground with his right foot slightly behind him. As he locked up with his opponent, he lunged forward, pushing off his right great toe, when it slipped backward, thereby hyperextending the big toe. He reports that he is now experiencing pain every time he moves through the push-off phase of gait. Upon observation, the athletic trainer notes slight swelling and redness on the plantar aspect of the first MTP joint. There is no obvious deformity; however, there is pain at the first MTP joint during palpation. The athlete has normal and full AROM.

1. Based on the MOI, what injury is most likely?
2. The patient has full AROM, but what ROM would you test to confirm your diagnosis?
3. What would be a positive indicator for this test, and how would you compare your results?

Follow-up: The athletic trainer diagnoses the injury as mild to moderate in grade.

1. Can the wrestler continue to participate in the tournament?
2. What would you recommend for acute treatment and management of this injury for the tournament?
3. The wrestler is from a visiting school; please list two or three things the athletic trainer should do before the athlete returns home.

ONE-IN-A-MILLION CASE STUDY

An athletic trainer is called onto the field to examine a 21-year-old man who is a collegiate football player who sustained an injury to his right foot. He describes his right foot in a fixed and fully plantarflexed position as another player landed on the back of his heel, thereby applying an axial load to the foot. Upon observation, the athletic trainer notices swelling over the dorsum of the foot, and, upon palpation, the athlete has considerable pain in the midfoot region over the first and second metatarsal heads. The athlete has full ROM; however, he is unable to bear weight.

1. Provide your differential diagnosis. List two or three potential injuries to either rule them in or out, based on the information provided.
2. Discuss your next course of action for diagnosis and acute treatment of this injury.

Follow-up: The athlete returns to the athletic training clinic the following day with dorsal to plantar, lateral, and medial oblique views (non–weight bearing) of his right foot that he received at the emergency room. The radiographs are negative for fracture; however, he is still unable to bear weight, and the swelling over the dorsum of his foot has markedly increased. Further, the pain over the first and second metatarsal heads has not improved and instead has become more localized. The athletic training staff take note of what appears to be a slight gap between the medial and intermediate cuneiforms on the radiograph.

1. How does this information inform your differential diagnosis?
2. What is your greatest concern at this point, and what is your next course of action, based on the information above?
3. Why is the type of radiograph that was obtained at the emergency room not the appropriate special test for this type of injury?
4. What can you do to improve special test results for this type of injury in the future?

WRAP-UP

Critical Thinking Questions

1. What are the strengths and weaknesses in the design of the medial longitudinal arch? In what ways might changes in the shape of the arch affect structures farther up the kinetic chain?
2. What role could the windlass mechanism play in rehabilitation? How could it be manipulated to target specific tissues and structures?
3. Given the location of the retrocalcaneal bursa, how might it affect your assessment of Achilles tendon injury in both acute and chronic conditions?

Pearls and Pitfalls

- **Trust your physical examination.**
  - Diagnostic imaging is a useful tool, but it can be expensive and time consuming. In many cases, a sound and thorough physical examination is sufficient when evaluating soft-tissue injury to the foot and ankle, as demonstrated previously in this chapter. Remember to use the Ottawa Ankle Rules when trying to determine whether imaging of the foot and/or ankle is truly necessary.
- **Special tests are the last step in HIPS for a reason.**
  - Special tests are useful diagnostic tools that too often become a crutch to young clinicians. In the HIPS evaluation method, special tests are performed after the history, inspection, and palpation have all occurred. By the time special tests are performed, you should already have a differential diagnosis in mind, and special tests can help confirm or refute your assessments. Always take into consideration the diagnostic accuracy of the test and what that means for your evaluation. Not all foot and ankle special tests are created equal.
- **Reassess lingering injuries.**
  - An often-overlooked pathology is anterior impingement in the ankle. When a patient sustains a lateral or syndesmotic ankle sprain, changes in the joint can lead to lingering symptoms, such as pain and pinching in the anterior ankle. Rather than continuing to treat the same injury to no avail, reassess the problem. Are there biomechanical changes or differences in arthrokinematics compared to the healthy limb? A proper assessment is the foundation of a treatment plan, and it is important to remember that injuries can evolve over time.

References

1. Nwawka OK, Hayashi D, Diaz LE, et al: Sesamoids and accessory ossicles of the foot: anatomical variability and related pathology. *Insights Imaging* 2013;4(5):581-593.
2. Dedmond BT, Cory JW, McBryde A, Jr.: The hallucal sesamoid complex. *J Am Acad Orthop Surg* 2006;14(13):745-753.
3. Maceira E, Monteagudo M: Subtalar anatomy and mechanics. *Foot Ankle Clin* 2015;20:195-221.
4. Irwin TA, Lien J, Kadakia AR: Posterior malleolus fracture. *J Am Acad Orthop Surg* 2013;21(1):32-40.
5. Welck MJ, Zinchenko R, Rudge B: Lisfranc injuries. *Injury* 2015;46(4):536-541.
6. Panchani PN, Chappell TM, Moore GD, et al: Anatomic study of the deltoid ligament of the ankle. *Foot Ankle Int* 2014;35:916-921.

7. Norkus SA, Floyd RT: The anatomy and mechanisms of syndesmotic ankle sprains. *J Athl Train*. 2001;36(1):68-73
8. Golano P, Vega J, de Leeuw PA, et al: Anatomy of the ankle ligaments: a pictorial essay. *Knee Surg Sports Traumatol Arthrosc* 2010;18(5):557-569.
9. Brage ME, Bennett CR, Whitehurst JB, Getty PJ, Toledano A: Observer reliability in ankle radiographic measurements. *Foot Ankle Int* 1997;18(6):324-329.
10. Brage ME, Rockett M, Vraney R, Anderson R, Toledano A: Ankle fracture classification: a comparison of reliability of three x-ray views versus two. *Foot Ankle Int* 1998;19(8):555-562.
11. Bontrager KL: *Textbook of Radiographic Positioning and Related Anatomy*. St. Louis, MO, Elsevier Mosby, 2014.
12. Vangsness CT, Carter V, Hunt T, Kerr R, Newton E: Radiographic diagnosis of ankle fractures: are three views necessary? *Foot Ankle Int* 1994;15(4):172-174.
13. Hedges JR, Anwar RAH: Management of ankle sprains. *Ann Emerg Med* 1980;9(6):298-302.
14. van Dijk CN, Mol BWJ, Lim LSL, Marti RK, Bossuyt PMM: Diagnosis of ligament rupture of the ankle joint: Physical examination, arthrography, stress radiography and sonography compared in 160 patients after inversion trauma. *Acta Orthop Scand* 1996;67(6):566-570.
15. Stiell IG, Greenberg GH, McKnight RD, Nair RC, McDowell I, Worthington JR: A study to develop clinical decision rules for the use of radiography in acute ankle injuries. *Ann Emerg Med* 1992;21:384-390.
16. Beckenkamp PR, Lin CWC, Macaskill P, Michaleff ZA, Maher CG, Moseley AM: Diagnostic accuracy of the Ottawa Ankle and Midfoot Rules: a systematic review with meta-analysis. *Br J Sports Med* 2017;51:504-10.
17. Nielson JH, Gardner MJ, Peterson MGE, et al: Radiographic measurements do not predict syndesmotic injury in ankle fractures: an MRI study. *Clin Orthop Relat Res* 2005;436:216-221.
18. Kerr R, Forrester DM, Kingston S: Magnetic resonance imaging of foot and ankle trauma. *Orthop Clin N Am* 1990;21(3):591-601.
19. Rosenberg ZS, Beltran J, Bencardino JT: MR imaging of the ankle and foot. *RadioGraphics* 2000;20(suppl_1):S153-S179.
20. Ekinci S, Polat O, Günalp M, Demirkan A, Koca A: The accuracy of ultrasound evaluation in foot and ankle trauma. *Am J Emerg Med* 2013;31(11):1551-1555.
21. Khoury V, Guillin R, Dhanju J, Cardinal É: Ultrasound of ankle and foot: overuse and sports injuries. *Semin Musculoskelet Radiol* 2007;11(2):149-161.
22. Rawool NM, Nazarian LN: Ultrasound of the ankle and foot. *Semin Ultrasound CT MR* 2000;21(3):275-284.
23. Starkey C, Ryan J: *Evaluation of Orthopedic and Athletic Injuries*, ed 2. Philadelphia, PA, FA David, 2002.
24. Astrom M, Arvidson T: Alignment and joint motion in the normal foot. *J Orthop Sports Phys Ther* 1995;22(5):216-222.
25. Hunt KJ, Hurwit D, Robell K, Gatewood C, Botser IB, Matheson G: Incidence and epidemiology of foot and ankle injuries in elite collegiate athletes. *Am J Sports Med* 2017;45:426-433.
26. Besse JL: Metatarsalgia. *Orthop Traumatol Surg Res* 2017;103(1S):S29-S39.
27. Di Caprio F, Meringolo R, Shehab Eddine M, Ponziani L: Morton's interdigital neuroma of the foot: a literature review. *Foot Ankle Surg* 2018;24(2):92-98.
28. Rodeo SA, O'Brien SJ, Warren RF, Barnes R, Wickiewicz TL: Turf toe: diagnosis and treatment. *Phys Sportsmed* 1989;17:132-147.
29. Goff JD, Crawford R: Diagnosis and treatment of plantar fasciitis. *Am Fam Phys* 2011;84:676-682.
30. Boakye L, Chambers MC, Carney D, Yan A, Hogan MCV, Ewalefo SO: Management of symptomatic plantar fasciitis. *Oper Tech Orthop* 2018;28:73-78.
31. Shah S, Thomas AC, Noone JM, Blanchette CM, Wikstrom EA: Incidence and cost of ankle sprains in United States emergency departments. *Sports Health* 2016;8:547-552.
32. Delahunt E, Bleakley CM, Bossard DS, et al: Clinical assessment of acute lateral ankle sprain injuries (ROAST): 2019 consensus statement and recommendations of the International Ankle Consortium. *Br J Sports Med* 2018;52:1304-1310.
33. Petscavage J, Baker SR, Clarkin K, Luk L: Overuse of concomitant foot radiographic series in patients sustaining minor ankle injuries. *Emerg Radiol* 2010;17:261-265.
34. Lötscher P, Lang TH, Zwicky L, Hintermann B, Knupp M: Osteoligamentous injuries of the medial ankle joint. *Eur J Trauma Emerg Surg* 2015;41(6):615-621.
35. Alshalawi S, Galhoum AE, Alrashidi Y, et al: Medial ankle instability: the deltoid dilemma. *Foot Ankle Clin* 2018;23(4):639-657.
36. Williams GN, Allen EJ: Rehabilitation of syndesmotic (high) ankle sprains. *Sports Health* 2010;2(6):460-470.
37. Klatte-Schulz F, Minkwitz S, Schmock A, et al: Different achilles tendon pathologies show distinct histological and molecular characteristics. *Int J Mol Sci* 2018;19(2):404.
38. Magnussen RA, Dunn WR, Thomson AB: Nonoperative treatment of midportion Achilles tendinopathy: a systematic review. *Clin J Sport Med* 2009;19(1):54-64.
39. Schiller J, DeFroda S, Blood T: Lower extremity avulsion fractures in the pediatric and adolescent athlete. *J Am Acad Orthop Surg* 2017;25(4):251-259.
40. Hendrix CL: Calcaneal apophysitis (Sever disease). *Clin Podiatr Med Surg* 2005;22(1):55-62.
41. Goost H, Wimmer MD, Barg A, Kabir K, Valderrabano V, Burger C: Fractures of the ankle joint: investigation and treatment options. *Dtsch Arztebl Int* 2014;111(21):377-388.
42. Welck MJ, Hayes T, Pastides P, Khan W, Rudge B: Stress fractures of the foot and ankle. *Injury* 2017;48(8):1722-1726.
43. Rizzone KH, Ackerman KE, Roos KG, Dompier TP, Kerr ZY: The epidemiology of stress fractures in collegiate student-athletes, 2004–2005 through 2013–2014 academic years. *J Athl Train* 2017;52:966-975.
44. Nazem TG, Ackerman KE: The female athlete triad. *Sports Health* 2012;4(4):302-311.
45. Langley B, Cramp M, Morrison SC: Clinical measures of static foot posture do not agree. *J Foot Ankle Res* 2016;9:45.
46. Nilsson MK, Friis R, Michaelsen MS, Jakobsen PA, Nielsen RO: Classification of the height and flexibility of the medial longitudinal arch of the foot. *J Foot Ankle Res* 2012;5(1):3.
47. Croy T, Koppenhaver S, Saliba S, Hertel J: Anterior talocrural joint laxity: diagnostic accuracy of the anterior drawer test of the ankle. *J Orthop Sports Phys Ther* 2013;43(12):911-919.
48. Hertel J, Denegar CR, Monroe MM, Stokes WL: Talocrural and subtalar joint instability after lateral ankle sprain. *Med Sci Sports Exerc* 1999;31(11):1501-1508.
49. Lynch SA: Assessment of the injured ankle in the athlete. *J Athl Train* 2002;37(4):406-412.

50. Schneiders A, Karas S: The accuracy of clinical tests in diagnosing ankle ligament injury. *Eur J Physiother* 2016;18(4) 245-253.
51. Schwieterman B, Haas D, Columber K, Knupp D, Cook C: Diagnostic accuracy of physical examination tests of the ankle/foot complex: a systematic review. *Int J Sports Phys Ther* 2013;8(4):416-426.
52. Slaughter AJ, Reynolds KA, Jambhekar K, David RM, Hasan SA, Pandey T: Clinical orthopedic examination findings in the lower extremity: correlation with imaging studies and diagnostic efficacy. *Radiographics* 2014;34(2):e41-e55.
53. Bahr R, Pena F, Shine J, et al: Mechanics of the anterior drawer and talar tilt tests: a cadaveric study of lateral ligament injuries of the ankle. *Acta Orthop Scand* 1997;68(5): 435-441.
54. Gaebler C, Kukla C, Breitenseher MJ, et al: Diagnosis of lateral ankle ligament injuries: comparison between talar tilt, MRI and operative findings in 112 athletes. *Acta Orthop Scand* 1997;68(3):286-290.
55. Rosen AB, Ko J, Brown CN: Diagnostic accuracy of instrumented and manual talar tilt tests in chronic ankle instability populations. *Scand J Med Sci Sports* 2015;25(2):e214-221.
56. Mulligan EP: Evaluation and management of ankle syndesmosis injuries. *Phys Ther Sport* 2011;12(2):57-69.
57. Alonso A, Khoury L, Adams R: Clinical tests for ankle syndesmosis injury: reliability and prediction of return to function. *J Orthopaed Sports Phys Ther* 1998;27(4): 276-284.
58. Sman AD, Hiller CE, Rae K, et al: Diagnostic accuracy of clinical tests for ankle syndesmosis injury. *Br J Sports Med* 2015;49(5):323-329.
59. Teitz CC, Harrington RM: A biomechanical analysis of the squeeze test for sprains of the syndesmotic ligaments of the ankle. *Foot Ankle Int* 1998;19(7):489-492.
60. Cimino WR: Tarsal tunnel syndrome: review of the literature. *Foot Ankle* 1990;11(1):47-52.
61. Datema M, Hoitsma E, Roon KI, Malessy MJA, Dijk JGV, Tannemaat MR: The Tinel sign has no diagnostic value for nerve entrapment or neuropathy in the legs. *Muscle Nerve* 2016;54(1):25-30.
62. Garras DN, Raikin SM, Bhat SB, Taweel N, Karanjia H: MRI is unnecessary for diagnosing acute achilles tendon ruptures: clinical diagnostic criteria. *Clin Orthop Relat Res* 2012;470(8):2268-2273.
63. Somford MP, Hoornenborg D, Wiegerinck JI, Nieuwe Weme RA: Are you positive that the Simmonds-Thompson test is negative?: a historical and biographical review. *J Foot Ankle Surg* 2016;55(3):682-683.
64. Moore MB: The use of a tuning fork and stethoscope to identify fractures. *J Athl Train* 2009;44(3):272-274.
65. Schneiders AG, Sullivan SJ, Hendrick PA, et al: The ability of clinical tests to diagnose stress fractures: a systematic review and meta-analysis. *J Orthopaed Sports Phys Ther* 2012;42(9):760-771.
66. Toney CM, Games KE, Winkelmann ZK, Eberman LE: Using tuning-fork tests in diagnosing fractures. *J Athl Train* 2016;51(6):498-499.

CHAPTER 6

Knee Joint

Kaitlyn Shank, MEd, ATC, CCRP
Joseph M. Hart, PhD, ATC, FACSM, FNATA

OVERVIEW

The knee joint is made up of the articulating femur, tibia, and patella bones. The knee is also made up of many soft-tissue structures, such as muscles, ligaments, joint capsule, and menisci, and delicate structures, such as the major nerve, artery, and vein that run through the posterior knee. This chapter will review not only the anatomy of the knee but also the pathophysiology and presentation of common injuries to these structures. Clinicians can use the skills discussed in this chapter to help effectively identify and treat common athletic knee injuries.

LEARNING OBJECTIVES

After completing this chapter, the reader will be able to do the following:

1. Identify all key components of a knee evaluation.
2. Obtain a thorough history, including key questions that may help provide clues to the structures of the knee that are injured.
3. Perform special tests that target specific structures of the knee.
4. Give appropriate referral and treatment instructions to a patient based on the evaluation.

FUN FACTS ABOUT THE KNEE

- The patella is the largest sesamoid bone in the body. A sesamoid bone is a bone that lies within a tendon or muscle.
- More than 50% of athletic injuries are lower extremity injuries, with the knee and ankle accounting for the most injuries.
- The cruciate ligaments have been known about since ancient Egypt, and their anatomy was described in the famous Smith Papyrus (3000 BC).

Introduction

The knee is a hinge joint that moves in all planes: in the frontal plane, through varus and valgus motion; the sagittal plane, through flexion and extension; and the transverse plane, through the rotation of the screw-home mechanism. The screw-home mechanism occurs during the last 30° of knee extension, where the tibia or femur rotates to achieve full extension. In open-chain motion, the tibia externally rotates, and in closed-chain movements, the femur internally rotates to accommodate for the incongruent (different size) condyles.[1-3]

The knee is a commonly injured joint in the athletic population. It is important, as a clinician, to understand the fundamentals of a clinical evaluation of the knee. The information in this chapter should be used to enable the clinician to complete a thorough evaluation of a knee injury and provide an appropriate treatment or referral.

Clinical Anatomy

Bones of the Knee

The knee joint is made up of the distal femur and the proximal tibia, which articulate with one another to allow flexion, extension, and rotation of the knee joint.[1] The third bone in the knee joint is the patella, which is a sesamoid bone that articulates with the femur.[4] The fibula is another bone in the knee joint, which articulates with the tibia.[1] The bony anatomy of the knee is shown in **Figure 6.1**.

Femur

The distal femur is composed of the medial and lateral condyles.[1] The condyles are convex structures that allow articulation with the tibia. The articular surfaces of both condyles have thick cartilage that allows for smooth motion against the tibia bone. When injury occurs, such as an articular cartilage lesion, the smooth translation between condyles is disrupted, which causes pain in the knee joint. Patients often report deep pain in the knee that they cannot touch.

Superior to the articulating surfaces of the medial and lateral condyles are the medial and lateral epicondyles. The epicondyles are palpable bony landmarks on either side of the knee joint. The medial epicondyle is the proximal attachment of the medial collateral ligament, and the lateral epicondyle is the proximal attachment of the lateral collateral ligament. The epicondyles may become tender to palpation when the iliotibial (IT) band causes irritation and inflammation around the lateral epicondyle or when injury occurs to either the medial or lateral collateral ligaments.

Tibia

The proximal tibia also has medial and lateral condyles, often referred to as the medial and lateral tibial plateaus.[1] The tibial plateaus are concave, which allows them to articulate with and cradle the convex femoral condyles to allow knee joint motion. Between the medial and lateral condyles of the tibia is the intercondylar eminence. The intercondylar eminence serves as the origin of the anterior cruciate ligament (ACL).[1] The superior medial and lateral condyles are known as the medial and lateral joint lines. These are important structures to include in palpation during an examination because they may be tender as a result of injury to the bone or nearby meniscus.

The tibial tuberosity is in the midline of the proximal tibia, distal to the joint line. This serves as the insertion point of the patellar tendon. The tibial tuberosity could be inflamed with injury to the patellar tendon. In pediatric populations, those with Osgood-Schlatter disease present with a very prominent tibial tuberosity because of the patellar tendon pulling on the bone while the child is growing.

Another bony prominence on the tibia is Gerdy tubercle, which lies on the lateral aspect of the proximal tibia and is the insertion point of the IT band. This prominence can become tender or inflamed with injury or tightness of the IT band.

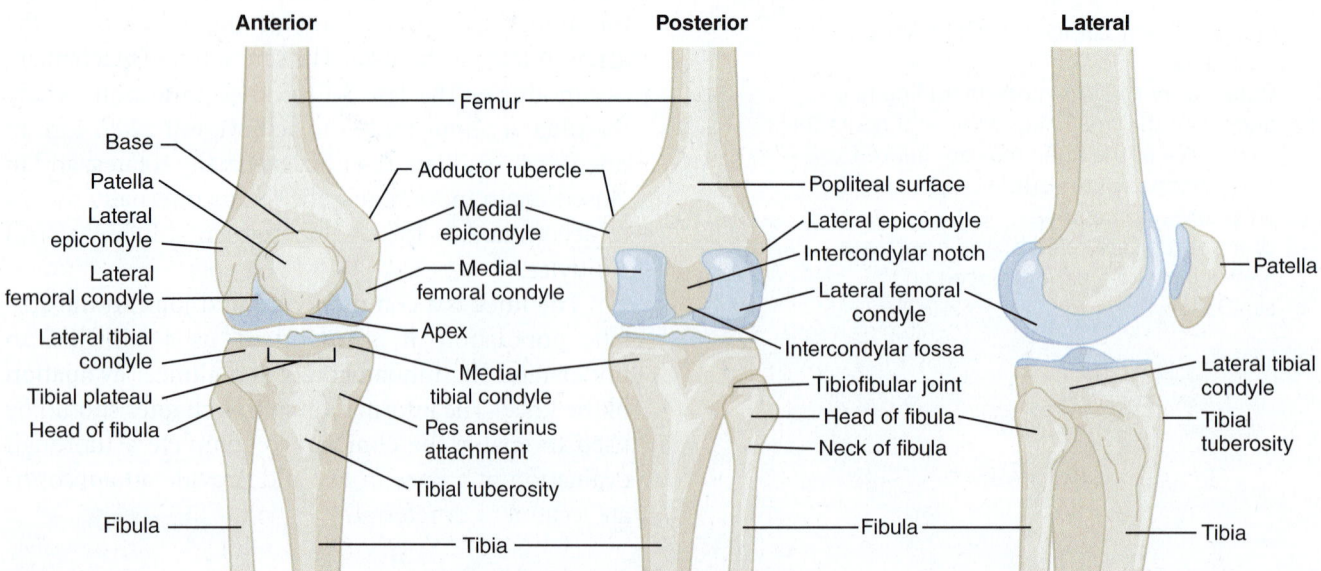

Figure 6.1 Drawing showing bony anatomy of the knee.

Patella

The patella is the largest sesamoid bone in the body.[4] It has thick articular cartilage that allows it to articulate with the femur's trochlear notch. The medial patellofemoral ligament inserts on the superior medial aspect of the patella to restrict lateral movement of the patella.

Fibula

The fibula articulates with the proximal tibia and serves as the distal attachment of the lateral collateral ligament.

Articulations and Ligamentous Support

Ligaments

The ACL originates on the intercondylar eminence of the tibia, runs laterally and posteriorly to insert on the lateral femoral condyle, and is responsible for preventing anterior translation and excessive anterolateral rotation of the tibia.[2,5] It is a commonly injured ligament, often from a plant-and-twist mechanism with the knee in flexion and the tibia externally rotated. The ACL is responsible for stabilizing the knee, and a deficient ACL could lead to wear and tear on other structures, such as the meniscus, if left unrepaired.[2,3]

The posterior cruciate ligament (PCL), originating on the posterior intercondylar area of the tibia and inserting on the lateral side of the medial femoral condyle, is responsible for preventing posterior translation of the tibia.[1] A PCL injury can occur from a posterior force on the tibia and is commonly known as the dashboard injury, as a result of the knee hitting the dashboard of a car during an accident.[2]

The lateral collateral ligament (LCL), also sometimes referred to as the fibular collateral ligament, resists varus knee joint movement. It originates on the lateral femoral epicondyle and inserts on the head of the fibula.[1] The LCL is a thin ligament that can be sprained or ruptured from excessive outward, varus force to the knee.[2]

The medial collateral ligament (MCL), also referred to as the tibial collateral ligament, resists valgus knee joint movement. It originates on the medial femoral epicondyle and inserts on the medial tibia, below the condyle.[1] The MCL is thicker and more membranous than the LCL. It is one of the most commonly injured ligaments in the knee as a result of inward, or valgus, force; injury to the MCL can cause laxity in the ligament, which is graded on a scale from I (minimal laxity) to III (great laxity, with minimal or no end point).[2,3,6]

The four aforementioned ligaments are shown in **Figure 6.2**, and details of ligament origin and insertion details are outlined in **Table 6.1**.

The IT band, although not a ligament, is a thick band of fascia on the lateral aspect of the knee originating at the iliac crest and tensor fascia lata muscle.[1] It inserts distal to the knee joint on the tibia, at Gerdy's tubercle.[1] The IT band has a strong connection of fascia to the quadriceps muscles and lateral patella. Because of this, tightness in the IT band may cause malalignment and poor biomechanics.

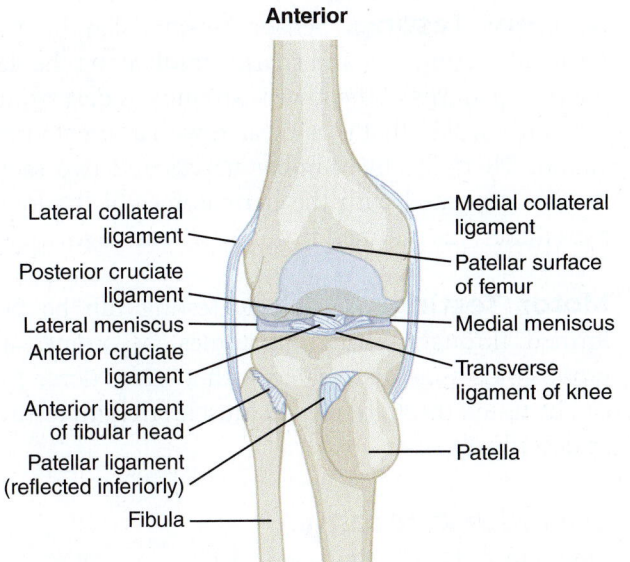
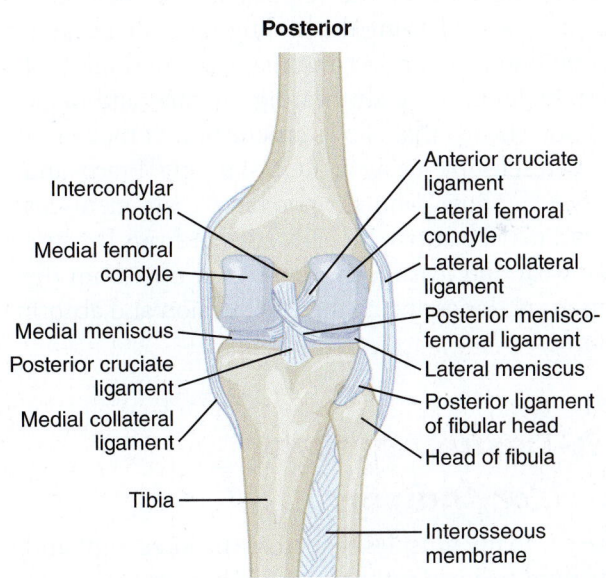

Figure 6.2 Drawing showing ligaments of the knee.

© Jones & Bartlett Learning

Table 6.1 Knee Ligament Origins and Insertions

Ligament	Origin	Insertion
Anterior cruciate ligament	Intercondylar eminence of the tibia	Lateral femoral condyle
Posterior cruciate ligament	Posterior intercondylar eminence of the tibia	Lateral side of the medial femoral condyle
Lateral collateral ligament	Lateral femoral epicondyle	Head of the fibula
Medial collateral ligament	Medial femoral epicondyle	Medial tibia
Iliotibial band	Iliac crest and tensor fascia lata muscle	Gerdy tubercle

Runners commonly experience distal knee pain caused by a tight IT band repetitively rubbing over the lateral femoral epicondyle.

Menisci

The medial meniscus is the larger of the two menisci. It is C shaped and is located on top of the articular surface of the medial condyle of the tibia. The lateral meniscus is smaller and more circular, located on top of the articular surface of the lateral condyle of the tibia. The medial and lateral menisci can been seen[1] in Figure 6.2.

The menisci are responsible for cushioning and attenuating forces through the knee joint. They are thick cartilage rings that can absorb and cushion load, preventing bone-on-bone articulation. A meniscal injury can be painful not only because of the tear itself but also because the load-bearing weight is not being properly absorbed by the menisci. Menisci are often surgically repaired, rather than removed (meniscectomy), because of the importance of their load absorption role.[3] During the healing stage after repair, it is important to protect the meniscus and allow it to heal by limiting weight-bearing activities and range of motion (ROM) that allows articulation of the femur and meniscus by using a ROM-limiting brace and crutches.[2,3] Those who do not have their meniscus repaired may be at risk for early osteoarthritis because of the wear and tear on the femur and tibia from the meniscus no longer being there to cushion and absorb the force.

Soft-Tissue Anatomy
Muscular Anatomy

There are many muscles that cross the knee joint and contribute to knee joint motion. These muscles are often grouped by muscle action. The extensors extend the knee when concentrically contracted, and the flexors flex the knee when concentrically contracted. There are other muscles, such as the adductors, that cross the knee joint, but they produce actions other than knee extension or flexion. All muscle origin, insertion, action, and innervations[1,2,7,8] are described in **Table 6.2**. They are also shown in **Figures 6.3**, **6.4**, and **6.5**.

Neurologic Anatomy

Patellar Tendon Reflex. A reflex is an involuntary action in response to a stimulus. A nerve is stimulated, and, rather than an action potential being initiated and sending a message to the brain, the stimulus is processed at the spinal level. This stimulation causes an involuntary movement by the associated muscle. The patellar tendon reflex is tested by hitting the patellar tendon, just inferior to the patella, while the knee is flexed and relaxed (bent over a table, for example).[2,3] A negative reflex could indicate a problem with the spinal cord.

Sensory Testing. Sensory testing can be performed by using dull and sharp stimuli along the dermatome patterns of the lower extremity. A dermatome is an area of skin that is associated with a spinal innervation. There are five lumbar nerves and two sacral nerves associated with the dermatomes of the lower extremities,[1] as outlined in **Table 6.3** and **Figure 6.6**.

Motor Testing. Neurologic testing can be performed through testing myotomes. Myotomes are groups of muscles associated with a spinal nerve that can be tested through manual muscle strength testing[1] as described in **Table 6.4**.

Vascular Anatomy

The popliteal vein and artery are located in the posterior knee (**Figure 6.7**). They are centered at the midline of the popliteal fossa and run alongside the tibial

Table 6.2 Muscular Anatomy

Muscle	Origin	Insertion	Action	Innervation	Palpation	Manual Muscle Test
Quadriceps						
Rectus femoris	AIIS				Palpate from the AIIS down the middle thigh, over the patella, and through the patellar tendon to the insertion on the tibial tuberosity.	Patient seated upright at the edge of the examination table with legs bent over the edge. Patient extends his or her knee straight out. Support hand is placed above the knee while pressure is applied to the distal tibia with the other hand.
Vastus lateralis	Greater trochanter and lateral linea aspera	Tibial tuberosity	Extends the knee	Femoral nerve	Palpate from the greater trochanter, down the lateral thigh, over the patella, and through the patellar tendon to the insertion on the tibial tuberosity.	
Vastus medialis	Medial linea aspera				Palpate from the superior medial thigh, down the medial aspect of the thigh, over the patella, and through the patellar tendon to the insertion on the tibial tuberosity.	
Vastus intermedius	Anterior surface of the femur				This muscle lies directly under the rectus femoris and cannot be palpated superficially.	

(continues)

Chapter 6 Knee Joint

Table 6.2 Muscular Anatomy *(continued)*

Muscle	Origin	Insertion	Action	Innervation	Palpation	Manual Muscle Test
Hamstrings						
Biceps femoris	Ischial tuberosity	Head of the fibula	Flexes the knee	Sciatic nerve	Palpate from the ischial tuberosity down the lateral aspect of the posterior thigh, and follow the tendon to the insertion, on the head of the fibula.	Patient lies prone on table with knee flexed to 45° and slightly externally rotated. Place support hand on posterior thigh, and push distal tibia toward the table with the other hand.
Semitendinosus		Pes anserinus			Palpate from the ischial tuberosity down the medial aspect of the posterior thigh, and follow the tendon to the insertion, on the pes anserinus.	
Semimembranosus		Posterior medial condyle of the tibia			Palpate from the ischial tuberosity down the medial aspect of the posterior thigh, and follow the tendon to the insertion, on the posterior medial condyle of the tibia (the medial tendon when differentiating against the semitendinosus).	Patient lies prone on table with knee flexed to 45° and slightly externally rotated. Place support hand on posterior thigh, and push distal tibia toward the table with the other hand.

Clinical Anatomy

Other Muscles

	Origin	Insertion	Action	Innervation	Palpation	Manual Muscle Test
Adductor magnus	Inferior ramus, ischial ramus, and ischial tuberosity	Linea aspera and adductor tubercle of the femur		Obturator nerve	Palpate as a unit from the ischial ramus/pubis, down the medial thigh. Adductor magnus insertion can be found superior to the medial femoral condyle, on the medial thigh (adductor tubercle).	Patient side lying on table with upper leg abducted and lower leg adducted. Support upper leg while applying pressure downward on lower leg, proximal to knee joint.
Adductor longus	Superior pubis	Middle third of linea aspera	Adducts the thigh			
Adductor brevis	Lateral inferior pubis ramus	Proximal linea aspera				
Gracilis	Inferior pubic symphysis	Anteromedial tibia, on pes anserinus	Adducts the leg, flexes the knee, and internally rotates the hip when knee is flexed		Palpate from the AIIS, down and across the anterior thigh (diagonal direction), to its insertion on the pes anserinus.	Patient side lying on table with upper leg abducted and lower leg adducted. Support upper leg while applying pressure downward on lower leg, proximal to the ankle joint.
Sartorius	Anterior superior iliac spine	Anteromedial tibia, on pes anserinus	Flexes the knee (also flexes, abducts, and externally rotates hip)	Femoral nerve	Palpate from the inferior pubic symphysis down the medial thigh, across the knee joint, to its insertion on the pes anserinus.	Patient lies supine on table with hip and knee flexed, with hip abduction and external rotation. Place your hand on proximal knee and proximal ankle. Apply pressure in the direction of hip extension, internal rotation, adduction, and knee extension.

(continues)

Chapter 6 Knee Joint

Table 6.2 Muscular Anatomy *(continued)*

Muscle	Origin	Insertion	Action	Innervation	Palpation	Manual Muscle Test
Gastrocnemius	Medial head: medial femoral condyle Lateral head: lateral femoral condyle	Posterior calcaneus via the Achilles tendon	Flexes knee and plantarflexes foot	Tibial nerve	Palpate from the posterior medial and lateral femoral condyles down the posterior tibia until insertion at the posterior calcaneus (via Achilles tendon) is reached.	Patient standing (possibly holding onto chair for stability). Instruct patient to rise up on toes, pushing body weight directly upward. Push down on shoulders.
Plantaris	Inferior lateral supracondylar ridge of femur	Posterior calcaneus via the Achilles tendon	Flexes knee and plantarflexes foot		This muscle is difficult to palpate because it lies under the gastrocnemius muscle. Palpation near the origin may be possible by palpating the posterior lateral femoral condyle.	
Popliteus	Lateral surface of the lateral femoral condyle	Proximal posterior tibia	Flexes and medially rotates the knee		This muscle cannot be isolated for palpation because it lies under the gastrocnemius.	Patient sits with knee flexed over the end of the table and tibia externally rotated. Hold the distal tibia and apply internal rotation force to the tibia.

AIIS, anterior inferior iliac spine.
All figures in table © Jones & Bartlett Learning.

Clinical Anatomy   **135**

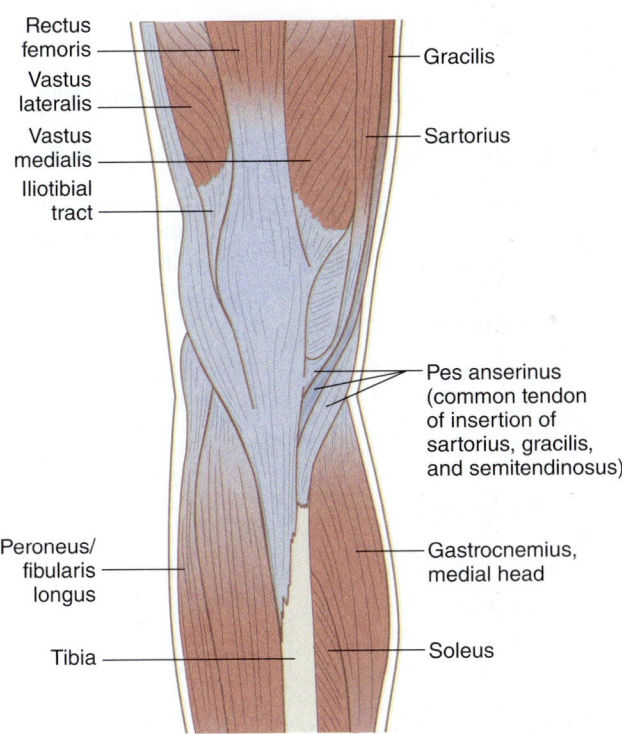

Figure 6.3 Drawing showing anterior view of knee muscles.

© Jones & Bartlett Learning

nerve. Many branches stem off the popliteal artery and vascularize the structures of the knee joint; they also continue on to serve the distal leg.[1] It is important to evaluate the vascular anatomy after a major knee injury by palpating for a pulse. In the knee, this

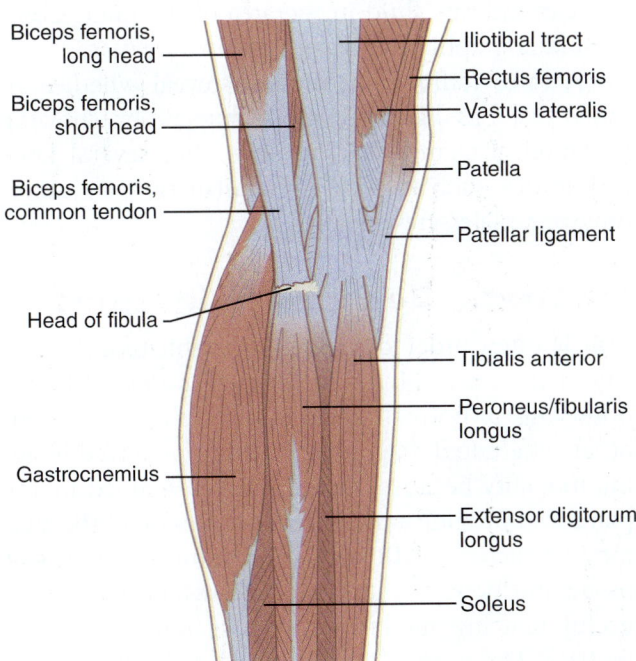

Figure 6.4 Drawing showing lateral view of knee muscles.

© Jones & Bartlett Learning

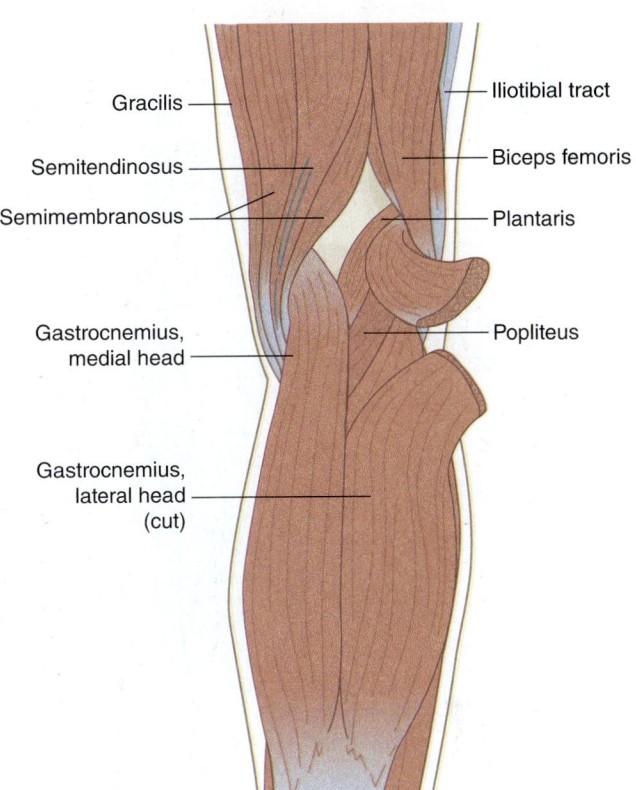

Figure 6.5 Drawing showing posterior view of knee muscles.

© Jones & Bartlett Learning

Table 6.3	Dermatomes Associated With the Knee
L3	Medial knee, medial calf
L4	Anterior knee
L5	Anterior-lateral and lateral knee
S1	Posterior lateral knee
S2	Posterior midline of knee

Table 6.4	Myotomes Associated With the Knee
L3, L4	Extension of the knee
L5, S1	Flexion of the knee

is done by placing the fingers in the posterior knee. It is important that the knee be flexed while trying to palpate the pulse because, by positioning the patient this way, it relaxes the posterior leg muscles, which would otherwise block access to the pulse. If the popliteal pulse cannot be assessed, another method of assessing the vascularity would be to assess distally. An intact distal pulse could indicate the blood is still being supplied to the distal leg, which would indicate that the popliteal vascular structures are likely

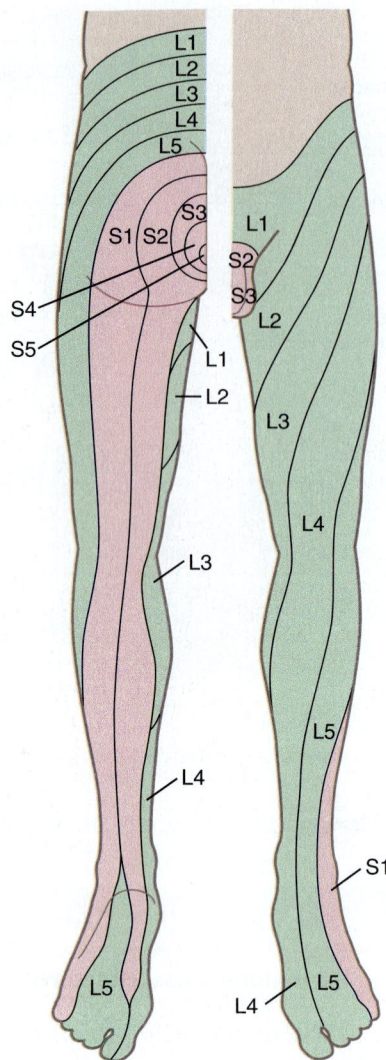

Figure 6.6 Drawing showing dermatome patterns of the lower extremities.
© Jones & Bartlett Learning

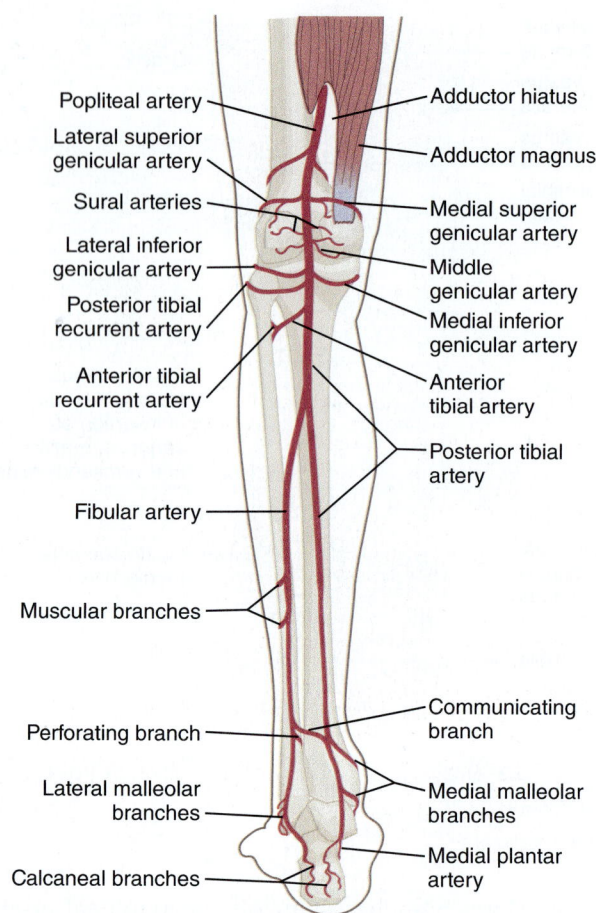

Figure 6.7 Drawing showing arteries of the posterior leg.
© Jones & Bartlett Learning

intact. The distal pulses that can be assessed are the posterior tibial pulse and the dorsal pedal pulse.[2] The posterior tibial pulse can be found just posterior to the medial malleolus, and the dorsal pedal pulse can be found on the top of the midfoot just lateral to the extensor hallucis longus tendon.

Overview of Radiology and Imaging

Radiograph

Radiographs are commonly taken of the knee to assess for abnormalities in the bone, such as a fracture, arthritis, myositis ossificans, patient alignment (mechanical or anatomic), patellar position and alignment, or even a tumor. They allow medical professionals to observe the integrity of the bony structures of the knee joint and can indicate fluid in the area of the joint. Common radiographic views are listed in **Table 6.5**.

A knee radiograph can also reveal whether an individual has had a previous surgery by showing postsurgical changes in the knee after several knee procedures, such as an ACL reconstruction, an osteotomy, or a plate/screw fixation.

Magnetic Resonance Imaging

MRI is often ordered to assess the soft-tissue integrity of the knee. Many doctors will order MRI after observing a normal knee radiograph to rule out other differential diagnoses. MRI is a preferred imaging modality because images can be obtained in any plane and provide a more detailed picture of the anatomic structures. MRI can show injury to both soft tissue and bone at the same time, which makes it a useful imaging modality to assess musculoskeletal injuries. Many knee injuries can be observed using MRI, such as a rupture of a ligament (ACL, PCL, MCL, or LCL), meniscus pathologies, articular cartilage injuries, and tendon/muscular injuries. MRI

Table 6.5 Common Radiographic Views of the Knee

Anterior-Posterior	Posterior-Anterior	Lateral	Sunrise	Long Leg
Used to assess the anterior knee and joint spaces	Used to assess the posterior knee and joint spaces	Used to assess medial knee and patellar position	Used to assess patellofemoral joint	Used to assess alignment of the knee (varus vs. valgus)

All photos courtesy of Kaitlyn Shank.

can be performed using different weighting to allow certain structures to stand out more than others. T1 weighting will show fat brighter and other structures darker, whereas T2 weighting will make structures, especially fluid, brighter in the image. Different weighting is ordered depending on the suspected injury, which would allow for the best view of the involved structure. In **Figure 6.8**, panel A is an example of T2 weighting, and panels B and C are examples of T1 weighting.

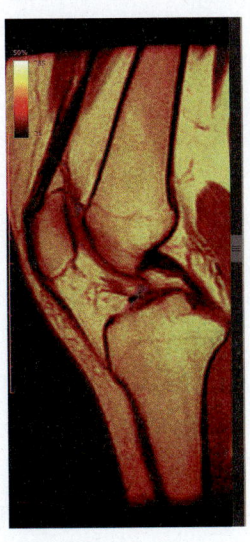
A

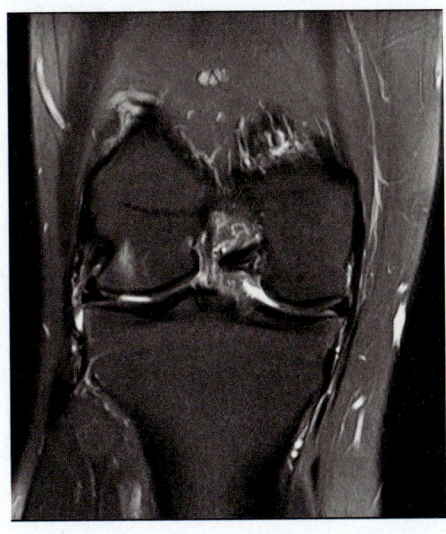
B

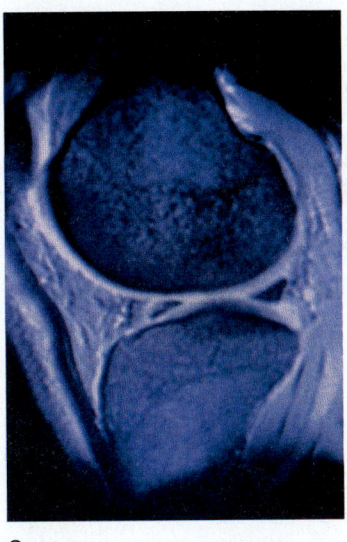
C

Figure 6.8 Radiographs showing T2 and T1 weighting. **A.** Anterior cruciate ligament tear. **B.** Articular cartilage defect. **C.** Meniscus tear.

A. springsky/Shutterstock; B. Courtesy of Kaitlyn Shank; C. edwardolive/Shutterstock.

Evaluation of the Knee

History

Taking a comprehensive history is one of the most important components of an evaluation. After taking a history, a clinician should be able to come up with a list of differential diagnoses for further assessment in his or her evaluation. The clinician's role during the history is to listen. Remember that the history is subjective, meaning this is how the patient observes and experiences the symptoms of the injury. It is helpful for a clinician to facilitate the conversation in such a way that the questions can help rule in or out particular injuries. Examples of these questions are presented in **Table 6.6**.

During the history portion of an evaluation, the clinician should be able to pick up on key words or phrases that can provide clues about the patient's potential injuries. Listed in **Table 6.7** are key terms that may indicate a particular injury.

It is important to avoid tunnel vision after taking a history and to keep an open mind. Rather than focusing on one specific injury, the clinician should make a refined list of differential diagnoses to keep all possibilities in consideration. Specifying one injury based on history alone may lead to the clinician making an inaccurate diagnosis of the injury; this could potentially cause the clinician to miss important information, such as a concomitant injury. As the evaluation continues, the list will be narrowed down by performing injury-specific assessments to rule in or out each of the differential pathologies.

Inspection

The inspection portion of an evaluation of the knee joint can be very telling. When inspecting the knee, the purpose is to look for deformity, discoloration, and swelling/effusion.

- Deformity
  - Patellar dislocation: An acute injury in which the patella has migrated (laterally) out of the trochlear notch.
  - Knee dislocation: An acute injury in which the femur or tibia is displaced from its normal position.

Table 6.6 Knee Evaluation Questions for Specific Injuries

Question	Clue
How fast did your knee swell up?	Fast (blood), possibly ACL; slow (synovial), possibly meniscus
Does your knee feel unstable?	Stabilizing ligament, such as ACL
Does your knee pop or catch?	Meniscus tear or loose body
Is the pain sharp or dull pain?	Sharp: possible fracture; dull: possible soft-tissue irritation, such as iliotibial band

ACL, anterior cruciate ligament.

Table 6.7 Key Words Used to Describe Knee Injuries

Injury	Key Words
Meniscal injury	Feeling a pop or catch when moving the knee while weight bearing or pain with deep squatting
Anterior cruciate ligament tear	Mechanism of injury of planting the foot and cutting, and then hearing a pop in the knee; feels unstable to walk
Chondromalacia patella	Pain feels deep under the patella, as if the patient cannot touch it
Loose body in joint	Knee locks when trying to move it; then, the patient has to readjust before continuing through range of motion
Fracture	Intense, sharp pain in a focal area
Iliotibial band syndrome	Popping or snapping on the lateral aspect of the knee

- Discoloration: Redness or ecchymosis
  - Redness, especially near a wound, may be indicative of an infection.
  - Ecchymosis is indicative of trauma to an area that has caused bleeding under the skin.
    - Deep red or purple discoloration can indicate severe bleeding, which may have been caused by a more severe injury that was fairly recent.
    - Green/yellow discoloration can indicate an older bruise that is now in its healing phase.
- Swelling/effusion
  - Joint effusion specifically occurs when there is injury inside the knee joint capsule. Injuries that may cause an effusion are ruptures of the cruciate ligaments, meniscal injuries, patellar subluxations or dislocations, and injuries to the articular cartilage. A joint effusion differs from regular knee swelling in that the inflammation is contained within the knee joint.
  - Swelling in the knee occurs outside of and more superficial to the joint capsule. For example, if the patellar tendon is injured and inflamed, there will be swelling around the tendon itself, which appears different than would a joint effusion.
- Range of motion
  - Active range of motion: ROM measurement of the knee with a goniometer is performed by having the patient lying supine on an examination table[7,9,10] (**Figure 6.9**). The stationary arm is aligned with the greater trochanter of the femur. The moving arm is then aligned with the lateral malleolus. The fulcrum of the goniometer is placed at the lateral knee, over the joint line. This can be seen in Figure 6.9. Knee extension is measured with the leg in extension; if needed, allow the patient's distal leg to hang off the table to assess for any hyperextension. To measure knee flexion, have the patient lay prone on an exam table, and have them flex their knee as much as they can.
  - Passive ROM: Passive ROM of the knee is achieved by the examiner holding the patient's leg and telling him or her to completely relax. The examiner can then move the knee into flexion and extension. When flexing the knee, there will likely be a soft, bouncy feel at the end of the ROM due to the musculature prohibiting the knee to flex farther. When assessing passive ROM knee extension, there will

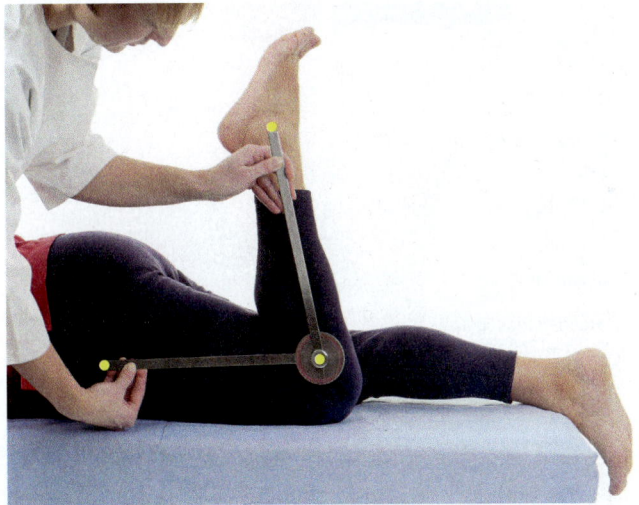

Figure 6.9 Photograph showing measurement of knee flexion and extension range of motion with a long-arm goniometer. The axis of the goniometer should be aligned with the knee joint axis of rotation (approximately at the lateral epicondyle). The stationary axis (proximal) should be in line with the greater trochanter and the moving axis (distal) aligned with the lateral malleolus. Yellow dots represent the location of bony landmarks to use during knee ROM measurement.

© pryzmat/Shutterstock

  also be a bouncy, soft end feel, but be aware that some patients will have hyperextension, where their knee extends past 0° of flexion. To assess for hyperextension, extend the patient's knee, and hold the distal tibia (or ankle) while supporting the posterior knee with the other hand. If the patient has hyperextension, the examiner will be able to pull up on the ankle while extending the knee and see the hyperextension.
  - Resistive ROM: Resistive ROM is performed by measuring muscular strength in a particular ROM. This is often performed by manual muscle testing, noted in Table 6.1. For a quick evaluation, break tests of the quadriceps and hamstrings can be performed while a patient is seated at the end of a treatment table. For a quadriceps break test, the patient would extend his or her knee fully and hold that position while the examiner would apply pressure downward, trying to flex the patient's knee. A hamstring break test can be done with the patient seated at the end of the table or lying prone. The patient would flex his or her knee 90° and hold that position while the examiner applies force to extend the patient's knee.

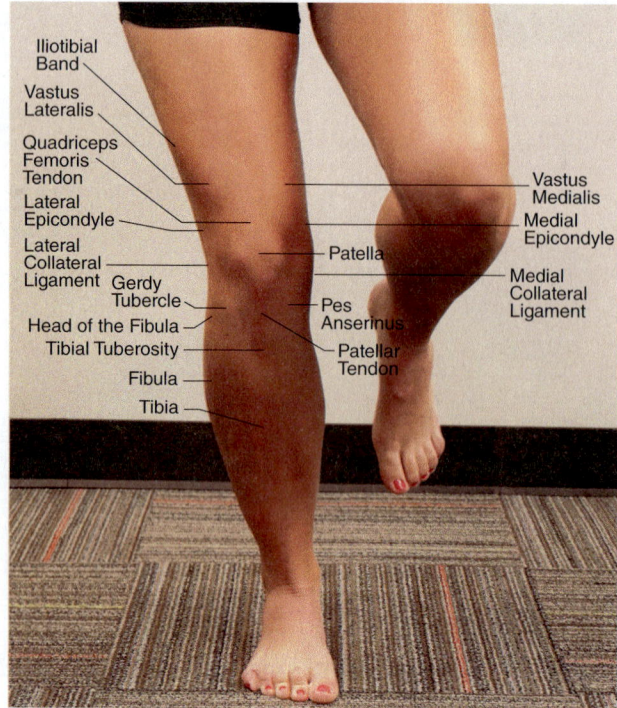

Figure 6.10 Clinical photograph showing common areas to palpate during a knee examination.
© Jones & Bartlett Learning

Quick Tips for Evaluations

- Check the scene, and make sure that play has stopped before entering the field.
- Assess for an emergency that would warrant emergency medical services, and call as soon as possible.
- Look for obvious, serious deformity in the knee, such as a dislocation.
- It is important to use time on field wisely and perform only the tests needed to determine whether it is safe to move the patient off the field.
- Recruit help in moving the patient in the safest way possible.
- Perform an abbreviated evaluation to determine whether it is safe for the patient to return to play.
- Treat the patient with ice if appropriate.
- Remember to notify the coach of the patient's playing status after your assessment.

Palpation

Palpation is performed by firmly pressing on different anatomic structures to find areas of tenderness or deformity. Using anatomic knowledge, the clinician can examine the palpable structures for tenderness. Note that palpation can be performed only on superficial structures. Key components to palpate during a knee examination are the bony landmarks, reviewed earlier in this chapter; the medial and lateral collateral ligaments; and the patellar tendon, quadriceps, and hamstring muscles. Finding tenderness in these areas is helpful in identifying the structures involved in the knee injury. **Figure 6.10** shows palpable landmarks of the anterior knee.

Special Tests

Special tests are performed to test targeted anatomic structures to assess integrity, pain, and end feel. Each special test in the knee has been developed to show a positive or negative result, which will then lead the clinician in making the most accurate diagnosis possible. The next section will discuss common athletic knee injuries and the special tests that should be done when assessing each injury.

Manual Muscle Testing

Manual muscle testing is an important component of a clinical evaluation. The manual muscle tests for each muscle are listed in Table 6.1. Distinguishing between different muscles can be very beneficial to a clinician's examination. Differentiating and testing each individual muscle allows for a more specific assessment, thus leading to a more accurate diagnosis. Note that, as a result of muscle weakness, it is important to further investigate the route of weakness. Although there may be injury in the muscle itself, it is possible that the injury is rooted more proximally—for example, in the spine if the injury is actually occurring at the spinal cord, but is observed through a myotome at the knee. Knee extension is associated with the L3 and L4 myotomes, and knee flexion is associated with the L5 and S1 myotomes.[1]

Neurologic Testing

Neurologic testing is performed when a nerve injury is a concern. As noted previously in this chapter, there are dermatome patterns on the skin that are associated with spinal nerves. To perform a neurologic test, clinicians often use an object with sharp and dull ends. Patients close their eyes and need to determine whether they are feeling a sharp or dull sensation as the clinician brushes the skin with one of the edges.[2] It is important to test all areas of skin, as there are five dermatome patterns that cover the knee (Table 6.2). Neurologic testing is also included in manual muscle testing. It is important to distinguish the root cause of muscular weaknesses as either muscular injury or spinal injury.

Vascular Assessment

The knee has a large artery and vein in the posterior midline of the joint. The popliteal artery is a supplier of blood to skin in the area of the knee as well as deeper branches of arteries that supply the lower leg. These delicate structures are important to consider when a patient has a traumatic knee injury. To assess the integrity of the popliteal artery, the clinician should check for a pulse in the posterior knee. Next, the clinician should passively flex the patient's knee slightly and then palpate deep in the midline of the posterior knee, in the popliteal fossa; this technique requires some practice, as the popliteal artery is a difficult pulse to find.[6] If there were injury to the popliteal vein, the lower leg would swell in response to the blood not being carried up the leg. Injury to either structure would require immediate medical attention. The integrity of the vascular structures also can be assessed by checking the posterior tibial pulse; dorsal pedal pulse; and, more distally, capillary refill on the toenails. If there are abnormalities in the distal exams after knee injury, it could indicate that there is injury to the vascular structures in the knee.

Additionally, it is important to note that the legs are an area of concern for blood clots, which sometimes develop in patients after surgery. If a blood clot is suspected, the test for the Homans sign can be performed. To do this, have the patient actively extend his or her knee; then, passively dorsiflex the patient's ankle and palpate the calf. A positive sign would be deep calf pain.

Pathologies of the Knee

ACL Injury

The ACL is a ligament inside the knee joint that primarily restricts anterior translation of the tibia.[2,3] It attaches anteriorly on the intercondylar notch of the tibia and posteriorly on the posterior lateral femoral condyle. The mechanism of injury for an ACL rupture (tear) occurs when the femur internally rotates while the tibia externally rotates[2,3] (**Table 6.8**). This usually occurs when a patient plants his or her foot and quickly changes direction. This mechanism of injury, combined with the patient hearing or feeling a pop, is usually a good indication of rupture of the ACL. While evaluating for an ACL tear, it is important to keep in mind the other structures that may have been injured during the traumatic event. Because of the traumatic mechanism of injury, ACL tears are commonly accompanied by other injuries in the knee joint, the most common being the meniscus. The combination of injury to the ACL, MCL, and lateral meniscus is known as the terrible triad injury.[3]

Evaluation

When evaluating a patient with injury to the ACL, an immediate effusion (intra-articular swelling) will likely occur. Effusion, in combination with pain, will prohibit the patient from returning to activity. Although the ACL itself cannot be palpated, palpation of the knee will confirm a joint effusion and may elicit pain near the attachment points of the ACL. ROM may be limited because of pain, joint effusion, or a possible displaced meniscus (that may accompany the ACL injury).

Special Tests

Lachman. The Lachman test is the gold standard special test in assessing for an ACL injury (**Figure 6.11**). The examination is performed by having the patient lie supine on a table with legs extended. The examiner should passively bend the knee to 20° to 30° of flexion with one hand around the tibia and the other around the femur. The examiner should then stabilize the femur and pull the tibia anteriorly. A positive test would be indicated by

Table 6.8 Anterior Cruciate Ligament Injury Quick Tips

Pathology	Description	Presentation (HIPS)	Special Tests/Imaging	Differential Diagnosis	5-Min Sideline Assessment Tips
ACL injury	Tear or rupture to the ACL	Contact or noncontact injury Plant, cut, twist mechanism Immediate effusion	Anterior drawer Lachman Pivot shift	Posterior cruciate ligament tear Meniscus tear	Take note of immediate effusion Try to perform Lachman or anterior drawer test

ACL, anterior cruciate ligament; HIPS, history, inspection, palpation, special tests.

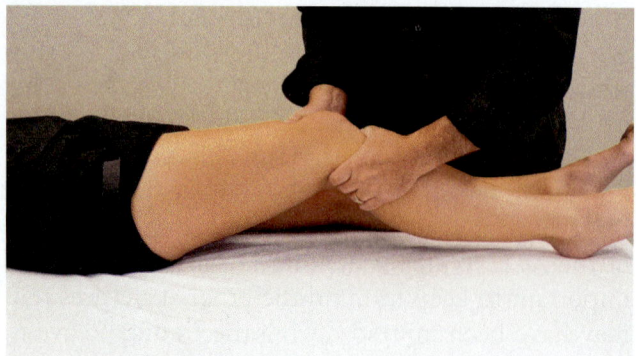

Figure 6.11 Clinical photograph showing the Lachman test.
© Jones & Bartlett Learning

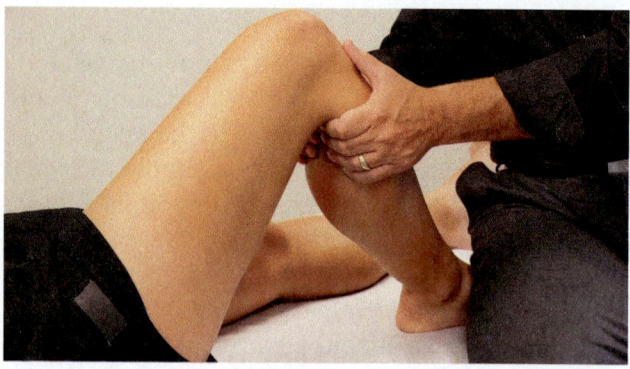

Figure 6.12 Clinical photograph showing the anterior drawer test.
© Jones & Bartlett Learning

extensive anterior translation of the tibia, without an end point. The normal end point of the ACL should be soft but abrupt. If the examiner cannot, for any reason, secure his or her hands around the patient's leg, there are alternative methods to performing this test. Examiners can add an object, such as a foam roller under the patient's thigh, to help maintain the 20° to 30° of flexion. The examiner can then stabilize the thigh against the object and use his or her other hand to pull anteriorly on the tibia.[9,10]

Anterior Drawer. The patient should be positioned supine, with the knee bent to 70° to 90° of flexion. The examiner then places both hands around the proximal tibia, with fingertips on the posterior tibia, and pulls the tibia forward. A positive test would be indicated by excessive anterior translation without an end feel.

It should be noted that this test can sometimes produce a false-positive result. Considering the patient's starting position is important to rule out a false-positive result. If the tibia's starting position is more than 1 cm posterior to the medial femoral condyle, there may be a PCL injury. By pulling the tibia forward and feeling excessive movement, the clinician may think that is a result of a positive anterior drawer test, when in fact the tibia's starting position is significantly more posterior because of the PCL tear such that pulling the tibia into neutral may trick the clinician into thinking that the anterior drawer test is positive[9,10] (**Figure 6.12**).

Pivot Shift. This test is difficult to do on a conscious patient because it is very painful and can cause the patient to guard the knee by contracting his or her muscles. This test is usually performed under anesthesia before the patient's reconstructive surgery. To perform the examination, the patient lies supine, with knees extended. The examiner's hands should be placed on the lateral knee and the distal tibia. The examiner then passively flexes the patient's knee while applying a valgus force. A positive test result would be indicated if there is a rotational "clunk" during the ROM. A negative test result would be a smooth glide throughout the ROM, but, as mentioned before, most conscious patients with ACL injury will guard the knee, leading to a false-negative test result.[9,10]

Imaging

Radiography. Radiography may be performed initially if the mechanism of injury is unknown or the clinician was not present during injury (**Figure 6.13**). A radiograph may show a lateral tibial avulsion (Segond fracture), which is commonly associated with an ACL tear.[3]

Magnetic Resonance Imaging. MRI will show the ACL tear itself (sagittal view) as well as bone bruising on the anterior femur and posterior tibia, which is commonly associated with an ACL tear (**Figure 6.14**).

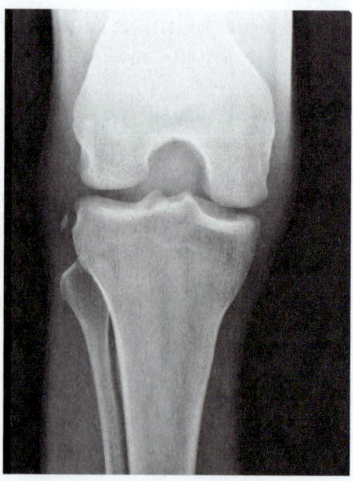

Figure 6.13 Radiograph showing Segond fracture.
Case courtesy of Dr Maulik S Patel, Radiopaedia.org, rID: 20287.

Pathologies of the Knee   **143**

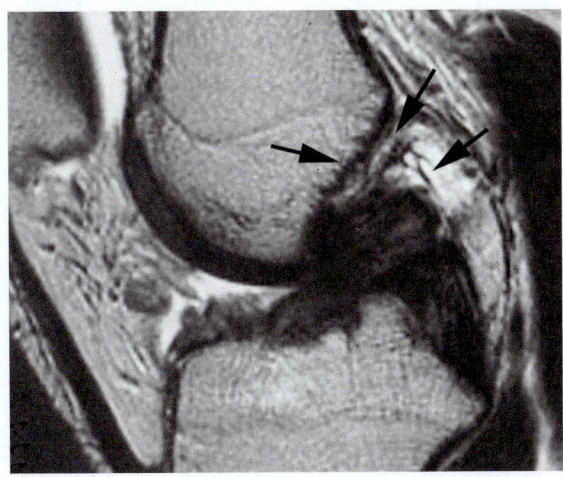

Figure 6.14 Anterior cruciate ligament tear shown on MRI.

Reproduced from Johnson TR, Steinbach LS. eds: *Essentials of Musculoskeletal Imaging*. Rosemont, IL, American Academy of Orthopaedic Surgeons, 2004.

Differential Diagnoses

- Quadriceps or patellar tendon injury
- PCL tear
- Meniscus injury

Treatment

Initial on-field treatment involves removal of the patient from activity and application of ice and a brace for stability. Patients will often want to use crutches to avoid weight bearing after initial injury.

During early treatment, it is important to reduce the effusion with ice and anti-inflammatory agents. The emphasis of rehabilitation should be on ROM, as most surgeons will not repair the ligament if the patient has not achieved full ROM after initial injury. Last, it is important to tone the quadriceps muscles because they often atrophy after an ACL injury.

Regarding surgical intervention, all active patients should be referred to an orthopaedic surgeon to discuss reconstruction of the ACL. Although not necessary, reconstruction will be required in most patients to achieve an active lifestyle in the future. Because of a lack of blood supply to the ligament, the ACL cannot repair itself; thus, it can only be replaced surgically using an autograft or allograft.

Rehabilitation

The rehabilitation process following an ACL tear is lengthy. It can take up to 6 months to gain enough strength in order to begin a return-to-sport–specific program. The lengthy rehabilitation may not allow him or her to return to sport participation for 8 to 12 months after surgery (**Table 6.9**).

PCL Injury

The PCL is primarily responsible for restricting posterior translation of the tibia. It has two bundles, the anterolateral and posteromedial, which run

Table 6.9 Example of Rehabilitation Guidelines After Anterior Cruciate Ligament Reconstruction

Phase	Rehabilitation Goals	Examples of Exercises
Phase I (immediately postoperative): Weeks 1–4	Weight bearing as tolerated with crutches for the first 2 weeks, then transition to normal gait Protect graft Control inflammation/swelling 0°–120° active range of motion as tolerated (avoid hyperextension)	Patellar mobilization Hamstring curls (for patellar tendon graft repair) Heel slides Quadriceps sets Gastrocnemius/soleus stretching Straight leg raises in all directions
Phase II: Weeks 4–10	Restore normal gait and stair climbing Maintain full extension and progress toward full flexion Increase hip, quadriceps, hamstring, and calf strength Increase proprioception	Closed kinetic chain strengthening, such as wall sits, step-ups, mini squats, and partial lunges. Range of motion exercises Stationary biking Elliptical machine
Phase III: Weeks 10–16	Full range of motion Improve strength to prepare for sport activity Protect patellofemoral joint Restore normal running mechanics	Introduce open kinetic chain exercises, with progression to eccentric exercises Running progression (weeks 12–16) Advanced hip, quadriceps, and hamstring strengthening Advanced proprioceptive exercises

(continues)

Table 6.9 Example of Rehabilitation Guidelines After Anterior Cruciate Ligament Reconstruction (continued)

Phase	Rehabilitation Goals	Examples of Exercises
Phase IV: Months 4–6	Symmetric performance between limbs Perform sport agility drills	Advanced strengthening Advanced proprioceptive exercises Agility exercises, including speed and change of direction
Phase V: Month 6 and beyond	Safe return to sport Maintain range of motion and strength Maintain and increase endurance	Progression to return to sport with sport-specific activities

Data from Miller MD, Hart JA, MacKnight JM: *Essential Orthopaedics*. Philadelphia, PA, Saunders/Elsevier, 2009; and Prentice W: *Principles of Athletic Training: A Guide to Evidence-Based Clinical Practice*. New York, NY, McGraw-Hill Education, 2016.

together from the posterior intercondylar notch of the tibia to the medial femoral condyle. Unlike the ACL, the PCL has a vascular supply and therefore has the potential to heal independently of surgical intervention. PCL injuries can result from several mechanisms of injury, such as contact with another person, trauma (dashboard injury) forcing the tibia posteriorly, or falling on a flexed knee while the ankle is in plantar flexion[2,6] (**Table 6.10**).

Evaluation

Patients with an injury to the PCL may report pain, swelling, and a feeling of instability in the knee. Observation of the knee may show an effusion (intra-articular swelling). The PCL cannot be palpated, but palpation of the knee may confirm joint effusion or pain near the PCL attachment sites. ROM may be painful and could be limited because of effusion.

Special Tests

Posterior Drawer. The patient should be positioned supine, with knee bent to 70° to 90° of flexion. The examiner then places both hands around the proximal tibia, with fingertips on the posterior tibia. The tibia needs to be reduced to neutral position before the examination is performed. Patients with a PCL injury will have an anatomic abnormality, where the tibia sits more than 1 cm posteriorly to the lateral femoral condyle. The examiner should bring the tibia forward into neutral position, then push the tibia posteriorly, toward the patient. A positive test would be indicated by excessive posterior translation without an end feel[9,10] (**Figure 6.15**).

Posterior Sag. As mentioned previously, the tibia sits more posterior than usual in patients with a deficient PCL, which can be observed by the posterior sag sign. To perform this test, the patient needs to lie

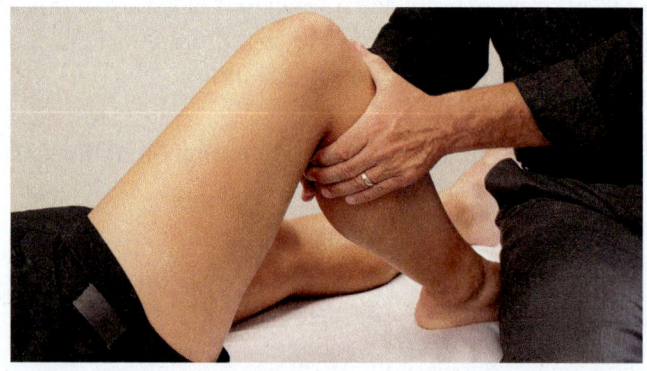

Figure 6.15 Clinical photograph showing the posterior drawer test.
© Jones & Bartlett Learning

Table 6.10 PCL Injury Quick Tips

Pathology	Description	Presentation (HIPS)	Special Tests/Imaging	Differential Diagnosis	5-Min Sideline Assessment Tips
PCL injury	Tear or rupture of the PCL	Dashboard injury Usually due to posterior force on tibia	Posterior drawer Posterior sag	Anterior cruciate ligament tear Posterolateral corner injury Tibial fracture	Effusion Try to perform posterior drawer test

PCL, posterior cruciate ligament; HIPS, history, inspection, palpation, special tests.

Pathologies of the Knee

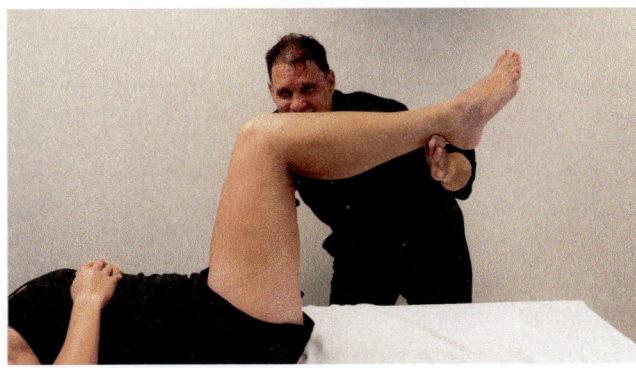

Figure 6.16 Clinical photograph showing the posterior sag test.
© Jones & Bartlett Learning

supine, with hips and knees flexed to 90°. The examiner should hold the patient's legs up to allow him or her to relax the muscles while in this position. A positive test will show the tibia "sagging" lower toward the table when compared to the other side[9,10] (**Figure 6.16**).

Imaging

Radiography. A radiograph may show a possible avulsion fracture that occurred at one of the attachment sites of the ligament. A stress radiograph can also be obtained to show the excessive posterior displacement of the tibia when the examiner is applying posterior force to it while the radiograph is obtained.

Magnetic Resonance Imaging. MRI will show a disrupted PCL and any other concomitant injury that may have occurred, such as a meniscus injury (**Figure 6.17**).

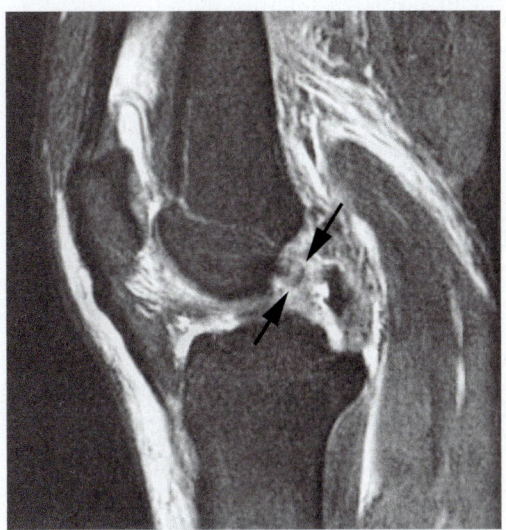

Figure 6.17 Posterior cruciate ligament tear shown on MRI.
Reproduced from Johnson TR, Steinbach LS. eds: *Essentials of Musculoskeletal Imaging*. Rosemont, IL, American Academy of Orthopaedic Surgeons, 2004.

Differential Diagnosis
- ACL tear
- Posterolateral corner injury
- Tibial fracture

Treatment
Initial on-field treatment involves removing the patient from activity and applying ice and compression.

During early treatment, it is important to reduce the effusion with ice, compression, and anti-inflammatory agents.

Not all patients who have PCL tears will be required to undergo surgery. The PCL has healing capabilities, whereas the ACL does not. Depending on the grade and severity of the tear, the patient may or may not need surgery. The patient should be referred to an orthopaedic surgeon to determine the need for surgery after imaging studies are performed.[3]

Rehabilitation
Therapy should focus on regaining stability in the joint through muscular strengthening, especially if the patient does not have surgery to repair the ligament. It is important to consider that patients who do not have surgery to repair the ligament may be placed at additional risk for arthritis because of the activity affecting an unstable joint. Stabilization and strengthening should be the focus of the rehabilitation plan.

MCL Injury
The MCL is the most commonly injured ligament in the knee. It lies outside of the knee joint, on the medial aspect of the knee joint, and restricts valgus knee motion. When valgus force is placed on the knee, it not only stresses and injures the MCL, but the lateral meniscus is often also injured because of the compressive forces to the lateral knee joint during valgus knee motion. MCL tears vary in grade and therefore can be treated both with or without surgery (**Table 6.11**).

Evaluation
The mechanism of injury for an MCL tear is valgus force to the knee, which is associated with pain and a possible "pop" sound or feeling. Because of the varying grades of MCL tear, it is possible that a patient can continue vigorous activity, despite having an injury to the MCL. Patients may or may not present with swelling after an injury or tear to the MCL. Swelling or tenderness can be palpated along the length of the MCL and/or medial knee and may cause limited ROM

Chapter 6 Knee Joint

Table 6.11 MCL Injury Quick Tips

Pathology	Description	Presentation (HIPS)	Special Tests/Imaging	Differential Diagnosis	5-Min Sideline Assessment Tips
MCL injury	Tear or rupture of the MCL	Mechanism of valgus knee force May be associated with a "pop" sound or feeling	Valgus stress test	Meniscus tear Anterior cruciate ligament tear Gracilis or sartorius tendon injury	Return to play will be determined by the grade of injury

MCL, medial collateral ligament; HIPS, history, inspection, palpation, special tests.

as a result of pain. It is important to be cautious when palpating areas on the bone where an avulsion of the MCL may have occurred. An avulsion of the MCL would result in pain and possible deformity either on the distal femur or proximal tibia.[2,3]

Special Tests

Valgus Stress Test. The patient lies supine, with knees extended. The examiner should position one hand on the distal tibia and the other around the posterior aspect of the knee. It is especially helpful if the examiner can palpate the medial joint line while performing the examination. The examination is performed with 30° of knee flexion as well as 0° of flexion to isolate the anterior and posterior aspects of the MCL, respectively (**Figures 6.18** and **6.19**). The examiner should position the patient's knee in the appropriate amount of knee flexion and then apply valgus force to the knee while stabilizing the distal tibia. The test would be positive if there is excessive motion/opening of the medial joint space.[9,10]

Imaging

Radiography. A radiograph could show an avulsion fracture of the tibia or femur associated with an MCL injury.

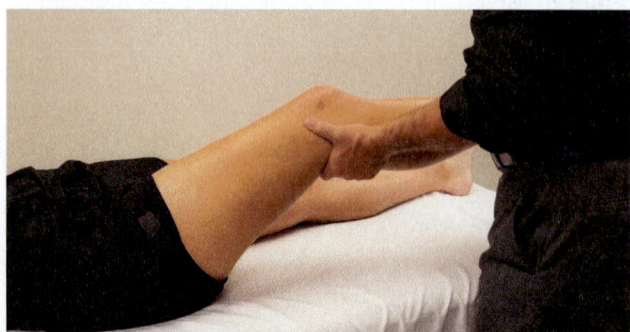

Figure 6.18 Clinical photograph showing valgus stress test being performed with knee in 30° of knee flexion.
© Jones & Bartlett Learning

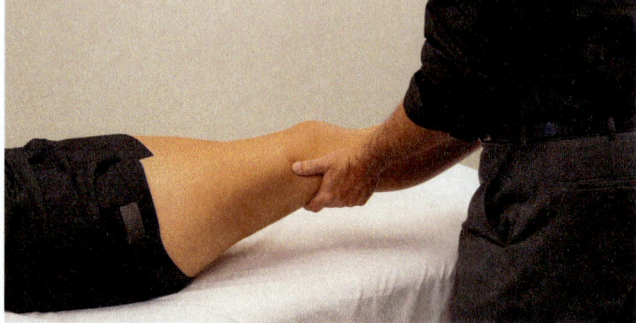

Figure 6.19 Clinical photograph showing valgus stress test being performed with knee in 0° of knee flexion.
© Jones & Bartlett Learning

Magnetic Resonance Imaging. MRI will show whether there is a tear in the MCL and also help determine its grade and severity (**Figure 6.20**).

Differential Diagnosis

- Meniscus tear
- ACL tear
- Gracilis or sartorius muscle injury (these tendons are close to the MCL insertion)

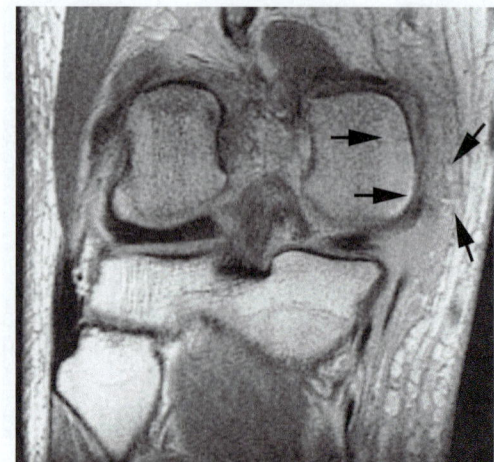

Figure 6.20 Medial collateral ligament tear on MRI.
Reproduced from Johnson TR, Steinbach LS. eds: *Essentials of Musculoskeletal Imaging*. Rosemont, IL, American Academy of Orthopaedic Surgeons, 2004.

Treatment

Treatment of a high-grade tear involves removing the patient from activity, applying ice, and elevating the knee. In the following days, the patient should wear a compression sleeve with a knee immobilizer while remaining weight bearing as tolerated.

For a low-grade tear, the patient can continue to play depending on the level of pain-free knee function. Patients can wear a brace during play for protection and comfort.

Rehabilitation

After the inflammatory response phase has passed, the focus should be on ROM and strengthening exercises. Depending on the grade and severity, return to play can take anywhere from 1 to 4 weeks.

LCL and Posterolateral Corner Injury

The LCL is located on the lateral aspect of the knee, outside of the knee joint, and primarily restricts varus stress. Much like MCL injuries, there are several grades of LCL tears, which are mostly treated nonsurgically. The posterolateral corner (PLC) is a bundle of ligaments posterior to the LCL that prevent external rotation of the tibia. The PLC is commonly injured during traumatic injuries where the ACL, PCL, or LCL are also injured[2,3] (**Table 6.12**).

Evaluation

LCL injuries can be either acute or chronic and can result from either noncontact or contact injury. A common mechanism of injury to the LCL is varus force on the knee joint. Patients may report pain on the lateral side of the knee in addition to instability. Chronic LCL injuries occur gradually but will also likely be accompanied by pain and instability. Upon observation of the knee, there may be swelling on the lateral aspect of the knee. Observing the alignment of the knee could be helpful when evaluating an LCL injury, which could present as genu varum. Palpation of the LCL may reveal swelling in the area or deformity of the ligament if there is an avulsion and will elicit pain. ROM may be limited because of pain if there is injury to the LCL or PLC. If there is injury to the PLC, there may be excessive tibial external rotation motion.[3]

Special Tests

Peroneal Nerve Assessment. The function of the peroneal nerve should be assessed because it is located very close to the LCL and could have been injured along with the ligament.

Varus Stress Test. The patient lies supine, with knees extended. The examiner should position one hand on the distal tibia and the other around the posterior aspect of the knee. It is especially helpful if the examiner can palpate the lateral joint line while performing the examination. The examination is performed with 30° of knee flexion as well as 0° of flexion. The examiner should position the patient's knee in the appropriate amount of knee flexion and then apply varus force to the knee while stabilizing the distal tibia. The test is positive if there is excessive motion/opening of the lateral joint space[9,10] (**Figure 6.21**).

Dial Test. The patient lies prone on the table with knee flexed. This test will be performed at 30° and 90° of flexion (**Figure 6.22**). With the knee flexed, the examiner externally rotates the tibia and compares motion bilaterally. PLC injury is suspected if there is increased external rotation at 30° of knee flexion. If there is increased external rotation at 90° of flexion, PLC injury is also suspected as well as a possible PCL injury.[3]

Imaging

Radiography. Radiographs could show an avulsion of the fibular head.

Table 6.12 Lateral Collateral Ligament Injury Quick Tips

Pathology	Description	Presentation (HIPS)	Special Tests/ Imaging	Differential Diagnosis	5-Min Sideline Assessment Tips
LCL injury	Tear or rupture of the LCL	Pain on lateral knee Mechanism of varus knee force	Varus stress test	Lateral meniscus tear Posterior cruciate ligament tear Fibula fracture	Return to play will depend on grade of sprain

LCL, lateral collateral ligament; HIPS, history, inspection, palpation, special tests.

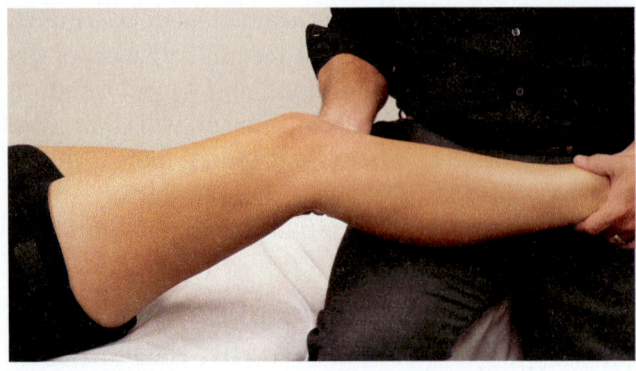 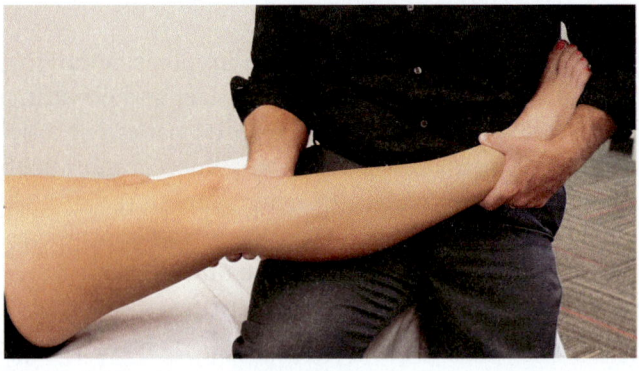

Figure 6.21 Clinical photographs showing the valgus stress test being performed. **A.** 30° of knee flexion. **B.** 0° of knee flexion.

© Jones & Bartlett Learning

Magnetic Resonance Imaging. MRI is recommended to confirm the ligament tear and rule out any other concomitant injuries.

Differential Diagnoses

- Lateral meniscus tear
- PCL tear
- Fibula fracture

Treatment

Acute treatment of a patient with LCL or PLC injury would include rest and ice to reduce inflammation. Immobilization in extension or slight flexion with toe touch or partial weight bearing should be followed for 2 to 4 weeks. Most patients with LCL injuries can be treated without surgery, but grade 3 injuries often require surgical repair. For nonsurgical treatment, rehabilitation should progress to include

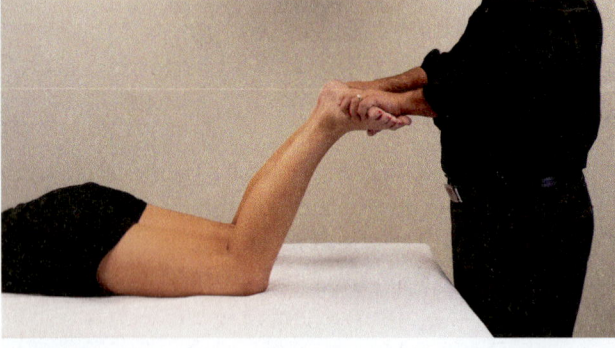

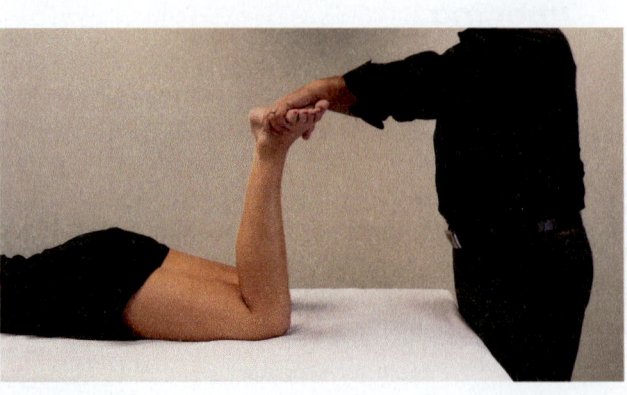

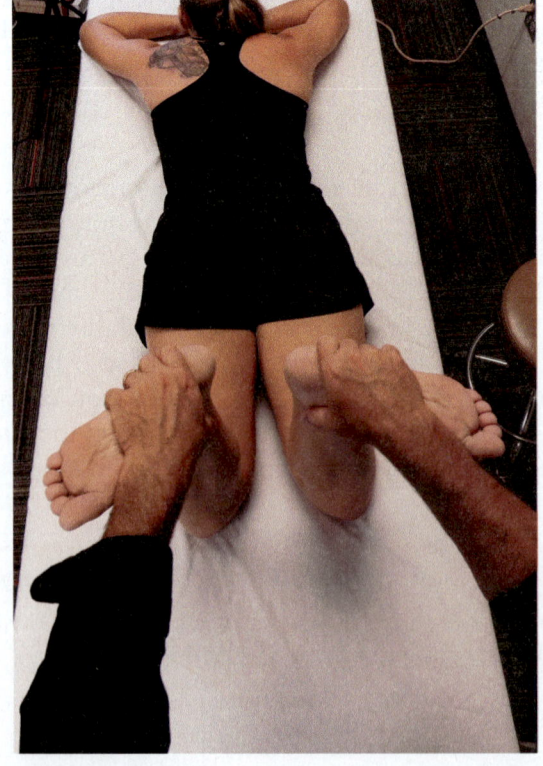

Figure 6.22 Clinical photographs showing the dial test being performed. **A.** 30° of knee flexion. **B.** 90° of knee flexion. **C.** Overhead view, 90° of knee flexion.

© Jones & Bartlett Learning

weight bearing and strengthening exercises to return to activity from 4 to 6 weeks after injury.[3]

Meniscus Tear

The menisci are two C-shaped structures made up of fibrocartilage that are responsible for absorbing and distributing load across the knee joint. Because of the limited blood supply, both the medial and lateral meniscus are limited in their ability to heal. Meniscus injuries usually require surgical intervention to either repair or cut out torn or degenerative meniscus tissue (meniscectomy) (**Table 6.13**).

Evaluation

The mechanism for meniscus injury is twisting or hyperflexion of the knee. Patients with meniscal pathology will report pain when twisting or bending the knee into deep flexion (especially during weight bearing). The patient may also report a popping, locking, or catching sensation in the knee.[2] Observation of the knee may appear normal with meniscus injury. Palpation of either meniscus is not possible because of its location on top of the tibia and inside the knee joint; however, it is possible that a patient may have tenderness along the medial or lateral joint line where the anterior menisci originate. ROM could be limited because of pain or mechanical limitations. Depending on the type of meniscus tear, meniscus tissue can flip and turn inside the knee joint. This torn tissue can cause a physical stop when moving the knee through a ROM.[3]

Special Tests

McMurray. The patient lies supine on the table. One of the examiner's hands should be placed on the distal tibia, and the other on the posterolateral knee with thumb and index fingers on the medial and lateral joint lines if possible. Start by passively flexing the knee and hip 90°. Slowly extend and flex the knee while the tibia is internally rotated and while applying a varus force on the knee joint. To test other areas of the meniscus, passively extend and flex the knee again, with the tibia in external rotation while applying a valgus force to the knee joint. A positive test would be a palpable "pop" or "clunk" on the joint line. This is the most specific meniscal test, but it is not very sensitive[9,10] (**Figure 6.23**).

Apley Compression/Distraction. These two tests are performed with the patient lying prone on a table, with knee bent at 90°. For compression, the examiner holds the distal tibia, applies pressure downward into the knee, and twists internally and externally. The distraction test is performed the exact same way, but the force is pulled up toward the ceiling rather than pushed down into the knee. A positive test would result in pain or mechanical symptoms with the compression test that resolve with the distraction test. If the patient is still symptomatic with the distraction test, this may indicate a ligamentous injury[9,10] (**Figure 6.24**).

Thessaly Test. The patient is standing on the ipsilateral leg, with knee flexed 20°. The contralateral leg is flexed to 90° to avoid contact with the floor. The examiner then holds the patient's hands to stabilize him or her as the patient rotates medially and laterally on the ipsilateral leg three times each way. A positive test would be indicated by pain, discomfort, or locking or catching in the knee joint[9,10] (**Figure 6.25**).

Squat Test. The patient squats as deeply as he or she can and then tries to walk forward while in a squatted position. A positive test would be indicated by pain or mechanical symptoms in the posterior knee. Anterior knee pain during this test may be indicative of a chondral injury on the patella or trochlea[9,10] (**Figure 6.26**).

Table 6.13 Meniscus Tear Quick Tips

Pathology	Description	Presentation (HIPS)	Special Tests/ Imaging	Differential Diagnosis	5-Min Sideline Assessment Tips
Meniscus tear	A tear in either the medial or lateral meniscus	Pain with twisting or deep flexion Clicking or catching sensation through range of motion	McMurray Apley compression/distraction Thessaly Squat	Loose body Osteochondritis dissecans Articular cartilage lesion Plica injury Fat pad impingement	Not applicable

HIPS, history, inspection, palpation, special tests.

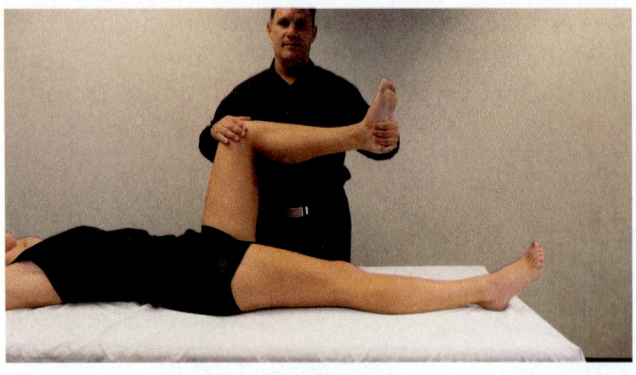
A

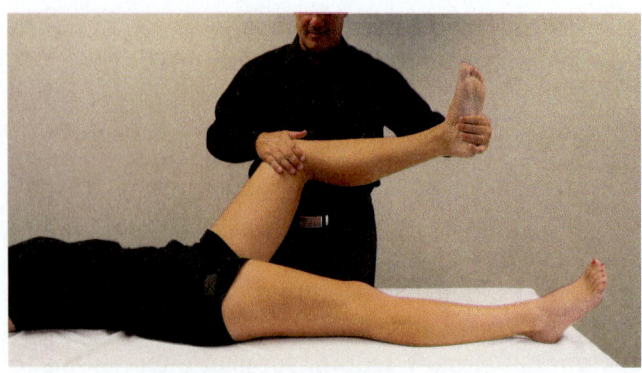
B

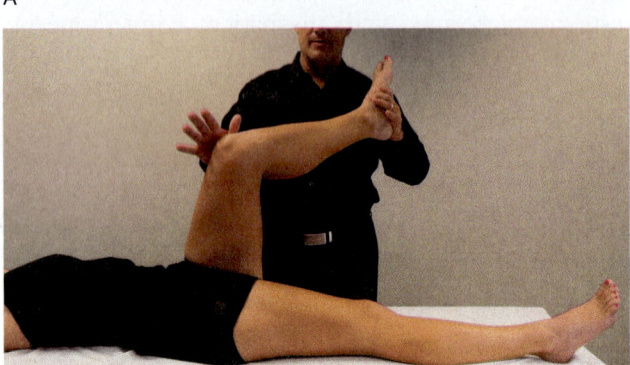
C

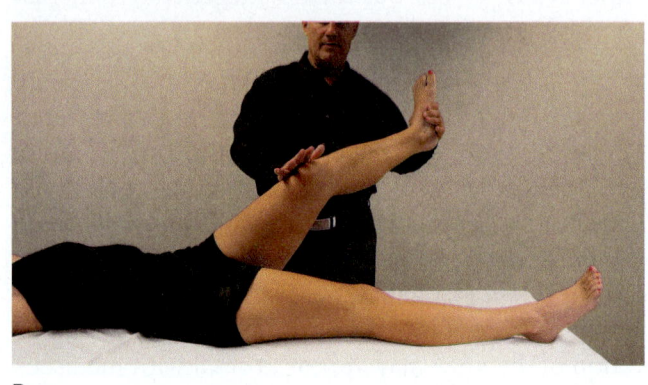
D

Figure 6.23 Clinical photographs showing the McMurray test being performed. **A.** Hip flexion, tibial internal rotation, and varus stress. **B.** Less hip flexion, tibial internal rotation, and increased varus stress on the knee. **C.** Hip flexion, tibial external rotation, and knee valgus stress. **D.** Less hip flexion, tibial external rotaion, and increased valgus stress on the knee.

© Jones & Bartlett Learning

Imaging

Radiography. Radiographs will appear normal.

Magnetic Resonance Imaging. MRI is the gold standard imaging technique to diagnose a meniscus injury. MRI would show a meniscus tear and the specific tear pattern (**Figure 6.27**).

Differential Diagnoses

- Loose body
- Osteochondritis dissecans
- Articular cartilage lesion
- Tibial plateau fracture
- Plica injury
- Fat pad impingement

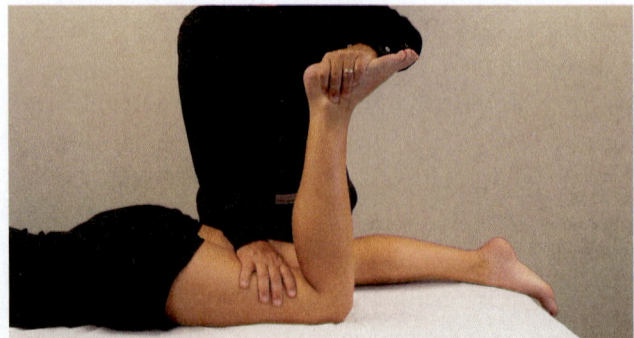

Figure 6.24 Clinical photograph showing the Apley compression/distraction test.

© Jones & Bartlett Learning

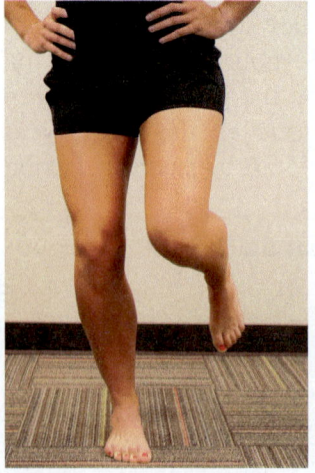
A

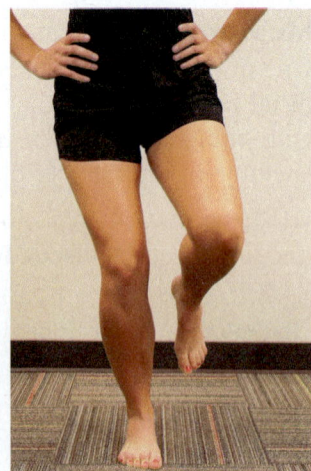
B

Figure 6.25 Clinical photographs showing the Thessaly test. **A.** Twisting on the support leg to rotate the femur externally. **B.** Twisting on the support leg to rotate the femur internally.

© Jones & Bartlett Learning

Pathologies of the Knee   151

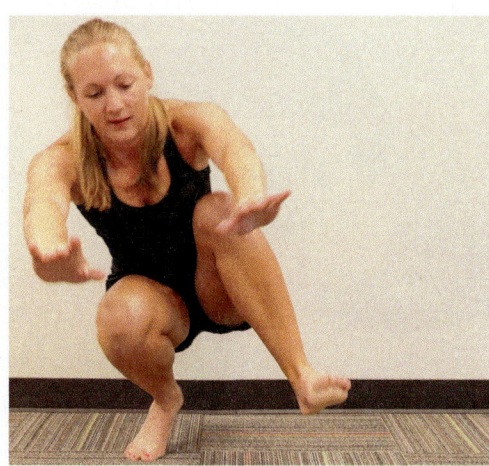

Figure 6.26 Clinical photograph showing the squat test.
© Jones & Bartlett Learning

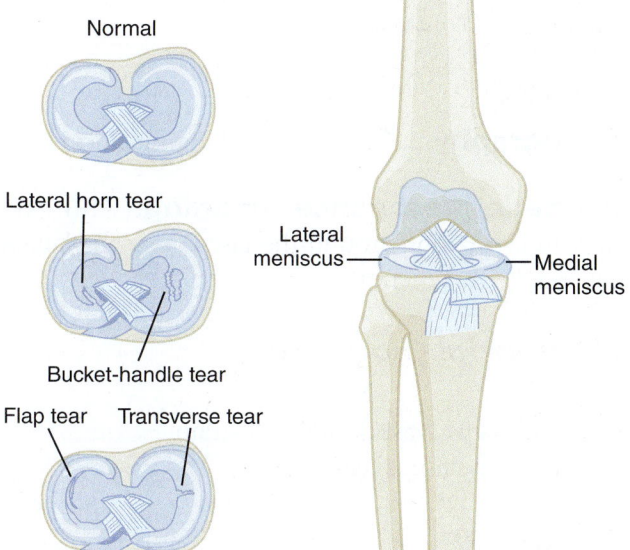

Figure 6.27 Drawings showing common meniscal tear patterns.
© Jones & Bartlett Learning

Treatment

For initial on-field treatment, remove the patient from activity and apply ice and compression. Patients with locked ROM because of a displaced meniscus should be referred to an orthopaedic surgeon as soon as possible.

Early treatment involves patient follow-up with an orthopaedic surgeon if symptoms do not resolve after nonsurgical treatment.

Surgical intervention is a common treatment for meniscal tears (**Figures 6.28** and **6.29**). A surgeon can either repair the meniscus or perform a meniscectomy, which is a procedure in which the torn parts of the meniscus are removed rather than stitched and repaired. A meniscus can be repaired only if the tear is located in the red zone, where there is blood supply in the area. In the area of the meniscus called the

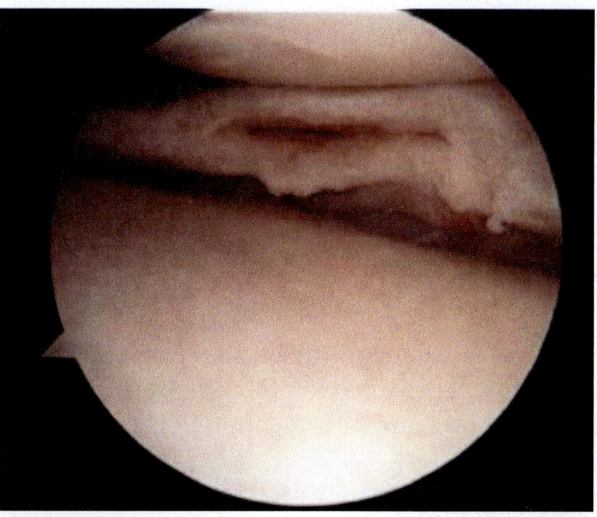

Figure 6.28 Arthroscopic view of a torn meniscus prior to repair.
Courtesy of Kaitlyn Shank.

white zone, where there is little to no circulation, a meniscectomy must be done. Meniscal repair is preferred over meniscectomy because it preserves the meniscus and, in doing so, preserves the cartilage and bone. Bone preservation is ideal in preventing osteoarthritis in the knee.[3]

Rehabilitation

Rehabilitation following a meniscus repair is lengthier than a meniscectomy because during a meniscectomy, structures are removed rather than repaired, so the healing time is much faster. Although this sounds appealing, the absence of a meniscus can potentially put the patient at risk for osteoarthritis or other joint damage because of the loss of cushion the meniscus provides.

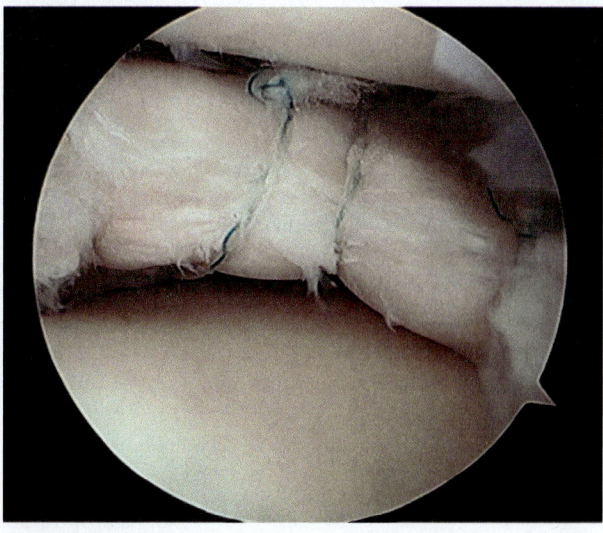

Figure 6.29 Arthroscopic view of a repaired meniscus tear.
Courtesy of Kaitlyn Shank.

IT Band Syndrome (Distal)

The IT band is a thick band of fascia that runs along the lateral aspect of the thigh from the iliac crest and tensor fascia lata muscle and inserts on the Gerdy tubercle. IT band friction syndrome can occur either proximally as the IT band rubs over the greater trochanter of the femur or distally as the IT band rubs against the lateral epicondyle of the femur (**Table 6.14**). Tightness in the IT band fascia can cause the tissue to rub on these bony structures and with repetitive motion (ie, running), which can cause irritation and inflammation in the area.

Evaluation

IT band syndrome at the knee is a chronic injury that develops over time from repetitive rubbing of the IT band tissue over the lateral epicondyle of the femur. Patients will report pain or aching over the lateral epicondyle that increases with activity when the knee is flexed and extended repetitively. Observation of the knee may appear normal, or there may be some inflammation over the lateral epicondyle. Palpation will elicit pain over the lateral aspect of the knee (lateral epicondyle) as well as possibly up the lateral thigh along the IT band. ROM may be limited because of pain, especially during knee extension.[2,3]

Special Tests

Noble. The patient is lying supine on the table, with hip and knee flexed to 90°. The examiner places pressure with his or her thumb over the IT band and lateral epicondyle and then extends and flexes the patient's knee. A positive test would be shown by pain or snapping in the area of palpation[9,10] (**Figure 6.30**).

Renne. Similar to the Noble test, but the patient is weight bearing and standing rather than lying down during the Renne test. The examiner places pressure

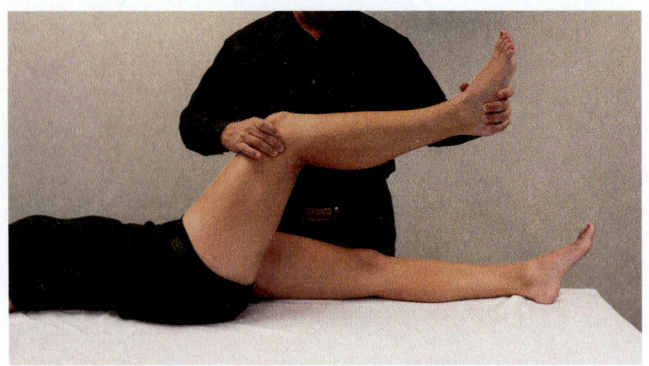

Figure 6.30 Clinical photograph showing the Noble test.
© Jones & Bartlett Learning

with his or her thumb over the IT band and lateral epicondyle and then instructs the patient to squat. A positive test result is pain or snapping in the area of palpation[9,10] (**Figure 6.31**).

Imaging

Radiography. Radiographs will appear normal.

Magnetic Resonance Imaging. MRI will show inflammation around the fascia near the lateral epicondyle of the femur.

Differential Diagnoses

- LCL tear
- Quadriceps (vastus lateralis) strain
- Lateral meniscus tear

Treatment

An IT band syndrome injury does not necessarily warrant removal from activity. Pain should be used as an indicator of whether the patient can continue activity. Extreme pain during activity should warrant removal from activity, whereas tolerable pain that does not inhibit the patient's function should not warrant cessation of activity.

Table 6.14 Iliotibial Band Syndrome Quick Tips

Pathology	Description	Presentation (HIPS)	Special Tests/ Imaging	Differential Diagnosis	5-Min Sideline Assessment Tips
IT band syndrome (distal)	Irritation of the IT band, usually associated with a tight IT band and repeated motion (such as running), which causes irritation/friction of surrounding structures	Aching pain on lateral femoral epicondyle Usually chronic Mostly seen in running athletes	Noble test Renne test	Lateral collateral ligament tear Quadriceps strain Lateral meniscus tear	Not applicable

HIPS, history, inspection, palpation, special tests; IT, iliotibial.

Pathologies of the Knee

pain syndrome (PFPS) is often identified as anterior knee pain, which can be caused by soft-tissue or bony pathologies (**Table 6.15**). These pathologies, whether tissue is tight, unstable, or abnormal, cause abnormal patellar tracking in the trochlear notch, which then results in pain and inflammation.

Evaluation

PFPS presents as recurring pain that flares up after sport or activity or, in severe cases, after activities of daily living, such as going up or down stairs. Patients will present with anterior knee pain, with pain increasing when the knee is moving through flexion and extension, especially during weight-bearing activities, such as squatting or getting up from a seated position. Observation of the knee will likely appear normal, with possible trace swelling around the patella. It is important, during evaluation, to observe the patient walking, so any patellar tracking abnormalities can be observed through the gait cycle. It can also be helpful to measure the patient's Q angle and alignment, which may be abnormal in patients with PFPS. Patients with PFPS will be tender to palpation around the anterior knee and undersurface of the patella. ROM may be limited in patients with PFPS. It is important to not only assess for pain but also to feel for crepitus in the patellofemoral joint while the patella is moved through flexion and extension of the knee. ROM of the patella itself can also be assessed. While the patient has his or her knee relaxed in full extension, the patella can be passively moved in all directions (medially, laterally, superiorly, and inferiorly) to assess for limited or excessive motion. Crepitus can also be noted during passive ROM of the patella.[2,3]

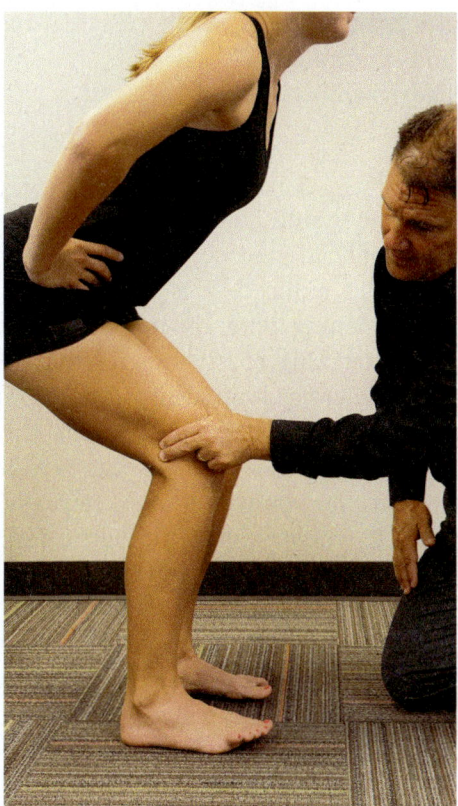

Figure 6.31 Clinical photograph showing the Renne test.
© Jones & Bartlett Learning

Initial treatment should include reducing inflammation and limiting activity that will involve repetitive motion of the IT band rubbing on the inflamed area. After the patient resumes full activity, it is important for him or her to make an effort to keep the fascia as loose as possible by undergoing a thorough rehabilitation program that includes stretching, foam rolling, and modalities such as ultrasound or heat therapy.[2,3]

Patellofemoral Pain Syndrome

Patellofemoral pain can be caused from abnormalities in the retropatellar (under the patella) or peripatellar (around the patella) areas of the knee. Patellofemoral

Special Tests

Clarke Test. The patient lies supine with knees extended and relaxed. The examiner cups his or her hand and places it superior to the patella so the

Table 6.15 Patellofemoral Pain Syndrome Quick Tips

Pathology	Description	Presentation (HIPS)	Special Tests/ Imaging	Differential Diagnosis	5-Min Sideline Assessment Tips
Patellofemoral pain syndrome	Pain caused by the patella tracking incorrectly through the trochlear groove	Pain on the anterior knee Crepitus when moving the knee through a range of motion	Q-angle measurement Clarke test	Patellar tendinitis Chondral lesion Quadriceps tendinitis Patellar instability	Not applicable

HIPS, history, inspection, palpation, special tests.

webbing of the hand is centered over the patella. The examiner pushes the patella inferiorly and holds it in that position and then instructs the patient to contract his or her quadriceps muscles. A positive test would be if the patient experiences pain with this test, indicating injury to the underside of the patella.[9,10]

Q-Angle Assessment. Have the patient stand in anatomic position. Using a goniometer, align the stationary arm with the anterior superior iliac spine along the anterior thigh and the moving arm with the tibial tubercle. The fulcrum should be over the anterior midline of the patella. Normal Q angle is 13° (±4°), with women having larger Q angles than men because women have wider hips[7,9,10] (**Figure 6.32**).

Imaging

Radiography. Radiographs may show patellar tilt, abnormal patella position, or areas of wear/arthritis.

Magnetic Resonance Imaging. MRI is not necessary for this pathology but if performed would show in detail the areas of inflammation and the areas of injury that are causing PFPS.

Differential Diagnoses

- Patellar tendinitis
- Chondral or cartilage lesion
- Quadriceps tendinitis
- IT band syndrome
- Patellar instability

Treatment

Initial treatment should focus on reducing inflammation through application of ice, rest, and NSAIDs. After inflammation has reduced, it is important to implement a strengthening program for weak quadriceps muscles and stretching of the muscles that are tight. Imagine the patella has four strings attached to it (for each quadriceps muscle). If the string on the lateral side is really tight, and the medial string is really loose (weak); the patella would not track centrally in the trochlear notch when moving through a ROM. The tension from each string (muscle) needs to be equalized for the patella to track correctly in the notch. Referral to an orthopaedic surgeon is necessary only after 4 to 6 weeks of unsuccessful nonsurgical management. Surgery is the last resort but can be done to release tight fascia or débride the patella.[2,3]

Patellar Instability

Patellar instability is a result of traumatic subluxation or dislocation of the patella. During a subluxation or dislocation event, the medial patellofemoral ligament (MPFL) is torn (**Table 6.16**). The MPFL is the primary restraint to lateral patellar motion, so a patient with an MPFL tear may subsequently have additional lateral patellar instability episodes. The chief complaint in patients with patellar instability will be instability or episodes of subluxation or dislocation, with or without pain.

Evaluation

Initial presentation of patella instability can be acute, subacute, or chronic. Patients may complain that they have had several episodes of instability in the past (chronic), or an injury may be evaluated as the patella is dislocated or has just been reduced (acute or subacute). Observation of the knee will show obvious deformity in an acute dislocation, where the patella will be outside of the trochlear notch, on the lateral side of the knee. In chronic cases, observation will be normal. Palpation findings will vary depending on the phase of injury. Obvious deformity will be palpated in an acute injury, and effusion and tenderness may be present in a subacute injury. Flexion and extension ROM will be very limited in an acute injury, where the patella is dislocated; the patient will be apprehensive to flex or extend his or her knee. In a subacute

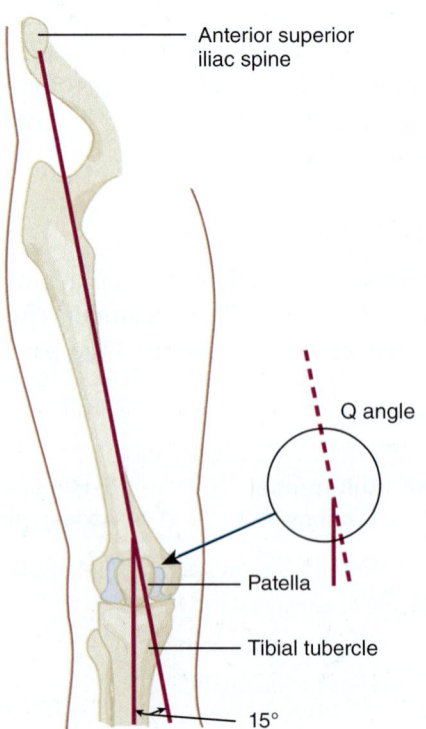

Figure 6.32 Drawing showing Q-angle measurement.

© Jones & Bartlett Learning

Table 6.16 Patellar Instability Quick Tips

Pathology	Description	Presentation (HIPS)	Special Tests/Imaging	Differential Diagnosis	5-Min Sideline Assessment Tips
Patellar instability	Includes patellar dislocation, subluxation, and the residual instability after such an episode	Dislocation: Obvious deformity of the patella laterally displaced Subluxation: Episode of the patella tracking outside of the trochlear groove, but not completely dislocating out of the joint	Lateral patellar apprehension J sign	Patellofemoral pain syndrome Loose body	To relocate a dislocated patella, passively extend the patient's knee, and the patella will be drawn back into the joint and relocated. Remove from activity and refer for further examination.

HIPS, history, inspection, palpation, special tests.

or chronic injury, flexion and extension ROM may be normal, but there will be excessive lateral patellar motion, which may cause the patient to tighten his or her quadriceps muscle to resist lateral patellar motion (apprehension).[2,3]

Special Tests

Lateral Patellar Apprehension. The patient is lying supine on the table with knees extended. The examiner stabilizes the lower leg with one hand, and with the other hand applies lateral pressure to the patella. This can be replicated with the knee bent to 45° as well. A positive examination is apprehension to the lateral motion, which can be confirmed by the patient suddenly flexing his or her quadriceps muscle to stop the lateral motion of the patella or the patient stating that he or she is uncomfortable with that motion.[9,10] The examiner should be cautious of false-positive results in patients who have excessive laxity, which will allow excessive lateral motion of the patella but will not induce apprehension (**Figure 6.33**).

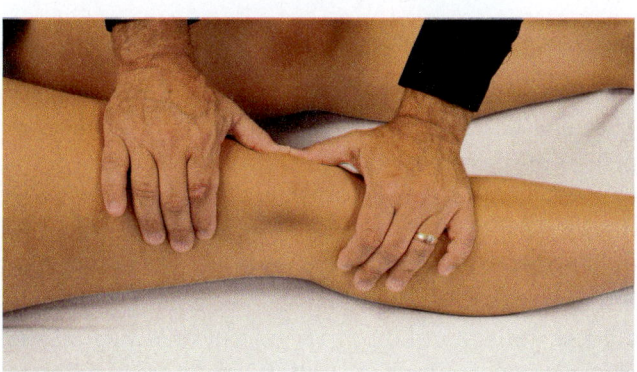

Figure 6.33 Clinical photograph showing the lateral patellar apprehension test.

© Jones & Bartlett Learning

J Sign. The patient is seated on the table with knees bent over the end at 90°. The examiner instructs the patient to extend his or her knee, while observing whether there is a sudden lateral patellar shift during extension. This finding would indicate a positive test.[9,10]

Imaging

Radiography. Radiographs could show bony abnormalities causing the instability, such as a shallow trochlear notch, as well as injury to the patella from the subluxation or dislocation event.

Magnetic Resonance Imaging. MRI could show effusion, MPFL injury, and cartilage injury from the traumatic event.

Differential Diagnoses

- PFPS
- Loose body

Treatment

Initial on-field treatment should include passively extending the patient's knee to reduce the patella if dislocated and then removing from activity and applying ice and rest. After an acute episode, the patient should be referred for imaging to observe injuries to surrounding structures that may have occurred during the event. Immobilization is not necessary but may be helpful in patients with substantial swelling.

Rehabilitation

Early rehabilitation will focus on reducing inflammation and resting the knee. Later rehabilitation focuses on strengthening the medial quadriceps muscle (vastus medialis) to help realign the patella in the trochlear notch.

Table 6.17 Patellar Tendinitis Quick Tips

Pathology	Description	Presentation (HIPS)	Special Tests/Imaging	Differential Diagnosis	5-Min Sideline Assessment Tips
Patellar tendinitis	Overuse injury commonly seen in jumping Irritation/inflammation of the patellar tendon from repetitive motion	Pain on patellar tendon Pain with explosive/jumping motion May see swelling along patellar tendon	None	Patellofemoral pain syndrome Prepatellar bursitis	Not applicable, as this is a chronic injury

HIPS, history, inspection, palpation, special tests.

Patients with recurrent instability episodes may wear a brace that helps keep the patella in place. If the patient continues to have instability episodes despite nonsurgical management, such as bracing and rehabilitation, surgery may be performed to stabilize the patella (MPFL reconstruction).

Patellar Tendinitis

Patellar tendinitis is a chronic overuse injury that usually results from repetitive flexion and extension of the knee (running or jumping). Patellar tendinitis is sometimes referred to as jumper's knee because of the mechanism of injury. This injury is common in patients who perform activities that involve repetitive jumping, such as basketball players. Patellar tendinitis is usually treated nonsurgically and rarely requires surgical intervention (Table 6.17).

Evaluation

Patellar tendinitis presents as pain and inflammation over the patellar tendon. Patients will complain that pain increases with jumping or running.[2] Observation may show swelling over the patellar tendon. Palpation may elicit pain over the patellar tendon or at the patellar tendon insertion (tibial tubercle). Knee flexion may be limited because the quadriceps muscles are tight or because of pain from stretching the patellar tendon during knee flexion.

Special Tests

Ensure the tendon is intact and not torn. Manual muscle testing can also be assessed for quadriceps group.

Imaging

Radiography. Radiographs should appear normal, although patella alta (high) or patella baja (low) can be noted.

Magnetic Resonance Imaging. MRI is not always necessary but can rule out a complete tear or other abnormalities associated with the injury.

Differential Diagnoses

- PFPS
- Prepatellar bursitis

Treatment

Initial treatment should consist of rest and removal from sport activity while completing a mild rehabilitation program until inflammation decreases. Progressive return-to-sport activity can begin after inflammation has subsided while maintaining a rehabilitation program that focuses on strengthening the hamstrings and gluteal muscles and stretching the quadriceps and hip flexors. Some patients find relief in wearing a knee strap (such as the Cho-Pat band by MEDI-DYNE) that goes around the distal knee and applies pressure on the patellar tendon (above the insertion). The strap is thought to help "move" the insertion point proximally and take stress and tension off the actual insertion point.

Summary

This chapter discussed the anatomy, injury mechanisms, and evaluation techniques of the knee joint (Table 6.18 presents a summary of special tests of the knee).[2,6,9-16] This information can be used by clinicians to evaluate patients with knee injuries. It is important to understand basic knee anatomy; having a good understanding of knee joint anatomy allows clinicians to understand where structures originate as well as the type of tissue that makes up the different structures. During an evaluation, it is important for clinicians to not only evaluate locally at the site

Table 6.18 Special Tests of the Knee

Test	Patient Position	Procedure	Positive Test	Implication	Evidence[a]
Lachman	Supine	Position hands to stabilize above and below the knee joint. Passively pull the tibia anteriorly while stabilizing the femur.	Excessive anterior displacement of the tibia	Anterior cruciate ligament rupture	Large positive likelihood ratio (27.3) and moderate negative likelihood ratio (0.15)
Anterior drawer	Supine with knee positioned in 70° to 90° of flexion, with foot flat on the table	Position hands around the proximal tibia, with thumbs resting on the tibial plateau; then pull the tibia anteriorly.	Excessive anterior displacement of the tibia	Anterior cruciate ligament rupture	Moderate positive likelihood ratio (5.2) and small negative likelihood ratio (0.43)
Pivot shift	Supine	Hold the patient's leg by placing hands on lateral knee and distal tibia. Passively flex the patient's knee while applying valgus force.	Rotational "clunk" during the rage of motion	Anterior cruciate ligament rupture	Large positive likelihood ratio (16) and moderate negative likelihood ratio (0.18)
Posterior drawer	Supine with knee positioned in 70° to 90° of flexion, with foot flat on the table	Position hands around the proximal tibia, with thumbs resting on the tibial plateau; then push the tibia posteriorly.	Excessive posterior displacement of the tibia	Posterior cruciate ligament rupture	Large positive likelihood ratio (90) and large negative likelihood ratio (0.10)
Posterior sag	Supine, with knees and hips flexed to 90°	Examiner holds the distal tibia parallel with the table and looks at tibia position from the side.	One tibia is sitting lower than the other while the patient is relaxed	Posterior cruciate ligament rupture	Large positive likelihood ratio (79) and small negative likelihood ratio (0.21)
Valgus stress	Supine	Examiner holds the patient's leg so that one hand is on the distal tibia and the other placed on the lateral knee to allow them to apply a valgus force to the knee. This examination is performed with both 0° and 30° of passive flexion.	Excessive valgus motion, compared to the contralateral side	Medial collateral ligament sprain or tear	Not applicable
Varus stress	Supine	Examiner holds the patient's leg so that one hand is on the distal tibia and the other placed on the medial knee to allow application of a varus force to the knee (may need to slightly abduct the leg to apply force). This examination is performed with both 0° and 30° of passive flexion.	Excessive varus motion, compared to the contralateral side	Lateral collateral ligament sprain or tear	Not applicable

(continues)

Table 6.18 Special Tests of the Knee (continued)

Test	Patient Position	Procedure	Positive Test	Implication	Evidence[a]
Dial	Prone, knees bent to 90° or 30°	Passively externally rotate tibia by externally rotating feet/ankles.	Excessive external rotation compared to contralateral side	Posterolateral corner injury	Small positive likelihood ratio (1.00) and small negative likelihood ratio (0.70)
McMurray	Supine	While palpating the joint line, passively flex the patient's knee while applying a varus force; then after the knee is flexed completely, passively extend the knee while applying a valgus force.	A palpable "pop" or "clunk" on the joint line	Meniscal pathology	Moderate positive likelihood ratio (3.7) and small negative likelihood ratio (0.20)
Apley compression/distraction	Prone, knees bent 90°	Hold the distal tibia and apply pressure downward into the knee; then internally and externally rotate the tibia. While maintaining the same hand position, pull upward and rotate the tibia internally and externally.	Pain, clicking, or popping with compression test and relief with the distraction test	Meniscal pathology	Small positive likelihood ratio (2.9) and small negative likelihood ratio (0.20)
Thessaly	Standing on ipsilateral leg with 20° of flexion and holding examiner's hands with contralateral knee bent to 90°	Patient actively twists on ipsilateral leg to rotate internally and externally	Pain, clicking, or popping while twisting	Meniscal pathology	Small positive likelihood ratio (1.08) and small negative likelihood ratio (0.87)
Squat (duck walk)	Patient is standing while squatting with maximal flexion	Instruct patient to walk forward while maintaining the deep squat.	Pain, clicking, or popping while walking	Meniscal pathology	Not applicable
Noble	Supine with ipsilateral hip and knee bent with 90° of flexion	Examiner palpates the IT band in the area of the femoral epicondyle and then instructs the patient to extend and flex the knee.	Pain or popping or snapping over the femoral epicondyle	IT band tightness (possibly indicative of friction syndrome)	Not applicable
Renne	Patient is standing on the ipsilateral leg	Patient is instructed to squat to 30° to 40° of flexion while examiner is palpating over the lateral femoral epicondyle.	Pain or popping or snapping over the lateral femoral epicondyle	IT band tightness (possibly indicative of friction syndrome)	Not applicable
Clarke	Supine, knee relaxed in extension	Examiner cups hand and places it so the webbing is superior to the patella. Examiner then applies an inferior force to push the patella inferiorly and then instructs the patient to contract the quadriceps muscles.	Pain under the patella	Patellofemoral injury: Injury to cartilage under the patella	Small positive likelihood ratio (1.94) and small negative likelihood ratio (0.69)

Test	Patient Position	Procedure	Positive Test	Implication	Evidence[a]
Lateral patellar apprehension	Supine, knee relaxed in extension	Examiner places hands above and below the patella, with thumbs on the medial aspect of the patella. Examiner then pushes with his or her thumbs to move the patella laterally while the patient is relaxed.	Excessive lateral patellar motion or apprehension from the patient (contraction of quadriceps muscles to pull patella back into a neutral position)	Lateral patellar instability	Small positive likelihood ratio (2.26) and small negative likelihood ratio (0.79)
J sign	Seated on a table with knees bent 90° over the edge	Patient actively extends his or her knee while examiner observes patellar position.	A sudden lateral patellar shift during extension range of motion	Patellar instability	Not applicable

[a] A positive likelihood ratio is the proportion of patients who test positive and actually have the injury. A negative likelihood ratio is the proportion of patients who test negative and do not have the injury.

of injury but also evaluate regionally at the structures surrounding the knee joint to assess for alignment issues or tightness in structures surrounding the knee that may cause pain to localize in a different area of the knee. A clinician must also think globally about the entire body and understand there could be a case, for example, where the injury is actually in the spine, possibly compressing a nerve and causing symptoms to present in the knee. There are many common knee injuries and mechanisms for these injuries, but each case will not present in the most common way. Clinicians can use the information in this chapter to develop an understanding and techniques for evaluating pathologies of the knee.

CASE STUDY 1

A 20-year-old female cross-country runner comes to you complaining of knee pain. She explains that this pain feels dull and achy and has been going on for about 2 weeks. She claims that it is getting worse, but she can continue to "run through the pain." She claims that she is experiencing some occasional "popping" when she is running, particularly as she flexes her knee. You ask her to point to her pain, and she traces a circle around the lateral aspect of her knee. There is no obvious swelling or deformity, and she has full ROM and strength. She has been applying ice to her knee after practice every day and takes naproxen twice per day.

1. What additional questions would you like to ask the patient about her knee?
2. What are your differential diagnoses at this point?
3. What special tests would you perform to help complete your evaluation?

CASE STUDY 2

You are covering a high school lacrosse game, when one of your players performs a cutting maneuver and then falls to the ground. You are called onto the field, where you find the boy holding his left knee and yelling in pain. You notice there is no obvious deformity, and you determine it is safe to move him off the field. The coach is waiting to hear from you on whether the boy can return to the game, so you need to perform a quick sideline evaluation.

1. What are some of your initial questions that you would ask this patient?
2. How do you deal with his teammates and coach hovering over you during your evaluation?
3. Where do you position the patient for an optimal examination on the sideline (note that there is no treatment table)?

After some initial questions, you learn that the patient stepped wrong while cutting, which made his knee twist; he tells you he heard a loud "pop" sound. You notice a large effusion developing as you are asking your questions. You begin your examination, and the knee is tender along the medial tibial joint line. He has limited ROM and strength because of the effusion and pain.

1. What are your differential diagnoses?
2. What special tests would you perform?
3. What do you tell the coach about the patient's participation in the game?
4. Because this patient is a minor, how would you tell a parent that this may be a serious injury that needs referral to an orthopaedic surgeon?

ONE-IN-A-MILLION CASE STUDY

During a high school football scrimmage, a talented quarterback was running during a play when the opposing player tackled his legs. The quarterback heard a loud pop and went down on the field. The athletic trainer immediately ran onto the field to find an obvious deformity: a knee dislocation.[17] This is a rare but extremely serious injury. Knee dislocations are considered potentially life threatening because of the important arteries in the knee that are providing the lower leg with blood. This was the case for the high school quarterback. The patient was immediately rushed to a hospital, where the popliteal artery assessment was initially misjudged. Through assessment at a second hospital, it was found that the patient's popliteal artery was ruptured, cutting off the blood supply to the lower leg. It is possible that the amount of time between initial injury and popliteal artery rupture diagnosis was the cause of the death of tissue in the lower leg. Without blood and oxygen supply, the tissue in the lower leg begins to die rapidly. In this case, there was no option but to amputate the leg above the knee. In rare cases such as this one, early action and referral are imperative.

1. Describe the role of the first responders in a case such as this.
2. What are some red flags that would warrant immediate referral in patients with knee injuries?
3. How can you assess for vascular injury after major knee trauma such as this?
4. What are some things an athletic trainer should have prepared (both procedurally and on the sideline) in case of a serious event such as this?

WRAP-UP

Critical Thinking Questions

1. Why is the screw-home mechanism important to knee joint kinematics?
2. Why does the quadriceps muscle atrophy after ACL reconstruction surgery? How do you manage this in your rehabilitation plan for the patient?
3. What are some key on-field assessments when examining a knee injury when determining whether a patient can return to play?
4. How could malalignment of the lower extremity affect load distribution and joint mechanics in the knee joint? How can you help correct some of these imbalances through rehabilitation?

Pearls and Pitfalls

- The terrible triad of knee injuries is rupture of the anterior cruciate ligament (ACL), medical collateral ligament (MCL), and lateral meniscus.
- Be careful of false-positive results on special tests. Anterior and posterior drawer tests can be deceiving if the position of the tibia is not neutralized before starting the test.
- The screw-home mechanism occurs during the last 30° of knee extension, where the tibia or femur rotates to achieve full extension due to the lateral femoral condyle being longer. In open-chain motion, the tibia externally rotates, and in closed-chain movements, the femur internally rotates. The rotation is necessary to achieve full

extension and accommodate for the different sized condyles.
- During a knee examination, differentiating between knee swelling and a knee joint effusion is very beneficial in helping determine which structures are injured. A knee effusion will occur only if there is injury to a structure inside the knee joint, such as the ACL, PCL, or meniscus. Swelling around the knee occurs when there is injury to a structure outside of the knee joint capsule.

References

1. Gilroy AM, MacPherson BR, Ross LM: *Atlas of Anatomy*. Stuttgart, Germany, Thieme, 2008.
2. Prentice W: *Principles of Athletic Training: A Guide to Evidence-Based Clinical Practice*. New York, NY, McGraw-Hill Education, 2016.
3. Miller MD, Hart JA, MacKnight JM: *Essential Orthopaedics* Philadelphia, PA, Saunders/Elsevier, 2009.
4. Sarin VK, Erickson GM, Giori NJ, Bergman AG, Carter DR: Coincident development of sesamoid bones and clues to their evolution. *Anat Rec* 1999;257(5):174-180.
5. Davarinos N, O'Neill B, Curtin W: A brief history of anterior cruciate ligament reconstruction. *Adv Orthopaed Surg* 2014. https://www.hindawi.com/journals/aos/2014/706042/citations/. Accessed September 13, 2019.
6. Hootman JM, Dick R, Agel J: Epidemiology of collegiate injuries for 15 sports: summary and recommendations for injury prevention initiatives. *J Athl Train* 2007;42(2):311-319.
7. Kendall FP: *Muscles: Testing and Function with Posture and Pain*, ed 5. Baltimore, MD, Lippincott Williams & Wilkins, 2010.
8. Hoppenfeld S: *Physical Examination of the Spine and Extremities*. New York, NY, Prentice/Hall International, Inc., 1990, p 16.
9. Konin JG: *Special Tests for Orthopedic Examination*. Thorofare, NJ, SLACK Incorporated, 2006.
10. Starkey C, Brown SD, Ryan JL: *Examination of Orthopedic and Athletic Injuries*, ed 3. Philadelphia, PA, Davis, 2010.
11. Wetters NG, Weber A, Wuerz TH, Schub DL, Mandelbaum BR: Mechanism of injury and risk factors for anterior cruciate ligament injury. *Operat Techniq Sports Med* 2015;24(1):2-6.
12. Benjaminse A, Gokeler A, Van der Schans CP: Clinical diagnosis of an anterior cruciate ligament rupture: a meta-analysis. *J Orthop Sports Phys Ther* 2006;36(5):267-288.
13. Swain MS, Henschke N, Kamper SJ, Downie AS, Koes BW, Maher CG: Accuracy of clinical tests in the diagnosis of anterior cruciate ligament injury: a systematic review. *Chiropr Man Therap* 2014;22:25.
14. Kopkow C, Freiberg A, Kirschner S, Seidler A, Schmitt J: Physical examination tests for the diagnosis of posterior cruciate ligament rupture: a systematic review. *J Orthop Sports Phys Ther* 2013;43(11):804-813.
15. Rinonapoli G, Carraro A, Delcogliano A: The clinical diagnosis of meniscal tear is not easy: reliability of two clinical meniscal tests and magnetic resonance imaging. *Int J Immunopathol Pharmacol* 2011;24(1 Suppl 2):39-44.
16. Nijs J, Van Geel C, Van der Auwera C, Van de Velde B: Diagnostic value of five clinical tests in patellofemoral pain syndrome. *Man Ther* 2006;11(1):69-77.
17. O'Brien K: An arm and a leg. *The New York Times Magazine*, September 2012, p MM18.

CHAPTER 7

Hip and Thigh

Maureen K. Dwyer, PhD, ATC

OVERVIEW

In this chapter, the relevant anatomy of the hip and surrounding structures as they relate to structure and function of the joint will be reviewed. Important components of the clinical evaluation process will be outlined, and descriptions of and examination findings for common pathologic conditions of the joint will be presented. In addition, actual cases of patients, outlining differential diagnosis metrics and identifying important clinical examination findings, will be reviewed.

LEARNING OBJECTIVES

After completing this chapter, the reader will be able to do the following:

1. Identify and locate structures of the musculoskeletal, articular, nervous, and vascular systems related to the hip and pelvis.
2. Understand the functional application of these anatomic structures (including muscular actions and innervations).
3. Apply knowledge of the anatomic structures and their functional application to evaluate and diagnose various pathologies seen in athletics.

FUN FACTS ABOUT THE HIP

- Although commonly referred to as a ball-and-socket joint, the hip more closely resembles a conchoid shape,[1] which results in a slightly incongruous joint.
- The altered geometry of the articulation is important for appropriate transmission of loads and regulating dynamic lubrication during weight-bearing activities.
- The incongruity of the joint's surfaces produces both rolling and gliding arthrokinematic motions, which may help distribute contact loads and prevent early joint wear.

Introduction

As the link between the axial skeleton and the lower extremity, the hip is designed to provide a high degree of stability and mobility to allow for proper functioning and performance during activities. Although not as common as injuries to other joints, pathologic conditions of the hip can be difficult to diagnose and result in significant impairments and functional limitations. Comprehensive knowledge of hip anatomy and mechanics, along with a thorough understanding of normal joint function, is important to identify pathologic conditions and determine effective treatments.

Clinical Anatomy

Skeletal Anatomy

The hip is a multiaxial joint formed by the articulation between the os coxae and femur. Each innominate bone is composed of three bones—the ilium, ischium, and pubis—that unite at the triradiate cartilage to form the acetabulum (**Figure 7.1**). Complete bony fusion of the three bones of the pelvis does not

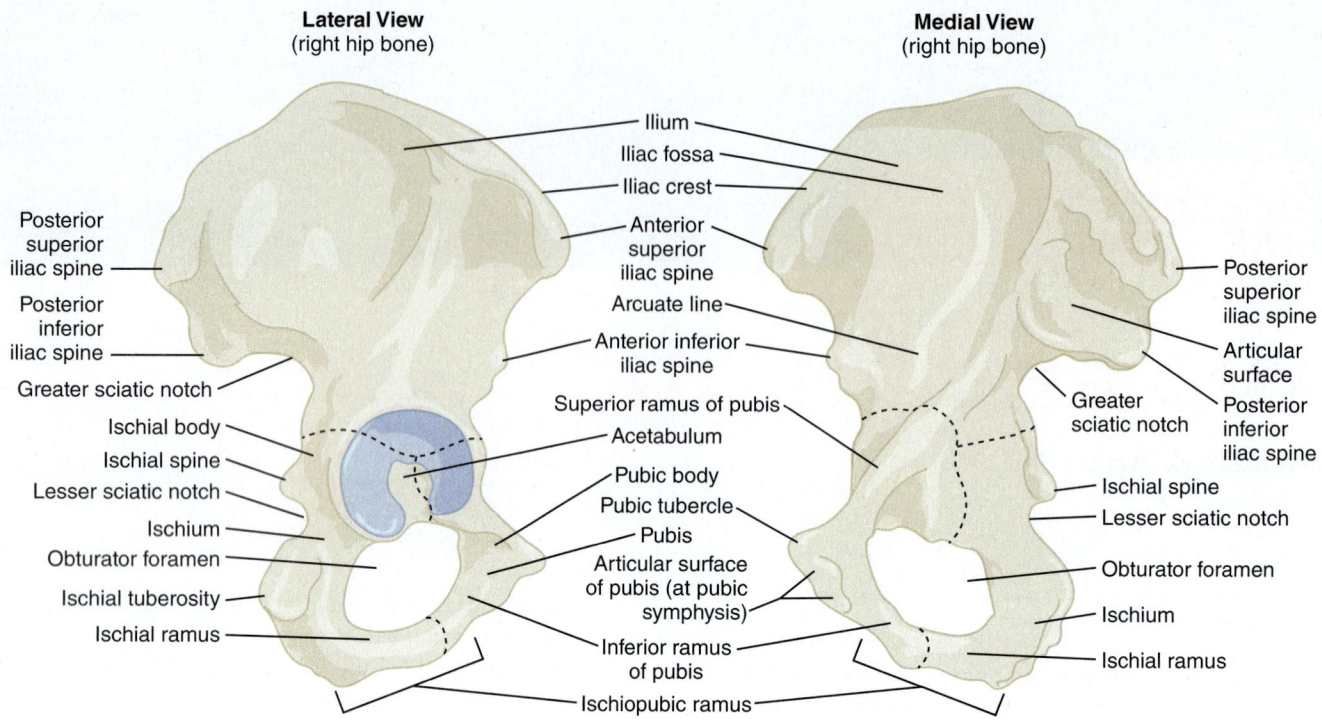

Figure 7.1 Drawings showing bony landmarks of the pelvis.
© Jones & Bartlett Learning

occur until adulthood.[2] The ilium is the largest of the three bones and forms the superior portion of the coxal bone. The ilium consists of a body and a wing. The wing is bordered by the large iliac crest along its superior margin, which extends to terminate anteriorly at the anterior superior iliac spine (ASIS) and posteriorly at the posterior superior iliac spine (PSIS). These three bony landmarks are easily palpated during the clinical examination and are important to assess for the presence of pelvic obliquities. Inferiorly along the anterior margin of the ilium is another bony prominence, the anterior inferior iliac spine, which serves as an important attachment point for the rectus femoris muscle. Posteriorly, the auricular surface of the ilium serves as the site of articulation with the sacrum to create the sacroiliac (SI) joint. Inferior to the PSIS, the posterior inferior iliac spine forms the superior border of the greater sciatic notch, through which the sciatic nerve travels to pass into the thigh. The sacrospinous ligament forms its inferior border and separates the greater and lesser sciatic foramen (**Figure 7.2**). The body of the ilium makes up the superoanterior portion of the acetabulum.

The ischium is a small, L-shaped bone that makes up the posterior margin of the pelvis (Figure 7.1). The ischium is composed of a body and two projecting rami, the superior and inferior ischial rami. The body enlarges posteriorly to form the ischial tuberosity, which is the attachment site for the hamstring muscle group. It is also the bone that supports the weight of the body during sitting. The two rami serve as important attachment sites for muscles.

The anterior margin of the os coxae is formed by the pubis (pubic bone) (Figure 7.1). The pubis consists of a body and two rami that connect it to the ilium superiorly and to the ischium inferiorly. The opening formed by the rami of the pubis and ischium is called the obturator foramen, an important anatomic landmark that serves as a conduit for arteries and nerves. The obturator foramen is covered by a strong membrane that provides surface area for muscle attachments (**Figure 7.3**). The two innominate bones articulate anteriorly at the pubic symphysis and are connected by strong ligaments.

The hip bone articulates with the femur at the concave acetabulum. The external border, or lunate surface, of the acetabulum is crescent moon shaped and covered with articular cartilage (**Figure 7.4**). The nonarticular central fossa serves as the attachment point for the ligamentum teres extending from the femoral head. The acetabulum is incomplete inferiorly, forming a notch that allows the passage of blood vessels and nerves into the central cavity of the joint. Attached to and extending the rim of the acetabulum is a ring of fibrocartilage called the acetabular labrum. The labrum is triangular in cross section,[3-5] connecting directly to the articular cartilage of the acetabulum (**Figure 7.5**). The labrum provides two key functions to help maintain normal hip mechanics: it enhances joint

Clinical Anatomy 165

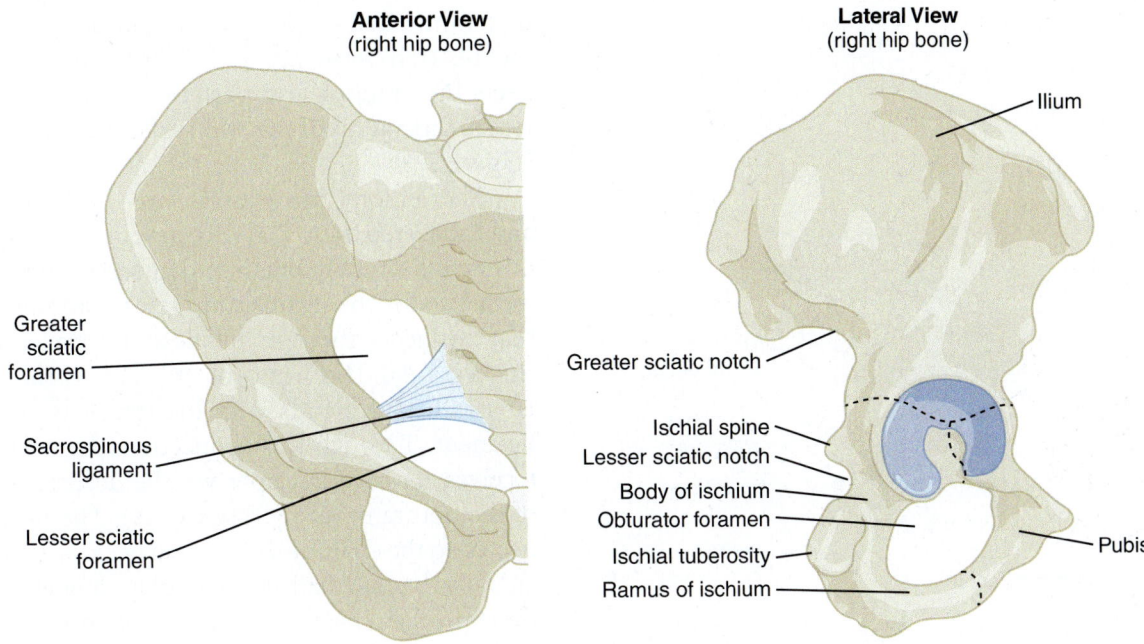

Figure 7.2 Drawings showing anterior and lateral views of the greater and lesser sciatic notch of the pelvis.
© Jones & Bartlett Learning

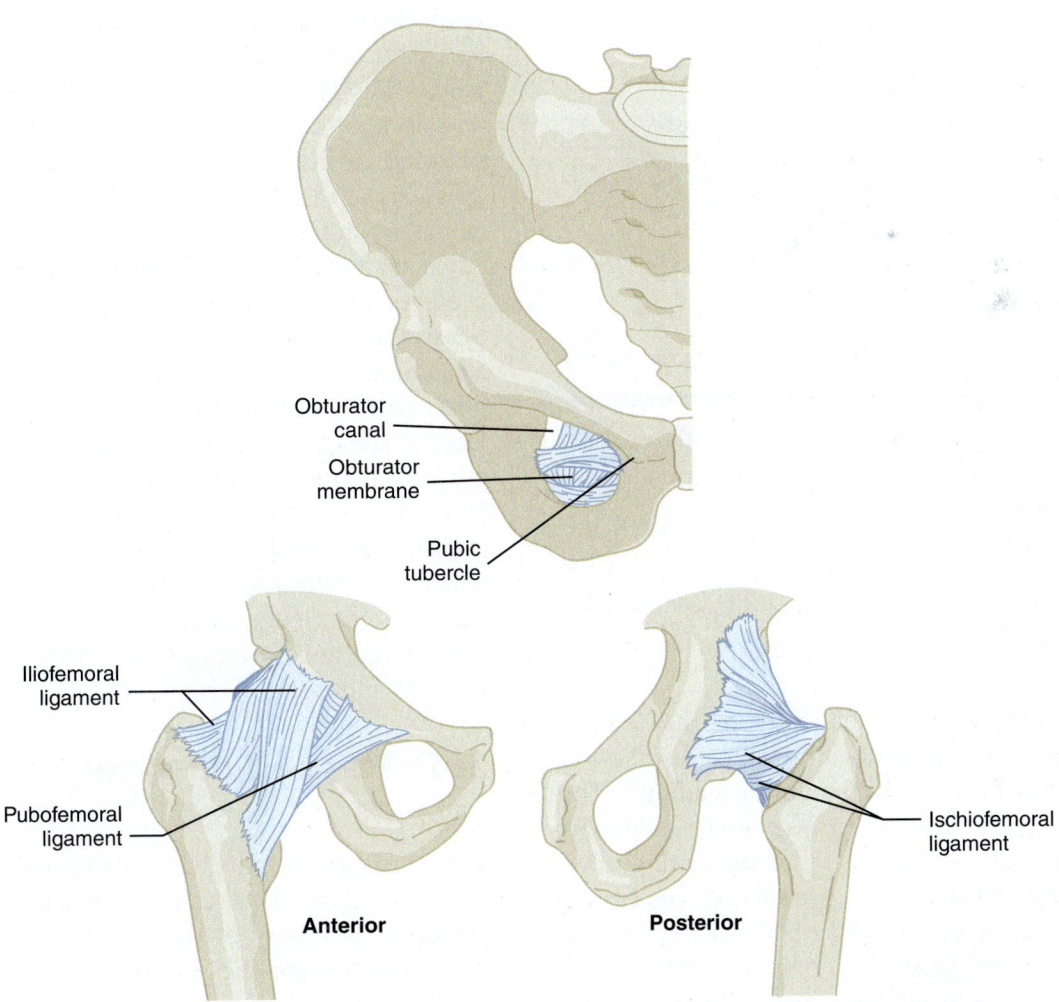

Figure 7.3 Drawings showing anterior and posterior views of the hip ligaments.
© Jones & Bartlett Learning

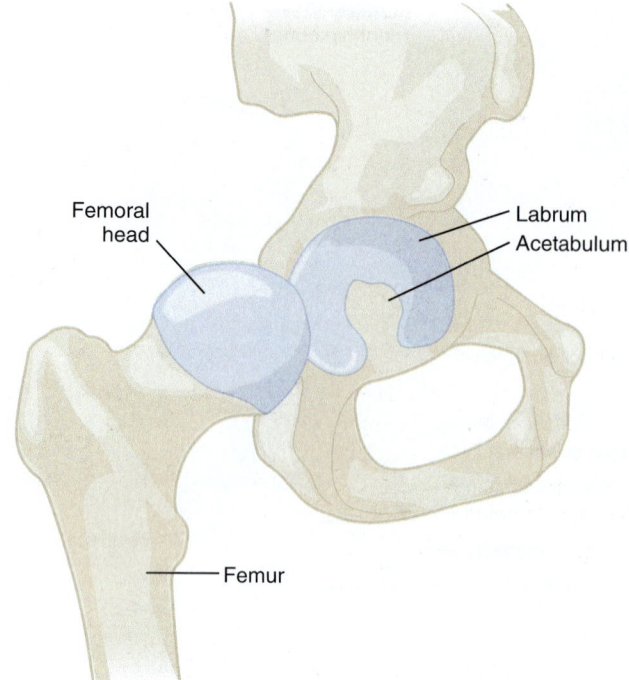

Figure 7.4 Drawing of the hip bone showing the acetabulum and labrum.

© Jones & Bartlett Learning

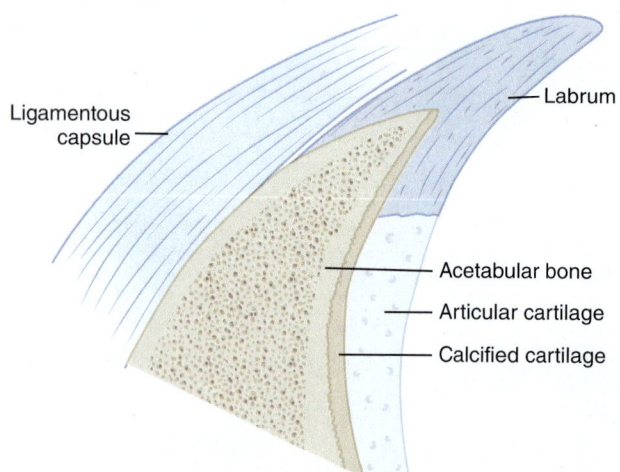

Figure 7.5 Drawing showing a cross section of the labrum.

© Jones & Bartlett Learning

is continued inferiorly across the acetabular notch by the transverse acetabular ligament, which connects the anterior and posterior lunate surfaces and resists separation of the two surfaces during loading[11] (Figure 7.4).

The femoral head forms two-thirds of a sphere and is covered with a layer of articular cartilage. At its center is a small depression that serves as the attachment site for the ligamentum teres, a round ligament that connects the femoral head to the acetabulum (Figure 7.4). The ligament attaches to the acetabular notch and blends with the transverse acetabular ligament. Through this connection, the femoral head receives its blood supply via the acetabular branch of the obturator artery (**Figure 7.6**). The head is connected to the shaft by the femoral neck, which is wider laterally than medially because of its angular extension down to the lesser trochanter. Superiorly, the neck is bordered by the large greater trochanter (**Figure 7.7**). Connecting the two trochanters anteriorly is the smooth intertrochanteric line and posteriorly is the rough intertrochanteric crest. These bony landmarks mark the border between the femoral neck and shaft and serve as important attachment sites for thigh and pelvic muscles. Appropriate orientation of the head and neck is important to enhance joint stability and preserve the health of the labrochondral surfaces. The long axis of the head and neck projects superomedially at an angle to the long axis of the obliquely oriented shaft (**Figure 7.8**). Normal head and neck offset averages $125°$[12] and allows for greater mobility as it places the head and neck more perpendicularly to the acetabulum in a neutral position. Reduced femoral offset could result in impingement of the joint's surfaces at the end ranges of motion.[13] The acetabulum is normally oriented $45°$ caudally and $15°$ anteriorly.[14] Normal acetabular anteversion averages $15°$ to $20°$[15] (**Figure 7.9**). Finally, the degree of acetabular depth, which determines femoral head coverage, is assessed via the center-edge angle of Wiberg. The normal center-edge angle averages $30°$, with angles smaller than $20°$ indicative of dysplasia.[16]

Soft-Tissue Anatomy

Ligaments

The hip is surrounded by a dense cylindrical capsule extending proximally from the anterior and posterior periphery of the acetabulum, external to the labrum. It attaches distally to the intertrochanteric line of the anterior femoral neck and posteriorly along a free border. The capsule enhances joint stability by preventing translation of the femoral

stability by increasing acetabular volume and femoral head coverage[3] and provides a pressurized seal of the central compartment of the hip during loading.[6,7] This seal helps prevent expression of synovial fluid from the central cavity of the joint, thus preventing direct contact of the articular cartilage surfaces.[8] The labrum is highly innervated, containing both nociceptors and mechanoreceptors.[9] However, only the external one-third of the labrum contains blood vessels, leaving most of the structure avascular[10] and limiting its healing ability following injury (Figure 7.5). The labrum

Clinical Anatomy 167

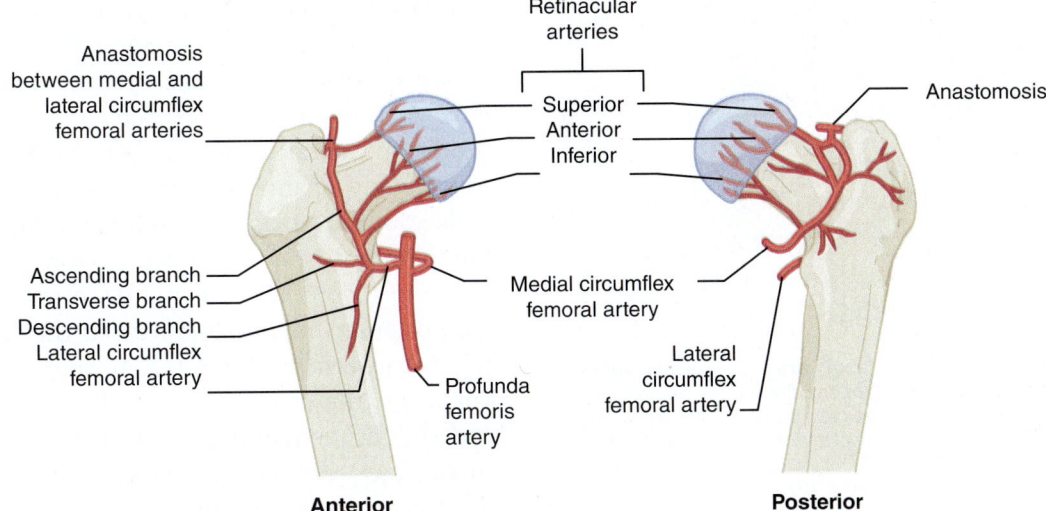

Figure 7.6 Drawings showing the vascular supply to the femoral head.
© Jones & Bartlett Learning

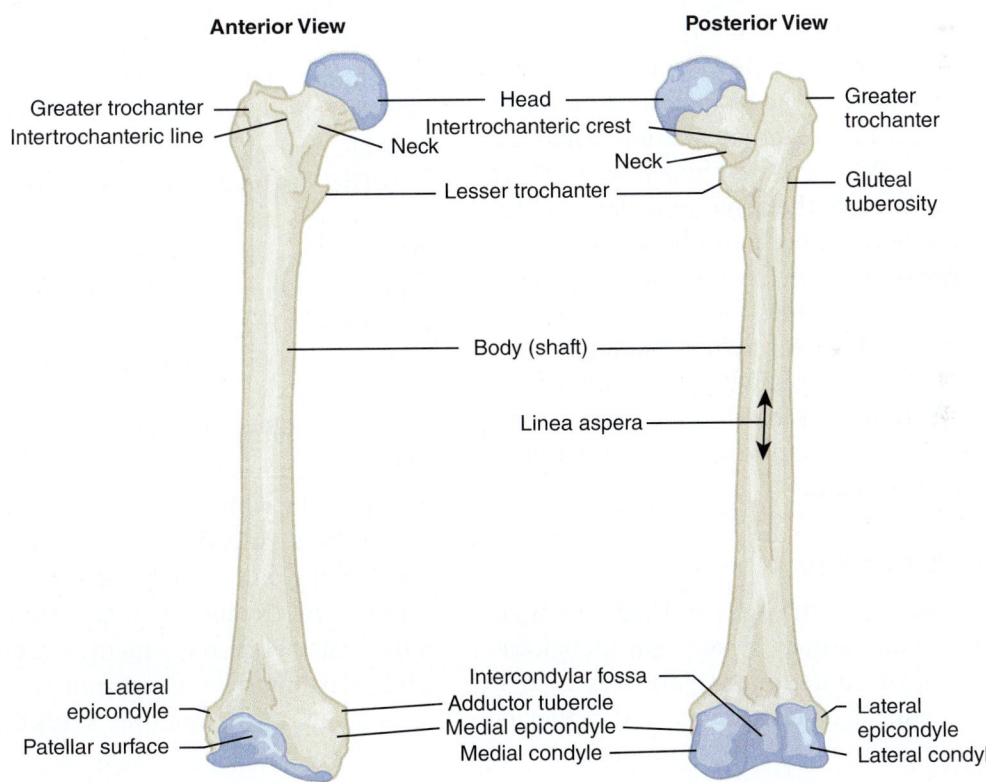

Figure 7.7 Drawings showing bony landmarks of the femur.
© Jones & Bartlett Learning

head in the acetabulum[17] and restraining free motion about the hip. Reinforcing the capsule are the three main ligaments that support the hip (**Figure 7.10**). Anteriorly, the Y-shaped iliofemoral ligament is the thickest[18] and strongest of the three.[19] The medial arm of the iliofemoral ligament is oriented vertically and connects the anterior inferior iliac spine (AIIS) to the distal anterior intertrochanteric line, whereas the lateral arm is directed more horizontally, originates slightly superior to the medial arm, and attaches to the anterior greater trochanter.[20] The iliofemoral ligament as a whole restricts external rotation,[20-23] whereas, in isolation, the lateral arm limits extension of the joint.[21] The ischiofemoral ligament extends from the ischial margin of the acetabulum to the greater trochanter of the femur. This ligament

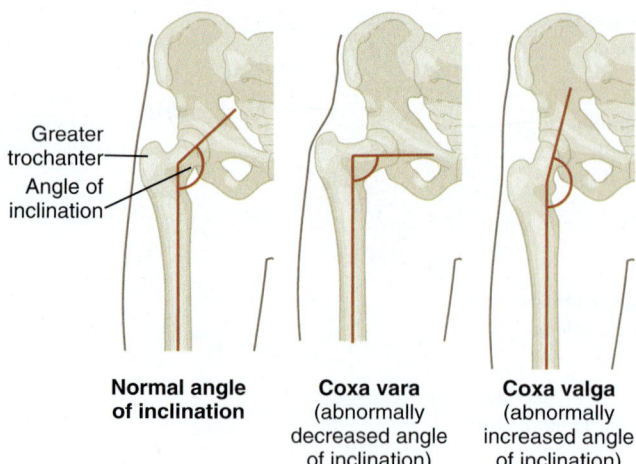

Figure 7.8 Drawings of the hip showing the angles of inclination.

© Jones & Bartlett Learning

provides support posteriorly and restricts internal rotation motion.[20,21] Inferiorly, the pubofemoral ligament resembles a sling, extending from the obturator crest of the pubic bone to the femoral neck, and acts to limit abduction and external rotation while the hip is extended.[20] Deep arcuate fibers from all three ligaments merge to form the zona orbicularis, which circumvents the femoral neck and helps to support the anterosuperior portion of the joint capsule.[24] The zona orbicularis provides the greatest contribution to resisting dislocation forces.[25] Although not a primary contributor to ligamentous stability of the hip, the ligamentum teres has been shown to prevent anteroinferior subluxation of the femoral head during squatting activities.[26,27]

Muscular Anatomy

The muscles that act on the hip and thigh are organized into four compartments based on their location and function: the anterior compartment, medial compartment, gluteal compartment, and posterior compartment. The anterior compartment consists of the sartorius, iliopsoas, quadriceps, and pectineus muscles (**Figure 7.11**). The origins, insertions, and innervations of these muscles are described in **Table 7.1**. The sartorius muscle is the longest muscle in the body, spanning from the ASIS to the medial surface of the tibia. The tendons of the gracilis and semitendinosus muscles merge with the sartorius to form a conjoined tendinous attachment called the pes anserinus. Also known as the "tailor's muscle" because it produces the movement of crossing one's legs, the sartorius acts to flex, laterally rotate, and abduct the femur at the hip. Because the sartorius crosses the knee, it can also assist with flexing the leg at the knee. Direct palpation of the sartorius muscle can be performed by placing a hand just distal and slightly medial to the ASIS while the patient actively flexes and laterally rotates the thigh. Electromyography (EMG) analysis revealed that the sartorius is most active during resisted flexion, abduction, and lateral rotation with the patient supine and this position should be used for manual muscle testing.[28]

The iliopsoas muscle complex is a composite of the iliacus, psoas major, and psoas minor muscles. The tendons of the iliacus and psoas major merge to form a conjoined tendon that attaches to the lesser trochanter of the femur (**Figure 7.12**). Together, these muscles are the prime flexor of the thigh at the hip and contribute to lateral rotation. The psoas major also contributes to stabilization of the lumbar spine.[29] The iliacus muscle can be palpated distal and medial to the ASIS while the patient is actively flexing the hip. Direct palpation of the psoas muscle is more challenging, but it can be performed. With the patient supine, the examiner's fingers are placed next to the umbilicus; while the patient is contracting his or her abdominal muscles, the examiner slides his or her fingers lateral to the midline. With the patient relaxed,

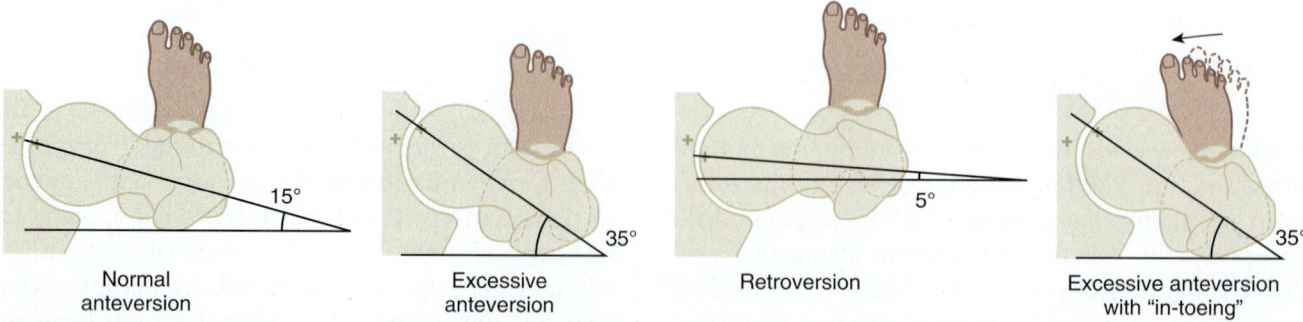

Figure 7.9 Drawings showing various degrees of anteversion and retroversion.

© Jones & Bartlett Learning

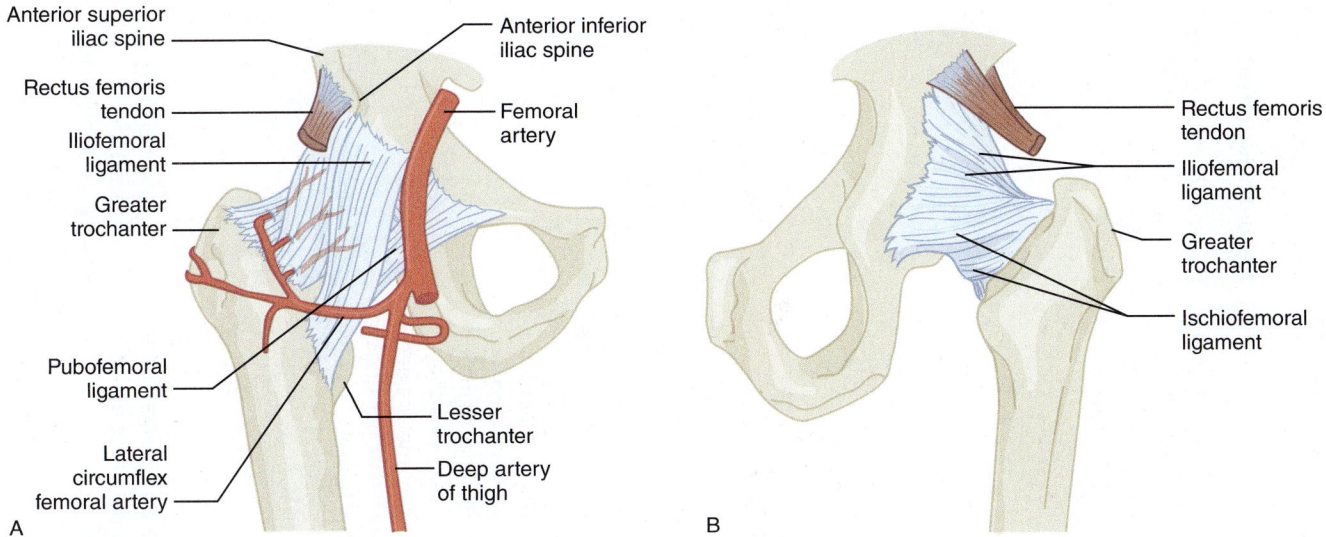

Figure 7.10 Drawings showing the hip ligaments. **A.** Anterior view. **B.** Posterior view.
© Jones & Bartlett Learning

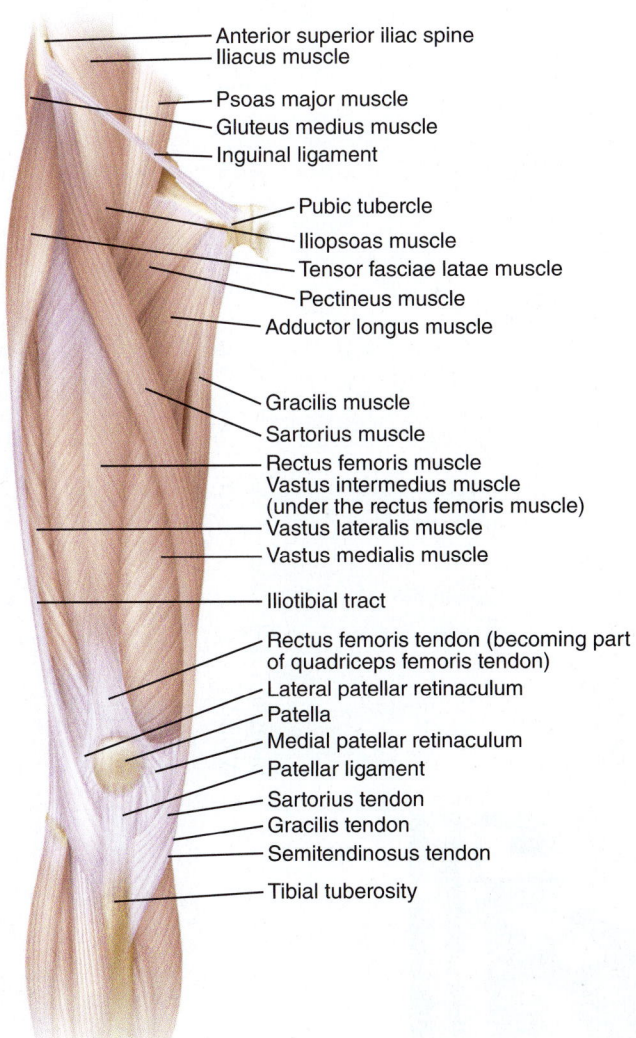

Figure 7.11 Drawing showing the anterior thigh muscles.
Reproduced from Armstrong AD, Hubbard MC. eds: *Essentials of Musculoskeletal Care*, ed 5. Burlington, MA, American Academy of Orthopaedic Surgeons, 2015.

the examiner slowly presses his or her fingers into the abdominal cavity until they are a couple of centimeters deep and then moves his or her fingers toward the spine to feel the psoas major.

If the patient is having difficulty relaxing, he or she should take a deep breath, and the examiner should begin pressing into the abdominal cavity while the patient exhales. Manual muscle testing for the iliopsoas muscle is performed by resisting hip flexion, with the knee straight, while the patient is in the supine position.

The quadriceps muscle group consists of four muscles: the vastus lateralis, vastus medialis, vastus intermedius, and rectus femoris (Figure 7.11). Of these, only the rectus femoris muscle crosses the hip, originating at the AIIS. As a group, the quadriceps muscles extend the leg at the knee, whereas the rectus femoris alone assists with hip flexion. The quadriceps muscles can be easily palpated along the anterior thigh. Manual muscle testing for the rectus femoris is best performed by resisting hip flexion while the patient is seated with the knee flexed to 90°.

The smallest muscle of the anterior compartment, the pectineus primarily functions to flex and adduct the thigh at the hip (Figure 7.11). EMG activity of the pectineus muscle was observed to be highest during hip flexion activities with moderate activity during exercises that required stabilization during static rotation.[30] Although a secondary internal rotation function has been suggested based on the muscle's anatomy, the recorded contribution of this muscle during static hip rotation exercises was negligent.[30]

The gluteal region is organized into superficial and deep muscles. The origins, insertions, and

Table 7.1 Muscles of the Anterior Compartment of the Thigh

Muscle	Origin	Insertion	Innervation	Palpation	Manual Muscle Test
Sartorius	ASIS and superior notch inferior to it	Superior part of medial surface of tibia	Femoral nerve	Palpated by placing a hand just distal and slightly medial to the ASIS while the patient actively flexes and laterally rotates the thigh	Patient seated with the hips and knees at 90°. Resistance applied to medial knee and medial distal tibia.
Iliopsoas					
Psoas major	Sides of T12–L5 vertebrae, intervertebral discs; transverse processes of L1–L5	Lesser trochanter of femur	Anterior rami L1–L3	With the patient supine, the examiner's fingers are placed next to the umbilicus, and, while the patient is contracting his or her abdominal muscles, the examiner slides his or her fingers lateral to the midline. With the patient relaxed, the examiner slowly presses his or her fingers into the abdominal cavity until they are a couple of centimeters deep and then moves his or her fingers toward the spine to feel the psoas major	Patient supine with the knee extended. Resistance applied at distal thigh.
Psoas minor	Sides of T12–L1 and IV disc	Pectineal line, iliopectineal eminence via iliopectineal arch	Anterior rami L1–L2	N/A	N/A
Iliacus	Iliac crest, iliac fossa, ala of sacrum, and anterior sacroiliac ligaments	Tendon of psoas major, lesser trochanter, and femur distal to it	Femoral nerve	Palpated distal and medial to the ASIS while the patient is actively flexing the hip	Patient supine with the knee extended. Resistance applied at distal thigh.

Clinical Anatomy

Quadriceps				
Vastus lateralis	Greater trochanter and lateral lip of linea aspera		Palpated along the lateral portion of the anterior thigh	Patient seated with the knee flexed to 90°. Resistance applied to shank while patient extends knee.
Vastus intermedius	Anterior and lateral surfaces of proximal femur		N/A	
Vastus medialis	Intertrochanteric line and medial lip of linea aspera	Conjoined tendon that attaches directly to the base of the patella and indirectly to the tibial tuberosity via the patellar ligament	Palpated along the medial portion of the anterior thigh	
Rectus femoris	AIIS		Palpated along the central portion of the anterior thigh	Patient seated with the knee flexed to 90°. Resistance applied to thigh while patient flexes hip.
			Femoral nerve	
Pectineus	Superior pubic ramus	Pectineal line of femur, just inferior to lesser trochanter	Palpated deep between the lateral and medial borders of the femoral triangle	Patient supine with knee extended. Resistance applied at distal thigh.
			Femoral nerve	

AIIS, anterior inferior iliac spine; ASIS, anterior superior iliac spine; N/A, not applicable.
All photos courtesy of Andrea Cripps and Matt Kutz.

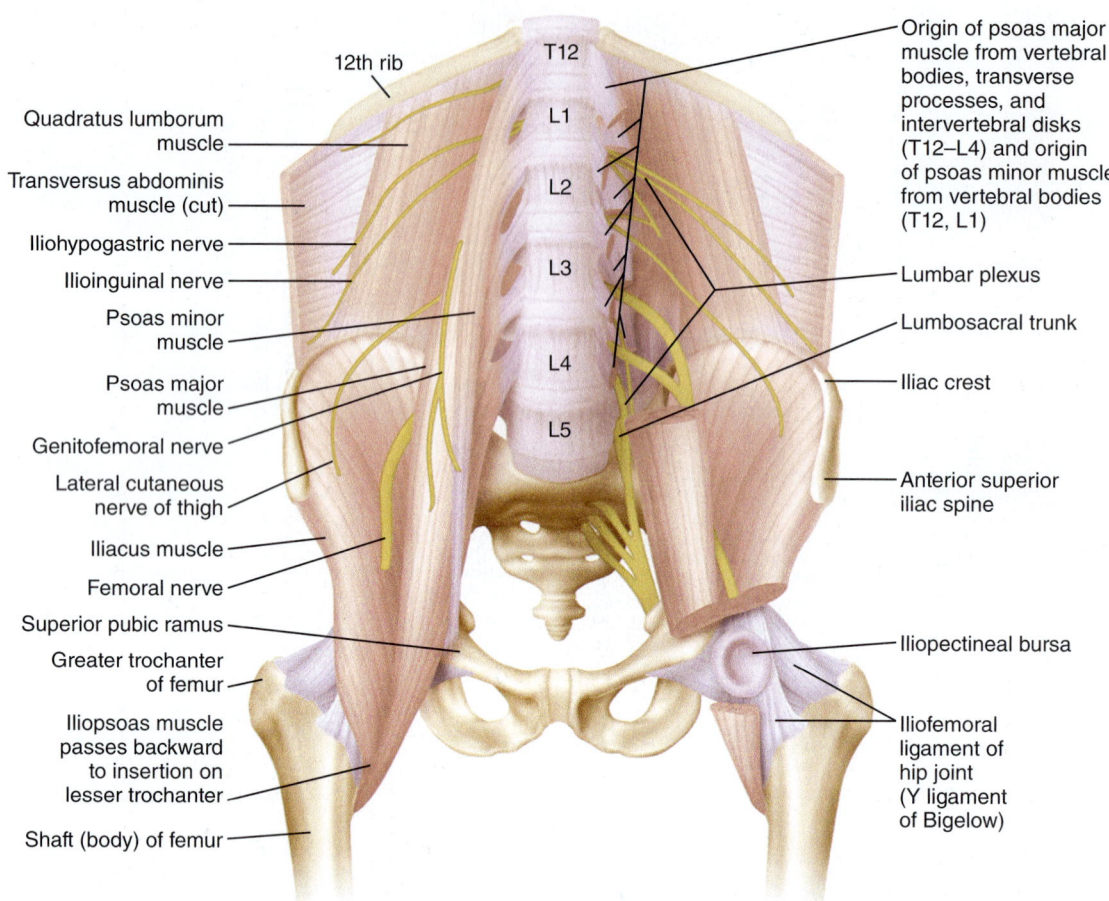

Figure 7.12 Drawing showing the anterior muscles of the pelvis.

Reproduced from Armstrong AD, Hubbard MC. eds: *Essentials of Musculoskeletal Care*, ed 5. Burlington, MA, American Academy of Orthopaedic Surgeons, 2015.

innervations of these muscles[31] are described in **Table 7.2**. The superficial muscles include the gluteus maximus and the three muscles that make up the pelvic deltoid: the gluteus minimus, gluteus medius, and tensor fascia lata (TFL) (**Figure 7.13**). The gluteus maximus is the strongest of the thigh muscles, acting to extend the thigh at the hip, especially from a seated position. It also assists in lateral rotation and thigh stabilization. The gluteus maximus muscle is easily palpated posteriorly of the buttock. Manual muscle testing is best examined during resisted thigh extension with the patient prone and the knee flexed to 90°.

The gluteus medius is a fan-shaped muscle that is separated into functionally distinct anterior, middle, and posterior parts. The anterior and middle fibers are oriented almost vertically, whereas the posterior fibers are more horizontal, parallel to the femoral neck[32] (**Figure 7.14**). EMG studies show phasic activation of the three parts of the gluteus medius muscle during gait, with the posterior segment demonstrating higher activity during the first 20% of the gait cycle and the anterior segment during mid-late stance phase.[32,33] Similar to the gluteus medius muscle, the gluteus minimus muscle is also divided into anterior and posterior parts, which function independently and phasically during the gait cycle.[34] The shift from posterior to anterior activation occurs as the body weight is propelled over the stance limb. Anatomic examinations revealed that fibers of the gluteus minimus muscle converge with the capsule on insertion, allowing it to assist with joint stabilization, especially when the thigh is extended.[35] Mechanically, the small gluteal muscles are at a disadvantage to act as the primary hip abductors; however, the vertically oriented fibers of the TFL provide this muscle with a better mechanical advantage to produce hip abduction[32] (**Figure 7.15**). EMG analysis supports this, as the gluteus medius exhibited minimal activity during isolated hip abductions, while the TFL showed intense activity.[32] As a result, the primary function of the gluteus medius and minimus muscles is pelvic stabilization during weight bearing, with the anterior portion of the gluteus medius assisting with pelvic

Table 7.2 Muscles of the Gluteal Compartment of the Thigh

Muscle	Origin	Insertion	Innervation	Palpation	Manual Muscle Test
Gluteus maximus	Ilium posterior to posterior gluteal line, dorsal surface of sacrum and coccyx, sacrotuberous ligament	Iliotibial tract, which inserts into lateral condyle of tibia; some fibers insert on gluteal tuberosity	Inferior gluteal nerve	Patient is prone. Palpated along the posterior buttock.	Resisted thigh extension with the patient prone and the knee flexed to 90°.
Gluteus medius	External surface of ilium between anterior and posterior gluteal lines, spanning from the ASIS to PSIS	Lateral surface of greater trochanter	Superior gluteal nerve	Patient is supine. Palpated at the proximal lateral ilium, along its insertion, inferior to the iliac crest.	The patient is in the side-lying position with the testing leg on top. Resistance to hip abduction is applied over the distal thigh.
Gluteus minimus	External surface of ilium between anterior and inferior gluteal lines, spanning from the AIIS to PIIS	Anterior surface of greater trochanter		N/A	
Tensor fascia lata	Ilium posterior to posterior gluteal line, dorsal surface of sacrum and coccyx, sacrotuberous ligament	Iliotibial tract, which inserts into lateral condyle of tibia; some fibers insert on gluteal tuberosity		Patient is supine. Palpated along the anterior iliac crest.	

(continues)

Table 7.2 Muscles of the Gluteal Compartment of the Thigh

Muscle	Origin	Insertion	Innervation	Palpation	Manual Muscle Test
Piriformis	Anterior surface of S2-S4	Superomedial surface of greater trochanter	Anterior rami S1-S2	Palpated by placing the thumb of one hand on the PSIS and the pinky of the same hand on the greater trochanter. The piriformis will be located at the level of the middle finger.	Patient is supine with the leg and thigh flexed to 90°. Resistance is applied to the lateral aspect of the knee while the patient externally rotates.
Obturator internus	Rami of obturator foramen and quadrilateral plate	Superomedial surface of greater trochanter	Nerve to obturator internus	N/A	
Superior gemellus	Ischial spine	Medial surface of greater trochanter			
Inferior gemellus	Ischial tuberosity	Medial surface of greater trochanter	Nerve to quadratus femoris	N/A	
Quadratus femoris	Lateral border of ischial tuberosity	Quadrate tubercle on intertrochanteric crest			

(continued)

AIIS, anterior inferior iliac spine; ASIS, anterior superior iliac spine; N/A, not applicable; PIIS, posterior inferior iliac spine; PSIS, posterior superior iliac spine.
Reproduced from Solomon LB, Lee YC, Callary SA, Beck M, Howie DW. Anatomy of piriformis, obturator internus and obturator externus: implications for the posterior surgical approach to the hip. *J Bone Joint Surg Br* 2010;92(9):1317-1324.
All photos courtesy of Andrea Cripps and Matt Kutz.

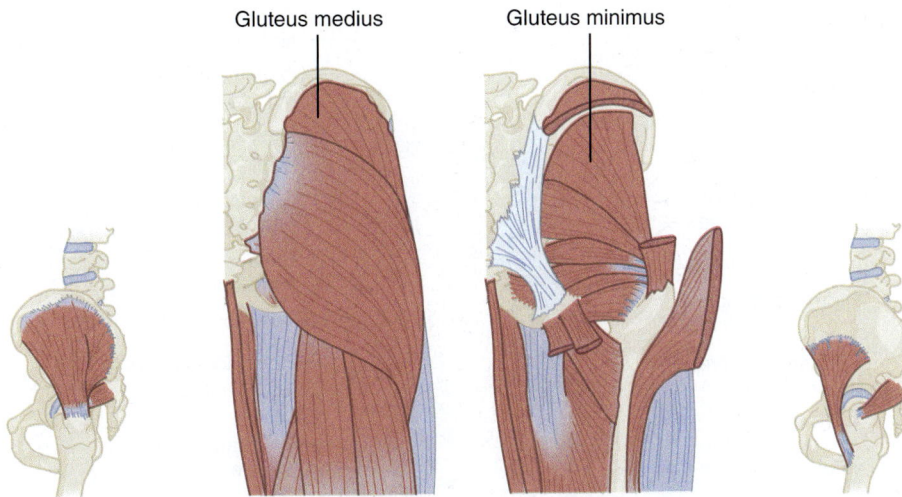

Figure 7.13 Drawings showing the muscles of the superficial gluteal compartments of the thigh. The figures on the left show the gluteus medius in isolation, and the figures on the right show the gluteus minimus in isolation.

© Jones & Bartlett Learning

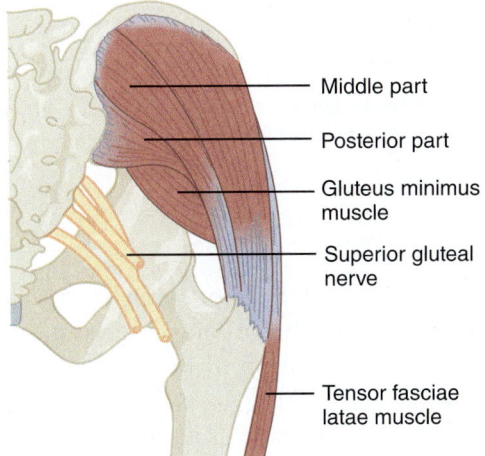

Figure 7.14 Drawing showing the functional segments of the gluteus medius.

© Jones & Bartlett Learning

rotation. The role of the gluteus medius and minimus in hip abduction is secondary, with the anterior fibers helping to initiate this motion before the TFL takes over.[32] The gluteus medius muscle can be palpated at the proximal lateral ilium, along its insertion, inferior to the iliac crest, whereas the TFL is best identified by palpating the anterior iliac crest. Manual muscle testing for the hip abductors is traditionally performed with the patient side lying and the testing leg on top. Resistance to hip abduction is applied over the distal thigh;[28] however, assessing muscle performance during resisted abduction in standing may be more functionally applicable.[36]

Often called the rotator cuff of the hip, the deep muscles of the gluteal compartment consist of the piriformis, obturator internus, superior and inferior

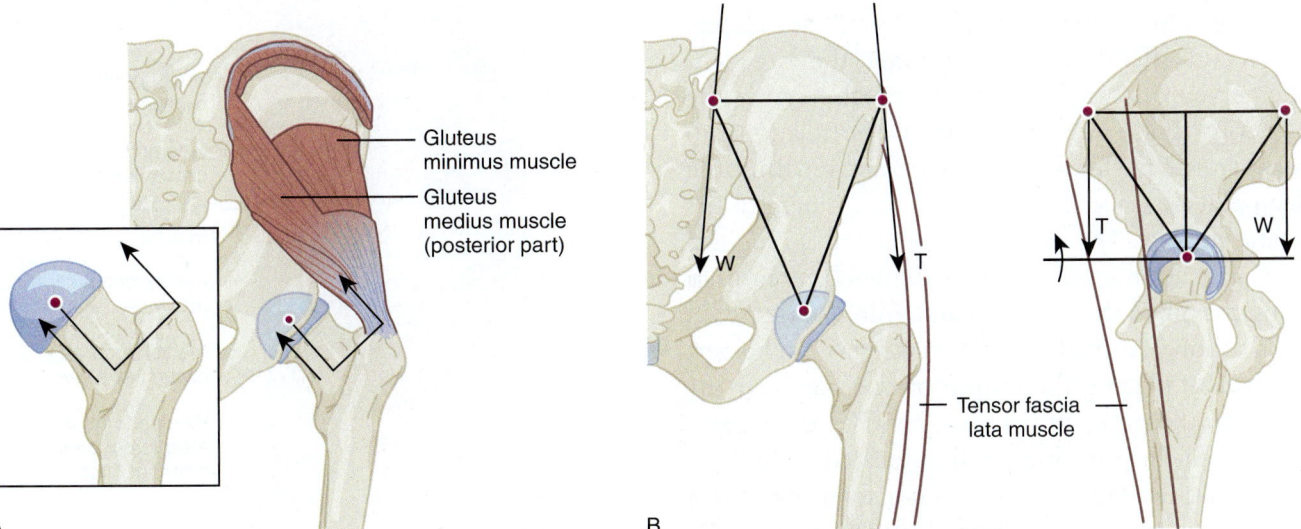

Figure 7.15 Drawing showing mechanical angles of the hip. **A.** Gluteus medius. **B.** Tensor fascia lata, where T is the resultant force of the tensor fascia lata muscle and the anterior part of the gluteus medius, and W is the body weight force.

© Jones & Bartlett Learning

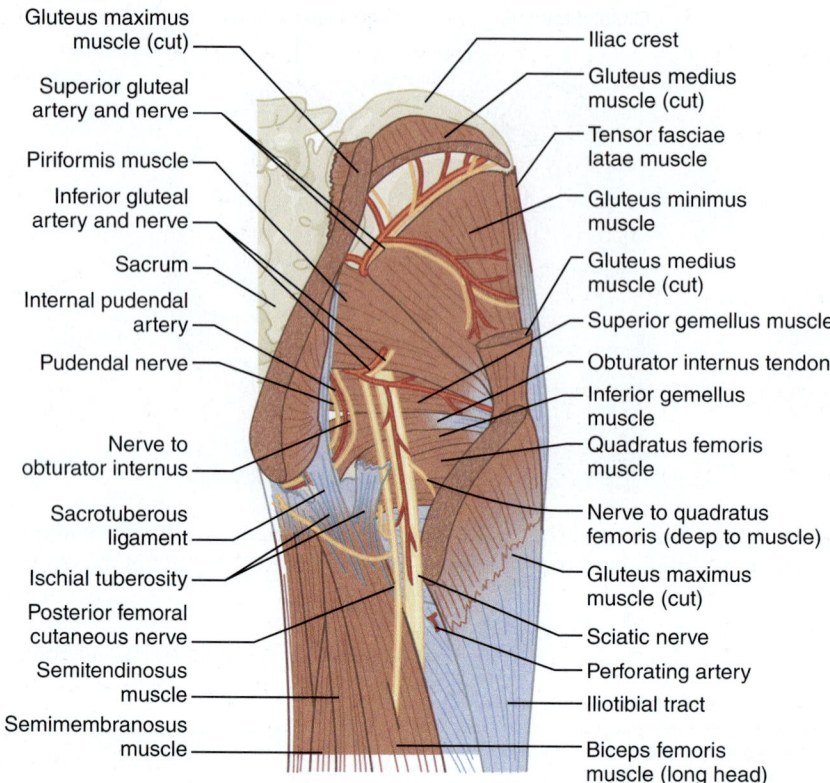

Figure 7.16 Drawing showing the muscles of the deep gluteal compartment.
© Jones & Bartlett Learning

gemelli, and quadratus femoris (**Figure 7.16**). Although small in size, the piriformis muscle is an important anatomic landmark and functional component of the hip. Originating from the anterior sacral vertebrae, the piriformis passes through the greater sciatic notch to reach the greater trochanter of the femur. In doing so, it serves as a border, with the superior gluteal nerve and vessels exiting superior to it and the inferior gluteal nerve and vessels exiting inferior to it (**Figure 7.17**). Lateral to the inferior gluteal nerve and inferior to the piriformis, the large sciatic nerve exits the greater sciatic notch to enter the posterior thigh. Any alteration in the relationship between the piriformis and sciatic nerve within the deep gluteal space can result in impingement of the sciatic nerve.[37] The piriformis exhibited its highest EMG activation levels during activities that required stabilization of the hip by maintaining static external rotation.[30] Palpation of the piriformis can be performed by placing the thumb of one hand on the PSIS and the pinky of the same hand on the greater trochanter. The piriformis will be located at the level of the middle finger. The obturator internus covers most of the internal obturator foramen, exiting the pelvis through the lesser sciatic notch (Figure 7.16). It exists as a tendon, which separates the bellies of the superior and inferior gemelli muscles. The three muscles form a conjoined tendon and function as a unit. Activation of the obturator internus has been shown during isometric hip abduction, extension, and external rotation torques.[38] The

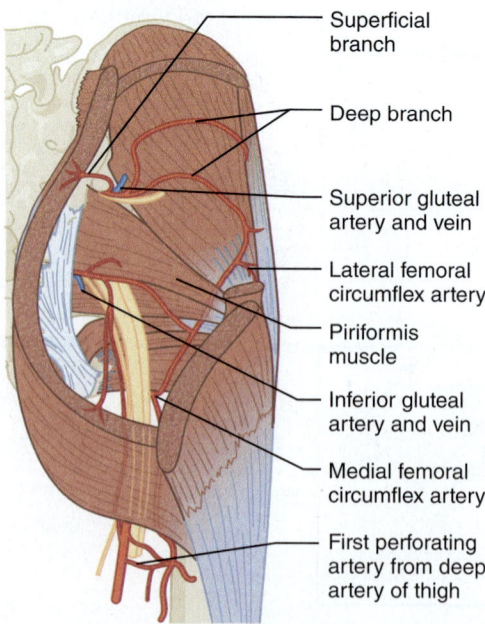

Figure 7.17 Drawing showing the structures comprising the greater sciatic foramen.
© Jones & Bartlett Learning

quadratus femoris also demonstrated high levels of activity during resisted external rotation.[39] Given the small moment arms of all the deep gluteal muscles, they most likely are not capable of producing large degrees of lateral rotation; however, their high level of activity during functional activities is likely demonstrative of their role in joint stabilization, as they contract to prevent subluxation of the femoral head in the acetabulum.[39]

The medial compartment of the hip consists of the gracilis, adductor longus, adductor brevis, adductor magnus, and obturator externus muscles (**Figure 7.18**). The origins, insertions, and innervations of these muscles are described in **Table 7.3**. The gracilis is the only medial compartment muscle to cross both the hip and knee and joins the sartorius and semitendinosus in attaching at the pes anserinus. Given its vertical orientation, the gracilis is not capable of producing large forces, acting more as a synergist to adduction of the thigh and flexion and medial rotation of the leg at the knee.

The adductor longus originates as a strong tendon from the body of the pubis, which can be easily observed and palpated during resisted adduction, especially when the leg is placed in a figure-of-4 position. Deep to the adductor longus lies the adductor brevis, the smallest of the adductor muscles. The adductor brevis is an important anatomic landmark, as the divisions of the obturator nerve pass anterior and posterior to it. The largest of the adductor muscles, the adductor magnus, has both an adductor and hamstring portion. The fibers of the adductor portion are oriented medially and originate from the rami of the pubis and ischium, whereas the fibers of the hamstring portion are more vertical and originate with the hamstring muscle group from the ischial tuberosity. The two portions function independently, mimicking their names. The hamstring portion of the adductor magnus is the only muscle of the medial compartment that is not innervated by the obturator nerve, receiving its innervation from the sciatic nerve. As a group, the adductor muscles function to adduct the thigh, with the adductor magnus most active during resisted adduction. The adductor group was found to produce the greatest force during supine adduction with the legs straight; however, resisted adduction with the hips flexed to 45° resulted in the highest level of EMG muscle activation.[40] These positions are recommended for use during manual muscle testing.

The final muscle of the medial compartment of the thigh is the obturator externus (Figure 7.18). Although it can be classified as a deep rotator of the hip because of its location and action, the obturator externus shares a common innervation with the muscles of the medial compartment, so it is often described with them. The obturator externus originates along the external border of the obturator foramen and passes sling-like under the femoral neck to attach to the trochanteric fossa. This anatomic orientation contributes to its primary function of stabilizing the femoral head in the acetabulum.[41]

The posterior compartment of the thigh comprises the hamstring muscles: the biceps femoris, semimembranosus, and semitendinosus (**Figure 7.19**). The origins, insertions, and innervations of these muscles are described in **Table 7.4**. The biceps femoris has both a long and a short head, with only the long head capable of acting to move both the hip and knee. The lateral long head of the biceps femoris and the two medial hamstring muscles share a strong tendinous origin off the ischial tuberosity. The short head of the biceps femoris originates along the linea aspera of the femur, combining with the long head to attach to the fibular head. The semitendinosus travels to the superior margin of the tibia to attach

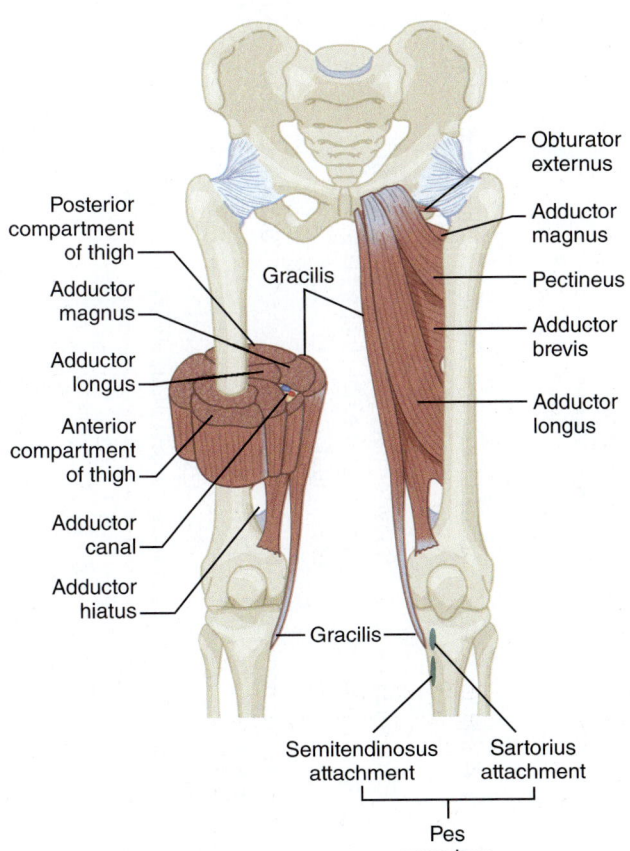

Figure 7.18 Drawing showing the muscles of the medial compartment of the thigh.

© Jones & Bartlett Learning

Table 7.3 Muscles of the Medial Compartment of the Thigh

Muscle	Origin	Insertion	Innervation	Palpation	Manual Muscle Test
Adductor longus	Body of the pubis, inferior to the pubic crest	Middle third of the medial lip of the linea aspera	Obturator nerve	Patient is supine with leg in a figure-of-4 position. Palpated along medial border of the proximal thigh.	Patient is supine with knee extended. Resistance along medial thigh while patient adducts.
Adductor brevis	Inferior ramus and body of pubis	Pectineal line and proximal part of the linea aspera	Obturator nerve	N/A	
Adductor magnus					
Adductor portion	Inferior ramus of pubis and ramus of ischium	Gluteal tuberosity, linea aspera, and medial supracondylar line	Obturator nerve	Patient is supine with knee extended. Palpated on the medial aspect of the thigh while applying resistance into hip adduction, feeling for the engagement of the musculature.	Patient is supine with knee extended. Resistance along medial thigh while patient adducts.
Hamstring portion	Ischial tuberosity	Adductor tubercle of the femur	Tibial part of the sciatic nerve		
Gracilis	Body and inferior ramus of pubis	Superior part of the medial surface of the tibia (pes anserinus)	Obturator nerve		
Obturator externus	External bony margin of the obturator foramen	Piriformis fossa	Obturator nerve	N/A	Tested with piriformis muscle.

Courtesy of Andrea Cripps and Matt Kutz.

Data from Solomon LB, Lee YC, Callary SA, Beck M, Howie DW. Anatomy of piriformis, obturator internus and obturator externus: implications for the posterior surgical approach to the hip. *J Bone Joint Surg Br* 2010;92(9):1317-1324.

Clinical Anatomy **179**

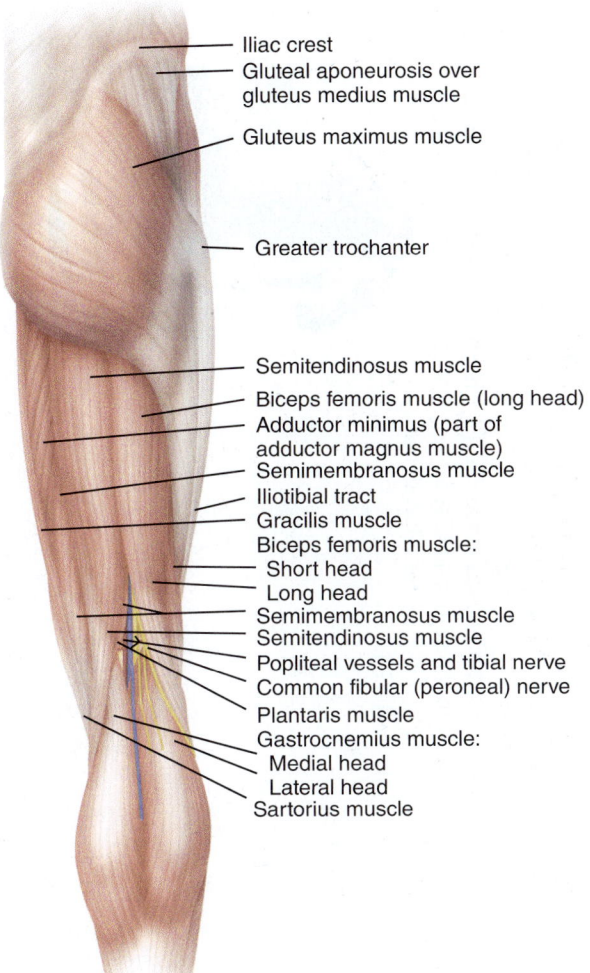

Figure 7.19 Drawing showing the muscles of the posterior compartment of the thigh.

Reproduced from Armstrong AD, Hubbard MC. eds: *Essentials of Musculoskeletal Care*, ed 5. Burlington, MA, American Academy of Orthopaedic Surgeons, 2015.

Neurologic Anatomy

The four main nerves innervating muscles of the hip and thigh are the femoral nerve anteriorly, the sciatic nerve posteriorly, the obturator nerve medially, and the gluteal nerves for the gluteal muscles (**Figure 7.20**). The femoral nerve is the largest branch of the lumbar plexus and travels from the abdominal cavity into the pelvis by passing deeply to the inguinal ligament. It then enters the femoral triangle, lateral to the femoral artery and vein (**Figure 7.21**). Upon entering the thigh, the femoral nerve branches to innervate the muscles of the anterior thigh.

The sciatic nerve, the largest nerve in the body, is the continuation of the sacral plexus and is really two nerves that share the same sheath: the tibial nerve and common fibular nerve, named for their paths and innervation in the leg. The sciatic nerve passes through the greater sciatic notch, inferior to the piriformis muscle, and travels deep to the gluteus maximus and posterior to the adductor magnus, separating into its two nerves approximately midway down the thigh. The sciatic nerve innervates no muscles in the gluteal region but supplies all the muscles in the posterior thigh, leg, and foot.

The obturator nerve arises from the lumbar plexus and passes into the lower pelvis, traveling through a hole in the obturator membrane known as the obturator canal. It then divides into anterior and posterior branches that travel with the adductor brevis to supply the muscles of the medial compartment (**Figure 7.22**).

The deep gluteal nerves originate from the sacral plexus, leaving the pelvis via the greater sciatic notch, either superior or inferior to the piriformis muscle. The superior gluteal nerve runs between the gluteus medius and minimus, innervating both muscles along with the TFL. The inferior gluteal nerve provides innervation to the gluteus maximus (**Figure 7.23**).

Testing for appropriate nerve function is performed by assessing both motor and sensory output along with reflexes. Sensory output is assessed by touching or tapping along the areas of innervation (**Figure 7.24**). The L1 nerve root provides sensory innervation to the buttock and proximal posterior thigh, whereas L2 supplies the lateral proximal thigh and L3 the medial and distal thigh. Sensory innervation to the leg is provided by L4–S1 nerve roots, with L4 supplying the medial leg and first toe, L5 supplying the lateral proximal leg and middle toes, and S1 supplying the distal lateral leg and fifth toe. Motor testing for the femoral nerve is performed by resisting knee flexion. Motor performance of the common fibular nerve is assessed by resisted

with the sartorius and gracilis at the pes anserinus. In contrast, the semimembranosus tendon attaches to the posterior medial tibial condyle. The hamstring muscles act to flex the leg at the knee and extend the thigh at the hip, but they cannot produce both movements at the same time. With the knee straight, they produce active extension of the hip, especially in a weight-bearing position. The biceps femoris also contributes to lateral rotation of a flexed knee, whereas the medial hamstrings contribute to medial rotation. The hamstrings can easily be palpated along the posterior thigh, with their tendons becoming most prominent against resisted knee flexion. Manual muscle testing for the hamstring muscles is performed with the patient prone and resistance provided against knee flexion. Medially or laterally rotating the leg during testing can help isolate the hamstring muscles.

Table 7.4 Muscles of the Posterior Compartment of the Thigh

Muscle	Origin	Insertion	Innervation	Palpation	Manual Muscle Test
Biceps femoris					
Long head	Ischial tuberosity		Tibial portion of sciatic nerve	Patient is prone. Palpated along the lateral portion of the posterior thigh.	Patient is prone. Resistance along the posterior shank while flexing the knee. Lateral rotation of the leg during testing can isolate the biceps femoris.
Short head	Lateral lip of linea aspera	Lateral side of the head of fibula; tendon is split by the lateral collateral ligament	Common fibular portion of sciatic nerve		
Semitendinosus		Medial surface of the superior part of the tibia (pes anserinus)		Patient is prone. Palpated along the medial portion of the posterior thigh. Semimembranosus tendon lies deep to the semitendinosus tendon and is better felt with the knee flexed.	Patient is prone. Resistance along the posterior shank while flexing the knee. Medial rotation of the leg during testing can isolate the medial hamstring muscles.
Semimembranosus	Ischial tuberosity	Medial condyle of tibia	Tibial portion of sciatic nerve		

All photos courtesy of Andrea Cripps and Matt Kutz.

Clinical Anatomy

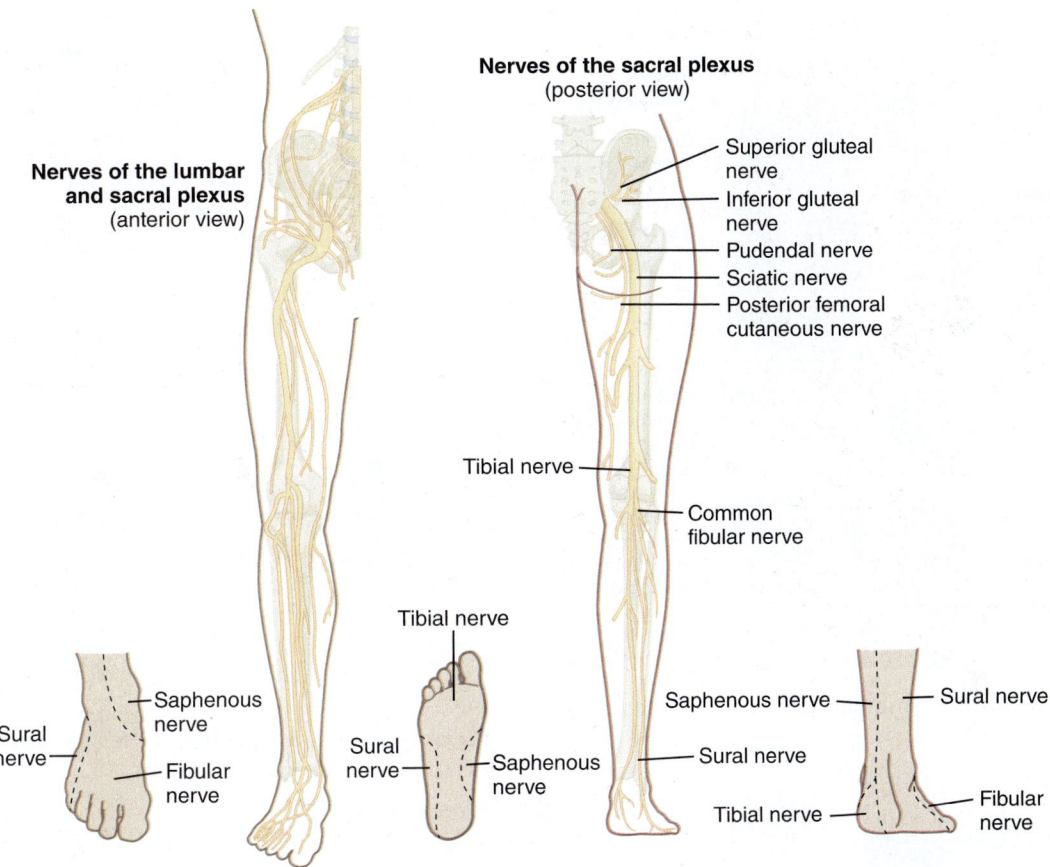

Figure 7.20 Drawings showing the nerves of the hip and thigh.
© Jones & Bartlett Learning

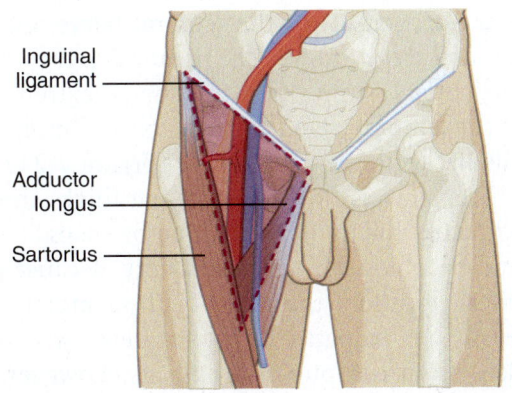

Figure 7.21 Drawing of the pelvis showing the femoral triangle.
© Jones & Bartlett Learning

dorsiflexion, whereas the tibial nerve is assessed by resisted plantar flexion. Reflex testing for L2–L4 is assessed with the patellar reflex and for S1 with the Achilles reflex (**Figure 7.25**).

Vascular Anatomy

The femoral artery is the direct continuation of the external iliac artery as it passes deeply to the inguinal ligament and enters the femoral triangle

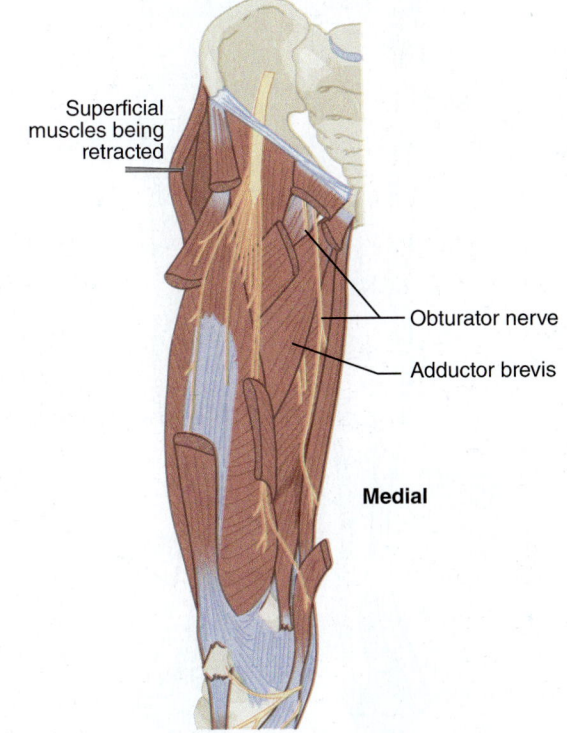

Figure 7.22 Drawing of the lower pelvis and thigh musculature showing the obturator nerve branches.
© Jones & Bartlett Learning

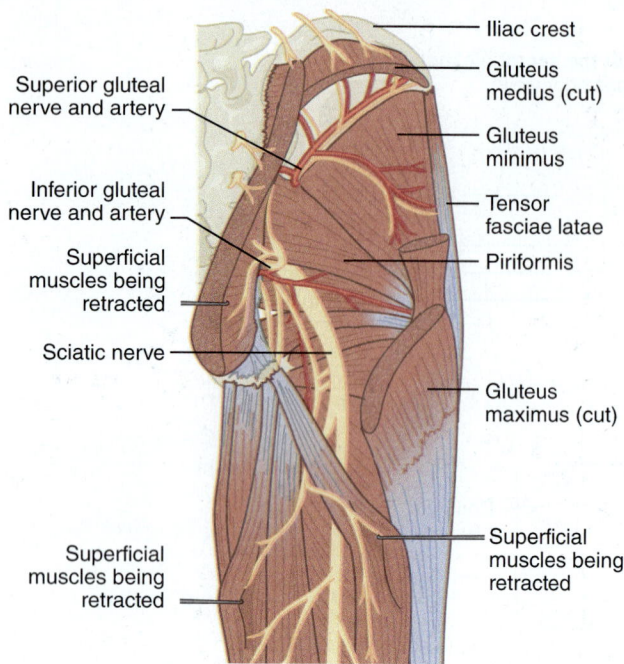

Figure 7.23 Drawing of the thigh musculature showing the gluteal nerves.

© Jones & Bartlett Learning

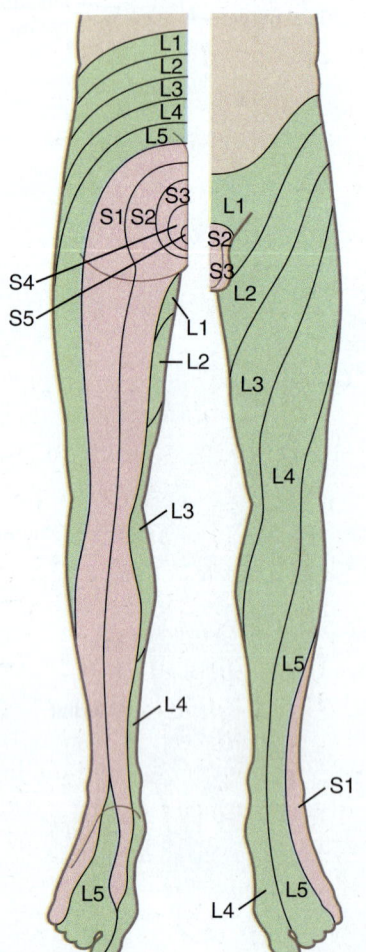

Figure 7.24 Drawing showing a map of the dermatomes of the lower extremities.

© Jones & Bartlett Learning

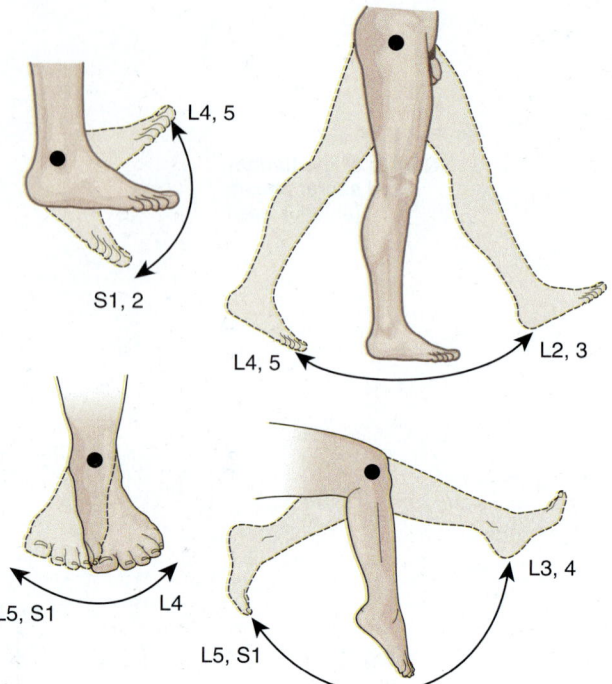

Figure 7.25 Drawing showing the myotomes and reflexes of the lower extremities.

© Jones & Bartlett Learning

(**Figure 7.26**). The femoral triangle is bordered laterally by the sartorius, medially by the adductor longus, and superiorly by the inguinal ligament. It is the main conduit for the femoral nerve and vessels to enter the thigh. The femoral artery is the primary blood supply for the lower extremity. It enters the femoral triangle lateral to the femoral vein and medial to the femoral nerve (Figure 7.21). The artery then travels down the medial thigh, through the adductor hiatus in the adductor magnus muscle, and becomes the popliteal artery. Because of its superficial location, the pulse of the femoral artery can easily be palpated approximately two fingerbreadths from the pubic symphysis; however, this also places the artery at risk for injury.

The femoral artery branches distal to the inguinal ligament to form the deep artery of the thigh, which passes down the posterior medial thigh to supply the muscles of the anterior compartment (Figure 7.26). Coming off the deep artery of the thigh are the medial and lateral circumflex arteries. The medial circumflex artery provides most of the blood supply to the femoral head and neck. Injury to this region can disrupt these vessels. The lateral circumflex artery passes laterally to supply the lateral muscles of the thigh.

The obturator artery is the continuation of the internal iliac artery (**Figure 7.27**). This artery passes

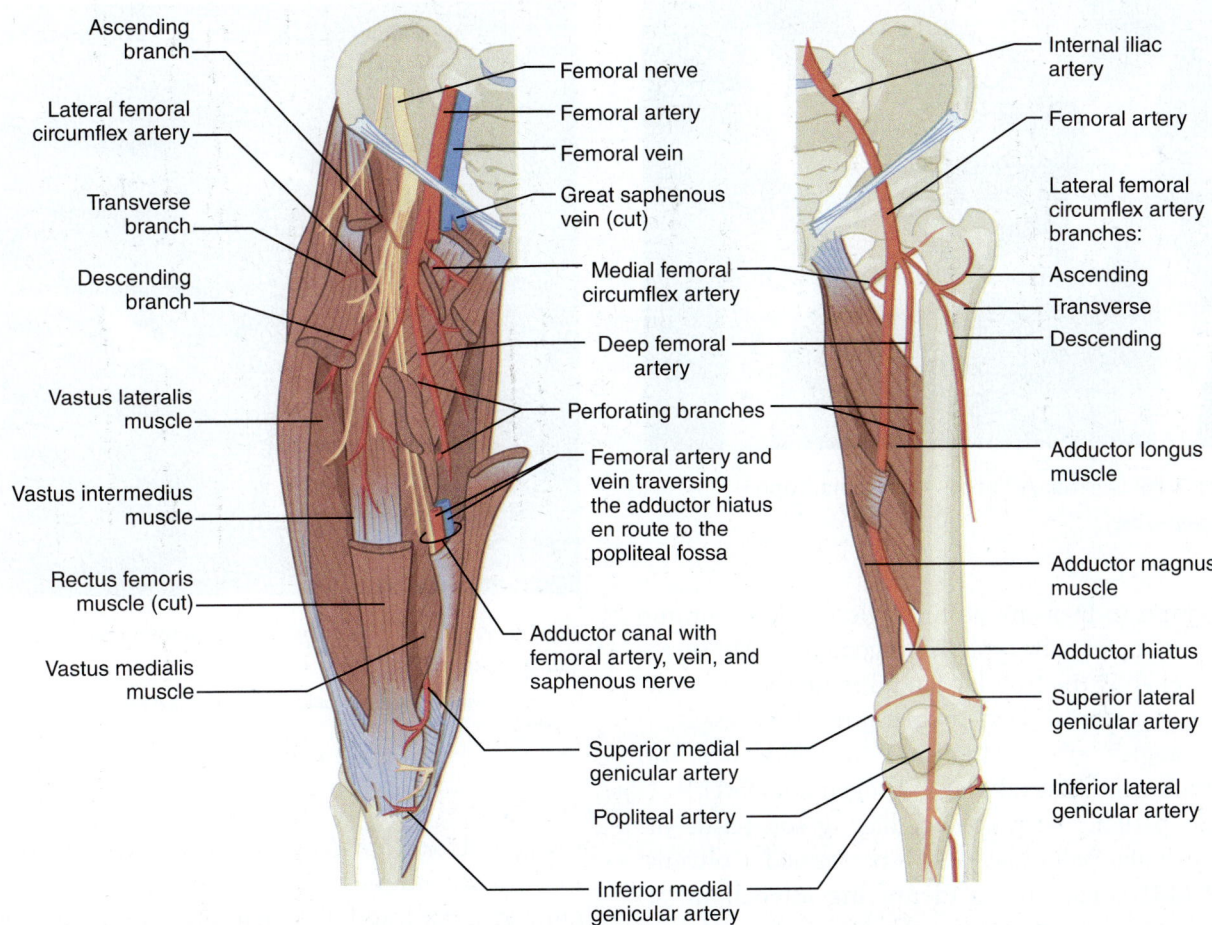

Figure 7.26 Drawings showing the vascular anatomy of the lower leg.

© Jones & Bartlett Learning

through the obturator membrane, with the obturator nerve and vein, and divides into anterior and posterior branches, which are bisected by the adductor brevis. The obturator artery provides blood supply to the muscles of the medial compartment.

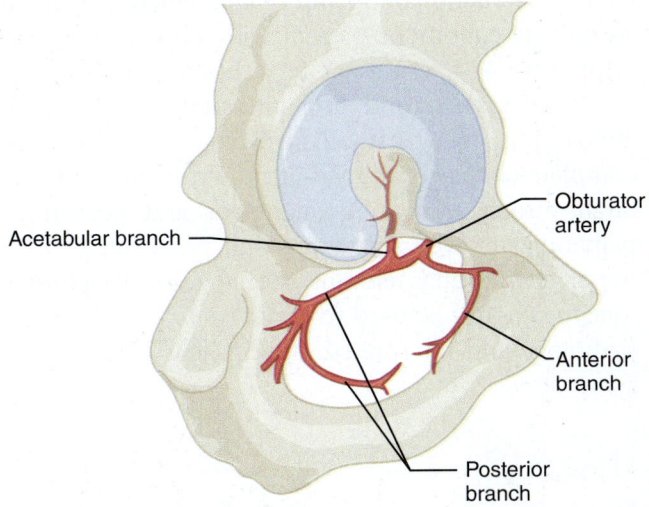

Figure 7.27 Drawing of the pelvis showing the obturator artery and its branches.

© Jones & Bartlett Learning

Overview of Radiology and Imaging

Plain radiographs are often the first imaging studies obtained for patients presenting with hip pain. Although fractures and dislocations can occur at the pelvis and femur, they are not common; thus, plain radiographs for this region are most useful in assessing joint morphology and degenerative changes. The type of radiographic imaging performed is dependent on the suspected pathology. Standard AP radiographs of the hip and pelvis are obtained to determine the presence of fractures, examine bony architecture, check for evidence of joint-space narrowing or changes to bone quality, and quantify femoral head coverage (**Figure 7.28**). Femoral head coverage is assessed by measuring the lateral center-edge angle (**Figure 7.29**). A lateral center-edge angle less than 20° is indicative of hip dysplasia, or a shallow hip socket, whereas lateral center-edge angle values greater than 35° indicate overcoverage, resulting in a pincer-type impingement.[42] The 45° Dunn view is the most appropriate

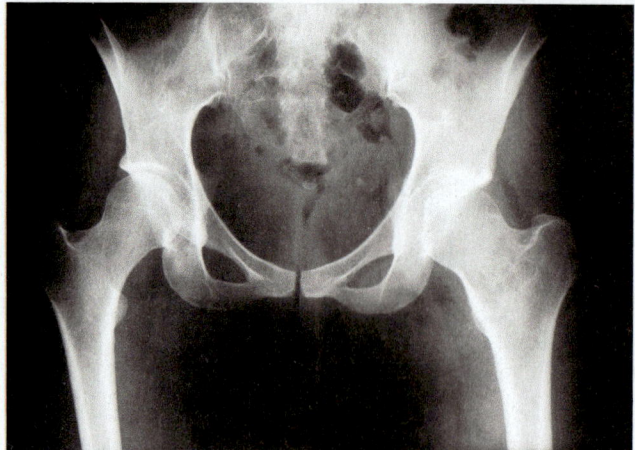

Figure 7.28 Normal AP pelvis view radiograph.
© Mediscan/Alamy Stock Photo

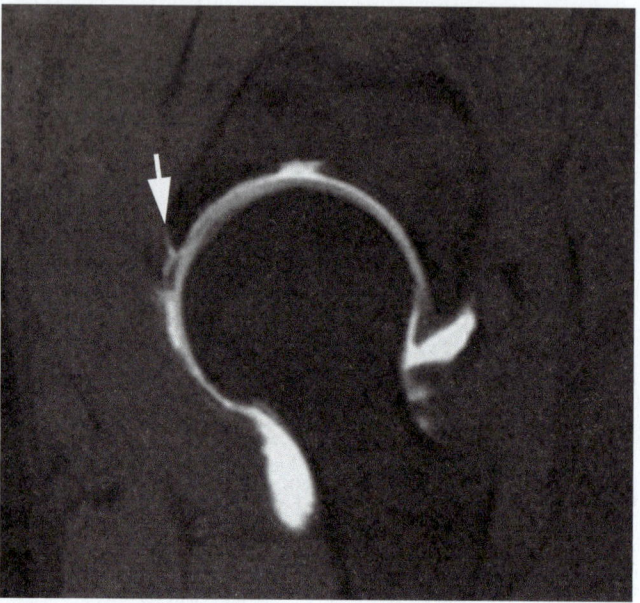

Figure 7.30 Magnetic resonance arthrogram showing a labral tear.
Reproduced from Johnson TR, Steinbach LS, eds: *Essentials of Musculoskeletal Imaging*. Rosemont, IL, American Academy of Orthopaedic Surgeons, 2004.

radiograph to measure alpha angle for determining the presence of cam-type impingement.[43] Although not as reliable, the frog-leg lateral radiographic view is also commonly used to measure alpha angle.[43] Alpha angles greater than 60° are indicative of cam-type femoroacetabular impingement (FAI).[44]

For patients suspected of having soft-tissue or intra-articular pathology, MRI is performed. Conventional MRI is effective at identifying osteochondral injuries, musculotendinous pathologies, and inflammation. Radial MRI is also the most accurate method to measure alpha angle for determining cam-type FAI.[43] However, magnetic resonance arthrography (MRA) is more appropriate to determine injuries to the labrochondral structures and the ligamentum teres and identify the presence of loose bodies and synovial chondromatosis[45,46] (**Figure 7.30**). MRA has limited value in the staging of articular cartilage lesions, with sensitivity reported to be less than 50% compared to arthroscopic findings.[46] Recent advances in MRI techniques, such as delayed gadolinium-enhanced MRI and T2* mapping, allow for a more in-depth analysis of the structure of articular cartilage.[47] These techniques have been shown to be effective at detecting early changes to the articular cartilage surfaces of patients with hip dysplasia and FAI.[48]

Evaluation of the Hip

Clinical evaluation of the hip can be difficult, as many pathologic conditions present with similar signs and symptoms. As a result, having a thorough knowledge of normal anatomy and mechanics of the hip is imperative to identifying pathologic changes in function. A complete clinical examination should include a thorough history, observing alignment and posturing, palpating involved structures, and performing functional testing and relevant special tests. Diagnostic imaging should be used to verify a suspected clinical pathology and interpreted only in lieu of presenting symptoms.

History

Because most injuries to the hip and pelvis are chronic in nature, acquiring a thorough and complete history is necessary for differential diagnosis of the cause of

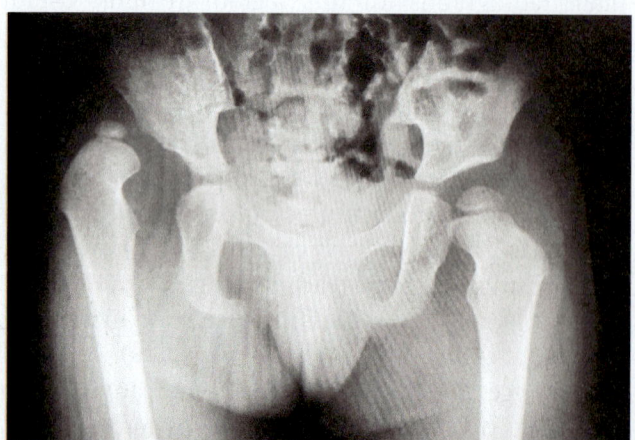

Figure 7.29 A radiograph showing hip dysplasia.
© Bunsinth-Nan-Pua/Shutterstock

the symptoms. The assessment should begin by asking the patient to provide details regarding his or her current symptoms. Can you describe your symptoms? Can you point to the specific affected area? When did your symptoms begin and how long have they been present? What factors exacerbate or alleviate your symptoms? Although not common, an acute episode of pain is often associated with a precipitating event. In these instances, it is important to ask the patient what happened and when it happened. For most patients with hip pain, there is no known precipitating event, with the presentation of symptoms occurring gradually over the course of time. If this is the case, identifying any changes to activity type or training regimen can help differentiate between conditions. Patients should also be asked to provide any previous history of the current condition or treatments undertaken for the hip, whether surgical or nonsurgical. Congenital abnormalities, such as Legg-Calvé-Perthes (LCP) disease or slipped capital femoral epiphysis (SCFE), cause alterations in joint mechanics and can lead to symptoms presenting in adulthood. LCP disease is a childhood disease whereby blood flow to the femoral head is temporarily disrupted, resulting in the bone breaking down and losing its shape. Although blood flow is often restored, the altered morphology of the femoral head can result in bone and cartilage injuries later in life. SCFE refers to a fracture of the growth plate of the femur, resulting in the femoral head slipping posteriorly to the neck. Surgical intervention is necessary to restore normal alignment.

Identifying the specific location of symptoms can help isolate their cause. Pain deep in the region of the anterior groin is most associated with intra-articular pathologies, including acetabular labral tears, degenerative changes, synovial pathologies, loose bodies, and avascular necrosis. More specific and localized pain in the anterior groin may indicate extra-articular conditions, such as hip flexor strains, iliopsoas snapping syndrome, or femoral stress fractures. Pain along the lateral thigh is often associated with greater trochanteric bursitis, iliotibial band syndrome, or abductor tendon tears. Posterior hip pain could be the result of muscle pathologies, such as piriformis syndrome and hamstring muscle tears; however, pain in this region is often the result of referred pain from the SI joint or low back.

Observation and Inspection

Given the girth surrounding the hip, direct observation of most acute injuries is challenging, with the exception of contusions, dislocations, or obvious fractures. Careful inspection of the hip and pelvis should be performed to rule these out and to identify any biomechanical alterations that could contribute to pathology. As the patient is describing the symptoms, it is important to note any visual indicators of pain. Is he or she avoiding loading the painful side? Is he or she altering standing/sitting position due to discomfort? Is he or she hesitant to touch the area? If possible, ask the patient to walk, assessing for the presence of an antalgic gait or obvious biomechanical abnormalities; for example, a toe-out gait could indicate the presence of femoral or acetabular anteversion, whereas excess trunk lean to the ipsilateral side may be indicative of gluteal muscle weakness.[49] Patients with gluteal muscle weakness lean to the painful or weak side because it shifts the center of gravity over the joint, thereby reducing the force required by the abductors to overcome gravity.

While the patient is standing, examine for any pelvic obliquity by assessing for bilateral equality of the height of the iliac crests, greater trochanters, ASIS, and PSIS (**Figure 7.31**). Gross assessment of the angle of inclination can be done by examining the relationship between the femur and tibia during standing. An increase in this angle, called coxa valga, could present as genu varum or a more lateral positioning of the patella. In contrast, a decrease in this angle, called coxa vara, could lead to genu valgum or medially placed "squinting" patella (**Figure 7.32**). Measurement of the angle of torsion can be performed with the patient

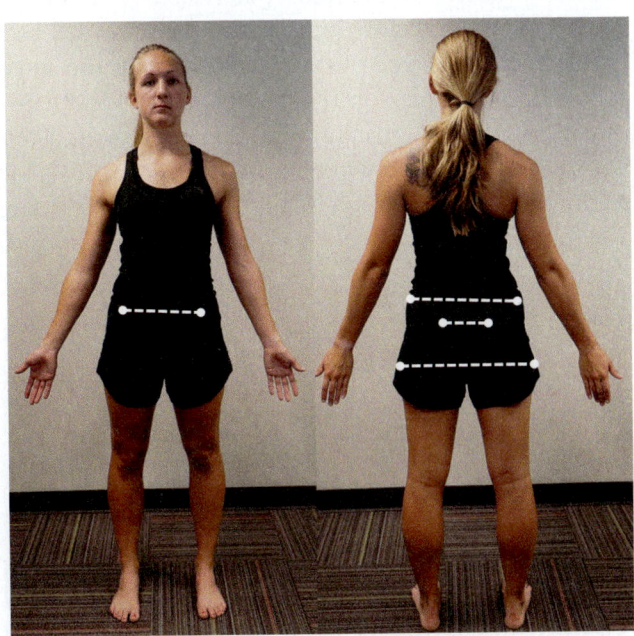

Figure 7.31 Photographs showing pelvic obliquity assessment.

© Jones & Bartlett Learning

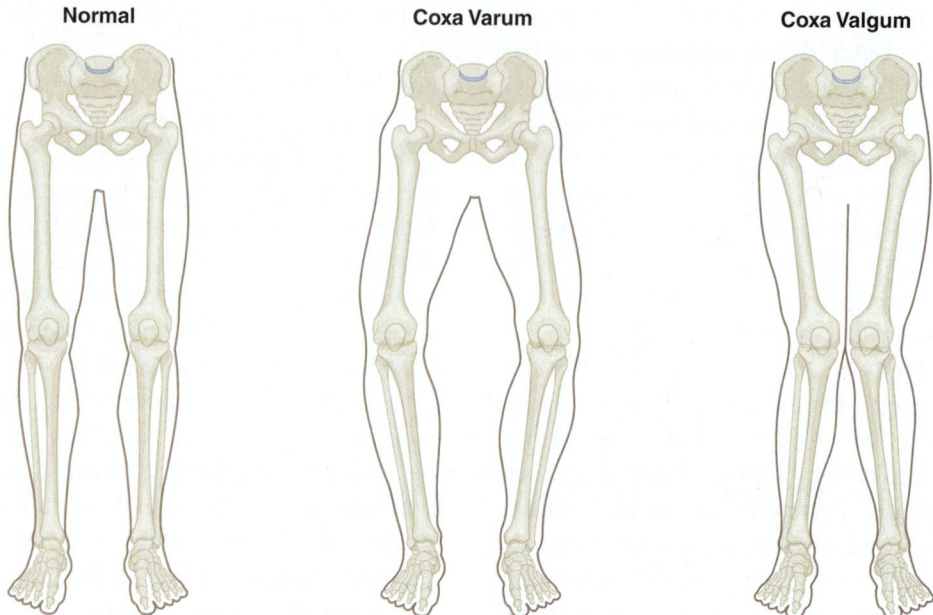

Figure 7.32 Drawings showing normal angulation of the hips and femurs, coxa varum, and coxa valgum.
© Jones & Bartlett Learning

lying prone. With the testing knee bent to 90°, rotate the thigh until the femur is in neutral, identified as the position in which the greater trochanter is most prominent. While this position is held, a second examiner measures the angle of the leg (**Figure 7.33**). Angles less than 15° indicate femoral retroversion, while angles larger than 15° represent anteversion.

Assessment of motion around the hip should be performed actively, passively, and against resistance. Normal active ranges of motion for all three cardinal planes are listed[50] in **Table 7.5**. Active range of motion for hip flexion should be performed with the knee flexed, as extending the knee would limit hip flexion due to tightness of the hamstring muscles. Active motion for flexion/extension should be performed while standing (**Figure 7.34**), for adduction/abduction while side lying (**Figure 7.35**),

Table 7.5 Average Normal Active Ranges of Hip Motion[a]

Motion	Average Peak Active Range of Motion
Hip flexion	121° (120° to 130°)
Hip extension	20°
Hip abduction	42°
Hip adduction	20° (20° to 30°)
Hip internal rotation	32°
Hip external rotation	32°

[a]Data from 1,683 subjects.
Reproduced from Roach KE, Miles TP. Normal hip and knee active range of motion: the relationship to age. *Phys Ther* 1991;71(9):656-665.

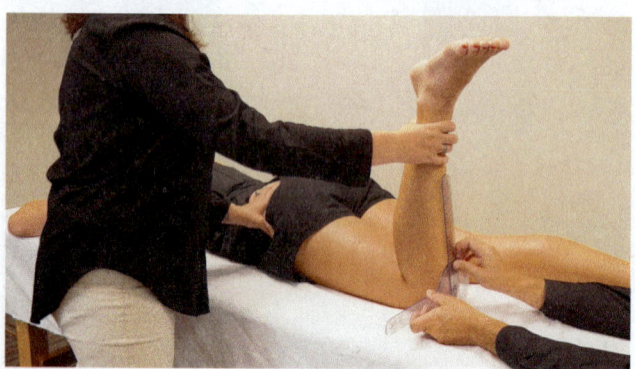

Figure 7.33 Clinical photograph demonstrating the angle of torsion (Craig test).
© Jones & Bartlett Learning

and for external/internal rotation while seated (**Figure 7.36**).

To measure passive hip flexion range of motion, the patient is supine. A hand is placed over the iliac crest to stabilize the pelvis. The hip is moved into flexion, and the knee is allowed to flex naturally from hamstring tension. The normal end feel of hip flexion is soft, as the thigh and abdominal muscles come together. Hip flexor tightness can also be assessed using the Thomas test (**Figure 7.37**). To perform this test, the patient is supine with the hips positioned at the end of the table and the legs hanging off the edge. The examiner places his or her hand under the lumbar region of the patient. The patient then

Evaluation of the Hip

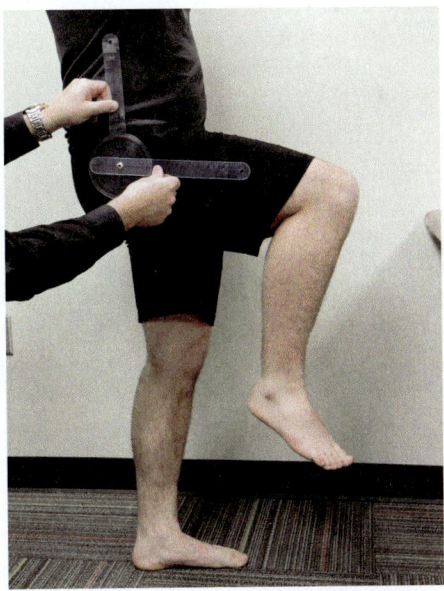

Figure 7.34 Clinical photograph demonstrating hip flexion range of motion.

Courtesy of Andrea Cripps and Matt Kutz.

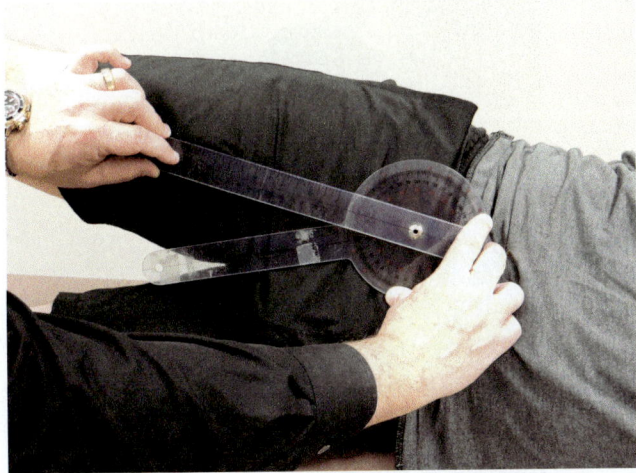

Figure 7.35 Clinical photograph demonstrating measurement of hip adduction/abduction range of motion.

Courtesy of Andrea Cripps and Matt Kutz.

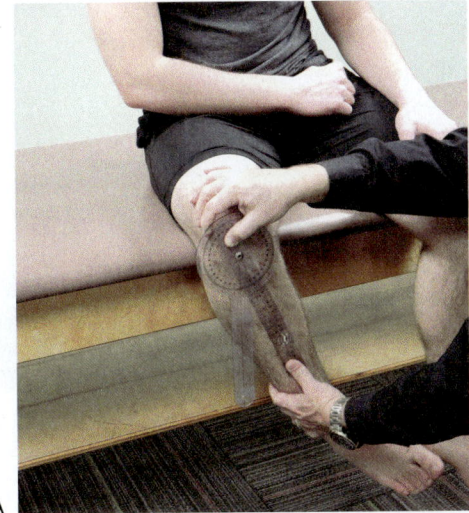

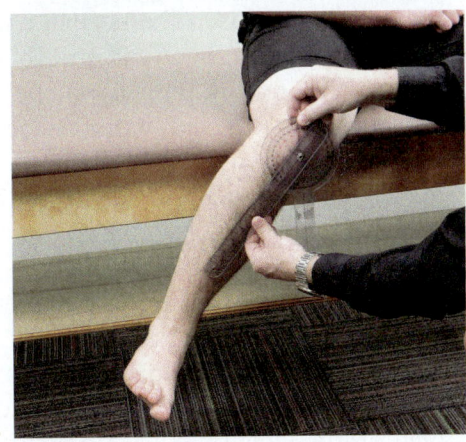

Figure 7.36 Clinical photographs showing external **(A)** and internal **(B)** range of motion of the hip.

Courtesy of Andrea Cripps and Matt Kutz.

Passive frontal plane hip motion is assessed with the patient in a side-lying position. For passive hip abduction, the testing limb is on top. With a hand stabilizing the pelvis to prevent lateral tilting, the leg is brought into abduction, keeping the

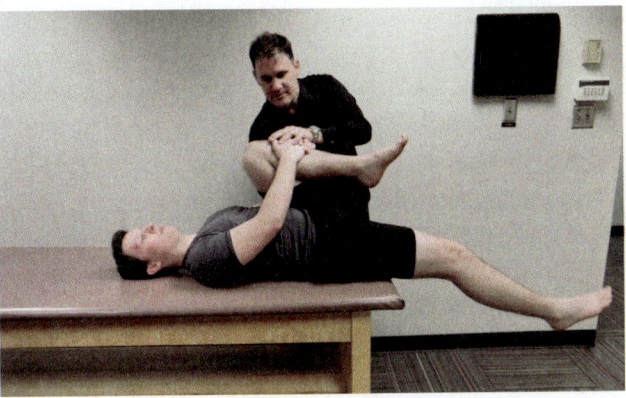

Figure 7.37 Clinical photograph demonstrating the Thomas test.

Courtesy of Andrea Cripps and Matt Kutz.

passively flexes the uninvolved limb to the chest, leaving the testing limb on the examination table. If the testing leg rises off the table, the test is positive for iliopsoas tightness. If the testing knee cannot be flexed to 90°, the test is positive for rectus femoris tightness. Hip extension is measured with the patient prone. A hand is placed over the sacrum to prevent the pelvis from rising off the table during testing. The hip is brought into extension, keeping the knee straight (**Figure 7.38**). The normal end feel is firm because of the tension of the anterior capsuloligamentous structures.

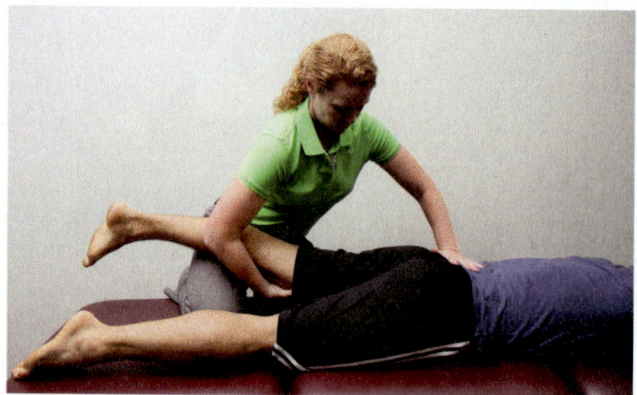

Figure 7.38 Clinical photograph demonstrating hip extension passive range of motion.

© Jones & Bartlett Learning

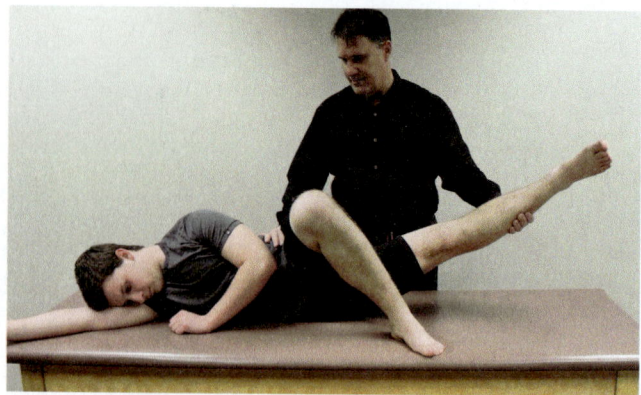

Figure 7.40 Clinical photograph demonstrating hip adduction passive range of motion.

Courtesy of Andrea Cripps and Matt Kutz.

knee straight (**Figure 7.39**). The normal end feel is firm because of ligamentous tension. To perform hip adduction, the testing limb is on the bottom. The contralateral leg is flexed, with the foot on the table in front of the testing leg. The pelvis is stabilized, and the leg is moved into adduction with the knee straight (**Figure 7.40**). The normal end feel is firm due to tension to the iliotibial band.

Passive hip rotation can be measured with the patient lying prone and the knees bent to 90°.[51] Internal rotation is assessed by having the patient let the shank fall out to the side, while controlling movement of the thigh off the table by putting pressure on the ipsilateral pelvis. External rotation is measured by straightening the contralateral limb and having the ipsilateral limb moved inward. Rotation is controlled by stabilizing the ipsilateral pelvis. The normal end feel for both internal and external rotation is firm, resulting from tension of the ligaments and small rotators of the hip (**Figure 7.41**).

Resisted hip flexion should be performed with the knee both flexed and extended to isolate iliopsoas and rectus femoris strength. To assess the iliopsoas muscle, the patient should be supine with the knee extended. With a hand over the ASIS to stabilize the pelvis, resistance is provided against the distal femur, proximal

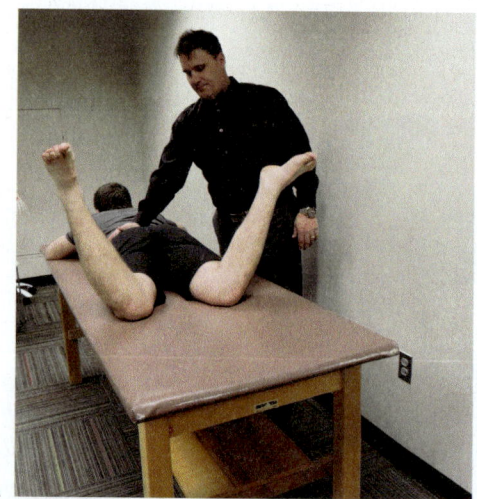

A

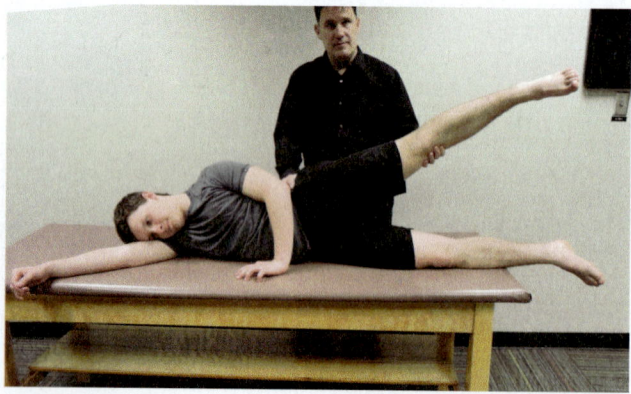

Figure 7.39 Clinical photograph demonstrating hip abduction passive range of motion.

Courtesy of Andrea Cripps and Matt Kutz.

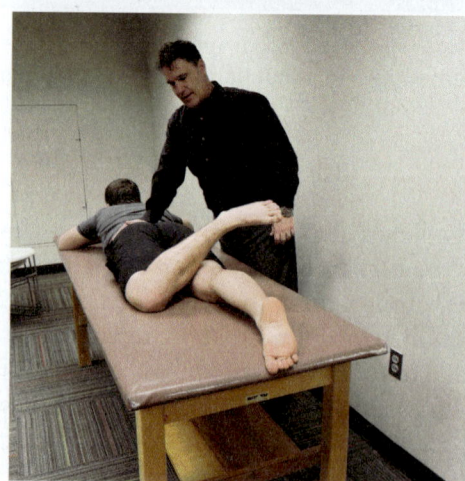

B

Figure 7.41 Clinical photographs demonstrating **(A)** internal and **(B)** external rotation passive range of motion.

Courtesy of Andrea Cripps and Matt Kutz.

to the knee, while the patient attempts to flex the hip (**Figure 7.42A**). For rectus femoris testing, the patient is seated with the knee bent to 90°. The examiner stabilizes the anterior pelvis and applies resistance to the distal femur while the patient attempts to flex the hip (**Figure 7.42B**). Resisted hip extension is also performed with the knee flexed and extended to isolate contributions from the hamstrings and gluteus maximus. To test the hamstrings, the patient is lying prone with the knee extended. The posterior pelvis is stabilized, and resistance is provided proximal to the popliteal fossa while the patient attempts to extend the hip (**Figure 7.43A**). For gluteus maximus testing, the patient is prone, and the knee is flexed to 90°. The posterior pelvis is again stabilized, and resistance is applied over the proximal posterior thigh while the patient attempts to extend the hip (**Figure 7.43B**).

Resisted hip adduction is performed with the patient lying on the affected side with the knee extended. The uninvolved limb is raised into abduction by the examiner. Resistance is applied over the medial femoral condyle while the patient attempts to bring the legs together into adduction (**Figure 7.44**). For hip abduction testing, the patient is lying on the unaffected side with the bottom leg knee slightly flexed. While the pelvis is stabilized over the iliac crest, resistance is provided over the lateral femoral condyle while the patient attempts to abduct the leg (**Figure 7.45**). Strength of the muscles of the pelvic deltoid can also be assessed using the Trendelenburg test. To perform this test, the patient is asked to raise the uninvolved leg off the ground by flexing the hip and knee to allow the foot to clear the ground. Once balanced, the patient is asked to raise the nonstance side of the pelvis as high as possible and hold for 30 seconds without leaning. The test is positive for

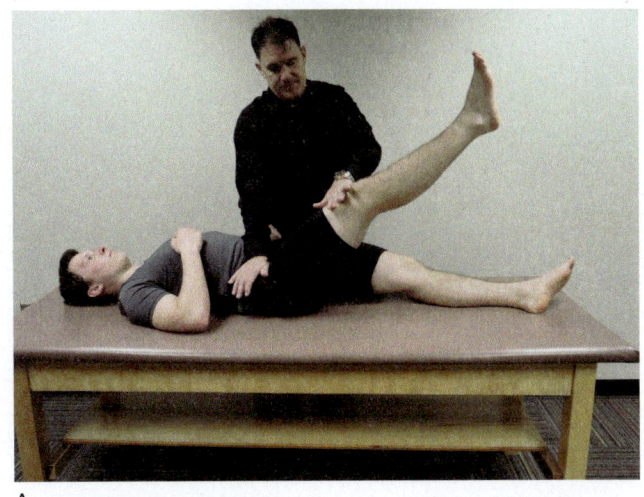

A

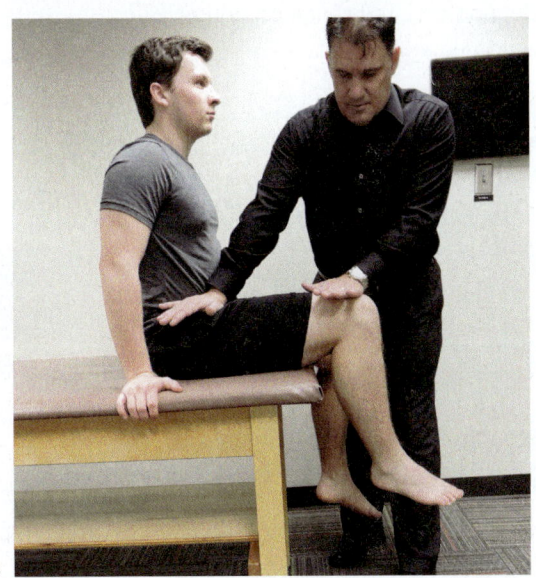

B

Figure 7.42 Clinical photographs demonstrating hip flexion resisted range of motion. **A.** Iliopsoas. **B.** Rectus femoris.

Courtesy of Andrea Cripps and Matt Kutz.

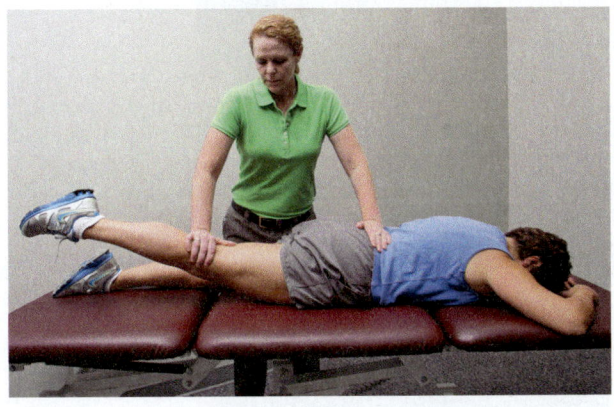

A

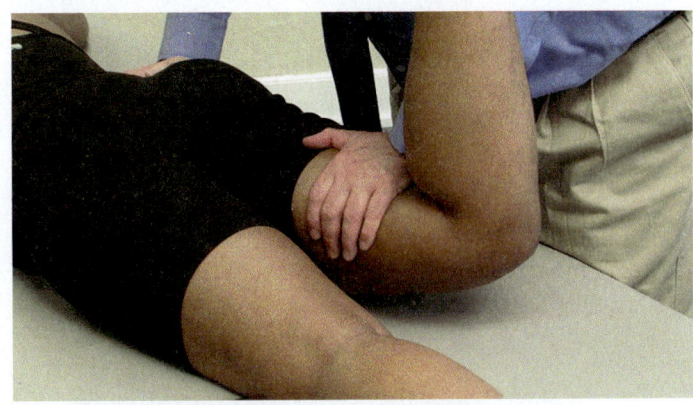

B

Figure 7.43 Clinical photographs demonstrating hip extension resisted range of motion. **A.** Hamstring muscles. **B.** Gluteus maximus.

A. © Jones & Bartlett Learning; **B.** Reproduced from Armstrong AD, Hubbard MC. eds: *Essentials of Musculoskeletal Care*, ed 5. Burlington, MA, American Academy of Orthopaedic Surgeons, 2015.

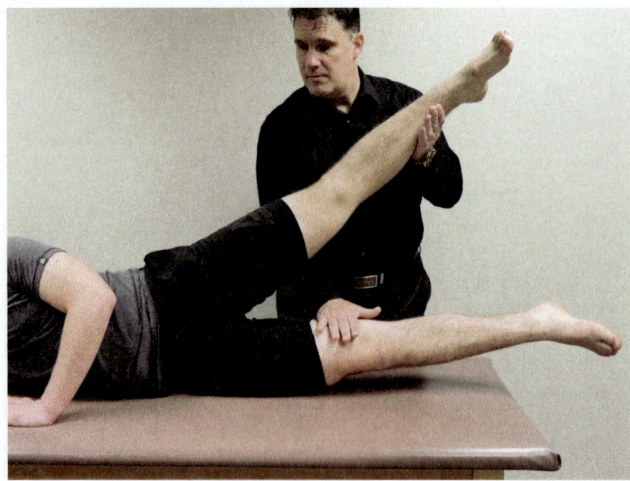

Figure 7.44 Clinical photograph demonstrating hip adduction resisted range of motion.

Courtesy of Andrea Cripps and Matt Kutz.

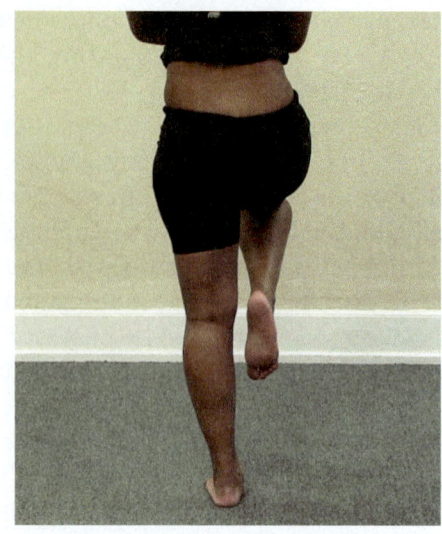

Figure 7.46 Clinical photograph demonstrating the Trendelenburg test.

Reproduced from Armstrong AD, Hubbard MC. eds: *Essentials of Musculoskeletal Care*, ed 5. Burlington, MA, American Academy of Orthopaedic Surgeons, 2015.

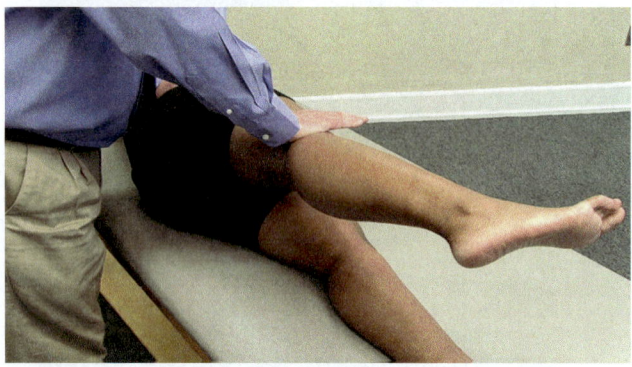

Figure 7.45 Clinical photograph demonstrating hip abduction resisted range of motion.

Reproduced from Armstrong AD, Hubbard MC. eds: *Essentials of Musculoskeletal Care*, ed 5. Burlington, MA, American Academy of Orthopaedic Surgeons, 2015.

weakness if the patient cannot achieve maximum elevation of the pelvis or cannot hold the position for 30 seconds[52] (**Figure 7.46**).

To assess resisted hip rotation, the patient is seated with the knees at 90°. For resisted internal rotation, the medial thigh is stabilized, and resistance is provided against the lateral distal leg as the patient attempts to internally rotate the femur (**Figure 7.47**). To assess external rotation, the lateral thigh is stabilized, and resistance is applied against the medial distal leg while the patient attempts to externally rotate the femur.

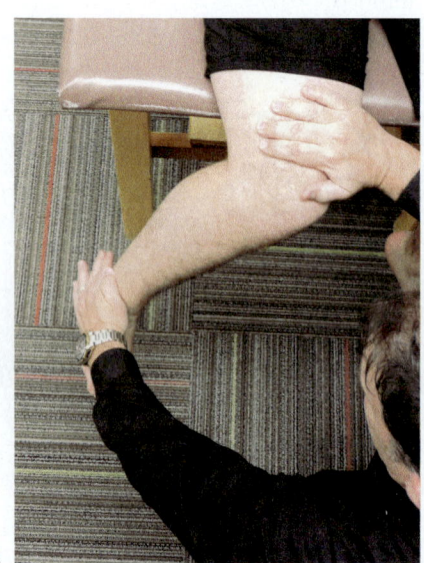
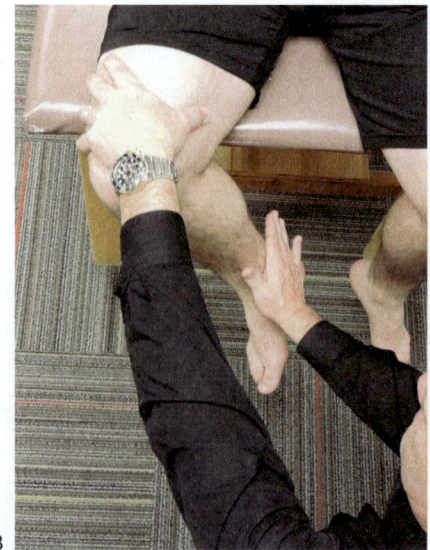

Figure 7.47 Resisted range of motion of the hip. **A.** Internal. **B.** External.

Courtesy of Andrea Cripps and Matt Kutz.

Neurologic Assessment

Testing for neurologic impairment should include sensory, motor, and reflex testing, as described previously (Figures 7.24 and 7.25). Pain and paresthesia in the lower extremity can be referred from nerve impingement at the vertebral level or impingement as the nerve courses through the gluteal and thigh region. Isolating the location and path of nerve symptoms can pinpoint their cause. For example, impingement of the sciatic nerve in the spine will result in pain and paresthesia that travels all the way down to the foot in the sensory regions provided by the S1–S2 nerve roots. In contrast, impingement of the sciatic nerve as it courses through the greater sciatic notch with the piriformis muscle usually results in neurologic symptoms that are isolated to the gluteal and posterior thigh region, rarely travelling distal to the knee.

Special Tests

Special tests are devised to assist with differentiating between potential causes of clinical symptoms. Other than a handful of tests designed to assess for muscle contracture, most of the special tests described for the hip are designed to rule in or out intra-articular pathology. Published studies examining diagnostic accuracy for special tests of the hip are lacking. Of the special tests designed to assess for muscle contracture, only the FAIR (flexion-adduction-internal rotation) test for diagnosing piriformis syndrome has been examined for its diagnostic utility (**Figure 7.48**). Compared to EMG measures of sciatic nerve function, the FAIR test demonstrated both high sensitivity and specificity, meaning that the results observed for a specific patient are accurate in detecting the pathology.[53] Numerous tests for detecting the presence of labral tears have been described in the literature and assessed for their diagnostic accuracy.[46,54-57]

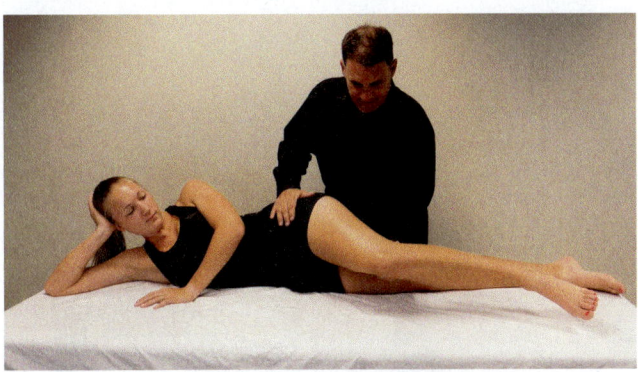

Figure 7.48 Clinical photograph demonstrating the FAIR (flexion-adduction-internal rotation) test.

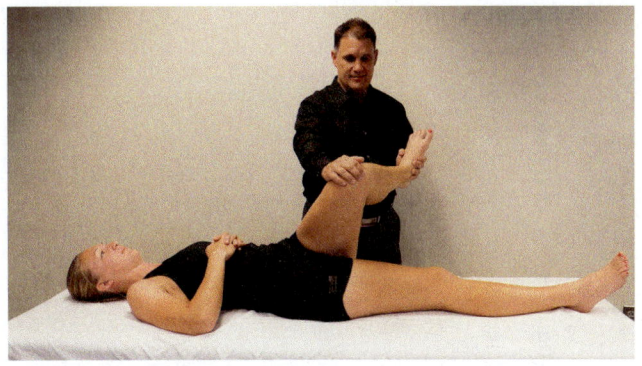

Figure 7.49 Clinical photograph demonstrating the FADDIR (flexion-adduction-internal rotation) test.

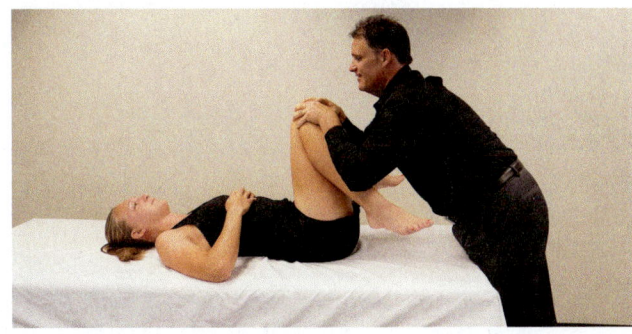

Figure 7.50 Clinical photograph demonstrating the flexion internal rotation test.

The flexion-adduction-internal rotation (FADDIR) test[46,55,56] (**Figure 7.49**) and flexion-internal rotation test[54,58] (**Figure 7.50**) have consistently demonstrated high sensitivity when compared to both MRA and arthroscopy; however, no test has been shown to be useful at ruling in the condition given that many studies examined only patients with confirmed labral tears. Therefore, it appears that the absence of clinical symptoms during these tests would occur only in the absence of intra-articular pathology.

A summary of special tests for the hip and thigh is presented in **Table 7.6**.

Common Hip Pathologies

Injuries to the hip and thigh are estimated to account for 4% to 6% of all injuries in sports,[59] but the prevalence of injuries to this region has been reported as high as 15% when examining individual sports, such as basketball and hockey.[60,61] Traditionally, hip pain has been identified as resulting from extra-articular injuries, such as coxa saltans, bursitis, and tendinitis;[24,62-66] however, with the advancement of diagnostic and evaluative tools, intra-articular injuries,

Table 7.6 Special Tests for the Hip and Thigh

Test	Patient Position	Procedure	Positive Test	Implication	Evidence
FADDIR	Supine	The examiner brings the involved hip into flexion and internal rotation and then moves the hip into adduction.	Re-creation of pain and/or mechanical clicking in the joint	Intra-articular pathology	High sensitivity; specificity is zero
Ober test	Side lying with affected limb on top	While stabilizing the pelvis, the examiner should abduct the leg as far as possible, flex the knee to 90°, and then extend the hip. Slowly release the patient's thigh.	The thigh remains abducted when the leg is released	External snapping hip syndrome	N/A
FAIR test	Side lying with affected limb on top	Stabilization is provided to ensure the pelvis is in a neutral position. The examiner passively flexes, adducts, and internally rotates the thigh of the involved hip. The examiner then stabilizes the hip with one hand and applies a distal load on the knee with the other hand.	Reproduction of radicular like symptoms or pain in the region where the sciatic nerve intersects with the piriformis muscle	Piriformis syndrome	High sensitivity and specificity
FABER test	Supine	The foot of the involved side is placed on the opposite knee. The hip is now in a position of flexion, abduction, and external rotation. To stress the SI joint, extend the range of motion by placing one hand on the flexed knee and the other hand on the ASIS of the opposite side and apply pressure.	Increased pain posteriorly or anterior hip/groin pain	Posterior pain: SI joint pathology Anterior pain: intra-articular pathology	N/A

Common Hip Pathologies

Test	Position	Description	Positive Finding	Indication	
Trendelenburg test	Standing	The patient is asked to raise the uninvolved leg off the ground by flexing the hip and knee to allow the foot to clear the ground. Once balanced, the patient is asked to raise the nonstance side of the pelvis as high as possible and hold for 30 seconds without leaning.	The patient cannot achieve maximum elevation of the pelvis or cannot hold the position for 30 seconds	Gluteal muscle weakness	N/A
Thomas test	Supine	The hips are positioned at the end of the table with the legs hanging off the edge. The examiner places his or her hand under the lumbar region of the patient. The patient then passively flexes the uninvolved limb to the chest, leaving the testing limb on the exam table.	If the testing leg rises off the table, the test is positive for iliopsoas tightness. If the testing knee cannot be flexed to 90°, the test is positive for rectus femoris tightness	Iliopsoas or rectus femoris tightness	N/A
Ipsilateral prone kinetic test	Prone	Examiner places one thumb on the PSIS and the other thumb on the sacrum parallel to it. Patient actively extends the leg on the same side.	PSIS does not move superiorly and laterally	Posteriorly rotated ilium	N/A

(continues)

Table 7.6 Special Tests for the Hip and Thigh *(continued)*

Test	Patient Position	Procedure	Positive Test	Implication	Evidence
Gapping test	Supine	Examiner crosses the arms and places the heel of his or her hands against each ASIS and pushes down and out with both arms.	Unilateral gluteal or posterior leg pain	Sprain of the anterior SI ligaments	Moderate sensitivity and low specificity
Approximation test	Side lying	Examiner's hands are placed over the upper part of the iliac crest, and a downward force is applied, pressing the pelvis toward the floor.	An increased feeling of pressure in the SI joints	Sprain of the posterior SI ligaments	N/A
SI rocking test	Supine	The iliac crests are exposed, and the examiner places both hands on the iliac crests, with the thumbs on the ASIS. The examiner applies a force, pushing the ASIS medially toward each other.	Pain in the SI joint	SI joint integrity	N/A

Courtesy of Andrea Cripps and Matt Kutz.

Common Hip Pathologies **195**

Prone knee bending test	Prone	Examiner passively flexes the patient's knee to end range and maintains it there for 45 seconds. The hip should not be rotated.	Pain in the anterior thigh or on the unilateral lumbar area, buttock, or posterior thigh	Anterior pain may indicate a tight/strained quadriceps muscle or neural tension of the femoral nerve. Posterior pain may indicate lumbar radiculopathy of L2–L3 nerve roots.	N/A
Gillet test	Standing	Examiner palpates the inferior aspect of the PSIS of the tested side with one hand and the S2 spinous process with the other. The patient flexes the hip past 90°.	The examiner should feel the PSIS move inferiorly and laterally relative to the sacrum. A positive test is when this motion is absent	SI joint hypomobility	High specificity; zero sensitivity
Straight leg raise test	Supine	Examiner passively flexes the patient's hip while maintaining the knee in full extension.	Patient reports reproduction of pain at 40° or less of hip flexion	Disc herniation	High sensitivity; low specificity

A. Straight leg raise. **B.** Well straight leg raise.

(continues)

Table 7.6 Special Tests for the Hip and Thigh

Test	Patient Position	Procedure	Positive Test	Implication	Evidence
Gaenslen test	Supine	The tested leg is moved into maximal flexion while the nontested leg is kept in extension. The examiner then places one hand on the anterior thigh of the nontested leg and the other hand on the knee of the tested leg to apply a flexion overpressure. The extended leg may also be placed off the table to create a greater force.	Presence of low back pain	SI joint pain	Moderate sensitivity; low specificity
Hip scoring test	Supine	The examiner passively flexes the hip to 90° with the knee bent to a comfortable position. The examiner then applies a compressive load down the shaft of the femur by pushing downward at the knee. While maintaining this compression, the examiner passively internally and externally rotates the femur in the acetabulum.	The reproduction of pain or presence of mechanical clicking in the joint	Possible intra-articular pathology	Moderate sensitivity; low specificity
Ely test	Prone	Flex the knee to 90° or greater; then, passively extend the hip.	Anterior and/or medial thigh pain	Irritation of the femoral nerve	N/A

(continued)

Common Hip Pathologies 197

	Supine	With the patient supine with the heels off the end of the exam table, the examiner holds the patient's feet together with hips and knees bent (A). The examiner places his or her thumbs over the medial malleoli while providing traction and instructs the patient to raise the hips upward (B) and then return them to the starting position (C).	Any difference in the final position of the thumbs	Leg length asymmetry	N/A
Weber–Barstow maneuver					
Leg length discrepancy	Supine	With legs in a neutral position, measure the distance from the ASIS to the medial malleoli of the ankle.	Unequal distances	Leg length discrepancy	N/A

Courtesy of Andrea Cripps and Matt Kutz.

© Jones & Bartlett Learning

(continues)

Table 7.6 Special Tests for the Hip and Thigh

Test	Patient Position	Procedure	Positive Test	Implication	Evidence
90-90 straight leg raise test	Supine	Hips and knees are flexed to 90°. Instruct patient to grasp behind both thighs to stabilize the hips and actively extend each knee separately.	Unable to extend the knee to within 20° of full extension	Hamstring muscle tightness	N/A

(continued)

Courtesy of Andrea Cripps and Matt Kutz.

ASIS, anterior superior iliac spine; N/A, not applicable; PSIS, posterior superior iliac spine; SI, sacroiliac.

such as lesions of the acetabular labrum and chondral injuries, are becoming increasingly recognized as a source of hip pain.[24,62,67-70] This section will outline the clinical evaluation presentation and diagnostic imagining findings specific to the most common hip conditions.

Muscle Injuries

Muscle injuries account for the highest percentage of all hip and thigh injuries, with incidence ranging from 25% to 53% of all injuries.[71,72] Muscle strains are the most commonly reported hip injury for all sports.[61,73] Adductor and hip flexor tears are the most commonly injured muscles in collegiate athletes,[73] whereas hamstring muscle tears are most prevalent in professional basketball players.[61] Muscle strains occur as a result of a sudden overstretching of the muscle, with mechanical models demonstrating that the muscle is most susceptible to injury during eccentric contractions.[74,75] The myotendinous junction is the most common site of injury. The hamstring muscles are most susceptible to injury during sprinting,[76] whereas adductor and rectus femoris injuries are most prevalent during sudden changes of direction or kicking.[77,78]

For adductor muscle strains, the mechanism of injury is commonly forced abduction with external rotation. The patient will present with acute pain in the adductor region and be unable to continue with activity. Clinical examination will reveal pain with palpation over the origin of the adductor longus and gracilis along with painful and reduced motion into adduction. In the case of an avulsion, there may be a palpable defect in the muscle proximally. MRI can provide information regarding the degree of muscle injury. Bony avulsions can be detected with a plain radiograph.

For rectus femoris muscle strains, a common mechanism is forceful stretching or contraction, often associated with an eccentric muscle contraction while the knee is flexed and hip is extended. The patient will present with pain in the anterior thigh and may recall feeling a tearing sensation. The pain is such that the patient is unable to continue with activity. Clinical examination will reveal pain with palpation over the anterior thigh in addition to painful or reduced motion. Although not common, a complete avulsion of the rectus femoris will present with a defect close to its origin on the AIIS. Avulsion fractures of the ASIS involving the sartorius muscle can also occur through a similar mechanism and present with similar findings. MRI is useful to determine the exact location and grade of the injury. Bony avulsions can be detected with a plain radiograph.

Hamstring muscle strains are usually the result of excessive stretching of the muscle at the terminal swing phase of gait. The biceps femoris is the most commonly injured of the hamstring muscles.[79] The patient will present with an acute onset of posterior thigh pain and may describe hearing a popping sound at the point of injury. Given that many hamstring injuries occur to the proximal tendon, the patient may complain of pain at the ischial tuberosity while sitting, be unable to continue activity, and may have difficulty with walking. Reinjury is common following hamstring muscle strains,[80] so it is important to ask the patient about any history of previous posterior thigh injuries. Clinical examination will reveal pain with palpation over the posterior thigh with a reduction in motion and strength testing in hip extension. Although not common, complete proximal hamstring ruptures or hamstring avulsions can occur, and, if so, there may be a palpable defect in the muscle. MRI is useful to isolate the affected muscle and stage the injury. Bony avulsions can be detected with a plain radiograph.

Muscle contusions are also a common occurrence of thigh pain, accounting for 12% of all injuries.[81] Contusions most often occur to the quadriceps muscles and are the result of a direct compressive force applied to the anterior thigh. The resulting injury is usually such that the patient cannot continue activity. The patient will present with acute onset of intense pain in the anterior thigh, along with pain with palpation. Ecchymosis will begin to develop over the next couple of days. Immediate treatment of muscle contusions is essential to preventing complications, including compartment syndrome or myositis ossificans.[81] As soon as possible, the knee of the involved limb should be flexed and immobilized at 120° for the first 24 to 48 hours.[82] Ice should be applied to assist with controlling the pain and swelling. Myositis ossificans is a benign ossifying lesion that can occur following trauma, with reported incidences after quadriceps contusion of 9% to 17%.[83] Factors that can contribute to the development of myositis ossificans include exposing the muscle to repetitive trauma before it is fully healed and inadequately controlling inflammation immediately following injury. The lesion usually forms 2 to 4 weeks following injury and can be palpated as the lesion ossifies within the muscle. Compartment syndrome should be suspected with severe contusions. Symptoms suggestive of compartment syndrome include excessive pain and taut swelling. One study reported that all patients with compartment syndrome reported pain with passive stretch and over one-half experienced paresthesia.[84] Ultrasonography is the preferred modality to characterize the hematoma and identify complications early.[85]

Intra-articular Pathology

Intra-articular pathology has become a more recognized source of hip pain in the past decade. Data from professional hockey players revealed that intra-articular pathology accounted for 11% of all hip and groin injuries, with acetabular labral tears being the most common diagnosis (69%).[60] Patients with intra-articular hip pathology will present with anterior hip/groin pain,[56,86,87] often accompanied by mechanical symptoms,[57] such as clicking and locking. The "C sign" is a common finding in patients with intra-articular injury. To describe the location of pain, the patient will hold the hand in a C shape and place it around the lateral hip at the level of the greater trochanter[88] (**Figure 7.51**). Most patients state that pain initially occurs during specific movements, usually a pivot or twisting motion; however, as time progresses, these episodes of pain become more frequent and result in continuous symptoms.[87] Patients may also report pain or an "uncomfortable" feeling during sitting and often will not be able to sit for long periods of time. In most cases, the onset of symptoms is insidious, with many patients unable to recall a specific aggravating event. The impingement, or FADDIR, test is the most valid clinical test for assessing intra-articular pathology (Figure 7.49). To perform the FADDIR test, the patient is supine. The examiner brings the involved hip into flexion and internal rotation and then moves the hip into adduction. Re-creation of pain and/or mechanical clicking in the joint is a positive test. MRA should be performed to confirm clinical suspicion of intra-articular pathology and help differentiate between extra-articular causes of anterior groin pain, such as adductor strains, athletic pubalgia, and iliopsoas tendinopathies (**Table 7.7**).

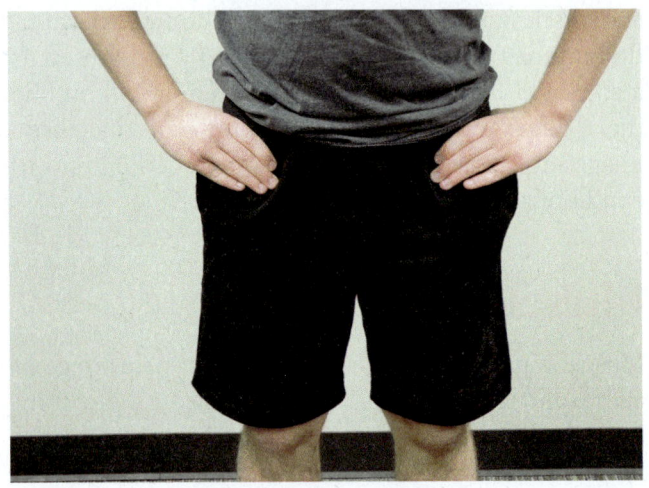

Figure 7.51 Photograph showing the C-shape location of pain.

Courtesy of Andrea Cripps and Matt Kutz.

Plain radiographs should also be obtained to determine the presence of altered bony morphology, such as FAI or dysplasia. Changes to bony morphology can alter loading patterns within the hip, predisposing it to degenerative changes of the labrochondral surfaces over time.[89,90] It is important to note that not all patients with morphologic changes will become symptomatic and not all patients with symptoms of intra-articular injuries will exhibit bony changes. Pain associated with FAI or dysplasia is the result of injury to the joint structures, such as the labrum, articular cartilage, or synovium. Symptomatic FAI is associated with either abnormal sphericity of the femoral head (cam type), excessive projection of the anterolateral acetabular rim (pincer type), or a combination of both (cam-pincer type). The impingement occurs when the hip is flexed and internally rotated, which forces contact between the femoral head and neck and acetabulum. Repetitive impingement, such as occurs during activities that require high degrees of flexion and rotation, can damage the labrum and labrochondral junction, which causes the resultant symptoms. Patients with FAI will often present with

Table 7.7 Intra-articular Pathology Quick Tips

Pathology	Description	Presentation (HIPS)	Special Tests/Imaging	Differential Diagnosis	5-Min Sideline Assessment Tips
Intra-articular pathology	Injury to the capsuloligamentous structures of the hip	Insidious onset, often atraumatic Anterior or groin pain; C shape Mechanical clicking	FADDIR test	Adductor strain Sports hernia Iliopsoas snapping syndrome	None

FADDIR, flexion adduction internal rotation; HIPS, history, inspection, palpation, special tests.

reduced internal rotation range of motion during clinical evaluation. Dysplasia is associated with a shallow hip socket, which can lead to instability of the joint. Dysplasia is common in athletes who participate in sports that require large ranges of motion, such as dancing and gymnastics. Patients with dysplasia will often demonstrate generalized laxity during clinical evaluation.

Snapping Hip Syndrome

The causes of snapping hip syndrome can be identified as internal, external, or intra-articular. Intra-articular snapping was discussed previously with regard to intra-articular pathology. Internal snapping hip syndrome involves migration of the iliopsoas tendon over the iliopectineal eminence when the leg is extended from a flexed position, which produces a painful snap (**Figure 7.52**). The pain described with internal snapping hip syndrome is attributed to iliopsoas bursitis or tendinopathy due to repeated rubbing. Common causes are muscle tightness, a thickened bursa, or an anteriorly rotated pelvis. Patients will complain of localized pain and tenderness to the anterior hip, and the snap can be reproduced clinically when moving from flexion to extension (**Table 7.8**). The tendon can be palpated deep to and medial or lateral of the femoral pulse. Tightness associated with the psoas muscle can be assessed by direct palpation, as described previously. Given the proximity of the iliopsoas tendon to the anterior hip, iliopsoas tendinopathy is often

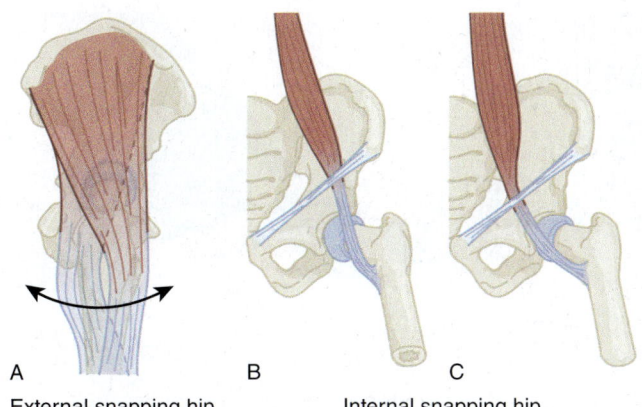

Figure 7.52 Drawings showing iliopsoas snapping syndrome. **A.** Hip muscle moving during flexion and extension. **B.** The starting position of the iliopsoas tendon. **C.** The snapped position of the iliopsoas tendon during hip extension.

© Jones & Bartlett Learning

associated with labrochondral injuries and can mimic their pain pattern. Differentiating between the two conditions can be difficult; however, pain due to involvement of the iliopsoas will be reproduced during direct palpation. Obtaining MRA images is helpful in ruling out intra-articular involvement.

External snapping hip syndrome refers to the snapping of the iliotibial band or gluteus maximus over the greater trochanter as the hip is extended. The snapping can be present with or without pain. The pain described with external snapping hip syndrome is often attributed to concomitant trochanteric bursitis or tendinopathy due to repeated rubbing.[91] In addition to the snapping, patients will complain

Table 7.8 Snapping Hip Syndrome Quick Tips

Pathology	Description	Presentation (HIPS)	Special Tests/ Imaging	Differential Diagnosis	5-Min Sideline Assessment Tips
Snapping hip syndrome	Internal: Tightness of the iliopsoas tendon External: Tightness of the iliotibial band	Internal: Localized pain and tenderness to the anterior hip. Snap can be reproduced clinically when moving from flexion to extension. External: Localized pain over the greater trochanter that is exacerbated with activity. Snap can be reproduced with active hip flexion while the patient is in a side-lying position.	Internal: Reproduction of snapping while palpating the tendon External: Ober test	Internal: Intra-articular pathology or iliopsoas strain External: Greater trochanter bursitis	None

HIPS, history, inspection, palpation, special tests.

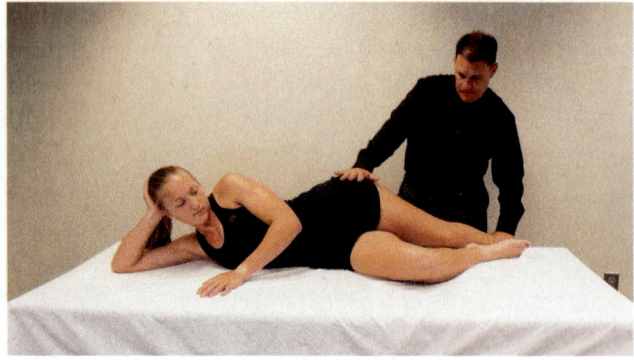

Figure 7.53 Clinical photograph demonstrating the Ober test.

© Jones & Bartlett Learning

of localized pain over the greater trochanter that is exacerbated with activity. The snapping can be reproduced clinically with active hip flexion while the patient is in a side-lying position.[92] Preventing the excursion of the tendon during testing by stabilizing the lateral thigh should negate the snapping.[93] To assess for tightness of the iliotibial band, Ober test can be performed (**Figure 7.53**). To perform this test, have the patient lie on his or her side with the involved leg uppermost. While stabilizing the pelvis, abduct the leg as far as possible, flex the knee to 90°, and then extend the hip. Slowly release the patient's thigh. If the iliotibial band is normal, the patient's thigh should drop to the adducted position. The test is positive if the thigh remains abducted when the leg is released. In difficult cases, diagnostic imaging may be required to isolate the cause of snapping. If so, ultrasonography is the preferred modality, as it allows for dynamic examination.[94]

Piriformis Syndrome

Piriformis syndrome is a condition in which the sciatic nerve is impinged by the piriformis muscle, resulting in pain and paresthesia in the posterior hip. Compression of the sciatic nerve can be due to anatomic variations in the relationship between the nerve and muscle (**Figure 7.54**), trauma to the muscle, muscle hypertrophy, muscle shortening, or altered femoropelvic biomechanics.[95] Patients will often complain of buttock pain with intermittent sciatica symptoms. Sciatica caused by impingement of the nerve at the piriformis usually will not extend past the posterior thigh and can help differentiate it from sciatica caused by impingement at the nerve root, which will extend down to the foot. A systematic review identified four key symptoms associated with a diagnosis of piriformis syndrome: buttock pain, increased pain with sitting, tenderness with palpation of the muscle near the greater sciatic notch, and pain and paresthesia with tension of the piriformis muscle[95] (**Table 7.9**). Tension of the piriformis muscle can be created using the FAIR test (Figure 7.48). To perform the FAIR test, the patient is side lying with the involved leg uppermost. Stabilization is provided to ensure the pelvis is in a neutral position. The examiner passively flexes, adducts, and internally rotates the thigh of the involved hip. The examiner then stabilizes the hip with one hand and applies a distal load on the knee with the other hand. Reproduction of radicular-like symptoms or pain in the region where the sciatic nerve intersects with the piriformis muscle indicates compression of the nerve. Pain without radicular symptoms could

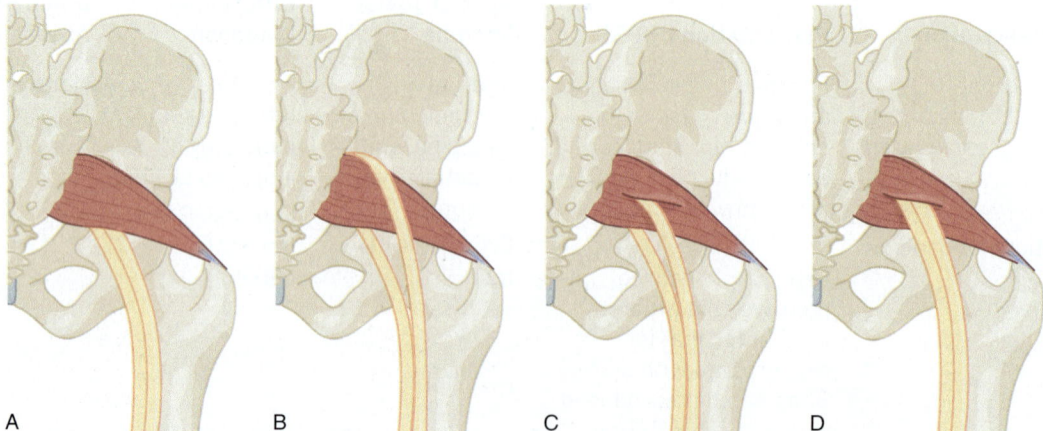

Figure 7.54 Drawings showing anatomic variations of the sciatic nerve. **A.** Normal anatomic alignment of the sciatic nerve. **B.** The sciatic nerve running around the piriformis. **C.** The sciatic nerve running through and under the piriformis. **D.** The sciatic nerve running through the piriformis.

© Jones & Bartlett Learning

Table 7.9 Piriformis Syndrome Quick Tips

Pathology	Description	Presentation (HIPS)	Special Tests/ Imaging	Differential Diagnosis	5-Min Sideline Assessment Tips
Piriformis syndrome	Compression of the sciatic nerve by the piriformis muscle	Buttock pain Increased pain with sitting Tenderness with palpation of the muscle near the greater sciatic notch Pain and paresthesia with tension of the piriformis muscle	FAIR test	Sciatica from impinged nerve roots Piriformis muscle injury	None

HIPS, history, inspection, palpation, special tests.

indicate tendinopathy of the muscle, but the diagnosis of piriformis syndrome is applicable only when neurologic symptoms are present. Imaging studies are not generally useful for diagnosing piriformis syndrome; however, in chronic cases that are not responding to treatment, magnetic resonance neurography may help identify anatomic variants of the relationship between the piriformis muscle and sciatic nerve.[96]

Hip Pointer

A hip pointer is a common injury in contact sports and refers to contusion of the iliac crest and surrounding tissue caused by a direct blow to the area (**Figure 7.55**). Patients will present with acute, intense pain over the iliac crest. The pain associated with hip pointers can be debilitating, leading to difficulty or an inability to walk (**Table 7.10**). Clinical examination will reveal pain with direct palpation and painful or limited motion. Ecchymosis will often develop. Imaging studies often are not warranted but may be appropriate to rule out fracture.

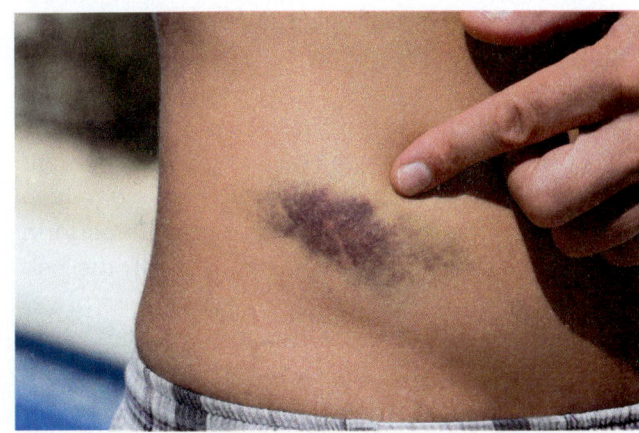

Figure 7.55 Photograph of a hip pointer injury.
© majivecka/Shutterstock

Table 7.10 Hip Pointer Quick Tips

Pathology	Description	Presentation (HIPS)	Special Tests/ Imaging	Differential Diagnosis	5-Min Sideline Assessment Tips
Hip pointer	Contusion of the iliac crest and surrounding tissue caused by a direct blow to the area	Acute intense pain over the iliac crest Pain with direct palpation Painful or limited motion	None	None	Assess the level of pain and inflammation. Assess ability to bear weight. If the patient cannot bear weight, provide crutches and ice. If the patient can bear weight, conduct a full functional assessment. If the patient is able to reenter competition, pad the area prior to return.

HIPS, history, inspection, palpation, special tests.

Stress Fractures

Stress fractures in an active population are most often due to overloading on the bone, where resorption rate exceeds the rate of bone growth,[97] such as occurs with a rapid increase in training. They are more common in endurance athletes, especially runners and military recruits. In the hip, stress fractures of the femoral neck have the highest incidence. Most femoral neck stress fractures occur along the medial aspect of the neck, perpendicular to the stress lines (**Figure 7.56**), and are the result of excessive compressive forces.[97] Fractures that occur along the superolateral neck are not as common in athletes but pose a higher nonunion risk, as they are the result of tensile forces. The clinician should inquire about any recent changes to training regimens or footwear, proper nutrition, and any previous history of fractures. The patient will complain of nonspecific anterior groin pain that worsens during activity; however, pain will often progress to constant if left untreated.[98] The fulcrum test can be used to help differentiate femoral neck stress fractures. To perform the fulcrum test, the patient is supine, with the pelvis level and square to the trunk. The examiner places one arm under the thigh of the involved limb. With the other hand, the examiner applies a downward load onto the knee of the involved limb. If the patient experiences pain in the femur with this test, it is indicative of a stress fracture to the bone. Additional diagnostic testing is required to confirm. Plain radiographs are not usually sufficient to identify stress fractures. MRI has been indicated as the gold standard for early detection of stress fractures.[97] A patient with a confirmed compression femoral neck stress fracture that is caught early should immediately cease training and undergo a period of immobilization followed by a conservative progressive rehabilitation program to return to activity. Any fracture evident on the tensile side of the neck or any displaced fracture should be treated surgically.[99]

Sacral stress fractures in athletes are not as common and are often insufficiency-type fractures; therefore, female athletes with relative energy deficiency in sports may be more prone to this type of stress fracture.[100] A complete history should include questions regarding training regimes, nutrition, menstrual cycles (as appropriate), and any previous history of fractures. Differential diagnosis can be difficult, as pain presentation is similar to that found with low back pain and buttock pain. The patient will complain of dull pain in the area of the low back and sacrum and will be point tender with direct palpation of the sacrum.[93] Pain may be elicited during physical tests for the sacrum, including the FABER (flexion-abduction-external rotation) test and SI joint maneuvers; however, no accurate clinical test exists for diagnosing sacral stress fractures.[100] The FABER test is performed with the patient supine. The foot of the involved side is placed on the opposite knee. The hip is now in a position of flexion, abduction, and external rotation. To stress the SI joint, extend the range of motion by placing one hand on the flexed knee and the other hand on the anterior superior iliac spine of the opposite side and apply pressure. If the patient complains of increased pain posteriorly, there may be pathology in the SI joint. Anterior hip/groin pain would continue to indicate hip involvement. To perform SI joint maneuver tests, the patient is supine with the pelvis level and square to the trunk. The examiner places one hand on each of the ASIS of the ilium. For distraction of the SI joint, the examiner applies a medial load onto each ASIS, pushing the ASIS toward the midline of the body. For compression of the SI joint, the examiner applies a lateral load onto each ASIS, pushing the ASIS away from the midline of the body. Pain during either test or reproduction of symptoms indicates SI joint pathology. Diagnostic imaging should be ordered if the clinical examination dictates it and a sacral stress fracture is suspected. Again, MRI is the gold standard for detecting sacral stress fractures.

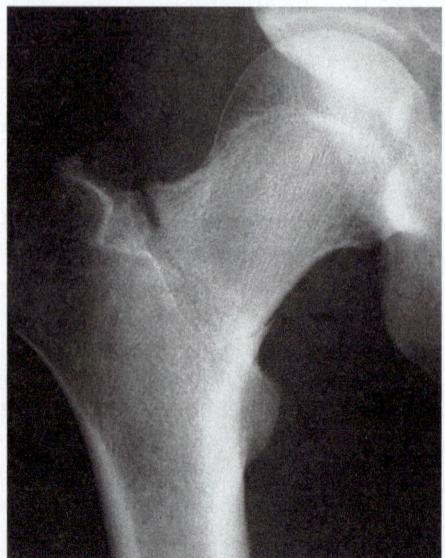

Figure 7.56 Radiograph showing a femoral stress fracture.

© Jones & Bartlett Learning

Pediatric Hip Diseases

SCFE is the most common adolescent hip pathology and occurs when the head of the femur slips distally in relation to the femoral neck at the growth plate[101] (**Figure 7.57**). SCFE usually develops during periods of rapid growth after the onset of puberty and is often unilateral. Patients will complain of an

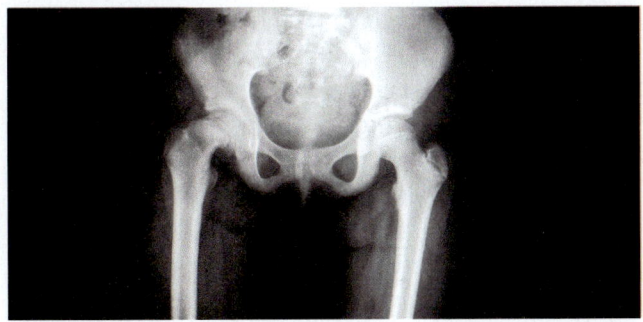

Figure 7.57 Radiograph showing slipped capital femoral epiphysis.
© Yok_onepiece/Shutterstock

insidious onset of pain, stiffness, and instability in the affected hip, which is exacerbated with activity. Motion at the hip will be limited, specifically in flexion, internal rotation, and abduction. Passive movement into flexion will often result in external rotation of the hip to allow for the femoral head to move through the acetabulum. Plain radiographs are indicated to diagnose and assess the degree of slippage. Treatment usually involves surgical stabilization of the epiphysis to prevent further slippage.

LCP disease involves idiopathic osteonecrosis of the femoral head at the epiphysis due to a disruption in blood supply. The cause of LCP disease is unknown, but may be associated with early participation in sports, such as gymnastics and dancing.[102] The disruption in blood supply arrests bone growth and leads to a flattening of the femoral head (**Figure 7.58**). Patients will initially present with a limp, the severity of which is dependent on the stage of the disease. Physical examination will reveal limited internal rotation and abduction of the hip with the leg extended.[103] Plain radiographs are essential to identify LCP disease early and prevent further damage. Bilateral frog-leg lateral radiographs provide the best views.[104] Initial treatment strategies include protected weight bearing, removal from physical activity, and NSAIDs. For patients who do not respond to initial treatment, surgical intervention is warranted to stabilize the femoral head and reorient it with the acetabulum.[105]

SI Joint Pathology

SI joint dysfunction is a term used to describe myriads of conditions that produce pain in and around the sacroiliac joint. Given the complex anatomy and mechanics of the SI joint, differential diagnosis of the cause of pain is difficult, with no clinical or imaging test that is sensitive or specific for the diagnosis. Differential diagnosis can include musculoskeletal pathologies, including hip disease, lumbar disk pain, radiculopathies, and fractures as well as nonmusculoskeletal pathologies, including infection, inflammation, and tumors.[106,107] A thorough history should include questions regarding the chronicity and type of pain, description of provocative maneuvers, and any previous history of back pain or injury or inflammatory conditions. The physical examination should include static assessment of pelvic symmetry in standing, including bilateral palpation of the ASIS, iliac crests, PSIS, greater trochanters, and gluteal fold. Leg-length symmetry should be determined. True leg length is measured from the ASIS to the medial malleolus, and any differences are the result of true bony inequality. Apparent leg length is measured from the umbilicus to the medial malleolus, with differences usually the result of pelvic obliquity.[107] Dynamic observation of asymmetry during gait and active ranges of motion for the spine and hip should be performed. Pelvic hypomobility can be assessed using either the Gillet test or ipsilateral prone kinetic test. To perform the Gillet test, the patient is standing. The examiner palpates the inferior aspect of the PSIS of the tested side with one hand and the S2 spinous process with the other and asks the patient to flex the hip past 90°. The PSIS should move inferiorly and laterally relative to the sacrum. Sacral hypomobility is present when this motion is absent. For the ipsilateral prone kinetic test, the patient is prone, and the examiner places one thumb on the PSIS and the other thumb on the sacrum parallel to it. The patient is instructed to actively extend the leg on the same side. The PSIS should move superiorly and laterally. Lack of this movement would indicate a posteriorly rotated ilium. Numerous physical tests have been described to determine the presence of SI joint dysfunction;

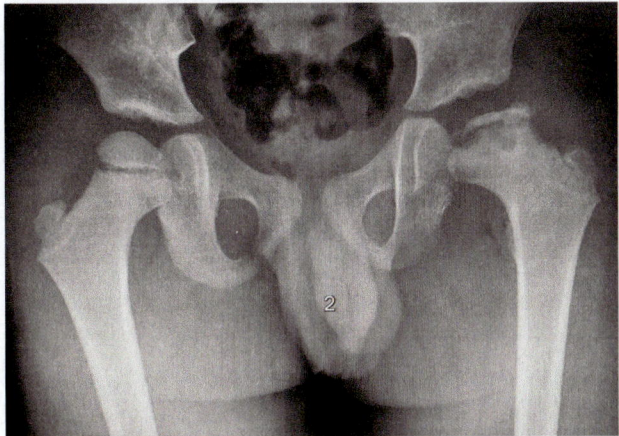

Figure 7.58 Radiograph showing Legg-Calvé-Perthes disease.
© Bunsinth-Nan-Pua/Shutterstock

however, no single test has been identified to reliably diagnose the condition.[106,108] Reproduction of pain during testing is indicative of a positive test. The most commonly used tests include the gapping test (SI compression test), Gaenslen test, SI distraction test, and FABER test.[109] The FABER test and SI compression/distraction tests have been described previously. To perform the Gaenslen test, the patient is supine, and the tested leg is moved into maximal flexion while the nontested leg is kept in extension. The examiner then places one hand on the anterior thigh of the nontested leg and the other hand on the knee of the tested leg to apply a flexion overpressure. The extended leg may also be placed off the table to create a greater force. The presence of pain in the low back area is indicative of SI joint dysfunction. Diagnostic accuracy is improved when three or more tests are positive.[106,110] Imaging studies are often not effective at identifying the specific cause of SI joint pain but can be useful to rule out more serious conditions.[111] Plain radiographs can help identify degenerative changes or fractures, and MRI can be used to identify soft-tissue pathology or inflammatory sacroiliitis.[112] The best diagnostic evidence supports the use of a single fluoroscopic-guided sacroiliac joint injection; a 75% or greater reduction in pain is indicative of a positive test for SI joint dysfunction.

Quick Tips for Evaluations for Pathology

On-field management of hip and thigh injuries mostly involves contusions and muscle strains. Although uncommon, hip dislocations or femur fractures represent medical emergencies.

- Hip pointer: Following a direct blow to the lateral hip, the patient will report intense, immediate pain over the area of the iliac crest. Pain and swelling can have a rapid onset. If the injury is severe enough, the patient may not be able to independently ambulate. In this case, he or she should be removed from competition, and ice should be applied immediately and often. Crutches should be provided until full pain-free weight bearing can be achieved. If the injury is mild, the patient should be removed from competition, and a complete functional evaluation should be performed. If the patient can return, then the injured area should be padded to complete the competition and treatment should commence immediately after.
- Quadriceps contusion: Following a direct blow to the anterior thigh, the patient will report immediate pain. If the injury is severe enough, he or she may not be able to continue competition. In this case, the patient should be assisted to the sideline, and treatment should commence immediately. The involved knee should be flexed to 120° and immobilized in that position while ice is applied. If the patient is able to continue competing without functional limitations, treatment should begin immediately after the end of the activity.
- Hip dislocation: Hip dislocations in athletics are extremely rare. When they do occur, the hip is most commonly dislocated posterior, and the hip will be in a shortened position in adduction and internal rotation. The patient will be in extreme pain and unable to move the limb. The patient should be immediately immobilized in the position in which he or she was found and distal sensory and vascular function should be assessed. The patient should be transported to the hospital immediately for further evaluation and reduction. Caution should be taken in trying to reduce a hip dislocation on the field. If reduction is not successful in the first one or two attempts, no further efforts should be made.
- Femoral fracture: Femoral fractures are also extremely rare but are easy to diagnose, as they result in deformity. A patient with a suspected femoral fracture should be immediately immobilized in the position in which he or she was found, and distal neurovascular function should be checked. The patient should be transported to the hospital immediately for further evaluation and treatment. Femoral fractures represent a medical emergency because of the close relationship between the femur bone and important vascular structures of the lower extremity, especially the femoral artery.

CASE STUDY 1

A 20-year-old woman who is an equestrian reported to the clinic with bilateral anterior hip and thigh pain, greater on the right than the left. She reports that she has been experiencing aching and occasional clicking in both hips for the past 6 to 9 months and the discomfort has not subsided with nonsurgical treatment, including rest, anti-inflammatory medication, and therapy. She describes daily pain located in the anterior groin crease, which

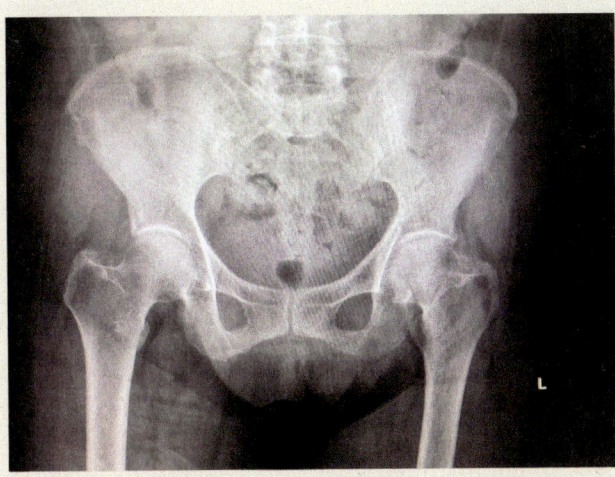

Figure 7.59 AP radiograph of the pelvis.
© Good Image Studio/Shutterstock

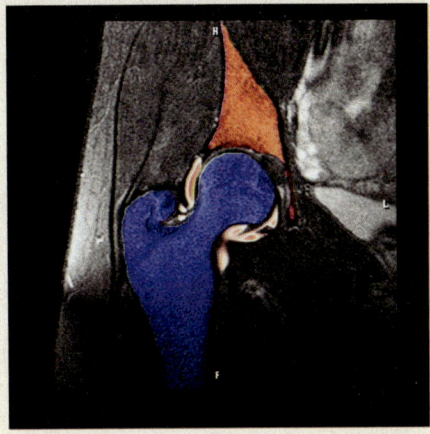

Figure 7.60 Magnetic resonance arthrography demonstrating labral tear.
© Living Art Enterprises/Science Source

increases with activity, especially while getting on and off her horse. She denies any numbness or tingling or pain in any other location. She has no previous history of hip pain or injury but has undergone bilateral fasciotomies to relieve posterior compartment syndrome in her legs. Clinical examination revealed normal heel-toe gait and no pain with spine motion. Range-of-motion measures for the right hip were 115° of hip flexion, full extension; 40° of abduction; 40° of external rotation; and 15° of internal rotation. She expressed mild discomfort at the extremes of flexion and internal rotation. Left-sided motion was normal, except for internal rotation, which was limited to 15° with minimal discomfort. AP radiograph of the pelvis revealed normal joint spaces with mild bilateral acetabular dysplasia (**Figure 7.59**). She was referred for additional imaging; MRA of her right hip revealed a mildly hypertrophic labrum anteriorly, which is consistent with mild dysplasia, and diffuse tearing of the anterior and anterosuperior labrum (**Figure 7.60**). There was also suspected mild articular cartilage thinning. Because of the patient's unrelenting pain and mechanical symptoms, arthroscopy of the right hip was performed. The arthroscopy confirmed the presence of the enlarged and torn anteromedial labrum along with a mild anteromedial acetabular articular cartilage lesion and reactive synovitis. Four months after surgery, she reported resolution of her pain and mechanical symptoms and was pain free during activity, including horseback riding.

1. What other conditions would you want to evaluate and rule out for a patient presenting with anterior groin pain and occasional clicking in the hip?
2. What is the biomechanical reason that mounting and dismounting the horse would exacerbate intra-articular hip pain?

CASE STUDY 2

A 26-year-old former baseball catcher presents to the clinic with primarily anterior right hip pain. He underwent an arthroscopic partial labral débridement 2 years ago and, until recently, has been symptom free. He describes an ache that is present constantly and intensifies with activity, to the point that he is unable to walk long distances without severe limping and pain. Clinical evaluation reveals pain during FADDIR testing but no reproduction of mechanical symptoms. His motion is limited in internal rotation, flexion, and adduction due to pain, not mechanical limits. Pelvic radiographs were normal without the presence of bony morphologic abnormalities. Alpha angle was 50°. Repeat MRA was not performed, as the diagnostic accuracy is limited in a hip that has undergone previous arthroscopy. The patient was referred for further biomechanical evaluation, which revealed an anteriorly rotated pelvis and an inability to rotate the pelvis during function. Hip flexion, internal rotation, and adduction range of motion increased when the pelvis was held in a posteriorly rotated position during testing. The patient was referred to a physical therapist who specializes in manual therapy and motor control. Three months later, the patient returned to the clinic. Follow-up evaluation revealed a neutrally aligned pelvis and normal hip range of motion in all planes. Gait was returned to normal, and the patient was pain free and able to return to high-level activity.

1. What were the clinical indicators that the patient's symptoms were externally caused and did not involve a reinjury to his intra-articular structures?
2. What are the biomechanics of pelvic-related hip impingement?

WRAP-UP

Critical Thinking Questions

1. What are the main evaluation findings that would help in the differential diagnosis of intra-articular versus extra-articular involvement?
2. What role does the pelvis play in normal hip function?
3. Although uncommon, what are the most important conditions to rule out with an on-the-field hip injury?

Pearls and Pitfalls

- Pathologies of the hip are often nonspecific and require an in-depth knowledge of anatomy to accurately diagnose.
- For any presentation of anterior hip pain, intra-articular involvement should be ruled out.
- Differentiating between pelvic and hip pain generators is crucial to identifying the true cause of hip symptoms. If specific muscle impairment is identified, further examination of biomechanical alignment and function is warranted to address the underlying cause.

References

1. Menschik F: The hip joint as a conchoid shape. *J Biomech* 1997;30(9):971-973.
2. Moore KL, Dalley AF, Agur AMR: *Clinically Oriented Anatomy*, ed 5. Philadelphia, PA, Lippincott Williams & Wilkins, 2006.
3. Tan V, Seldes RM, Katz M, Freedhand AM, Klimkiewicz JJ, Fitzgerald RH: Contribution of acetabular labrum to articulating surface area and femoral head coverage in adult hip joints: an anatomic study in cadavera. *Am J Orthop* 2001;30(11):809-812.
4. Lecouvet FE, Vande Berg BC, Malghem J, et al: MR imaging of acetabular labrum: variations in 200 asymptomatic hips. *Am J Roentgen* 1996;167:1025-1028.
5. Won Y-Y, Chung I, Chung N, Song K: Morphological study on the acetabular labrum. *Yonsei Med J* 2003;44(5):855-862.
6. Hlavacek M: The influence of the acetabular labrum seal, intact articular superficial zone and synovial fluid thixotropy on squeeze-film lubrication of a spherical synovial joint. *J Biomech* 2002;35:1325-1335.
7. Ferguson SJ, Bryant JT, Ganz R, Ito K: An in vitro investigation of the acetabular labral seal in hip joint mechanics. *J Biomech* 2003;36(2):171-178.
8. Ferguson SJ, Bryant JT, Ganz R, Ito K: The influence of the acetabular labrum on hip joint cartilage consolidation: a poroelastic finite element model. *J Biomech* 2000;33(8):953-960.
9. Kim YT, Azuma H: The nerve endings of the acetabular labrum. *Clin Orthop Relat Res* 1995;320:17-181.
10. Peterson W, Peterson F, Tillman B: Structure and vascularization of the acetabular labrum with regard to the pathogenesis and healing of labral lesions. *Arch Orthop Trauma Surg* 2003;123:283-288.
11. Lohe F, Eckstein F, Sauer T, Putz R: Structure, strain and function of the transverse acetabular ligament. *Acta Anat* 1996;157:315-323.
12. Boese CK, Dargel J, Oppermann J, et al: The femoral neck-shaft angle on plain radiographs: a systematic review. *Skelet Radiol* 2016;45(1):19-28.
13. Notzli HP, Wyss TF, Stoecklin CH, Schmid MR, Treiber K, Hodler J: The contour of the femoral head-neck junction as a predictor for the risk of anterior impingement. *J Bone Joint Surg Br* 2002;84(4):556-560.
14. Anda S, Svenningsen S, Dale LG, Benum P: The acetabular sector angle of the adult hip determined by computed tomography. *Acta Radiol Diagn (Stockh)* 1986;27(4):443-447.
15. Tonnis D, Heinecke A: [Decreased acetabular anteversion and femur neck antetorsion cause pain and arthrosis. 1: Statistics and clinical sequelae]. *Z Orthop Ihre Grenzgeb* 1999;137(2):153-159.
16. Larson CM, Moreau-Gaudry A, Kelly BT, et al: Are normal hips being labeled as pathologic: a CT-based method for defining normal acetabular coverage. *Clin Orthop Relat Res* 2015;473(4):1247-1254.
17. Smith M, Costic R, Allaire R, Schilling P, Sekiya J: A biomechanical analysis of the soft tissue and osseous constraints of the hip joint. *Knee Surg Sports Traumatol Arthrosc* 2014;22(4):946-952.
18. Philippon MJ, Michalski MP, Campbell KJ, et al: A quantitative analysis of hip capsular thickness. *Knee Surg Sports Traumatol Arthrosc* 2015;23(9):2548-2553.
19. Hewitt JD, Glisson RR, Guilak F, Vail TP: The mechanical properties of the human hip capsule ligaments. *J Arthroplasty* 2002;17(1):82-89.
20. Martin HD, Savage A, Braly B, Palmer I, Beall DP, Kelly BT: The function of the hip capsular ligaments: a quantitative report. *Arthroscopy* 2008;24(2):188-195.
21. Wagner F, Negrao J, Campos J, et al: Capsular ligaments of the hip: anatomic, histologic, and positional study in cadaveric specimens with MR arthrography. *Radiology* 2012;263(1):189-198.
22. Myers CA, Register BC, Lertwanich P, et al: Role of the acetabular labrum and the iliofemoral ligament in hip stability: an in vitro biplane fluoroscopy study. *Am J Sports Med* 2011;39:85S-91S.
23. Domb B, Philipon M, Giordano B: Arthroscopic capsulotomy, capsular repair, and capsular plication of the hip: relation to atraumatic instability. *Arthroscopy* 2013;29(1):162-173.

24. Torry MR, Schenker ML, Martin HD, Hogoboom D, Philippon M: Neuromuscular hip biomechanics and pathology in the athlete. *Clin Sports Med* 2006;25:179-197.
25. Ito H, Song Y, Lindsey DP, Safran MR, Giori NJ: The proximal hip joint capsule and the zona orbicularis contribute to hip joint stability in distraction. *J Orthop Res* 2009;27(8):989-995.
26. Martin RL, Palmer I, Martin HD: Ligamentum teres: a functional description and potential clinical relevance. *Knee Surg Sports Traumatol Arthrosc* 2012;20(6):1209-1214.
27. Kivlan B, Richard Clemente F, Martin RL, Martin HD: Function of the ligamentum teres during multi-planar movement of the hip joint. *Knee Surg Sports Traumatol Arthrosc* 2013;21(7):1664-1668.
28. Bernard J, Beldame J, Van Driessche S, et al: Does hip joint positioning affect maximal voluntary contraction in the gluteus maximus, gluteus medius, tensor fasciae latae and sartorius muscles? *Orthop Traumatol Surg Res* 2017;103(7):999-1004.
29. Santaguida PL, McGill SM: The psoas major muscle: a three-dimensional geometric study. *J Biomech* 1994;28(3):339-345.
30. Giphart JE, Stull JD, Laprade RF, Wahoff MS, Philippon MJ: Recruitment and activity of the pectineus and piriformis muscles during hip rehabilitation exercises: an electromyography study. *Am J Sports Med* 2012;40(7):1654-1663.
31. Solomon LB, Lee YC, Callary SA, Beck M, Howie DW: Anatomy of piriformis, obturator internus and obturator externus: implications for the posterior surgical approach to the hip. *J Bone Joint Surg Br* 2010;92(9):1317-1324.
32. Gottschalk F, Kourosh S, Leveau B: The functional anatomy of tensor fasciae latae and gluteus medius and minimus. *J Anat* 1989;166:179-189.
33. Semciw AI, Pizzari T, Murley GS, Green RA: Gluteus medius: an intramuscular EMG investigation of anterior, middle and posterior segments during gait. *J Electromyogr Kinesiol* 2013;23(4):858-864.
34. Semciw AI, Green RA, Murley GS, Pizzari T: Gluteus minimus: an intramuscular EMG investigation of anterior and posterior segments during gait. *Gait Posture* 2014;39(2):822-826.
35. Beck M, Sledge JB, Gautier E, Dora CF, Ganz R: The anatomy and function of the gluteus minimus muscle. *J Bone Joint Surg Br* 2000;82(3):358-363.
36. Norcross MF, Blackburn JT, Goerger BM: Reliability and interpretation of single leg stance and maximum voluntary isometric contraction methods of electromyography normalization. *J Electromyogr Kinesiol* 2010;20(3):420-425.
37. Hernando MF, Cerezal L, Perez-Carro L, Abascal F, Canga A: Deep gluteal syndrome: anatomy, imaging, and management of sciatic nerve entrapments in the subgluteal space. *Skelet Radiol* 2015;44(7):919-934.
38. Hodges PW, McLean L, Hodder J: Insight into the function of the obturator internus muscle in humans: observations with development and validation of an electromyography recording technique. *J Electromyogr Kinesiol* 2014;24(4):489-496.
39. Semciw AI, Freeman M, Kunstler BE, Mendis MD, Pizzari T: Quadratus femoris: an EMG investigation during walking and running. *J Biomech* 2015;48(12):3433-3439.
40. Lovell GA, Blanch PD, Barnes CJ: EMG of the hip adductor muscles in six clinical examination tests. *Phys Ther Sport* 2012;13(3):134-140.
41. Gudena R, Alzahrani A, Railton P, Powell J, Ganz R: The anatomy and function of the obturator externus. *Hip Int* 2015;25(5):424-427.
42. Tannast M, Hanke MS, Zheng G, Steppacher SD, Siebenrock KA: What are the radiographic reference values for acetabular under- and overcoverage? *Clin Orthop Relat Res* 2015;473(4):1234-1246.
43. Hipfl C, Titz M, Chiari C, et al: Detecting cam-type deformities on plain radiographs: what is the optimal lateral view? *Arch Orthop Trauma Surg* 2017;137(12):1699-1705.
44. Sutter R, Dietrich TJ, Zingg PO, Pfirrmann CW: How useful is the alpha angle for discriminating between symptomatic patients with cam-type femoroacetabular impingement and asymptomatic volunteers? *Radiology* 2012;264(2):514-521.
45. Byrd JT, Jones KS: Diagnostic accuracy of clinical assessment, magnetic resonance imaging, magentic resonance arthrography, and intra-articular injection in hip arthroscopy patients. *Am J Sports Med* 2004;32(7):1668-1674.
46. Keeney JA, Peelle MW, Jackson J, Rubin D, Maloney WJ, Clohisy JC: Magnetic resonance arthrography versus arthroscopy in the evaluation of articular hip pathology. *Clin Orthop Relat Res* 2004;429:163-169.
47. Sutter R, Zanetti M, Pfirrmann CW: New developments in hip imaging. *Radiology* 2012;264(3):651-667.
48. Domayer SE, Mamisch TC, Kress I, Chan J, Kim YJ: Radial dGEMRIC in developmental dysplasia of the hip and in femoroacetabular impingement: preliminary results. *Osteoarthritis Cartilage* 2010;18(11):1421-1428.
49. Inman VT: Functional aspects of the abductor muscles of the hip. *J Bone Joint Surg* 1947;29(3):607-619.
50. Roach KE, Miles TP: Normal hip and knee active range of motion: the relationship to age. *Phys Ther* 1991;71(9):656-665.
51. Moreside JM, McGill SM: Quantifying normal 3D hip ROM in healthy young adult males with clinical and laboratory tools: hip mobility restrictions appear to be plane-specific. *Clin Biomech* 2011;26(8):824-829.
52. Hardcastle P, Nade S: The significance of the Trendelenburg test. *J Bone Joint Surg* 1985;67-B(5):741-746.
53. Fishman L, Dombi G, Michaelsen C, et al: Piriformis syndrome: diagnosis, treatment, and outcome: a 10-year study. *Arch Phys Med Rehabil* 2002;83:295-301.
54. Hase T, Ueo T. Acetabular labral tear: arthroscopic diagnosis and treatment. *Arthroscopy* 1999;15(2):138-141.
55. Leunig M, Werlen S, Ungersbock A, Ito K, Ganz R. Evaluation of the acetabular labrum by MR arthrography. *J Bone Joint Surg Br* 1997;79(2):230-234.
56. Burnett SJ, Della Rocca GJ, Prather H, Curry M, Maloney WJ, Clohisy JC: Clinical presentation of patients with tears of acetabular labrum. *J Bone Joint Surg* 2006;88:1448-1457.
57. Narvani A, Tsiridis E, Kendall S, Chaudhuri R, Thomas P: A preliminary report on prevalence of acetabular labrum tears in sports patients with groin pain. *Knee Surg Sports Traumatol Arthrosc* 2003;11:403-408.
58. Chan YS, Lien LC, Hsu HL, et al: Evaluating hip labral tears using magnetic resonance arthrography: a prospective study comparing hip arthroscopy and magnetic resonance arthrography diagnosis. *Arthroscopy* 2005;21(10):1250.
59. Prather H, Colorado B, Hunt D: Managing hip pain in the athlete. *Phys Med Rehabil Clin N Am* 2014;25(4):789-812.
60. Epstein DM, McHugh M, Yorio M, Neri B: Intra-articular hip injuries in national hockey league players: a descriptive epidemiological study. *Am J Sports Med* 2013;41(2):343-348.
61. Jackson TJ, Starkey C, McElhiney D, Domb BG: Epidemiology of hip injuries in the National Basketball Association: a 24-year overview. *Orthop J Sports Med* 2013;1(3):2325967113499130.
62. Lewis CL, Sahrmann SA: Acetabular labral tears. *Phys Ther* 2006;86:110-121.

63. Anderson K, Strickland S, Warren R: Hip and groin injuries in athletes. *Am J Sports Med* 2001;29(4):521-533.
64. Troum OM, Crues JV: The young adult with hip pain: diagnosis and medical treatment, circa 2004. *Clin Orthop Relat Res* 2004;418:9-17.
65. Braly B, Beall DP, Martin HD: Clinical examination of the athletic hip. *Clin Sports Med* 2006;25:199-210.
66. Adkins S, Filger R: Hip pain in athletes. *Am Fam Physician* 2000;61(7):2109-2118.
67. McCarthy JC, Noble P, Schuck M, Wright J, Lee JA: The role of labral lesions to development of early degenerative hip disease. *Clin Orthop Relat Res* 2001;393:25-37.
68. Bohannon Mason J: Acetabular labral tears in the athlete. *Clin Sports Med* 2001;20(4):779-790.
69. Narvani A, Tsiridis E, Tai C, Thomas P: Acetabular labrum and its tears. *Br J Sports Med* 2003;37:207-211.
70. McCarthy JC, Noble P, Aluisio FV, Schuck M, Wright J, Lee JA: Anatomy, pathologic features, and treatment of acetabular labral tears. *Clin Orthop Relat Res* 2003;406:38-47.
71. Ueblacker P, Muller-Wohlfahrt HW, Ekstrand J: Epidemiological and clinical outcome comparison of indirect ('strain') versus direct ('contusion') anterior and posterior thigh muscle injuries in male elite football players: UEFA Elite League study of 2287 thigh injuries (2001-2013). *Br J Sports Med* 2015;49(22):1461-1465.
72. Edouard P, Branco P, Alonso JM: Muscle injury is the principal injury type and hamstring muscle injury is the first injury diagnosis during top-level international athletics championships between 2007 and 2015. *Br J Sports Med* 2016;50(10):619-630.
73. Kerbel YE, Smith CM, Prodromo JP, Nzeogu MI, Mulcahey MK: Epidemiology of hip and groin injuries in collegiate athletes in the United States. *Orthop J Sports Med* 2018;6(5):2325967118771676.
74. Lovering RM, Hakim M, Moorman CT, III, De Deyne PG: The contribution of contractile pre-activation to loss of function after a single lengthening contraction. *J Biomech* 2005;38(7):1501-1507.
75. Garrett WE, Safran MR, Seaber A, Glisson RR, Ribbeck BM: Biomechanical comparison of stimulated and nonstimulated skeletal muscle pulled to failure. *Am J Sports Med* 1987;15(5):448-454.
76. Liu H, Garrett WE, Moorman CT, Yu B: Injury rate, mechanism, and risk factors of hamstring strain injuries in sports: a review of the literature. *J Sport Health Sci* 2012;1(2):92-101.
77. Serner A, Mosler AB, Tol JL, Bahr R, Weir A: Mechanisms of acute adductor longus injuries in male football players: a systematic visual video analysis. *Br J Sports Med* 2019;53(3):158-164.
78. Eckard TG, Padua DA, Dompier TP, Dalton SL, Thorborg K, Kerr ZY: Epidemiology of hip flexor and hip adductor strains in National Collegiate Athletic Association Athletes, 2009/2010-2014/2015. *Am J Sports Med* 2017;45(12):2713-2722.
79. Hoskins W, Pollard H: The management of hamstring injury—Part 1: Issues in diagnosis. *Man Ther* 2005;10(2):96-107.
80. Orchard J, Best TM: The management of muscle strain injuries: an early return versus the risk of recurrence. *Clin J Sport Med* 2002;12(1):3-5.
81. Trojian TH: Muscle contusion (thigh). *Clinics Sports Med* 2013;32(2):317-324.
82. Aronen JG, Garrick JG, Chronister RD, McDevitt ER: Quadriceps contusions: clinical results of immediate immobilization in 120 degrees of knee flexion. *Clin J Sport Med* 2006;16(5):383-387.
83. Ryan JB, Wheeler JH, Hopkinson WJ, Arciero RA, Kolakowski KR: Quadriceps contusions: West Point update. *Am J Sports Med* 1991;19(3):299-304.
84. Mithofer K, Lhowe DW, Vrahas MS, Altman DT, Altman GT: Clinical spectrum of acute compartment syndrome of the thigh and its relation to associated injuries. *Clin Orthop Relat Res* 2004(425):223-229.
85. Megliola A, Eutropi F, Scorzelli A, et al: Ultrasound and magnetic resonance imaging in sports-related muscle injuries. *Radiol Med* 2006;111(6):836-845.
86. O'Leary JA, Berend K, Vail TP: The relationship between diagnosis and outcome in arthroscopy of the hip. *Arthroscopy* 2001;17(2):181-188.
87. Fitzgerald RH. Acetabular labrum tears: diagnosis and treatment. *Clin Orthop Relat Res* 1995;311:60-68.
88. Byrd JWT: *Operative Hip Arthroscopy*, ed 2. New York: Springer; 2005.
89. Harris MD, Anderson AE, Henak CR, Ellis BJ, Peters CL, Weiss JA: Finite element prediction of cartilage contact stresses in normal human hips. *J Orthop Res* 2012;30(7):1133-1139.
90. Chegini S, Beck M, Ferguson SJ: The effects of impingement and dysplasia on stress distributions in the hip joint during sitting and walking: a finite element analysis. *J Orthop Res* 2009;27(2):195-201.
91. Flato R, Passanante GJ, Skalski MR, Patel DB, White EA, Matcuk GR, Jr: The iliotibial tract: imaging, anatomy, injuries, and other pathology. *Skelet Radiol* 2017;46(5):605-622.
92. Lewis CL. Extra-articular snapping hip: a literature review. *Sports Health* 2010;2(3):186-190.
93. Battaglia PJ, D'Angelo K, Kettner NW: Posterior, lateral, and anterior hip pain due to musculoskeletal origin: a narrative literature review of history, physical examination, and diagnostic imaging. *J Chiropr Med* 2016;15(4):281-293.
94. Lee KS, Rosas HG, Phancao JP: Snapping hip: imaging and treatment. *Semin Musculoskelet Radiol* 2013;17(3):286-294.
95. Hopayian K, Danielyan A: Four symptoms define the piriformis syndrome: an updated systematic review of its clinical features. *Eur J Orthop Surg Traumatol* 2018;28(2):155-164.
96. Lewis AM, Layzer R, Engstrom JW, Barbaro NM, Chin CT: Magnetic resonance neurography in extraspinal sciatica. *Arch Neurol* 2006;63(10):1469-1472.
97. Tins BJ, Garton M, Cassar-Pullicino VN, Tyrrell PN, Lalam R, Singh J: Stress fracture of the pelvis and lower limbs including atypical femoral fractures: a review. *Insights Imaging* 2015;6(1):97-110.
98. Biz C, Berizzi A, Crimi A, Marcato C, Trovarelli G, Ruggieri P: Management and treatment of femoral neck stress fractures in recreational runners: a report of four cases and review of the literature. *Acta Biomed* 2017;88(4 S):96-106.
99. Jacobs JM, Cameron KL, Bojescul JA: Lower extremity stress fractures in the military. *Clin Sports Med* 2014;33(4):591-613.
100. Wagner D, Ossendorf C, Gruszka D, Hofmann A, Rommens PM: Fragility fractures of the sacrum: how to identify and when to treat surgically? *Eur J Trauma Emerg Surg* 2015;41(4):349-362.

101. Karkenny AJ, Tauberg BM, Otsuka NY: Pediatric hip disorders: slipped capital femoral epiphysis and Legg-Calve-Perthes disease. *Pediatr Rev* 2018;39(9):454-463.
102. Larson AN, Kim HK, Herring JA: Female patients with late-onset Legg-Calve-Perthes disease are frequently gymnasts: is there a mechanical etiology for this subset of patients? *J Pediatr Orthop* 2013;33(8):811-815.
103. Skaggs DL, Tolo VT. Legg-Calve-Perthes disease. *J Am Acad Orthop Surg* 1996;4(1):9-16.
104. Cook PC: Transient synovitis, septic hip, and Legg-Calve-Perthes disease: an approach to the correct diagnosis. *Pediatr Clin North Am* 2014;61(6):1109-1118.
105. Divi SN, Bielski RJ. Legg-Calve-Perthes disease. *Pediatr Ann* 2016;45(4):e144-149.
106. Eskander JP, Ripoll JG, Calixto F, et al: Value of examination under fluoroscopy for the assessment of sacroiliac joint dysfunction. *Pain Physician* 2015;18(5):E781-786.
107. Brolinson PG, Kozar AJ, Cibor G. Sacroiliac joint dysfunction in athletes. *Curr Sports Med Rep* 2003;2(1):47-56.
108. van der Wurff P, Buijs EJ, Groen GJ: A multitest regimen of pain provocation tests as an aid to reduce unnecessary minimally invasive sacroiliac joint procedures. *Arch Phys Med Rehabil* 2006;87(1):10-14.
109. McKenzie-Brown AM, Shah RV, Sehgal N, Everett CR: A systematic review of sacroiliac joint interventions. *Pain Physician* 2005;8(1):115-125.
110. Szadek KM, van der Wurff P, van Tulder MW, Zuurmond WW, Perez RS: Diagnostic validity of criteria for sacroiliac joint pain: a systematic review. *J Pain* 2009;10(4):354-368.
111. Simopoulos TT, Manchikanti L, Singh V, et al: A systematic evaluation of prevalence and diagnostic accuracy of sacroiliac joint interventions. *Pain Physician* 2012;15(3):E305-344.
112. Tuite MJ: Sacroiliac joint imaging. *Semin Musculoskelet Radiol* 2008;12(1):72-82.

UNIT III

Upper Extremity Evaluation

CHAPTER 8	Wrist and Hand	215
CHAPTER 9	Elbow	273
CHAPTER 10	Shoulder	337
CHAPTER 11	Abdomen and Thorax	413
CHAPTER 12	Spine	503
CHAPTER 13	Head and Face	579

CHAPTER 8

Wrist and Hand

Sara D. Rynders, MPAS, PA-C

OVERVIEW

This chapter will introduce the reader to the complexities of hand and wrist anatomy and provide education on the observation, evaluation, and diagnosis of commonly encountered injuries. In-depth discussion of these topics will produce an appreciation for the delicate nature of the fingers, hands, and wrists and establish a foundation for a knowledgeable and detailed evaluation of the injured patient.

LEARNING OBJECTIVES

After completing this chapter, the reader will be able to do the following:

1. Identify the bones, joints, muscles, and nerves of the wrist and hand.
2. Perform testing of the three main nerves to the hand.
3. Obtain an accurate and detailed history of a hand or wrist injury or complaint.
4. Assemble a differential diagnosis based on symptoms and location.
5. Demonstrate an in-depth understanding of common wrist and hand conditions.
6. Know special tests for various conditions and what positive and negative results indicate.
7. Understand how to initially evaluate for and manage an injury at the sideline and when to refer to a physician.

FUN FACTS ABOUT THE WRIST AND HAND

- Cracking knuckles does NOT cause arthritis.
- Approximately one-fourth of the brain's motor cortex is devoted solely to the movement of the hand.
- Chimpanzees and monkeys have opposable thumbs to the index finger, but only humans can oppose the thumb across the palm because of the ulnar opposition motion afforded by the fourth and fifth carpometacarpal joints.
- The arc of finger flexion follows a spiral pattern (not circular) because of the varying lengths of the phalanges, and this spiral mimics the Fibonacci sequence commonly seen in nature.

Introduction

The wrist and hand are arguably the most anatomically elegant and biomechanically complicated sets of joints in the human body. Evolved from the weight-bearing structures of phylogenetic ancestors, these articulations have developed into complex structures capable of the finest pincer grasp and strongest composite grip. The wide range of abilities that the hands and wrists permit can be observed in the ethereal mastery of a concert pianist, the gravity-defying finger strength of a rock climber, and the unyielding grip necessary of a world-class weight lifter. None of these activities would be possible without the beautifully orchestrated myriad of movements provided by the hands and wrists.

Clinical Anatomy

Bones of the Wrist and Hand

The skeletal anatomy of the hands and wrists includes, listed from proximal to distal, the distal radius and distal ulna, eight carpal bones, five metacarpal bones, five proximal phalanges, four middle phalanges, and five distal phalanges.

Phalanges and Metacarpals

The distal phalanx serves as the insertion point for the common extensor tendon dorsally and the flexor digitorum profundus tendon volarly. The end of the bone fans out into a structure called the tuft. The nailbed adheres to the distal phalanx tuft.

The middle phalanx is present in all digits except the thumb. It serves as the insertion point for the flexor digitorum superficialis tendon volarly.

The proximal phalanx is the largest of the phalanges. The lumbrical and palmar and dorsal interosseous muscles attach to the base of the proximal phalanx.

The metacarpal bones are made up of a base, shaft, neck, and rounded head. They provide a frame upon which the small hand muscles attach for fine motor movements. The palmar and dorsal interosseous muscles originate from the metacarpal shafts. The smallest-diameter metacarpal is the fourth metacarpal bone. The commonly injured metacarpal is the fifth metacarpal at the level of the neck, commonly referred to as a boxer's fracture.

Carpals

There are eight uniquely shaped carpal bones that make up the wrist: the scaphoid, lunate, triquetrum, pisiform, trapezium, trapezoid, capitate, and hamate. The bones are divided into rows called the proximal carpal row (scaphoid, lunate, triquetrum, pisiform) and distal carpal row (trapezium, trapezoid, capitate, and hamate).

The scaphoid is a peanut-shaped bone that lies on the radial side of the wrist and articulates with the radius at the scaphoid fossa. The bone has proximal and distal poles and a bony protuberance volarly called the scaphoid tubercle. The scaphoid bone articulates with the lunate bone by way of the scapholunate (SL) ligament. The scaphoid, lunate, and triquetrum move as a singular unit in the uninjured wrist. The scaphoid bone has a unique retrograde blood supply. This is important to remember when assessing scaphoid fractures, as they are prone to osteonecrosis.

The lunate is a C-shaped bone that articulates with the head of the capitate distally and the radius at the lunate fossa proximally.

The triquetrum makes up the ulnarmost bone of the proximal carpal row.

The pisiform is a pea-shaped bone that is technically a sesamoid bone. It articulates volarly with the triquetrum but is otherwise embedded within the extensor carpal ulnaris tendon.

The trapezium bone is a saddle-shaped bone that articulates with the thumb metacarpal. Its unique shape allows for the exceptional rotational movement of the thumb ray.

The trapezoid articulates with the trapezium, scaphoid, and capitate.

The capitate is the largest of the carpal bones and sits centrally in the wrist. Its rounded proximal head articulates with the concave surface of the lunate bone.

The hamate is a unique bone for its volar bony protuberance, called the hook of the hamate. The hook serves to protect the adjacent ulnar artery and deep motor branch of the ulnar nerve. The hook is prone to injury from a fall on an outstretched hand.

Distal Radius

The distal aspect of the radius is a sloped structure composed of the radial styloid, scaphoid fossa, and lunate fossa. The ulnar aspect of the distal radius has a slight concave curvature called the sigmoid notch to accommodate the head of the distal ulna. The volar surface of the bone is smooth, with a gently sloping flare as it approaches the radiocarpal articulation. The square, flat pronator quadratus originates here. On the dorsal surface of the bone there is a longitudinal groove and accompanying tubercle called the Lister tubercle that serves as a fulcrum around which the extensor pollicis longus tendon passes.

Distal Ulna

The distal ulna is a short, cylindrical structure with a small bony protuberance called the ulnar styloid. The distal ulna is designed to rotate during supination and pronation of the forearm and articulates with the lunate and triquetrum as well as the sigmoid notch of the distal radius.

Articulations and Ligamentous Support

Each articulation is named for the bones proximal to and distal to the joint and are always named in a proximal-to-distal fashion. For example, the articulation between a carpal bone (proximal) and a metacarpal bone (distal) is called the carpometacarpal (CMC) joint. The articulation between a metacarpal bone and a phalanx is called the metacarpophalangeal (MCP) joint (**Figure 8.1**).

There are a multitude of small, intricate ligaments in the hand, wrist, and fingers that contribute to the stability and elegant biomechanics of the joints. It is imperative for the athletic trainer to know and understand the anatomy and function of several key structures: the ulnar collateral ligament (UCL) of the thumb

Clinical Anatomy **217**

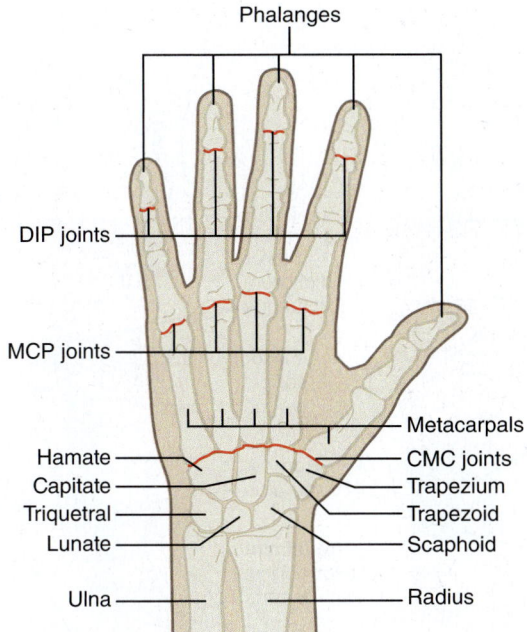

Figure 8.1 Drawing showing the bones and joints of the hand and wrist.

CMC, carpometacarpal; DIP, distal interphalangeal; MCP, metacarpophalangeal.
© Jones & Bartlett Learning

MCP joint, the SL and lunotriquetral (LT) ligaments of the wrist, and the triangular fibrocartilage complex (TFCC) of the distal radioulnar joint (DRUJ). The form and function of these three particular structures will be described further later in this chapter.

Distal Radioulnar Joint

The DRUJ describes the articulation between the distal radius and the head of the distal ulna. The head of the ulna rotates within the radial sigmoid notch to permit forearm supination and pronation. The joint is primarily stabilized by the radioulnar ligaments.

Radiocarpal Joint

The radiocarpal joint refers to the articulation of the distal radius with the proximal row of carpal bones (scaphoid, lunate, and triquetrum). More specifically, the joint can be divided into the radioscaphoid articulation, radiolunate articulation, and ulnotriquetral articulation. The joint can be accessed for injections and aspirations from the dorsal wrist between the third and fourth extensor compartments.

Intercarpal Joints

The carpal bones are divided into proximal and distal carpal rows. The proximal carpal row moves as a unit because of the attachments of the SL ligament and LT ligament. The articulation between the proximal and distal carpal rows is called the midcarpal joint. There is a small amount of motion that normally occurs at this joint during hand and wrist movements, but in certain conditions of laxity the midcarpal joint can become unstable.

CMC Joints

The CMC joints are generally referred to numerically based on their location from radial to ulnar. The first CMC joint lies at the base of the thumb and is a saddle-shaped joint that allows for a circumferential arc of thumb motion. The fourth and fifth CMC joints are also slightly mobile to allow for ulnar opposition of the ring and small fingers. This function is important for grip strength and accomplishing thumb opposition.

MCP Joint

The MCP joint is located between the rounded head of the metacarpal and the concave base of the proximal phalanx. The radial collateral ligaments (RCLs) and UCLs as well as the well-matched bowl-in-cup articular configuration provide good joint stability.

Interphalangeal Joints

The interphalangeal (IP) joints exist between the proximal and middle phalanx and the middle and distal phalanx. There are two IP joints in each finger, but the thumb has only one IP joint between the proximal phalanx and distal phalanx. The IP joints are buttressed volarly by the fibrocartilaginous volar plate and are resistant to varus and valgus stress by the RCLs and UCLs.

Soft-Tissue Anatomy

Muscular Anatomy

The athletic trainer should also have comprehensive knowledge of the extrinsic (originating from outside the region of the joint) and intrinsic (originating from within the region of the joint) muscles and tendons of the wrist and hand (**Figures 8.2** and **8.3**, and **Tables 8.1**, **8.2**, and **8.3**). Muscles and tendons that originate more proximally in the forearm are responsible for most gross hand motion, such as flexing and extending the digits, but it is the small, intrinsic muscles of the hand that work synergistically with those extrinsic muscles to provide finely controlled movements and more than one movement at a time. Consider the posture of holding a pencil: the fingers are flexed; the thumb is flexed, abducted, and slightly opposed; and the wrist is slightly extended. This is a perfect example of the

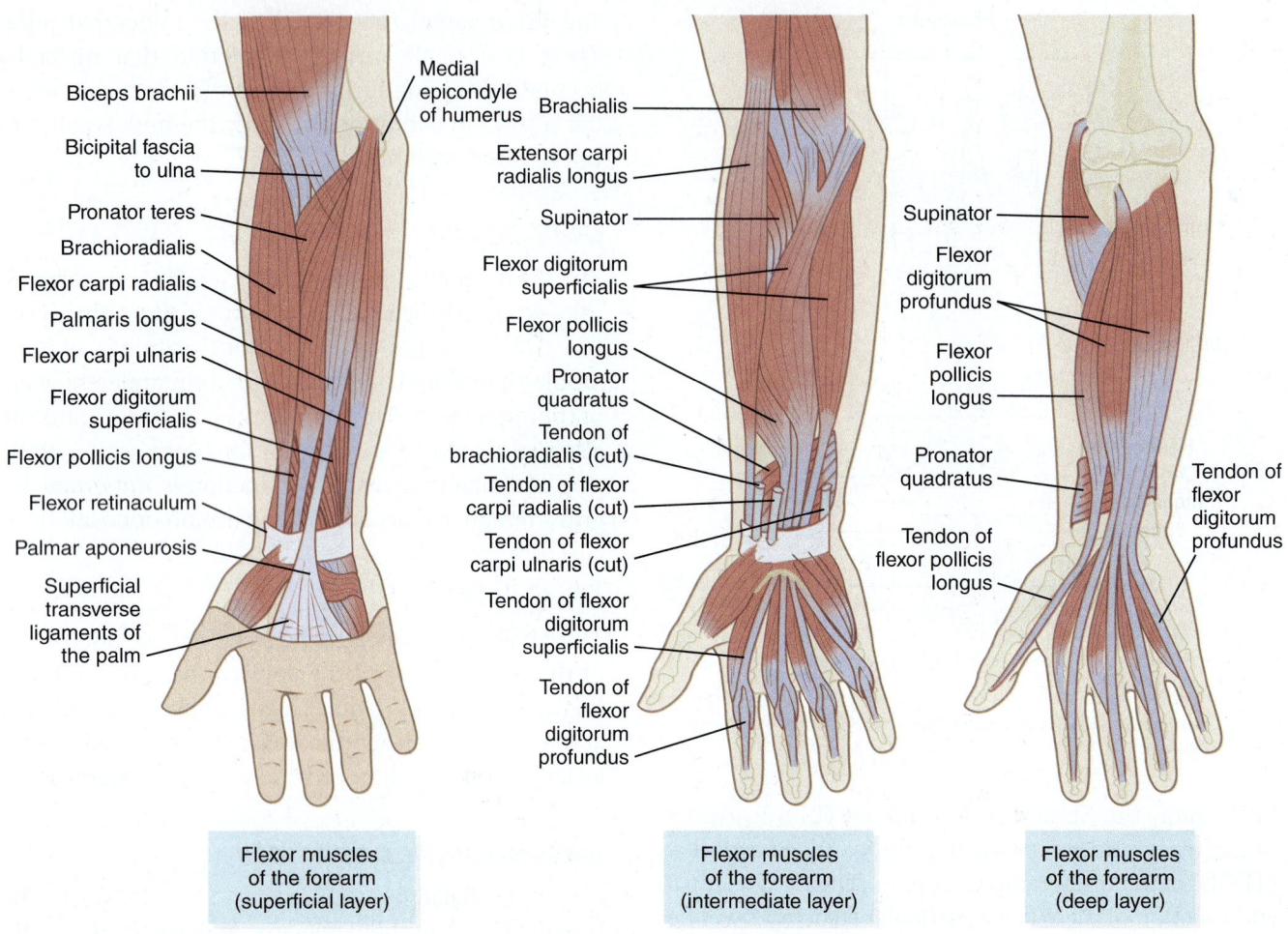

Figure 8.2 Drawings showing flexor muscles and tendons of the wrist and hand.
© Jones & Bartlett Learning

complexity of motions that must occur in order to perform even the most basic hand functions.

More important than remembering the origin of individual muscles and tendons is remembering their insertion sites. This is because most injuries involving tendons in the hand will occur at their insertion point distally, such as a mallet finger injury (extensor tendon rupture) and jersey finger (flexor tendon rupture). Additionally, close attention should be paid to the extensor hood mechanism in the finger (**Figure 8.4**). Note that the extensor tendon divides in the finger and intercalates with the intrinsic muscles of the hand. This will be important during discussion of mallet finger and central slip injuries later in the text.

Neurologic Anatomy

The three nerves responsible for motor and sensory innervation to the hand are the terminal branches of the median, ulnar, and radial nerves. The median nerve divides in the forearm into the median nerve proper and the anterior interosseous nerve (AIN). The radial nerve divides in the forearm into the posterior interosseous nerve and the superficial sensory radial nerve. The terminal branches of the median and ulnar nerves contain sensory fibers for sensation in the hand as well as motor fibers to the intrinsic hand muscles. The terminal sensory branches of the median and ulnar nerves subdivide into common digital nerves and digital nerves as they move distally. The terminal branch of the radial nerve provides no motor innervation to the intrinsic hand muscles but does provide sensation to the dorsal hand (**Figure 8.5**). Cervical nerves C6, C7, and C8 provide the dermatomal distribution to the hand and wrist (**Table 8.4**) and cranial nerves C6, C7, C8, and T1 provide the myotomal distribution (**Table 8.5**).

Vascular Anatomy

The arterial supply to the hand is provided by the beautifully redundant palmar arch system. Fed by the radial and ulnar arteries at the wrist, the arch

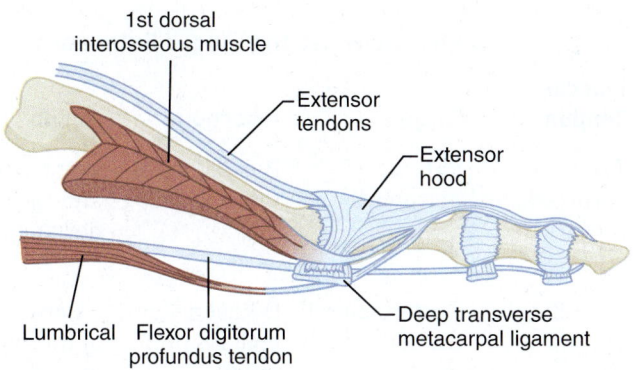

Figure 8.4 Drawing showing the extensor hood of the finger.
© Jones & Bartlett Learning

system ensures dual supply of blood to the fingers and thumb such that, if one artery or one arch is compromised, the other will provide complementary flow (**Figure 8.6**).

Overview of Radiology and Imaging

Radiography

The fingers, hand, and wrist can be imaged separately or as a group, depending on what structures need to be visualized. It is best practice to image the most specific region of injury whenever possible—for example,

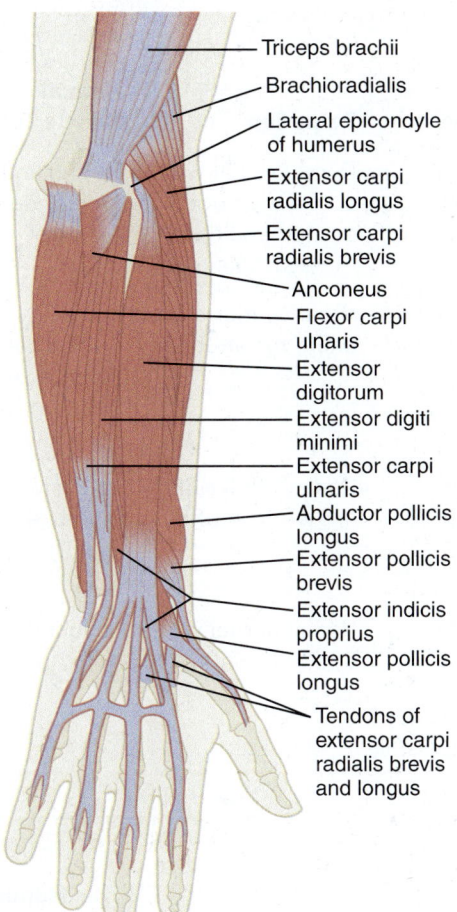

Figure 8.3 Drawing showing the extensor muscles and tendons of the wrist and hand.
© Jones & Bartlett Learning

Table 8.1 Extrinsic Wrist and Finger Extensors

Muscle/Tendon	Origin	Insertion	Action	Nerve	Palpation	Manual Muscle Test
Extensor digitorum communis	Lateral epicondyle	Extensor hood of digits	Finger extension	PIN of radial nerve	Dorsal hand and wrist	Extend second to fifth digits
Extensor digitorum minimi	Lateral epicondyle	Extensor hood of small finger	Accessory fifth finger extension	PIN of radial nerve	Dorsal fifth finger MCP joint	Extend fifth digit
Extensor indicis proprius	Posterolateral distal ulna	Extensor hood of index finger	Accessory index finger extension	PIN of radial nerve	Dorsal index MCP joint	Extend second digit
Extensor carpi ulnaris	Lateral epicondyle	Fifth metacarpal base	Wrist extension and ulnar deviation	PIN of radial nerve	Dorsal-ulnar wrist just distal and ulnar to the ulnar styloid	Extend and ulnarly deviate the wrist
Extensor carpi radialis longus	Lateral supracondylar ridge of humerus	Base of second metacarpal	Wrist extension and radial deviation	Radial nerve	Dorsal radial wrist at the base of the second and third metacarpals	Extend and radially deviate the wrist

(continues)

Table 8.1 Extrinsic Wrist and Finger Extensors (continued)

Muscle/Tendon	Origin	Insertion	Action	Nerve	Palpation	Manual Muscle Test
Extensor carpi radialis brevis	Lateral epicondyle	Base of third metacarpal	Wrist extension and radial deviation	PIN of radial nerve	Dorsal radial wrist at the base of the second and third metacarpals	Extend and radially deviate the wrist
Extensor pollicis longus	Posterolateral distal ulna and interosseous membrane	Dorsal distal phalanx of thumb	Extension of thumb interphalangeal joint	PIN of radial nerve	Ulnar border of anatomic snuffbox	Thumb interphalangeal joint extension Lift thumb off flat table
Extensor pollicis brevis	Radial shaft	Dorsal base of proximal phalanx of thumb	Extension of thumb MCP joint	PIN of radial nerve	Radial border of anatomic snuffbox	Extension of thumb MCP joint
Abductor pollicis longus	Proximal dorsal radius and ulna	Radial base of the thumb metacarpal	Thumb abduction	PIN of radial nerve	Radial border of anatomic snuffbox	Abduct thumb

MCP, metacarpophalangeal; PIN, posterior interosseous nerve.

Table 8.2 Extrinsic Wrist and Finger Flexors

Muscle/Tendon	Origin	Insertion	Action	Nerve	Palpation	Manual Muscle Test
Flexor digitorum profundus	Proximal interosseous membrane and anterior ulna	Volar distal phalanx of digits two through five	Flexion of DIP joint of digits two through five	Index and middle finger: AIN from median nerve Ring and small finger: Ulnar nerve	Volar middle and distal phalanx	Block flexion at middle phalanx and flex at DIP joint
Flexor digitorum superficialis	Medial epicondyle, coronoid process, and medial border of radius	Bifurcates at proximal phalanx; inserts on volar middle phalanx of digits two through five	Flexion of PIP joint digits two through five	Median nerve	Volar palm	Hold other digits in extension and flex digit at PIP joint
Flexor pollicis longus	Anterior shaft of radius and interosseous membrane	Volar distal phalanx of thumb	Flexion of the thumb interphalangeal joint	AIN of median nerve	Volar thumb at proximal phalanx and distal phalanx	Flex thumb at IP joint
Flexor carpi radialis	Medial epicondyle	Volar base of second and third metacarpals	Wrist flexion	Median nerve	Volar radial wrist	Flex wrist
Flexor carpi ulnaris	Medial epicondyle and proximal medial shaft of olecranon process and ulna	Fifth metacarpal base, pisiform, and hamate	Wrist flexion and ulnar deviation	Ulnar nerve	Volar ulnar wrist	Flex and ulnarly deviate wrist

AIN, anterior interosseous nerve; DIP, distal interphalangeal; IP, interphalangeal; PIP, proximal interphalangeal.

Table 8.3 Intrinsic Hand Muscles

Muscle/Tendon	Origin	Insertion	Action	Nerve	Palpation	Manual Muscle Test
Abductor pollicis brevis	Scaphoid tubercle and flexor retinaculum	Base of thumb proximal phalanx and extensor pollicis longus tendon	Thumb abduction	Recurrent branch of median nerve	Thenar eminence	Thumb abduction
Flexor pollicis brevis	Flexor retinaculum and trapezium tubercle	Volar base of thumb proximal phalanx	Flexion of thumb MCP joint	Ulnar and median nerve	Thenar eminence	Flex thumb MCP joint
Adductor pollicis	Volar carpal bones and volar second and third metacarpal base	Ulnar side of thumb proximal phalanx base	Thumb adduction	Ulnar nerve	Thenar eminence	Adduct thumb
Opponens pollicis	Flexor retinaculum and trapezium tubercle	Radial side of thumb metacarpal	Thumb opposition	Recurrent branch of median nerve	Thenar eminence	Oppose thumb
Abductor digiti minimi	Pisiform, pisohamate ligament, and flexor retinaculum	Base of fifth finger proximal phalanx and extensor hood	Fifth digit abduction	Ulnar nerve	Hypothenar eminence	Abduct fifth digit
Flexor digiti minimi	Hood of hamate and flexor retinaculum	Base of fifth finger proximal phalanx	Fifth finger MCP joint flexion	Ulnar nerve	Hypothenar eminence	Flex fifth finger MCP joint
Opponens digiti minimi	Hood of hamate and flexor retinaculum	Ulnar border of fifth metacarpal shaft	Fifth finger opposition	Ulnar nerve	Hypothenar eminence	Oppose fifth finger
Dorsal interosseous muscles	Metacarpal shafts	Base of proximal phalanges and extensor hood	Finger abduction	Ulnar nerve	Between metacarpal bones, dorsal hand	Abduct fingers
Palmar interosseous muscles	Metacarpal shafts	Base of proximal phalanges and extensor hood	Finger adduction	Ulnar nerve	Between metacarpal bones, deep	Adduct fingers
Lumbricals	Flexor digitorum profundus tendon in palm	Radial base of proximal phalanges	Flex MCP joints and extend PIP joints	First and second: median nerve Third and fourth: ulnar nerve	Palm; deep	Flex MCP joints and extend PIP joints

MCP, metacarpophalangeal; PIP, proximal interphalangeal.

a finger injury necessitates a finger radiograph as opposed to a hand radiograph. In this way the examiner may visualize as much detail as possible on the image. PA, lateral, and oblique views are appropriate screening radiographs for the finger, hand, and wrist joints (**Figures 8.7**, **8.8**, and **8.9**).

Additionally, specific radiographic views of a region may be ordered based on the suspected

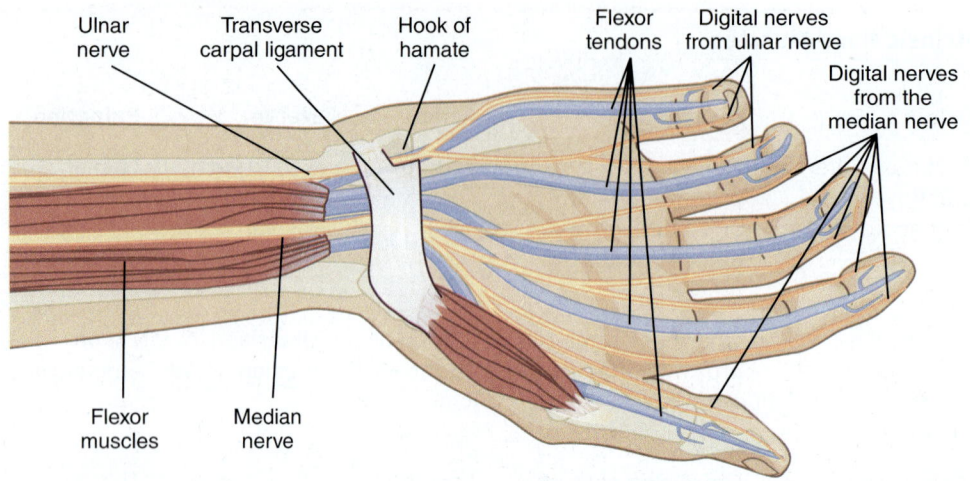

Figure 8.5 Drawing showing the nerves of the wrist and hand.
© Jones & Bartlett Learning

Table 8.4 Sensory Testing of Nerve Root Dermatomes

Nerve Root	Testing Location on Hand
C6	Thumb
C7	Index and middle fingers
C8	Ring and small fingers

Table 8.5 Motor Testing of Nerve Root Myotomes

Nerve Root	Test
C6	Brachioradialis reflex (wrist extension)
C7	Triceps reflex
C8	Finger flexion (grip strength)
T1	Finger abduction/adduction

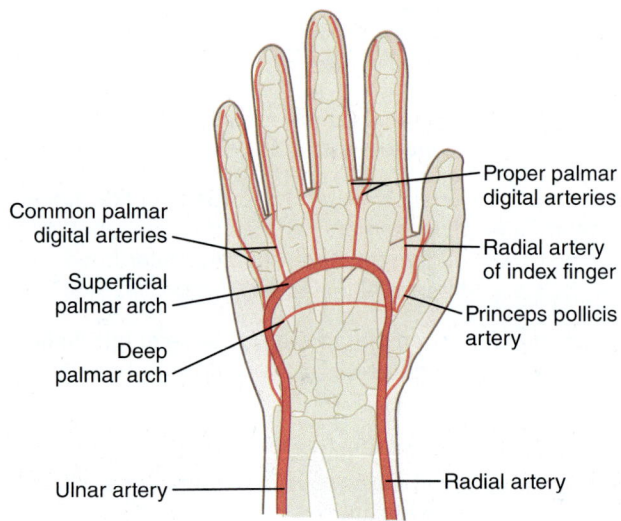

Figure 8.6 Drawing showing the deep and superficial palmar arch system.
© Jones & Bartlett Learning

diagnosis. Unsupported lateral views of the finger are helpful to evaluate mallet finger injuries. The wrist joint has several ancillary views that can be used based on the suspected injury. A scaphoid view, sometimes called an ulnar deviation view, helps to elongate the scaphoid in the PA plane to evaluate for scaphoid fractures (**Figure 8.10**). A PA clenched fist view of the wrist requires the patient to make a tightly clenched fist while the radiograph is taken. This causes the capitate to compress the SL ligament and is helpful to evaluate for SL ligament tears. Of note, a clenched fist view should always be compared to the uninjured wrist to evaluate for normal physiologic widening of the SL interval.

Magnetic Resonance Imaging

MRI is an ancillary test that should be used only when other methods of diagnosis, such as physical examination and plain radiographs, are not definitive. Depending on the zone of injury, the region of the MRI study should be specified to the finger, hand, or wrist, as specific coils can be used to increase the level of detail seen in the image. MRI can be useful to identify tendon injuries and tendinitis, SL ligament tears or triangular fibrocartilage tears in the wrist, and occult (previously unseen) scaphoid fractures in the patient with anatomic snuffbox tenderness and a normal radiograph. Indications and pathology-specific MRI findings will be discussed later in the chapter.

Overview of Radiology and Imaging **223**

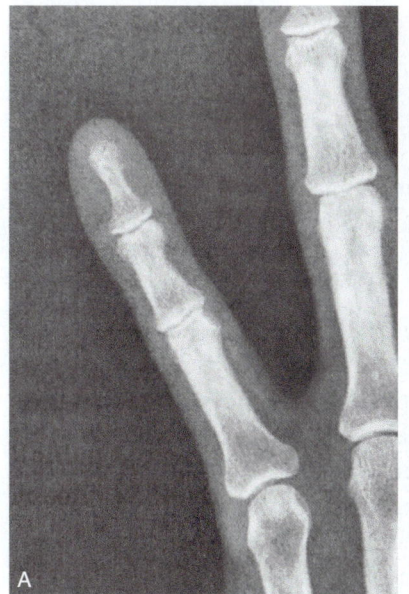
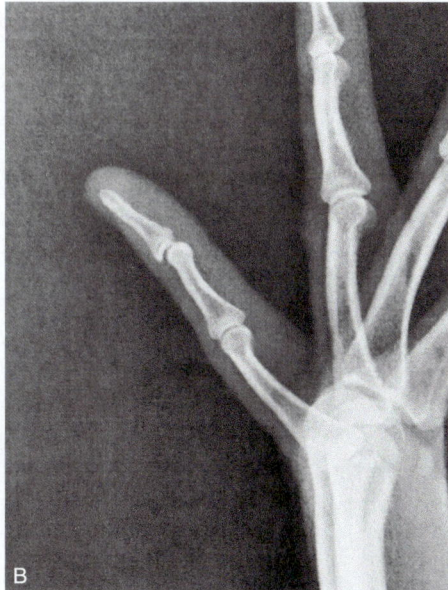
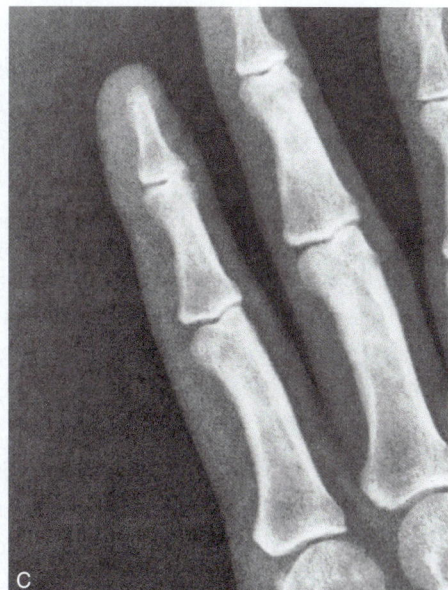

Figure 8.7 Radiographs of the finger. **A.** PA view. **B.** Lateral view. **C.** Oblique view.
Courtesy of Sara Rynders.

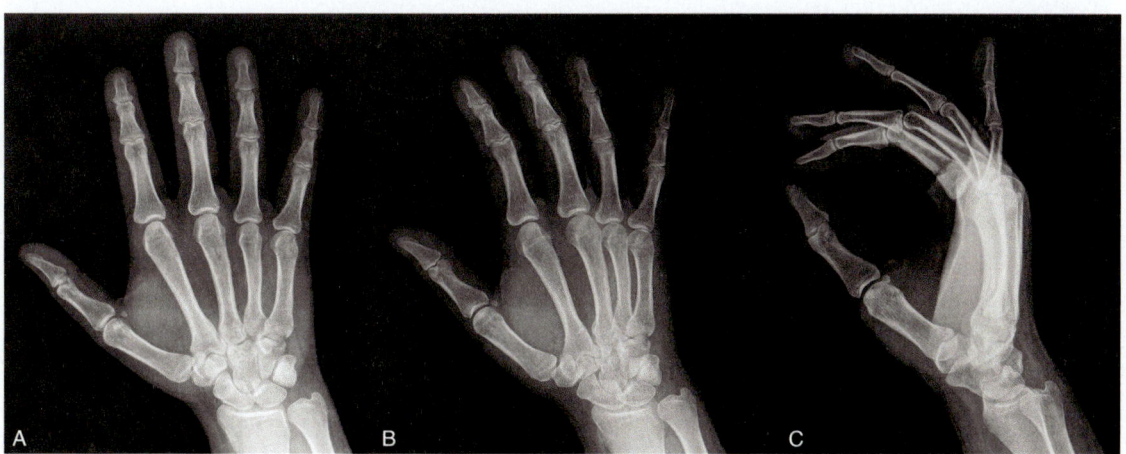

Figure 8.8 Radiographs of the hand. **A.** PA view. **B.** Oblique view. **C.** Lateral view.
© Radiologist/E+/Getty Images

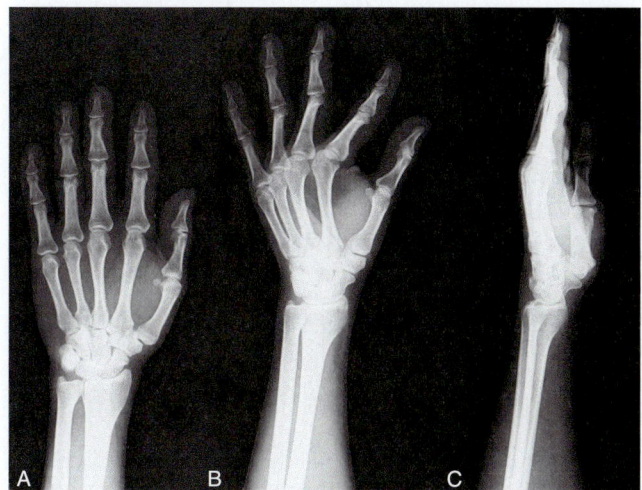

Figure 8.9 Radiograph of the wrist. **A.** PA view. **B.** Lateral view. **C.** Oblique view.
© Kitawan/Shutterstock

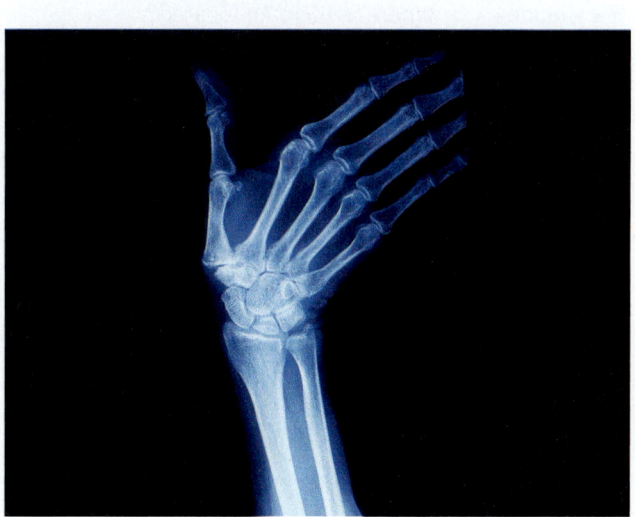

Figure 8.10 Radiograph showing the scaphoid, or ulnar deviation, view of the wrist.
© Yok_onepiece/Shutterstock

Ultrasonography

Nonvascular ultrasonography, also known as musculoskeletal ultrasonography, can be a very useful tool in the diagnosis of hand and wrist injuries. Unfortunately, the availability of the test, the paucity of radiologists trained to perform the test, and variability of results from provider to provider mean that only certain centers are regularly performing this examination. When it is available, ultrasonography can be a quick and noninvasive method of diagnosing tendon ruptures and thumb UCL injuries.

Computed Tomography

CT is usually used to assess bony structures and bony architecture of the finger, hand, and wrist. Most commonly, CT scans are used to characterize fracture patterns in order to determine the need for surgery and assist with surgical planning.

Evaluation of the Hand and Wrist

History

Completing a thorough history of the complaint is absolutely essential to establishing an accurate diagnosis. The most important components of a good history are (1) establishing *when* the injury occurred or the pain began; (2) the *mechanism of injury*, if known; and (3) the *location* of the pain. The interviewer should ask open-ended questions and give the patient time and space to tell his or her story. After listening, the interviewer should use investigative questioning to fill in the missing pieces and gather additional information. Consider the mnemonic OPQRST to remember the core questions of a health interview (**Table 8.6**). Specifically, inquire whether there was a fall and, if so, the degree of force associated with the fall. Was there a fall

Table 8.6 Mnemonic for Core Interview Questions

O = Onset	• What were you doing when the symptoms started? • Describe the position of the finger, hand, or wrist when the injury occurred. • Was it a sudden or gradual onset?	• Sudden onset of pain suggests a traumatic injury, such as a fracture or tendon or ligament rupture. • Gradual onset suggests a more chronic condition, such as tendinitis.
P = Provocative or Palliative	• What makes the symptoms better and what makes them worse? • What position makes the pain occur?	• Wrist pain with rotational movements (such as opening a doorknob) can suggest injury to the triangular fibrocartilage. • Wrist pain with weight bearing in extension can suggest an injury to the scapholunate ligament.
Q = Quality	• Is the pain sharp and shooting or dull and achy? • It is constant or intermittent?	• Pain from tendinitis tends to radiate from a central area. • Pain from a fracture or sprain tends to localize.
R = Region and Radiate	• Where is the pain located? • Can you point to the area of pain with one finger? • If a line is drawn exactly down the center of the wrist, is the pain on the ulnar or radial side? • Does the pain radiate?	• Asking the patient to point to the area of pain is one of the single most effective ways of narrowing a differential diagnosis. • Approximately 50% of wrist problems can be ruled out by asking on which side of the wrist the pain occurs, radial or ulnar. • Pain around the thumb metacarpophalangeal joint should be suspicious for an ulnar collateral ligament injury. • Pain and tenderness at the anatomic snuffbox is highly suggestive of a scaphoid fracture, even in the setting of negative radiographs.
S = Severity	• How severe is the pain? • Is it keeping you awake at night? • Are you able to perform general activities of daily living?	• Pain level is a subjective measure of injury severity. Asking whether the patient is able to sleep, get dressed, make meals, etc., helps to better understand the level of injury severity and interference in daily life.
T = Time	• How long has the condition been going on? • How has it changed over time: better, worse, or the same?	• Chronic, overuse-type injuries will have a more gradual onset, and the patient may not know an exact date or time that the condition started. • Pain from a fracture will likely improve over time. Pain from an overuse injury will likely worsen over time.

Table 8.7 Sample of Clinical Deductions Based on Possible Responses

Radial-Side Wrist Pain	Ulnar-Side Wrist Pain	Dorsal Wrist Pain	Volar Wrist Pain	Jammed Finger
Scaphoid fracture Scapholunate ligament injury de Quervain tenosynovitis Intersection syndrome Extensor carpi radialis brevis/extensor carpi radialis longus insertional tendinitis Flexor carpi radialis tendinitis Distal radius fracture Ganglion cyst Preiser disease (osteonecrosis of the scaphoid)	Triangular fibrocartilage complex tear Ulnocarpal impaction syndrome Distal radioulnar joint instability Extensor carpi ulnaris tendinitis Flexor carpi ulnaris tendinitis Hook of hamate fracture Distal ulnar fracture Cubital tunnel syndrome Ulnar artery thrombosis Lunotriquetral ligament tear Pisotriquetral joint arthritis Triquetral fracture Fifth metacarpal base fracture Fifth carpometacarpal joint fracture-dislocation Kienböck disease (osteonecrosis of the lunate)	Extensor tendinitis Scapholunate tear	Flexor carpi ulnaris or flexor carpi radialis tendinitis Carpal tunnel syndrome	Mallet finger Proximal interphalangeal joint sprain Central slip injury/boutonniére deformity Thumb ulnar collateral ligament tear

from a height or while running? High-energy mechanisms tend to have a higher degree of injury severity. Also note what activities the patient may be doing repetitively that could lead to overuse syndromes, such as tendinitis.

Inspection

Silently observe the patient and the injury during the interview portion of the visit. An acutely injured finger, hand, or wrist will likely demonstrate obvious edema (swelling) and possible ecchymosis (bruising, depending on the acuity of the injury). Note where the edema and ecchymosis are located to help narrow down the differential diagnosis (**Table 8.7**). The patient with a severe injury or fracture may be guarding the area and not moving it voluntarily. Also, a significantly injured finger will often exhibit a flexed, sausage like posture. Pathologies that are more chronic in nature, such as tendinitis, will often have more subtle outward findings, if not a completely normal appearance.

After observing for erythema (redness), edema (swelling), and ecchymosis (bruising), the examiner needs to perform an osteokinematic assessment. Normal range of motion (ROM) for the hand and wrist joints is listed in **Table 8.8**. Note whether the finger joints appear reduced on inspection and, if dislocated, in which direction. It is also very important to look for and document any lacerations, puncture wounds, abrasions, or open wounds. Fractures are classified as open or closed based on whether the skin barrier overlying the zone of injury has been violated. Open fractures necessitate immediate medical attention and prompt use of intravenous antibiotics in order to prevent infection.

Table 8.8 Finger and Wrist Normal ROM

Wrist flexion/extension	70°/80°
Wrist supination/pronation	80°/80°
Wrist radial/ulnar deviation	20°/30°
Finger metacarpophalangeal joint flexion/extension	90°/−20°
Finger proximal interphalangeal joint flexion/extension	100°/0°
Finger distal interphalangeal joint flexion/extension	80°/0°
Thumb metacarpophalangeal joint flexion/extension	55°/0°
Thumb interphalangeal joint flexion/extension	80°/−15°

ROM, range of motion.

Palpation

The next step in evaluation is always palpation. Ask the patient to point with one finger to the area that hurts the most and then begin the palpation examination on structures just adjacent to that area. The clinician should gently but deliberately palpate specific anatomic landmarks and document areas of tenderness. Is there tenderness specific to the metacarpal shaft, MCP joint, or CMC joint? Is there tenderness over the anatomic snuffbox, radial styloid, or Lister tubercle? There is a high concentration of structures in a small area in the hand and wrist. A picture of the underlying anatomy should constantly run through the clinician's head as the exam is carried out. Also, always palpate a joint above and below the zone of injury to evaluate for any additional or previously unrecognized injuries.

Special Tests

After palpation, consider whether there are any additional special tests to perform to further differentiate the diagnosis or qualify a suspected diagnosis. If a joint injury is suspected, the ligamentous support of the joint should be evaluated. MCP and proximal interphalangeal (PIP) joints should be gently placed under varus and valgus stress to evaluate for ligamentous laxity of the collateral ligaments. If a finger or wrist tendon injury is suspected, each tendon should be tested individually. Specific tests will be explained in detail later in this chapter. Also, assess the patient's strength against resistance, as this can not only identify weakness but also produce pain in an injured or inflamed tendon.

After special tests, perform and document a neurologic examination of the hand. For an examination to be considered complete, both motor and sensory testing are necessary of the median, ulnar, and radial nerves. A quick baseline assessment is easy to perform. Ask the patient whether he or she is able to feel light touch in the fingertips of the index (median nerve) and small fingers (ulnar nerve) and the dorsal surface of the thumb (radial nerve). Next, test the motor component of each nerve by asking the patient to flex the fingers into a fist (median nerve), abduct and adduct the fingers (ulnar nerve), and extend the wrist and thumb into a thumbs up gesture (radial nerve). If a more detailed neurologic examination is necessary because of concern for nerve injury, use a two-point discrimination testing disk (**Figure 8.11**). This test will determine whether the patient has normal sensation (6- to 7-mm two-point discrimination or less) or whether sensation is abnormal and the patient has lost protective sensation to pain and temperature (8 mm or more). Ask the patient to close his or her eyes while carefully alternating between one point and two points on the disk. Start at an 8-mm width and decrease until the patient cannot discriminate between two points and one point. Test on both

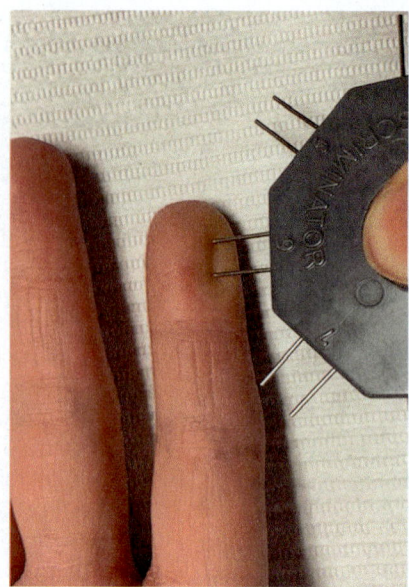

Figure 8.11 Clinical photograph showing two-point discrimination test.
Courtesy of Sara Rynders.

the radial and ulnar aspects of each digit to isolate individual digital nerves. Ask the patient to report whether and when he or she feels two points or one point on the fingertips. Record the width at which the patient can discriminate between two points.

Last, examine and document the vascular status of the hand and wrist. Palpate the radial artery at the wrist. The artery should have a distinct, bounding feel. Additionally, a capillary refill test can be performed. Pinch the patient's fingertips firmly and then release. Observe that they will blanch white to red, and count the number of seconds it takes to return to red. Normal perfusion has a capillary refill time of less than 2 seconds. Last, the patency of the radial and ulnar arteries can be assessed using the Allen test (**Figure 8.12**). This test is useful to determine whether there is a blockage in one of the arteries or the patient has a dominant arterial blood flow to the palmar arch system. Place the thumbs firmly over the volar wrist, one on the ulnar artery and the other over on the radial artery, completing occluding blood flow to the hand. Ask the patient to pump his or her fist to drain the venous system in the capillary beds. Note that the hand turns white. Next, release the thumb overlying the radial artery. Observe the hand to see whether redness returns to the palm and digits. If the hand remains white, then the patient has an ulnar artery occlusion or ulnar artery-dominant blood flow to the hand. Repeat the test, only this time release the thumb overlying the ulnar artery. Document the findings.

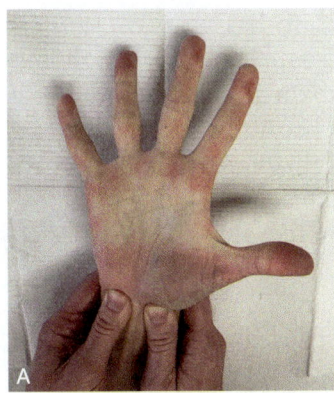 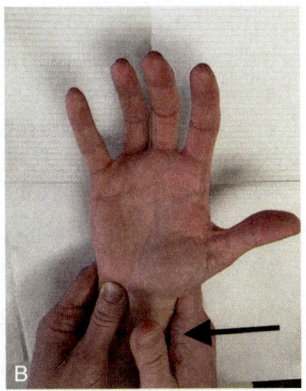 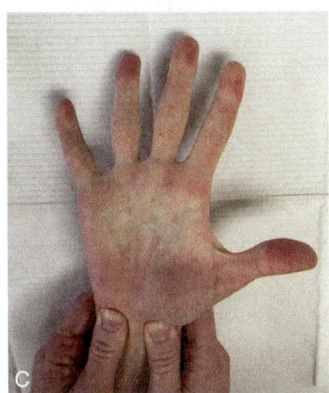 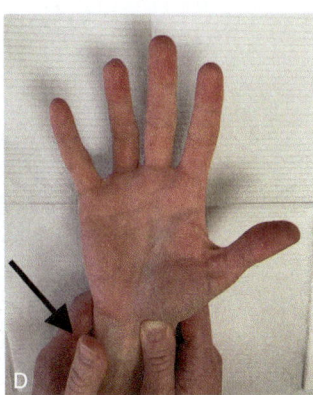

Figure 8.12 Clinical photographs showing the Allen test. **A.** The clinician occludes the patient's radial and ulnar arteries while the patient opens and closes the fist to exsanguinate the hand. **B.** The clinician's thumb over the radial artery is released and blood is allowed to flow. If the radial artery is patent, the palm will turn pink. **C.** The radial and ulnar arteries are occluded a second time while the patient opens and closes the fist to exsagunate the hand. **D.** The thumb over the ulnar artery is released and blood is allowed to flow. If the ulnar artery is patent, the palm will turn pink.

Courtesy of Sara Rynders.

Conditions Causing Radial-Side Wrist Pain

Scaphoid Fracture

The scaphoid, sometimes called the navicular, is the most commonly fractured carpal bone in the wrist, accounting for up to 70% of all carpal fractures.[1] The most common mechanism of injury is a fall onto an outstretched hand with the wrist hyperextended (**Table 8.9**). Scaphoid fractures are more common in high-impact sports, such as football and basketball; it is thought that 1 in 100 college football players will sustain a scaphoid fracture during their college career.[2] Despite its relative frequency of occurrence, fractures of the scaphoid are among the most commonly missed injuries on initial evaluation. Up to 25% of patients with a scaphoid fracture will have negative radiographs on initial examination.[1] The clinician needs to maintain a high level of suspicion for proper follow-up and diagnosis of these injuries.

The scaphoid bone has a unique blood supply. Fed by branches of the radial artery, the scaphoid bone receives its blood supply in a retrograde fashion, from distal to proximal (**Figure 8.13**). This is significant because fractures that occur in the waist and proximal third of the scaphoid put the proximal portion of the bone at high risk for osteonecrosis due to interruption in the already tenuous blood supply. If a scaphoid fracture goes unrecognized and untreated, numerus case series have demonstrated that the patient has a 10% risk of fracture nonunion (higher for displaced fractures) and a 13% to 50% risk for osteonecrosis of the scaphoid, early-onset

Table 8.9 Scaphoid Fracture Quick Tips

Pathology	Description	Presentation (HIPS)	Special Tests/ Imaging	Differential Diagnosis	5-Min Sideline Assessment Tips
Scaphoid fracture	Fracture of the scaphoid bone	Sudden onset of radial-side wrist pain, usually after a fall onto an outstretched hand	Tenderness at the anatomic snuffbox Obtain scaphoid-view radiographs and possibly an MRI	Scapholunate ligament injury de Quervain tenosynovitis Intersection syndrome Extensor carpi radialis brevis/ extensor carpi radialis longus insertional tendinitis Flexor carpi radialis tendinitis Distal radius fracture Ganglion cyst Preiser disease (osteonecrosis of the scaphoid)	If pain or tenderness at the anatomic snuffbox is present, remove the patient from play, apply a splint, and obtain further radiograph evaluation

HIPS, history, inspection, palpation, special tests.

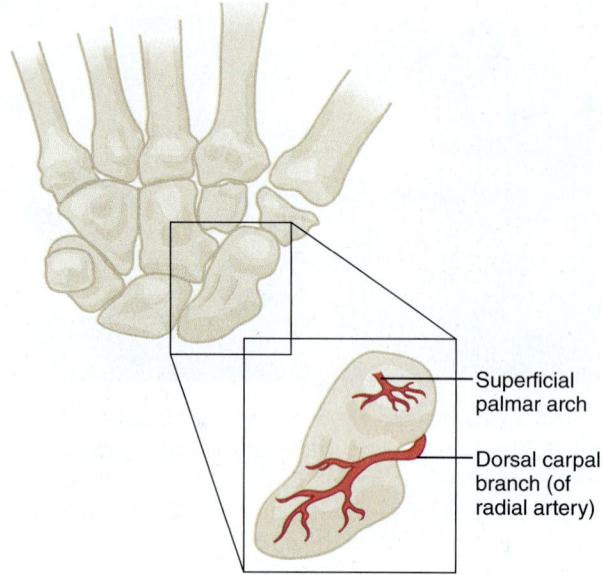

Figure 8.13 Drawing showing the blood supply of the scaphoid bone.
© Jones & Bartlett Learning

and progressive wrist arthritis, and chronic wrist pain with progressive loss of motion.[3]

Scaphoid fractures can occur at the waist (or middle of the bone), the distal pole (or tubercle), or the proximal pole (**Figure 8.14**). Noting the fracture location and whether the fracture is displaced is important in determining the need for surgical intervention, the risk for nonunion, and the potential healing time. All displaced scaphoid fractures require surgical correction. A nondisplaced fracture of the distal third or tubercle of the scaphoid bone has a 95% chance of healing with proper cast immobilization, and union takes approximately 6 to 8 weeks.

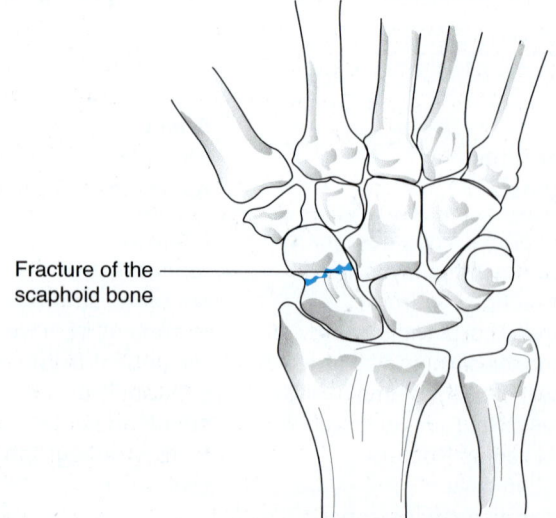

Figure 8.14 Drawing showing the scaphoid fracture pattern.
© Jones & Bartlett Learning

A middle-third waist fracture has an 80% to 90% chance of healing without surgical intervention and takes 8 to 12 weeks. A proximal pole fracture has a very high risk of nonunion because of its location and tenuous blood supply and therefore is almost always considered a fracture to be managed with surgery.[1]

A scaphoid fracture should always be suspected in a patient who sustains a fall and reports wrist pain. Typically, the pain will occur immediately, but occasionally a patient will not realize or admit to the pain until several hours or even days later. In some circumstances, the pain is mild, and the patient may not report the injury for several weeks, noting progressive wrist stiffness with pain. Occasionally, the patient will report feeling a painful "pop" at the time of injury. The patient may describe the wrist pain as diffuse about the radiocarpal joint or localized to the radial side of the wrist. The pain will occur or increase with all wrist motions, and the patient may report a diminished ability to flex and extend the wrist.

Careful inspection of the wrist will reveal edema over the radial side of the wrist, often both dorsally and volarly. Ecchymosis may be present radially and volarly. Alternatively, the wrist may have a very normal appearance if the patient presents weeks after the injury.

Examine the wrist with the patient in a seated position facing the examiner. Ask the patient to perform active ROM of the wrist to the point of discomfort or pain. ROM testing will reveal reduced flexion, extension, and radial and ulnar deviation. Notate the end points of all motion and which positions cause pain. Next, palpate the anatomic snuffbox for tenderness. This area is located at the recess created by the abductor pollicis longus (APL) and extensor pollicis brevis (EPB) tendons and the extensor pollicis longus tendon at the radial base of the thumb. It is anatomically superficial to the scaphoid bone (**Figure 8.15**). Also, palpate the scaphoid tubercle volarly on the wrist. This can be identified by following the flexor carpi radialis (FCR) tendon to the wrist crease until a bony prominence is encountered. Slightly extending the wrist can make the tubercle more prominent for palpation. Tenderness at these locations is pathognomonic for a scaphoid fracture. Note both tender and nontender findings.

> **Note**
>
> Tenderness at the anatomic snuffbox is thought to have a sensitivity of 85% and a specificity of 29% for scaphoid fracture. Tenderness at the scaphoid tubercle is thought to have a sensitivity of 95% and a specificity of 74%.[4]

Conditions Causing Radial-Side Wrist Pain

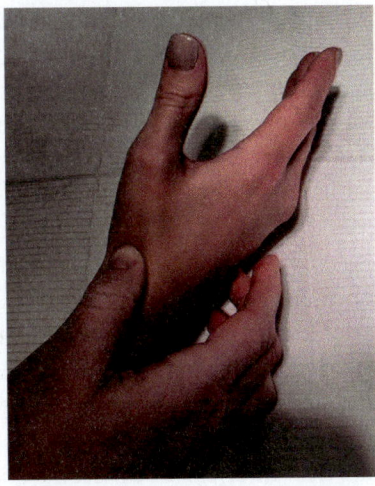

Figure 8.15 Clinical photograph showing the palpation of the anatomic snuffbox.

Courtesy of Sara Rynders.

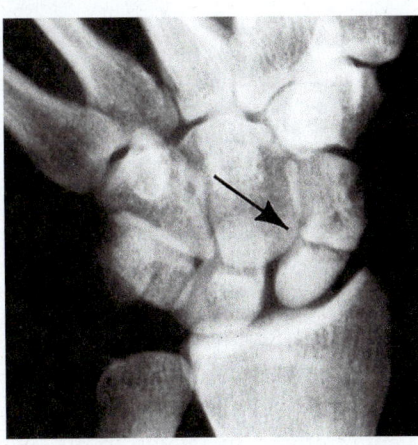

Figure 8.16 Radiograph showing the scaphoid view of the wrist demonstrating a nondisplaced transverse scaphoid waist fracture (arrow).

Reproduced from Armstrong AD, Hubbard MC, eds: *Essentials of Musculoskeletal Care*, ed 5. Burlington, MA, American Academy of Orthopaedic Surgeons, 2015.

Additionally, a thorough examination of ancillary structures should be performed. Deliberately palpate and ask about tenderness at the distal radius and radial styloid, DRUJ, ulnar styloid, and TFCC. Palpate the thumb CMC joint, metacarpal, and MCP joint looking for additional injuries. Palpate the hook of hamate, as it can be injured during a fall on the hand. Palpate the joint distal to the zone of injury. Palpate the forearm for tenderness and examine the elbow joint. Make a point to palpate the radial head at the elbow, as it is commonly injured during a fall on an outstretched hand. Note additional areas of concern or tenderness.

Radiographic imaging should be obtained for all patients with wrist pain after a fall. PA; lateral; oblique; and scaphoid, or ulnar deviation, views should be obtained. The ulnar deviation view will elongate the scaphoid and place it into an extended position on the film, which will improve the ability to identify and characterize a fracture (**Figure 8.16**). As previously mentioned, up to 25% of scaphoid fractures are not visible or not identified on initial radiographs. If there is clinical suspicion for a scaphoid fracture but radiographs are negative, the patient should be immobilized in a thumb spica splint, and a secondary set of films should be obtained in 1 to 2 weeks. If radiographs remain negative but there is persistent radial-side wrist pain and/or hasty return to play is necessary, MRI of the wrist can be ordered. The current literature suggests that MRI has a 98% sensitivity, 99% specificity, and 96% accuracy for identifying scaphoid fractures.[5] CT can also be used to detect and characterize scaphoid fractures, though it is not as useful at detecting occult fractures. Frequently, CT can be used to evaluate for healing of the scaphoid fracture prior to return to play.

The clinician should consider and evaluate for the following alternative injuries in the patient presenting with radial-side wrist pain: distal radius fracture, other carpal bone fracture, de Quervain tenosynovitis or other extensor tendinitis, SL ligament tear, thumb metacarpal base fracture (Bennett fracture), and FCR tendinitis or rupture. Careful and deliberate physical examination in conjunction with plain radiographs will help to narrow the spectrum of possible clinical diagnoses.

The clinician must be diligent to always consider scaphoid fracture in the differential diagnosis in the patient with wrist pain, particularly if a patient sustains a wrist injury but wants to dismiss it as simply a wrist sprain without a proper workup. Missing these injuries can have devastating consequences. Early-onset wrist arthritis, chronic wrist pain, and loss of motion can be debilitating. Surgical techniques and recovery times can be simple and straightforward in an acutely diagnosed fracture but quickly turn to complex reconstructions and even wrist fusion procedures when diagnosis is delayed.

Five-Minute Sideline Assessment

Assess any player with wrist pain ranging from mild to severe for this condition. Remove any gloves, equipment, tape, or supportive devices from the wrist prior to evaluation. First, inspect for gross deformity of the wrist that could indicate a major fracture or dislocation. Ask the patient to point to the area of pain. Palpate the anatomic snuffbox and scaphoid tubercle. Place the wrist through ROM to assess for pain. If tenderness is identified or pain is produced, remove the patient from play. If available, apply a thumb spica splint and await radiographic assessment before allowing return to play.

de Quervain Tenosynovitis and Intersection Syndrome

de Quervain tenosynovitis is an inflammatory condition of the APL and EPB tendons at the level of the radial styloid of the wrist, first described by the Swiss-born surgeon Dr. Fritz de Quervain in 1895. Often called a stenosing tenosynovitis because of the constricting tendencies of the fibro-osseous sheath, this condition is frequently caused by a combination of narrowing within the tendon's canal and friction of the tendons from overstretch or overuse. It is more frequently encountered in racket sports, weight lifting, rowing, and golfing, and it occurs more often in females[6] (**Table 8.10**).

The extensor tendons are divided into six individual compartments at the level of the wrist (**Figure 8.17**). Each compartment has its own synovial sheath that bathes the tendons in synovial fluid and allows for smooth tendon gliding. The EPB and APL tendons are contained within the first extensor compartment. The tendons lie within a fibro-osseous sheath continuous with the extensor retinaculum that tethers them to a groove in the radial styloid, creating a biomechanical pulley as they travel distally to the thumb. Under normal conditions, the tendons are bathed in a small amount of synovial fluid; however, when the tendons become irritated because of injury or repetitious activity, specifically repetitive thumb abduction and wrist ulnar deviation, the fluid surrounding the tendons increases and creates a narrowing of the space within the tunnel. As friction increases, the tendon lining becomes inflamed, hence the name stenosing tenosynovitis. Additionally, normal anatomic variants exist in which there is an extra slip of the APL tendon or an additional longitudinal septum within the canal. These conditions can result in even less space within the fibro-osseous sheath and predispose the patient to this inflammatory condition.

A similar but altogether different condition is termed intersection syndrome. Intersection syndrome is also an inflammatory condition at the level of the wrist, but it occurs more proximally on the wrist at the intersection of the first and second extensor compartments (**Figure 8.18**). It is encountered less often than de Quervain tenosynovitis. In this condition, there is no stenosing effect from a fibro-osseous tunnel. Instead, it is thought to be caused by repetitive activity that creates an area of friction and subsequently inflammation where the first and second extensor compartments overlap. Intersection syndrome can occur independent of or simultaneously

Table 8.10 de Quervain Tenosynovitis and Intersection Syndrome Quick Tips

Pathology	Description	Presentation (HIPS)	Special Tests/ Imaging	Differential Diagnosis	5-Min Sideline Assessment Tips
de Quervain tenosynovitis	Inflammation of the first extensor compartment tendons (abductor pollicis longus and extensor pollicis brevis)	Usually a gradual onset of radial-side wrist pain worse with thumb abduction and wrist ulnar deviation	Finkelstein test	Scapholunate ligament injury Intersection syndrome Scaphoid fracture Extensor carpi radialis brevis/extensor carpi radialis longus insertional tendinitis Flexor carpi radialis tendinitis Distal radius fracture Ganglion cyst Preiser disease (osteonecrosis of the scaphoid)	Not applicable
Intersection syndrome	Inflammation of the intersection of the first and second extensor compartments	Pain, tenderness, and crepitus in the distal-radial third of the forearm	Not applicable	As above, de Quervain tenosynovitis	Not applicable

HIPS, history, inspection, palpation, special tests.

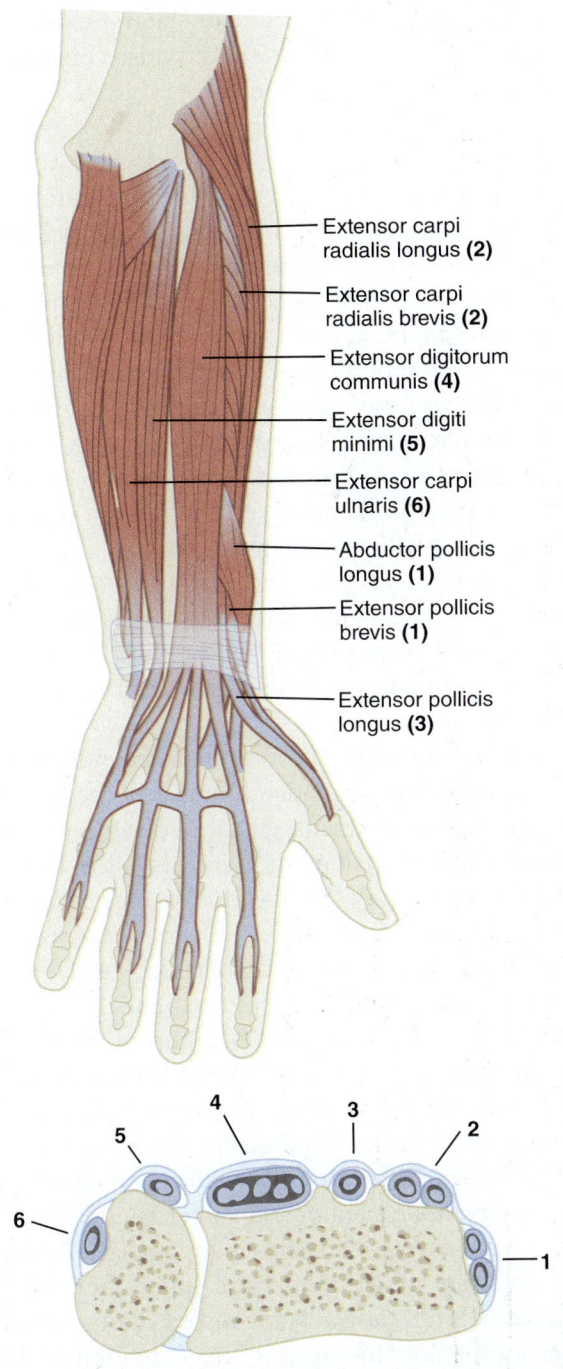

Figure 8.17 Drawing showing the anatomy of the extensor compartments of the wrist.

© Jones & Bartlett Learning

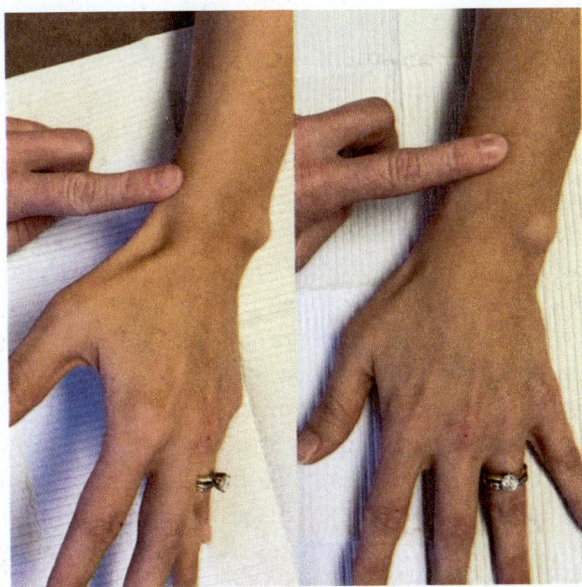

Figure 8.18 Clinical photograph showing the palpation of the first extensor compartment (left) at the radial styloid and palpation of the intersection of the first and second extensor compartment more proximally and dorsally (right).

Courtesy of Sara Rynders.

with de Quervain tenosynovitis, and an astute clinician should always evaluate for both.

The patient presenting with de Quervain tenosynovitis and/or intersection syndrome will report a gradual onset of radial-side wrist pain over weeks to months. He or she may remember an exact moment when the condition started. Initially, the pain will occur only with thumb abduction activities, but, as the condition progresses, the patient will also report pain at rest. The patient may report an underlying dull ache along the radial wrist and thumb with intermittent sharp, shooting pain with thumb or wrist motion.

Specific to de Quervain tenosynovitis, the patient may report the presence of a firm, small nodule on the radial side of the wrist that represents an accumulation of synovial fluid from the underlying inflamed tendon sheath, also known as a ganglion cyst. These nodules are not always present, however. Less often, the patient may report a "catching" or "locking" of the thumb indicating a triggering-like condition that occurs when the inflamed tendon attempts to glide in the fibro-osseous tunnel but becomes temporarily entrapped due to its size.

Examine the wrist with the patient in a seated position facing the examiner. Upon inspection of the patient's wrist, there may be a noticeable area of swelling near the radial styloid. Observe for any signs of trauma or masses in the region, such as ganglion cysts. Ask the patient to place the thumb and wrist through active ROM. When de Quervain tenosynovitis is present, pain will be experienced with thumb abduction and opposition and ulnar deviation. Next, evaluate for triggering of the first extensor compartment by asking the patient to flex and extend the thumb at the IP joint and observe for any locking or catching. Next, firmly palpate the first extensor compartment over the radial styloid. This area will be exquisitely tender to palpation in de Quervain tenosynovitis. Last, evaluate for any palpable firm nodules along the first extensor compartment consistent with ganglion cysts.

The most widely used physical exam test to diagnose de Quervain tenosynovitis is the Finkelstein test. Interestingly, there are no known studies to evaluate the specificity and sensitivity of this test as of this writing, though it is universally used and considered very reliable for diagnosing de Quervain disease. There is also some variation noted in the literature on exactly how the test is being performed in clinical practice. For the purpose of this text, the most common technique of performing the Finkelstein test is described here. First, have the patient form a fist with the thumb tucked under the fingers. Ask him or her to relax the wrist. The examiner then places the wrist in neutral and passively ulnarly deviates the wrist (**Figure 8.19**). The patient with de Quervain tenosynovitis will experience discomfort with this maneuver.

The examination is not complete until the athletic trainer evaluates for intersection syndrome. Exam findings specific to intersection syndrome are tenderness to palpation over the intersection of the first and second compartments on the dorsal-radial distal forearm. Pain can be reproduced with wrist extension and thumb abduction, and palpation of the intersection during this motion may elicit palpable crepitus (grinding, popping, crunching sensation).

It is very important to always evaluate for concomitant intersection syndrome in the patient with de Quervain tenosynovitis and radial-side wrist pain. When intersection syndrome occurs simultaneously with de Quervain tenosynovitis, both conditions must be addressed in order for the patient to improve.

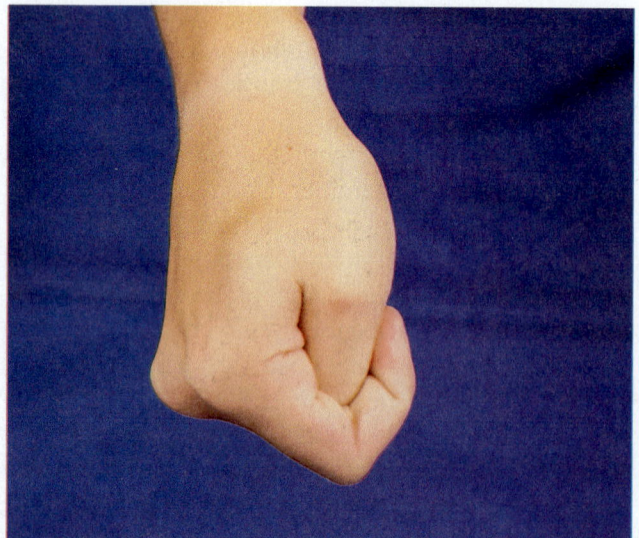

Figure 8.19 Clinical photograph showing the Finkelstein test.
© Jones & Bartlett Learning

Persistent radial-side wrist pain after treatment for de Quervain tenosynovitis should raise concern for a missed intersection syndrome.

When documenting findings of these two conditions, it is imperative to document both the positive and negative physical examination findings. For example, in a patient with isolated de Quervain tenosynovitis, it is important to document that the patient had "tenderness over the first extensor compartment and a positive Finkelstein test" and "no tenderness at the intersection of the first and second extensor compartments with no crepitus noted." This proves that the examiner evaluated for both conditions.

A set of screening radiographs may be appropriate to help delineate a differential diagnosis. Radiographs will appear normal in the setting of de Quervain tenosynovitis and intersection syndrome. Evaluate for alternative injuries, such as a radial styloid fracture or scaphoid fracture and, in an older athletic population, radiocarpal arthritis and first CMC joint arthritis.

MRI can be used to confirm a suspected diagnosis or evaluate for a differential diagnosis in the patient in whom conservative management of de Quervain tenosynovitis or intersection syndrome has failed. However, MRI is not necessary for diagnosis of these conditions.

Initial treatment of de Quervain tenosynovitis includes rest, activity modification or avoidance, NSAIDs, and a thumb spica splint. Therapeutic modalities, such as ultrasonography or iontophoresis, are widely used as well, though their efficacy is unproven. If the patient fails to achieve symptom relief after several weeks of conservative measures, it is widely accepted that a cortisone injection into the first extensor compartment or at the intersection of the first and second extensor tendons is appropriate. Additionally, splinting in a thumb spica splint after injection may be helpful. Researchers studied the use of injections and splints for treating this condition in 1991. They found 67% improvement with injection alone, 57% improvement with injection and a splint, and a 19% improvement with only a splint.[6] The patient's symptoms should improve or resolve over the 4 to 6 weeks following injection, and he or she should be able to return to a full level of play. A biomechanical evaluation of his or her athletic activity may be warranted to prevent recurrence. If the patient's symptoms fail to improve after conservative care and cortisone injections, surgical release of the fibro-osseous sheath overlying the first extensor compartment may be warranted. Results are excellent after release, with return to full play around 4 to 6 weeks. Surgical intervention for intersection syndrome is rare.

Table 8.11 Comparing de Quervain Tenosynovitis and Intersection Syndrome

	de Quervain Tenosynovitis	Intersection Syndrome
Location	First extensor compartment at the level of the radial styloid	Intersection of the first and second extensor compartments more proximal on the wrist
Finkelstein test	Positive	Negative
Pain	Occurs with independent thumb abduction, thumb opposition, and wrist ulnar deviation	Occurs with simultaneous thumb abduction and wrist extension
Additional findings	Check for ganglion cysts or triggering	Palpate for crepitus at the intersection

The entire differential diagnosis of radial-side wrist pain should be evaluated for during physical examination. Recall the differential diagnosis of radial-side wrist pain reviewed in **Table 8.11**. Palpation of the anatomic snuffbox; SL interval; and extensor carpi radialis brevis and extensor carpi radialis longus tendon insertions on the second CMC joint, first CMC joint, FCR tendon, and scaphoid tubercle all should be included in the examination.

Distal Radius Fractures

Fractures of the distal end of the radius are one of the most common fractures to occur in the upper extremity (**Table 8.12**). Most often, this fracture occurs because of a fall on an outstretched hand. The incidence of distal radius fractures has a bimodal distribution, with peak incidence in patients younger than 18 years and older than 65 years.[7] When a distal radius fracture occurs in a younger person, there is a 23% chance that the injury occurred during play or sports activities. When the injury occurs in an older person, there is often an association with gait instability or bone fragility due to osteoporosis.[8,9]

Fractures of the distal radius may occur in several configurations, and developing a basic knowledge of bone anatomy and fracture descriptors is key to identifying, describing, and understanding these injuries. The distal aspect of the radius bone is made up of the epiphysis (articular end of the bone), the metaphysis (the wide area of the bone between the epiphysis and the shaft), and the diaphysis (shaft of the bone). The radial styloid is also an aspect of the distal radius, lying laterally and distally on the bone. When describing a fracture, the first descriptor is always displaced or nondisplaced. Any fracture that has even a small amount of movement away from its original position is considered displaced. The second descriptor is intra-articular or extra-articular. If the fracture enters the joint space of the radiocarpal joint, it is intra-articular; if it remains outside the joint, it is extra-articular. The third descriptor is the location of the fracture on the distal radius, for example, the radial styloid or metaphysis. In the fracture shown in **Figure 8.20**, the description would be a "displaced, extra-articular fracture of the metaphysis of the left distal radius. A displaced ulnar styloid fracture is also present."

There are several classification systems for distal radius fractures and several named fractures. The two most frequently encountered fracture patterns are the Colles fracture and Smith fracture. A Colles fracture is a dorsally angulated fracture, whereas

Table 8.12 Radius Fracture Quick Tips

Pathology	Description	Presentation (HIPS)	Special Tests/ Imaging	Differential Diagnosis	5-Min Sideline Assessment Tips
Distal radius fractures	Fracture of the distal end of the radius bone	Acute onset of wrist pain after an impact, such as falling on an outstretched hand	Obtain radiographs	Scapholunate ligament injury Scaphoid fracture	If severe pain and wrist deformity are present, remove the patient from play, splint the wrist, and obtain radiographs

HIPS, history, inspection, palpation, special tests.

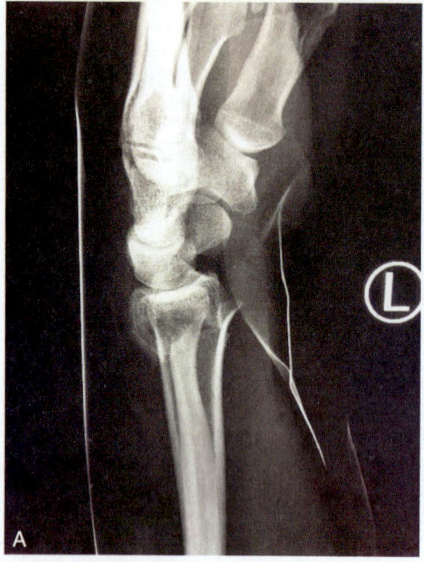 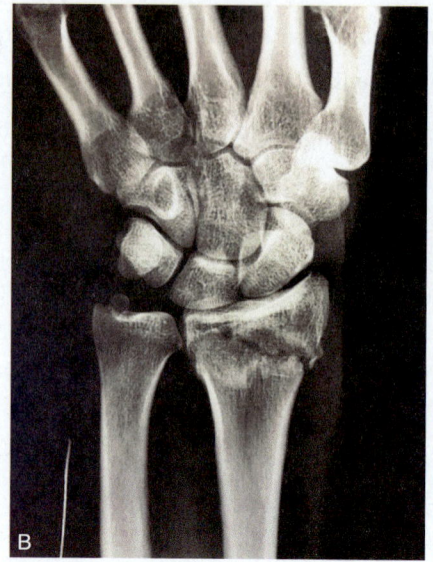 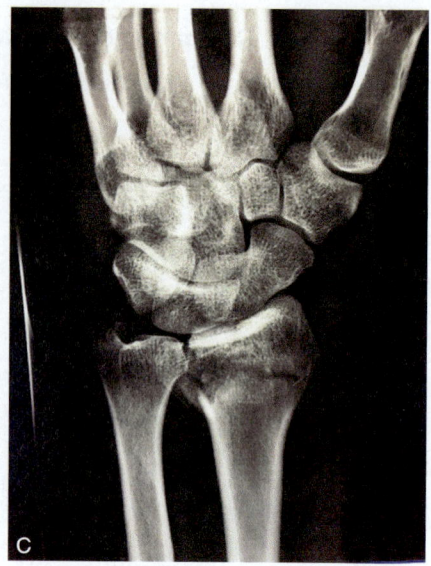

Figure 8.20 Radiographs showing a distal radius fracture. **A.** Lateral view. **B.** Oblique view. **C.** PA view.
Courtesy of Sara Rynders.

a Smith fracture is a volarly angulated fracture. An orthopaedic surgeon will carefully examine a patient's radiographs to check various measurements and angles to characterize the fracture and determine its severity.

The patient presenting with a distal radius fracture will always report an event that can be related to the onset of symptoms. The clinician should inquire how the patient fell or had contact with another player or surface and ask about the position of the wrist during the impact. The patient may report feeling a "pop" or giving way in the wrist at the time of injury. The patient will also report relatively severe pain in the affected wrist and may be supporting, protecting, or guarding the affected wrist with the opposite hand. The patient will be reluctant to move the wrist, and even slight motion will cause severe pain. In displaced fractures, there may be a deformity noted at the wrist joint causing the wrist to look bent like a fork. Ask the patient whether he or she feels any numbness or tingling distally in the fingertips, as occasionally a displaced distal radius fracture can cause compression, contusion, or stretching of the median nerve.

Examination of the patient with a distal radius fracture may occur on the field, on the sideline, or in the athletic training clinic after injury. The wrist should be examined with the patient in a seated position facing the examiner. An aggressive physical examination is not necessary in the presence of severe pain, as a screening set of radiographs will provide the definitive diagnosis. Inspect the wrist for deformity, edema, and ecchymosis. Inspect for any abrasions or open wounds. Ask the patient to point to the area of pain in order to better localize it. Ask the patient to move the fingers through gentle active flexion and extension. If this can be accomplished without severe pain, then ask the patient to move the wrist through gentle active flexion and extension. In the presence of a distal radius fracture, the patient will be apprehensive or have severe pain with wrist motion and possibly even with finger motion. If the patient does not exhibit severe pain, palpate the distal radius and note whether there is bony tenderness present. A distal radius fracture will have tenderness to palpation. Next, perform a thorough neurovascular examination. Ask the patient whether he or she is able to feel light touch in the fingertips of the volar thumb, index and middle fingers (median nerve); ulnar side of the ring finger and small finger (ulnar nerve); and dorsal surface of the thumb (radial nerve). Next, test the motor component of each nerve by asking the patient to flex the fingers into a fist (median nerve), abduct and adduct the fingers (ulnar nerve), and extend the thumb into a thumbs-up gesture (radial nerve). Note the capillary refill of the digits, which normally takes less than 2 seconds.

Also perform a cursory evaluation of the forearm, elbow, and hand/fingers for ancillary injuries. Palpate the major bony landmarks of the joints and perform active ROM of the elbow and digits, noting any additional areas of injury or tenderness.

Immediate stabilization of the wrist is necessary for support and pain control. Splint the wrist in a comfortable neutral position, elevate, and apply ice. Obtain radiographs as soon as possible. Three standard views of the wrist should be obtained: PA, lateral, and oblique to evaluate for the presence of a fracture. Occasionally, a CT scan will be ordered by a physician to better understand the bony architecture of the fracture and its intra-articular components for surgical planning.

After the fracture has been characterized on radiographs, a treatment plan can be developed. A significantly displaced fracture may require the physician to perform immediate closed reduction using a local anesthetic or with conscious sedation. Nondisplaced or mildly displaced fractures do not require immediate reduction and can be splinted in a short arm or sugar tong splint. The need for surgical intervention will be determined by the orthopaedic surgeon. Surgery for a displaced fracture with no neurologic findings could potentially be delayed 1 to 2 weeks to the end of the season, depending on the type of sport (noncontact), position played and hand dominance, performance level of the patient, and the timing of the injury relative to the sport's season. The risks and benefits of continued protected participation should be discussed with the patient. A patient with a nondisplaced fracture that does not require surgical intervention should not participate in sport, as the risk of further displacement of the fracture could turn a nonsurgical problem into a surgical one.

Nondisplaced fractures of the distal radius can be managed in a cast for 4 to 6 weeks, with frequent radiographs to monitor for fracture displacement. ROM exercises for the elbow and fingers should be initiated immediately to reduce edema and prevent stiffness. After 4 to 6 weeks of cast wear, the patient can transition to intermittent splinting and start wrist ROM and stretching. Active strengthening can occur at the 6- to 8-week point, and return to play can occur when there is evidence of fracture healing and painless functional ROM is present.

Displaced distal radius fractures can be managed with outpatient surgery. Frequently, a volar approach with a volar locking plate is used, but complex or comminuted fractures may require additional and/or alternative surgical techniques to attain anatomic fracture reduction (**Figure 8.21**). The goal of every surgical technique is to attain anatomic fracture reduction, as this is the only variable proven to be associated with better functional outcomes and reduced risk of long-term arthritis. Early mobilization of the wrist may be an option after surgery, but no correlation between early mobilization and better outcomes or earlier return to play has been shown.[10] Bone quality, fixation techniques, and fracture complexity must be taken into account when contemplating early mobilization. Discussion with the surgeon regarding postoperative rehabilitation recommendations is imperative.

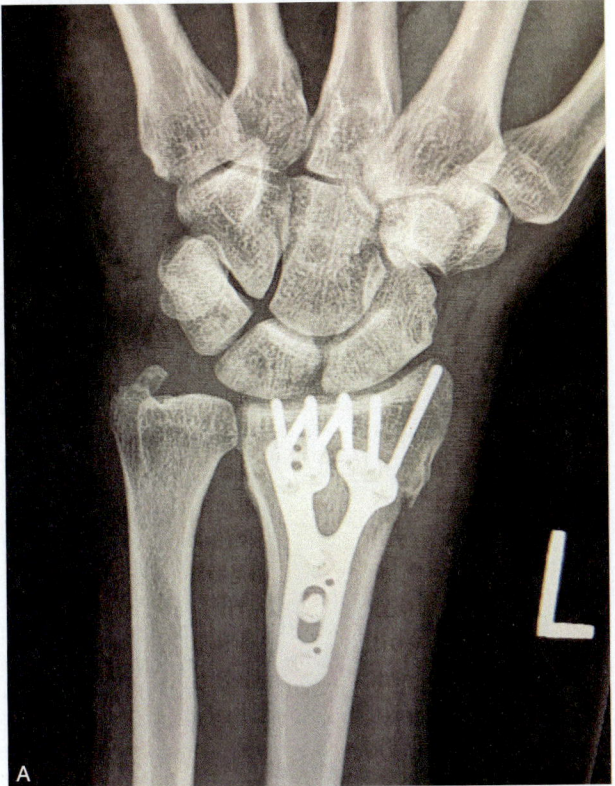 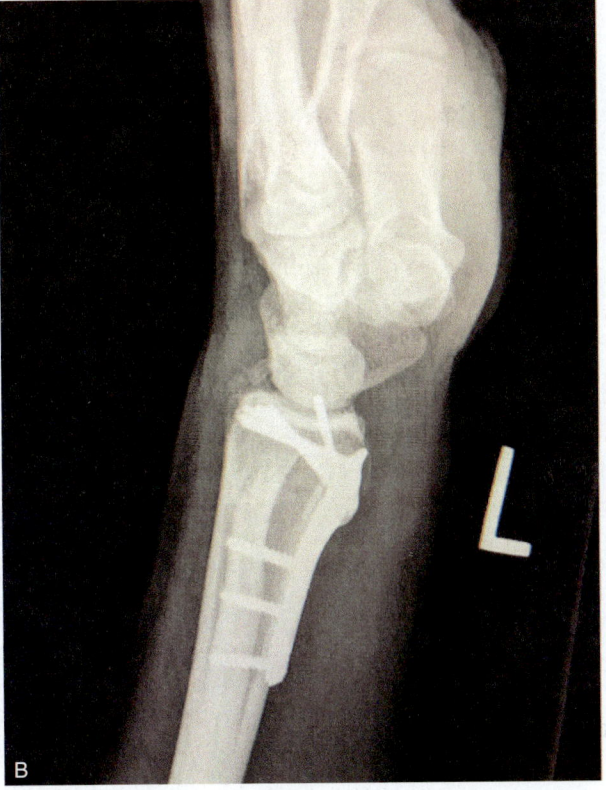

Figure 8.21 Postoperative radiographs of the same patient as shown in Figure 8.20 after treatment with a volar locking plate. **A.** PA view. **B.** Lateral view.

Courtesy of Sara Rynders.

Outcomes after distal radius fractures is an area of study that requires additional research with large prospective trials. Current consensus is that functional outcomes and satisfaction are directly related to younger age, higher activity level, and low fracture complexity. In general, most patients do well after these injuries when appropriately treated. Anatomic alignment of intra-articular fracture components, regardless of type of treatment used, is associated with better outcomes. In a small study of 27 patients with displaced distal radius fractures treated with surgery with a volar plate system, significant gains in ROM were obtained within the first 3 months of surgery. Supination and pronation returned to 92% within 3 months of surgery and wrist flexion and extension and grip strength returned to 87% to 90% and 94%, respectively, at 1 year after surgery.[11]

The differential diagnosis of a distal radius fracture includes any wrist pathology that can be associated with sudden onset of pain. This includes fractures of the ulna; fractures of the carpus, including scaphoid fracture and SL or LT ligament injuries; or wrist capsular sprain. In the presence of radiographs devoid of a fracture, all these entities should be accounted for.

> **Five-Minute Sideline Assessment**
>
> The patient with acute-onset wrist pain should be removed from play immediately. Note any wrist deformity or open wounds. If the wrist is obviously deformed or an open fracture is identified, a splint should be applied and immediate medical attention sought. Otherwise, ask the patient to point to where the pain is and whether he or she is able to flex and extend the wrist. Tenderness over the distal radius and severe pain with attempted wrist motion are highly suggestive of a fracture. Apply a splint to the wrist and obtain radiographs. Apply ice and elevate the wrist immediately.

SL and LT Ligament Injury

SL and LT ligament injuries are two of the most complicated conditions to diagnose and treat in orthopaedic surgery (Table 8.13). Nonetheless, if missed or inappropriately treated, the consequences can be devastating. Progressive loss of wrist motion, swelling, pain, and irreversible wrist arthritis can occur if these injuries are overlooked. This section will place emphasis on the more commonly encountered SL ligament injury but will also touch briefly on injuries of the LT and a condition called perilunate fracture-dislocation.

A brief review of carpal anatomy and wrist kinematics is necessary to understand the pathomechanics that occur with wrist ligament injuries. The SL and LT are considered to be intrinsic ligaments of the wrist because they lie within the wrist joint itself. The SL ligament (sometimes referred to as the scapholunate interosseous ligament) is a stout, C-shaped ligament that connects the scaphoid and the lunate bones. It is considered a primary stabilizer of the wrist joint. The SL ligament has three distinct segments: dorsal, proximal (or membranous), and volar. The most important segment for the SL ligament's integrity is the dorsal segment, which is the thickest and strongest component of the ligament. The LT ligament connects the lunate, and the triquetrum is strongest at its volar segment.

Together, the SL and the LT function to form a connected row of bones called the proximal carpal row that, under normal conditions, will move in a synchronous manner as a unit. In the uninjured wrist, the lunate is held in a neutral position by the opposing forces transmitted through the SL and LT ligaments. The SL has a flexion moment arm, and the LT has an extension moment arm. During wrist flexion and radial deviation, the scaphoid flexes, bringing

Table 8.13 Scapholunate and Lunotriquetral Ligament Injury Quick Tips

Pathology	Description	Presentation (HIPS)	Special Tests/ Imaging	Differential Diagnosis	5-Min Sideline Assessment Tips
SL and LT ligament injury	Partial or complete tear of the SL or LT ligament	Usually generalized wrist pain after an impact or fall on an outstretched hand	Watson scaphoid shift test for SL injuries LT ligament shift test for LT injuries	Scaphoid fracture Scapholunate ligament injury Extensor carpi radialis brevis/ extensor carpi radialis longus insertional tendinitis Distal radius fracture Ganglion cyst Preiser disease (osteonecrosis of the scaphoid)	Evaluate for palpable wrist tenderness. If pain is severe, the wrist can be splinted, and the patient may be able to return to play

HIPS, history, inspection, palpation, special tests; LT, lunotriquetral; SL, scapholunate.

with it the lunate and triquetrum, therefore flexing the entire proximal row as a unit. During wrist extension and ulnar deviation, the scaphoid and proximal row extend as a unit. This is the result of the interconnections provided by the SL and LT.

When the SL is compromised, the proximal carpal row no longer moves as a unit. The scaphoid naturally falls into flexion over the radioscaphocapitate ligament, whereas the lunate is subjected to the unopposed extension force of the LT and falls into an extension deformity called dorsal intercalated segment instability deformity. Biomechanical forces that would normally be transmitted through the SL are dispersed to the extrinsic wrist ligaments, causing undue strain and abnormal carpal motion. This is important because, over time, a predictable pattern of arthritis develops in the wrist called scapholunate ligament advanced collapse (**Figure 8.22**).

Classification of SL injuries is based on the type of instability present (dynamic versus static) and the acuity of the injury (acute, subacute, or chronic). It is sufficient for the clinician to know that SL tears can be partial or complete and may present early or late after injury.

The athletic trainer should ask the patient how the injury occurred and when the pain started. Was the injury recent or remote? SL or LT injuries typically occur from a fall on an outstretched hand, a sudden axial load on the wrist, or a collision with another player. The pain from a ligament tear may be reported along a spectrum from mild to severe. Ask the patient where the pain occurs. Classically, an SL tear will produce dorsoradial-side wrist pain, and an LT tear will produce dorsal-ulnar wrist pain. A patient may think he or she just sprained the wrist, and an astute athletic trainer should always consider the diagnosis of SL or LT tear in this scenario. Frequently, but not always, the patient will report feeling a "pop" in the wrist at the time of injury or a "popping" sensation with wrist motion after the injury has occurred. The patient may report that the wrist feels weak, especially when attempting to perform a push-up.

Inspection of an acutely injured wrist may reveal dorsal wrist edema or ecchymosis. No obvious deformity will be present with an intrinsic ligament tear. Ask the patient to perform wrist ROM and document the ranges. Often, motion will be noticeably limited in flexion, extension, and radial and ulnar deviation.

The patient should be seated at an examination table, and the examiner should be seated across from him or her. Examination of the wrist should begin with palpation. First, palpate for tenderness over the SL ligament. This is performed in the soft spot in the wrist located between the third and fourth extensor compartments, 1 cm distal to the Lister tubercle. Tenderness in this interval is suggestive of an SL tear (**Figure 8.23**). Next, evaluate the integrity of the SL ligament by performing the Watson scaphoid shift test. Ask the patient to place the elbow of the affected

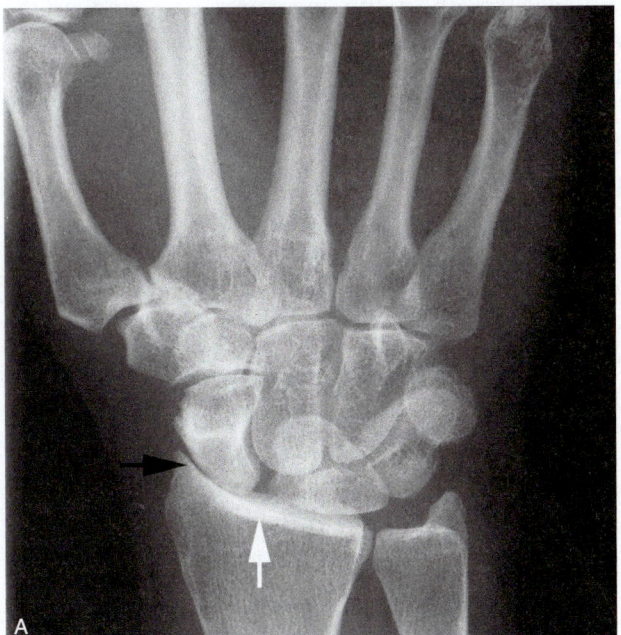
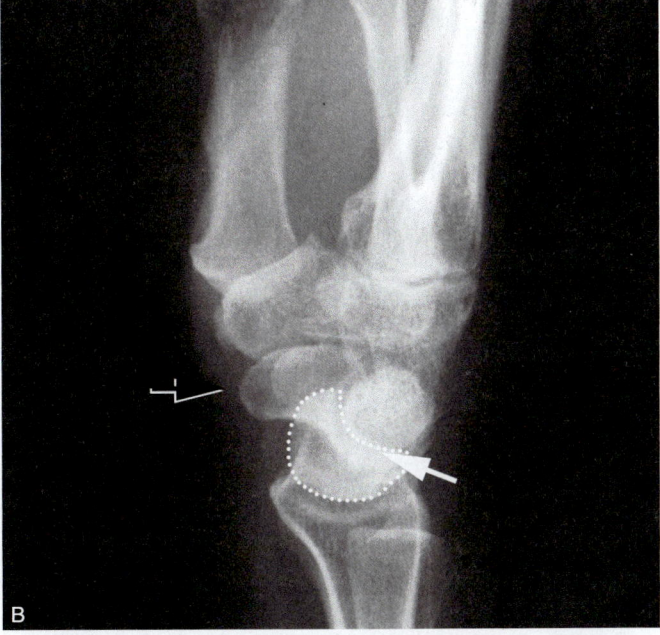

Figure 8.22 Radiographs of a wrist affected by scapholunate advanced collapse. **A.** PA view. The black arrow represents early arthritis affecting the radial styloid with beaking. The white arrow indicates static widening of the scapholunate interval. **B.** Lateral view. The lunate extends relative to the scaphoid (arrows).

Reproduced from Johnson TR, Steinbach LS, eds: *Essentials of Musculoskeletal Imaging*. Rosemont, IL, American Academy of Orthopaedic Surgeons, 2004.

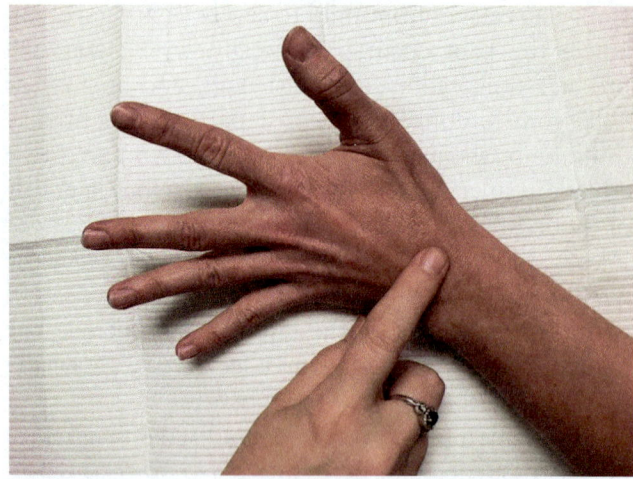

Figure 8.23 Clinical photograph showing the palpation of the scapholunate interval.

Courtesy of Sara Rynders.

> **Note**
>
> The Watson scaphoid shift test has a sensitivity of 48% and a specificity of 67% for detecting SL injuries.[12] The test should be compared to the uninjured side. Patients can have bilateral ligamentous laxity, which makes this test unreliable in some cases.

wrist on the table, as if he or she were going to arm wrestle. The athletic trainer places one hand on the radial aspect of the wrist and, with the thumb, applies direct, constant pressure over the scaphoid tubercle. The patient relaxes the wrist, and the athletic trainer then passively moves the wrist from ulnar to radial deviation while keeping constant pressure over the scaphoid tubercle. A palpable and frequently painful "clunk" is felt when the scaphoid contacts the dorsal rim of the radius, and a positive test should raise suspicion for an SL tear (**Figure 8.24**).

A thorough examination of the wrist should also include palpation over the anatomic snuffbox and distal radius as well as the TFCC. Document a thorough neurovascular examination with particular attention paid to the median nerve, which can be injured during a fall on an outstretched hand.

SL injuries should be evaluated with a very specific set of radiographs read by an orthopaedic surgeon or radiologist. The usual PA, lateral, and oblique views should be accompanied by a set of PA stress views of both the affected and unaffected wrists. For a PA stress view, the patient clenches the fist while the radiograph is obtained, which creates an axial force across the wrist that drives the capitate bone against the SL ligament. In the setting of an SL tear, the space between the scaphoid and the lunate (called the SL interval) may appear widened on the PA view, greater than 3 mm (**Figure 8.25**). It is important to compare the PA neutral and stress views with the same views of the uninjured wrist because some patients may have a naturally wide SL interval. The clinician will also be obtaining measurements and angles of the lateral views to determine the SL angle. A normal SL angle is between 30° and 60°.

Advanced imaging of the wrist may be a useful tool to help evaluate for an SL or LT tear. In a review of SL diagnosis and management, a 71% sensitivity, 88% specificity, and 84% accuracy were noted in the diagnosis of SL tears on MRI with or without contrast.[13] A 95% sensitivity and an 86% specificity of identifying SL tears with CT arthrography have been reported.[14] In all cases, the values are compared against the gold standard of diagnosis, which is currently wrist arthroscopy.

> **Note**
>
> The gold standard diagnostic tool for SL injuries is a wrist arthroscopy.

To date, diagnostic wrist arthroscopy is the best way to see the SL ligament and evaluate for static and dynamic instability. During arthroscopy, the ligament is directly seen and manipulated with a probe

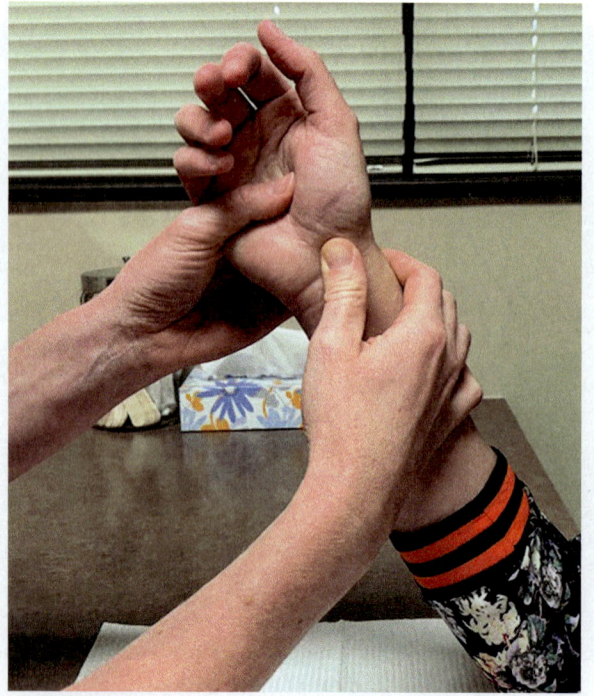

Figure 8.24 Clinical photograph showing the Watson scaphoid shift test.

Courtesy of Sara Rynders.

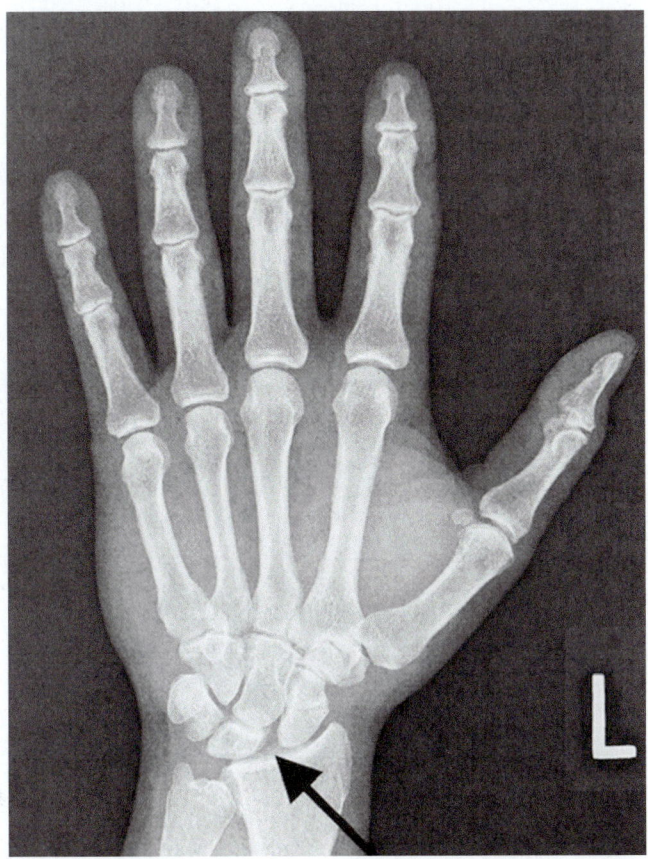 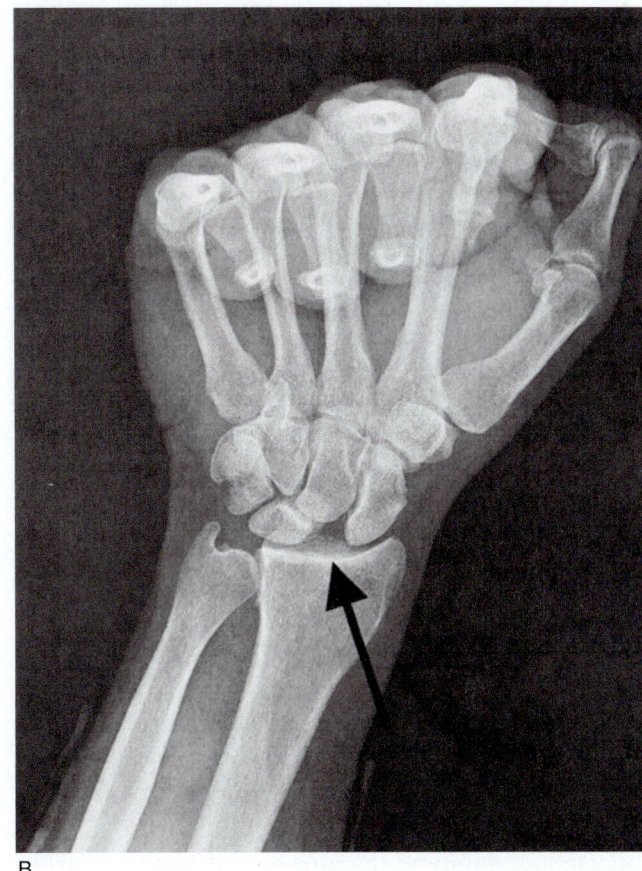

Figure 8.25 Radiographs of a scapholunate (SL) injury. **A.** Neural PA radiograph with borderline SL widening. **B.** PA clenched fist view with SL interval widening.

Courtesy of Sara Rynders.

to determine whether there is a complete tear or gapping. In some cases of stable partial tears, the SL ligament can be débrided. In cases of complete tears or unstable gapping, a variety of surgical options exist, with the goal to repair or stabilize the SL and prevent progression of arthritis.

The differential diagnosis of SL ligament tears includes any injury that causes radial-side wrist pain, such as distal radius fracture, radial styloid fracture, first CMC or scaphotrapeziotrapezoid joint arthritis, de Quervain tenosynovitis, other carpal fracture, or even a TFCC tear. All of these entities should be considered and narrowed down via history, physical examination, and appropriate ancillary testing.

There is a wide range of management options for tears of the SL. Stable partial tears can be managed with a period of 4 to 6 weeks of cast immobilization, whereas complete chronic tears may require complex ligament reconstructions that require months of rehabilitation. The outcome of return to play, level of play, and wrist mobility after SL injury is highly dependent on the degree of the SL tear, type of surgical procedure performed (if any), and whether the injury is identified early or late. In general, if a patient has a mild injury, such as a stable partial tear that can be treated with a cast or limited arthroscopic débridement, the anticipated outcome is good for achieving baseline wrist motion and return to play after 4 to 8 weeks. If a ligament repair or reconstruction is required, nearly all cases result in permanent loss of some wrist motion. Return to play will be determined by the type of sport and position played and may take 3 to 6 months.

Early and accurate diagnosis of SL ligament injuries is paramount to a patient receiving an appropriate diagnosis and treatment. Without treatment, this condition can result in permanent and devastating wrist arthritis within 10 years of injury. In a patient with persistent wrist pain, radiographs can sometimes be normal; a wrist sprain is never just a wrist sprain until a complete evaluation for an SL injury is performed.

In addition to the more commonly encountered SL ligament injury, the clinician should be aware of LT ligament tears and perilunate injuries. Injury to the LT ligament can present similarly to an SL tear,

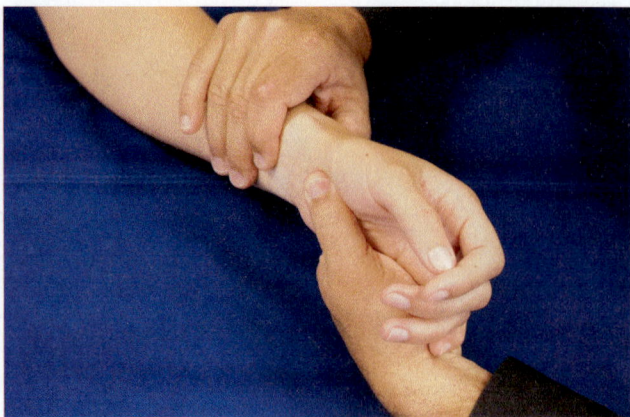

Figure 8.26 Clinical photograph showing the lunotriquetral shear test.
© Jones & Bartlett Learning

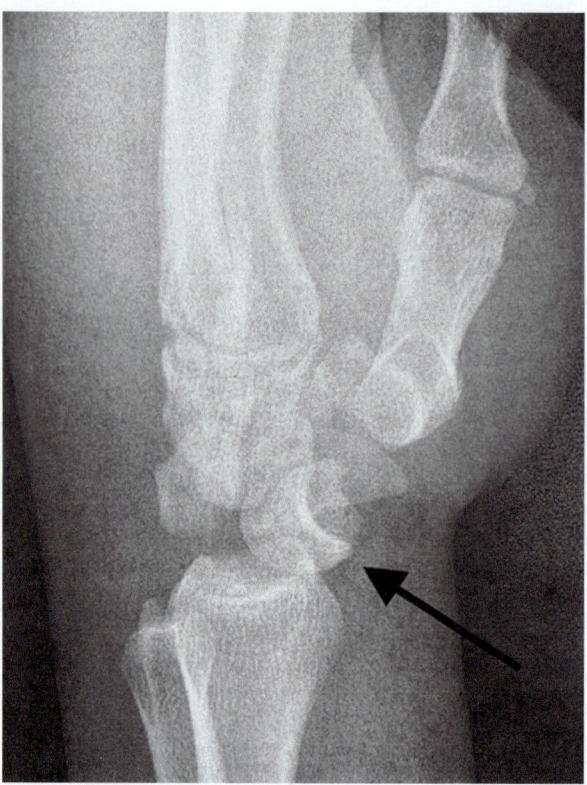

Figure 8.27 Lateral radiograph showing the perilunate dislocation on a lateral radiograph. Note the anterior dislocation of the lunate in this perilunate dislocation injury (arrow).
Courtesy of Sara Rynders.

but the location of the pain will be slightly more ulnar. The LT can be palpated between the fourth and fifth extensor compartments, just distal to the radiocarpal joint. Tenderness over this interval is suggestive of an LT tear. Additionally, the LT shear test can be performed. During this test, the patient sits across the table from the athletic trainer with the affected extremity in the arm-wrestle position on the table. The examiner places one thumb dorsally over the lunate and applies pressure to stabilize it. With the other thumb, the examiner applies an opposing volar pressure over the pisiform. A positive test occurs when the maneuver produces pain, crepitus, and laxity (**Figure 8.26**). The test is sensitive but not very specific for an LT tear, as there is a long list of problems that can cause ulnar-side wrist pain.

A perilunate injury refers to a condition where the SL ligament is disrupted and the zone of injury continues through the capitolunate joint and the LT ligament. The lunate may remain reduced in the capitolunate joint, or it may dislocate volarly outside of the wrist through a rent in the joint capsule (**Figure 8.27**). A variation of this injury is called the transscaphoid perilunate fracture-dislocation, in which the zone of injury occurs through the scaphoid bone instead of the SL ligament and continues around to the LT ligament. This variety of injuries generally requires a high-energy trauma, such as a fall from a height or high-velocity contact with another object or player. These injuries are usually severely painful. Because the lunate bone can dislocate volarly, it can impinge on the median nerve. If this injury is suspected, it is supremely important to assess the status of the median nerve. If the lunate is found to be dislocated, it is imperative to achieve an emergent reduction by an orthopaedic surgeon.

Five-Minute Sideline Assessment

SL ligament injury is nearly impossible to accurately diagnose on the sideline. The patient will report a fall or contact with another player and may report that he or she sprained his or her wrist. The patient may report a "pop," but not always. In the scenario of a patient reporting wrist pain on the field, perform a cursory evaluation for any open injuries and assess finger and wrist ROM. Palpate bony landmarks for tenderness that could raise suspicion for a fracture. If the player occupies an unskilled position and has minimal wrist pain with a normal neurovascular examination, it is not inappropriate to tape or splint the wrist until a thorough assessment can be performed at the end of play.

Conditions Causing Ulnar-Side Wrist Pain

TFCC Injury

The TFCC, as its name suggests, is a complex of structures located on the ulnar side of the wrist between the head of the ulna and the carpus (**Table 8.14**). The complex is made up of a fibrocartilage disk,

Conditions Causing Ulnar-Side Wrist Pain

Table 8.14 Triangular Fibrocartilage Complex Injury Quick Tips

Pathology	Description	Presentation (HIPS)	Special Tests/Imaging	Differential Diagnosis	5-Min Sideline Assessment Tips
TFCC injury	Partial or complete tearing of the complex of structures on the ulnar side of the wrist called the TFCC	Acute or gradual onset of ulnar-side wrist pain Occasionally associated with clicking or locking	Ulnar fovea sign test Ulnar grind test Piano key test	Ulnocarpal impaction syndrome DRUJ instability Extensor carpi ulnaris tendinitis Flexor carpi ulnaris tendinitis Hook of hamate fracture Distal ulnar fracture Cubital tunnel syndrome Ulnar artery thrombosis Lunotriquetral ligament tear Pisotriquetral joint arthritis Triquetral fracture Fifth metacarpal base fracture Fifth carpometacarpal joint fracture-dislocation Kienböck disease (osteonecrosis of the lunate)	Tenderness over the TFCC ulnarly; evaluate for gross DRUJ instability or frank dislocation

DRUJ, distal radioulnar joint; HIPS, history, inspection, palpation, special tests; TFCC, triangular fibrocartilage complex.

the volar and dorsal distal radioulnar ligaments, a meniscus homolog, volar ulnocarpal ligaments, and the floor of the extensor carpi ulnaris (ECU) tendon subsheath (**Figure 8.28**). The TFCC serves two main purposes: it is a major stabilizing structure of the DRUJ and is a load-bearing structure that carries approximately 20% of the axial load of the wrist. Much like the meniscus in the knee, the TFCC is vulnerable to tears that can result in a range of symptoms, from completely asymptomatic to a painful, lax, and grossly unstable wrist.

The most important anatomic feature to remember about the TFCC is its blood supply. The peripheral portion of the TFCC is vascularized, whereas the central portion is largely avascular (**Figure 8.29**). This is significant in determining the healing potential of a TFCC tear. Tears that occur in the periphery of the TFCC are amenable to healing and surgical repair because of the presence of small blood vessels. Tears that occur in the central portion of the TFCC lack adequate blood supply for healing and therefore require débridement, not repair, if symptomatic.

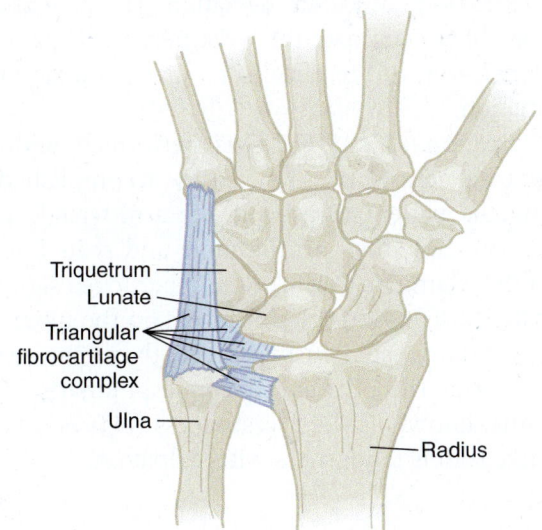

Figure 8.28 Drawing showing the triangular fibrocartilage complex anatomy.

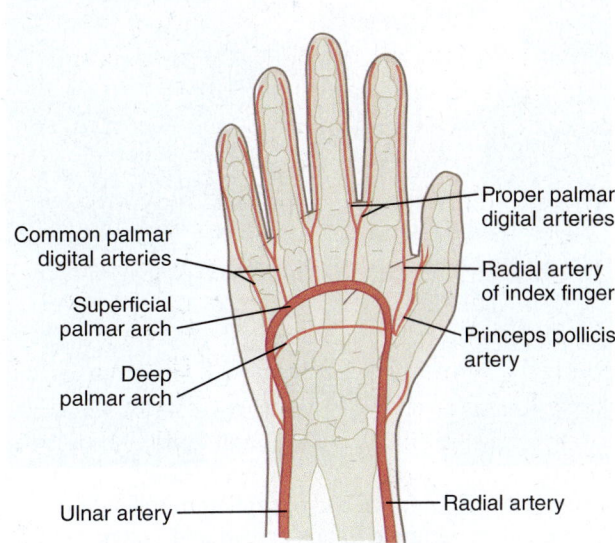

Figure 8.29 Drawing showing the triangular fibrocartilage complex vascularity.

Tears of the TFCC can occur acutely or develop gradually over time. Any activity that involves axial loading of the wrist, repetitive ulnar deviation, or twisting of the wrist can place a patient at risk for this injury, as can a fall on an outstretched hand. TFCC injuries occur slightly more often in sports such as gymnastics because of the impactful loading on the wrist.

Additionally, specific anatomic features can predispose a patient to a TFCC tear. A condition termed positive ulnar variance occurs when the distal ulna is more than 4 mm longer relative to the distal radius (**Figure 8.30**). This condition can occur as the result of a normal congenital variant or be acquired due to a condition that causes the radius to shorten, such as after a distal radius fracture that healed in a shortened position or with growth arrest of the radial physis during childhood. Regardless of the cause, the longer position of the distal ulna creates increased axial load across the TFCC and may predispose it to injury. A longer distal ulna can even cause impaction of the distal ulna directly through the TFCC and onto the carpus, a condition termed ulnocarpal impaction syndrome. Although it is important for the clinician to be aware of these two predisposing factors for TFCC tears, the presence of these conditions does not automatically mean that a patient will go on to have future problems with the TFCC.

TFCC tears are classified into Palmer type 1 and type 2 tears. Type 1 tears are considered traumatic lesions and can occur in the central portion of the TFCC (more common) or the periphery. Type 2 tears are considered degenerative lesions that occur over the course of time and result in thinning of the fibrocartilage disk until a central perforation occurs.[15] A complete schematic of Palmer classification of TFCC tears is shown in **Figure 8.31**.

The patient with a TFCC tear will present with ulnar-side wrist pain. Ask where the pain is located and if the pain is worse with weight bearing in extension (push-up position); when making a power grip; or with rotational wrist motion, such as opening a doorknob. Inquire whether there was a specific injury, such as a fall or twisting type injury, or pain has developed gradually over time. Inquire whether there is a "popping" or "clicking" sensation or a sense that the wrist is dislocating. Additionally, consider risk factors that can predispose to positive ulnar variance by asking whether the patient has ever had a previous wrist injury, such as a broken wrist as a child.

Inspection of the wrist with a TFCC injury will often reveal a normal appearance. In an acute injury, there may be some generalized edema over the ulnar side of the wrist. Note the position of the ulnar styloid and whether it appears prominent compared to the uninjured site.

Observe the wrist ROM. There will often, but not always, be pain and limitation with wrist flexion, extension, and ulnar deviation. The patient may not be able to supinate the wrist because of pain and apprehension, or the distal ulna may subluxate with supination.

Palpation of the TFCC is performed with the wrist in a neutral position, easily accomplished by asking the patient to assume the arm-wrestle position with the elbow on the table and seated across from the examiner. Perform the ulnar fovea sign test: Palpate the TFCC in the soft recess on the ulnar side of the wrist located just distal to the ulnar styloid and between the ECU and flexor carpi ulnaris (FCU) tendons, known as the foveal recess (**Figure 8.32**). A positive sign is tenderness with palpation.

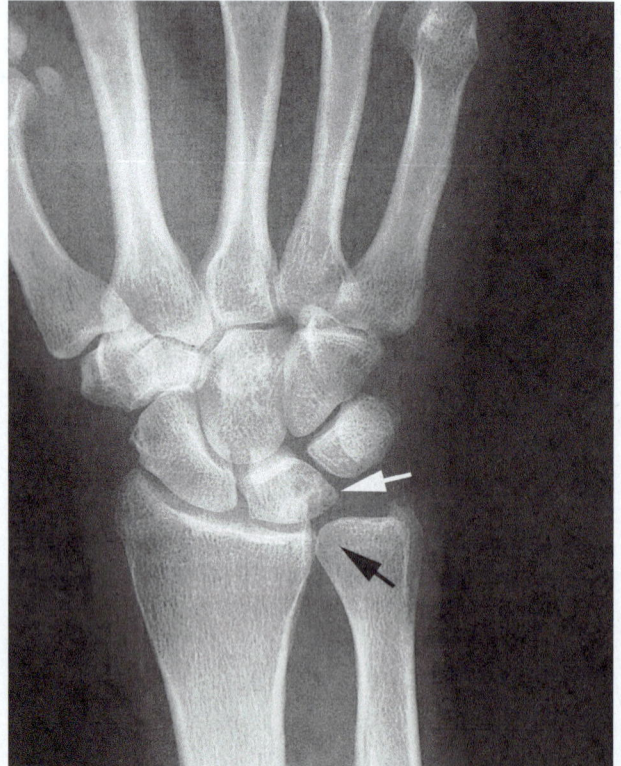

Figure 8.30 PA neutral radiograph demonstrating ulnar positive variance (black arrow) and lucency in the lunate suggestive of ulnocarpal impaction syndrome (white arrow).

Reproduced from Johnson TR, Steinbach LS, eds: *Essentials of Musculoskeletal Imaging*. Rosemont, IL, American Academy of Orthopaedic Surgeons, 2004.

> **Note**
>
> Pain at the ulna fovea is 95.2% sensitive and 86.5% specific for a TFCC tear.[16]

Conditions Causing Ulnar-Side Wrist Pain

	Clinical DRUJ Instability	Involved TFCC Component		TFCC Healing Potential	Status of DRUJ Cartilage	Treatment
		Distal	Proximal			
Class 1: Repairable distal tear 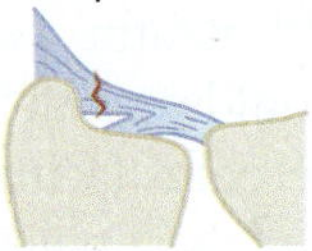	None or Slight	Torn	Intact	Good	Good	Repair Suture (Ligament to Capsule)
Class 2: Repairable complete tear 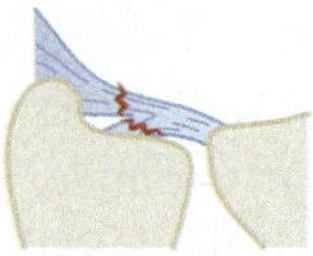	Mild or Severe	Torn	Torn	Good	Good	Repair Foveal Refixation
Class 3: Repairable proximal tear 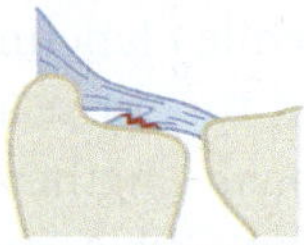	Mild or Severe	Intact	Torn	Good	Good	
Class 4: Nonrepairable 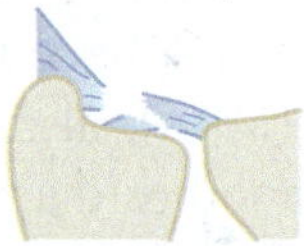	Severe	Torn	Torn	Poor	Good	Reconstruction Tendon Graft
Class 5: Arthritic DRUJ 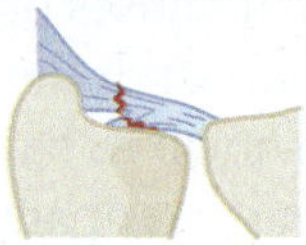	Mild or Severe	§	§	§	Poor	Salvage Arthroplasty or Joint Replacement

Figure 8.31 Chart showing the Palmer classification of triangular fibrocartilage complex tears.

DRUJ, distal radiolunar joint; TFCC, triangular fibrocartilage complex.
© Jones & Bartlett Learning

Next, perform the ulnar grind test. With the patient's affected wrist in neutral, the examiner places his or her hand into the patient's as if the two were going to shake hands. With the other hand, the examiner stabilizes the forearm. Then, the examiner places the patient's wrist into extension and applies an axial load with the wrist in ulnar deviation (**Figure 8.33**). This creates an axial load across the

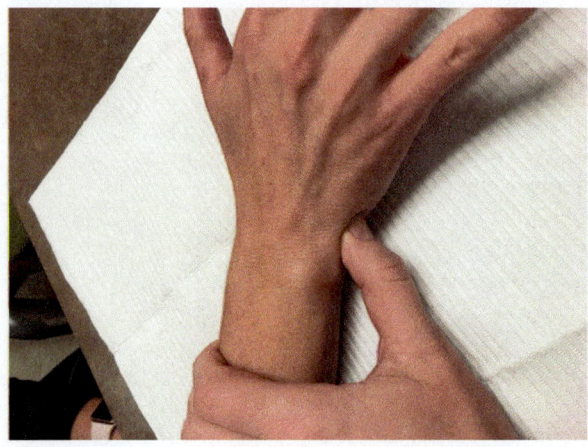

Figure 8.32 Clinical photograph showing palpation of the triangular fibrocartilage complex.

Courtesy of Sara Rynders.

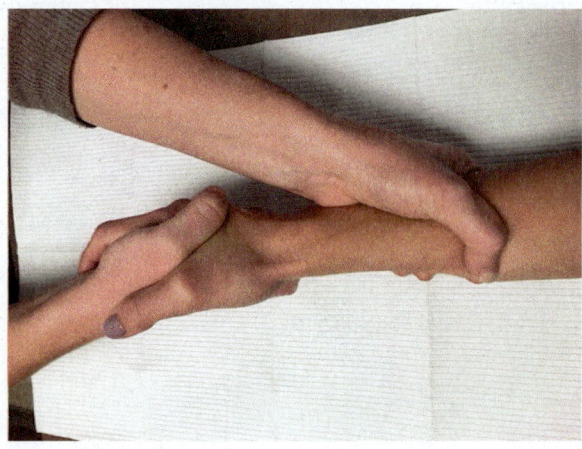

Figure 8.33 Clinical photograph showing the ulnar grind test.

Courtesy of Sara Rynders.

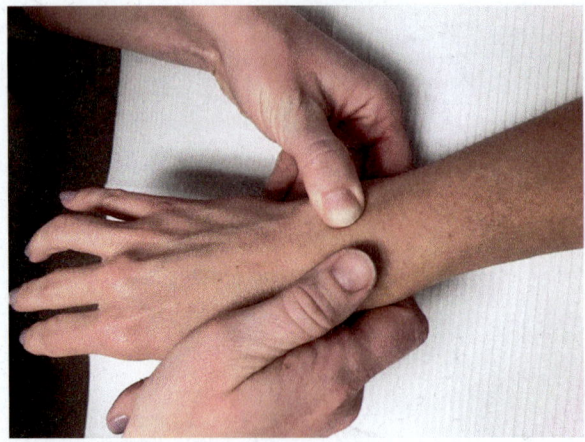

Figure 8.34 Clinical photograph showing the piano key test for distal radioulnar joint instability.

Courtesy of Sara Rynders.

TFCC and will be painful in the presence of a TFCC tear. Last, test the DRUJ for instability. Palpate the DRUJ with the wrist in pronation and perform the piano key test. The examiner places one hand on the radius and with the other applies dorsal to volar pressure over the distal ulna (**Figure 8.34**). Then, the test is performed on the unaffected wrist for comparison of laxity. In the presence of DRUJ instability, there will be increased motion and/or pain produced with this test. In severe cases of DRUJ instability, there may be a clunk or frank dislocation of the distal ulna from the DRUJ.

The wrist examination is not complete until additional structures on the ulnar side of the wrist are palpated and their condition documented. Palpate the ECU and FCU tendons and perform a strength against resistance test. Palpate the pisotriquetral joint and the hook of hamate in the palm. Palpate the SL interval and the LT joint and evaluate for instability or pain. Palpate the hand metacarpals and the forearm, looking for additional injuries.

Plain radiographs of the wrist should be ordered, and particular attention should be paid to the ulnar styloid, DRUJ, and ulnar carpus. In addition to the standard lateral and oblique views, obtain a PA neutral view of the wrist. A PA neutral view can be obtained by abducting the shoulder to 90° and flexing the elbow to 90° with the palm facing down. A comparison PA neutral view of the unaffected wrist should also be obtained. Performing a neutral view allows an accurate measurement of the length of the distal ulna relative to the distal radius. The examiner should note the length of ulnar variance, if it differs from the unaffected wrist, and if the DRUJ is reduced on the lateral view (**Figure 8.35**). The patient may also perform the PA neutral view while clenching the fist. This increases axial load across the wrist and can be helpful to evaluate for functional lengthening of the distal ulna and widening of the DRUJ, indicative of DRUJ instability.[17]

Plain radiographs will frequently be normal. Magnetic resonance arthrography (MRA), also known as an MRI with arthrography, is another diagnostic tool that can be used to diagnose and characterize TFCC tears as well as evaluate for other causes of ulnar-side wrist pain. MRA is MRI with contrast dye injected into the joint. This study has been shown to have superior accuracy in detecting TFCC tears compared to traditional MRI.[18] Despite the improved accuracy of MRA, the gold standard of diagnosis for TFCC tears remains direct visualization with wrist arthroscopy.

Initial management of TFCC tears without DRUJ instability centers around taping, splinting, and activity modification. Cortisone injections can also be used for symptomatic treatment of chronic tears. In one study of 84 patients with TFCC tears, 57% showed improvement after 4 weeks of nonsurgical treatment and did not require surgery for repair or débridement.[19]

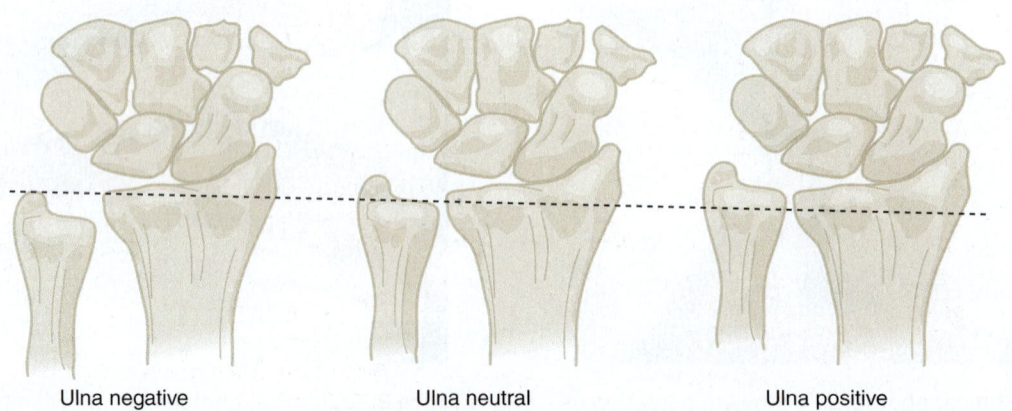

Ulna negative   Ulna neutral   Ulna positive

Figure 8.35 Drawings showing ulnar variance that can be seen on a PA neutral radiograph.

The differential diagnosis of ulnar-side wrist pain includes ECU tendinitis; FCU tendinitis; fracture of the distal ulna or radius; fracture of the pisiform, triquetrum, hamate, or fifth metacarpal base; or LT tear. The athletic trainer should consider all of these diagnoses throughout the evaluation process.

> **Five-Minute Sideline Assessment**
>
> Have a high clinical suspicion for a TFCC tear in any patient with ulnar-side wrist pain. A quick sideline evaluation should include a general inspection of the wrist to evaluate whether the distal ulna has dislocated from the DRUJ, which should be treated urgently. A dislocated ulna will present with a prominent ulnar styloid and severe pain. Motion of the wrist will be completely limited by pain and guarding. In milder presentations of this condition, the patient will have ulnar-side wrist pain, possibly clicking or limitation to supination ROM, and tenderness at the foveal recess on examination.

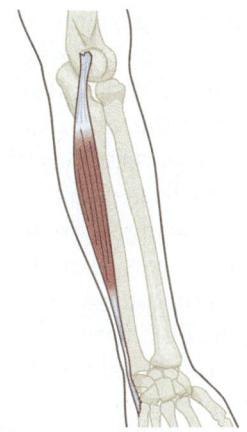

Figure 8.36 Drawing showing the anatomy of the extensor carpi ulnaris tendon.
© Jones & Bartlett Learning

ECU Tendon Injury

The evaluation of the patient presenting with ulnar-sided wrist pain should always include a thorough examination of the ECU tendon at the wrist (**Table 8.15**). The ECU tendon originates from the elbow at the lateral epicondyle and travels down the ulnar side of the forearm, terminally inserting onto the dorsal aspect of the fifth metacarpal base (**Figures 8.36** and **8.37**). At the level of the wrist, the

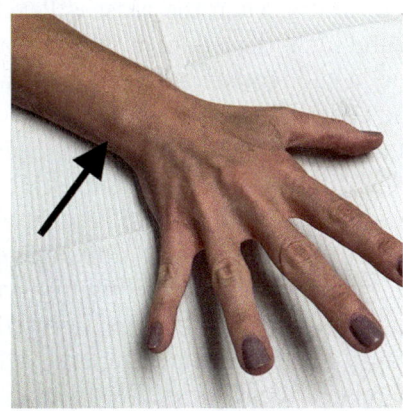

Figure 8.37 Clinical photograph showing the surface anatomy location of the extensor carpi ulnaris tendon.
Courtesy of Sara Rynders.

Table 8.15 Extensor Carpi Ulnaris Tendon Injury Quick Tips

Pathology	Description	Presentation (HIPS)	Special Tests/ Imaging	Differential Diagnosis	5-Min Sideline Assessment Tips
ECU tendinitis	Inflammation and possible subluxation of the ECU tendon at the level of the wrist	Gradual onset of ulnar-side wrist pain Snapping or popping present if ECU is subluxating	None	Ulnocarpal impaction syndrome Distal radioulnar joint instability ECU tendinitis Triangular fibrocartilage complex tear Hook of hamate fracture Distal ulnar fracture Cubital tunnel syndrome Ulnar artery thrombosis Lunotriquetral ligament tear Pisotriquetral joint arthritis Triquetral fracture Fifth metacarpal base fracture Fifth carpometacarpal joint fracture-dislocation Kienböck disease (osteonecrosis of the lunate)	Not applicable

ECU, extensor carpi ulnaris; HIPS, history, inspection, palpation, special tests.

tendon travels within a bony groove on the ulnar styloid and is held in place by a fibro-osseous sheath, or circumferential band of tissue, that compartmentalizes the tendon and stabilizes it during wrist motion. The ECU tendon is important for wrist extension and ulnar deviation as well as stabilization of the wrist during power grip. During supination, the ECU tendon lies dorsal to the axis of motion and therefore exerts a large extension force on the wrist. When the wrist is pronated, the ECU tendon lies volar relative to the axis of motion and contributes less to wrist extension and more to ulnar deviation.[20] Athletic activities such as tennis, baseball, hockey, golf, and rugby can cause a spectrum of pathology to the ECU tendon from inflammation (tendinitis) to instability and, rarely, attritional tendon rupture. The ECU is most vulnerable to injury when the wrist is flexed during supination and ulnar deviation, or when the tendon is placed under a sudden lateral force when engaged in an isometric contraction.[21]

The clinician should inquire as to the location of the pain and how or when it started. The patient presenting with ECU tendinitis will report ulnar-side wrist pain that may be sharp or dull. There may be a particular event related to the onset of symptoms, and most commonly symptoms will present gradually over time. The patient may report a sharp pain specifically related to wrist extension and ulnar deviation or a continuous dull, achy pain over the ulnar side of the wrist, even at rest. The athletic trainer should also inquire whether the patient experiences any painful catching, popping, or snapping on the ulnar side of the wrist. The patient experiencing ECU tendon instability may often feel the tendon slide or snap in and out of the fibro-osseous groove of the ulnar styloid.

The athletic trainer will observe the ulnar side of the wrist and note any edema. Inflammation within the ECU tendon sheath can often be observed in thin individuals. As the patient pronates and supinates the wrist, observe the position of the ECU tendon as it relates to the ulnar styloid. A tendon that subluxates will be observed sliding in and out of the fibro-osseous tunnel.

Conduct an examination with the patient seated across the examination table with the arm in the neutral position. Palpate the ECU tendon on the ulnar side of the wrist both in its groove along the distal ulna and at its insertion on the dorsal fifth metacarpal base. Tenderness will be present in cases of injury or inflammation. Ask the patient to extend and ulnarly deviate the wrist while the examiner applies a flexion and radial counterforce. Pain and giving way

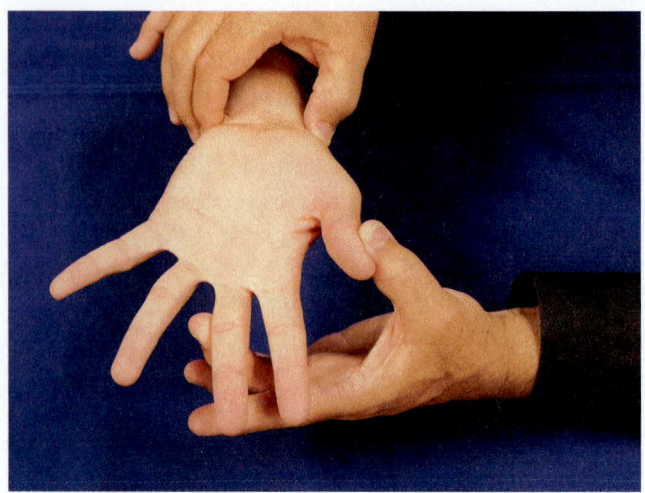

Figure 8.38 Clinical photograph showing the extensor carpi ulnaris synergy test.
© Jones & Bartlett Learning

is suggestive of ECU tendinitis. Additionally, the ECU synergy test is a means of differentiating intra-articular and extra-articular sources of ulnar-side wrist pain, therefore helping to identify ECU tendinitis. To perform this test, the patient places the elbow on the examination table flexed at 90°. The forearm is supinated so that the palm is facing the patient. The patient is asked to radially abduct the thumb while the examiner places resistance against the thumb and middle finger with one hand and palpates the ECU tendon with the other to confirm muscle activation (**Figure 8.38**). Pain at the ECU is indicative of ECU tendinitis.[22]

> **Note**
>
> The ECU synergy test has been found to be 73.7% sensitive and 85.7% specific in detecting problems with the ECU.[23]

Next, evaluate for ECU tendon instability. With the arm in the arm-wrestle position, elbow flexed at 90° and resting on the table, the athletic trainer places the index finger and thumb on either side of the tendon at the level of the ulnar styloid. The patient is instructed to rotate the wrist through pronation and supination while the examiner palpates for subluxation or dislocation of the tendon through the arc of motion (**Figure 8.39**).

The wrist examination is not complete until additional structures on the ulnar side of the wrist are palpated and their condition documented. Palpate the FCU tendon and perform a strength against

Conditions Causing Ulnar-Side Wrist Pain

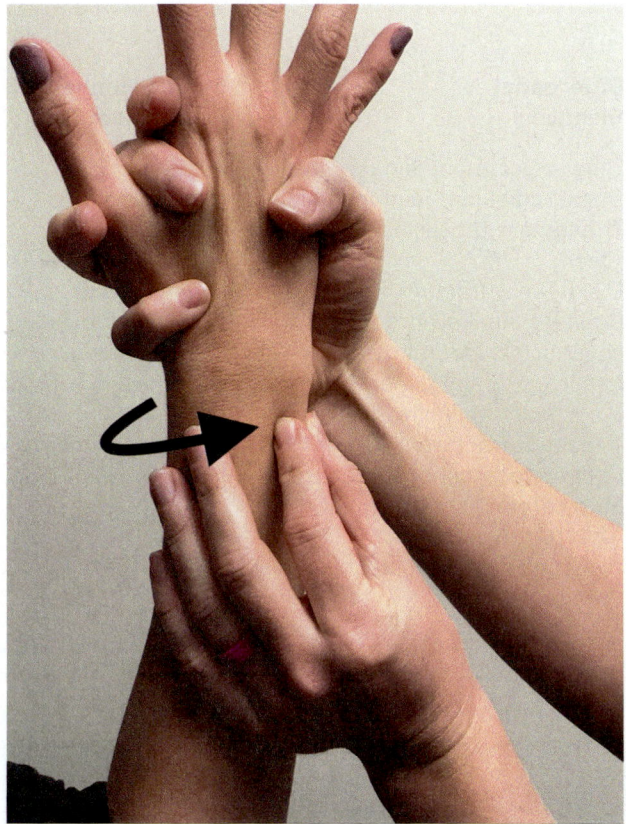

Figure 8.39 Clinical photograph showing palpation of the extensor carpi ulnaris tendon for subluxation.
Courtesy of Sara Rynders.

resistance test. Palpate the TFCC at the ulnar fovea and perform additional testing for TFCC tears. Palpate the pisotriquetral joint and the hook of hamate in the palm. Palpate the LT joint and evaluate for instability or pain. Palpate the hand metacarpals and the forearm, looking for additional injuries.

A standard series of PA, lateral, and oblique screening wrist radiographs should be performed to rule out other causes of ulnar-side wrist pain. Radiographs will appear normal in the presence of ECU tendinitis or ECU instability.

MRI can play a role in the identification of ECU tendinitis but should be used only when the diagnosis is uncertain. There are more than 10 anatomic structures that can contribute to ulnar-side wrist pain, so when the examiner cannot be sure of the clinical diagnosis of ECU tendinitis or the patient has failed to respond to nonsurgical management of ECU tendinitis, MRI can be used to confirm the diagnosis or to help to differentiate between causes of ulnar-side wrist pain.

Rest, taping, splinting in 30° of extension and ulnar deviation, anti-inflammatory medications, and therapeutic modalities are mainstays of initial treatment of ECU tendinitis. Cortisone injections can also be performed sparingly to relieve inflammation. Chronic instability of the ECU tendon often needs to be managed surgically. Rehabilitation goals of ROM and strength should be 80% of the uninjured side before return to play is recommended.[24]

The differential diagnosis of ECU tendinitis is ECU instability; TFCC tear; DRUJ instability; ulnocarpal impaction syndrome; FCU tendinitis; pisotriquetral joint arthrosis; Kienböck disease; LT ligament tear; fracture of the ulnar styloid, triquetrum, fifth metacarpal base, or hamate; or ulnar nerve lesion.

Five-Minute Sideline Assessment

Quick palpation of the ECU tendon can be performed on the sideline, as can the ECU synergy test. Pain with these maneuvers can help to localize the injured area to the ECU tendon. Also, observe the ECU tendon for subluxation out of the fibro-osseous groove of the distal ulna during wrist rotation. Remember, ECU tendinitis has a more chronic, insidious onset of symptoms, whereas acute disruption of the ECU subsheath can present with acute pain and may be difficult to assess on the sideline. Radiographs are an appropriate diagnostic tool to help rule out other, more serious injuries and help determine whether it is safe for the patient to return to play.

Hook of Hamate Fracture

A fracture of the hook of hamate, while not frequently encountered in the general population, does tend to occur more commonly in racket or club-type sports (**Table 8.16**). The hamate bone lies on the ulnar aspect of the wrist in the distal row of carpal bones. A bony protuberance emerges from the volar aspect of the bone, termed the hook of hamate, which serves as a bony protector for the ulnar artery and the deep motor branch of the ulnar nerve and as a biomechanical fulcrum around which the ulnar-most flexor tendons pass (**Figure 8.40**). Because of the hook's proximity to these major structures, a fracture can cause secondary ulnar nerve injury or flexor tendon injury. In one literature review of 127 hook of hamate fractures, a 15% incidence of tendon rupture was reported.[25] The blood supply of the hook is variable. A nutrient vessel exists from the base of the hamate, but perhaps up to 71% of the population does not have a blood vessel that enters through the distal tip of the hook. This is significant because it could account for the high rate of fracture nonunions seen in the hook of hamate.[26]

Table 8.16 Hook of Hamate Fracture Quick Tips

Pathology	Description	Presentation (HIPS)	Special Tests/ Imaging	Differential Diagnosis	5-Min Sideline Assessment Tips
Hook of hamate fracture	Fracture of the bony hook of the hamate bone	Sudden or insidious onset of volar-ulnar hand pain Can occur after an impact from a racket or club handle or a fall on an outstretched hand	Hook of hamate pull test	Ulnocarpal impaction syndrome Distal radioulnar joint instability Triangular fibrocartilage complex tear Distal ulnar fracture Cubital tunnel syndrome Ulnar artery thrombosis Lunotriquetral ligament tear Pisotriquetral joint arthritis Triquetral fracture Fifth metacarpal base fracture Fifth carpometacarpal joint fracture-dislocation Kienböck disease (osteonecrosis of the lunate)	Assess for point tenderness directly of the hook of hamate and have a high level of suspicion if pain is associated with numbness or tingling in the ring and small fingers

HIPS, history, inspection, palpation, special tests.

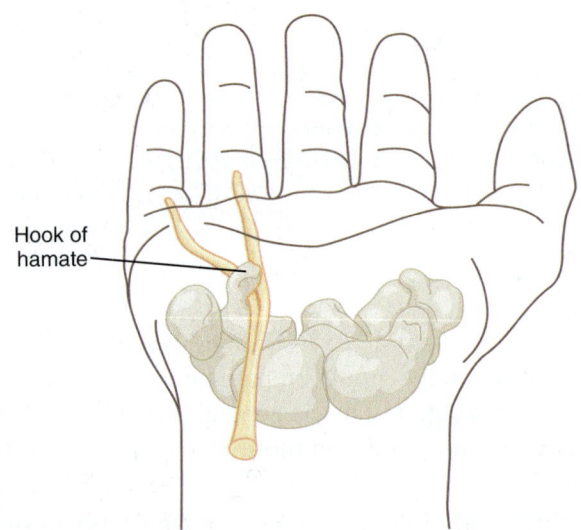

Figure 8.40 Drawing showing the hook of hamate.
© Jones & Bartlett Learning

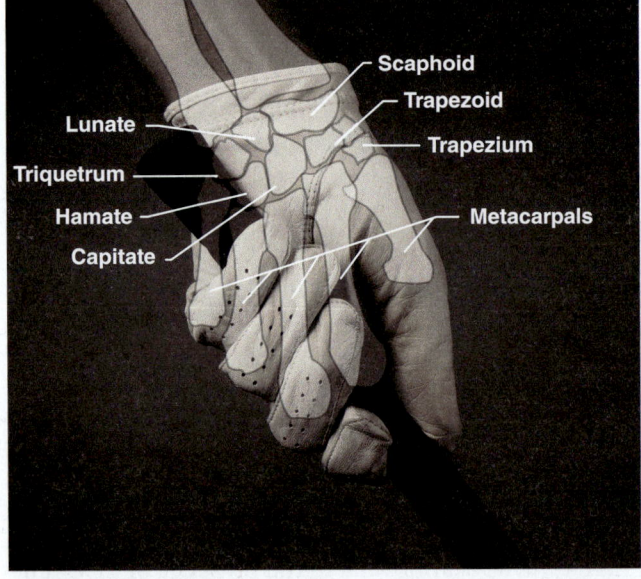

Figure 8.41 Position of golf club against the hook of hamate.
© Steve Cukrov/Shutterstock.

Although the incidence of hook of hamate fractures is not known, it is more commonly encountered in sports such as golf, baseball, racquetball, or tennis. This is because the bony protuberance is vulnerable to injury from a forceful impact from the end of a bat, racket, or golf club (**Figure 8.41**). The wrist closer to the handle is more often affected. The nondominant hand is more vulnerable in golfers and baseball players, whereas the dominant hand is more often affected in tennis and racquetball players.[1] A hook of hamate fracture can also occur due to a fall on an outstretched hand. There is a paucity of reports and research in the literature about hook of hamate fractures. This is in part because the injury often goes unrecognized or presents late. Regardless of this fact, or perhaps because of it, it is absolutely essential that the clinician be able to evaluate for and treat this injury.

The patient with a hook of hamate fracture will report volar-ulnar hand pain, but the mechanism of injury could be recent or remote. The athletic trainer should ask the patient how long the pain has been present and whether there was a specific event that triggered the pain. Did the golfer's club make contact with the ground during a swing? Did the baseball player's bat make impact on the hand on a forceful hit? Frequently, the patient will not be able to pinpoint the exact location of the pain but instead will describe a vague area over the base of the palm. The patient may report edema in the case of acute injury but not with remote injury. Next, query about injury to adjacent structures. It is essential to ask the patient whether he or she has any weakness in the hand given that the motor branch of the ulnar nerve lies in close proximity to the hook of hamate. Also ask about numbness or tingling in the ring and small fingers, as the superficial sensory branch of the ulnar nerve may be symptomatic. Inquire about snapping or crepitus with flexion and extension of the fingers, as the ulnar flexor tendons run past the hook and can be irritated or even injured with a fracture.

Physical examination of the patient with a hook of hamate fracture will reveal point tenderness to palpation over the hook of hamate in the palm. This is located 2 cm distal and radial to the more easily palpable pisiform (**Figure 8.42**). Rarely, crepitus or mobility of the fractured hook can be felt. Assess sensation in the fingers with emphasis on the ulnar nerve distribution. Sometimes, there is tingling or decreased sensation reported in the small finger and ulnar aspect of the ring finger. Perform a Tinel test over the ulnar nerve at the level of the Guyon canal (space between the pisiform and hook of hamate). The test is positive if numbness and tingling are reproduced or worsened in the ulnar nerve distribution. Also, test the motor branch of the ulnar nerve by asking the patient to abduct and adduct the fingers against resistance and perform a grip test. If weakness is present, injury or irritation to the ulnar motor branch is suspected. Assess the flexion and extension of the digits, with focus on the ring and small fingers. If there is an inability to flex the digits or pain, snapping, or crepitus is present, consider injury or inflammation of the flexor tendons. Finally, assess the vascular status of the hand by checking capillary refill in the digits and performing an Allen test to evaluate for blood flow through the radial and ulnar arteries. Although extremely rare, if an impact occurred in the palm that is of sufficient enough force to break the hook of hamate, it could also cause damage to the ulnar artery and lead to an ulnar artery thrombosis. When the artery is unharmed, the Allen test will reveal patent radial and ulnar circulation to the digits. If the ulnar artery is occluded, the digits will not perfuse when the ulnar artery is tested for patency.

The hook of hamate pull test has been used to help identify hook of hamate fractures on physical examination. To perform this test, the patient is seated across the table from the examiner with the affected hand on the exam table, palm up. The examiner places the patient's wrist in extreme ulnar deviation. The patient closes the fingers into flexion, and the examiner tries to extend the ring and small fingers from the DIP joints against resistance from the patient. A positive test will elicit moderate to extreme pain at the hook of hamate with this maneuver (**Figure 8.43**). In a small sample of five

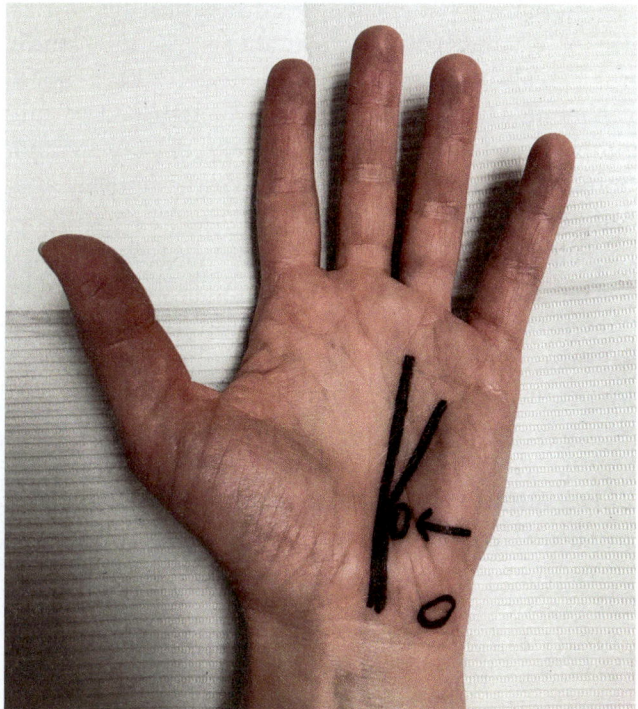

Figure 8.42 Clinical photograph showing the surface anatomy location of the hook of hamate.

Courtesy of Sara Rynders.

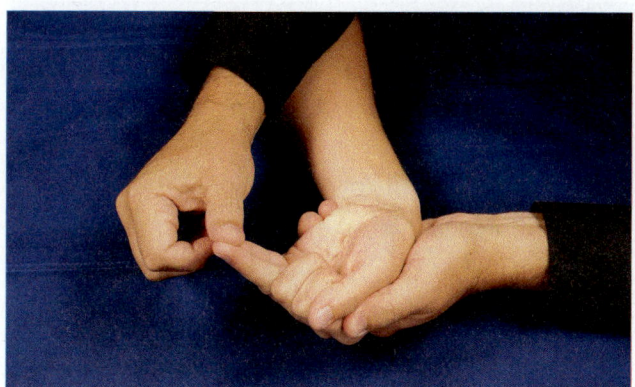

Figure 8.43 Clinical photograph showing the hook of hamate pull test.

© Jones & Bartlett Learning

patients, this test was sensitive for a hook of hamate fracture 100% of the time, but its specificity has not yet been tested.[27]

The examiner should complete the patient's examination by evaluating for tenderness at adjacent structures, including the TFCC, pisiform, and pisotriquetral joint; first CMC joint; scaphoid tubercle; and FCU and FCR tendons. Also, test the patient for cubital tunnel syndrome if paresthesias are present in the fingers.

If a hook of hamate fracture is suspected, the examiner should obtain a standard set of wrist radiographs plus specific views. Although this fracture will usually be missed on standard PA, lateral, and oblique wrist radiographs, obtaining these images is still recommended for complete radiographic evaluation of the wrist. When evaluating for hook of hamate fractures, the examiner must obtain a radiographic view devoted solely to viewing the bony protuberance of the hamate. This can be accomplished two ways. The first radiographic view is the carpal tunnel view and has been found to be 40% to 50% sensitive for identifying hook of hamate fractures (**Figure 8.44**). The second radiographic view is the supinated, oblique view, which has been found to have a variable 5% to 100% sensitivity rate.

As evidenced by the wide range of radiograph sensitivity rates for identifying this fracture, it is important to remember that radiographs, regardless of view, are only approximately 31% sensitive in detecting hook of hamate fractures compared to the more reliable CT scan.[28] CT of the wrist has been found to be 100% sensitive, 94% specific, and 97% accurate in diagnosis of hook of hamate fractures and is therefore the diagnostic test of choice for identifying these injuries[29] (**Figure 8.45**).

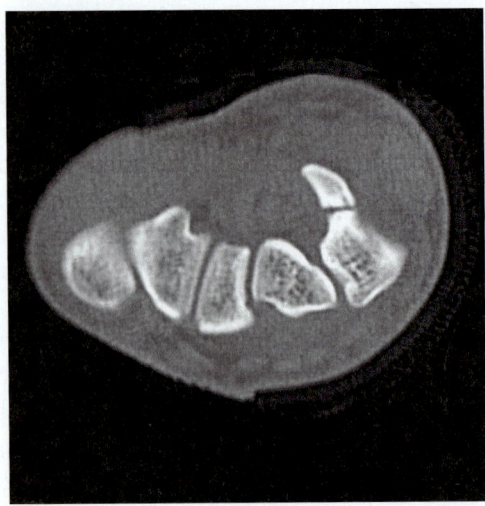

Figure 8.45 Radiograph showing supinated oblique view of hook of hamate fracture.

Reproduced from Johnson TR, Steinbach LS, eds: *Essentials of Musculoskeletal Imaging*. Rosemont, IL, American Academy of Orthopaedic Surgeons, 2004.

Treatment of hook of hamate fractures depends largely on the location of the fracture, age of the fracture, and whether it is displaced. An acute nondisplaced fracture may heal with 6 to 8 weeks of cast immobilization. Displaced or chronic fractures will likely require surgery for excision of the hook because of its tendency toward nonunion. Generally favorable results are seen with excision of the hook of hamate, and most patients will be able to return to previous level of play with little pain or discomfort. Occasionally, a patient will need to adjust his or her grip or wear a padded glove after surgery. A study of 11 high-level patients who underwent a hook of hamate excision showed that all returned to full sports participation within 6 weeks of surgery and scored 0 on the Disabilities of the Arm, Shoulder and Hand questionnaire.[30]

Differential diagnosis of hook of hamate fractures includes soft-tissue contusion, TFCC tear, FCU or FCR tendinitis, pisiform fracture or pisotriquetral arthritis, cubital tunnel syndrome, ulnar tunnel syndrome, or ulnar artery thrombosis.

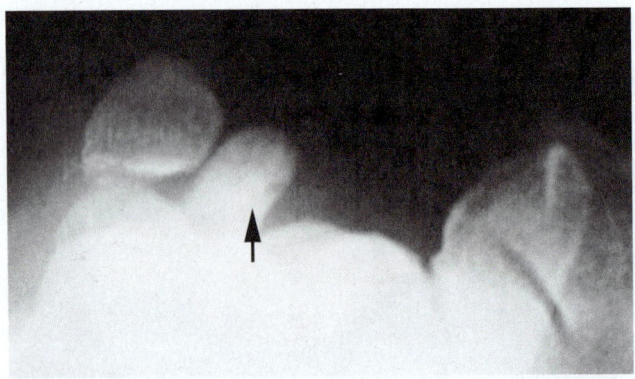

Figure 8.44 Radiograph showing carpal tunnel view of hook of hamate fracture (arrow).

Reproduced from Johnson TR, Steinbach LS, eds: *Essentials of Musculoskeletal Imaging*. Rosemont, IL, American Academy of Orthopaedic Surgeons, 2004.

Five-Minute Sideline Assessment

The clinician must have a high level of suspicion for this injury. If a patient falls on an outstretched hand or experiences a high-impact injury from a racket, bat, or club, palpating of the hook of hamate in the palm for tenderness is the single most useful tool on the field. Players will often try to play through this injury or present late with chronic hand pain. A thorough radiographic evaluation is necessary for diagnosis.

Conditions of the Hand and Fingers

Fractures of the Base of the Thumb: Bennett Fracture and Rolando Fracture

It could be argued that the thumb is the single most evolved structure in the human body. Capable of nearly 360° of rotational mobility, the thumb also flexes, extends, abducts, adducts, and opposes, accounting for up to 40% of human hand function.[31] It is an essential structure for basic tasks, such as pinching and gripping, but also allows the performance of complicated fine motor skills. A fracture of the thumb can have devastating consequences to hand function if not treated properly.

Two of the most commonly encountered fractures in the thumb are the Bennett fracture and the Rolando fracture (**Table 8.17**). These fractures are caused by a fall resulting in an axial load with an abduction force on the thumb. Both fractures occur at the base of the metacarpal and involve the first CMC joint, but there are subtle differences in their characteristics. A Bennett fracture is an intra-articular fracture of the first metacarpal base where a small volar-ulnar fragment remains reduced and the remainder of the metacarpal base subluxates off the trapezium. The volar-ulnar base is held reduced by the attachment of the anterior oblique ligament (formerly called the beak ligament), and the metacarpal base is subluxated because of the pull created by the insertion of the abductor pollicis brevis tendon (**Figure 8.46**). A Rolando fracture is an intra-articular fracture of the first metacarpal base with more than one fracture fragment, causing a comminuted Y- or T-fracture pattern. Because these fractures affect the articular surface of the first CMC joint, there is the potential for the development of posttraumatic arthritis, loss of motion, and chronic pain if the congruity of the joint surface is not restored. These fractures are considered unstable and require surgical correction.

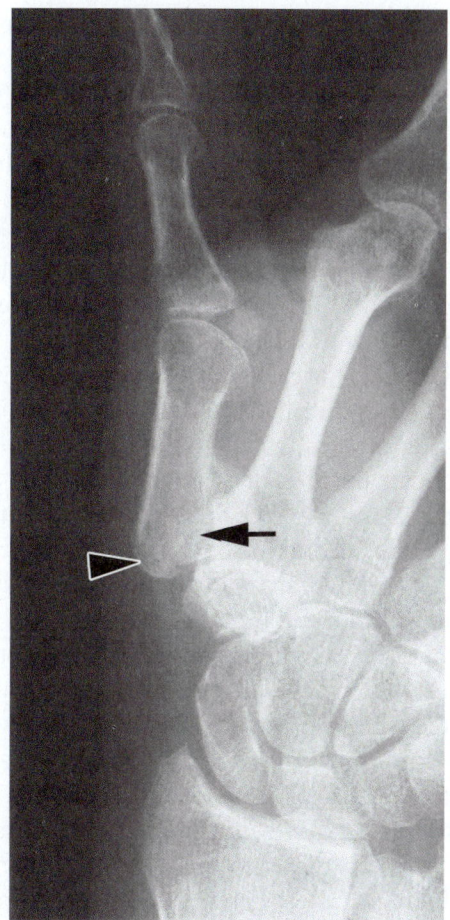

Figure 8.46 Radiograph showing a Bennett fracture. The arrowhead is pointing to the subluxated first metacarpal. The arrow is pointing to the Bennet fracture fragment attached to the anterior oblique ligament.

Reproduced from Johnson TR, Steinbach LS, eds: *Essentials of Musculoskeletal Imaging*. Rosemont, IL, American Academy of Orthopaedic Surgeons, 2004.

The patient with a Bennett or Rolando fracture will report a fall onto the thumb with subsequent severe thumb pain. Pain will occur with any attempt at thumb motion. Observation will reveal edema and prominence or fullness about the thumb base at

Table 8.17 Bennett and Rolando Fractures Quick Tips

Pathology	Description	Presentation (HIPS)	Special Tests/ Imaging	Differential Diagnosis	5-Min Sideline Assessment Tips
Bennett fracture and Rolando fracture	Intra-articular fractures of the base of the first metacarpal	Sudden onset of pain and possible deformity at the base of the thumb	Radiographs of the thumb	Scaphoid fracture Thumb phalanx fracture Distal radius fracture Scapholunate ligament injury	Assess for pain and deformity at the base of the thumb; splint and obtain radiographs

HIPS, history, inspection, palpation, special tests.

the level of the first CMC joint. Check for any open wounds or abrasions. Inspection of the thumb reveals tenderness to palpation over the base of the thumb metacarpal and first CMC joint. The patient will have a reluctance or inability to abduct, adduct, or oppose the thumb, but flexion and extension of the thumb MCP and IP joints will be preserved. The athletic trainer should test the thumb's sensation to light touch distally and capillary refill, both of which are usually normal with this injury.

Additional injuries to adjacent structures should be evaluated for. Palpate the thumb MCP joint to assess for tenderness, and stress the MCP joint's UCL and RCL for pain or laxity. Perform the same assessment at the IP joint. Also palpate the distal radius and radial styloid, second through fourth metacarpals, and the remaining carpal bones for any tenderness that could indicate additional injuries.

Radiography of the thumb is the diagnostic tool of choice. Obtain PA, lateral, and oblique views of the affected thumb. Note on the radiographs whether there are one or more fracture fragments and subluxation of the metacarpal base off the trapezium.

CT can be used to better visualize the metacarpal base for intra-articular step-offs or to characterize the nature of the fracture fragments to determine the need for surgery or surgical planning.

Reduction of Bennett and Rolando fractures requires axial traction, palmar abduction, and pronation while applying pressure over the metacarpal base. Almost all of these fractures require surgical intervention to reduce and restore the integrity of the metacarpal base. Surgical management may involve closed reduction and percutaneous pinning or open reduction and internal fixation. Regardless of the method used, the goal is to align the fracture fragments, create a congruent joint line without step-offs, and reduce the subluxated metacarpal. Surgery, followed by 4 to 6 weeks of cast immobilization and therapy, usually allows the patient to return to the original level of play by 6 to 8 weeks. Outcomes after appropriate treatment are generally good given that the thumb's multiplanar ROM can usually make up for any acquired stiffness.[32]

Differential diagnosis of Bennett and Rolando fractures includes extra-articular fracture of the thumb metacarpal or fracture patterns of the thumb metacarpal base that do not result in subluxation. Additionally, consider contusion or sprain, thumb MCP joint UCL or RCL injury, scaphoid fracture, radial styloid or distal radius fracture, or flexor or extensor tendon injury. All of these injuries should be considered when evaluating pain at the base of the thumb.

> **Five-Minute Sideline Assessment**
>
> The patient with a Bennett or Rolando fracture will report severe onset of pain after a fall on the thumb. The patient may guard the thumb, and any motion will cause severe pain at the base of the thumb. Assess for the area of tenderness over the base of the thumb and quickly assess for any open injuries. Check flexor and extensor tendon function distally in the thumb at the IP joint and perform a cursory neurovascular examination. Splint the thumb in a position of comfort until radiographs can be obtained.

Metacarpal Fractures

Fractures of the metacarpal bones are commonly encountered injuries in sports and account for 18% of all upper extremity fractures in the general population.[33] These fractures tend to occur from a direct blow onto the hand (such as being stepped on), a sudden axial load on the metacarpal head (such as punching an object), or a sudden twisting motion (such as a finger caught in equipment). The fracture may occur at the metacarpal head, neck, shaft, or base. It may be open or closed, intra-articular or extra-articular, and displaced or nondisplaced. The most frequently encountered metacarpal fracture is the boxer's fracture, which refers to a fifth metacarpal neck fracture. These fractures, like most metacarpal fractures, tend to angulate with the apex dorsally due to the forces exerted by the intrinsic and extrinsic hand muscles (**Table 8.18**).

The patient presenting with a metacarpal fracture will report a severe, sudden onset of hand pain that is frequently associated with an injurious event. The patient will usually report dorsal hand pain and limited motion due to the pain or swelling.

Inspection of the injured hand will often reveal marked edema and ecchymosis. Evaluate for any open injuries or abrasions. There may be a visible deformity on the dorsum of the hand due to the angulation of the underlying bone fracture. There may also be a loss of the normal contour of the metacarpal head at the MCP joint due to the angulation that has occurred more proximally. This is most evident when the patient makes a fist. It is also important to assess for abnormal alignment of the digits, as an angulated or rotated metacarpal will result in angulation or rotation of the digit distally.

Begin the examination seated across the table from the patient. Ask the patient to flex and extend the digits to the best of his or her ability. Note any stiffness, loss of motion, or abnormal crossover of

Conditions of the Hand and Fingers

Table 8.18 Metacarpal Fractures Quick Tips

Pathology	Description	Presentation (HIPS)	Special Tests/ Imaging	Differential Diagnosis	5-Min Sideline Assessment Tips
Metacarpal fractures	Fracture of the metacarpal bone	Sudden onset of pain and possible deformity in the hand after an impact or fall	Radiographs of the hand	Contusion Wrist ligament injury	Assess for bony tenderness over the metacarpals. If present, splint and obtain radiographs

HIPS, history, inspection, palpation, special tests.

the fingers through this motion (**Figure 8.47**). Next, palpate the metacarpal bones, identifying not only which metacarpal is tender but also where along the bone the tenderness occurs: the head, shaft, or base. Perform a basic neurovascular examination, which is usually found to be normal, as well as palpation of the digits and wrist to assess for any additional injuries.

Obtain a standard set of PA, lateral, and oblique hand radiographs. It is important to obtain three different views in order to visualize the angulation, rotation, and displacement of the metacarpal fracture. The clinician should be familiar with how to name and describe a metacarpal fracture. The first descriptor is always about fracture displacement, either displaced or nondisplaced. Next, identify whether the fracture is intra-articular or extra-articular. Then, identify which metacarpal bone is affected, first through fifth, and the type of fracture pattern seen, transverse, oblique, spiral, or comminuted. Last, describe the fracture location on the bone:

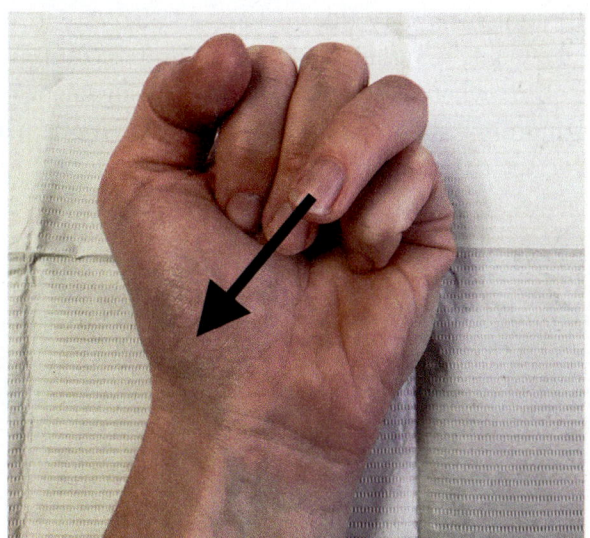

Figure 8.47 Clinical photograph showing the abnormal crossover of the fourth finger due to a metacarpal fracture.
Courtesy of Sara Rynders.

head, neck, shaft, or base (**Figure 8.48**). Be sure to assess adjacent bones for additional fractures.

CT may be used in a limited fashion, particularly in the setting of metacarpal base fractures that cannot be well visualized on standard radiographs because of the overlapping nature of the CMC joints. CT can help in better understanding the fracture pattern characteristics and aid in surgical planning.

Metacarpal fractures can be managed with cast immobilization or surgery. Generally, nondisplaced and minimally displaced or angulated fractures can be managed in a splint or cast for 4 to 6 weeks. Return to unrestricted play is anticipated between 6 and 8 weeks, though a patient may be able to play in a protective cast earlier, depending on severity of the fracture, amount of healing seen on radiographs, and whether the position is skilled or unskilled. Displaced fractures or multiple metacarpal fractures require surgical management with either temporary pins or a plate and screw fixation. The time to return to play with surgical management is equal to that of nonsurgical management. Most metacarpal fractures heal without complication, and a patient can expect to return to his or her full level of play without limitations.

The differential diagnosis of a metacarpal fracture includes a fracture of the carpus or phalanges and a contusion or soft-tissue injury.

Five-Minute Sideline Assessment

The patient with a metacarpal fracture will report sudden onset of hand pain after some type of impact on the hand. Quickly assess for any open wounds or abrasions and identify the location of the pain. Evaluate for any noticeable deformity on the dorsum of the hand or a loss of prominence of the metacarpal head. Ask the patient to flex and extend the digits and note whether there is severe pain, angulation, or crossover rotation through the motion. Stabilize the hand in a splint and obtain radiographs for definitive diagnosis.

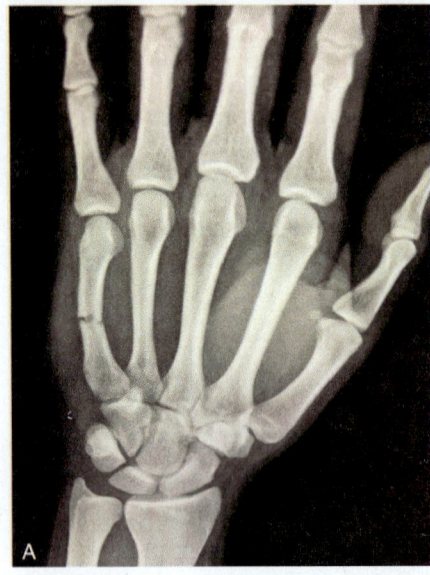 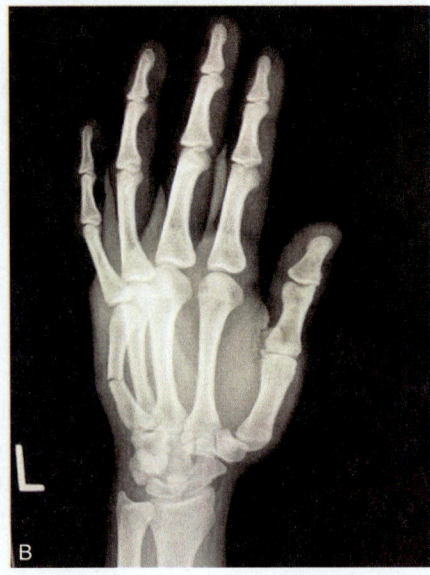 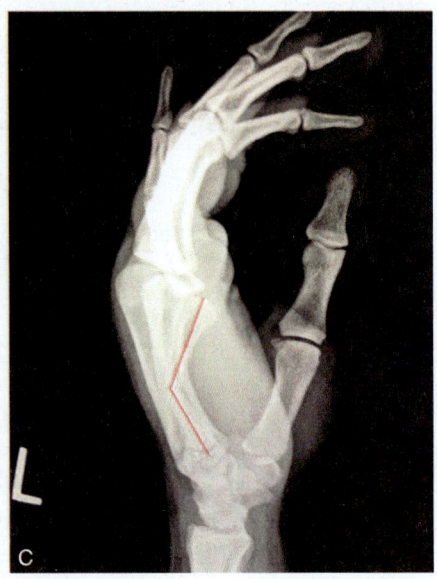

Figure 8.48 Radiographs of the hand demonstrating a left fifth metacarpal transverse shaft fracture with approximately 50° of volar angulation. **A.** PA radiograph. **B.** Oblique radiograph. **C.** Lateral radiograph.

Courtesy of Sara Rynders.

Thumb UCL Injuries

The UCL of the thumb MCP joint (referred to as the thumb UCL) is a very important structure for thumb stability, pinch grasp, and key pinch. Sprains and ruptures of the thumb UCL are commonly encountered in sports such as skiing, basketball, and football. The thumb UCL is particularly vulnerable to injury for several reasons. First, the thumb's naturally extended and abducted position on the hand means that it is more likely than any other digit to be hyperabducted by forceful contact with a ball or another player or when falling on an outstretched hand. Second, the bony architecture of the MCP joint does not provide much for inherent joint stability; instead, the joint's stability is conferred by the RCLs and UCLs, volar plate, and dorsal joint capsule (**Table 8.19**).

The thumb UCL is a stout ligament located on the ulnar aspect of the MCP joint that is composed of the proper and accessory collateral ligaments. It originates on the head of the thumb metacarpal and inserts in a fanlike manner on the base of the thumb proximal phalanx (**Figure 8.49**). It lies deep to the adductor aponeurosis, which is important because in some circumstances the UCL tears and the ruptured flap displaces above the adductor aponeurosis, a condition called a Stener lesion. The term skier's thumb refers to an acutely injured UCL, whereas the term gamekeeper's thumb refers to a chronic condition of UCL laxity and MCP joint instability due to long-standing strain on the ligament. A variation of acute thumb UCL injury can occur when a bony avulsion of the ligament off the thumb proximal phalanx occurs, instead of a tear within the substance of the ligament.

Table 8.19 Ulnar Collateral Ligament Injuries Quick Tips

Pathology	Description	Presentation (HIPS)	Special Tests/ Imaging	Differential Diagnosis	5-Min Sideline Assessment Tips
Thumb UCL injuries	Partial or complete tear of the thumb UCL at the MCP joint	Acute: sudden onset of pain, weakness, and laxity of the thumb MCP joint Chronic: gradual onset of pain and laxity of the thumb MCP joint	Stress of the UCL in flexion and extension	Phalanx or metacarpal fracture MCP joint dislocation Radial collateral ligament sprain Capsular sprain Contusion Tendon injury	Assess for tenderness over the ulnar side of the thumb MCP joint. If present, splint and obtain radiographs prior to stress testing the ligament

HIPS, history, inspection, palpation, special tests; MCP, metacarpophalangeal; UCL, ulnar collateral ligament.

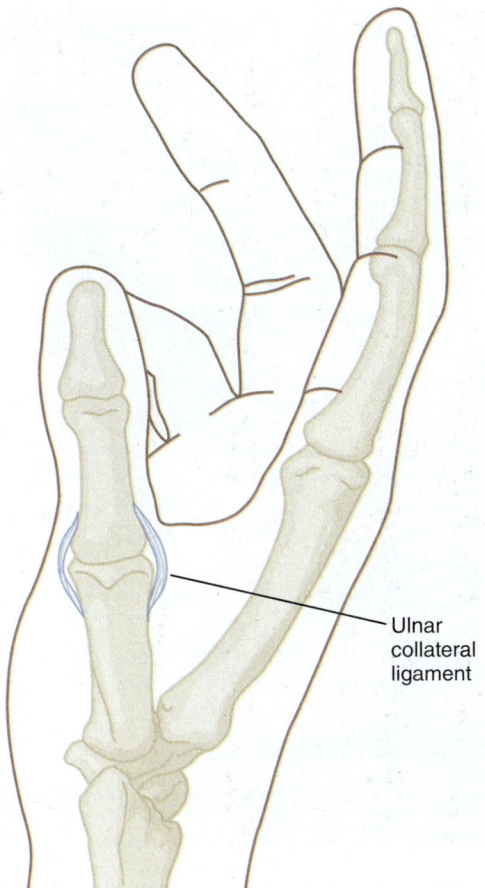

Figure 8.49 Drawing showing the anatomy of the thumb ulnar collateral ligament.

© Jones & Bartlett Learning

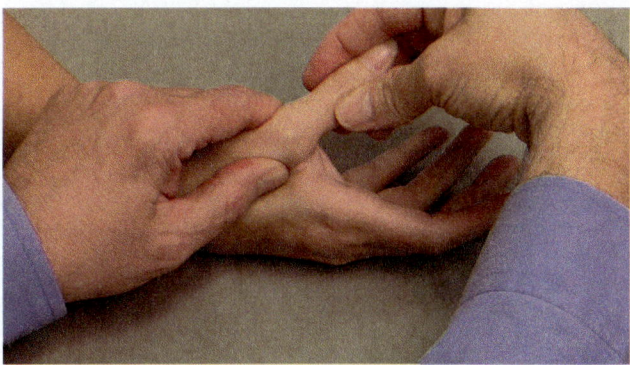

Figure 8.50 Clinical photograph showing stress testing of the thumb ulnar collateral ligament.

Reproduced from Armstrong AD, Hubbard MC, eds: *Essentials of Musculoskeletal Care*, ed 5. Burlington, MA, American Academy of Orthopaedic Surgeons, 2015.

The patient with an acutely injured thumb UCL will report a sudden onset of ulnar-side thumb pain localized to the MCP joint. He or she may report a fall or impact on the hand during which the thumb was hyperabducted. Occasionally, the patient will report feeling a "pop" or a subluxation/dislocation type event. The patient will note that the thumb is minimally painful until he or she tries to put any pressure on the thumb tip, such as with a pinch grasp or key pinch. This action will cause acute pain.

On examining the thumb, the athletic trainer may notice fullness about the ulnar aspect of the thumb MCP joint. It is essential to visualize both the injured and the uninjured thumb simultaneously to compare and contrast the appearance. The injured thumb may be held in a slightly abducted posture. However, in the cases of mild sprains and incomplete tears, the appearance of the thumb may be quite normal and equal to the uninjured side.

Examination of the patient with a thumb UCL tear should start with asking the patient to localize the pain. Palpate the thumb UCL on the ulnar aspect of the MCP joint. A ligament sprain will have tenderness on palpation. Next, test the integrity of the thumb UCL. Stabilize the thumb metacarpal with one hand and with the other apply a valgus stress to the proximal phalanx (**Figure 8.50**). Perform this maneuver with the MCP joint in full extension and in 30° of flexion; in this way, both the accessory and proper collateral ligaments, respectively, are isolated and tested for laxity. Pain and/or laxity with this stress test indicates a UCL sprain. It will take time and practice to become comfortable with the feel of this test. A local anesthetic block around the ligament can be performed prior to testing if the patient has too much pain to accurately evaluate the laxity of the thumb UCL.

Additionally, the examiner can determine the *severity* of the ligament sprain with this same maneuver. Making the determination between a stable partial tear and an unstable complete tear is important, as it guides treatment. There is some controversy in the current literature about just how much laxity during stress testing is indicative of a complete tear. It has been found that both proper technique and comparison to the uninjured thumb are necessary to help determine abnormal laxity in the thumb UCL. False-positive test results for complete ligament injury have been identified when the thumb was examined in pronation and false-negative test results for complete ligament injury when the thumb was examined in supination.[34] Mindful examination of the patient is essential.

It is generally accepted that laxity of a thumb UCL of 30° or more at the MCP joint is indicative of a complete ligament tear.[35] Additionally, it is suggested that a difference of more than 10° to 15° of laxity compared to the uninjured thumb is indicative of a complete tear. However, there can be normal variation between bilateral thumbs that makes this interpretation confusing. One study of the laxity

Table 8.20 Grades of Ulnar Collateral Ligament Tears Determined by Stress Testing

Grade 1	Pain but no laxity.
Grade 2	Pain, some laxity, but a definite end point is present. This usually signifies a partial tear.
Grade 3	Pain and gross laxity with no definitive end point.

Data from Avery III DM, Inkellis ER, Carlson MG: Thumb collateral ligament injuries in the athlete. *Curr Rev Musculoskelet Med* 2017;10:28-37.

of bilateral thumb UCLs of uninjured individuals found that 34% of patients had variable laxity from one side to the other. Therefore, perhaps a more reliable indicator of a complete UCL tear on physical examination is the absence of a firm end point on stress testing.[36] When valgus stress is applied to the thumb UCL, the proximal phalanx will have a continuous abduction motion without a palpable stopping point. When this occurs, the examiner can be confident that a complete UCL tear is present.

A grading system for thumb UCL tears has been established and may be useful to help differentiate partial versus complete tears[37] (**Table 8.20**).

A standard set of thumb radiographs that include PA, lateral, and oblique views is always obtained to identify alternative injuries or fractures. There is some controversy in the literature surrounding whether to perform stress testing of a thumb UCL prior to obtaining radiographs. Some think that stress testing an unrecognized bony avulsion fracture could result in further displacement of the bone fragment; others think a stress examination is always necessary, regardless of the presence of a bony injury. The author's preferred method is to assess for tenderness at the UCL on initial physical examination and then obtain a set of screening radiographs prior to stress testing. If a large bony avulsion fragment is identified, stress testing may not be indicated, as the severity of the injury and the subsequent stability of the joint are determined by the displacement of the bony fragment and its potential to heal, not by ligamentous laxity (**Figure 8.51**). If no avulsion fracture is present or only a small sliver of bony avulsion is seen within the tissues, stress testing is performed to assess the ligament's integrity.[38] A set of stress radiographs may help to determine the angle of laxity compared to the uninjured thumb. These radiographs may be obtained after initial screening radiographs to determine that there is no bony component and should be compared to the uninjured thumb.

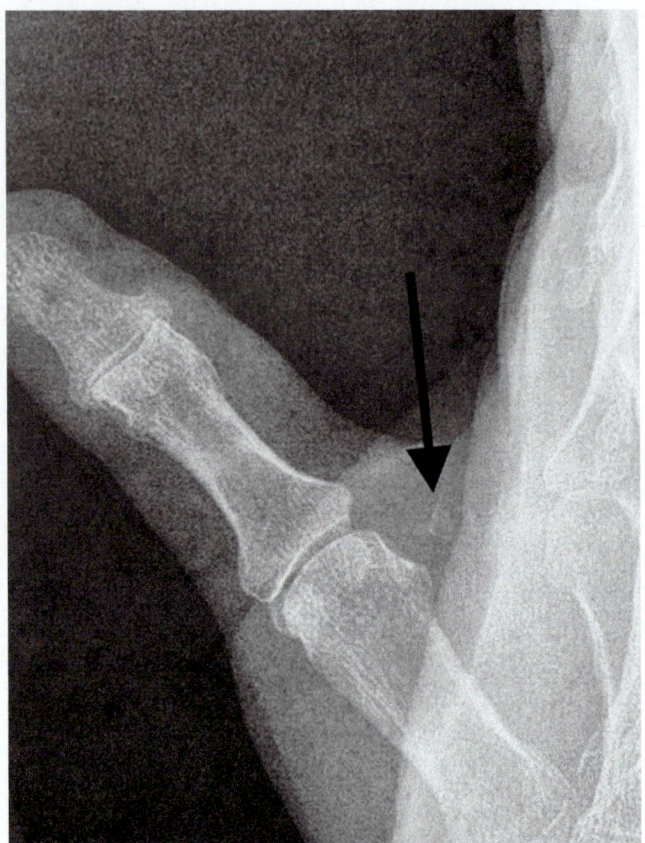

Figure 8.51 Radiograph of the thumb with a displaced ulnar collateral ligament avulsion fracture (arrow).
Courtesy of Sara Rynders.

MRI or ultrasonography of the thumb UCL is useful to differentiate partial from complete ligament tears when physical examination is inconclusive. These studies can also help to determine the presence of a Stener lesion. A recent literature review reported that ultrasonography was 76% sensitive and 81% specific at identifying complete UCL tears.[39] MRI has been shown to be superior to ultrasonography at identifying UCL injuries and is 100% specific and sensitive.[40]

Treatment of UCL injuries is determined by the instability of the joint. If the UCL is determined to be a grade 1 or 2 injury—that is, a partial tear without laxity—the patient is treated with continuous thumb spica casting or splint immobilization for 4 weeks followed by 2 additional weeks of splint immobilization and ROM. Frequently, patients in unskilled positions can play through this injury with proper protection techniques. In the presence of a grade 3, or complete, ligament tear, surgical repair is recommended. This can be performed using a wide variety of techniques, including direct ligament repair or suture anchor technique. Chronic, unstable injuries may require a more complex reconstruction using tendon grafts. Recovery after surgery can take 6 to 8 weeks.

After surgery, patients can expect to regain ROM of the MCP joint to 80% to 90% of the uninjured thumb and pinch and grip strength within 5% to 10% of the uninjured side.[41]

The differential diagnosis of thumb UCL injuries includes RCL injuries, volar plate or capsular injuries of the thumb MCP joint, fracture or dislocation of the thumb proximal phalanx or metacarpal, Bennett or Rolando fractures, and contusion of the thenar eminence. Sprains and ruptures of the thumb UCL are injuries that should not be missed, as chronic laxity of the ligament results in chronic pain, instability, and early onset of arthritis.

Five-Minute Sideline Assessment

The patient with a thumb UCL injury will report a sudden hyperextension or abduction force on the thumb, such as "my thumb bent backward." The patient will report pain around the thenar eminence of the thumb and the MCP joint. The clinician should perform an immediate evaluation to palpate for tenderness at the ulnar aspect of the thumb MCP joint. If the area is tender, a set of screening radiographs should be performed prior to stress testing to evaluate for an avulsion fracture. If the patient participates in a non-skilled position, it is possible for the thumb to be taped, splinted, and protected for immediate return to play prior to a thorough evaluation.

Finger PIP Joint Injuries

Injury to the finger PIP joint is a commonly encountered occurrence in sports and activity. There are myriad injuries that may occur due to falls, twists, lacerations, crush injuries, impact from equipment or contact with another player, or forceful finger gripping. This section will focus on three of the most commonly encountered PIP joint injuries with emphasis on thorough examination of the joint.

The PIP joint is a hinge joint with a normal ROM from 0° to 100°. It is stabilized by the bony contour of the convex proximal phalanx condyles within the concave middle phalanx facets as well as by collateral ligaments and a stout fibrocartilaginous volar plate (**Figure 8.52**). Finger movement is accomplished through a complex set of intrinsic and extrinsic hand muscles. Speaking plainly, flexion of the PIP joint occurs due to the pull of the flexor digitorum superficialis (FDS) tendon, which inserts in a bifurcated fashion at the base of the middle phalanx (**Figure 8.53**). Extension of the PIP joint occurs due to the extensor hood mechanism of the finger and in particular the insertion of the extensor digitorum communis tendon's central slip on the dorsal base of the middle phalanx (**Figure 8.54**).

Frequently, injury to the PIP joint is incorrectly disregarded as a jammed finger; however, this term describes a mechanism of injury and does nothing to define the actual structural derangement of the injured digit. Is the collateral ligament sprained? Is the volar plate disrupted? From this moment forward, the clinician will be able examine and describe the exact anatomic injury to the PIP joint.

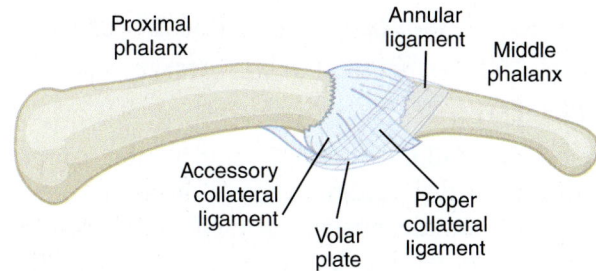

Figure 8.52 Drawing showing the anatomy of the proximal interphalangeal joint.

© Jones & Bartlett Learning

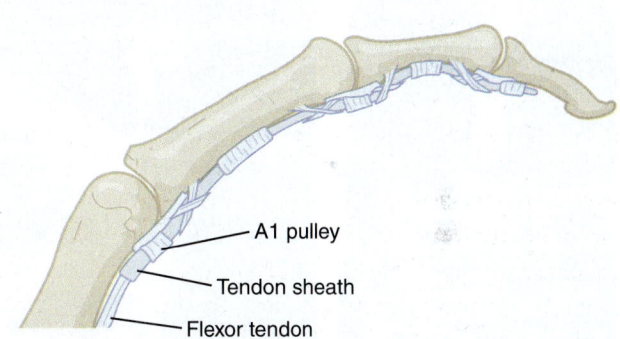

Figure 8.53 Drawing showing the flexor tendon anatomy.

© Jones & Bartlett Learning

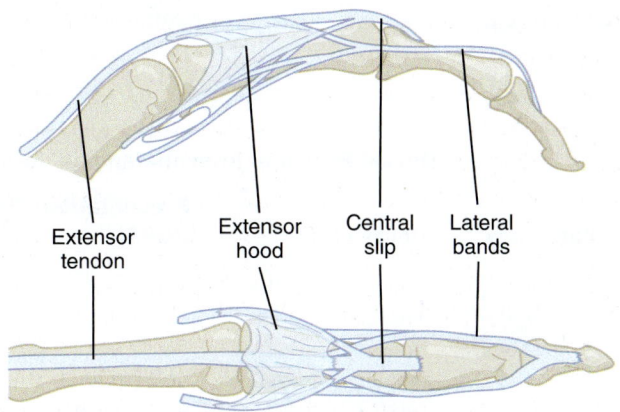

Figure 8.54 Drawing showing the extensor tendon anatomy.

© Jones & Bartlett Learning

Dorsal PIP Joint Dislocations and Volar Plate Avulsion Fractures

Dorsal dislocation of the PIP joint is more common than a volar dislocation. A dorsal dislocation occurs when the middle phalanx is displaced dorsal relative to the proximal phalanx (**Figure 8.55**). This can occur from a hyperextension mechanism combined with a sudden axial force, such as when the fingertip is struck by a ball. The injury may present as a frank dislocation, called a bayonet position, or as a subtle hyperextension of the joint appreciated on examination or radiograph (**Table 8.21**).

Concomitant periarticular fractures can also occur with a dislocation. The volar plate attaches to the middle phalanx and acts as a check against hyperextension of the PIP joint. When the finger is forcibly hyperextended, stress is placed across the volar plate, and it can rupture, sometimes pulling a small piece

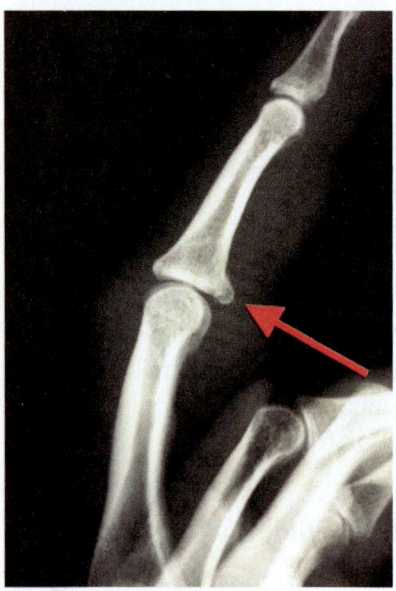

Figure 8.56 Lateral radiograph showing a volar plate avulsion fracture (arrow).
Courtesy of Sara Rynders.

of bone off of the volar base of the middle phalanx. When present, these injuries are visible on radiographs (**Figure 8.56**).

PIP Joint Fracture-Dislocations

PIP joint fracture-dislocations can be very complex and difficult injuries to treat successfully (**Table 8.22**). Frequently, the joint becomes impacted, as the base of the middle phalanx splits on the head of the proximal phalanx. This fracture pattern is called a pilon fracture. All PIP joint fracture-dislocations should be taped and splinted in a position of comfort and referred to an orthopaedic surgeon.

Central Slip Injury

The central slip is the term used to describe the central extensor mechanism of the finger that terminates at the PIP joint. It arises from the extensor digitorum

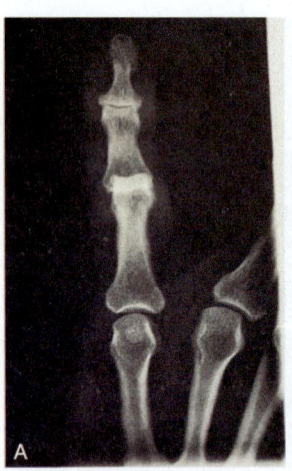 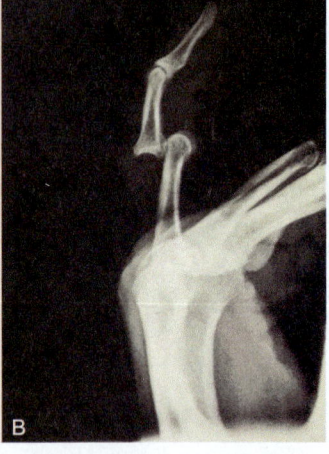

Figure 8.55 Radiographs of a dorsal proximal interphalangeal joint dislocation. **A.** PA view of the finger demonstrating overlap of the middle phalanx on the proximal phalanx. **B.** Lateral view of the finger demonstrating a dorsally dislocated middle phalanx.
Courtesy of Sara Rynders.

Table 8.21 Dorsal Proximal Interphalangeal Joint Dislocation and Volar Plate Avulsion Fractures Quick Tips

Pathology	Description	Presentation (HIPS)	Special Tests/ Imaging	Differential Diagnosis	5-Min Sideline Assessment Tips
Dorsal PIP joint dislocations	Dislocation of the PIP joint in which the middle phalanx displaces dorsal relative to the proximal phalanx	Sudden onset of pain and deformity of the affected finger	Obtain finger radiographs	PIP joint sprain Phalanx fracture Contusion Central slip injury	Assess for PIP joint deformity. Attempt reduction if no open wounds are present and patient will tolerate; otherwise, splint and seek immediate care

HIPS, history, inspection, palpation, special tests; PIP, proximal interphalangeal.

Table 8.22 Proximal Interphalangeal Joint Fracture-Dislocation Quick Tips

Pathology	Description	Presentation (HIPS)	Special Tests/ Imaging	Differential Diagnosis	5-Min Sideline Assessment Tips
PIP joint fracture-dislocations	Impaction-type fracture of the proximal phalanx into the base of the middle phalanx	Sudden onset of finger pain and PIP joint swelling; inability to flex or extend without pain	Obtain finger radiographs	PIP joint sprain PIP joint dislocation Central slip injury Phalanx fracture	Assess for pain and inability to flex or extend at the PIP joint. Splint and obtain radiographs

HIPS, history, inspection, palpation, special tests; PIP, proximal interphalangeal.

communis tendon. Injury to the central slip of the finger can result from a sudden flexion force on the PIP joint, a volar PIP joint dislocation (which is less common), or direct laceration (**Table 8.23**). Central slip injuries may present with an obvious inability to extend at the PIP joint, such as after a laceration, or may present weeks after injury as a subtle flexion deformity at the PIP joint. If left untreated, the unopposed flexion forces across the volar PIP joint drive it into flexion while hyperextension forces at the DIP joint terminal extensor tendon contract the finger PIP joint into a flexed posture known as a boutonniére deformity (**Figure 8.57**). Injury to the central slip requires prompt recognition and extension splinting of the PIP joint. Surgical repair of the central slip is sometimes indicated.

The patient with an injury to the PIP joint will report a moment when the finger was forcibly hyperextended, twisted, stepped on, or jammed. Frequently, fingers are injured by the impact of a ball off the end of the digit while attempting a catch. The patient will localize the pain to the PIP joint of the digit and may report swelling or bruising in the finger.

The examiner should immediately inspect for any open injuries or lacerations. Observe the general alignment of the digit and whether there is any angular or rotational deformity present that could suggest fracture or dislocation. Frequently, the PIP joint will appear noticeably larger than its uninjured counterparts and will have obvious ecchymosis after injury. One truly unforgettable situation is an acutely dislocated PIP joint, in which the finger will be observed to be grossly out of alignment. If the digit is appropriately aligned, the patient should

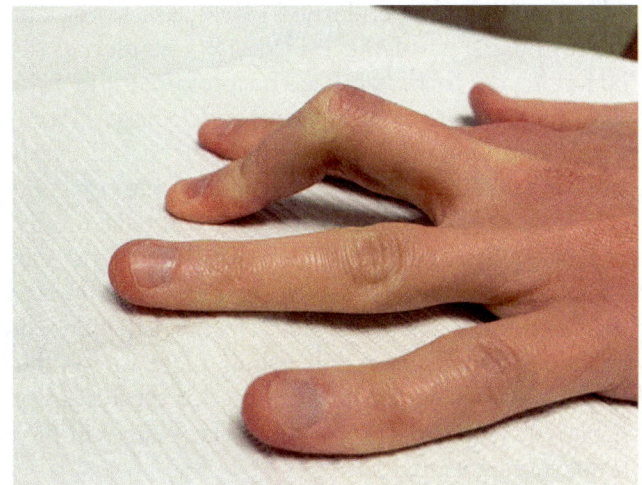

Figure 8.57 Picture showing the pathomechanics of a boutonniére deformity. Note the flexed PIP joint and extended DIP joint.

Courtesy of Sara Rynders.

Table 8.23 Central Slip Injury Quick Tips

Pathology	Description	Presentation (HIPS)	Special Tests/ Imaging	Differential Diagnosis	5-Min Sideline Assessment Tips
Central slip injury	Stretch or rupture of the extensor tendon central slip at its insertion on the dorsal middle phalanx	Sometimes subtle; can occur with a sudden flexion force, volar PIP joint dislocation, or direct laceration	Elson test	PIP joint sprain PIP joint dislocation Phalanx fracture	Assess for finger deformity or open injuries; if present remove from play for further evaluation

HIPS, history, inspection, palpation, special tests; PIP, proximal interphalangeal.

flex and extend the digit as much as comfortably possible and the ROM measurements recorded. An injured PIP joint will often have decreased ROM due to pain and swelling. A central slip injury will have a loss of full extension at the PIP joint.

General examination of the injured digit always begins with palpation for tenderness. Deliberate palpation of specific structures of the PIP is paramount to a good examination. Consider the mantra "bone, ligament, tendon" when examining a finger to ensure the evaluation of all important structures. Palpate the proximal, middle, and distal phalanx for tenderness. Palpate the MCP, PIP, and DIP joints independently for tenderness. Next, assess the collateral ligaments of the PIP joint for tenderness or laxity. To do this, stabilize the proximal and middle phalanx with a thumb and index finger. Apply a varus and valgus stress to the joint in full extension and 30° of flexion and note any pain or laxity (**Figure 8.58**). A sprained PIP joint will have tenderness over the affected collateral ligament and may have laxity on stress testing in flexion. A grossly unstable joint will have laxity in both flexion and extension. Next, assess the volar plate for tenderness by palpating the volar aspect of the PIP joint. A patient with an injury to the volar plate will have tenderness with palpation.

Assess the tendons that cross the PIP joint. Examine the flexor tendons of the finger by asking the patient to place his or her hand on the examination table with the palm up. First test the flexor digitorum profundus (FDP) tendon by placing one finger over the volar middle phalanx to block it and ask the patient to flex the DIP joint. Then, test the FDS tendon by holding the uninvolved fingers in full extension on the examination table and asking the patient to flex the finger at the PIP joint (**Figure 8.59**). If a

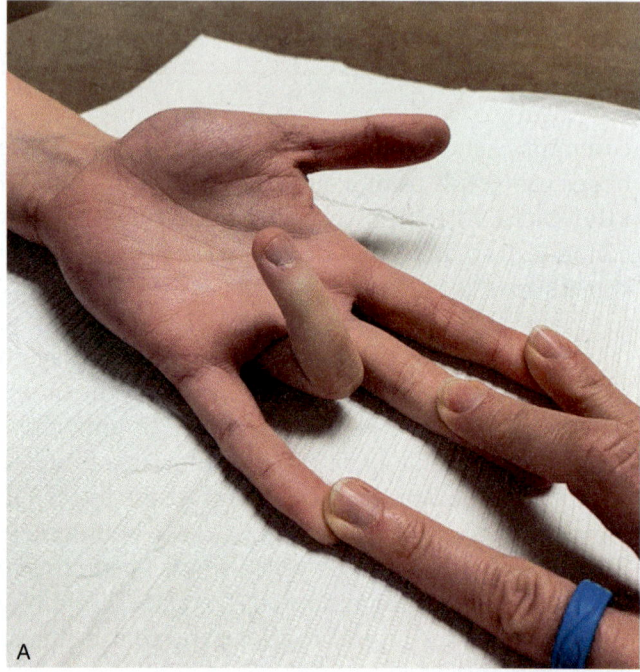

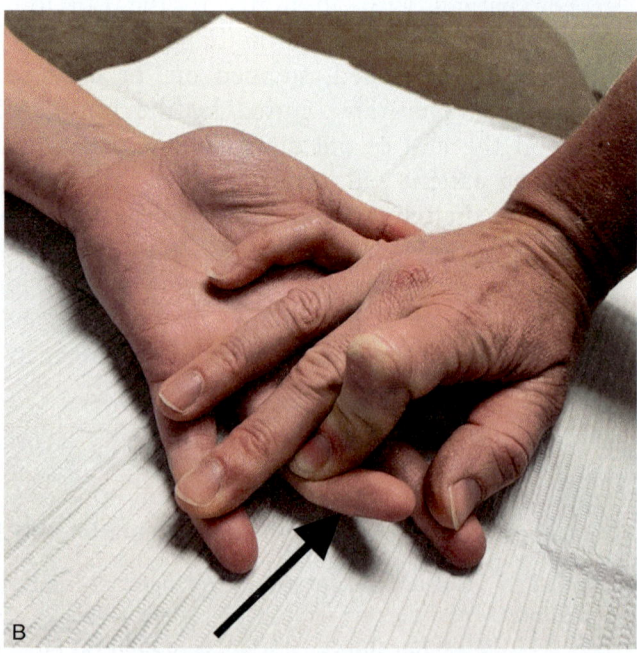

Figure 8.59 Clinical photograph showing the testing of the flexor tendons of the fingers. **A.** Testing of the flexor digitorum superficialis tendon. **B.** Testing of the flexor digitorum profundus tendon.

Courtesy of Sara Rynders.

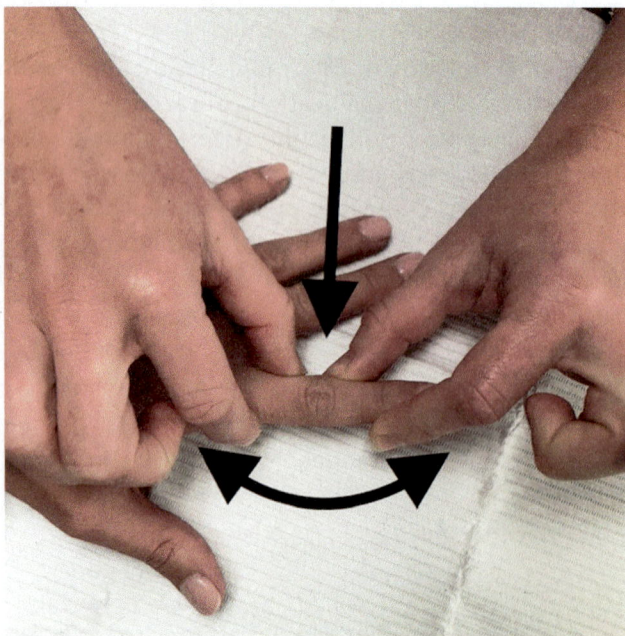

Figure 8.58 Clinical photograph showing the testing of the collateral ligaments of the proximal interphalangeal joint.

Courtesy of Sara Rynders.

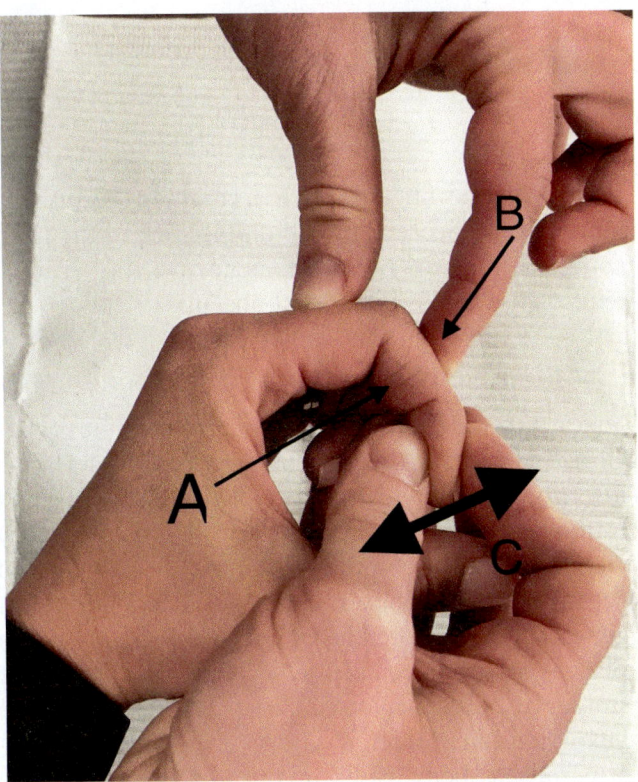

Figure 8.60 Clinical photograph showing the Elson test. **A.** Patient actively extends at proximal interphalangeal joint. **B.** Clinician resists active extension. **C.** Clinician passively flexes and extends at the distal interphalangeal (DIP) joint. A positive test, indicating a central slip rupture, occurs when the DIP joint goes into rigid extension during the test and passive DIP joint motion is not possible.

Courtesy of Sara Rynders.

flexor tendon is injured, the respective joint will not flex upon testing.

Next, examine the extensor tendon insertion at the DIP joint. Ask the patient to actively extend the digit at the PIP joint and note any loss of extension. It is important to remember the anatomy of the extensor mechanism of the finger; finger extension may still be intact even when the central slip is injured because the patient can still extend through an intact terminal extensor tendon at the DIP joint. To isolate the central slip insertion, perform the Elson test (**Figure 8.60**). Ask the patient to flex the fingers into a loose fist position. The examiner places a thumb over the dorsal middle phalanx to block extension. Ask the patient to actively extend against the examiner's thumb. With the other hand, the examiner attempts to passively flex and extend the digit at the DIP joint. If the DIP joint is supple to passive motion, the patient is actively extending through the central slip, and it can be considered intact. However, if the DIP joint becomes rigid in extension during this maneuver, the patient is attempting to extend the PIP joint through the terminal extensor tendon, and the central slip is likely ruptured.

Last, a neurovascular examination is essential in order to perform a complete evaluation. Assess capillary refill and ask the patient whether he or she can feel sensation to light touch on the ulnar and radial aspects of the fingertip and the sensation feels normal compared to other unaffected digits. Often, transient paresthesias may be present when a finger PIP joint is dislocated due to the tension placed across the digital nerves. Sensation should return to normal after the PIP joint is reduced.

It is absolutely necessary to obtain radiographs of an injured PIP joint to evaluate for fracture, dislocation, or subluxation. Obtain PA, lateral, and oblique views of the injured digit. Radiographs of the hand often do not provide enough detail, and a small avulsion fracture could be missed.

Advanced MRI can assess the central slip and volar plate. MRI can be used to augment physical examination but may not be necessary for diagnosis.

An acutely dislocated finger should be reduced immediately. After a thorough neurovascular examination is performed and documented, a local anesthetic should be applied around the digital nerves at the base of the digit to aid with pain control prior to reduction. For dorsal dislocations, the examiner uses his or her thumb to apply a constant dorsal pressure over the prominent middle phalanx, while simultaneously pulling longitudinal traction and slight flexion until the middle phalanx reduces into the PIP joint. For lateral dislocations, the examiner applies longitudinal traction to the digit and constant pressure over the middle phalanx in the lateral position. Postreduction radiographs should be obtained to confirm reduction and rule out fractures. It is prudent to reexamine the PIP joint for stability after reduction. Test each collateral ligament for stability in extension and 30° of flexion. If the ligaments give a firm end point, the joint is stable. Then, ask the patient to flex and extend the digit through ROM. If the joint remains reduced through ROM, the finger may be buddy taped and full ROM can be started immediately. If the joint re-dislocates during ROM, an extension blocking aluminum splint can be applied in a position that keeps the joint reduced. This flexed position also approximates the volar plate for healing. An orthopaedic surgeon should be consulted to monitor gradual return to full motion.

If the examiner has difficulty reducing the joint, it is possible that the volar plate has become interposed into the PIP joint and is blocking the reduction. In this instance, an orthopaedic surgeon should be consulted, as multiple repeated attempts at reduction are not recommended. Occasionally, surgical reduction is necessary.

If a volar plate avulsion fracture is present on radiograph, it is necessary to quantify the fracture's size and amount of displacement. Nonsurgical management with splinting is indicated if the PIP joint is reduced, the fracture encompasses less than 40% of the middle phalanx joint surface, and the fracture is nondisplaced in 30° of PIP joint flexion. An aluminum splint in 30° of dorsal block should be applied, and repeat imaging studies should be obtained to ensure proper alignment of the fracture. Finger extension can gradually be increased by 10° weekly until full ROM is achieved. Return to play is anticipated approximately 6 weeks after the injury or sooner for unskilled positions. If the fracture does not meet the aforementioned criteria, surgical fixation may be required.[41]

If a central slip injury is identified, the patient's PIP joint should be continuously splinted in full extension for approximately 6 weeks. The patient should undergo therapy for DIP joint flexion, and an orthopaedic surgeon should be consulted. It takes 10 to 12 weeks for the central slip to heal and ROM to be achieved.

The most common complication of injury to the PIP joint is stiffness. Patients may also experience chronic PIP joint enlargement or nodularity due to formation of a posttraumatic scar. If a central slip rupture is missed, a boutonniére deformity may develop. If a volar plate injury is not properly treated, a contracture of the PIP joint may develop. Complex PIP joint fracture-dislocations are prone to the development of posttraumatic arthritis. Luckily, with proper identification and treatment, most patients treated for minor PIP joint sprains have full return of motion and function within 4 to 6 weeks of injury.

> **Five-Minute Sideline Assessment**
>
> Quickly assess the finger for any lacerations or open wounds. Observe any gross deformity of the digit that could indicate a fracture or dislocation; if present, obtain a radiograph and reduce the dislocation as described previously. If the finger appears well aligned, ask the patient to flex and extend the digit to the extent to which he or she is comfortable. Perform a thorough assessment for tenderness and stress test the collateral ligaments to check for gross instability. If finger motion is preserved and the PIP joint is stable on testing, the finger can be buddy taped for comfort, and play can be resumed. Thorough examination with radiographic testing should be performed after play has terminated.

Finger Tendon Injuries: Jersey Finger and Mallet Finger

Injuries to the fingertips are a common occurrence in athletics. This section will discuss two of the most common fingertip injuries that involve the terminal tendon insertions at the distal phalanx.

Jersey Finger

Jersey finger is a term used to describe an avulsion or closed rupture of the FDP tendon from its terminal insertion on the volar aspect of the distal phalanx (**Figure 8.61**). The term refers to the mechanism by which this injury commonly occurs: the FDP tendon ruptures from its bony attachment when a flexed finger is suddenly, forcibly extended, such as when a player grabs the neck of a jersey and the other player suddenly pulls away as in football and rugby. The flexor tendon, under traction force from the forearm muscle belly, pulls in one direction, and the bone is pulled in the other direction by the jersey (**Table 8.24**). The ring finger is the most commonly involved digit.

The patient with a jersey finger injury will report a sudden event, such as grabbing a jersey or getting a finger caught in equipment, and subsequently will notice an inability to flex the tip of the injured finger. Frequently, the patient will report feeling a "pop" or burning sensation in the finger at the time of injury. Occasionally, the patient will report feeling

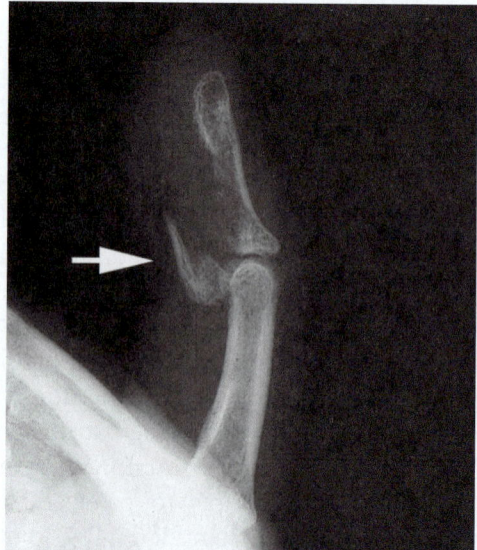

Figure 8.61 Lateral radiograph of a jersey finger (arrow).

Reproduced from Johnson TR, Steinbach LS, eds: *Essentials of Musculoskeletal Imaging*. Rosemont, IL, American Academy of Orthopaedic Surgeons, 2004.

Finger Tendon Injuries: Jersey Finger and Mallet Finger

Table 8.24 Jersey Finger Quick Tips

Pathology	Description	Presentation (HIPS)	Special Tests/Imaging	Differential Diagnosis	5-Min Sideline Assessment Tips
Jersey finger	Flexor digitorum profundus tendon rupture from its insertion on the distal phalanx	Occurs after a sudden resisted force on a flexed DIP joint Inability to flex the DIP joint of the finger	Attempt active flexion of an isolated DIP joint	Finger sprain Fracture Mallet finger	Assess the patient's ability to perform isolated DIP joint flexion. If unable to flex at the DIP joint, splint the digit in flexion and refer for orthopaedic evaluation

DIP, distal interphalangeal; HIPS, history, inspection, palpation, special tests.

pressure or discomfort along the course of the tendon into the palm.

The clinician will observe the affected digit to be resting in an extended position at the DIP joint (**Figure 8.62**). This is due to the unopposed extension force from the extensor tendon dorsally. There may be some edema or ecchymosis noted at the volar distal or middle phalanx. Note any open injuries that could indicate a tendon laceration, instead of a tendon rupture.

Examination of the digit should begin with palpation. Palpate the digit along the course of the flexor tendon, starting distally at its insertion site and working into the palm; note any tenderness. Often, the patient will report tenderness over the volar distal phalanx near the DIP joint and possibly at the level of the tendon stump. Palpate for any firm masses in the digit or the palm that could indicate the level of the ruptured tendon, though this is not always possible. Next, examine the flexor tendons of the finger. Ask the patient to place his or her hand on the examination table with the palm up. The examiner places one finger over the volar middle phalanx to block it and asks the patient to flex the DIP joint. If a jersey finger is present, the patient will not be able to flex at the DIP joint. Next, the examiner holds the uninvolved fingers in full extension on the examination table and asks the patient to flex the finger at the PIP joint. Note that a patient with a jersey finger will be able to flex the PIP joint because the FDS tendon remains intact. Finally, perform a neurovascular examination of the fingertip, including capillary refill and sensation to light touch, on the radial and ulnar borders of the digit. The neurovascular examination should be normal.

Obtain PA, lateral, and oblique views of the affected hand. A radiograph of the affected hand is essential for two reasons: First, it can help to rule out alternative diagnoses, such as a fingertip fracture, and, second, it is sometimes possible to identify the level of the retracted tendon stump if a small fleck of bone remains attached to the tendon and is visible on radiograph. Larger avulsion fractures may also be identified on radiograph.

Ultrasonography or MRI may be useful tools to help confirm the injury and identify the level of tendon retraction. Knowing the level of tendon retraction guides treatment recommendations and can limit the amount of surgical dissection and time. Neither modality is proven more reliable, though ultrasonography results can be variable if the sonographer is inexperienced.

Unlike extensor tendons, flexor tendons are under a considerable amount of tension, even at rest. Therefore, when a flexor tendon is ruptured, it is prone to retraction away from the injury site. There are three types of FDP avulsions as classified

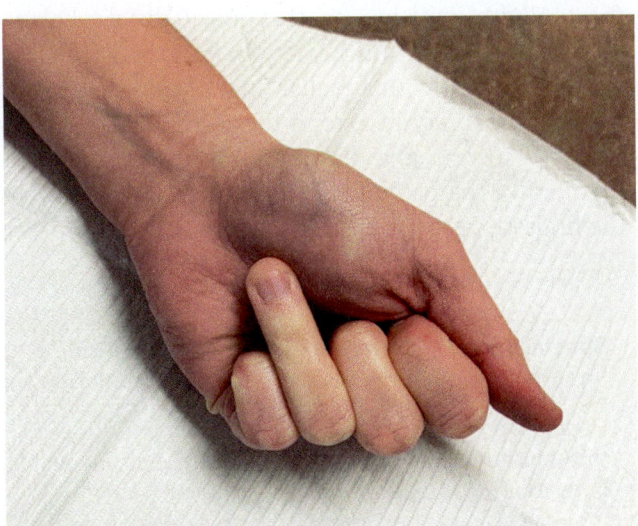

Figure 8.62 Photograph showing the loss of distal interphalangeal (DIP) joint flexion on inspection. Note the DIP joint extension when this patient with a jersey finger injury makes a fist.

Courtesy of Sara Rynders.

by Leddy and Packer. Type 1 injuries occur when the tendon ruptures from its insertion and retracts into the palm; these injuries require surgical repair within 7 to 10 days due to the loss of blood supply to the tendon. Type 2 injuries are most common and occur when the tendon ruptures and retracts to the level of the PIP joint. Surgical treatment can be delayed if necessary for a patient to complete a competition or season. Type 3 injuries occur when a bony avulsion is present. Generally, the bony prominence prevents the tendon from retracting past the level of the A4 pulley. These injuries must be treated as fractures and require immediate surgical repair.[42] If a jersey finger is discovered late, complex or staged tendon reconstruction may be necessary.

Complex hand therapy is necessary following a flexor tendon repair. Several protocols exist and are used based on surgeon preference. Patients can expect to return to play by 8 to 12 weeks after repair if they can demonstrate painless functional ROM and grip strength greater than or equal to 80% of the uninjured hand. Common side effects of injury and repair are stiffness and tendon adhesions, some of which require repeat surgical attention. Adherence to a prescribed therapeutic protocol is paramount to a good recovery.

The differential diagnosis of a jersey finger injury is fracture, tendon rupture or laceration at a different level, or nerve lesion resulting in loss of finger flexion. The clinician should be able to perform a thorough and specific examination of the affected finger to specify the exact structure that has been injured.

Mallet Finger

Mallet finger refers to an avulsion or rupture of the terminal extensor tendon at its insertion on the dorsum of the distal phalanx (**Table 8.25**). These injuries typically occur when the distal phalanx is forcibly flexed while the distal phalanx is actively extended, such as jamming the end of the finger on an object

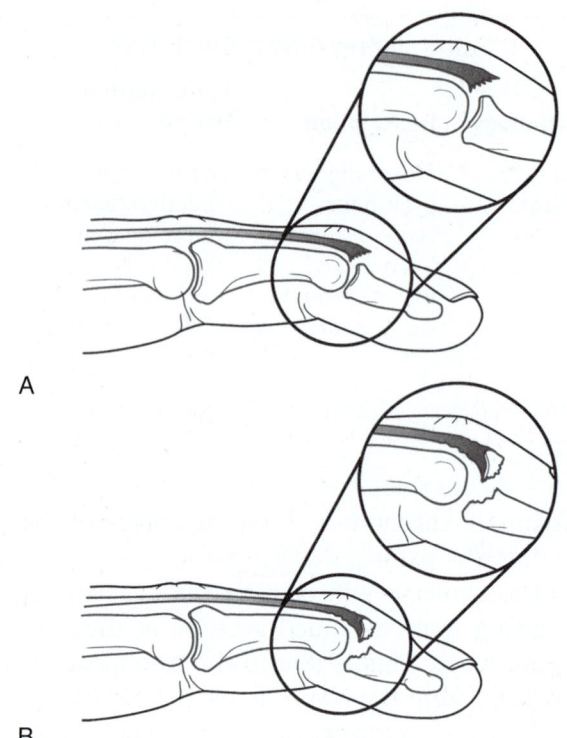

Figure 8.63 A. Drawing of a soft-tissue mallet finger injury caused by a rupture of the extensor tendon. **B.** Drawing of a soft-tissue mallet finger injury caused by an avulsion.

Reproduced from Johnson TR, Steinbach LS, eds: *Essentials of Musculoskeletal Imaging.* Rosemont, IL, American Academy of Orthopaedic Surgeons, 2004.

or ball. These injuries are common in ball-handling and contact sports. A mallet finger injury may occur as an isolated rupture of the extensor tendon, termed soft-tissue mallet finger, or as an avulsion fracture of the tendon's insertion on the dorsal distal phalanx, termed bony mallet finger (**Figure 8.63**).

The patient with a mallet finger injury will report a sudden inability to extend the distal phalanx and a flexed posture of the distal phalanx at the DIP joint. Frequently, the patient will remember an event when the fingertip was jammed or forcibly flexed. He or she

Table 8.25 Mallet Finger Quick Tips

Pathology	Description	Presentation (HIPS)	Special Tests/ Imaging	Differential Diagnosis	5-Min Sideline Assessment Tips
Mallet finger	Rupture of the terminal extensor tendon from its insertion on the dorsal distal phalanx	Patient reports he or she jammed the finger Distal phalanx is in a flexed position with inability to actively extend at the DIP joint	Radiographs to evaluate for bony injury	Finger sprain Fracture Jersey finger	Observe for flexed position of the distal phalanx. Splint in extension and evaluate the digit after play

HIPS, history, inspection, palpation, special tests.

will mention that he or she has not been able to extend the distal phalanx since that time and may report pain or burning pain over the dorsal DIP joint.

The clinician will observe the affected digit to be resting in a flexed position at the DIP joint. This is due to the unopposed flexion force from the FDP tendon volarly. There may be some edema or ecchymosis noted at the dorsal distal or middle phalanx. Note any open injuries that could indicate a tendon laceration instead of a tendon rupture. Also, note whether an injury has occurred to the nail plate or nail bed, such as a bruise, called a subungual hematoma.

Begin the examination by noting the degree of flexion at the DIP joint. With the finger in full extension at the MCP and PIP joints, ask the patient to try to actively extend the finger at the DIP joint. A patient with a mallet finger injury will not be able to actively extend the DIP joint. Palpate the DIP joint and distal phalanx for tenderness, as the patient may have soreness over the dorsal DIP joint. Also, check the FDS and FDP tendons as previously described in this section. The flexor tendons should be fully intact. Perform a thorough neurovascular examination, including capillary refill and sensation to light touch, on the radial and ulnar borders of the digit, which should be normal and intact in the setting of a mallet finger.

Obtain PA, unsupported lateral and oblique views of the affected digit. A true lateral view is essential, as careful inspection of the DIP joint on lateral radiographs will determine treatment options. The DIP should not be passively extended while the radiograph is obtained so that subluxation of the distal phalanx can be appreciated if present. A mallet finger injury will appear as a flexed distal phalanx on the lateral radiograph. First, evaluate the distal phalanx for presence of a bony avulsion fracture from the dorsal rim. If present, measure the amount of fragment displacement and note whether the joint line has been disrupted. Next, evaluate for volar subluxation of the distal phalanx off the head of the middle phalanx (**Figure 8.64**).

Advanced imaging is not necessary for the diagnosis and management of mallet finger injuries.

Most mallet finger injuries can be managed nonsurgically with a prolonged course of 6 to 12 weeks of continuous DIP joint extension splinting or serial DIP joint extension casting (**Figure 8.65**). Bony mallet finger injuries usually unite within 6 to 8 weeks, whereas soft-tissue mallet finger injuries take somewhere between 8 and 12 weeks to heal. However, if there is subluxation of the distal phalanx, a displaced fracture, and/or a fracture fragment that encompasses 40% of the joint line or more, the mallet finger injury will

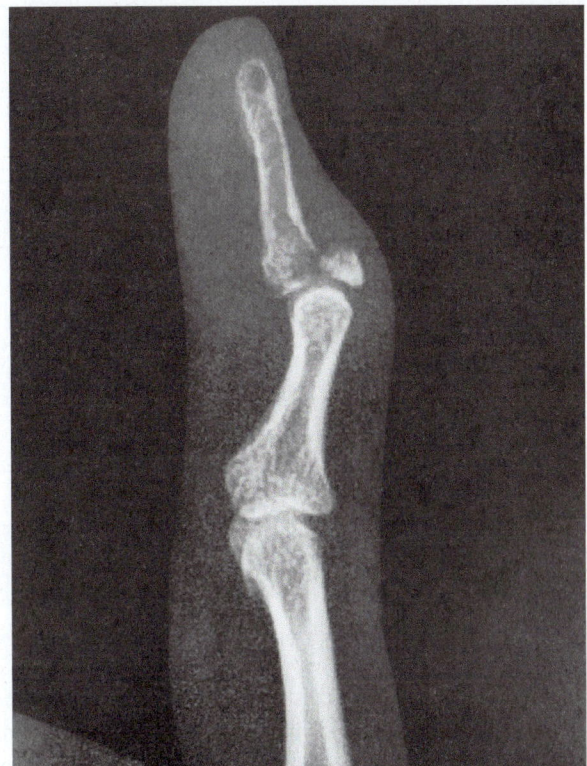

Figure 8.64 Radiograph of a bony mallet finger with volar subluxation of the distal phalanx.

Courtesy of Sara Rynders.

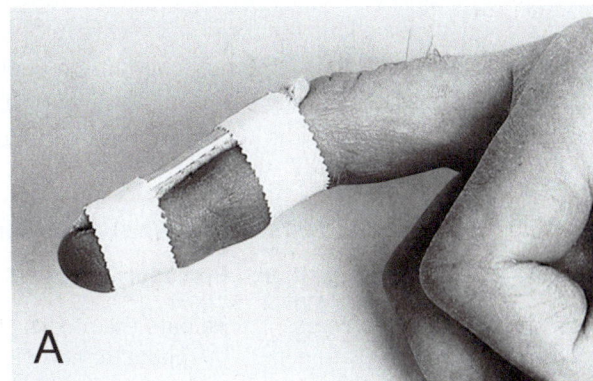
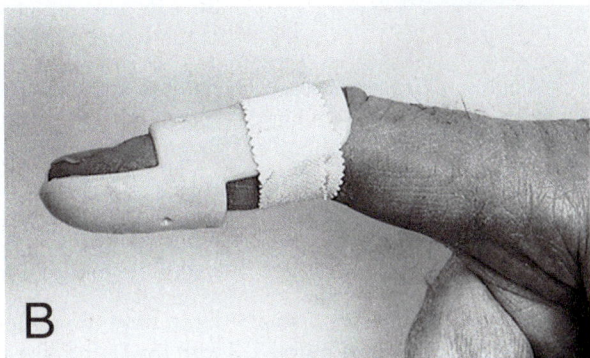

Figure 8.65 A and **B**, Photographs of extension splinting of a mallet finger injury.

Reproduced from Armstrong AD, Hubbard MC, eds: *Essentials of Musculoskeletal Care*, ed 5. Burlington, MA, American Academy of Orthopaedic Surgeons, 2015.

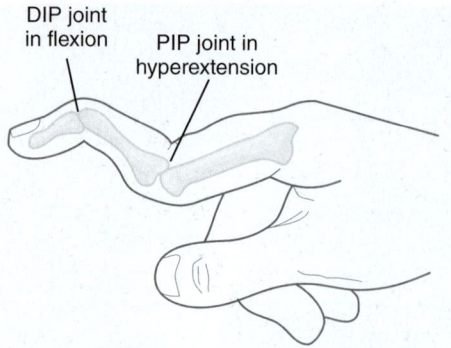

Figure 8.66 Drawing showing a swan-neck deformity.
DIP, distal interphalangeal; PIP, proximal interphalangeal.
© Jones & Bartlett Learning

require surgical management for tendon repair or fracture reduction and pinning.

If a mallet finger injury goes untreated or undertreated or fails to respond to prolonged splinting, a swan-neck deformity may develop (**Figure 8.66**). A swan-neck deformity occurs when the terminal extensor tendon is disrupted and the DIP joint falls into flexion. The lateral bands of the extensor mechanism compensate to provide extension of the digit but, in doing so, cause hyperextension of the PIP joint. If left untreated, this deformity can become permanent and interfere with the ability to flex the digit.

With appropriate treatment, mallet finger injuries have a good to excellent outcome for return to play and full hand function. Delaying treatment of soft-tissue mallet fingers for up to 1 month after injury has not been shown to affect the tendon's ability to heal.

Therefore, treatment of soft-tissue mallet finger injuries can be delayed if necessary to complete a competition or season. Additionally, many players can continue their sport even with the application of the extensor splint, as it does not interfere with most hand function.

It is not uncommon for the patient to have a residual extensor lag of up to 10° to 15° after appropriate treatment. This occurs more often with soft-tissue mallet finger injuries because the extensor tendons heal in a slightly stretched or lengthened position. This small amount of residual extensor lag is usually inconsequential and would be of concern only if a swan-neck deformity developed.

Five-Minute Sideline Assessment

If a patient reports an injury to the fingertip, assess for any obvious deformity, such as flexion of the DIP joint consistent with a mallet finger injury. If the finger is held in extension, ask the patient to actively flex the digit, and test the FDP and FDS tendons independently. If the patient is unable to flex at the DIP joint, a jersey finger is the likely diagnosis. In either scenario, if there are no open injuries and the patient is not experiencing severe pain, the DIP joint can be splinted or taped in extension for protection, and the patient can resume play. Thorough examination, including radiographs, should occur immediately upon the completion of the game.

A summary of the special tests for the wrist and hand can be found in **Table 8.26**.

Table 8.26 Special Tests for the Wrist and Hand

Test	Patient Position	Procedure	Positive Test	Implication	Evidence
Anatomic snuffbox tenderness	Seated across from examiner, hand on table	Palpate the recess created by the abductor pollicis longus and extensor pollicis brevis tendons and the extensor pollicis longus tendon at the radial base of the thumb.	Pain during palpation	Scaphoid fracture	85% sensitive and 29% specific for scaphoid fracture
Scaphoid tubercle tenderness	Seated across from examiner, hand on table	Palpate the scaphoid tubercle at the volar-radial base of the wrist. It can be identified by following the flexor carpi radialis tendon distally until a bony prominence is encountered. Place the wrist in slight extension to make the tubercle more prominent.	Pain during palpation	Scaphoid fracture	95% sensitive and 74% specific
Finkelstein test	Seated across from examiner with hand on table	First, have the patient form a fist with the thumb tucked under the fingers. Ask him or her to relax the wrist. The clinician then places the wrist in neutral and passively, ulnarly deviates the wrist.	Pain and apprehension	de Quervain tenosynovitis	Not reported

Test	Patient Position	Procedure	Positive Test	Implication	Evidence
Watson scaphoid shift test	Patient seated across examination table with elbow resting on table, hand elevated in the air (arm-wrestle position)	The clinician places one hand on the radial aspect of the wrist and, with the thumb, applies direct, constant pressure over the scaphoid tubercle. The patient relaxes the wrist, and the clinician then passively moves the wrist from ulnar to radial deviation while keeping constant pressure over the scaphoid tubercle.	A palpable and frequently painful "clunk" is felt when the scaphoid contacts the dorsal rim of the radius	Probable scapholunate ligament tear	48% sensitive and 67% specific for scapholunate injuries
LT shear test	Patient seated across examination table with elbow resting on table, hand elevated in the air (arm-wrestle position)	The clinician places one thumb dorsally over the lunate and applies pressure to stabilize it. With the other thumb, the clinician applies an opposing volar pressure over the pisiform.	Pain, crepitus, and laxity	LT tear	Sensitive, but not very specific, for LT tears
Ulna fovea sign	Patient seated across table from examiner, hand on table	Palpate the TFCC in the soft recess on the ulnar side of the wrist located just distal to the ulnar styloid and between the extensor carpi ulnaris and flexor carpi ulnaris tendons, known as the foveal recess.	Tenderness at the ulnar fovea	TFCC tear	95.2% sensitive and 86.5% specific for a TFCC tear
Ulnar grind test	Patient seated across table from examiner	With the patient's affected wrist in neutral, the examiner places his or her hand into the patient's as if the two were going to shake hands. With the other hand, the examiner stabilizes the forearm. Then, the examiner places the patient's wrist into extension and applies an axial load with the wrist in ulnar deviation. This creates an axial load across the TFCC.	Pain with testing	TFCC tear	
Piano key test	Patient seated across table from examiner	The examiner places one hand on the radius and, with the other, applies dorsal to volar pressure over the distal ulna. Then, the test is performed on the unaffected wrist for comparison of laxity.	Increased motion, laxity, or pain with testing	Distal radioulnar joint instability related to TFCC tear	
Hook of hamate pull test	Patient is seated across table from examiner with palm up	The examiner places the patient's wrist in extreme ulnar deviation. The patient closes the fingers into flexion, and the examiner tries to extend the ring and small fingers from the DIP joints against resistance from the patient.	Moderate to extreme pain at the hook of hamate (ulnar volar palm)	Hook of hamate fracture	Possibly 100% sensitive; specificity not tested

(continues)

Table 8.26 Special Tests for the Wrist and Hand (continued)

Test	Patient Position	Procedure	Positive Test	Implication	Evidence
UCL stress test	Patient seated across from examiner	Stabilize the thumb metacarpal with one hand and, with the other, apply a valgus stress to the proximal phalanx. Perform this maneuver with the metacarpophalangeal joint in full extension and in 30° of flexion.	Pain without laxity, pain and laxity, laxity alone	Pain without laxity can indicate a partial UCL tear; pain and laxity can indicate a high-grade partial or complete UCL tear; laxity without pain may indicate a chronic injury	Highly variable and likely related to examiner's experience
Elson test	Patient seated across from examiner	Ask the patient to flex the fingers into a loose fist position. The examiner places a thumb over the dorsal middle phalanx to block extension. Ask the patient to actively extend against the examiner's thumb. With the other hand, the examiner attempts to passively flex and extend the digit at the DIP joint.	DIP joint becomes rigid in extension during the maneuver	Central slip injury	

DIP, distal interphalangeal; LT, lunotriquetral; TFCC, triangular fibrocartilage complex; UCL, ulnar collateral ligament.

CASE STUDY 1

A 21-year-old, right-handed man who is a hurdler misses his last hurdle, stumbles, and falls during the final event of his state championship. He gets up after the fall but is holding his right wrist in pain. He presents to the athletic trainer covering the event. He states that the only thing that hurts is his right wrist, and he points to the radial side.

1. What do you do first? What is the differential diagnosis?
2. What should be included in the examination?
3. What is the first line of treatment?
4. What radiographic views should be obtained?

Six days later, the patient is seen in the orthopaedic clinic. The provider removes the splint and performs an examination. The patient continues to report tenderness at the anatomic snuffbox and now has mild edema on the radial side of the wrist. The provider repeats a series of wrist radiographs (**Figure 8.67**).

1. What is the diagnosis?

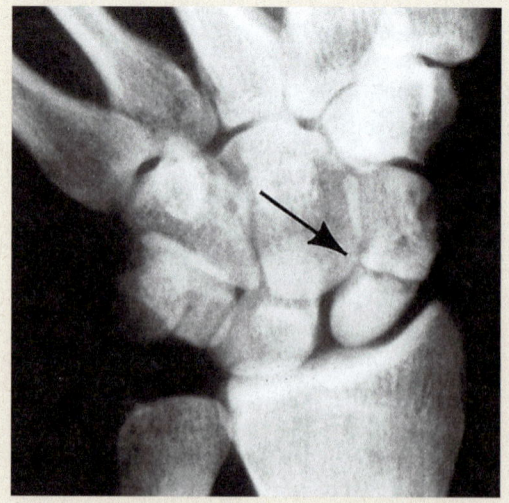

Figure 8.67 Radiograph of the wrist shows a nondisplaced scaphoid fracture (arrow).

Reproduced from Armstrong AD, Hubbard MC, eds: *Essentials of Musculoskeletal Care*, ed 5. Burlington, MA, American Academy of Orthopaedic Surgeons, 2015.

CASE STUDY 2

A 19-year-old, left-handed man who is a linebacker is at football practice doing tackle drills when he is observed to be holding his right middle finger and shaking his hand after a hard hit. He does not seek evaluation during practice.

Later that day, he is in the athletic training room and asks the athletic trainer to look at his right middle finger. He states that he is not really sure what he did to it but he thinks he may have jammed it during drills earlier that day.

The clinician asks the patient to localize the area of pain, and he points to the right middle finger PIP joint. The athletic trainer observes the right hand and notices that the right middle finger PIP joint is noticeably larger than the other digits. There is edema present and a small amount of ecchymosis volarly. There are no open injuries or abrasions. The finger is held in a slightly flexed posture at the PIP joint.

1. What is the differential diagnosis?

The clinician refers the patient for a finger radiograph. PA, lateral, and oblique views of the middle finger are obtained. The PIP joint is noted to be in approximately 30° of flexion, but the joint is reduced. A small, minimally displaced 1-mm avulsion fracture is seen on the lateral radiograph (**Figure 8.68**).

1. What is the diagnosis?

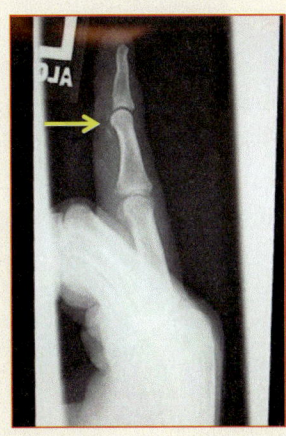

Figure 8.68 Lateral radiograph of the injured finger (arrow).

Reproduced from Avery DM, Rodner CM, Edgar CM: Sports-related wrist and hand injuries: a review. *J Orthop Surg Res* 2016;11(1):99.

ONE-IN-A-MILLION CASE STUDY

A 22-year-old left-handed college baseball catcher experiences acute right-hand pain after catching a hard pitch in his gloved hand during a game. He is evaluated in the dugout and is able to flex and extend the digits and has a normal neurovascular examination. There are no open injuries. There is tenderness in the palm and at the volar base of the right middle finger. His hand pain is severe enough that he cannot tolerate catching with the right hand, and he is pulled from the game. The athletic trainer applies ice to the right hand.

After the game, he is examined in the athletic training room. His right palm is observed to be mildly edematous and ecchymotic. There is some edema limiting the motion of the index, middle, and ring finger MCP joints. He has full MCP joint extension to 0° and MCP joint flexion to approximately 60° in the affected digits. He has tenderness to palpation along the middle finger volar proximal phalanx, volar MCP joint, and palm. There is no tenderness of the finger DIP and PIP joints. There is no tenderness to palpation over the remainder of the digits, thumb, or wrist.

The patient is sent for PA, lateral, and oblique radiographic views of the hand (**Figures 8.69** and **8.70**).

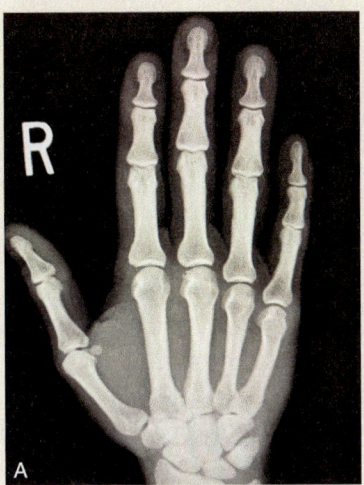 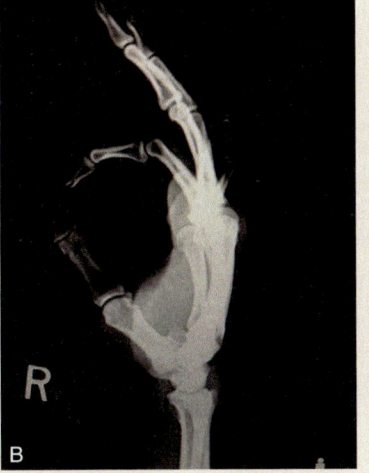 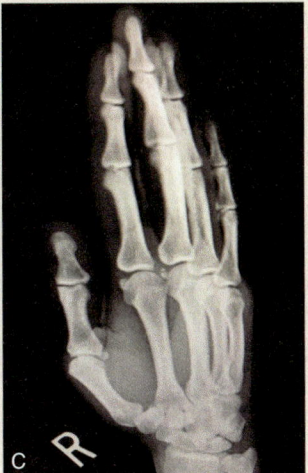

Figure 8.69 Radiographs of the injured hand. **A.** PA view. **B.** Lateral view. **C.** Oblique view.

Courtesy of Sara Rynders.

Chapter 8 Wrist and Hand

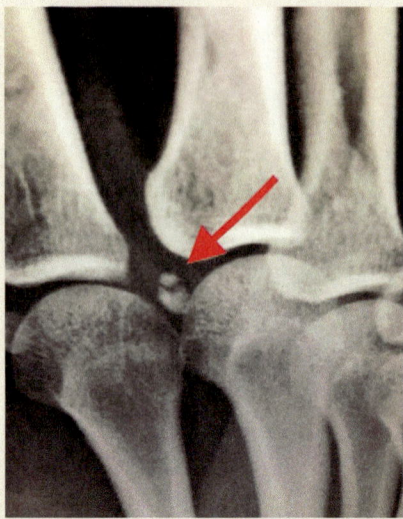

Figure 8.70 Magnified oblique radiograph view of the fractured sesamoid bone at the base of the middle finger (arrow).

Courtesy of Sara Rynders.

1. What is the differential diagnosis?
2. What are some red flags that would warrant immediate surgical intervention?
3. How could you assess the integrity of the neurovascular systems in the hand?
4. Describe the anatomic variations that occurred in this case which led to the injury.

WRAP-UP

Critical Thinking Questions

1. What three main nerve branches provide innervation to the hand?
2. Why are fractures of the scaphoid so important to diagnose and properly treat?
3. What is the difference between de Quervain tenosynovitis and intersection syndrome?
4. What is the most reliable way to diagnose TFCC tears?
5. What is the difference between a jersey finger and a mallet finger?

Pearls and Pitfalls

- In any patient who presents with negative radiographs and persistent anatomic snuffbox tenderness, the thumb should be placed in a spica splint and reevaluation for a scaphoid fracture performed within 2 weeks.
- A sprained wrist should be evaluated for injury to the intrinsic wrist ligaments, specifically the scapholunate ligament and the lunotriquetral ligament.
- Always check for intersection syndrome when evaluating a patient for de Quervain tenosynovitis.
- Hook of hamate fractures have a high rate of nonunion. Always have a high level of suspicion for this injury and evaluate with a CT scan if physical examination and radiographs are inconclusive.
- Always evaluate for rotational or angular deformity of the fingers through ROM in the setting of a metacarpal fracture.
- Stress testing of the thumb UCL can take time to become comfortable with. Performing a local anesthetic block can help. MRI or ultrasonography can also help to determine whether the ligament has a

partial or complete tear if the physical examination is inconclusive.
- A jammed finger is never just a jammed finger. Always evaluate individual structures to tailor treatment recommendations.
- Jersey fingers *always* require surgery. Mallet fingers *may* require surgery if surgical criteria are met.

References

1. Geissler WB, Slade JF: Fractures of the carpal bones, in Wolfe SW, Hotchkiss RN, Pedersen WC, Kozin SH, eds: *Green's Operative Hand Surgery*, ed 6. Philadelphia, PA, Elsevier, 2011, pp 639-708.
2. Rettig AC, Ryan RO, Stone JS: Epidemiology of hand injuries in sports, in Strickland JW, Rettig AC, eds: *Hand Injuries in Athletes*. Philadelphia, PA, WB Saunders, 1992, pp 37-48.
3. Steinmann SP, Adams JE: Scaphoid fractures and non-unions: diagnosis and treatment. Instructional lecture. *J Orthop Sci* 2006;11:424-431.
4. Ghane MR, Rezaee-Zavareh MS, Emami-Meibodi MK, Dehghani V: How trustworthy are clinical examinations and plain radiographs for diagnosis of scaphoid fractures? *Trauma Monthly* 2016;21(5):E23345.
5. Ring D, Lozano-Calderon S: Imaging for suspected scaphoid fractures. *JHS* 2008;33A:954-957.
6. Weiss A-P, Akelman E, Tabatabai M: Treatment of de Quervain's disease. *JHS* 1994;19A(4):595-598.
7. Karl JW, Olson PR, Rosenwasser MP: The epidemiology of upper extremity fractures in the United States, 2009. *J Orthop Trauma* 2015;29:242-244.
8. Wood AM, Robertson GA, Rennie L, Caesar BC, Court-Brown CM: The epidemiology of sports-related fractures in adolescents. *Injury* 2010;41:834-838.
9. Nellans KW, Kowalski BS, Chung KC: The epidemiology of distal radius fractures. *Hand Clin* 2012;28(2):113-125.
10. Lichtman DM, Randipsingh RR, Boyer MI, et al: Treatment of distal radius fractures. *J Am Acad Orthop Surg* 2010;18:180-189.
11. Dillingham C, Horodyski M, Struk AM, Wright T: Rate of improvement following volar plate open reduction and internal fixation of distal radius fractures. *Adv Orthop* 2011;2011:565642.
12. Ruston J, Konan E, Sorene E: Diagnostic accuracy of clinical examination and magnetic resonance imaging for common articular wrist pathology. *Acta Orthop Belg* 2013;79(4):375-380.
13. Kuo CE, Wolfe SW: Scapholunate instability: current concepts in diagnosis and management. *J Hand Surg* 2008;33A:998-1013.
14. Bille B, Harley B, Cohen H: A comparison of CT arthrography of the wrist to findings during wrist arthroscopy. *J Hand Surg* 2007; 32A:834-841.
15. Palmer AK: Triangular fibrocartilage complex lesions: a classification. *J Hand Surg* 1989;14:594-606.
16. Tay SC, Tomita K, Berger RA: The "ulnar fovea sign" for defining ulnar wrist pain: an analysis of sensitivity and specificity. *J Hand Surg* 2007;32A:438-444.
17. Tomaino MM: The importance of the pronated grip x-ray view in evaluating ulnar variance. *J Hand Surg* 2000;25A(2):352-357.
18. Lee YH, Choi YR, Kim S, Song HT, Suh JS: Intrinsic ligament and triangular fibrocartilage complex (TFCC) tears of the wrist: comparison of isovolumetric 3D-THRIVE sequence MR arthrography and conventional MRI image at 3T. *Magn Reson Imaging* 2013;31(2):221-226.
19. Park MJ, Jagadish A, Yao J: The rate of triangular fibrocartilage injuries requiring surgical intervention. *Orthopedics* 2010; 33(11):806.
20. Horii E, An KN, Linscheid RL: Excursion of prime wrist tendons. *J Hand Surg* 1993;18A(1):83-90.
21. Campbell D, Campbell R, O'Connor P, Hawkes R: Sports-related extensor carpi ulnaris pathology: a review of functional anatomy, sports injury and management. *Br J Sports Med* 2013;47:1105-1111.
22. Ruland R, Hogan C: The ECU synergy test: an aid to diagnose ECU tendonitis. *J Hand Surg* 2008;33A:1777-1782.
23. Sato J, Yoshinori I, Hideo N: Diagnostic performance of the extensor carpi ulnaris (EDU) synergy test to detect sonographic ECU abnormalities in chronic dorsal ulnar-sided wrist pain. *J Ultrasound Med* 2016;35:7-14.
24. Topper SM, Wood MB, Linscheid RL: Athletic injuries of the wrist, in Cooney WP, Linscheid RL, Dobyns JH, eds: *The Wrist: Diagnosis and Operative Treatment*. St Louis, MO, Mosby, 1998, pp 1031-1074.
25. Milek MA, Boulas HJ: Flexor tendon ruptures secondary to hook of hamate fractures. *J Hand Surg* 1990;15(5):740-744.
26. Failla JM: Hook of the hamate vascularity: vulnerability to osteonecrosis and non-union. *J Hand Surg* 1993;18:140-147.
27. Wright TW, Moser WM, Sahajpal DT: Hook of hamate pull test. *J Hand Surg* 2010;35A:1887-1889.
28. Kato H, Nakamura R, Horii E, et al: Diagnostic imaging for fracture of the hook of hamate. *Hand Surg* 2000;5(1):19-24.
29. Andersen R, Radmer S, Sparmann M, et al: Imaging of hamate bone fractures in conventional x-rays and high-resolution computed tomography: an *in vitro* study. *Invest Radiol* 1999;34(1):46-50.
30. Devers BN, Douglas KC, Naik RD, et al: Outcomes of hook of hamate excision in high-level amateur athletes. *J Hand Surg* 2013;38(1):72-76.
31. Moran SL, Berger RA: The biomechanics of hand trauma: what you need. *Hand Clin* 2003;19:17-31.
32. Rivlin M, Fei W, Mugdal CS: Bennett fracture. *J Hand Surg* 2015;40:1667-1668.
33. Chung KC, Spilson SV: The frequency and epidemiology of hand and forearm fractures in the United States. *J Hand Surg* 2001;26:908-915.
34. Mayer SW, Rush DS, Leversedge FJ: The Influence of thumb metacarpophalangeal joint rotation on the evaluation of ulnar collateral ligament injuries: a biomechanical study in a cadaver model. *J Hand Surg* 2014;39(3):474-479.
35. Heyman P, Gelberman RH, Duncan K, Hipp JA: Injuries of the ulnar collateral ligament of the MCP joint: biomechanical and prospective clinical studies on the usefulness of valgus stress testing. *Clin Orthop Relat Res* 1993;292:165-171.
36. Malik AK, Morris T, Chou D, Sorene E, Taylor E: Clinical testing of ulnar collateral ligament injuries in the thumb. *J Hand Surg Eur* 2009;34:363-366.

37. Avery DM III, Inkellis ER, Carlson MG: Thumb collateral ligament injuries in the patient. *Curr Rev Musculoskelet Med* 2017;10:28-37.
38. Hintermann B, Holzach PJ, Schutz M, Matter P: Skier's thumb: the significance of bony injuries. *Am J Sports Med* 1993;21:800-804.
39. Papandreau RF, Fowler T: Injury at the thumb UCL: is there a Stener lesion? *J Hand Surg* 2008;33(10):1882-1884.
40. Hergan K, Mittler C, Oser W: Ulnar collateral ligament: differentiation of displaced and nondisplaced tears with US and MR imaging. *Radiology* 1995;194(1):65-71.
41. Merrell G, Slade JF: Dislocations and ligament injuries in the digits, in Wolfe SW, Hotchkiss RN, Pedersen WC, Kozin SH, eds: *Green's Operative Hand Surgery*, ed 6. Philadelphia, PA, Elsevier, 2011, pp 291-332.
42. Leddy JP, Packer JW: Avulsion of the profundus tendon insertion in athletes. *J Hand Surg* 1977;2:66-69.

CHAPTER 9

Elbow

Natalie L. Myers, PhD, ATC, PES
Aaron D. Sciascia, PhD, ATC, PES, SMTC

OVERVIEW

The elbow complex is composed of three joints: the humeroulnar joint, the humeroradial joint, and the proximal radioulnar joint. The elbow is characterized as a trochoginglymoid joint. The joint is surrounded by muscular and ligamentous structures that provide dynamic and static stability. Because the elbow is an active joint, a detailed evaluation process to accurately diagnose a patient is critical to care. Time should be taken to rule in or out the presence of pathology. A detailed evaluation should include a thorough history; inspection; and physical examination, including range of motion, muscular strength, special tests, and vascular and neurologic assessments.

LEARNING OBJECTIVES

After completing this chapter, the reader will be able to do the following:

1. Describe the clinical anatomy of the elbow.
2. Describe commonly accepted techniques and procedures for evaluation of the common elbow injuries. These techniques and procedures include the following: (a) taking a history, (b) inspection, (c) palpation, and (d) special tests.
3. Perform a clinical history and examination of the elbow.
4. Determine the clinical usefulness of varying diagnostic techniques during the elbow examination.

FUN FACTS ABOUT THE ELBOW JOINT

- Is it true that every part of your body is the same size as another part? Maybe so, as apparently the foot is approximately the same length as the distance between the elbow and the wrist.
- Have you ever hit your elbow in just the right spot and felt numbness or tingling into the hand? You hit your funny bone, but the "funny" thing is, it is not a bone; it is actually the ulnar nerve. Some believe it is a play on the word *humorous*, as the long bone in the upper arm is named the humerus.
- It is impossible for people with structurally normal joints to touch the lips to the elbow.

Introduction

The elbow is one of the most active joints within the appendicular skeleton, as any activity required from the hand involves movement from the elbow. Consequently, the elbow is left vulnerable to traumatic and atraumatic syndromes, inflammatory disorders, and neuropathies. A detailed clinical history and examination will help clinicians form differential diagnoses that will aid in the final clinical diagnostic process. Although traumatic events can occur at the elbow, it is not unlikely for atraumatic episodes to be the source of pain and dysfunction that result in the inability of the patient to participate in work, sport, daily activities of living, or any life roles that are deemed necessary for the individual. As with other joints in the upper limb, cervical spine pathology must be ruled out as a source of distal pain as the

Clinical Anatomy

Bones of the Elbow

The elbow complex comprises three bones: the distal humerus, the proximal radius, and the proximal ulna.

The Distal Humerus

The distal humeral shaft transitions to the medial and lateral supracondylar ridges. Distal to the ridges are the medial and lateral epicondyles. The medial epicondyle is the more prominent bony landmark of the two and serves as a point of attachment for the ulnar collateral ligament and the flexor-pronator mass. The lateral epicondyle serves as the origin of the lateral ligament complex and the extensor-supinator muscle mass. The condyles are the most distal bony landmarks of the humerus, and they form the articular surfaces of the capitulum laterally and the trochlea medially. Anteriorly, the radial fossa and coronoid fossa accommodate the radial head and coronoid process of the ulna during flexion (**Figure 9.1**). Posteriorly, the olecranon fossa accommodates the olecranon process of the ulna during extension[1] (Figure 9.1A).

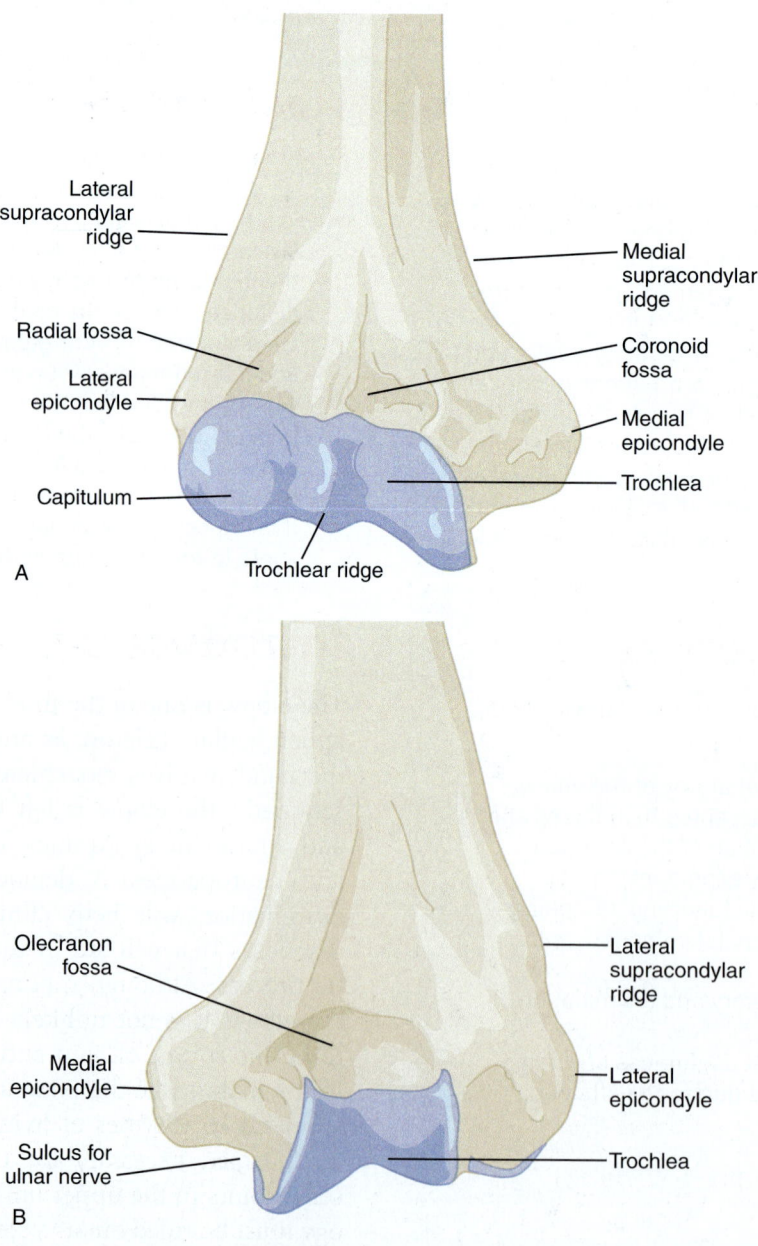

Figure 9.1 Drawings showing the anatomy of the right distal humerus. **A.** Anterior anatomy. **B.** Posterior anatomy.

© Jones & Bartlett Learning

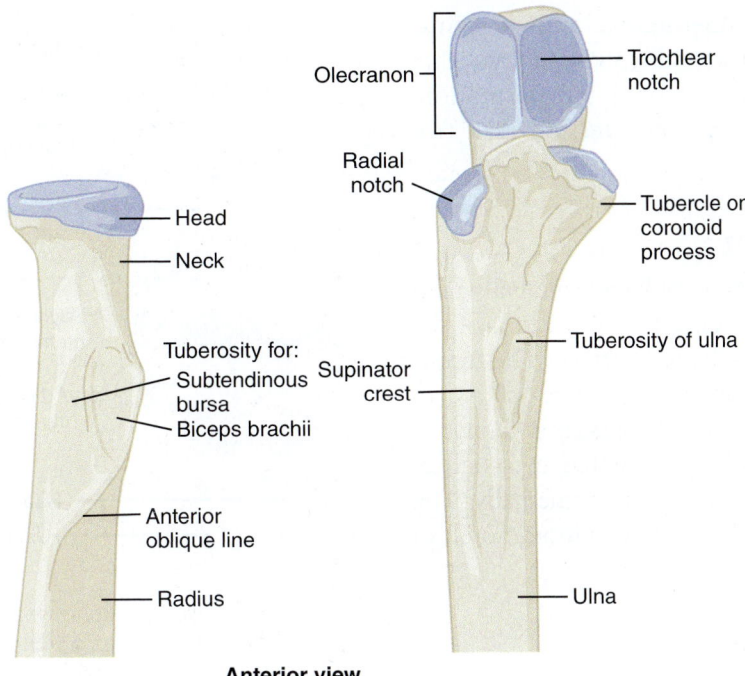

Figure 9.2 Drawings showing anterior anatomy of the proximal radius and ulna.
© Jones & Bartlett Learning

The Proximal Radius

The proximal radius consists of the radial head, which is cylindrical in its shape with a concave surface to accommodate the convex capitulum during joint movement. The medial portion of the radial head also articulates with the radial notch of the ulna. Distal to the radial head, the proximal radius narrows to form the neck of the radius. The radial tuberosity is found on the medial aspect of the distal radial neck and serves as an insertion point for the distal biceps tendon[1] (**Figure 9.2**).

The Proximal Ulna

The proximal ulna is home to the olecranon process (**Figure 9.3**), which is the attachment site for the distal triceps tendon. The concave anterior surface of the olecranon is known as the greater sigmoid notch (incisura semilunaris, or trochlear notch) and articulates with the trochlea, providing essential stability for the joint.[2] Toward the distal aspect of the sigmoid notch is a pointed prominence known as the coronoid process, which serves as the insertion point for the brachialis tendon and oblique cord ligament. Lateral to the coronoid process is the radial notch of the ulna (lesser semilunar notch, or lesser sigmoid notch). On the lateral aspect of the proximal ulna (distal to the radial notch) is the supinator crest. This bony landmark serves as the attachment point for the lateral ulnar collateral ligament.[1]

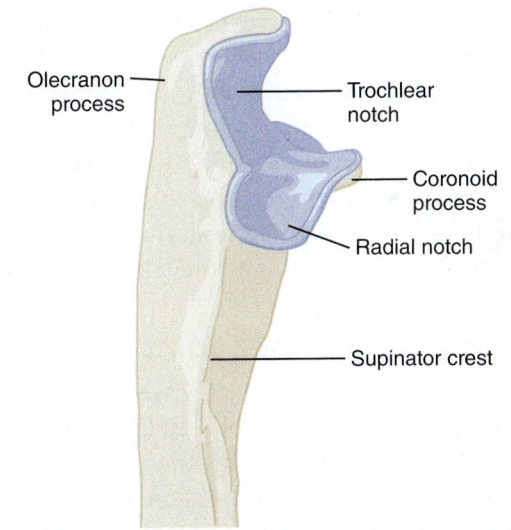

Figure 9.3 Drawing showing lateral view of the right proximal ulna.
© Jones & Bartlett Learning

Articulations and Ligamentous Support

The elbow complex is composed of three joints: the humeroulnar joint, the humeroradial joint, and the proximal radioulnar joint. The humeroulnar joint is generally described as a hinge or ginglymus joint allowing for both flexion and extension. However, some believe it is more appropriately described as a modified hinge joint, as small amounts of external and internal rotation occur during extreme flexion and extension.[3] The humeroradial and proximal radioulnar joints are trochoid (pivot) joints that allow for axial rotation or a pivoting type of motion. Consequently, the elbow is characterized as a trochoginglymoid joint.[2]

Humeroulnar Joint

The surface of the trochlea is larger medially and projects more distally than the lateral portion of the trochlea and has a pulley-shaped surface. The trochlea is covered by articular cartilage over an arc of 300°. The trochlea has a center depression, known as the trochlear groove, which is oriented in a helical manner from anterolaterally to posteromedially. The trochlea articulates with the greater sigmoid notch of the proximal ulnar.

Humeroradial Joint

The capitulum is spheroidal in shape and covered by hyaline cartilage, which is 2 mm thick on the capitulum's anterior surface. The capitulum articulates with the radial head. The trochleocapitellar groove, between the trochlea and capitulum, is a point of articulation for the rim of the radial head.[1] This radial head articulates with this groove during flexion, pronation, and supination. This groove's axis is internally rotated (5° to 7°) in relation to the humeral epicondyles. In relation to the humeral axis, the condyles are oriented 30° anterior and exhibit an approximately 6° to 8° valgus tilt.[4,5]

Proximal Radioulnar Joint

Hyaline cartilage covers the concave portion of the proximal radius, and 240° of articular cartilage on the radial head articulates with the ulna. Therefore, the anterolateral third of the radial head (120°) is without cartilage, making it more susceptible to fracture.[1] The head and neck of the radius are not colinear with the rest of the radius and form an angle of 15° with respect to the shaft of the radius.[1]

The coronoid and olecranon processes comprise the proximal ulna. These two bony landmarks make up the saddle-shaped, ellipsoid articular surface of the sigmoid notch. The middle portion of the sigmoid notch is without articular cartilage but instead is covered by fatty tissue. The greater sigmoid notch has an arc of approximately 190° and opens 30° posterior to the long axis of the ulna. The lesser sigmoid notch has an arc of approximately 70° and articulates with the radial head to allow for pronation and supination.

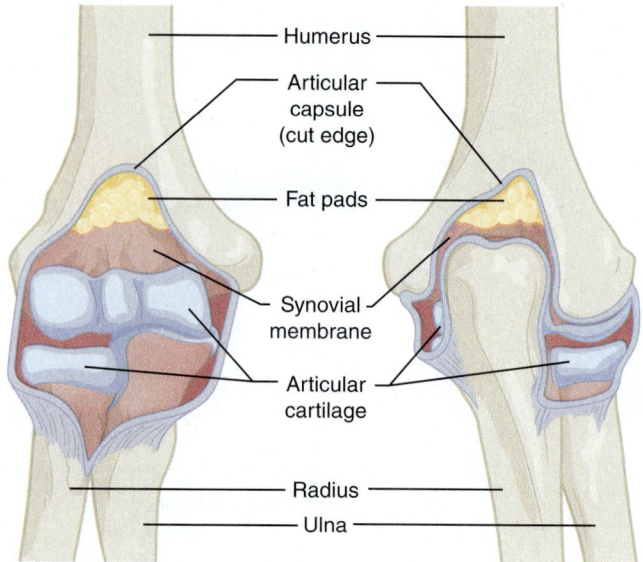

Figure 9.4 Drawings showing anterior and posterior view of the elbow joint capsule.

© Jones & Bartlett Learning

Elbow Joint Capsule

The elbow's joint capsule surrounds all three joint articulations and originates proximal to the coronoid and radial fossa. Distally, the capsule attaches laterally to the annular ligament and medially to the anterior rim of the coronoid process. Posteriorly, the capsule originates just above the olecranon fossa and distally along the supracondylar ridges of the humerus. The capsule also attaches along the medial and lateral rims of the sigmoid notch (**Figure 9.4**). The anterior portion of the capsule will be taut during elbow extension and lax during elbow flexion.[1]

Ulnar Collateral Ligament

The ulnar collateral ligament (UCL) is fan shaped and located on the ulnar side of the elbow; it consists of three separate bundles: anterior, posterior, and transverse (**Figure 9.5**). The anterior bundle of the UCL originates at the anteroinferior medial epicondyle and inserts on the sublime tubercle (medial aspect of the coronoid process).[6] The anterior bundle has two distinct bands: anterior and posterior.[7] The anterior band is taut and serves as the primary valgus stabilizer from 30° to 90° of flexion, and the posterior band is taut and serves as the primary valgus stabilizer from 90° to 120° of flexion.[8-10]

It is important to note that the anterior bundle consists of distinct collagen bundles within the layers of the capsule; however, the bundle has an additional ligament complex superficial to the capsular layers of

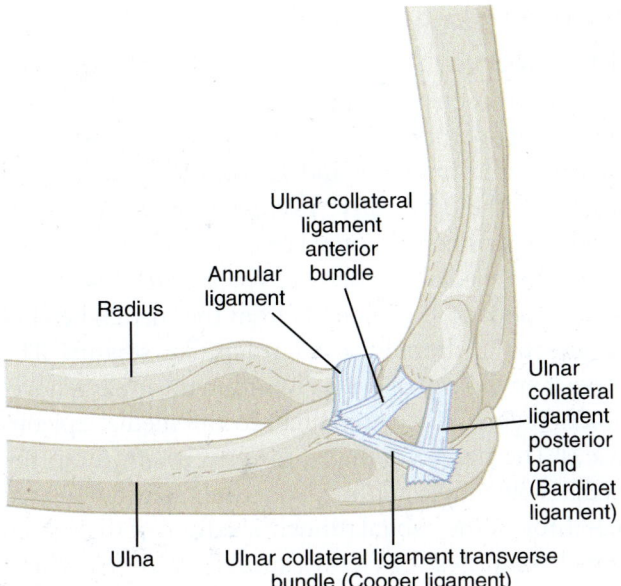

Figure 9.5 Drawing showing anatomy of the ulnar collateral ligament complex.

© Jones & Bartlett Learning

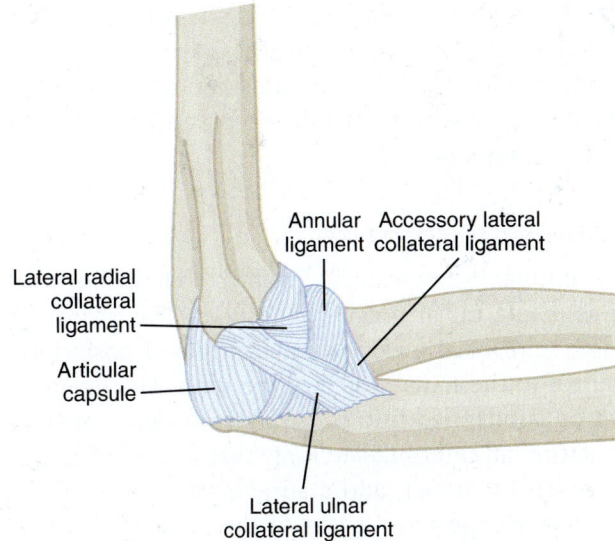

Figure 9.6 Anatomy of the lateral ligament complex.

© Jones & Bartlett Learning

the elbow that merge with the flexor muscle mass.[11] The mean length of the anterior bundle is approximately 27 mm, with a width of 4 to 5 mm.[12] The posterior bundle of the ligament (Bardinet ligament) is entirely contained within the layers of the capsule; it originates from the medial epicondyle and inserts along the medial margin of the trochlear notch.[2,5] This bundle is best defined in approximately 90° of flexion and has an average width of 5 to 6 mm.[11] The transverse bundle (ligament of Cooper) originates from the medial olecranon and inserts into the anteromedial aspect of the coronoid process, making it the only bundle that does not cross the elbow joint; therefore, this bundle offers no support to valgus stress. However, it does impart some medial support to the trochlear notch.

Lateral Ligament Complex

The lateral ligament complex (LLC) consists of four ligaments: the radial collateral ligament, the lateral ulnar collateral ligament, the accessory lateral collateral ligament, and the annular ligament. Unlike the UCL, individual variations among these ligaments are common (**Figure 9.6**).

Radial Collateral Ligament

The radial collateral ligament (RCL) originates from the lateral epicondyle and inserts into the annular ligament; it is poorly distinguished from the lateral joint capsule. The average length of the ligament is 20 mm with a width of 8 mm. The superficial portion of the ligament provides an origin point for the supinator muscle. Because the origin of the RCL is close to the axis of rotation, the ligament undergoes very little change during flexion and extension and remains relatively taut.[13]

Lateral Ulnar Collateral Ligament

The lateral ulnar collateral ligament (LUCL) originates from the lateral epicondyle and inserts into the tubercle at the crest of the supinator on the ulna. Additionally, the LUCL blends with the fibers of the annular ligament. Researchers dissecting cadaver specimens have found that the LUCL loosens during extension and tightens during elbow flexion.[14] The function of this ligament is to provide lateral stability of the elbow, preventing posterolateral rotatory instability. In the early 1990s, it was thought that the LUCL was the main structure to restrain posterolateral instability.[15] However, there is much debate regarding whether this ligament represents the main stabilizer against posterolateral rotatory forces. Several authors have found that posterolateral rotatory instability occurs only after the transection of both the LUCL and the RCL.[16,17] As such, the LLC as a whole contributes to elbow stability.

Accessory Lateral Collateral Ligament

The accessory lateral collateral ligament originates from the inferior margin of the annular ligament and inserts into the tubercle of the supinator crest.

This ligament is taut when varus stress is applied to the elbow. Flexion and extension movements do not appear to alter the ligament's position and length. Its function is to further stabilize the annular ligament during varus stress.[1]

Annular Ligament

The annular ligament encircles and stabilizes the radial head in the radial notch of the ulna. The ligament's origin and insertion occur anteriorly and posteriorly relative to the radial notch of the ulna. The ligament can be subdivided into three layers: a deep capsular structure, an intermediate layer that forms the annular ligament proper, and a superficial portion.[18] The anterior and posterior parts of the ligament become taut during extreme supination and pronation movements, respectively.[18]

There are two other ligaments that help stabilize the proximal radioulnar joint: the quadrate ligament and oblique cord. The quadrate ligament originates at the inferior edge of the radial notch and inserts into the radial neck. Some authors suggest that the ligament stabilizes the radioulnar joint by limiting spin of the radial head during supination and pronation.[19] The oblique cord is a bundle of fibrous tissue that runs on the ulna to an area just below the bicipital tuberosity of the radius. Its function remains uncertain in the literature, but it has been theorized the ligament limits supination movement.[20]

Soft-Tissue Anatomy

The elbow is surrounded by four primary muscle groups that help provide dynamic stability to the three elbow joints. The elbow flexors consist of the biceps brachii, brachialis, and brachioradialis. The elbow extensors consist of the triceps brachii and anconeus. The forearm flexor pronators (all originating from the medial epicondyle) consist of the pronator teres, flexor carpi radialis, palmaris longus, and flexor carpi ulnaris. Last, the forearm extensors consist of the extensor carpi radialis longus, extensor carpi radialis brevis, extensor digitorum communis, and extensor carpi ulnaris. An in-depth understanding of clinical anatomy allows for an organized and thoughtful examination procedure. Individual muscles surrounding the elbow joint should be palpated and assessed based on the origin and insertion of the muscles (**Table 9.1**). Note that manual muscle testing (MMT) should be performed in a gravity-dependent position and involve concentric and eccentric contractions.

Neurologic Anatomy

Ulnar Nerve. The ulnar nerve originates from cervical nerve roots C8 and T1 and continues into the medial cord of the brachial plexus. The nerve descends medial to the humerus and is considered a nerve of passage in the upper arm. The nerve passes under the arcade of Struthers, located approximately 8 cm proximal to the medial epicondyle. The arcade of Struthers is a fascial band that extends from the medial head of the triceps to the medial intermuscular septum. The nerve then travels superficially within the ulnar groove, which begins 3.5 cm proximal to the medial epicondyle.[21] The nerve continues to run posteriorly to the medial epicondyle and medially to the olecranon process through the cubital tunnel. The floor of the cubital tunnel comprises the elbow capsule and posterior and transverse ligaments of the ulnar collateral ligament. The roof of the tunnel is formed by the flexor carpi ulnaris (FCU) fascia and Osborne ligament (medial epicondyle to the olecranon process).[22] As the nerve exits the cubital tunnel, it passes between the two heads of the FCU into the forearm and travels down the medial side of the ulna. While in the forearm, the ulnar nerve has been traditionally described as giving off two motor branches: the first to the FCU and the second to the flexor digitorum profundus (FDP).[23] However, several researchers have identified innervation of the FCU and FDP to be done by multiple branches (range between 1 and 6 and 1 and 2, respectively).[24-27] The motor branch of the ulnar nerve is thought to innervate the medial half of the FDP, whereas the anterior interosseous nerve (AIN; branch of the median nerve) innervates the lateral half of the muscle. The nerve supplies two sensory branches in the forearm: the palmar cutaneous branch and the dorsal cutaneous branch. The palmar branch innervates the skin on the medial portion of the palm whereas the dorsal branch innervates the fifth and one-half of the fourth digits, and the associated dorsal area of the hand.

At the wrist, the ulnar nerve travels superficially to the flexor retinaculum (forms the roof of the carpal tunnel) and enters the hand through the Guyon canal. The canal is formed by two carpal bones (the pisiform and the hamate). In the hand, the ulnar nerve divides into two terminal branches: the superficial sensory branch and the deep motor branch. The superficial branch supplies the palmar surface of the fifth and one-half of the fourth digits. The deep motor branch separates from the ulnar nerve proper and travels through the Guyon canal, innervating the muscles of the hypothenar eminence, lumbricals (four and five),

Table 9.1 Clinical Anatomy of Muscles Surrounding the Elbow Joint

Muscle	Origin	Insertion	Action	Nerve Root Innervation	Palpation	Manual Muscle Test	Figure of Manual Muscle Test
Biceps brachii, long head	Supraglenoid tubercle of scapula	Radial tuberosity	Elbow flexion, elbow supination, assists with shoulder flexion	Musculocutaneous C5, C6	1. Have the patient seated with the forearm supinated 2. Clinician palpates the anterior arm. Ask patient to flex the elbow to elicit a muscle contraction	Patient will be seated with the arm resting by side with the forearm supinated. Clinician stabilizes proximal to the elbow with one hand while the other hand will provide a resistance distal to the elbow. The clinician will ask the patient to flex the elbow through the complete range of motion against resistance	*Courtesy of Andrea Cripps and Matt Kutz.*
Biceps brachii, short head	Coracoid process	Aponeurosis into forearm	Elbow flexion, elbow supination, assists with shoulder flexion	Musculocutaneous C5, C6	1. Have the patient seated with the forearm supinated 2. Clinician palpates the anterior arm. Ask patient to flex the elbow to elicit a muscle contraction	Patient will be seated with the arm resting by side with the forearm supinated. Clinician stabilizes proximal to the elbow with one hand while the other hand will provide a resistance distal to the elbow. The clinician will ask the patient to flex the elbow through the complete range of motion against resistance	*Courtesy of Andrea Cripps and Matt Kutz.*
Brachialis	Distal half of anterior surface of the humerus	Coronoid process of ulna	Elbow flexion	Musculocutaneous C5, C6	1. Have the patient seated with the forearm pronated and the elbow at 90° 2. Clinician palpates medial and lateral to the distal biceps brachii muscle belly. Have patient resist elbow flexion when forearm is pronated. Note that the brachialis is deep to the biceps brachii	Patient will be seated with the arm resting by side with the forearm pronated. Clinician stabilizes proximal to the elbow with one hand while the other hand will provide a resistance distal to the elbow. The clinician will ask the patient to flex the elbow through the complete range of motion against resistance	© Jones & Bartlett Learning.

(continues)

Table 9.1 Clinical Anatomy of Muscles Surrounding the Elbow Joint *(continued)*

Muscle	Origin	Insertion	Action	Nerve Root Innervation	Palpation	Manual Muscle Test	Figure of Manual Muscle Test
Pronator teres	Humeral head: medial supracondylar ridge of humerus. Ulnar head: medial side of the coronoid process of ulna	Midway along the lateral surface of the radius	Elbow pronation, assists with elbow flexion	Median C6, C7	1. Have patient seated with the elbow in 90° of flexion and forearm supinated 2. Clinician palpates the medial supracondylar ridge and moves distally and laterally (toward the radius) in a diagonal pattern along the muscle belly. May ask the patient to resist pronation during palpation	Patient will be sitting with the elbow flexed to 90° by the torso. Clinician will hold the elbow to the patient's side with one hand while the other hand will provide a resistance proximal to the wrist. The clinician will ask the patient to pronate the forearm through the complete range of motion against resistance	
Flexor carpi radialis	Anteroinferior aspect of medial epicondyle	Second and third metacarpals	Wrist flexion, assists with radial deviation and elbow flexion	Median C6, C7	1. Have the patient seated with the forearm supinated 2. Clinician has the patient perform flexion and radial deviation of the wrist while palpating the muscle belly 3. Proximal palpation at the medial epicondyle. Note that proximally this tendon will blend with the common flexor tendon of the elbow	Patient is seated with the forearm supinated and resting on a table. Clinician stabilizes proximal to the wrist with one hand while the other hand will provide a resistance distal to the wrist. The clinician will ask the patient to flex the wrist through the complete range of motion against resistance	

© Jones & Bartlett Learning

Muscle	Origin	Insertion	Action	Innervation	Palpation	Muscle Testing
Flexor carpi ulnaris	Humeral head: medial epicondyle Ulnar head: medial olecranon, and posterior border of the ulna	Pisiform bone and fifth metacarpal	Wrist flexion and ulnar deviation, assists with elbow flexion	Ulnar C8, T1	1. Have the patient seated with the forearm supinated 2. Clinician has the patient perform flexion and ulnar deviation of the wrist while palpating the muscle belly 3. Proximal palpation at the medial epicondyle. Note that proximally this tendon will blend with the common flexor tendon of the elbow	Patient is seated with the forearm supinated and resting on a table Clinician stabilizes proximal to the wrist with one hand while the other hand will provide a resistance distal to the wrist The clinician will ask the patient to flex the wrist through the complete range of motion against resistance
Triceps brachii, long head	Infraglenoid tuberosity of scapula	Posterior surface of olecranon process of ulna	Elbow extension	Radial C7, C8	1. Have patient prone with the arm/forearm hanging off the table 2. Clinician palpates the proximal posterior upper arm with the elbow extended	Patient will be prone with the shoulder in 90° of abduction Clinician stabilizes proximal to the elbow with one hand while the other hand will provide a resistance distal to the elbow The clinician will ask the patient to extend the elbow through the complete range of motion against resistance
Triceps brachii, medial head	Distal two-thirds of medial and posterior humerus	Posterior surface of olecranon process of ulna	Elbow extension	Radial C7, C8	1. Have patient prone with the arm/forearm hanging off the table 2. Clinician palpates proximal to the medial and lateral epicondyles (deep to long head and lateral head)	Patient will be prone with the shoulder in 90° of abduction Clinician stabilizes proximal to the elbow with one hand while the other hand will provide a resistance distal to the elbow The clinician will ask the patient to extend the elbow through the complete range of motion against resistance

Courtesy of Andrea Cripps and Matt Kutz

(continues)

Table 9.1 Clinical Anatomy of Muscles Surrounding the Elbow Joint *(continued)*

Muscle	Origin	Insertion	Action	Nerve Root Innervation	Palpation	Manual Muscle Test	Figure of Manual Muscle Test
Triceps brachii, lateral head	Upper half of posterior humerus	Posterior surface of olecranon process of ulna	Elbow extension	Radial C7, C8	1. Have patient prone with the arm/forearm hanging off the table 2. Clinician palpates proximal lateral two-thirds of upper arm	Patient will be prone with the shoulder in 90° of abduction Clinician stabilizes proximal to the elbow with one hand while the other hand will provide a resistance distal to the elbow The clinician will ask the patient to extend the elbow through the complete range of motion against resistance	*Courtesy of Andrea Cripps and Matt Kutz.*
Brachioradialis	Lateral supracondylar ridge	Radial styloid process	Elbow flexion, assists with pronation and supination	Radial C5, C6	1. Have the patient seated with the elbow at 90° and the thumb toward the ceiling 2. Clinician has the patient resist elbow flexion while palpating the proximal lateral forearm	Patient will be seated with the arm resting by side with the thumb toward the ceiling Clinician stabilizes proximal to the elbow with one hand while the other hand will provide a resistance distal to the elbow The clinician will ask the patient to flex the elbow through the complete range of motion against resistance	© Jones & Bartlett Learning
Extensor carpi radialis longus	Lateral supracondylar ridge	Second metacarpal	Wrist extension and radial deviation and assists with elbow flexion	Radial C6, C7	1. Have the patient seated with the elbow at 90° and the thumb toward the ceiling 2. Clinician palpates posterior to the brachioradialis and asks the patient to extend the wrist while palpating the muscle belly	Patient is seated with the forearm pronated and resting on a table Clinician stabilizes proximal to the wrist with one hand while the other hand will provide a resistance distal to the wrist The clinician will ask the patient to extend the wrist through the complete range of motion against resistance	*Courtesy of Andrea Cripps and Matt Kutz.*

Clinical Anatomy 283

Anconeus	Posterior lateral epicondyle	Lateral aspect of olecranon process and upper dorsal surface of ulna	Elbow extension	Radial C7, C8	1. Have patient seated or standing 2. Clinician palpates lateral to proximal posterior border of the ulna	Patient will be prone with the shoulder in 90° of abduction Clinician stabilizes proximal to the elbow with one hand while the other hand will provide a resistance distal to the elbow The clinician will ask the patient to extend the elbow through the complete range of motion against resistance
Supinator	Lateral epicondyle of humerus, radial collateral ligament, and supinator crest of ulna	Proximal and middle third of radius	Elbow supination	Posterior Interosseous C5, C6	1. Have patient seated with the elbow extended and the forearm pronated 2. Clinician palpates distal to the radial head along the proximal shaft of the radius while resisting supination	Patient will be supine or seated with the elbow flexed and the fist closed Clinician will hold the shoulder in flexion with one hand while the other hand will provide a resistance proximal to the wrist The clinician will ask the patient to supinate the forearm through the complete range of motion against resistance

(continues)

Table 9.1 Clinical Anatomy of Muscles Surrounding the Elbow Joint

Muscle	Origin	Insertion	Action	Nerve Root Innervation	Palpation	Manual Muscle Test	Figure of Manual Muscle Test
Pronator quadratus	Distal portion of shaft of ulna	Distal portion of shaft of radius	Elbow pronation	Anterior Interosseous C8, T1	1. Have patient seated with the elbow in 90° of flexion and forearm supinated 2. Clinician palpates along lateral shaft of distal ulna (deep to the flexor mass) while resisting pronation. Note, the muscle runs diagonally toward the distal radial shaft	Patient will be sitting with the elbow flexed to 90° by torso Clinician will hold the elbow to the patient's side with one hand while the other hand will provide a resistance proximal to the wrist The clinician will ask the patient to pronate the forearm through the complete range of motion against resistance	

(continued)

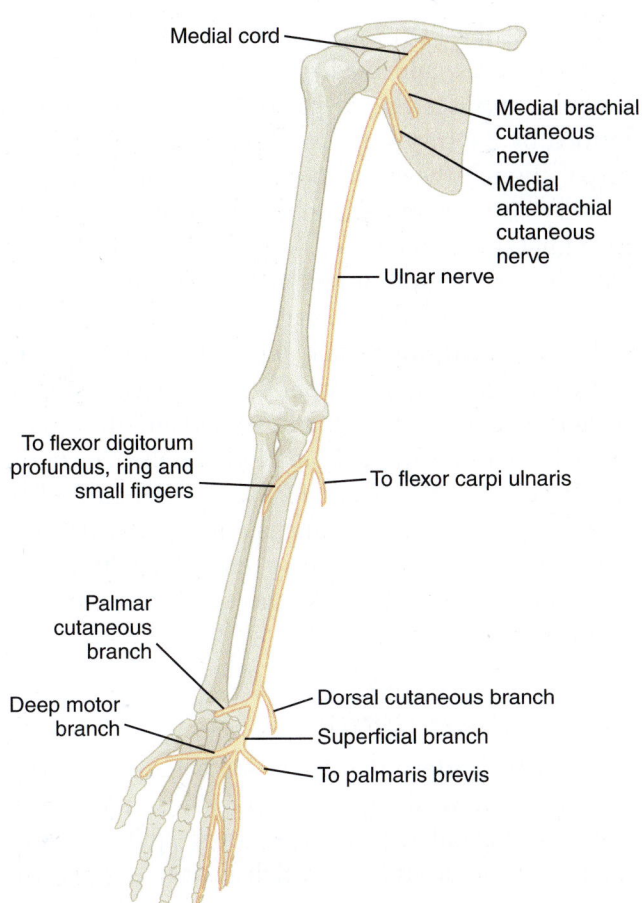

Figure 9.7 Drawing showing pathway of the ulnar nerve.
© Jones & Bartlett Learning

interossei, adductor pollicis (deep head), and flexor pollicis brevis (deep head).[28] It is important to note that anatomic variations of this nerve may be present in certain cases[28,29] (**Figure 9.7**).

Radial Nerve. The radial nerve originates from cervical nerve roots C5–T1 and continues into the posterior cord of the brachial plexus. As the radial nerve enters the upper arm, it passes anterior to the long head of the triceps brachii and lies within the posterior shaft of the humerus, on average 124 mm below the posterior tip of the acromion.[30] Most often, the nerve lies on the medial head of the triceps as it travels posteriorly on the humerus and then exits the posterior shaft of the humerus an average of 126 mm proximal to the lateral epicondyle. The radial nerve is never within 100 mm of either epicondyle.[30] As the nerve enters the elbow, it lies anterior to the capitulum.[31] On average 1.8 cm distal to the capitulum, the nerve branches into sensory (superficial radial nerve [SRN]) and motor (posterior interosseous nerve [PIN]) nerves.[32]

The SRN descends the lateral forearm along the lateral border of the brachioradialis and becomes subcutaneous at its middle third. Innervation of the SRN has been shown to be variable. A study done on 20 cadaver forearms found that the SRN innervated the posterior surface of the lateral 2.5 digits in 45% of the specimens, with 30% innervating the posterior surface of the lateral 3.5 digits and the associated palm area.[33] The PIN travels through the radial tunnel, passing beneath the supinator arch and penetrating the deep head of the supinator, to enter the posterior compartment of the forearm.[34] The floor of the radial tunnel consists proximally of the radiocapitellar joint and distally of the deep head of the supinator muscle. As the nerve continues through the tunnel and reaches the radial neck, the roof consists of recurrent vessels of the radial artery (leash of Henry). The PIN continues through the tunnel and passes beneath the proximal edge of the supinator (arcade of Froshe). The PIN then exists the tunnel, spawning several different branches responsible for innervating the extensor complex of the elbow wrist and hand. The nerve terminates in the fourth dorsal compartment to give sensory branches to the dorsal wrist.[35] Traditionally, the radial nerve proper has been thought to innervate the brachioradialis, extensor carpi radialis longus, extensor carpi radialis brevis, and anconeus; the PIN is responsible for the supinator, extensor carpi ulnaris, abductor pollicis longus, extensor pollicis longus, extensor pollicis brevis, extensor indicis proprius, extensor digitorum communis, and extensor digitorum minimus. However, it is important to understand that several authors have challenged these innervations, as the extensor carpi radialis longus and brevis have been shown to have branches from the PIN[36,37] (**Figure 9.8**).

Median Nerve. The median nerve is formed by portions of both the medial and lateral cord of the brachial plexus and has contributions from the entire plexus (C5–T1). The nerve is a nerve of passage within the upper arm, with all of its motor and sensory distributions below the elbow. The nerve runs deep to the short head of the biceps and lateral to the brachial artery. At the mid upper arm, it crosses to the medial side of the brachial artery and descends into the cubital fossa. Within the cubital fossa, the nerve lies deep to the bicipital aponeurosis and medial to the brachial artery. As the nerve travels distally, it adheres to the under surface of the flexor digitorum superficialis (FDS) and is superficial to the FDP. At the junction of the two heads of the pronator, the anterior interosseous nerve (AIN) arises as

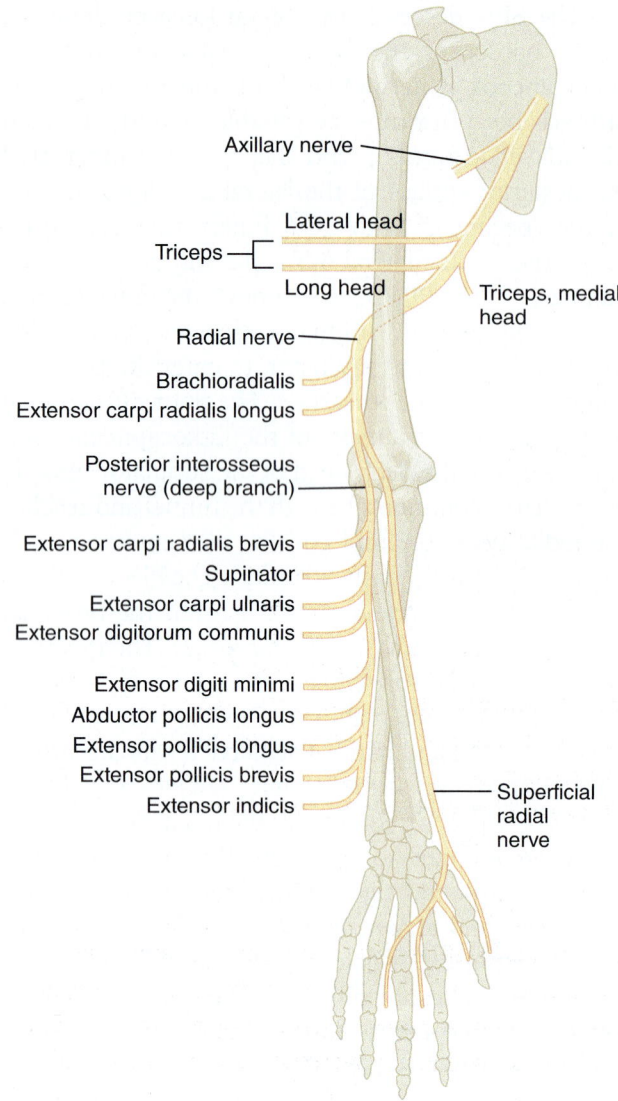

Figure 9.8 Drawing showing the pathway of the radial nerve.
© Jones & Bartlett Learning

a branch of the median nerve. The AIN travels deep alongside the anterior interosseous artery (a branch of the ulnar artery) and positions itself anterior to the interosseous membrane before terminating as sensory fibers to the anterior capsule of the carpals.

The AIN innervates the flexor pollicis longus, pronator quadratus, and the second and third digits of the FDP. The median nerve proper innervates the pronator teres, palmaris longus, and flexor carpi radialis. The median nerve gives off the palmar cutaneous branch approximately 4 to 5 cm proximal to the wrist (at the ulnar side of the flexor carpi radialis).[35] The palmar cutaneous branch divides into both radial (supplies skin at base of thenar eminence) and ulnar branches (supplies part of the lateral palm). As the median nerve travels down the forearm, it enters the carpal tunnel. The carpal tunnel is home to the four tendons of the FDP, four tendons of the FDS, flexor pollicis longus, and median nerve. The floor of the tunnel comprises the carpal bones, and the roof is formed by the transverse carpal ligament. Within the carpal tunnel, the nerve divides into three terminal branches: the lateral branch (supplies the thumb and the radial side of the index finger); the medial branch (supplies the middle finger and radial aspect of the ring finger); and the recurrent motor branch that innervates the flexor pollicis brevis (superficial head), abductor pollicis brevis, opponens pollicis, abductor pollicis (superficial head), and second and third lumbricals.[35] The recurrent branch of the median nerve has been shown to have location variability when examined in cadaver specimens. Previous researchers have found the branch to arise distal to the tunnel in some specimens and within the tunnel in others[38,39] (**Figure 9.9**).

Vascular Anatomy

The brachial artery descends down the upper arm anteriorly and medially to the brachialis muscle. Just distal to the radial head, the artery splits into the ulnar and radial arteries, which continue down the forearm. The ulnar artery passes deep to the pronator teres, flexor carpi radialis, palmaris longus, and FDS. As the artery enters the hand, it joins the superficial palmar branch of the radial artery. The artery has several different branches: anterior ulnar recurrent artery, posterior ulnar recurrent artery, and the common interosseous artery. Both the anterior and posterior ulnar recurrent arteries are located distal to the cubital fossa, giving off the first two medial branches of the ulnar artery. These arteries ascend to anastomose with the inferior and superior ulnar collateral arteries.[40] The common interosseous artery is located distal to the cubital fossa and is the first lateral branch of the ulnar artery.[40] The common interosseous artery divides into the anterior and posterior interosseous arteries. These two arteries are located distal to the radial tuberosity. The anterior interosseous artery runs anteriorly to the interosseous membrane and pierces the membrane just proximal to the pronator quadratus before anastomosing with the posterior interosseous artery. The posterior interosseous artery descends deep between the extensor carpi ulnaris and the extensor digiti minimi and ends by joining with the anterior interosseous artery. The posterior interosseous artery gives rise to the posterior interosseous recurrent artery within the proximal elbow. The posterior interosseous recurrent artery is located between the lateral epicondyle and the olecranon process, and runs deep to the anconeus, to anastomose with the middle collateral artery.[40]

As the radial artery crosses the elbow, it lies beneath the brachioradialis and travels into the anatomic snuffbox. The artery ends in the hand by anastomosing with the deep branch of the ulnar artery, completing the deep palmar arch.[40] The artery gives off a major branch, known as the radial recurrent artery, and is a lateral branch of the radial artery arising distal to the cubical fossa. The artery ascends, superficial to the supinator; appears between the brachioradialis and brachialis; and anastomoses with the radial collateral artery.[40] **Figure 9.10** provides a visual representation of the arterial anatomy of the distal upper arm, forearm, and hand.

The veins of the upper limb are divided into superficial and deep vessels. The deep veins accompany and lie on either side of the arteries and are connected to the superficial vessels by perforating veins. There are three major superficial veins of the upper limb, all arising from the dorsum of the hand as a dorsal arch: the cephalic vein, basilic vein, and median cubital vein.[40] The cephalic vein ascends laterally through the forearm, passing anteriorly to the elbow. As it passes the elbow, it travels proximally between the deltoid and pectoralis major and terminates by joining with the axillary vein just distal to the clavicle.[40] The basilica vein travels along the medial aspect of the forearm into the upper arm to join with the brachial vein. The median cubital

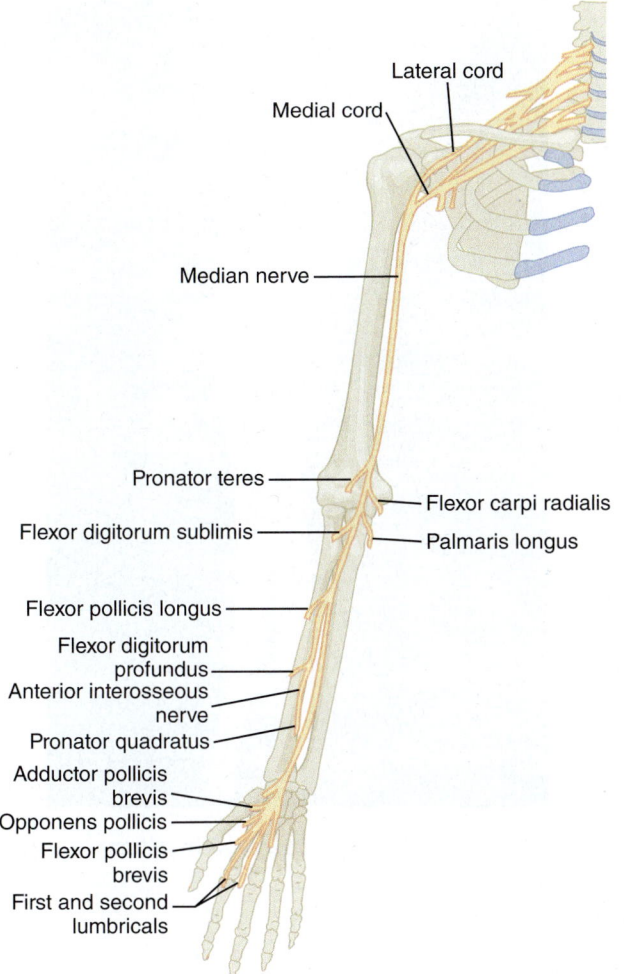

Figure 9.9 Drawing showing pathway of the median nerve.
© Jones & Bartlett Learning

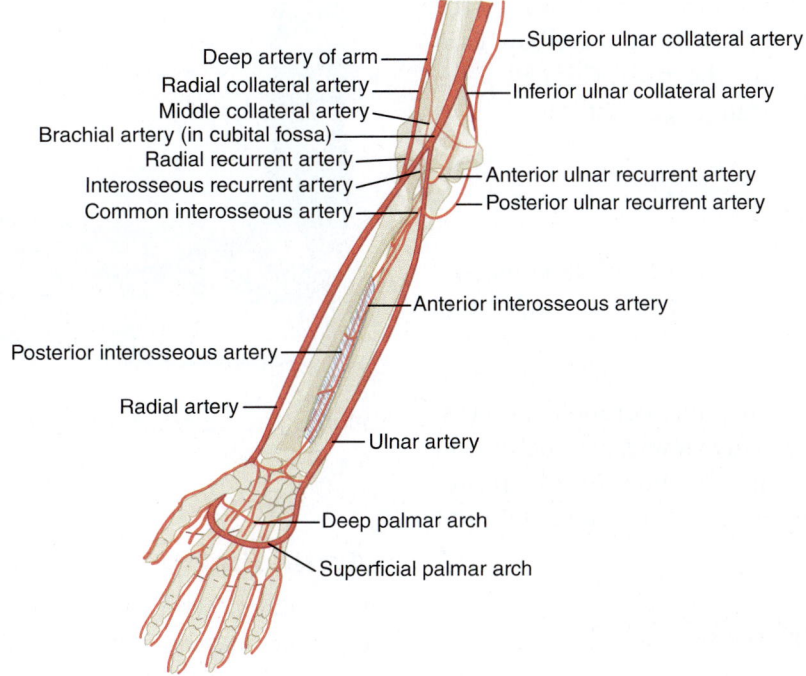

Figure 9.10 Drawing showing arterial anatomy of the forearm and hand.
© Jones & Bartlett Learning

vein joins the cephalic and basilica veins anterior to the elbow.[40]

Overview of Radiology and Imaging

Diagnostic imaging is often integrated into the examination process in the sports medicine field. As a clinician, it is important to use clinical judgment in determining when to order a specific test and the significance of any abnormal test findings. More and more researchers are showing that pathologic changes are present in asymptomatic people;[41,42] thus, treating the patient and not the scan should be of upmost importance to a clinician. Orchard et al suggest that "Imaging should be considered only after a provisional clinical diagnosis is reached, and only if it will influence management."[43] Consequently, clinicians must be equipped with the knowledge needed to understand and interpret common imaging techniques used in sports medicine.

Common Radiographic Views

There are several different radiographic views that can be executed, depending on the clinical findings of the examination. The two most common are the AP view and the lateral view.

The AP View

The AP view is the preferred method for assessing the medial and lateral epicondyles while the elbow is in an anatomic position with the patient seated. This view also allows the clinician to see joint articulations (**Figure 9.11**).

The Lateral View

The lateral view occurs with the shoulder in 90° of abduction with the elbow at a 90° angle resting on the table with the thumb pointing upward (**Figure 9.12**). This position allows the clinician to examine the humeroulnar joint, coronoid process, and olecranon process. This view is also helpful in identifying joint effusion. The anterior and posterior fat pads will be raised from the humerus if joint effusion is present.[44]

The Supracondylar AP View

This view assesses the integrity of the supracondylar ridges of the humerus and can be taken in either full or partial elbow flexion with the patient standing.

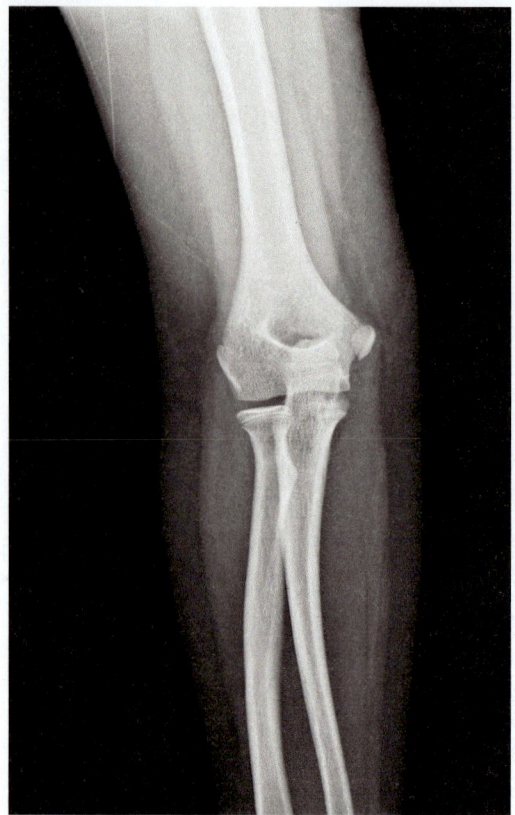

Figure 9.11 AP radiographic view of the elbow.
© Richman Photo/Shutterstock

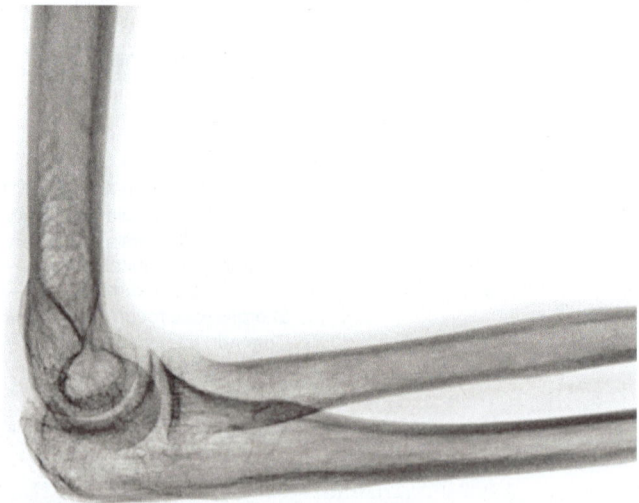

Figure 9.12 Lateral radiographic view of the elbow.
© samunella/Shutterstock

Acute Flexion AP View

For patients who cannot fully straighten the elbow, this view may be implemented and is a modification to the AP projection view. It most often comprises two views that concentrate on the distal humerus and the proximal forearm anatomy.

Inferior-Superior View

This view is appropriate for patients in elbow flexion greater than 90°, which allows for clear imaging of the olecranon process, distal humerus, and proximal forearm anatomy.

Coyle View

This view is often ordered when there is suspicion of a radial head fracture. It is an axial view projection with the elbow at 45° to 90° of flexion.

Common MRI Views and Injuries

Patient position is the first aspect to consider when using MRI. Most often, the patient will be positioned supine with the arm in anatomic position. The field of view should cover the distal humeral metaphysis to the bicipital tuberosity. Imaging should be performed in all three planes: axial, sagittal, and frontal.

Bone

MRI can be used to diagnose radial head fractures, which can be accompanied by persistent pain and joint effusion. MRI is also helpful in the diagnosis of osteochondrosis and osteochondral defect. Osteochondrosis most often affects the capitulum as a developmental form of osteonecrosis (Panner disease) and osteochondral defect, affecting the bone and cartilage of the capitulum.

Muscle and Tendons

The common flexor and extensor tendons are best evaluated in the frontal or axial planes of the MRI. Changes in tendon diameter should be monitored with respect to medial and lateral epicondylitis. The biceps and triceps tendons are best evaluated from the sagittal or axial planes. Partial tearing of the biceps can be difficult to visualize on MRI due to difficulty locating the bicipitoradial bursa. However, when this bursa is inflamed, it is easily identifiable and is often accompanied by partial tearing of the distal biceps tendon.[45]

Ligament Integrity

The ligaments of the elbow can be viewed using advanced imaging modalities, such as MRI. The sensitivity and specificity in the diagnosis of UCL injuries using MRI are 57% and 100%, respectively.[46] MRI may be used for accurate diagnosis of complete UCL tears. The use of MRI for assessment of the LLC has generated controversy. Early research suggests that MRI pulsed sequence is effective in the diagnosis of the proximal rupture of the LUCL, which is characteristic of posterolateral rotatory instability.[47] Depending on the type of pulsed sequence MRI, Carrino et al[48] found a wide range of success in the diagnosis of LUCL tears in cadaver models (range of 38% to 88%). It has been suggested that the "LUCL does not exist as a distinct structure and the LUCL generates many artifacts that can be confused with ligamentous rupture."[49] Therefore, MRI may not be reliable for the diagnosis of LUCL injuries. However, complete disruption of the LLC will more than likely be evident on an MRI.

Nerves

Nerve changes are best evaluated within the axial plane. The ulnar nerve is the largest and most superficial nerve of the elbow, making it the most easily visible on MRI. It can easily be identified within the cubital tunnel, which acts as a potential compression site.[45] Although not as superficial at the elbow, the radial and median nerves can still be viewed with MRI. When evaluating any nerve with MRI, one must be aware of denervation changes in muscles.

Other Imaging Options

Diagnostic ultrasonography, commonly referred to as musculoskeletal ultrasonography, is becoming increasingly popular within sports medicine to help with the diagnosis of pathology. Structures at the elbow are convenient to ultrasound assessment and often include UCL tears, ulnar neuropathy, biceps tendon ruptures, golfer's elbow, and tennis elbow. The sensitivity and specificity for UCL, ulnar nerve entrapment, and epicondylitis range from 86% to 100%.[50] Diagnostic ultrasonography units range in cost, depending on purchase decisions, such as portable versus line units; however, some authors believe that substituting ultrasonography for other imaging modalities (when appropriate) will result in large cost savings.[51]

Evaluation of the Elbow

Prior to conducting a thorough history as part of the evaluation process, clinicians should have the patient complete a patient-reported outcome measure to help determine self-perceived level of function. A variety of outcome measures can be used on patients with elbow conditions to help identify self-reported function, pain, and psychosocial components. For example, the Disabilities of the Arm, Shoulder and Hand (DASH); the Quick Disabilities of the Arm, Shoulder and Hand (QuickDASH); the Oxford Elbow Score; the Patient-Rated Tennis Elbow Evaluation (PRTEE); the American Shoulder and Elbow Surgeons (ASES) elbow form; and the Kerlan-Jobe Orthopaedic Clinic Shoulder and Elbow Score are options.

History

Gathering a patient history is an important part of the examination process and is most often the first interaction between the clinician and patient. The history-taking portion of the assessment allows the clinician to engage with the patient. The clinician should allow the patient to speak freely as to why he or she is in the office and the chief complaints being experienced. It is important that the patient feels comfortable discussing relevant information with the clinician. If the clinician lacks interpersonal skills, is not engaging, rushes the patient during history discussion, or lacks respect, then the quality of the visit and information gathered will likely suffer. The clinician holds the key for either negative or positive patient interaction. A successful history not only incorporates essential dialogue between the clinician and patient, but it also allows the clinician to gauge the personality of the patient, determine how the patient is responding to the health condition, and establish differential diagnoses. Last, the history should be used to rule out all nonmusculoskeletal-related problems. These are often referred to as red flags. Red flags most often represent cancer or cardiovascular, pulmonary, or severe neurologic trauma.

A thorough elbow history should incorporate both the abilities and the barriers of the patient. The clinician should address self-reported impairments, activity and participation levels, and environmental and personal factors. Be sure to discuss the patient's occupation (if any), sport involvement, hand dominance, location and severity of pain, onset of symptoms, and duration of symptoms. Last, it is important to recognize that pain is multidimensional and complex and patients will have different pain experiences. Clinicians should consider incorporating components from the biopsychosocial approach to health care and the International Classification of Functioning, Disability and Health as a guide during the evaluation process.

Faciliatory Questions

1. *I see on your chart you are experiencing elbow pain; can you elaborate on how you hurt your elbow?* This type of question allows the patient to express to the clinician his or her main concerns and promotes rapport between the patient and clinician. Based on the patient response, you can follow up with more specific questions if not divulged in the initial conversation.
2. *What was the mechanism of injury for this particular injury?* This line of questioning will help to determine whether the patient is suffering more acute versus chronic impairments. Did the patient fall on an outstretched hand or directly on the elbow, or perhaps started to develop the symptoms from repetitive activity?
3. *Do you have a previous history of surgery or trauma to this area or any other area in the body?* Previous elbow surgeries can often result in nerve trauma due to superficial pathways around the elbow.[52] Often, elbow symptoms can be a result of cervical or shoulder trauma; therefore, ruling out proximal pathology can help eliminate possible differential diagnoses.

Self-Reported Impairment Questions

1. *Can you describe the pain or any symptoms that you are experiencing?* The type of pain being experienced may help differentiate among pain generators, such as bone, muscle, tendon, capsule, nerve, or vascular. Clinicians should also inquire about any locking, popping, or clicking that is experienced by the patient. These types of symptoms can often be a result of loose bodies or changes to the joint. Additional pain questions should include questions related to severity and timing.
2. *Have you experienced any abnormal sensations throughout the arm prior to or after the related injury?* This line of questioning will help determine whether the patient is suffering from abnormal nerve distribution patterns. Document any presence of numbness or tingling that is different from the asymptomatic side.
3. *Have your symptoms changed or progressed since initial injury?* This question may help determine long-term outcomes of the patient. A patient presenting with persistent issues may need to be guided differently from a patient whose symptoms are improving but are not completely resolved.

Activity and Participation Level Questions

1. *What is your occupation?* Work-related or sport-related repetitive stress may lend itself to tendinopathy-based pathology. Individuals who participate in sports, particularly overhead sports, naturally put physical demands on the elbow. Identifying where in the swinging or throwing phase symptoms occur can help determine involved structures. If the patient does participate in overhead sports activity, it is also important to inquire about changes in equipment.
2. *What are you able to do and unable to do?* The clinician should document hand dominance and determine if the condition is interfering with the day-to-day function of the patient.
3. *Has your activity been altered due to your symptoms?* Health quality of life can become diminished in patients who are not able to participate in their normal routine.

Environment and Personal Factor Questions

1. *How old is the patient?* In pediatric patients, bony integrity needs to be considered because growth plates are not fully closed.
2. *Do you experience any stress related to work/sport, and, if so, do you have a strong social support*

Possible Clinical Deductions Based on Patient Responses

Clinician Question	Patient Response	Possible Clinical Deduction
Can you elaborate on how you hurt your elbow?	I was lifting weights (biceps curls with forearm rotation) and felt a pain in my elbow on my dominant side	Possibility of biceps or supinator muscle strain
Do you have a previous history of surgery or trauma to this area or any other area in the body?	Distal biceps repair 1.5 years ago	Possibility of reinjury to biceps tendon Possibility of medial or lateral antebrachial cutaneous nerve injury
Can you describe the pain or any symptoms that you are experiencing?	I have a dull pain in the front of my elbow	Possibility of supinator muscle strain Possibility of biceps tendon strain or rupture
Are you experiencing any abnormal sensations throughout?	I have numbness on the front and side of my forearm	Possibility of medial or lateral antebrachial cutaneous nerve injury; could be a result of initial surgery
Have your symptoms changed or progressed since the initial injury?	The pain has gotten better from when it first happened	Possibility of biceps tendon rupture
What is your occupation?	Construction worker	Manual labor intensive; constant use of upper limbs
What activities are you able and unable to do?	I am able to do tasks with my nondominant hand for work, such as hammer and drill I am no longer able to lift weights on the dominant arm	Still working, but has had to make changes due to dysfunction in the dominant arm
Have your activities been altered due to the symptoms?	Yes, I am unable to use the arm because it is difficult to bend it	Biceps tendon rupture
How old are you?	Male, 40 years of age	Biceps ruptures are most common in middle-aged men, and this patient has a previous history of biceps tendon repair
Are you under stress related to work, and if so do you have a strong social support network to help counteract some of the unwarranted stress?	I am the sole provider for my family, so ceasing work at this time is not an option; however, the elbow is affecting the quality of my work. My boss is willing to adjust the manual work demands while still keeping me on payroll	Support from employer and seems to be in good spirits overall

network to help counteract some of the unwarranted stress? Psychosocial factors can contribute to the way patients perceive and generate pain and should therefore be considered.

Inspection

Inspection of the elbow joint is similar to that of other upper limb joints. The clinician should observe the patient's static and dynamic posture during activities, such as standing, walking, and sitting, and in the sit-to-stand position while noting the activity at the elbow. The posture of the cervical spine, thoracic spine, scapula, and shoulder should be observed. Carrying angle should be assessed on both extremities, and the clinician should be aware of any flexion or extension contractures. The carrying angle of the elbow is formed between the long axis of the humerus and ulna when the elbow is in full extension. Because of the distal orientation of the trochlea compared to the capitulum, in full extension the forearm appears to be in an abducted position, or valgus posture. The normal carrying angle ranges between 10° and 18° for both men and women.[53]

However, some patients might present with excessive cubital valgus or varus (**Figure 9.13**).

The presence of scars, ecchymosis, swelling, cysts, hypertrophy, and atrophy must be considered and may help differentiate between acute and chronic conditions. Last, changes in muscle contour and symmetry can often be seen in those with muscle ruptures, particularly to the distal biceps and triceps.

Palpation

Palpation helps the clinician differentiate between structural damage to inert and/or contractile tissue. The clinician must be respectful of the patient during palpation maneuvers and should educate the patient on the structures being examined. Clinicians must understand and be able to recognize bony, ligamentous, arterial, nervous, and soft-tissue anatomy in order to carry out a thorough palpation examination. Remember, it may be difficult to palpate some bony anatomy of the elbow; this is dependent on individual muscle mass of the patient. **Table 9.2** provides palpatory strategies based on anatomic locations for inert tissue structures at the elbow. Muscle palpatory strategies are described in Table 9.1.

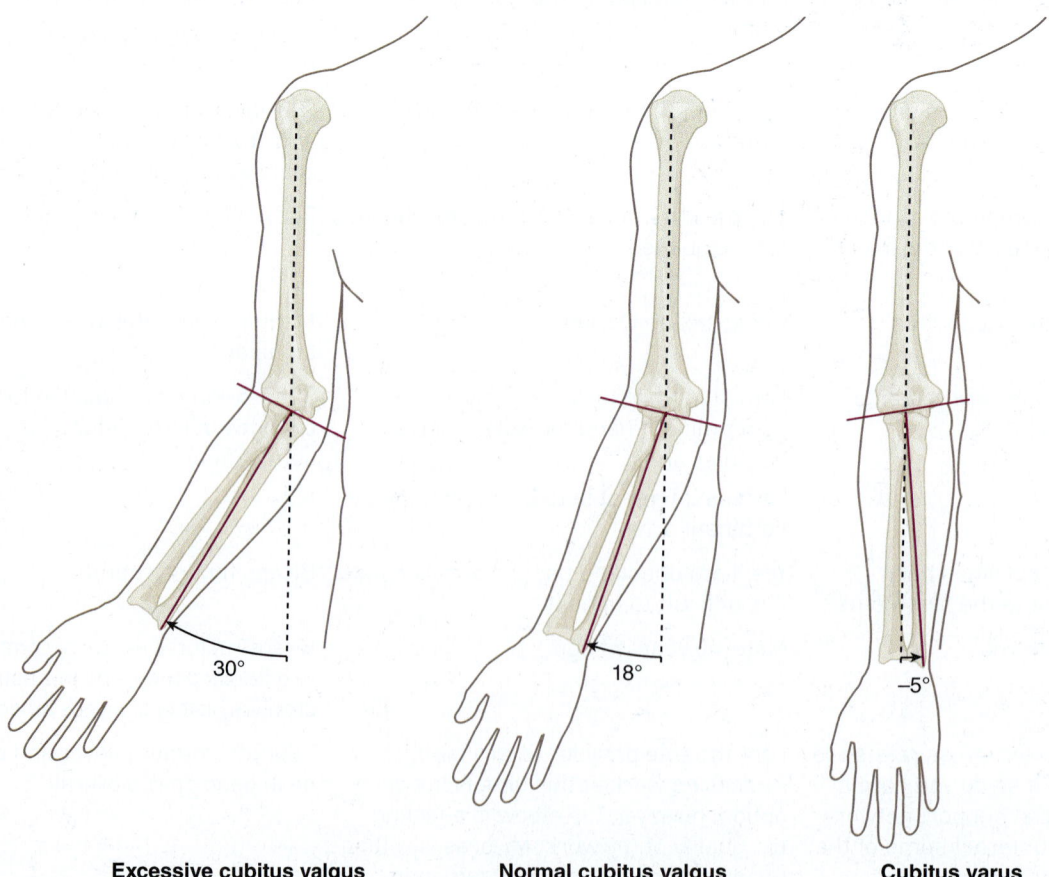

Excessive cubitus valgus   **Normal cubitus valgus**   **Cubitus varus**

Figure 9.13 Drawings showing carrying angle of the elbow.

Table 9.2 Inert Tissue Palpatory Strategies of the Elbow

Anterior Structures	Palpation	Origin	Insertion
Distal humerus	1. Have the patient seated with the forearm supinated 2. Clinician palpates the anterior arm along the length of the biceps until the antecubital fossa is reached	Not applicable	Not applicable
Brachial artery	1. Have the patient seated with the forearm supinated 2. Clinician palpates medial to the biceps tendon within the antecubital fossa	Not applicable	Not applicable
Median nerve	1. Have the patient seated with the forearm supinated 2. Clinician palpates medial to the biceps tendon within the antecubital fossa	Not applicable	Not applicable
Medial Structures	**Palpation**	**Origin**	**Insertion**
Medial epicondyle of the humerus	1. Have the patient seated with the forearm supinated 2. Clinician palpates down the medial border of the triceps until a bony prominence is felt on the medial distal humerus	Not applicable	Not applicable
Medial supracondylar ridge of the humerus	1. Have the patient seated with the forearm supinated 2. Clinician palpates the medial epicondyle and moves proximal until off the medial epicondyle	Not applicable	Not applicable
Ulnar nerve	1. Have the patient seated with the forearm supinated 2. Clinician palpates below the medial epicondyle into a groove known as the ulnar groove. The ulnar nerve travels through this groove	Not applicable	Not applicable
Ulnar collateral ligament (anterior bundle)	1. Have the patient seated with the forearm supinated 2. Clinician palpates below the medial epicondyle and over the joint space	Anteroinferior medial epicondyle	Sublime tubercle
Ulnar collateral ligament (posterior bundle)	1. Have the patient seated with the forearm supinated 2. Clinician palpates below the medial epicondyle and over the joint space	Medial epicondyle	Trochlear notch
Ulnar collateral ligament (transverse bundle)	1. Have the patient seated with the forearm supinated 2. Clinician palpates below the medial olecranon and just distal on the ulna	Medial olecranon	Anteromedial aspect of the coronoid process
Posterior Structures	**Palpation**	**Origin**	**Insertion**
Olecranon process	1. Have the patient seated with the forearm neutral 2. Clinician palpates down the posterior upper arm until bony prominence is felt on distal humerus	Not applicable	Not applicable
Olecranon bursae	1. Have the patient seated with the forearm neutral 2. Clinician palpates the olecranon process while feeling for fluid, swelling, or thickening of bursa 3. A healthy bursa is often nonpalpable	Not applicable	Not applicable
Lateral Structures	**Palpation**	**Origin**	**Insertion**
Lateral epicondyle of the humerus	1. Have the patient seated with the forearm neutral 2. Clinician palpates down the lateral border of the triceps until a bony prominence is felt on the lateral distal humerus	Not applicable	Not applicable
Lateral supracondylar ridge of the humerus	1. Have the patient seated with the forearm neutral 2. Clinician palpates the lateral epicondyle and moves proximal until off the lateral epicondyle	Not applicable	Not applicable

(continues)

Table 9.2 Inert Tissue Palpatory Strategies of the Elbow (continued)

Lateral Structures	Palpation	Origin	Insertion
Radial head	1. Have the patient supine with the forearm pronated 2. Clinician palpates the lateral epicondyle and moves distal across the joint space onto the radial head 3. Have the patient rotate the forearm to feel the radial head under the finger	Not applicable	Not applicable
Radial collateral ligament	1. Have the patient seated with the forearm pronated 2. Clinician palpates below the lateral epicondyle and over the joint space	Lateral epicondyle	Annular ligament and lateral joint capsule
Lateral ulnar collateral ligament	1. Have the patient seated with the forearm pronated 2. Clinician palpates below the lateral epicondyle and over the joint space	Lateral epicondyle	Tubercle at the crest of the supinator on the ulna and the annular ligament
Accessory lateral collateral ligament	1. Have the patient seated with the forearm pronated 2. Clinician palpates the inferior radial head	Inferior margin of the annular ligament	Tubercle of the supinator crest
Annular ligament	1. Have the patient seated with the forearm pronated 2. Clinician palpates over the radial head	Anterior radial notch of the ulna	Posterior radial notch of the ulna

Pathologies of the Elbow

The elbow is a trochoginglymoid joint that is susceptible to a variety of pathologies. These pathologies can be categorized as muscle based, ligamentous based, bone based, or neurologic based with either traumatic or atraumatic origins.

Muscle-Based Pathology

Lateral Epicondylalgia

Pain at or around the lateral elbow has been classified as lateral epicondylitis (inflammation of the lateral epicondyle), lateral epicondylosis (disease of the lateral epicondyle), lateral epicondylalgia (pain over the lateral epicondyle) (Table 9.3), lateral elbow tendinopathy

Table 9.3 Lateral Epicondylalgia Quick Tips

Pathology	Description	Presentation (HIPS)	Special Tests/Imaging	Differential Diagnosis	5-Min Sideline Assessment Tips
Lateral epicondylalgia	Pain at or around the lateral elbow	History: Typically, from repetitive movements Inspection: Alterations in resting posture Palpation: Common extensor tendon and lateral epicondyle Special tests: Range of motion not typically affected. Wrist extension may yield weakness	Cozen, Maudsley, Mills, and Polk tests Imaging warranted only with distal humeral fracture or another elbow fracture	Elbow fracture (radial head or distal humerus fracture) PLRI Radial tunnel syndrome	Most often driven from repetitive activity; inquire about MOI and length of pain Rule out fracture, PLRI, and dislocation Palpate over lateral epicondyle Wrist extension and grip strength assessment

HIPS, history, inspection, palpation, special tests; MOI, mechanism of injury; PLRI, posterolateral rotatory instability.

(tendon injury with no signs of inflammation), and, most commonly, tennis elbow.[54-57] The original name of epicondylitis was derived based on the occurrence of pain at or around the lateral epicondyle with initial suggestions of wrist extensor inflammation as being the cause of the pain.[58] However, various studies have identified an absence of inflammatory cells and/or proximal wrist extensor tendon degradation during histologic examination.[59-61] These findings led to the development of the terms lateral elbow tendinopathy and lateral epicondylosis. However, because the hallmark clinical finding is pain over the lateral epicondyle and/or proximal pain with active wrist extension, and that the lateral epicondyle itself is rarely inflamed, it has been posited that the term lateral epicondylalgia be used because the suffix *algia* means pain and the other terms can be used only with histologic verification[56] (**Figure 9.14**). Lateral elbow pain has been previously shown to frequently occur in recreational tennis players, hence the term tennis elbow.[55,62,63] The mechanism of injury has been suggested to be based on suboptimal levels of physiology (decreased muscle and cardiovascular fitness), volume (increased exposures and repetitious use of the arm), poor mechanics (hyperflexing or hyperextending the wrist during stroke play), and a combination of these mechanics.[64-66] Recent epidemiologic data have revealed that lateral epicondylalgia has a 1% to 10% prevalence rate and that occupational factors can lead to the development of the condition.[67] Of interest is that the occupational data suggest that the incidence of lateral epicondylalgia in workers rivals that of recreational tennis players, with incidences as high as 12% being reported.[68] Furthermore, physical impairments or deficits similar to those noted to lead to the condition in tennis players (postural issues, repetitive movements, and increased body mass index) have been identified in the working population.[68,69] These findings suggest that a comprehensive clinical examination that looks at both local and distant factors within the body should be performed in order to identify not only the what (lateral epicondylalgia) but also the why (causative factors for the epicondylalgia).

Outcome Measures. The DASH as well as the condensed version (QuickDASH) have been found to be useful for assessing patient perception of elbow function with lateral epicondylalgia. However, there is a patient-reported outcome measure specific to lateral epicondylalgia, known as the PRTEE.[70] The PRTEE is a 15-item disability questionnaire, meaning higher scores equate to greater levels of perceived disablement. The questionnaire has excellent psychometric properties for both laborers and nonlaborers with lateral epicondylalgia, and it correlates with the DASH.[70,71]

Specific History Questions. Subjectively, a history assessment that homes in on the mechanistic causes may assist the clinician with identifying the pathology. In particular, the following history items should be noted:

- Age: Due to the degradation of tissue and/or occupational causes, lateral epicondylalgia tends to arise more commonly in the fourth through sixth decades of life.[68] This is not to say that individuals younger than 40 to 60 years will not experience the condition, only that the condition is more frequent in these age ranges.
- Does the patient participate in activities (recreational or occupational) involving repetitious manipulation and arm movements known to lead to lateral elbow pain?
- Is pain elicited with active or forceful wrist extension?
- Is pain elicited with active or forceful forearm pronation and/or supination?
- Is pain elicited during and/or after gripping activities?
- Is the pain described as "deep" or "localized" to the proximal soft tissue on the lateral aspect of the forearm?
- Does the patient describe hand weakness with gripping activities?

Inspection. Posture is being identified as a factor related to lateral epicondylalgia[68] and has long been suggested as a concern in upper extremity dysfunction.[72-74] Clinicians should observe for alterations in resting posture, noting any spinal (excessive kyphotic or lordotic curves, forward head positioning), scapular

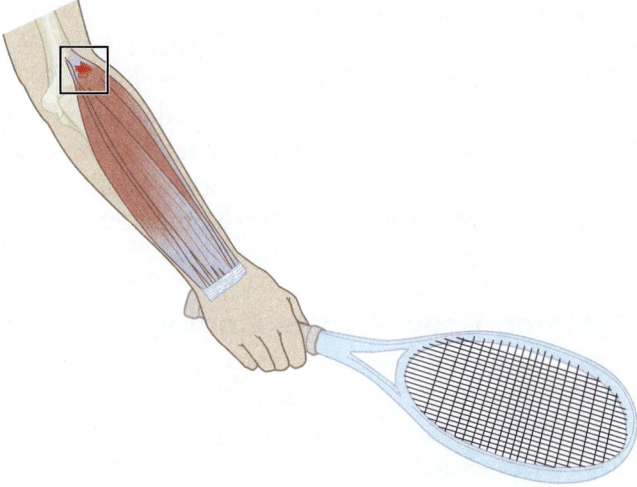

Figure 9.14 Anatomic drawing showing the location of lateral epicondylalgia.

(medial border or inferior angle prominence at rest), or shoulder (anteriorly and/or inferiorly positioned) abnormalities. Traditional inflammatory signs are likely absent; therefore, absence of redness, skin warmth, or swelling is common. Finally, maneuvers can be performed that assess deficits distant to the lateral elbow, including hip or leg stability and strength. Previous authors have noted the interrelated design of the body, termed the kinetic chain, where the anatomic segments work and fail as a unit.[75-81] It is possible that core and/or lower extremity deficiencies could be contributing to the lateral elbow pain, as hip weakness can increase loads and stresses on the elbow.[65] One option to assess these areas is to look at single-leg standing balance ability via the Trendelenburg maneuver and a single-leg squat.[78] In a standing balance test, the patient is asked to stand on one leg with no other verbal cue. Deviations, such as a Trendelenburg posture or internally or externally rotating the weight-bearing limb indicate, inability to control the posture and suggest proximal core weakness (**Figure 9.15**).

The single-leg squat would be the next progressive evaluation if the standing balance test is done well. Assuming the same starting point as the standing balance test, the patient is asked to do repetitive partial quarter to half squats with no other verbal cues. The patient may present with one or more of four possible deviations. First, the patient may perform only a one-third squat. This posture does not require high levels of abductor muscle activation. The one-half squat will more readily demonstrate any existing abductor muscle weakness. Second, the patient may use the arms for balance or go into an exaggerated flexed trunk

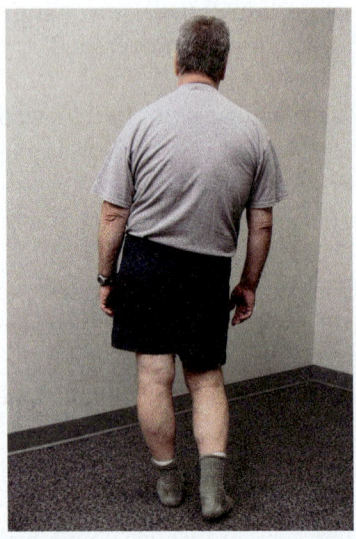
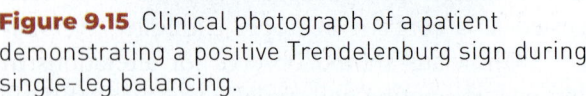

Figure 9.15 Clinical photograph of a patient demonstrating a positive Trendelenburg sign during single-leg balancing.

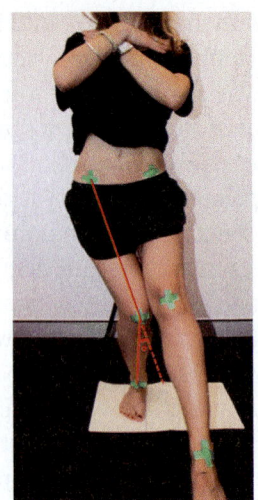

Figure 9.16 Clinical photograph of a patient demonstrating valgus knee positioning indicating dynamic hip muscle weakness.

Reproduced from Wyndow N, De Jong A, Rial K, et al: Foot and ankle mobility and the frontal plane projection angle in asymptomatic controls. *J Foot Ankle Res* 2015;8(Suppl 2):O43.

position. This excessive flexion forces the lower extremity into a falsely negative, optimally aligned position as the body attempts to balance on the descent phase of the squat. Third, the patient's knee may move into an exaggerated valgus position on descent. This would suggest that a proximal deficiency in strength and stability is present. Finally, the patient may dynamically rotate the leg as a unit on the descent phase of the squat. This has also been termed corkscrewing due to the rotary motion that occurs during this maneuver (**Figure 9.16**). Presence of any or all of these deviations is indicative of poor proximal control of the lower extremity.

Palpation. Palpation of the lateral elbow structures is recommended and should include the proximal common extensor tendon, the lateral epicondyle, and lateral joint line. Tenderness of any of these structures may suggest lateral epicondylalgia; however, tenderness alone should not lead to the clinical conclusion of the condition. Localized tenderness could be a spurious finding, so combining tenderness with the history-specific items and the other examination components will help in the development of a more accurate diagnosis.

Common Special Tests Findings. Range of motion at the elbow is not typically affected. Manual muscle testing of the muscles that act directly on the elbow will likely not reveal any strength deficits. However, muscle testing of the wrist extensors may reveal deficiencies in strength or tension-elicited pain. It should be noted that manual muscle testing cannot differentiate between strength loss from histologic tendon changes and tension-elicited pain. Furthermore, dynamometer-assessed grip strength has been shown to be more discriminatory between elbows with lateral epicondylalgia and those without the condition.[82] Thus, grip strength testing is the recommended method of strength testing. It is uncommon to elicit neurologic deficits or have the patient report paresthesia related to the radial or median nerve. Specific special tests for this condition can be found in the orthopaedic special tests section of this chapter.

Standard imaging, such as radiography, would be warranted only if a distal humeral fracture or other elbow-specific fracture were suspected. Because lateral epicondylalgia is a muscle-based pathology, radiographs will not have strong clinical value. Advanced imaging modalities, such as MRI or CT, are rarely used. Musculoskeletal diagnostic ultrasonography has been shown to have some clinical value. When diagnostic ultrasonography has been shown to identify a common extensor tendon cross-section area ≥32 mm² and a thickness of approximately 4 mm, there was a strong correlation with the presence of lateral epicondylalgia.[83]

Medial Epicondylalgia

Similar to lateral epicondylalgia, medial elbow pain has experienced the same nomenclature conundrum. For consistency and accuracy, medial epicondylalgia is the recommended term for clinical identification of medial elbow pain (**Table 9.4**). When diagnostic imaging or surgical options designed to verify the presence or absence of inflammation or tendon changes are available, more appropriate diagnoses, such as tendinopathy or tendinosis, can be provided.

In contrast to its lateral counterpart, medial epicondylalgia does not occur with as great a frequency, with reports suggesting an overall prevalence of approximately 1%. However, working populations can see incidences of approximately 5%.[67] The mechanism of injury for medial epicondylalgia has been thought to be repetitive eccentric loading of the muscles conducting wrist flexion and forearm pronation combined with valgus overload at the elbow.[84] This mechanistic description of the injury correlates with the activities of overhead athletes where the arm position between late cocking to deceleration can stress the medial elbow.[85,86] The mechanism also relates to the term golfer's elbow because breakdown of proper mechanics during the golf swing (typically, valgus stress with excessive degrees of freedom at the wrist) can cause medial-sided elbow pain.

Mimicking the pathophysiology of lateral epicondylalgia, repetitive stress on the common flexor tendon eventually results in degradation. Histology assessments have revealed tendon change over time via an inflammatory cascade.[87] Stress applied to the tendon repetitively creates an inflammatory response. Continuous activity results in continuous stress being applied to an already inflamed tendon, creating an increase in fibroblasts, vascular hyperplasia (tissue enlargement), and disorganized and immature collagen.[87] These negative responses lead to abnormal tendon changes that ultimately present with pain and an

Table 9.4 Medial Epicondylalgia Quick Tips

Pathology	Description	Presentation (HIPS)	Special Tests/ Imaging	Differential Diagnosis	5-Min Sideline Assessment Tips
Medial epicondylalgia	Pain at or around the medial elbow	History: Typically, from repetitive movements Inspection: Alterations in resting posture Palpation: Common flexor tendon and medial epicondyle Special tests: Range of motion not typically affected. Wrist flexion may yield weakness	Polk and golfer's elbow tests Imaging warranted only with distal humeral fracture or another elbow fracture	UCL injury Fracture (olecranon or distal humerus) Cubital tunnel syndrome	Most often driven from repetitive activity; inquire about MOI and length of pain Rule out fracture, dislocation, UCL sprain, and carpal tunnel syndrome Palpate over medial epicondyle and proximal flexor tendon Wrist flexion and grip strength assessment

HIPS, history, inspection, palpations special tests; MOI, mechanism of injury; UCL, ulnar collateral ligament.

inability to perform repetitive activity. Although the condition can begin with an inflammatory response, most symptoms appear after the inflammatory response has ceased and typically occur with greater chronicity.

Outcome Measures. No specific outcome measure has been developed or used for medial epicondylalgia. It is reasonable to suggest that traditional upper extremity regional tools, such as the DASH or QuickDASH, could be used for patients with this condition. It should be noted that evidence exists that has identified less pain and dysfunction with medial epicondylalgia compared to lateral epicondylalgia.[88]

Specific Questions. Subjectively, a history assessment that homes in on the mechanistic causes may assist the clinician with identifying the pathology. In particular, the following history items should be noted:

- Age: Due to the degradation of tissue and/or occupational causes, medial epicondylalgia is common for individuals 40 years of age and older.[84]
- Does the patient participate in activities (recreational or occupational) involving repetitious manipulation and arm movements known to lead to medial elbow pain?
- Is pain elicited with active or forceful wrist flexion?
- Is pain elicited with active or forceful forearm pronation and/or supination?
- Is pain elicited during and/or after gripping activities?
- Is the pain described as "deep" or "localized" to the proximal soft tissue on the medial aspect of the forearm?
- Does the patient describe hand weakness with gripping activities?

Inspection. Similar to the inspections suggested for lateral epicondylalgia, assessments of posture and lower extremity physical function are important for identifying potential kinetic chain deficits that may contribute to the medial elbow pain. Possible assessment of throwing, serving, swing, or labor mechanics may also help identify potential causes of excessive stress on the medial elbow, especially if the patient participates in baseball, tennis, golf, and/or manual labor occupations.

Palpation. Palpation of the medial elbow structures is recommended and should include the proximal common flexor tendon, medial epicondyle, and medial joint line. Tenderness of any of these structures may suggest medial epicondylalgia; however, tenderness alone should not lead to the clinical conclusion of the condition. Localized tenderness could be a spurious finding, so combining tenderness with the history-specific items and other examination components will help in the development of a more accurate diagnosis.

Common Special Tests Findings. Range of motion is not typically affected. MMT of the muscles that act directly on the elbow will likely not reveal any strength deficits. However, muscle testing of the wrist flexors may reveal deficiencies in strength or tension-elicited pain. It should be noted that MMT cannot differentiate between strength loss from histologic tendon changes and tension-elicited pain. It is uncommon to elicit neurologic deficits or have the patient report paresthesia related to the ulnar or median nerve. Specific special tests for this condition can be found in the orthopaedic special tests section of this chapter.

Standard imaging, such as radiography, would only be warranted if a distal humeral fracture or other elbow-specific fracture were suspected. Because medial epicondylalgia is a muscle-based pathology, radiographs will not have strong clinical utility. Advanced imaging modalities, such as MRI or CT, are also rarely used. Musculoskeletal diagnostic ultrasonography has been shown to have clinical value, with a strong positive likelihood ratio of 12 and negative likelihood ratio of 0.05.[89]

Distal Biceps Rupture

Distal ruptures of the biceps brachii are similar to the epicondylalgia conditions in that they occur primarily in individuals 40 years of age and older.[90,91] This particular elbow pathology affects males more often than females.[92] However, unlike lateral and medial epicondylalgia, which are considered overuse injuries, distal ruptures of the biceps brachii occur traumatically (**Figure 9.17**). The injury primarily occurs at the tendon's insertion on the radial tuberosity of the radius[90] (**Table 9.5**).

Eccentric load upon a flexed elbow, such as sudden forced extension that may occur when attempting to move or lift heavy objects, catching heavy objects from above, or bracing the body via the arm when falling (ie, grabbing a stair rail when falling down a flight of stairs), is the recognized mechanism of distal biceps ruptures.[90,91] It is possible that the anatomic construct of the elbow joint and surrounding area may contribute to the cause of distal biceps ruptures. For example, three vascular zones were identified in

Pathologies of the Elbow **299**

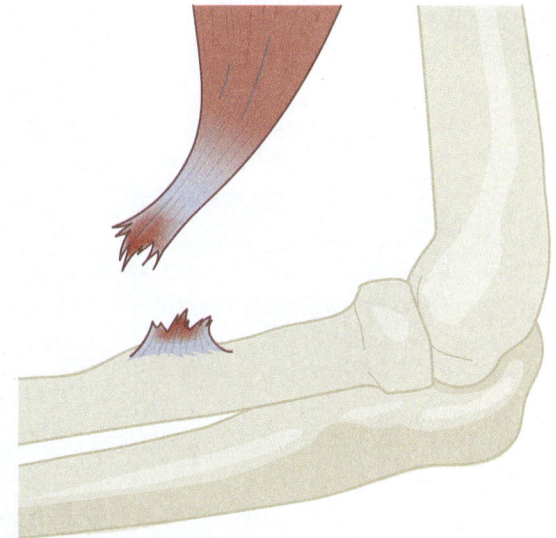

Figure 9.17 Drawing showing distal biceps tendon rupture.
© Jones & Bartlett Learning

the distal biceps tendon via advanced imaging.[93] In between the proximal and distal zones, which had adequate blood supply, a hypovascular zone was identified. Additionally, a 50% reduction in the radioulnar joint at the radial tuberosity occurred when subjects were moved from full supination to full pronation. This so-called mechanical impingement during these movements and the identification of a tendinous zone with inadequate blood supply were suggested to contribute to distal biceps tendon ruptures.[93] Furthermore, recent work has identified that both smoking and elevated body mass index are factors associated with an increased risk of sustaining this injury.[92]

Outcome Measures. Although specific studies have not directly examined the applicability of region-specific patient-reported outcome measures for outcomes related to distal biceps tendon ruptures, surgical and nonsurgical studies have utilized the DASH, ASES, and PRTEE.[94,95]

Specific Questions. The traumatic nature of the injury typically results in distinct clinical features. The clinician identifies the following history items:

- Age and sex: As noted earlier, males aged 40 years and older have the greatest risk of sustaining a distal biceps rupture.
- Was the patient attempting to move or lift heavy objects, catch a heavy object from above, or brace the body via the arm when falling?
- Was the dominant arm involved?[96]
- Was there a "snap" or other audible sound heard around the location of the elbow?
- Was a "pop" or other similar sensation felt at the time of injury around the location of the elbow?
- Does the patient smoke?
- Is the patient's body mass index elevated?
- Does the patient report cramping in the arm during supination or other forearm actions?

Inspection. Due to the traumatic nature of the injury, patients who sustained a distal biceps tendon

Table 9.5 Biceps Rupture Quick Tips

Pathology	Description	Presentation (HIPS)	Special Tests/ Imaging	Differential Diagnosis	5-Min Sideline Assessment Tips
Distal biceps rupture	Tear of the distal tendon at its insertion point on the radial tuberosity	History: Typically, occur from traumatic event, audible pop Inspections: Deformity and inflammation Palpation: Absence of distal tendon with complete tears Special tests: Difficulty/inability to flex elbow Weakness with elbow flexion and supination	Test battery: Biceps crease index and biceps crease ratio MRI is the gold standard for evaluating distal bicep tendon injury	Elbow fracture	Most often driven from single traumatic event Rule out fracture Will be palpable deformity at the distal biceps tendon (complete ruptures) Elbow flexion and extension range of motion Elbow flexion and forearm pronation strength assessment

HIPS, history, inspection, palpation, special tests.

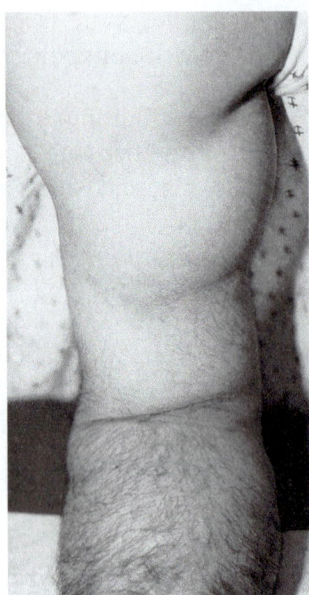

Figure 9.18 Clinical photograph of distal biceps tendon rupture.

Reproduced from Armstrong AD, Hubbard MC. eds: *Essentials of Musculoskeletal Care*, ed 5. Burlington, MA, American Academy of Orthopaedic Surgeons, 2015.

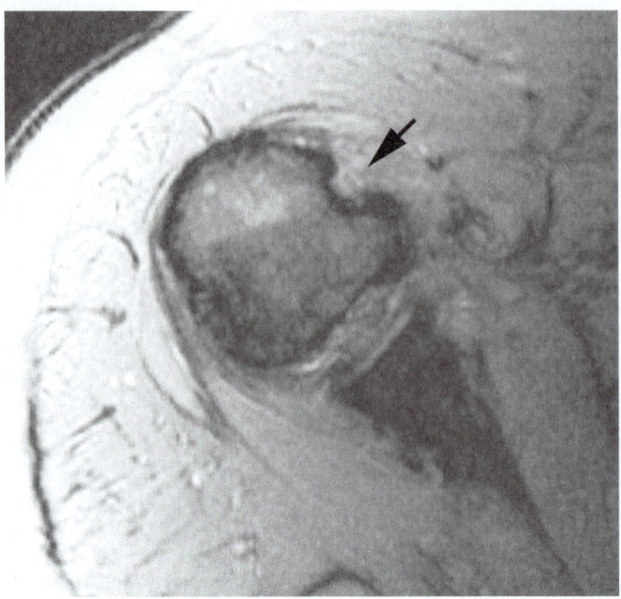

Figure 9.19 Magnetic resonance image showing a biceps tendon rupture.

Reproduced from Johnson TR, Steinbach LS. eds: *Essentials of Musculoskeletal Imaging*. Rosemont, IL, American Academy of Orthopaedic Surgeons, 2004.

rupture often present with evident ecchymosis (**Figure 9.18**) but may also have signs of inflammation, such as pain and swelling. It has been noted that subacute and chronic distal biceps tendon injuries may present with a loss of contour in the muscle due to atrophy.[97]

Palpation. Pain and tenderness over the affected area, specifically the radial tuberosity, antecubital fossa, distal third of the biceps muscle, and muscle belly, are possible. It has been noted that pain tends to dissipate quickly with this injury, especially with complete ruptures. As such, weakness with elbow flexion and supination may serve as a better indicator that an injury took place.[98]

Common Special Tests Findings. Range of motion will be affected in most cases, with a limitation of both elbow flexion and extension. Both motions are often limited and painful. MMT may reveal weakness of elbow flexion and forearm supination. Testing for both flexion and supination should be performed in all three positions of the forearm (pronation, neutral, and supination). In some cases, a maximum MMT grade of 3/5 will be recorded. However, in cases of partial rupture, it is possible the patient can resist some manual overpressure applied by the clinician, resulting in a grade of 4/5 or 5/5. It is uncommon to elicit neurologic deficits or for the patient to report paresthesia. Specific special tests for this condition can be found under the orthopaedic special tests section of this chapter.

MRI is considered the gold standard for evaluating the distal biceps tendon for injury (**Figure 9.19**). Advanced imaging modalities, such as MRI, can help visualize the existence of fluid in and around the affected area, tendon integrity, and presence or absence of the tendinous attachment to the radial tuberosity.[97,99] Attempts at using diagnostic ultrasonography are ongoing and beginning to show promise as an additional diagnostic modality.[100,101]

Ligamentous-Based Pathology

UCL Injury

Most clinicians are familiar with injuries to the UCL because of the increased incidence of injury that has been occurring to this structure the past 15 years. Greater frequency has been seen in professional and high school sports, with baseball and other overhead sports having the most recorded injuries.[102,103] Of note, elbow pain, especially medial-sided pain, occurs with greater frequency in overhead athletes as age increases, ranging from 20% to 30% at age 10 years to over 50% at age 14 years and older.[104-106]

Activities that place the elbow in a position where valgus stress occurs by design increase the loads placed on the UCL (**Table 9.6**). The repetitious nature of overhead sports and some manual labor activities essentially create a situation where the UCL can be injured at any time (**Figure 9.20**). The high loads and stresses reach and sometimes exceed the known load capacities of the UCL.[107]

Table 9.6 Ulnar Collateral Ligament Pathology Quick Tips

Pathology	Description	Presentation (HIPS)	Special Tests/Imaging	Differential Diagnosis	5-Min Sideline Assessment Tips
Ulnar collateral ligament injury	Pain and tenderness on the medial joint line	History: Typically, occur from repetitive overload Inspection: Alterations in resting posture Palpation: Tenderness to the medial joint line, medial epicondyle, or common flexor tendon Special tests: Elbow range of motion may not be affected. Assess glenohumeral motion	Moving valgus stress test	Medial epicondylalgia Fracture (olecranon or distal humerus) Cubital tunnel syndrome	Greater frequency in overhead sports; inquire about MOI during activity and area of pain Rule out medial epicondylalgia and fracture Palpate over medial joint line Perform moving valgus stress test Possible neurologic deficits/symptoms specific to ulnar nerve

HIPS, history, inspection, palpation, special tests; MOI, mechanism of injury.

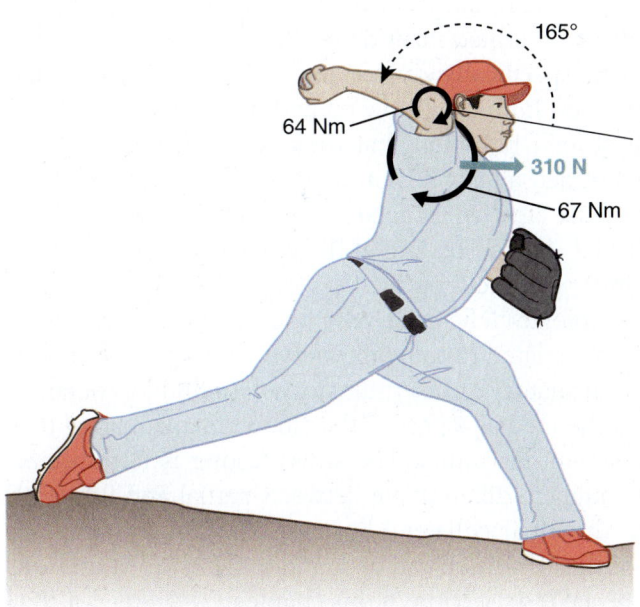

Figure 9.20 Drawing showing an example of overhead activity with valgus stress.
© Jones & Bartlett Learning

The concern is that the static and dynamic restraints of the medial elbow are not plentiful, with primary stabilization coming mainly from the UCL and joint capsule statically and the flexor carpi ulnaris, FDS, and pronator teres complex dynamically.[107] These limited restraints, when stressed repeatedly, eventually reach a limit and become injured. In order to reduce the incidence of this injury, the kinetic chain segments should be optimized, such as having optimal leg, hip, and trunk strength/stability; scapular stability and positioning; and muscle endurance.[65,108] Therefore, identifying the existence of a UCL injury is only one aspect of the examination. The other aspect should identify other structures that may be impaired.

Outcome Measures. Instruments, such as the DASH, QuickDASH, and ASES, may be used to assess patient self-reported physical function. However, these instruments are primarily focused on gauging a patient's ability to perform activities of daily living. The Kerlan-Jobe Orthopaedic Clinic Shoulder and Elbow Score may be useful for overhead athletes, with data existing for professional baseball, swimming, and collegiate-level athletes.[109-111] Another instrument that may be applicable would be the Patient-Specific Function Scale, as this questionnaire allows the patient to write down the exact activities or tasks that he or she has difficulty with due to the injury.[112]

Specific History Questions. The traumatic nature of the injury typically results in distinct clinical features; however, the clinician should gather a complete history for the subjective portion of the examination. The following history items should be noted:

- Was the patient performing an overhead task at the time of injury? This could be overhead sport or manual labor related.
- How often does the patient participate in overhead activities? Is overplaying or overtraining occurring?

- Does the patient report "looseness" of the elbow during overhead tasks or tasks involving forward elevation of the arm?
- Does the patient report medial elbow pain during overhead tasks or tasks involving forward elevation of the arm?
- Does the patient have pain during the acceleration phase of throwing?[113]
- How long has the dysfunction been present? This is important because pain is typically not present with chronic, long-standing injury to the UCL.
- Does the patient report numbness, tingling, and/or burning from the elbow to the fingers, especially into the fourth and fifth digits?
- Was the dominant arm involved?
- Was a "pop" or other similar sensation felt at the time of injury around the location of the elbow?

Inspection. Similar to the inspections suggested for lateral epicondylalgia, assessments of posture and lower extremity physical function are important for identifying potential kinetic chain deficits that may contribute to the UCL injury. Possible assessment of throwing, serving, swing, or labor mechanics may also help identify potential causes of excessive stress on the medial elbow, especially if the patient participates in baseball, tennis, javelin, and/or manual labor occupations.

Palpation. Palpation of the medial elbow structures is recommended and should include the proximal common flexor tendon, medial epicondyle, and medial joint line. Tenderness of any of these structures may suggest involvement of the UCL, especially tenderness over the medial joint line directly. Tenderness alone should not lead to the clinical conclusion of the condition. Localized tenderness could be a spurious finding; therefore, combining tenderness with the history-specific items and other examination components, such as pain and instability, with special testing will help develop a more accurate diagnosis. An additional area of palpation should be the superior and posterior aspects of the medial condyle and the olecranon fossa. These areas are important to include to determine whether not only tenderness exists but possible paresthesia.

Common Special Tests Findings. Range of motion at the elbow is not typically affected, and pain is often not a common complaint in chronic cases. Pain with activity can exist but often in the acute stages of the injury. Recent work has also suggested that an increase in injury risk occurs to overhead athletes when glenohumeral internal rotation deficit and total arc of motion are decreased on the dominant throwing arm[114-116] (**Figure 9.21**). In addition, osteologic changes at the glenohumeral joint have been found to be present in those with UCL trauma.[117] Muscle testing of the elbow as part of the examination assessing UCL integrity has not been reported to be a diagnostic finding. However, it has been reported that overhead athletes can demonstrate rotator cuff weakness, specifically during internal and external rotation, on both the throwing and nonthrowing arms.[118] It should be noted that these strength deficits were identified after the UCL was known to be injured, so a cause and effect relationship has not been established. Muscle testing of the elbow (flexion or extension) will likely be unaffected. It is possible to elicit neurologic deficits or have the patient report paresthesia related to the ulnar nerve. Stress testing can be confirmatory or discriminatory, with findings of laxity on the medial aspect of the elbow often equating to a ligamentous injury. The stress testing is not specific enough to differentiate between partial and full tears of the ulnar collateral ligament. Specific special tests for this condition can be found under the orthopaedic special tests section of this chapter.

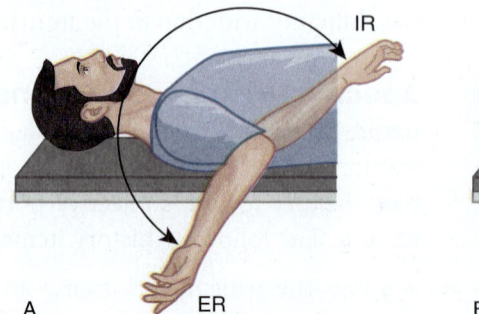 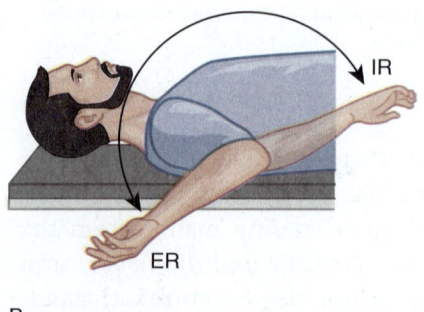

Figure 9.21 Drawings demonstrating total arc of motion **(A)** and glenohumeral internal rotation deficit **(B)**.

ER, external rotation; IR, internal rotation.

Advanced imaging modalities, such as MRI or magnetic resonance arthrography, would be recommended for visualizing injury to the UCL.

MRI can help rule in UCL injury, with clinical utility values being reported as infinite for the positive likelihood ratio, but it is not ideal for ruling out the injury (negative likelihood ratio of 0.43).[46] Conversely, magnetic resonance arthrography is ideal because it has strong positive and negative likelihood ratios (infinity and 0.08, respectively), and it has the added bonus of excellent interrater reliability.[119,120] Plain radiographs will not be of much help for determining UCL pathology in the skeletally mature individual; however, adolescent baseball players could present with UCL symptoms, but, in actuality, they may have Little Leaguer's elbow (apophysitis of the medial epicondyle). Radiographs will verify if apophysitis is present (**Figure 9.22**).

Posterolateral Rotatory Instability

Posterolateral rotatory instability (**Figure 9.23**) of the elbow occurs when the radius and ulna rotate externally in relation to the distal humerus, leading to posterior displacement of the radial head relative to the capitulum[15] (**Table 9.7**).

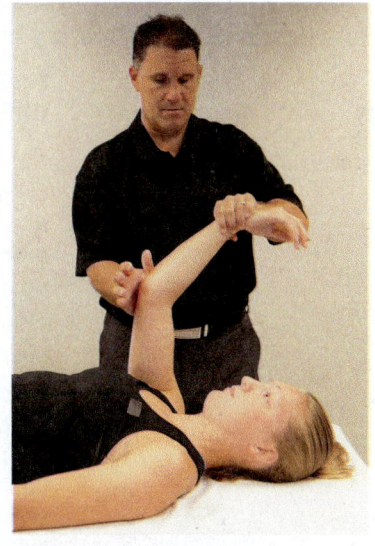

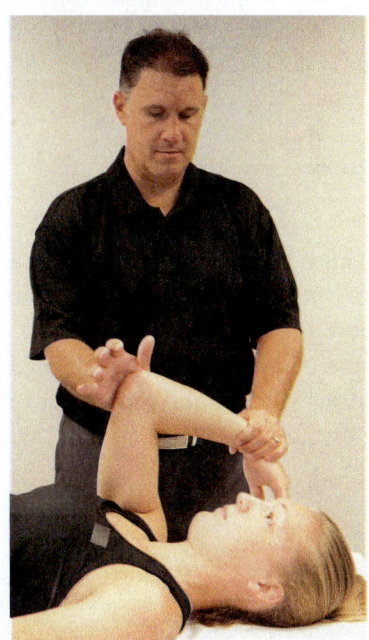

B

Figure 9.23 Clinical photographs performing the posterolateral rotatory instability special test. **A.** The patient's arm and elbow are flexed to 90° with the forearm supinated. **B.** The clinician grasps the wrist and forearm and passively flexes the elbow while applying valgus and axial stresses with supination.

© Jones & Bartlett Learning

Essentially, the LLC becomes disrupted either following dislocation (Figure 9.24A) (most common), radial head fractures, or coronoid fractures or from chronic cubitus varus of the elbow.[121] Due to the traumatic mechanism, this injury is nondiscriminatory because it does not have increased prevalence based on age, sex, or activity. However, patients who have experienced nursemaid's elbow (**Figure 9.24**), a condition classified as radial head dislocation/subluxation as a result of an applied traction of the arm away from

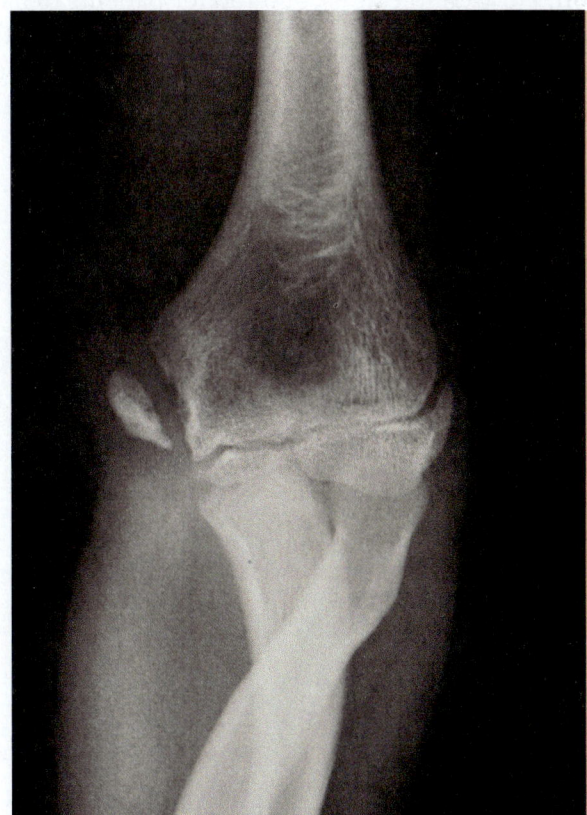

Figure 9.22 Radiograph demonstrating Little Leaguer's elbow.

© Scott Camazine/Science Source

Table 9.7 Posterolateral Rotatory Instability Pathology Quick Tips

Pathology	Description	Presentation (HIPS)	Special Tests/ Imaging	Differential Diagnosis	5-Min Sideline Assessment Tips
Posterolateral rotatory instability	Disruption of lateral elbow complex following trauma	History: Typically, occur from traumatic mechanism Inspection: Alterations in load-bearing positions Palpation: Tenderness to the lateral joint line, lateral epicondyle, or common extensor tendon Special tests: Elbow range of motion and muscle strength may not be affected	Lateral pivot shift or posterolateral rotatory drawer tests	Lateral epicondylalgia Elbow fracture (radial head or distal humerus)	Often traumatic and accompanied with a dislocation or fracture Palpate over lateral joint line Closed kinetic chain tasks may elicit loosening of the elbow

HIPS, history, inspection, palpation, special tests.

the body, may later in life have resultant posterolateral rotatory instability. It should be noted that nursemaid's elbow and posterolateral rotatory instability are not the same condition. The instability is the result or consequence, whereas the radial head injury is what led to the instability.

Patients with this condition can experience symptoms with and without loss of physical function. For example, it is common for patients to have difficulty performing closed-chain tasks with the arm.[121] The axial loading that is required to perform tasks, such as using the arms to push up the

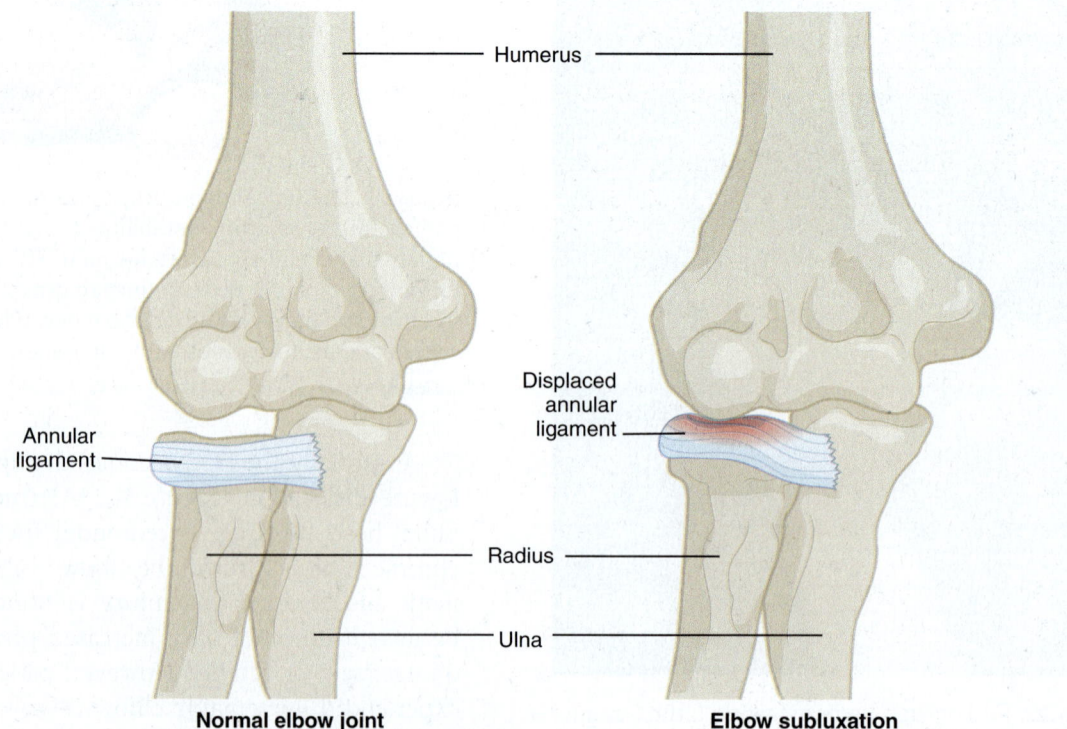

Figure 9.24 Drawings showing the location of nursemaid's elbow.

body when rising from a chair, becomes compromised due to the lack of stability at the elbow.[122] It has been noted that the diagnosis is clinically made using the patient's subjective information, clinical special testing for laxity, and ultimately testing integrity under anesthesia.[121]

Outcome Measures. No specific disease-oriented outcome measure has been developed or utilized exclusively for posterolateral rotatory instability. It is reasonable to suggest that traditional upper extremity regional tools, such as the DASH or QuickDASH, could be used for patients with this condition.

Specific History Questions. The following history items should be noted:

- Does the patient have a history of trauma involving the elbow?
- Did the patient have previous elbow surgery? It is possible for posterolateral rotatory instability to arise following relocation or fixation following a dislocation and following excision and/or extensive débridement of the lateral extensor mass.[123]
- Does the patient report "looseness" of the elbow during closed-chain tasks or other types of axial loading?
- Does the patient describe the elbow as "unstable," meaning the elbow "gives out" with activity?
- Does the patient report lateral elbow pain during closed-chain tasks or other types of axial loading?
- Was a "pop" or other similar sensation felt at the time of injury around the location of the elbow?
- Does a "pop," "click," or "catch" occur with activity?

Inspection. In most instances, the patient will not have any clear observational findings that will suggest posterolateral rotatory instability is present. Following management of an elbow fracture (distal humerus, radial head, or olecranon), patients should be assessed for instability in load-bearing positions.

Palpation. Palpation of the lateral elbow structures is recommended and should include the proximal common extensor tendon, lateral epicondyle, lateral joint line, and radial head. Because symptoms are typically elicited with load-bearing tasks, tenderness alone may not provide a clear answer as to whether or not posterolateral rotatory instability is present.

Common Special Tests Findings. Range of motion is not typically affected. Similar to the assessment of the UCL, muscle testing of the elbow may not assist the clinician in making the diagnosis of posterolateral rotatory instability. Patients with chronic instability may present with some elbow muscle weakness, but this would likely be secondary and not diagnostic of the condition. It is possible to elicit neurologic deficits or have the patient report paresthesia related to the radial nerve from the lateral elbow down to the first/second digits. Instability in load-bearing (axial-loaded) activities is a hallmark finding of this injury. Specific special tests for this condition can be found under the orthopaedic special tests section of this chapter.

Although this is a ligamentous-based pathology, imaging has not been shown to be completely helpful in identifying the injury. Plain radiography can sometimes help identify abnormalities of the key bony components (coronoid process, radial head, and/or capitulum) and may show an avulsion fracture of the origin or insertion of the LLC.[121] Advanced imaging modalities, such as MRI, have shown inconclusive evidence, with one study finding a perfect correlation between positive clinical tests and abnormalities seen on MRI[47] and others finding a much weaker relationship between the clinical and imaging results.[120,124]

Bone-Based Pathology

Fracture or Dislocation

Dislocation of the elbow is characterized as separation or disarticulation of the ulna and humerus. The injury often occurs when an individual attempts to brace himself or herself when falling from a height. As the hand contacts the ground, the ulna and humerus separate, forcing the ulna posteriorly. The traumatic nature of the injury may result in concomitant injury to various other elbow structures, including the annular ligament, radial head or coronoid process (fracture), and/or UCL.

Three primary types of fracture occur at the elbow: distal humerus fractures (**Figure 9.25**), radial head fractures (**Figure 9.26**), and olecranon fractures (**Figure 9.27**). Distal humerus fractures are relatively rare in skeletally mature individuals, representing only 2% of adult fractures,[125] but occur at a greater frequency in adolescent populations (10 to 14 years of age).[126] When a fracture does occur, the mechanism is often an impact injury of the ulna onto the capitulum and/or trochlea with the elbow flexed or extended.[125,127] Partial fractures of the lateral or medial condyle can occur and be contributed to indirect trauma to an extended elbow when it is positioned in either valgus or varus. Of particular interest is that these fractures

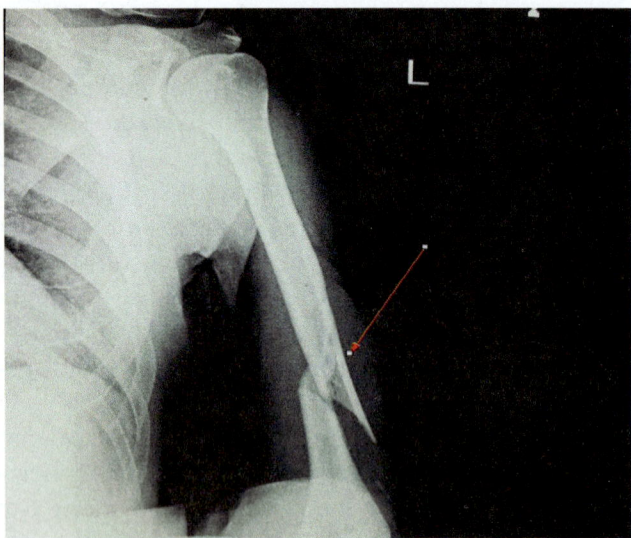

Figure 9.25 Radiograph showing distal humerus fracture (arrow).

© Richman Photo/Shutterstock

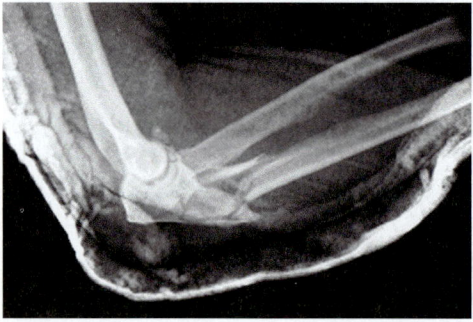

Figure 9.27 Radiograph showing an olecranon process fracture.

Reproduced from Armstrong AD, Hubbard MC. eds: *Essentials of Musculoskeletal Care*, ed 5. Burlington, MA, American Academy of Orthopaedic Surgeons, 2015.

can also result in injury to the static restraints opposite the injured side of the elbow. This suggests that either UCL injury or posterolateral rotatory instability can occur following this type of fracture.

A more common elbow bony disruption would be fractures involving the radial head. It has been noted that radial head fractures represent approximately one-third of all elbow fractures.[128] Similar to distal humerus fractures, high levels of trauma, often involving axial load to the forearm, are the classic mechanism of injury for these types of fractures. The axial load forces the radial head to compress against the capitulum of the humerus, resulting in bony injury. This mechanism is nondiscriminatory, meaning that there is no specific population that experiences these fractures more so than another.

Olecranon fractures are relatively common;[129] however, they tend to occur primarily in pediatric/adolescent and geriatric populations.[130] These types of fractures can be sustained from direct trauma to the olecranon or via an axially loaded mechanism, but they may also occur from contraction of the triceps brachii during high-trauma mechanisms.[130]

Outcome Measures. No specific disease-oriented outcome measure has been developed or used exclusively for elbow fractures. It is reasonable to suggest that traditional upper extremity regional tools, such as the DASH or QuickDASH, could be used for patients with any of the various elbow fracture types.

Specific History Questions. The following history items should be noted:

- Does the patient have a history of trauma involving the elbow?
- If yes, did the trauma involve a direct blow to the elbow or an axially loaded mechanism?
- Does the patient report difficulty fully flexing or extending the elbow?
- Does the patient have difficulty pronating or supinating the elbow?
- Does the patient report pain at rest or with elbow motion?
- Was a "pop" or other similar sensation felt at the time of injury around the location of the elbow?

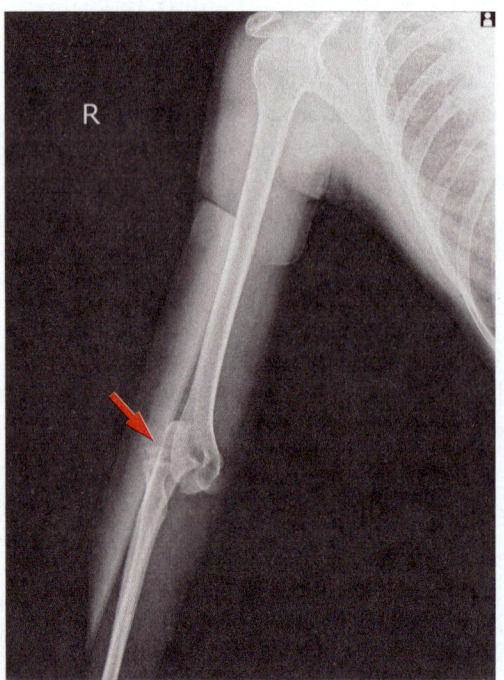

Figure 9.26 Radiograph showing radial head fracture (arrow).

© Richman Photo/Shutterstock

Inspection. Traditional signs of inflammation and acute trauma may be observed, including deformity, swelling, and ecchymosis. Patients may self-support the affected arm in order to avoid painful movements.

Palpation. Due to the traumatic mechanisms that can cause the various types of fracture at the elbow, it is suggested that all bony and soft-tissue structures be assessed. These structures would include the medial and lateral epicondyles, common flexor and extensor tendons, distal biceps and triceps tendons, antecubital fossa, olecranon process, olecranon fossa, and radial head. The axial-loaded mechanism may result in hand and wrist injury as well, so palpation and assessment of these distal structures are recommended.[130,131]

Common Special Tests Findings. A limited range of motion may exist either because of pain or disruption of the skeletal construct. Muscle testing of the elbow (flexion or extension) may not be able to be performed because of pain and/or the disrupted skeletal anatomy. If it can be performed, muscle testing may appear weak due to pain or disruption of the bony construct. It is possible to elicit neurologic deficits or have the patient report paresthesia related to any of the elbow nerves. It is crucial that vascular integrity be assessed at the distal portion of the extremity. Specific special tests for this condition can be found under the orthopaedic special tests section of this chapter.

Standard radiographs can be helpful in identifying the extent of the injury for the various types of elbow fractures. AP, lateral, oblique, and internal oblique views are recommended for distal humerus fractures.[126] Advanced imaging modalities, such as CT, are not typically ordered immediately following a traumatic elbow injury unless the fracture type is complex, such as a comminuted type of fracture.[125,126] Advanced imaging can be used later if soft-tissue integrity needs to be assessed.

AP and lateral radiographs serve as standard imaging for both radial head and olecranon fractures as well. It has been noted that it is common for a nondisplaced radial head fracture to not be seen clearly or immediately with plain radiographs.[131] A possible suggestive finding of radial head fracture could be the identification of an enlarged posterior fat pad, which may be visible with the lateral radiographic view.[131] This finding could suggest a radial head fracture is present because the posterior fat pad is within the capsule but outside the synovium. The visible posterior fat pad could mean that a hemarthrosis exists within the joint. It has been suggested that the lateral radiograph is critical for determining fracture severity, displacement, and concomitant bony injuries.[130]

Neurologic-Based Pathology
Cubital Tunnel Syndrome

Cubital tunnel syndrome typically arises from two sources: extended or prolonged sustained elbow flexion or following traumatic elbow injury (**Table 9.8**). Examples of sustained elbow flexion activities include sleeping with the elbows flexed either across the chest or under the body (sleeping prone with arms under the chest or pillow) and repeated and habitual mobile

Table 9.8 Cubital Tunnel Pathology Quick Tips

Pathology	Description	Presentation (HIPS)	Special Tests/ Imaging	Differential Diagnosis	5-Min Sideline Assessment Tips
Cubital tunnel syndrome	Compression of the ulnar nerve	History: Can occur from traumatic or repetitive mechanism Inspection: May not have clear observational findings Palpation: Medial elbow structures recommended for palpation, but often not tender Special tests: Neurologic symptoms to ulnar distribution may be common	Pressure provocation test or nerve conduction velocity tests	Medial epicondylalgia Fracture (olecranon or distal humerus) Ulnar collateral ligament injury	Can be acute or chronic episode; inquire about MOI and when symptoms occur Rule out medial epicondylalgia and UCL injury Palpate over ulnar groove Wrist flexion strength assessment Dermatome and peripheral nerve distribution assessment

HIPS, history, inspection, palpation, special tests; MOI, mechanism of injury; UCL, ulnar collateral ligament.

device use.[132] The syndrome arises due to compression of the ulnar nerve along its anatomic pathway due to a tensioning of the nerve and reduction of the pathway space each time the elbow is flexed from traction, muscle contraction, or muscle compression.[133,134] Overhead activities and occupations requiring repetitive use of the arms can also lead to ulnar nerve symptoms at the elbow.

Outcome Measures. No specific disease-oriented outcome measure has been developed or used exclusively for cubital tunnel syndrome. It is reasonable to suggest that traditional upper extremity regional tools, such as the DASH or QuickDASH, could be utilized for patients with elbow-related neurologic conditions.

Specific History Questions

- Does the patient participate in activities (recreational or occupational) involving repetitious manipulation and arm movements known to require repetitious elbow flexion?
- Does the patient describe hand weakness with gripping activities?
- Does the patient describe motor control issues with activities of daily living due to an inability to fully utilize the hand?
- Does the patient report intermittent or constant paresthesia from the elbow to the hand?
- Does the patient report paresthesia in the fourth and fifth digits?
- Does the patient have a history of trauma, such as an elbow fracture?
- Does the patient have a history of immobilization of the shoulder or elbow?

Inspection. In most instances, the patient will not have any clear observational findings that will suggest cubital tunnel syndrome is present. It is possible that a more proximal cause, such as postural deficits or scapular dyskinesis, could be driving the elbow symptoms. Considering that the nerves at the elbow originate from the cervical vertebrae and resultant brachial plexus, altered posture or scapular positioning could be placing traction on the nerves, thus leading to the neurologic complaints. It is recommended that an assessment for cervical and shoulder impairments be performed to rule out a proximal cause to the distal elbow condition.

Palpation. Palpation of the medial elbow structures is recommended and should include the proximal common flexor tendon, medial epicondyle, medial joint line, olecranon fossa, and antecubital fossa. Tenderness and/or pain is not the typical report but rather an exacerbation of paresthesia at the medial elbow or down into the fourth and fifth digits.

Common Special Tests Findings. Range of motion will likely be unaffected. Muscle testing of the elbow (flexion or extension) will likely be uncompromised. Positions of prolonged elbow flexion tend to arouse the neurologic/paresthesia symptoms specific to the ulnar nerve. The patient will report these symptoms anywhere from the medial elbow to the fourth/fifth digits.

In most cases, standard radiographs or advanced imaging studies are not necessary unless it is suspected that injury to the skeletal anatomy, UCL, or other soft-tissue structure could be creating the cubital tunnel symptoms. Diagnostic electromyography or nerve conduction velocity tests could help determine whether the neurologic symptoms are coming from proximal or distal locations.

Olecranon Bursitis

Olecranon bursitis is one of the more common yet poorly studied elbow conditions (**Table 9.9**). By definition, the condition is characterized by inflammation of the bursa; however, it is more accurately characterized as an increase in fluid within the bursal cavity.[135] It has been commonly taught that bursal tissue is a fluid-filled sac, yet this too is an incomplete description. Bursal tissue is an enclosed sac of fluid, but it is covered externally by a synovial membrane that serves to decrease friction between the olecranon process and skin during active elbow motion.[136] The classic mechanism of injury for developing bursitis has been noted to be repetitive microtrauma (aseptic); however, numerous cases of bacterial contamination (septic) have also been noted to occur.[137-140] Unfortunately, there is a moderate amount of overlap regarding the presentation of both aseptic and septic versions, which makes clinical diagnosis of the exact version of the condition difficult.[141]

Specific History Questions

- Have you recently experienced a fall directly onto your elbow?
- Do you perform an activity or task that requires you to repeatedly bend and straighten your elbow?
- Have you scraped or cut your elbow recently? (This is important to ask in order to determine whether a possible foreign body may be present, creating an inflamed or infectious state.)

Table 9.9 **Olecranon Pathology Quick Tips**

Pathology	Description	Presentation (HIPS)	Special Tests/ Imaging	Differential Diagnosis	5-Min Sideline Assessment Tips
Olecranon bursitis	An increase in fluid within the bursal cavity	History: Can occur from aseptic or septic trauma Inspection: Noticeable pronounced area of fluid directly over the olecranon process, which can present as deformity Palpation: Olecranon process Special tests: Rule out bacterial presence	None	Olecranon process fracture	Visual observation often reveals a noticeable pronounced area of fluid directly over the olecranon process Palpate over olecranon for temperature changes and tenderness

HIPS, history, inspection, palpation, special tests.

- Have you received a diagnosis of diabetes, gout, rheumatoid arthritis, alcoholism, or human immunodeficiency virus? (Higher incidences of olecranon bursitis have been associated with these conditions.[135])

Inspection. Visual inspection would reveal a noticeable pronounced area of fluid directly over the olecranon process. In cases of possible infection, erythema may also be present.

Palpation. If swelling is present over the olecranon process, clinicians should attempt to qualitatively note whether the protrusion is soft, firm, or hard. An assessment of tissue temperature is recommended to determine whether inflammation or infection is present. If infected, tenderness may be present during palpation. Although pain may be present, in most instances this occurs at the end range of active motion due to increased pressure beneath the skin. Typically, range of motion is not grossly affected by the presence of this condition, but it may be limited in the presence of sepsis.

Common Special Tests Findings. No special or stress tests exist for this condition. However, if it is suspected that infection is present, clinicians may assess the patient's temperature to determine whether fever is present. Referral should be considered to rule out the presence of bacteria.

Special Tests

The special tests portion of the evaluation process incorporates range of motion, muscle strength, neurologic screening, and special test assessment. All of these components, along with a detailed history, observation, and palpation, will help aid in the clinical diagnosis process when evaluating the elbow.

Range of Motion

Osteokinematic assessment examines the movement of bones that can be seen during different planes of motion (frontal, sagittal, and transverse). Several key points must be understood when executing the osteokinematic assessment: (1) planes of motion, (2) axis of rotation, and (3) degrees of freedom. There are three cardinal plans of motion within the body: frontal, sagittal, and transverse. Joint movement occurs parallel to the plane of motion; however, the axis of rotation is oriented perpendicular to the plane. The degrees of freedom represent how many planes of motion that are allowed at a particular joint. For example, the sagittal plane divides the body in left and right halves; thus, elbow flexion and extension at the humeroulnar joint occur in the sagittal plane around a medial to lateral axis accounting for one degree of freedom. The humeroradial joint allows for supination and pronation within the transverse plane. As with any joint motion, measuring active and passive elbow range of motion using a goniometer or an inclinometer is a reliable method for quantifying osteokinematic motion.[142] **Table 9.10** describes the ranges of motion at the humeroulnar, humeroradial, and proximal radioulnar joints, along with the goniometry alignment for each joint motion. Active range of motion should be performed prior to passive range of motion to help assess the patient's willingness to move the joint.

Arthrokinematics describes movement within a joint at the joint surfaces that cannot be seen with the eye. This type of motion combines three fundamental

Table 9.10 Testing Methods for Elbow Passive Range of Motion and Normative Values Among Different Sex and Age Groups

Testing Position	Stationary Arm	Fulcrum	Moving Arm	Normative Data[a]							
				Males				Females			
				2–8 y	9–19 y	20–44 y	45–69 y	2–8 y	9–19 y	20–44 y	45–69 y
Flexion											
Supine with the arm flat and supinated next to the torso. To allow for full elbow extension, place a towel proximal to the elbow.	Lateral midline of humerus	Lateral epicondyle	Lateral midline of the radius, using the radial styloid process as a reference	151° (151–152)	148° (147–150)	145° (144–146)	143° (142–145)	153° (152–154)	150° (149–151)	150° (149–151)	148° (147–149)
Extension											
Supine with the arm flat and supinated next to the torso. To allow for full elbow extension, place a towel proximal to the elbow.	Lateral midline of humerus	Lateral epicondyle	Lateral midline of the radius, using the radial styloid process as a reference	2° (1–4)	5° (4–7)	1° (0–2)	1° (−2–0)	7° (5–8)	6° (5–8)	5° (4–6)	4° (3–5)
Pronation											
Sitting with arm by the side and elbow flexed to 90° with thumb toward the ceiling.	Parallel to the anterior midline of the humerus	Laterally and proximally to the ulnar styloid process	Across the dorsal aspect of the forearm just proximal to the styloid process of the radius and ulna	80° (79–80)	80° (79–82)	77° (76–78)	78° (77–79)	85° (83–86)	81° (80–83)	82° (81–83)	81° (80–82)
Supination											
Sitting with arm by the side and elbow flexed to 90° with thumb toward the ceiling.	Parallel to the anterior midline of the humerus	Medially and proximally to the ulnar styloid process	Across the ventral aspect of the forearm just proximal to the styloid process	86° (85–88)	88° (86–90)	85° (84–86)	82° (81–84)	94° (91–96)	90° (88–92)	91° (90–92)	87° (86–88)

[a]Normative data presented as mean (95% confidence interval).
Modified from Soucie JM, Wang C, Forsyth A, et al: Range of motion measurements: reference values and a database for comparison studies. *Haemophilia* 2011;17(3):500-507.

movements: roll, spin, and glide. Most movement within a joint involves a combination of all three of these motions. The bones at the joint surface are either concave or convex. The concave or convex surfaces of the bones allow joints to fit with one another. This is known as joint congruency.

Joint congruency is maximal when a joint is in a closed-packed position, meaning joint surfaces have maximum contact with each other and the ligaments and capsule holding the joint together are taut. Thus, the joint exhibits maximal stability. In contrast, the open-packed position (resting position) describes joint incongruency, in which the ligaments and capsule are lax.

Capsular patterns should be implemented into the passive range of motion assessment, as these patterns help determine whether the joint capsule may be the culprit of restricted range of motion.[143] Each joint has its own capsular pattern in which one motion is more limited/restricted than the next.

Joint end feels should be assessed during the passive range of motion examination and are defined as the extreme passive movement of a joint that transmits a specific sensation in the clinician's hands.[143] The sensation is felt at the end range of joint motion. End feels can be both normal and abnormal; thus, it is important for the clinician to understand what a normal end feel for each joint should feel like. Joint congruency, capsular patterns, and end feels for each joint at the elbow are described in **Table 9.11**.

Muscle Strength Evaluation

There are different ways that muscle strength can be evaluated in the clinic. Most often, muscle strength is evaluated subjectively using a combination of resisted isometric muscle testing, break testing, and MMT. Resisted isometric testing is most often applied midrange of joint motion, and the patient is asked to hold the position against the clinician's resistance without moving the joint. Similar to this type of testing is the break test, in which a clinician provides resistance at the end range of joint motion. These types of testing are advantageous for patients who have pain during joint movement and are hesitant to resist muscle movement throughout a designated range of motion. It has been suggested that certain patterns are present following isometric muscle testing and may help the clinician differentiate between inert or contractile tissue involvement (**Table 9.12**).

A complete description of MMT can be found in Table 9.1. MMT allows the clinician to subjectively gauge the integrity of muscles throughout a specific range of motion. A common grading system is 0–5. Table 9.1 MMT describes gravity-dependent positions, whereas **Table 9.13** provides the clinician with gravity-eliminated positions that should be considered during MMT 0–2.

Table 9.12 Patterns of Muscle Testing Findings With Associated Tissue Involvement

Findings	Possible Tissue Involvement
Strong and painless contraction	No neurologic deficit
Strong and painful contraction	Lesion of tested muscle or tendon
Weak and painless contraction	Disorder of nervous system, complete rupture of muscle or tendon
Weak and painful contraction	Fracture, partial rupture of muscle or tendon

Table 9.11 Elbow Joint Congruency, Capsular Pattern, and End Feel

Joint	Closed-Packed Position	Open-Packed Position	Capsular Pattern	Normal End Feel
Humeroulnar	Full extension and supination	Elbow flexion: 70° Supination: 10°	Greater limitation in flexion than extension	Flexion: Soft-tissue approximation Extension: bone to bone
Humeroradial	Elbow flexion: 90° Supination: 5°	Full extension and supination	Greater limitation in flexion than extension, followed by limitations in supination and then pronation	
Proximal radioulnar	Supination: 5°	Elbow flexion: 70° Supination: 35°	Equal limitation of supination and pronation	Pronation and supination: bone to bone

Table 9.13	Elbow Testing Positions for Gravity-Eliminated Positions
Motion	**Gravity-Eliminated Position**
Elbow flexion	
Elbow extension	
Supination	
Pronation	
Wrist flexion	
Wrist extension	

All figures in table courtesy of Natalie L. Myers.

Neurologic Testing
Reflex Testing

Deep tendon reflex testing helps the clinician determine lower motor neuron dysfunction at the level of the spinal nerve roots. During the elbow examination, the cervical nerve roots should be assessed through testing the biceps brachii, brachioradialis, and triceps brachii reflex using a reflex hammer. Based on the motor response elicited from the reflex test, the clinician should categorize the response as normal, hyperreflexive (increased or exaggerated contraction), hyporeflexive (delayed contraction), or absent (no contraction).[144] It is important to compare reflexes bilaterally so the clinician can determine what a normal response is for that particular patient. Previous researchers have determined that patients with diminished upper limb reflexes are five times more likely to have abnormal electrodiagnostic findings.[145] **Table 9.14** describes in detail the reflex portion of the neurologic assessment.

Sensory Testing

Sensory testing focuses on testing both dermatomal patterns and peripheral nerve innervation. A dermatome is an area of the skin innervated by a single spinal nerve root. It is important to remember that the area innervated by the nerve root is larger than that innervated by the peripheral nerve (**Figure 9.28**). The clinician is often screening for radiculopathies or myelopathies when testing dermatomal patterns for sensory changes. Due to the overlapping of proximal dermatome fields, it is critical to test the distal segment of the dermatome.

To perform dermatomal testing, the patient must be informed of all testing procedures. The patient should identify the type of sensation he or she is experiencing: numbness, sharp/dull pain, tingling, or pins/needles. The patient should be in a seated position and light touch used to assess any sensory changes. First, the patient (with eyes open) is instructed to reveal any differences in light touch between the affected area and a nonaffected area (on same limb or different limb). Next, the patient is asked to close the eyes; the same steps are repeated in order to determine the extent of sensory loss. Following light touch testing, other methods of sensory testing may be employed; they include the pinprick (sharp versus dull pain), temperature (cold versus hot sensation), vibration, and two-point discrimination testing (often used with the fingers). Dermatomal patterns are shown in **Figure 9.29**.

Table 9.14 Reflex Testing at the Elbow

Reflex	Site of Testing	Picture of Testing	Normal Response	Cervical Nerve Root Contributions
Biceps brachii	Distal bicep tendon		Elbow flexion	C5[a]–C6
Brachioradialis	Proximal brachioradialis tendon		Elbow flexion and sometimes supination; also, may elicit only observable brachioradialis twitch	C5–C6[a]
Triceps brachii	Distal triceps tendon		Elbow extension	C6–T1, C7[a]

[a] Indicates primary level.
All figures in table © Jones & Bartlett Learning.

Myotome Testing

Myotomal testing focuses on evaluating the motor function of a group of muscles. A myotome is a group of muscles supplied by a single nerve root. Weakness of a myotome may be suggestive of nerve root trauma, whereas gross atrophy or multisegmental-level weakness is likely suggestive of myelopathy or peripheral nerve injury.

To perform myotomal testing, the clinician must inform the patient of all testing procedures. It is important for the clinician to understand that he or she is evaluating the strength of muscle(s) during an isometric contraction, not whether pain was caused during muscle contraction. The clinician will place the patient in a comfortable position while stabilizing the limb appropriately and will provide resistance against the patient for 5 seconds trying to break his or her position (break test). All tests should be performed bilaterally for appropriate comparison. Myotomal testing specific to upper quarter nerve roots is described in **Table 9.15**. When appropriate, a patient reporting to a clinician with elbow pathology should undergo all dermatomal and myotomal testing; these tests should not be isolated to just the nerve roots associated with elbow function.

Vascular Assessment

Vascular trauma around the elbow is uncommon but can appear following disruption to the elbow joint in forms of fractures or dislocations. In addition, patients who report a history of diabetes, thrombosis, abnormal vital signs, dizziness, or lightheadedness should

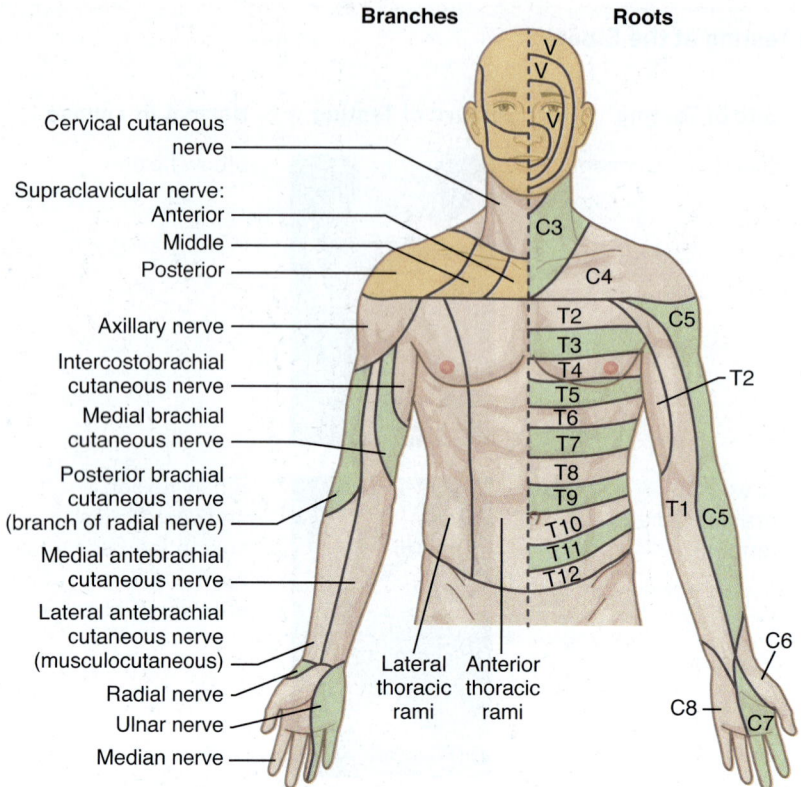

Figure 9.28 Drawing showing nerves of the sensory examination.
© Jones & Bartlett Learning

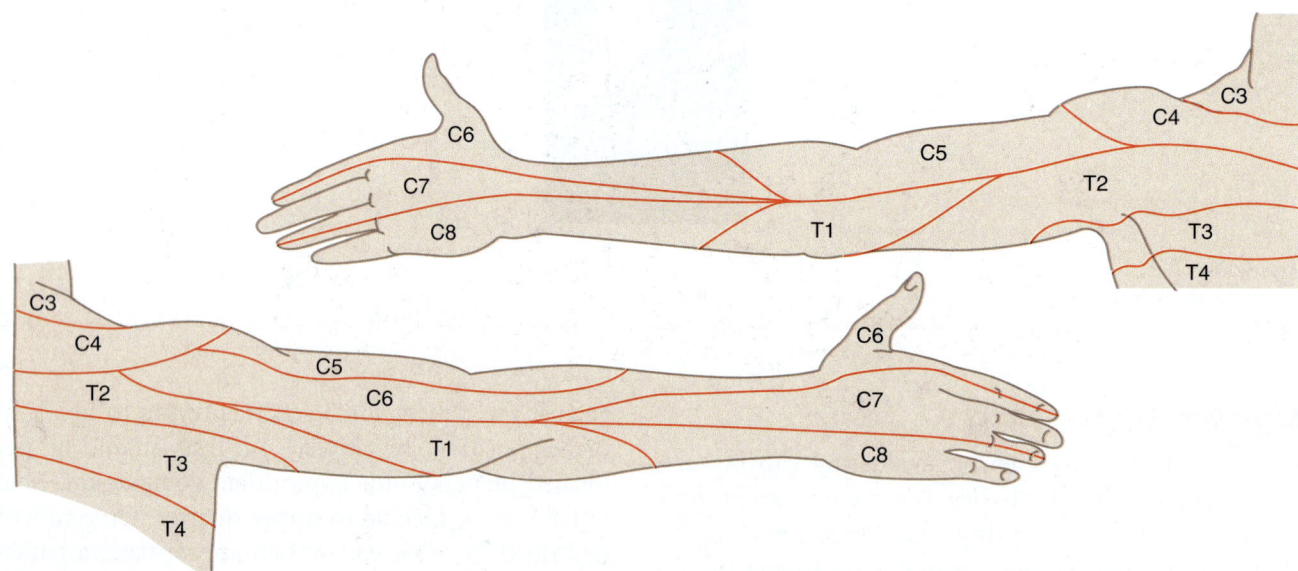

Figure 9.29 Drawing showing dermatomes of the upper limb.
© Jones & Bartlett Learning

undergo a vascular assessment, as these may be red flags indicating serious vascular disorders. Clinicians should examine the major arteries of the arm for pulse intensity, rate, rhythm, and tenderness.[146] To examine the brachial artery, the patient should be seated with the forearm supported by the table. The arm will be slightly abducted with the elbow flexed and supinated. The clinician will then palpate the brachial artery just medial to the biceps tendon in the cubital fossa with the second and third digits (**Figure 9.30A**). For the radial artery, the patient's forearm is supported on a table with the forearm in a neutral position. The clinician will palpate the radial artery on the dorsal side of the distal lateral forearm with the second and third digits (**Figure 9.30B**).

Special Tests 315

Table 9.15 Myotomal Testing for the Upper Quarter

Spinal Nerve Root	Motion Tested	Picture of Testing
C1	Cervical flexion	
C2	Cervical extension	
C3	Cervical lateral flexion	
C4	Scapular elevation	
C5	Shoulder abduction	
C6	Elbow flexion and wrist extension	

(continues)

Table 9.15 Myotomal Testing for the Upper Quarter *(continued)*

Spinal Nerve Root	Motion Tested	Picture of Testing
C7	Elbow extension and wrist flexion	
C8	Finger flexion and thumb extension	
T1	Finger abduction	

All figures in table courtesy of Natalie L. Myers.

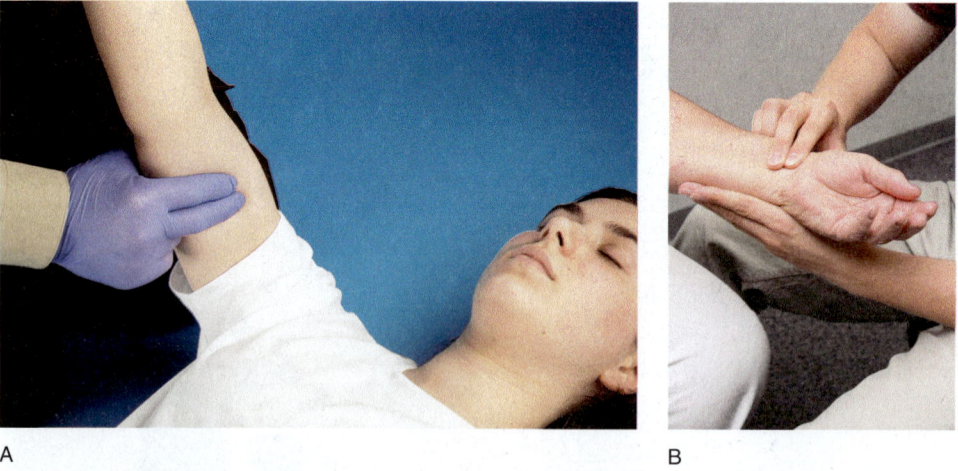

Figure 9.30 Photographs showing palpation for brachial artery pulse **(A)** and radial artery pulse **(B)**.
© Jones & Bartlett Learning

Orthopaedic Special Tests

Special tests should be performed when the clinician has a clear picture of the patient's presentation. Special tests help confirm a diagnosis; they are considered one part of the examination process and should be treated as such. A clinician should not depend only on the findings from special tests with respect to a clinical diagnosis. Clinicians should perform only special tests that are relevant to the patient's presentation to help confirm a diagnosis.[122,147-168] Consequently, understanding the diagnostic accuracy associated with special tests allows clinicians to make evidence-based decisions as to which special tests have the greatest clinical utility. These special tests are described in **Table 9.16**.

Table 9.16 Special Tests

Test	Pathology	Performance	Positive Finding	Sensitivity	Specificity	Positive Likelihood Ratio	Negative Likelihood Ratio	Evidence
Cozen test	Lateral epicondylalgia	Patient: Seated Limb position: Elbow 90° flexion, forearm pronated, wrist in full extension and radial deviation (hand fisted) Clinician: Grasp elbow and palpate lateral epicondyle; resist active wrist extension	Pain over lateral epicondyle and common extensor tendon	0.84	0	0.84	Inf.	Saroja et al[148]
Maudsley test (third digit extension test)	Lateral epicondylalgia	Patient: Seated Limb position: Elbow 90° flexion, forearm pronated with hand flat on table Clinician: Place pad of finger on fingernail of third digit of patient and resist active extension of finger	Pain over lateral epicondyle and common extensor tendon	0.88	0	0.88	Inf.	Saroja et al[148]
Mill test	Lateral epicondylalgia	Patient: Seated Limb position: Elbow extended; forearm pronated Clinician: Stabilize elbow while palpating lateral epicondyle; passively move wrist into flexion	Pain over lateral epicondyle and common extensor tendon	0.53	1.00	Inf.	0.47	Saroja et al[148]

(continues)

Table 9.16 Special Tests

Test	Pathology	Performance	Positive Finding	Sensitivity	Specificity	Positive Likelihood Ratio	Negative Likelihood Ratio	Evidence
Polk test	Lateral epicondylalgia	Patient: Seated. Limb position: Elbow flexed and forearm pronated while grasping a 5-lb object (A). Test: The patient is instructed to lift the object up (B)	Pain over lateral epicondyle and common extensor tendon	NR	NR	NR	NR	No evidence exists for this test
	Medial epicondylalgia	Patient: Seated. Limb position: Elbow flexed and forearm supinated while grasping a 5-lb object (A). Test: The patient is instructed to lift the object up (B)	Pain over medial epicondyle and common flexor tendon	NR	NR	NR		

(continued)

Orthopaedic Special Tests

Test	Condition	Procedure	Positive findings				Study
Golfer's elbow test	Medial epicondylalgia	Patient: Seated Limb position: Elbow extended and forearm supinated Clinician: Grasp elbow and resist active wrist flexion	Pain over medial epicondyle and common flexor tendon	NR	NR	NR	
Bicipital aponeurosis flex test	Biceps tendon rupture	Patient: Seated Limb position: Elbow extended, wrist flexed, and forearm supinated Clinician: With one hand on wrist and one finger on antecubital fossa, actively resist elbow flexion while palpating the medial, anterior, and lateral portions of the fossa	Lack of sharp edges medially suggests bicipital aponeurosis injury or possibly distal biceps tendon rupture	100	90	10	0	ElMaraghy and Devereaux[153]
Biceps crease interval	Biceps tendon rupture	Patient: Seated Limb position: Elbow flexed to 90° Clinician: Stabilize wrist with one hand and place first two fingers on antecubital fossa. Passively extend the elbow and supinate forearm. Using a writing instrument, mark flexion crease in antecubital fossa. Add a second mark at the start of the distal biceps curve	Crease interval >6 cm between the marks suggestive of distal biceps tendon rupture	92	100	Inf.	0.08	ElMaraghy et al[154]
				88	50	1.8	0.2	Devereaux and ElMaraghy[155]

(continues)

Table 9.16 Special Tests (continued)

Test	Pathology	Performance	Positive Finding	Sensitivity	Specificity	Positive Likelihood Ratio	Negative Likelihood Ratio	Evidence
Biceps crease ratio	Biceps tendon rupture	Repeat the same procedure for measuring the biceps crease interval on the uninvolved arm	Ratio >1.2 between the arms suggestive of distal biceps tendon rupture	96	80	4.8	0.05	ElMaraghy et al[154]
Biceps squeeze test	Biceps tendon rupture	Patient: Seated Limb position: Forearm in slight pronation resting in lap with elbow flexed 60° to 80° Clinician: Grasp muscle belly of biceps in one hand and the musculotendinous portion with the other	Lack of forearm supination as the biceps is squeezed with both hands	100	67	3	0	Ruland et al[156]
Hook test	Biceps tendon rupture	Patient: Seated Limb position: Elbow flexed to 90° and forearm supinated Clinician: Place finger under biceps tendon from lateral aspect of antecubital fossa	Lack of tendon to "hook" finger around equates to full tear. Painful test equates to partial tear	100 81	100 100	Inf. Inf.	0 0.2	O'Driscoll et al[157] Devereaux and ElMaraghy[155]

Passive forearm pronation	Biceps tendon rupture	Patient: Seated Limb position: Elbow flexed 90° with forearm supinated Clinician: Support elbow with one hand and grasp forearm with other; passively pronate forearm	Loss of visible and palpable movement of the biceps muscle belly going from proximal to distal	95	100	Inf.	0.05	Devereaux and ElMaraghy[155]
Supination–pronation test	Biceps tendon rupture	Patient: Standing Limb position: Both arms abducted 90° and both elbows flexed 60° to 70° Test: Patient actively pronates and supinates forearms	Lack of movement of biceps belly suggests distal biceps tendon rupture	100	NR	NR	NR	Metzman and Tivener[158]
Test battery: biceps crease index, hook test, passive forearm pronation	Biceps tendon rupture			100	50	2	0	ElMaraghy et al[154]
Test battery: biceps crease index, biceps crease ratio	Biceps tendon rupture			96	80	4.8	0.05	Devereaux and ElMaraghy[155]

(continues)

Table 9.16 Special Tests (continued)

Test	Pathology	Performance	Positive Finding	Sensitivity	Specificity	Positive Likelihood Ratio	Negative Likelihood Ratio	Evidence
Moving valgus stress test	Ulnar collateral ligament injury	Patient: Seated Limb position: Arm abducted to 90° with elbow in maximal flexion (A) Clinician: Standing behind patient, grasp wrist with one hand and apply valgus stress to elbow with other hand. Quickly extend the patient's elbow while maintaining the valgus stress (B)	Pain produced when moving the elbow from flexion to extension with maximum pain between 120° and 70°	100	75	4	0	O'Driscoll et al[159]
Valgus stress test (pain) Valgus stress test (laxity)	Ulnar collateral ligament injury	Patient: Seated Limb position: Elbow extended with supinated forearm Clinician: With one hand grasping the wrist and the other hand over the lateral elbow, apply valgus stress to the elbow. Repeat at 20° to 30° flexion	Pain or laxity medially with valgus stress (possible compression pain laterally)	65 19	50 100	1.3 Inf.	0.7 0.8	O'Driscoll et al[159] O'Driscoll et al[159]

Milking maneuver	Ulnar collateral ligament injury	Patient: Seated Limb position: Arm abducted to 90° with 90° elbow flexion and neutral forearm Clinician: Standing behind patient, grasp thumb of involved arm with one hand and apply valgus stress to lateral elbow. Pull on thumb moving arm into forced external rotation	Pain medially with the valgus stress	NR	NR	NR	NR	No evidence exists for this test
Lateral pivot shift test (awake) Lateral pivot shift test (anesthesia)	Posterolateral rotatory instability	Patient: Supine Limb position: Arm and elbow flexed to 90°, forearm supinated (A) Clinician: Grasping the wrist and forearm, passively flex elbow while applying valgus and axial stresses with supination (B)	Apprehension Visible or palpable "clunk" or dimple above radial head	38 100	NR NR	NR NR	NR NR	Regan and Lapner[122] Regan and Lapner[122]

(continues)

Table 9.16 Special Tests (continued)

Test	Pathology	Performance	Positive Finding	Sensitivity	Specificity	Positive Likelihood Ratio	Negative Likelihood Ratio	Evidence
Posterolateral rotatory drawer test	Posterolateral rotatory instability	Patient: Seated. Limb position: Arm resting in lap (A). Clinician: Stabilize humerus with one hand and grasp lateral elbow with other hand, then pull forearm posterolaterally (B)	Apprehension or dimple above radial head	NR	NR	NR	NR	No evidence exists for this test
Prone push-up test	Posterolateral rotatory instability	Patient: Prone with chest on table. Limb position: Arms abducted beyond shoulder width, elbows flexed 90°, and forearms supinated (A). Test: Patient pushes body up off table (B)	Apprehension as elbow moves into extension. Radial head dislocation could occur, equating to a positive test	88	NR	NR	NR	Regan and Lapner[122]

Chair push-up test	Posterolateral rotatory instability	Patient: Seated Limb position: Arms abducted beyond shoulder width, elbows flexed 90°, and forearms supinated (A) Test: Patient pushes body up out of chair (B)	Apprehension as elbow moves into extension. Radial head dislocation could occur, equating to a positive test	88	NR	NR	NR	Regan and Lapner[122]
Tabletop relocation test	Posterolateral rotatory instability	Patient: Standing in front of table Limb position: Hands on table edge (A) Test: Patient performs a modified push-up (B) Clinician: Apply pressure with thumb to radial head (C) and instruct patient to perform a second modified push-up (D). Remove thumb from patient's arm while patient stays in a partially flexed position	Pain and apprehension at 40° of flexion. Relief of pain as clinician stabilizes radial head. Pain and apprehension return when clinician removes hand from radial head	100	NR	NR	NR	Arvind and Hargreaves[162]

(continues)

Table 9.16 Special Tests *(continued)*

Test	Pathology	Performance	Positive Finding	Sensitivity	Specificity	Positive Likelihood Ratio	Negative Likelihood Ratio	Evidence
Elbow flexion test	Fracture	Patient: Seated Test: Patient actively attempts to flex both elbows	Limited motion compared to uninvolved arm	64	100	Inf.	0.36	Darracq et al[163]
	Cubital tunnel syndrome	Patient: Seated Limb position: Shoulder flexion to 60° to 80° with elbows fully flexed, forearms pronated, and wrists extended Test: Hold position for 3 minutes	Reproduction of paresthesia	93 75	NR 99	NR 75	NR 0.25	Buehler and Thayer[164] Novak et al[165]
Elbow pronation test	Fracture	Patient: Seated Test: Patient actively attempts to pronate both forearms	Limited motion compared to uninvolved arm	34	100	Inf.	0.66	Darracq et al[163]

Test	Condition	Procedure	Determination of Positive Test	Sensitivity	Specificity	+LR	Studies
Elbow supination test	Fracture	Patient: Seated Test: Patient actively attempts to supinate both forearms	Limited motion compared to uninvolved arm	43	97	14	0.58	Darracq et al[163]
Elbow scratch test	Cubital tunnel syndrome	Patient: Seated Limb position: Arm at side and humerus in external rotation with elbow flexed to 90° Clinician: Resist external rotation while scratching the area of the ulnar nerve	Weakness of external rotation	69	99	69	0.31	Cheng et al[166]
Pressure provocation test	Cubital tunnel syndrome	Patient: Seated Limb position: Arm resting in lap (A) Clinician: Grasp forearm around elbow with pressure over ulnar nerve; move arm into 20° flexion and supination. Hold 1 minute (B)	Reproduction of paresthesia	89 46 60	98 99 NR	45 46 NR	0.11 0.54 NR	Novak et al[165] Cheng et al[166] Beekman et al[167]

(continues)

Table 9.16 Special Tests (continued)

Test	Pathology	Performance	Positive Finding	Sensitivity	Specificity	Positive Likelihood Ratio	Negative Likelihood Ratio	Evidence
Tinel sign	Cubital tunnel syndrome	Patient: Seated Limb position: Arm at side and elbow flexed to 90° Clinician: Supporting arm at wrist, tap the path of the ulnar nerve	Reproduction of paresthesia	70 54 62	NR 99 NR	NR 54 NR	NR 0.46 NR	Novak et al[165] Cheng et al[166] Beekman et al[167]

Inf., infinity; NR, not reported.
All figures in table © Jones & Bartlett Learning.

Summary

The elbow is a complex joint that involves a detailed evaluation process to make an accurate diagnosis. It is important that the patient gain the trust of the clinician during the evaluation process. The clinician should remain detailed in the evaluation process to differentiate between different structures that may be involved. It is important to remember that patients may present differently during the evaluation process, so it is imperative to connect with the patient and listen to his or her chief complaints and goals moving forward. Although there are a variety of conditions/injuries that can occur to the elbow, it is recommended that clinicians rule in or out the presence of injury by pathologic category (muscle based, ligamentous based, bone based, or neurologic based). Most diagnoses will be guided by the information derived from the patient's history, especially because the clinical utility of existing special tests is not overwhelmingly strong.

CASE STUDY 1

A 20-year-old female right-handed collegiate softball player in her junior year who plays the outfield position presents with elbow pain. The patient has a prior history of right medial elbow pain during the start of her sophomore-year season. The elbow pain did resolve with physical therapy; however, she reinjured her elbow during the last game of her sophomore season. She felt pain while she was throwing a ball from center field to the second baseman. She felt a pop in her arm with immediate pain. There was swelling on the medial side of her right elbow. After the pop was felt, she did not continue throwing, but she did continue to bat. She returned home for summer break and did some physical therapy; however, she has returned for her junior year and the pain is still present.[169]

- Physical examination findings
    - Patient characteristics: Body mass index, 25 kg/m^2; pulse, 70 beats per minute; blood pressure, 110/69 mm Hg
    - Medical history: previous history of medial elbow pain, chronic low back pain
    - Medications: NSAIDs (minor relief)
    - Radiography: None
    - Outcome measure: Severe disability on the Kerlan-Jobe Orthopaedic Clinic Shoulder and Elbow Score
    - Other concerns:
        a. Reported pain on medial epicondyle and proximal common flexor group
        b. No significant swelling at time of reevaluation
        c. Right and left elbow flexion: 150°
        d. Right elbow extension: 0°
        e. Left elbow extension: 5° hyperextension
        f. Normal wrist range of motion
        g. Passive range of motion elicited end range pain with both flexion and extension with normal end feels
        h. Normal elbow strength bilaterally: biceps, triceps, wrist flexors and extensors (MMT: 5/5)
        i. Right shoulder external rotation 3/5 versus 5/5 on left
        j. Negative Tinel sign
        k. Positive moving valgus stress test
        l. Palpation-elicited medial elbow pain
        m. Normal neurologic examination

1. List three differential diagnoses (DD) that may be contributing to the patient's current status. Provide a rationale for each DD.
2. What additional history questions would you deem necessary to ask in this particular scenario? Would you implement an outcome measure as part of your assessment? If so, which outcome would you distribute to the patient and why?
3. Determine the appropriate physical examination components that you as a clinician would include as part of your assessment on this patient. Examples: range of motion, strength testing.

CASE STUDY 2

A 50-year-old right-handed man who plays recreational tennis reports to the clinic with right elbow pain. The pain has been persistent for the past 3 months. The pain started after a weekend-long tournament. Patient has been playing tennis for the past year in competitive United States Tennis Association leagues. He recently switched to a

(continues)

one-handed backhand from a two-handed backhand. The pain has progressively intensified over the past week from a 4/10 to an 8/10 on the Numeric Pain Rating Scale. The patient is no longer able to participate in tennis-related activity. Upon initial injury, he attended physical therapy for 1 month with no relief in his symptoms.

- Physical examination findings
    - Patient characteristics: body mass index, 30 kg/m^2; pulse, 80 beats per minute; blood pressure, 130/85 mm Hg
    - Medical history: Previous history of elbow pain on his left side that resolved on its own
    - Medications: NSAIDs (minor relief), corticosteroid injection after failed physical therapy. Injection relieved symptoms for 1 month, which enabled him to continue playing tennis.
    - Radiography: None
    - Outcome measure: Severe disability on PRTEE
    - Other concerns:
        a. Reported pain worst in the morning and aggravated by opening doors, carrying groceries, and brushing his teeth
        b. Chief complaint is stiff, achy, and sometimes throbbing pain
        c. Denies numbness and tingling in the upper limb
        d. No swelling at elbow compared to the contralateral side
        e. All active range of motion at the elbow was normal
        f. Wrist flexion and extension were both limited due to pain
        g. Passive range of motion was limited at end range of wrist flexion due to pain with a reproduction of symptoms
        h. Normal elbow strength bilaterally: biceps and triceps (MMT: 5/5)
        i. Wrist extension and grip strength (4/5) with pain on lateral elbow
        j. Positive Cozen test
        k. Mill test was inconclusive in that it was uncomfortable but did not produce pain at the lateral epicondyle
        l. The common extensor origin was tender to direct palpation as was the extensor carpi radialis brevis

1. List three DDs that may be contributing to the patient's current status. Provide a rationale for each DD.
2. What additional history questions would you deem necessary to ask in this particular scenario? Would you implement an outcome measure as part of your assessment? If so, which outcome would you distribute to the patient and why?
3. Why is it important to note the change in backhand mechanics in this particular scenario? Could changing from a two-handed backhand to a one-handed backhand play a role in injury development?
4. Determine the appropriate physical examination components that you as a clinician would include as part of your assessment on this patient. Examples: range of motion, strength testing.

ONE-IN-A-MILLION CASE STUDY

An 11-year-old boy in general good health began complaining of numbness and paresthesia in his hand that began 9 months ago. He was born in India and was delivered full term via cesarean section. The patient lived in India until he was 5 years old and then moved to the United States with his family. Prior to the symptoms arising, the patient spent 6 weeks in India visiting family. At 5 months, his hand strength was continuously worsening, and he had pain over the right medial elbow, forearm, wrist, and thumb. He had no history of cervical dysfunction or injury, neurologic diseases, or any recent illnesses (viral or otherwise). His medical history was unremarkable, and his immunizations were up to date. On physical examination, the right ulnar nerve was determined to be enlarged via palpation over the medial epicondyle. His ability to distinguish "sharp" sensation was diminished in the ulnar distribution of the hand as well as in the dorsum of the hand. Myotomal assessment revealed severe ulnar palsy with minimal function of intrinsic hand muscles innervated by the ulnar nerve and significant weakness in the FDP to the fourth and fifth digits with associated clawing. Median and radial motor function was normal.

MRI confirmed the thickened ulnar nerve. Nerve conduction studies revealed an absent right ulnar sensory and motor potential of the first dorsal interosseous muscle. The motor potential of the abductor digiti minimi muscle was significantly reduced, and the radial sensory potential was also significantly reduced. Electromyography studies revealed significant abnormal spontaneous activity and no voluntary motor unit activation in the ulnar-innervated forearm and intrinsic musculature of the hand.

WRAP-UP

Critical Thinking Questions

1. You are asked to evaluate a 20-year-old female javelin thrower who has elbow pain and numbness. She reports medial elbow tingling that radiated into the hand with hard throwing. She denies previous history of elbow pain but has a history of low back pain. Upon palpation, the patient is tender on the flexor pronator muscle mass, medial epicondyle, and ulnar groove. Which condition or conditions might you suspect and why? What special tests would you use to differentiate involved structures?
2. Identify the end feels you may find when performing a passive range of motion assessment in patients with the following suspected pathologies:
   - UCL stress test for suspected tear
   - Osteophyte with elbow flexion
   - Biceps rupture with elbow extension
3. Consider the scenario of a retired professional male golfer returning to golf after a 2-year hiatus. The patient has medial elbow pain. There is pain and stiffness in the morning with wrist movement, making activities of daily living difficult. There is also pain at the elbow during the driving and pitching swing. What history questions would you ask this patient in order to determine three to four differential diagnoses?
4. A college baseball pitcher reports numbness into the hand during pitching. He is predominantly a side-arm pitcher, and you have worked with this individual in the past on his pitching mechanics. You suspect that he has ulnar nerve pathology. What neurologic tests would you perform to rule in your suspicion? What common sensory deficiencies would the patient present with? In addition, which specific branch of the ulnar nerve could be affected?
5. While attending a gymnastics competition, you notice that a young girl around the age of 15 years falls awkwardly onto her hand. You are on the first row of bleachers, so you are able to hear and see the medical attention that this young girl is receiving. She is in immense pain because she has dislocated her elbow. You overhear the clinicians state the distal radial pulse is absent. Everyone is aware that this is a medical emergency; however, the parents of the child are not present. The clinicians want to call an ambulance, but the coach is saying that she can get her to the hospital faster than the ambulance could. Would you allow the coach to transport this athlete to the hospital, or do you wait for the ambulance to arrive? Explain the rationale behind your answer.

Pearls and Pitfalls

- Review the anatomy of the elbow: bony, ligamentous, neurologic, and vascular.
- Engage in a conversation with your patient during the history portion of the assessment. Understand the importance of active listening and the interaction needed between clinician and patient to create a positive experience for the patient.
- All findings from the examination process should be considered when discussing a final diagnosis with a patient.

References

1. Morrey BF: *The Elbow and Its Disorders*. Philadelphia, PA, Saunders, 2009.
2. Guerra JT: Clinical anatomy, histology, & pathomechanics of the elbow in sports. *Oper Tech Sports Med* 1996;4(2):69-76.
3. Morrey BF, Askew LJ, Chao EY: A biomechanical study of normal functional elbow motion. *J Bone Joint Surg Am* 1981;63(6):872-877.
4. Alcid JG, Ahmad CS, Lee TQ: Elbow anatomy and structural biomechanics. *Clin Sports Med* 2004;23(4):503-517, vii.
5. Fornalski S, Gupta R, Lee TQ: Anatomy and biomechanics of the elbow joint. *Tech Hand Up Extrem Surg* 2003;7(4):168-178.
6. Frangiamore SJ, Moatshe G, Kruckeberg BM, et al: Qualitative and quantitative analyses of the dynamic and static stabilizers of the medial elbow: an anatomic study. *Am J Sports Med* 2018;46(3):687-694.
7. Yoshida M, Goto H, Takenaga T, et al: Anterior and posterior bands of the anterior bundle in the elbow ulnar collateral ligament: ultrasound anatomy. *J Shoulder Elbow Surg* 2017;26(10):1803-1809.
8. Morrey BF, An KN: Articular and ligamentous contributions to the stability of the elbow joint. *Am J Sports Med* 1983;11(5):315-319.

9. Schwab GH, Bennett JB, Woods GW, Tullos HS: Biomechanics of elbow instability: the role of the medial collateral ligament. *Clin Orthop Relat Res* 1980(146):42-52.
10. Callaway GH, Field LD, Deng XH, et al: Biomechanical evaluation of the medial collateral ligament of the elbow. *J Bone Joint Surg Am* 1997;79(8):1223-1231.
11. Timmerman LA, Andrews JR: Histology and arthroscopic anatomy of the ulnar collateral ligament of the elbow. *Am J Sports Med* 1994;22(5):667-673.
12. Morrey BF, An KN: Functional anatomy of the ligaments of the elbow. *Clin Orthop Relat Res* 1985(201):84-90.
13. Stroyan M, Wilk KE: The functional anatomy of the elbow complex. *J Orthop Sports Phys Ther* 1993;17(6):279-288.
14. Hackl M, Bercher M, Wegmann K, Muller LP, Dargel J: Functional anatomy of the lateral collateral ligament of the elbow. *Arch Orthop Trauma Surg* 2016;136(7):1031-1037.
15. O'Driscoll SW, Bell DF, Morrey BF: Posterolateral rotatory instability of the elbow. *J Bone Joint Surg Am* 1991;73(3):440-446.
16. Cohen MS, Hastings H 2nd: Rotatory instability of the elbow. The anatomy and role of the lateral stabilizers. *J Bone Joint Surg Am* 1997;79(2):225-233.
17. McAdams TR, Masters GW, Srivastava S: The effect of arthroscopic sectioning of the lateral ligament complex of the elbow on posterolateral rotatory stability. *J Shoulder Elbow Surg* 2005;14(3):298-301.
18. Martin BF: The annular ligament of the superior radio-ulnar joint. *J Anat* 1958;92.
19. Spinner M, Kaplan EB: The relationship of the ulnar nerve to the medial intermuscular septum in the arm and its clinical significance. *Hand* 1976;8(3):239-242.
20. Patel BA: Form and function of the oblique cord (chorda obliqua) in anthropoid primates. *Primates* 2005;46(1):47-57.
21. Karatas A, Apaydin N, Uz A, Tubbs R, Loukas M, Gezen F: Regional anatomic structures of the elbow that may potentially compress the ulnar nerve. *J Shoulder Elbow Surg* 2009;18(4):627-631.
22. Granger A, Sardi JP, Iwanaga J, et al: Osborne's ligament: a review of its history, anatomy, and surgical importance. *Cureus* 2017;9(3):e1080.
23. Backhouse KM: *Nerve Supply in the Arm and Hand*, Philadelphia, PA, WB Saunders, 1981.
24. Paulos R, Leclercq C: Motor branches of the ulnar nerve to the forearm: an anatomical study and guidelines for selective neurectomy. *Surg Radiol Anat* 2015;37(9):1043-1048.
25. Marur T, Akkin SM, Alp M, et al: The muscular branching patterns of the ulnar nerve to the flexor carpi ulnaris and flexor digitorum profundus muscles. *Surg Radiol Anat* 2005;27(4):322-326.
26. Sunderland S, Hughes ES: Metrical and non-metrical features of the muscular branches of the ulnar nerve. *J Comp Neurol* 1946;85:113-125.
27. Tubbs RS, Custis JW, Salter EG, Blount JP, Oakes WJ, Wellons JC 3rd: Quantitation of and landmarks for the muscular branches of the ulnar nerve to the forearm for application in peripheral nerve neurotization procedures. *J Neurosurg* 2006;104(5):800-803.
28. Bonnel F, Vila RM: Anatomical study of the ulnar nerve in the hand. *J Hand Surg Br* 1985;10(2):165-168.
29. Oh CS, Won HS, Lee KS, Chung IH, Kim SM: Anatomic variation of the innervation of the flexor digitorum profundus muscle and its clinical implications. *Muscle Nerve* 2009;39(4):498-502.
30. Guse TR, Ostrum RF: The surgical anatomy of the radial nerve around the humerus. *Clin Orthop Relat Res* 1995(320):149-153.
31. Hackl M, Lappen S, Burkhart KJ, Neiss WF, Muller LP, Wegmann K: The course of the median and radial nerve across the elbow: an anatomic study. *Arch Orthop Trauma Surg* 2015;135(7):979-983.
32. Low CK, Chew JT, Mitra AK: A surgical approach to the posterior interosseous branch of the radial nerve through the brachioradialis—a cadaveric study. *Singapore Med J* 1994;35(4):394-396.
33. Auerbach DM, Collins ED, Kunkle KL, Monsanto EH: The radial sensory nerve: an anatomic study. *Clin Orthop Relat Res* 1994(308):241-249.
34. Cha J, York B, Tawfik J: Posterior interosseous nerve compression. *Eplasty* 2014;14:ic4.
35. Mazurek MT, Shin AY: Upper extremity peripheral nerve anatomy: current concepts and applications. *Clin Orthop Relat Res* 2001(383):7-20.
36. Abrams RA, Ziets RJ, Lieber RL, Botte MJ: Anatomy of the radial nerve motor branches in the forearm. *J Hand Surg Am* 1997;22(2):232-237.
37. Branovacki G, Hanson M, Cash R, Gonzalez M: The innervation pattern of the radial nerve at the elbow and in the forearm. *J Hand Surg Br* 1998;23(2):167-169.
38. Kozin SH: The anatomy of the recurrent branch of the median nerve. *J Hand Surg Am* 1998;23(5):852-858.
39. Papathanassiou BT: A variant of the motor branch of the median nerve in the hand. *J Bone Joint Surg Br* 1968;50(1):156-157.
40. Agur ADA: *Grant's Atlas of Anatomy*, ed 11. Baltimore, MD, Lippincott Williams & Wilkins, 2005.
41. Girish G, Lobo LG, Jacobson JA, Morag Y, Miller B, Jamadar DA: Ultrasound of the shoulder: asymptomatic findings in men. *AJR Am J Roentgenol* 2011;197(4):W713-719.
42. Nakashima H, Yukawa Y, Suda K, Yamagata M, Ueta T, Kato F: Abnormal findings on magnetic resonance images of the cervical spines in 1211 asymptomatic subjects. *Spine (Phila Pa 1976)* 2015;40(6):392-398.
43. Orchard J, Reed J, Anderson F: The use of diagnostic imaging in sports medicine. *Med J Aust* 2005;183(9):482-486.
44. Newberg AH: The radiographic evaluation of shoulder and elbow pain in the athlete. *Clin Sports Med* 1987;6(4):785-809.
45. Sampath SC, Sampath SC, Bredella MA: Magnetic resonance imaging of the elbow: a structured approach. *Sports Health* 2013;5(1):34-49.
46. Timmerman LA, Schwartz ML, Andrews JR: Preoperative evaluation of the ulnar collateral ligament by magnetic resonance imaging and computed tomography arthrography. Evaluation in 25 baseball players with surgical confirmation. *Am J Sports Med* 1994;22(1):26-31; discussion 32.
47. Potter HG, Weiland AJ, Schatz JA, Paletta GA, Hotchkiss RN: Posterolateral rotatory instability of the elbow: usefulness of MR imaging in diagnosis. *Radiology* 1997;204(1):185-189.
48. Carrino JA, Morrison WB, Zou KH, Steffen RT, Snearly WN, Murray PM: Lateral ulnar collateral ligament of the elbow: optimization of evaluation with two-dimensional MR imaging. *Radiology* 2001;218(1):118-125.
49. Terada N, Yamada H, Toyama Y: The appearance of the lateral ulnar collateral ligament on magnetic resonance imaging. *J Shoulder Elbow Surg* 2004;13(2):214-216.
50. De Smet AA, Winter TC, Best TM, Bernhardt DT: Dynamic sonography with valgus stress to assess elbow ulnar

51. Parker L, Nazarian LN, Carrino JA, et al: Musculoskeletal imaging: medicare use, costs, and potential for cost substitution. *J Am Coll Radiol* 2008;5(3):182-188.
52. Hsu SH, Moen TC, Levine WN, Ahmad CS: Physical examination of the athlete's elbow. *Am J Sports Med* 2012;40(3):699-708.
53. Beals RK: The normal carrying angle of the elbow: a radiographic study of 422 patients. *Clin Orthop Relat Res* 1976(119):194-196.
54. Alfredson H, Pietila T, Jonsson P, Lorentzon R: Heavy-load eccentric calf muscle training for the treatment of chronic achilles tendinosis. *Am J Sports Med* 1998;26(3):360-366.
55. Nirschl RP: Soft-tissue injuries about the elbow. *Clin Sports Med* 1986;5(4):637-652.
56. Waugh EJ: Lateral epicondylalgia or epicondylitis: what's in a name? *J Orthop Sports Phys Ther* 2005;35(4):200-202.
57. Yuan J, Wang MX, Murrell GAC: Cell death and tendinopathy. *Clin Sports Med* 2003;22(4):693-702.
58. Morris H: The rider's sprain. *Lancet* 1882;120:133-134.
59. Alfredson H, Ljung BO, Thorsen K, Lorentzon R: In vivo investigation of ECRB tendons with microdialysis technique—no signs of inflammation but high amounts of glutamate in tennis elbow. *Acta Orthop Scand* 2000;71(5):475-479.
60. Chard MD, Cawston TE, Riley GP, Gresham GA, Hazleman BL: Rotator cuff degeneration and lateral epicondylitis: a comparative histological study. *Ann Rheum Dis* 1994;53(1):30-34.
61. Potter HG, Hannafin JA, Morwessel RM, DiCarlo EF, O'Brien SJ, Altchek DW: Lateral epicondylitis: correlation of MR imaging, surgical, and histopathologic findings. *Radiology* 1995;196(1):43-46.
62. Gruchow HW, Pelletier D: An epidemiologic study of tennis elbow: incidence, recurrence, and effectiveness of prevention strategies. *Am J Sports Med* 1979;7(4):234-238.
63. Nirschl RP: Tennis elbow. *Orthop Clin North Am* 1973;4(3):787-800.
64. Descatha A, Dale AM, Jaegers L, Herquelot E, Evanoff B: Self-reported physical exposure association with medial and lateral epicondylitis incidence in a large longitudinal study. *Occup Environ Med* 2013;70:670-673.
65. Kibler WB, Sciascia AD: Kinetic chain contributions to elbow function and dysfunction in sports. *Clin Sports Med* 2004;23(4):545-552.
66. Nirschl RP, Ashman ES: Elbow tendinopathy: tennis elbow. *Clin Sports Med* 2003;22(4):813-836.
67. Shiri R, Viikari-Juntura E, Varonen H, Heliovaara M: Prevalence and determinants of lateral and medial epicondylitis: a population study. *Am J Epidemiol* 2006;164:1065-1074.
68. Shiri R, Viikari-Juntura E: Lateral and medial epicondylitis: role of occupational factors. *Best Pract Res Rheumatol* 2011;25(1):43-57.
69. Herquelot E, Bodin J, Roquelaure Y, et al: Work-related risk factors for lateral epicondylitis and other cause of elbow pain in the working population. *Am J Ind Med* 2012;56(4):400-409.
70. MacDermid JC: Update: the patient-rated forearm evaluation questionnaire is now the patient-rated tennis elbow evaluation. *J Hand Ther* 2005;18(4):407-410.
71. Newcomer KL, Martinez-Silvestrini JA, Schaefer MP, Gay RE, Arendt KW: Sensitivity of the patient-rated forearm evaluation questionnaire in lateral epicondylitis. *J Hand Ther* 2005;18(4):400-406.
72. Lukasiewicz AC, McClure P, Michener L, Pratt N, Sennett B: Comparison of 3-dimensional scapular position and orientation between subjects with and without shoulder impingement. *J Orthop Sports Phys Ther* 1999;29(10):574-586.
73. Sciascia A, Cromwell R: Kinetic chain rehabilitation: a theoretical framework. *Rehabil Res Pract* 2012;2012:1-9.
74. Yamamoto A, Takagishi K, Kobayashi T, et al: The impact of faulty posture on rotator cuff tears with and without symptoms. *J Shoulder Elbow Surg* 2015;24:446-452.
75. Bouisset S, Zattara M: A sequence of postural movements precedes voluntary movement. *Neurosci Lett* 1981;22:263-270.
76. Hirashima M, Kadota H, Sakurai S, Kudo K, Ohtsuki T: Sequential muscle activity and its functional role in the upper extremity and trunk during overarm throwing. *J Sports Sci* 2002;20:301-310.
77. Hirashima M, Yamane K, Nakamura Y, Ohtsuki T: Kinetic chain of overarm throwing in terms of joint rotations revealed by induced acceleration analysis. *J Biomech* 2008;41:2874-2883.
78. Kibler WB, Press J, Sciascia AD: The role of core stability in athletic function. *Sports Med* 2006;36(3):189-198.
79. Putnam CA: Sequential motions of body segments in striking and throwing skills: description and explanations. *J Biomech* 1993;26:125-135.
80. Sciascia AD, Thigpen CA, Namdari S, Baldwin K: Kinetic chain abnormalities in the athletic shoulder. *Sports Med Arth Rev* 2012;20(1):16-21.
81. Zattara M, Bouisset S: Posturo-kinetic organisation during the early phase of voluntary upper limb movement. 1. Normal subjects. *J Neurol Neurosurg Psychiatr* 1988;51:956-965.
82. Blanchette MA, Normand MC: Impairment assessment of lateral spicondylitis through electromyography and dynamometry. *J Can Chiropr Assoc* 2011;55(2):96-106.
83. Lee MH, Cha JG, Jin W, et al: Utility of sonographic measurement of the common tensor tendon in patients with lateral epicondylitis. *Am J Radiol* 2011;196:1363-1367.
84. Amin NH, Kumar NS, Schickendantz MS: Medial epicondylitis: evaluation and management. *J Am Acad Orthop Surg* 2015;23:348-355.
85. Elliott B, Fleisig G, Nicholls R, Escamillia R: Technique effects on upper limb loading in the tennis serve. *J Sci Med Sport* 2003;6(1):76-87.
86. Fleisig GS, Barrentine SW, Escamilla RF, Andrews JR: Biomechanics of overhand throwing with implications for injuries. *Sports Med* 1996;21:421-437.
87. Regan W, Wold LE, Coonrad R, Morrey BF: Microscopic histopathology of chronic refractory lateral epicondylitis. *Am J Sports Med* 1992;20:746-749.
88. Pienimäki TT, Siira PT, Vanharanta H: Chronic medial and lateral epicondylitis: a comparison of pain, disability, and function. *Arch Phys Med Rehabil* 2002;83(3):317-321.
89. Park GY, Lee SM, Lee MY: Diagnostic value of ultrasonography for clinical medial epicondylitis. *Arch Phys Med Rehabil* 2008;89(4):738-742.
90. Sarda P, Qaddori A, Nauschutz F, Boulton L, Nanda R, Bayliss N: Distal biceps tendon rupture: current concepts. *Injury* 2013;44(4):417-420.
91. Safran MR, Graham SM: Distal biceps tendon ruptures: incidence, demographics, and the effect of smoking. *Clin Orthop Rel Res* 2002;404:275-283.
92. Kelly MP, Perkinson SG, Ablove RH, Tueting JK: Distal biceps tendon ruptures: an epidemiological analysis using a large population database. *Am J Sports Med* 2015;43(8):2012-2017.

93. Seiler JG III, Parker LM, Chamberland PD, Sherbourne GM, Carpenter WA: The distal biceps tendon: two potential mechanisms involved in its rupture: arterial supply and mechanical impingement. *J Shoulder Elbow Surg* 1995;4(3):149-156.

94. Grewal R, Athwal GS, MacDermid JC, et al: Single versus double-incision technique for the repair of acute distal biceps tendon ruptures: a randomized clinical trial. *J Bone Joint Surg Am* 2012;94(13):1166-1174.

95. Freeman CR, McCormick KR, Mahoney D, Baratz M, Lubahn JD: Nonoperative treatment of distal biceps tendon ruptures compared with a historical control group. *J Bone Joint Surg Am* 2009;91:2329-2334.

96. Shukla DR, Morrey BF, Thoreson AR, An KN: Distal biceps tendon rupture: an in vitro study. *Clin Biomech (Bristol, Avon)* 2012;27(3):263-267.

97. Virk MS, DiVenere J, Mazzocca AD: Distal biceps tendon injuries: treatment of partial and complete tears. *Op Tech Sports Med* 2014;22:156-163.

98. Alentorn-Geli E, Assenmacher AT, Sanchez-Sotelo J: Distal biceps tendon injuries: a clinically relevant current concepts review. *EFORT Open Rev* 2016;1:316-324.

99. Festa A, Mulieri PJ, Newman JS, Spitz DJ, Leslie BM: Effectiveness of magnetic resonance imaging in detecting partial and complete distal biceps tendon rupture. *J Hand Surg Am* 2010;35(1):77-83.

100. Lobo Lda G, Fessell DP, Miller BS, et al: The role of sonography in differentiating full versus partial distal biceps tendon tears: correlation with surgical findings. *Am J Roentgenol* 2013;200(1):158-162.

101. Konin GP, Nazarian LN, Walz DM: US of the elbow: indications, technique, normal anatomy, and pathologic conditions. *Radiographics* 2013;33(4):E125-E147.

102. Petty DH, Andrews JR, Fleisig GS, Cain EK: Ulnar collateral ligament reconstruction in high school baseball players: clinical results and injury risk factors. *Am J Sports Med* 2004;32(5):1158-1164.

103. Erickson BJ, Gupta AK, Harris JD, et al: Rate of return to pitching and performance after Tommy John surgery in Major League Baseball pitchers. *Am J Sports Med* 2014;42:536-543.

104. Lyman S, Fleisig GS, Waterbor JW, et al: Longitudinal study of elbow and shoulder pain in youth baseball pitchers. *Med Sci Sports Exerc* 2001;33(11):1803-1810.

105. Lyman S, Fleisig G, Andrews JR, Osinski ED: Effect of pitch type, pitch count, and pitching mechanics on risk of elbow and shoulder pain in youth baseball pitchers. *Am J Sports Med* 2002;30:463-468.

106. Fleisig GS, Andrews JR, Cutter GR, et al: Risk of serious injury for young baseball pitchers: A 10-year prospective study. *Am J Sports Med* 2011;39(2):253-257.

107. Lin F, Kohli N, Perlmutter S, Lim D, Nuber GW, Makhsous M: Muscle contribution to elbow joint valgus stability. *J Shoulder Elbow Surg* 2007;16:795-802.

108. Kibler WB, Morgan CD, Sciascia AD: Kinetic chain deficits and their association with elbow MCL injury in overhead athletes, Keystone, CO American Orthopaedic Society for Sports Medicine Annual Meeting. In:2009.

109. Wymore L, Fronek J: Shoulder functional performance status of National Collegiate Athletic Association swimmers. *Am J Sports Med* 2015;43(6):1513-1517.

110. Kraeutler MJ, Ciccotti MG, Dodson CC, Frederick RW, Cammarota B, Cohen SB: Kerlan-Jobe Orthopaedic Clinic overhead athlete scores in asymptomatic professional baseball pitchers. *J Shoulder Elbow Surg* 2012;22:329-332.

111. Alberta FG, ElAttrache NS, Bissell S, et al: The development and validation of a functional assessment tool for the upper extremity in the overhead athlete. *Am J Sports Med* 2010;38(5):903-911.

112. Stratford P, Gill C, Westaway M, Binkley J: Assessing disability and change on individual patients: a report of a patient specific measure. *Physiother Can* 1995;47(4):258-263.

113. Ciccotti MG, Atanda A Jr, Nazarian LN, Dodson CC, Holmes L, Cohen SB: Stress sonography of the ulnar collateral ligament of the elbow in professional baseball pitchers: a 10-year study. *Am J Sports Med* 2014;42:544-551.

114. Wilk KE, Macrina LC, Fleisig GS, et al: Loss of internal rotation and the correlation to shoulder injuries in professional baseball pitchers. *Am J Sports Med* 2011;39(2):329-335.

115. Wilk KE, Macrina LC, Fleisig GS, et al: Deficits in glenohumeral passive range of motion increase risk of shoulder injury in professional baseball pitchers: a prospective study. *Am J Sports Med* 2015;43(10):2379-2385.

116. Dines JS, Frank JB, Akerman M, Yocum LA: Glenohumeral internal rotation deficits in baseball players with ulnar collateral ligament insufficiency. *Am J Sports Med* 2009;37(3):566-570.

117. Meyer J, Garrison JC, Conway JE: Baseball players with an ulnar collateral ligament tear display increased nondominant arm humeral torsion compared with healthy baseball players. *Am J Sports Med* 2017;45(1):144-149.

118. Garrison JC, Johnston C, Conway JE: Baseball players with ulnar collateral ligament tears demonstrate decreased rotator cuff strength compared to healthy controls. *Int J Sports Phys Ther* 2015;10(4):476-481.

119. Schwartz ML, al-Zahrani S, Morwessel RM, Andrews JR: Ulnar collateral ligament injury in the throwing athlete: evaluation with saline-enhanced MR arthrography. *Radiology* 1995;197:297-299.

120. Carrino JA, Morrison WB, Zou KH, Steffen RT, Snearly WN, Murray PM: Noncontrast MR imaging and MR arthrography of the ulnar collateral ligament of the elbow: prospective evaluation of two-dimensional pulse sequences for detection of complete tears. *Skeletal Radiol* 2001;30:625-632.

121. Charalambous CP, Stanley JK: Posterolateral rotatory instability of the elbow. *J Bone Joint Surg Br* 2008;90B:272-279.

122. Regan W, Lapner PC: Prospective evaluation of two diagnostic apprehension signs for posterolateral instability of the elbow. *J Shoulder Elbow Surg* 2006;15:344-346.

123. McKee MD, Schemitsch EH, Sala MJ, O'Driscoll SW: The pathoanatomy of lateral ligamentous disruption in complex elbow instability. *J Shoulder Elbow Surg* 2003;12:391-396.

124. Grafe MW, McAdams TR, Beaulieu CF, Ladd AK: Magnetic resonance imaging in diagnosis of chronic posterolateral rotatory instability of the elbow. *Am J Orthop* 2003;32:501-503.

125. Begue T: Articular fractures of the distal humerus. *Orthop Traumatol Surg Res* 2014;100:S55-S63.

126. Popkin CA, Rosenwasser KA, Ellis HB: Pediatric and adolescent t-type distal humerus fractures. *JAAOS Glob Res Rev* 2017;1(8):e040.

127. Ring D, Jupiter JB, Gulotta K: Articular fractures of the distal part of the humerus. *J Bone Joint Surg Am* 2003;85A:232-238.

128. Pike JM, Athwal GS, Faber KJ, King GJ: Radial head fractures: an update. *J Hand Surg Am* 2009;34:557-565.
129. Rommens PM, Kuchle R, Schneider RU, Reuter M: Olecranon fractures in adults: factors influencing outcome. *Injury* 2004;35:1149-1157.
130. Wiegand L, Bernstein J, Ahn J: Fractures in brief: olecranon fractures. *Clin Orthop Rel Res* 2012;470:3637-3641.
131. Pappas N, Bernstein J: Fractures in brief: radial head fractures. *Clin Orthop Rel Res* 2010;468:914-916.
132. Trehan SK, Parziale JR, Akelman E: Cubital tunnel syndrome: diagnosis and management. *Med Health RI* 2012;95(11):349-352.
133. Werner CO, Ohlin P, Elmqvist D: Pressures recorded in ulnar neuropathy. *Acta Orthop Scand* 1985;56(5):404-406.
134. Apfelberg DB, Larson SJ: Dynamic anatomy of the ulnar nerve at the elbow. *Plast Reconstruc Surg* 1973;51(1):79-81.
135. Blackwell JR, Hay BA, Bolt AM, Hay SM: Olecranon bursitis: a systematic overview. *Shoulder Elbow* 2014;6(3):182-190.
136. Reilly JP, Nicholas JA: The chronically inflamed bursa. *Clin Sports Med* 1987;6(2):345-370.
137. Canoso JJ, Yood RA: Reaction of superficial bursae in response to specific disease stimuli. *Arthritis Rheum* 1979;22(12):1361-1364.
138. Herrera FA, Meals RA: Chronic olecranon bursitis. *J Hand Surg Am* 2011;36(4):708-709; quiz 710.
139. Pien FD, Ching D, Kim E: Septic bursitis: experience in a community practice. *Orthopedics* 1991;14(9):981-984.
140. Stell IM: Septic and non-septic olecranon bursitis in the accident and emergency department—an approach to management. *J Accid Emerg Med* 1996;13(5):351-353.
141. Reilly D, Kamineni S: Olecranon bursitis. *J Shoulder Elbow Surg* 2016;25(1):158-167.
142. Soucie JM, Wang C, Forsyth A, et al: Range of motion measurements: reference values and a database for comparison studies. *Haemophilia* 2011;17(3):500-507.
143. Cyriax J: *Textbook of Orthopaedic Medicine: Diagnosis of Soft Tissue Lesions*, ed 8. London, UK, Balliere Tindall, 1983.
144. Mayo Clinic: *Clinical Examinations in Neurology*, ed 6. St Louis, MO, Mosby, 1991.
145. Lauder TD, Dillingham TR, Andary M, et al: Predicting electrodiagnostic outcome in patients with upper limb symptoms: are the history and physical examination helpful? *Arch Phys Med Rehabil* 2000;81(4):436-441.
146. Hill SR: *Clinical Methods: The History, Physical, and Labratory Examinations*, ed 3. Boston, MA, Butterworths, 1990.
147. Cozen K: The painful elbow. *Ind Med Surg* 1962;31:369-371.
148. Saroja G, Aseer AL, Sai V: Diagnostic accuracy of provocative tests in lateral epicondylitis. *Int J Physiother Res* 2014;2(6):815-823.
149. Fairbank SM, Corlett RJ: The role of the extensor digitorum communis muscle in lateral epicondylitis. *J Hand Surg Br* 2002;27(5):405-409.
150. Mills GP: The treatment of tennis elbow. *Br Med J* 1928:12-13.
151. Polkinghorn BS: A novel method for assessing elbow pain resulting from epicondylitis. *J Chiro Med* 2002;3(1):117-121.
152. Magee DJ. *Orthopedic Physical Assessment*, vol 5. St Louis, MO: Saunders Elsevier; 2008.
153. ElMaraghy A, Devereaux M. The "bicipital aponeurosis flex test": evaluating the integrity of the bicipital aponeurosis and its implications for treatment of distal biceps tendon ruptures. *J Shoulder Elbow Surg* 2013;22:908-914.
154. ElMaraghy A, Devereaux M, Tsoi K: The biceps crease interval for diagnosing complete distal biceps tendon ruptures. *Clin Orthop Rel Res* 2008;466:2255-2262.
155. Devereaux MW, ElMaraghy AW: Improving the rapid and reliable diagnosis of complete distal biceps tendon rupture: a nuanced approach to the clinical examination. *Am J Sports Med* 2013;41:1998-2004.
156. Ruland RT, Dunbar RP, Bowen JD: The biceps squeeze test for diagnosis of distal biceps tendon ruptures. *Clin Orthop Rel Res* 2005;437:128-131.
157. O'Driscoll SW, Goncalves LB, Dietz P: The hook test for distal biceps tendon avulsion. *Am J Sports Med* 2007;35(11):1865-1869.
158. Metzman LS, Tivener KA: The supination-pronation test for distal biceps tendon rupture. *Am J Orthop* 2015;44(10):E361-E364.
159. O'Driscoll SW, Lawton RL, Smith AM: The "moving valgus stress test" for medial collateral ligament tears of the elbow. *Am J Sports Med* 2005;33(2):231-239.
160. Jobe FW, Kvitne RS: Elbow instability in the athlete. *Instr Course Lect* 1991;40:17-23.
161. O'Driscoll SW, Jupiter JB, King GJ, Hotchkiss RN, Morrey BF: The unstable elbow. *Instr Course Lect* 2001;50:89-102.
162. Arvind CH, Hargreaves DG: Tabletop relocation test: a new clinical test for posterolateral rotatory instability of the elbow. *J Shoulder Elbow Surg* 2006;15:707-708.
163. Darracq MA, Vinson DR, Panacek EA: Preservation of active range of motion after acute elbow trauma predicts absence of elbow fracture. *Am J Emerg Med* 2008;26(7):779-782.
164. Buehler MJ, Thayer DT: The elbow flexion test. A clinical test for the cubital tunnel syndrome. *Clin Orthop Rel Res* 1988;233:213-216.
165. Novak CB, Lee GW, Mackinnon SE, Lay K: Provocative testing for cubital tunnel syndrome. *J Hand Surg Am* 1994;19(5):817-820.
166. Cheng CJ, Mackinnon-Patterson B, Beck JL, Mackinnon SE: Scratch collapse test for evaluation of carpal and cubital tunnel syndrome. *J Hand Surg Am* 2008;33(9):1518-1524.
167. Beekman R, Schreuder AH, Rozeman CA, Koehler PJ, Uitdehaag BM: The diagnostic value of provocative clinical tests in ulnar neuropathy at the elbow is marginal. *J Neurol Neurosurg Psychiatry* 2009;80(12):1369-1374.
168. Tinel J: The "tingling sign" in peripheral nerve lesions. In: Spinner M, ed. *Injuries to the Major Branches of Peripheral Nerves of the Forearm*, 2 ed. Philadelphia, PA, WB Saunders, 1978, pp 8-13.
169. Roberts E: *Physical Therapy Treatment in the Conservative Management of a Full-Thickness Ulnar Collateral Ligament Tear: A Case Report*. The University of Iowa's Institutional Repository, Physical Therapy & Rehabilitation Science, University of Iowa, 2017.

CHAPTER 10

Shoulder

Mark R. Lafave, PhD, CAT(C)
Breda H.F. Eubank, PhD, CAT(C)

OVERVIEW

The shoulder complex is one of the more complicated body regions to evaluate because of the number of bones, articulations, muscles, nerves, and blood vessels that allow it to function. In addition, the proximity of the shoulder to the neck region adds a layer of complexity to understanding the kinetic chain and pathology that overlap between these two regions.

LEARNING OBJECTIVES

After completing this chapter, the reader will be able to do the following:

1. Review and identify key bones, articulations, nerves, blood vessels, and muscles involved with the shoulder complex.
2. Introduce and apply specific testing relevant to injuries and pathology associated with shoulder injuries.
3. List and link common history questions associated with common shoulder injuries and pathology.
4. List and link common observations, posture, or shoulder position to shoulder injuries and pathology.
5. Apply typical range of motion (ROM) (active and passive) of the shoulder complex and identify which joints are responsible throughout the ROM.
6. Apply manual muscle testing (also known as isometric resisted testing) to major shoulder motions and further isolate muscles through manual muscle testing or special testing.
7. Apply special testing for various shoulder injuries and pathology.
8. Identify specific anatomic structures that are involved with shoulder injuries and pathology and be able to palpate those tissues.

FUN FACTS ABOUT THE SHOULDER

- The "socket" (glenoid fossa) of the shoulder is actually more flat than deep, and consequently the humeral head moves against a relatively flat surface.
- The sternoclavicular joint is the only bony articulation of the arm to the body.
- Due to the relative lack of bony articulations and shallow socket, the shoulder depends on muscular support for stability more than most other joints.
- The shoulder is one of the body's most mobile joints.

Introduction

The shoulder complex is attached to the appendicular skeleton through its clavicular attachment to the sternum (**Figure 10.1**). The rest of the shoulder complex is held in place by its muscular attachments; those permit function and act in a manner comparable to guy-wires on a bridge. This design allows for greater function and range of motion (ROM) typically required for athletic endeavors, but it also leaves the shoulder complex susceptible to a greater number of injuries.

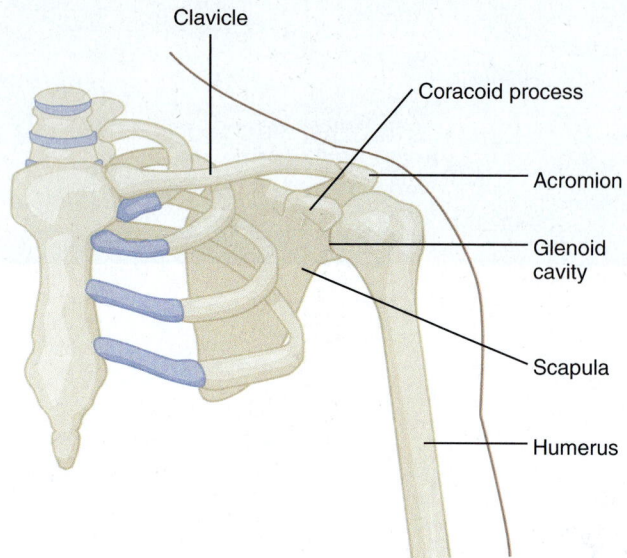

Figure 10.1 Drawing showing the bony attachment of the shoulder.

© Jones & Bartlett Learning

houses major nerves and blood vessels that must be considered when evaluating the upper extremity, neck, and shoulder region.

Clinical Anatomy

Skeletal Anatomy

The three primary bones in the shoulder region are the scapula, humerus, and clavicle. Bones in proximity through articular attachments are the manubrium and sternum proximally and the radius and ulna distally. The first and second ribs are also important bones and can serve as a potential cause of shoulder pathology. Key landmarks of the scapula include the acromion process, the glenoid fossa, the coracoid process, the spine of the scapula, the medial border of the scapula, the lateral border of the scapula, and the apex of the scapula. Key landmarks of the humerus include the bicipital groove, the greater tuberosity, the lesser tuberosity, the deltoid tuberosity, and the head of the humerus. **Figure 10.3** details the anatomy of the shoulder, including the muscles and bones.

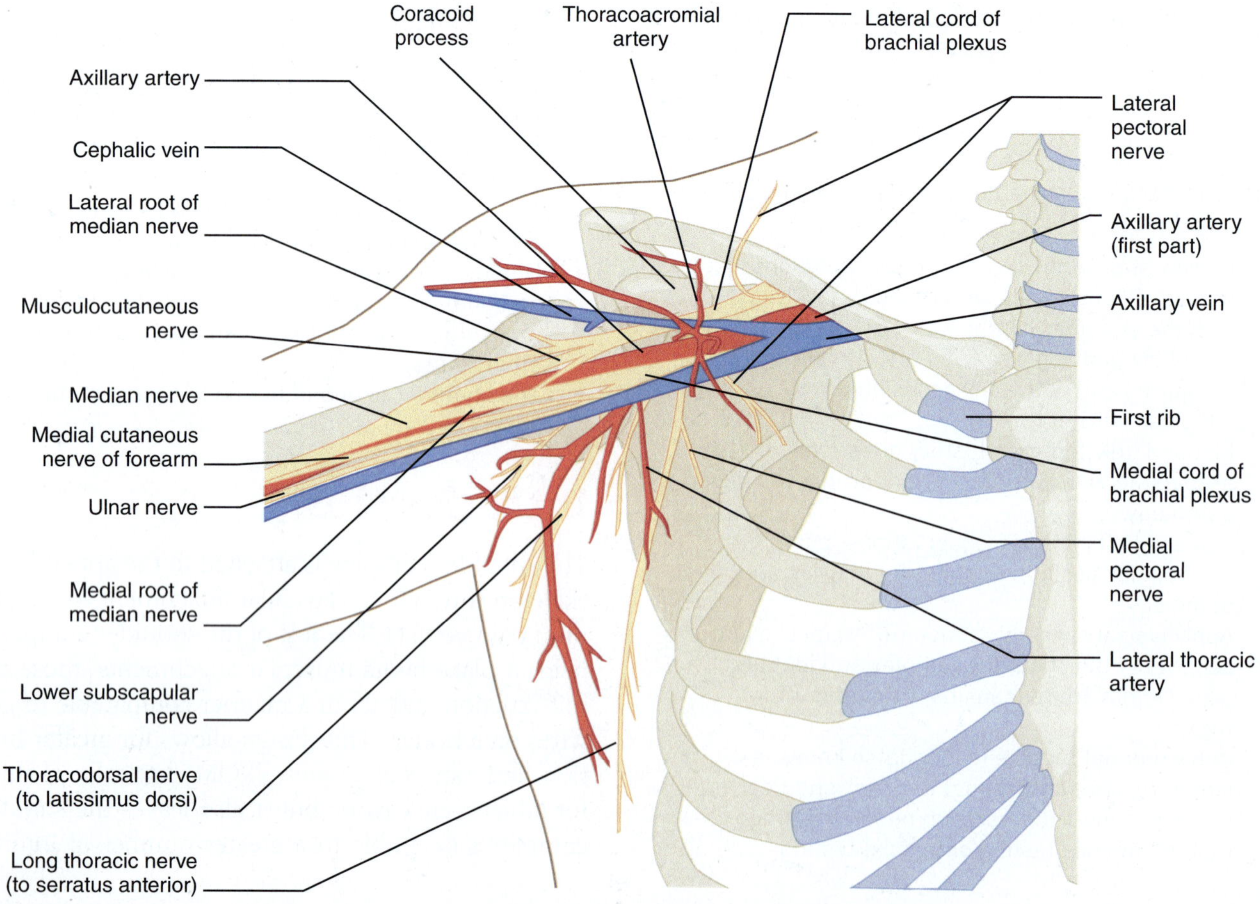

The shoulder region is also home to an important anatomic region called the axilla (**Figure 10.2**). The axilla (or armpit region) is important clinically because it

Figure 10.2 Drawing of the axilla showing nerves and blood vessels.

© Jones & Bartlett Learning

Clinical Anatomy

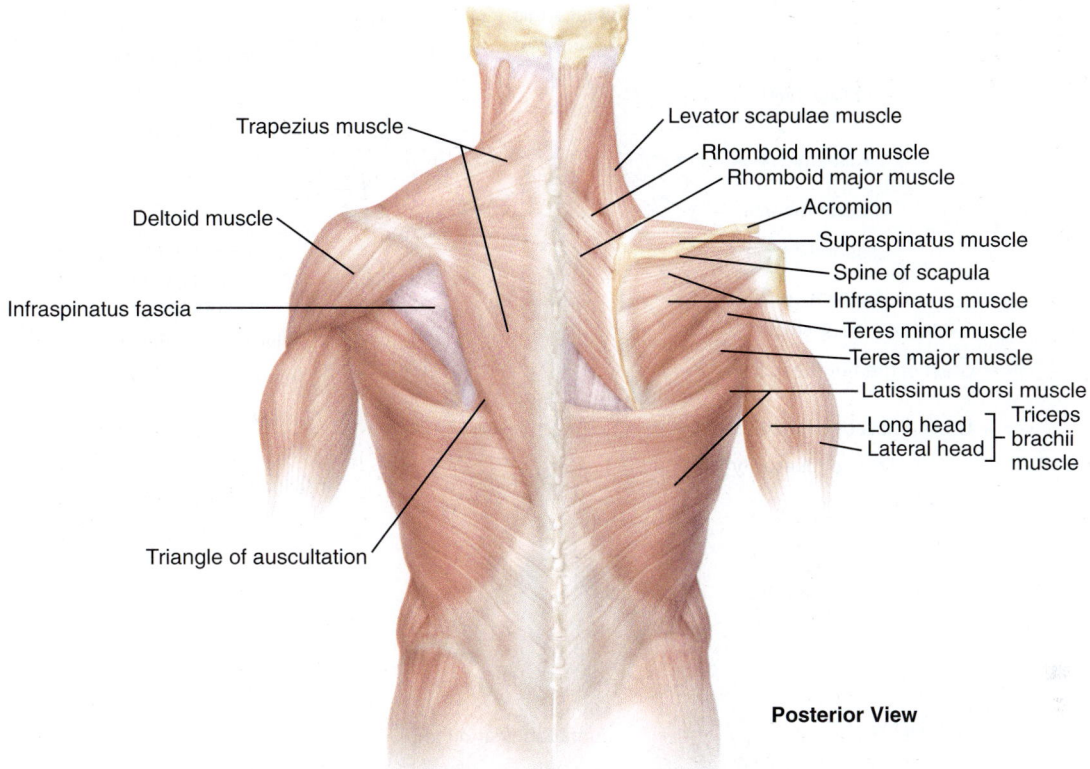

Posterior View

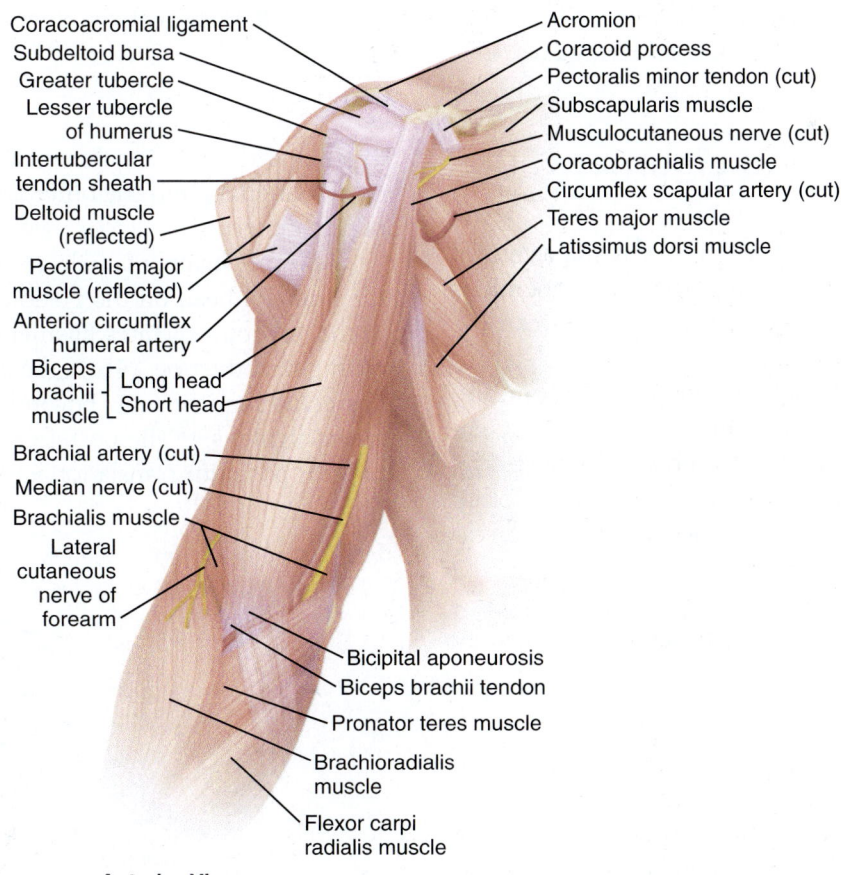

A   Anterior View

Figure 10.3 Drawings showing the anatomy of the shoulder. **A.** Muscle anatomy of the shoulder (posterior and anterior views). (Continued)

Reproduced from Armstrong AD, Hubbard, MC. eds: *Essentials of Musculoskeletal Care*, ed 5. Burlington, MA, American Academy of Orthopaedic Surgeons, 2015.

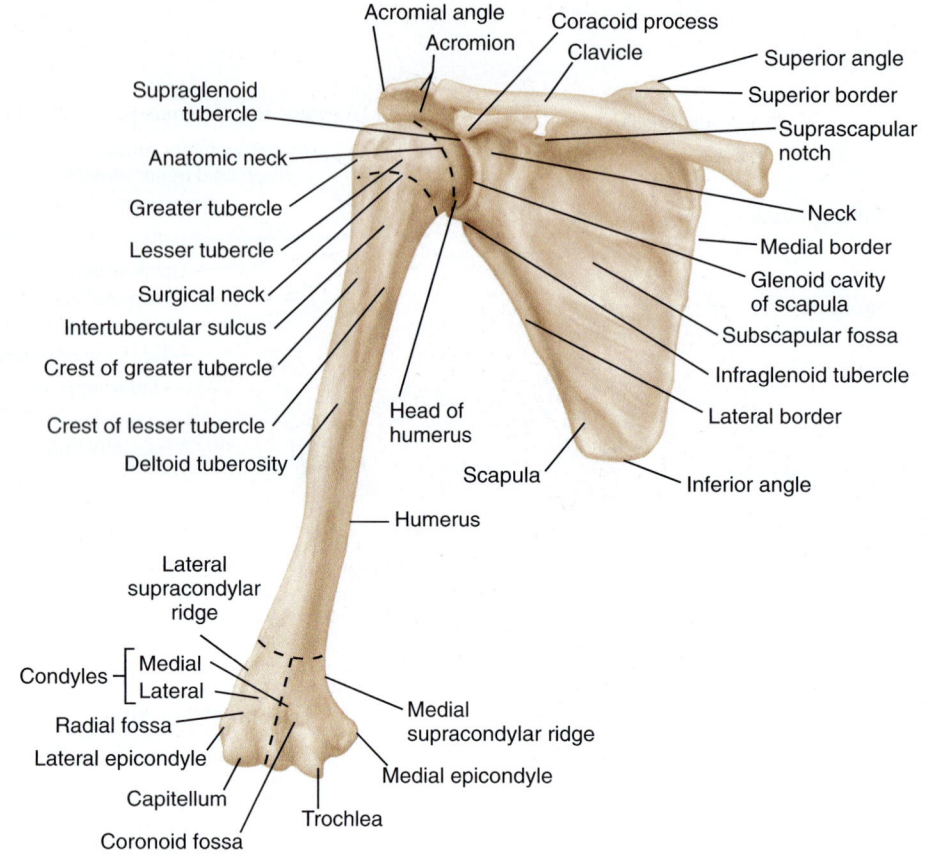

Figure 10.3 (Continued) Drawings showing the anatomy of the shoulder. **B.** Bony anatomy of the shoulder.

Reproduced from Armstrong, AD, Hubbard, MC. eds: *Essentials of Musculoskeletal Care*, ed 5. Burlington, MA, American Academy of Orthopaedic Surgeons, 2015.

Articulations and Ligamentous Support

The shoulder complex is a region that is characterized by a number of articulations that facilitate tremendous movement and requires synchronization between the glenohumeral (GH), acromioclavicular (AC), sternoclavicular (SC), and scapulothoracic joints. Technically, the scapulothoracic articulation is not a true articulation because it does not have two bones connected by fibrous or synovial structures, such as those in the other shoulder joints (ie, GH, AC, and SC). However, the scapulothoracic joint is a unique articulation between the scapula and ribs two through seven of the thorax. Ligaments are separated by the specific joint or articulation.

The GH Joint

The GH joint is a ball-and-socket synovial joint with a fibrous capsule that has reinforcement from the superior, middle, and inferior ligaments to provide stability (**Figure 10.4**). The glenoid labrum is an articular fibrocartilaginous disk that helps to deepen the socket on the surface of the glenoid fossa. The glenoid labrum (**Figure 10.5**) is intimately linked to a fibrous capsule with one attachment on the glenoid fossa outer boundary and the other attachment at the neck of the humerus.[1]

All three ligaments help to support translation of the humeral head on the glenoid fossa.[1] The position of the GH joint dictates ligament tautness. In neutral or slight abduction (45°), the superior and middle ligaments become taut. Beyond 45°, the inferior ligament tightens.[1-3] The posterior capsule and ligament prevent posterior translation and medial rotation.[1]

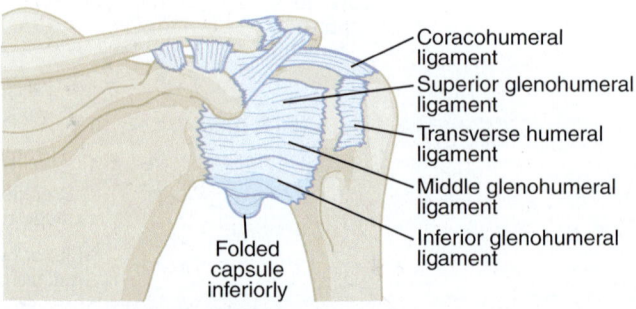

Figure 10.4 Drawing showing the glenohumeral joint and its ligaments.

© Jones & Bartlett Learning

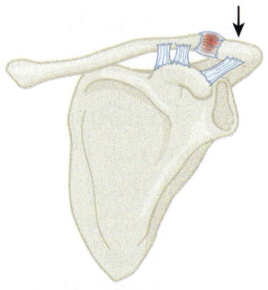
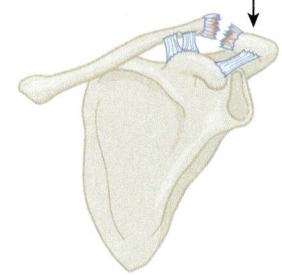
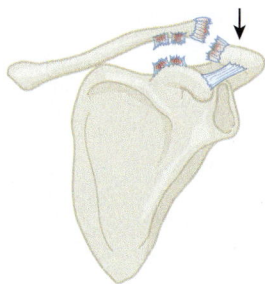

Type I

Pathology
Sprained AC ligaments; normal CC ligaments

Examination
Pain and swelling over the AC joint without a visible deformity

Radiography
Normal

Type II

Pathology
Disruption of the AC ligaments; sprained CC ligaments

Examination
Distal clavicle is unstable to horizontal stress; pain over the CC interspace

Radiography
Widened AC joint and slight elevation of the clavicle (<25%)

Type III

Pathology
Disruption of the AC and CC ligaments

Examination
Distal clavicle is unstable to horizontal and vertical stress; reducible

Radiography
Moderate elevation of the clavicle (25% to 100%)

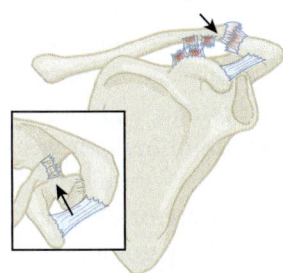
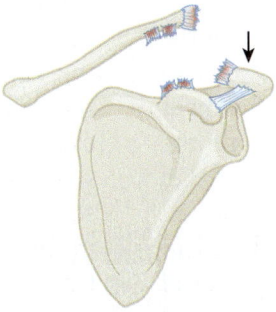
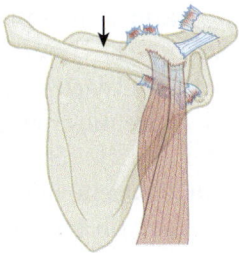

Type IV

Pathology
Posterior displacement into or through the trapezius muscle

Examination
Not reducible

Radiography
Axillary view shows posterior displacement

Type V

Pathology
Rupture of the deltotrapezial fascia

Examination
Clavicle palpable subcutaneously; not reducible

Radiography
Distal clavicle is elevated (>100% to 300%)

Type VI

Pathology
Inferior displacement of the distal clavicle under the conjoined tendon

Examination
Associated with rib fractures and neurovascular injury

Radiography
Clavicle is in a subacromial or subcoracoid position

Figure 10.5 Drawings showing the six types of glenoid labrum pathology.
AC, acromioclavicular; CC, coracoclavicular.

© Jones & Bartlett Learning

The Acromioclavicular Joint

The AC joint (**Figure 10.6**) is classified as a plane synovial joint because it articulates two relatively flat ends of two bones and facilitates mostly a gliding motion in multiple directions to support GH motion. The two ends of the articulating bones are supported by an articular disk rather than hyaline cartilage.[1,3] The AC joint itself has a fibrous capsule surrounding its articulations to mostly prevent superior movement of the clavicle on the scapula or acromion. However, the primary support for this joint actually comes from two external ligaments that attach the coracoid process of the scapula to the inferior side of the clavicle: the coracoclavicular (CC) ligaments. Those ligaments are called the conoid and trapezoid ligaments because of their shapes and adjoining bony protuberances.

The Sternoclavicular Joint

The SC joint (**Figure 10.7**) is a saddle synovial joint that has three degrees of freedom supporting GH motion.[1,2] Its primary articulation occurs between the medial end of the clavicle and the manubrium of the sternum. A secondary articulation occurs at the costochondral junction of the first rib. There are four ligaments that support this joint: anterior, posterior,

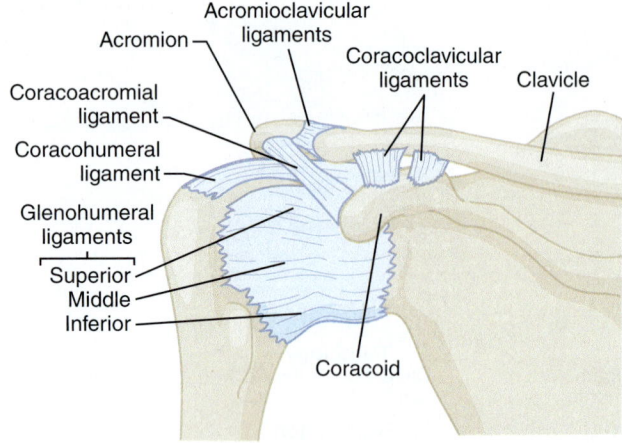

Figure 10.6 Drawing showing the acromioclavicular joint and its ligaments.

© Jones & Bartlett Learning

Soft-Tissue Anatomy

Muscular Anatomy

The muscles of the shoulder girdle are described in **Table 10.1** (and are shown in Figure 10.3A). The table includes proximal and distal attachments, common nerve innervation as well as where and how to palpate the muscle. A unique feature of the table is that it also includes a brief description of how to perform the manual muscle test (MMT) of the referenced muscle.

Neurologic Anatomy

There are some shoulder conditions or pathologies that present in a manner similar to a shoulder problem but are, in fact, not shoulder problems. The central cause of the shoulder pain or dysfunction is actually coming from the innervating segments, such as the spinal cord or nerve roots that are responsible for the nerve supply to the shoulder region. A scan or screening of the cervical region may be important in cases where neurologic signs or symptoms present, such as tingling, numbness, or weakness. Part of this scanning examination should include reflex testing in the upper extremity or dermatome, and myotome testing. If reflex, dermatome, or myotome testing is positive, further investigation of the cervical spine is necessary.

interclavicular, and costoclavicular. The anterior and posterior ligaments are attached to the surfaces of the clavicle and manubrium, which prevent anterior and posterior translation. The interclavicular ligament links the right and left clavicles superiorly along the manubrium, thus preventing superior or cephalad movement of either clavicle relative to one another.[1] The costoclavicular ligament links the distal end of the clavicle to the first rib and its associated costal cartilage. This ligament prevents a superior glide and rotation of the clavicle from the first rib.

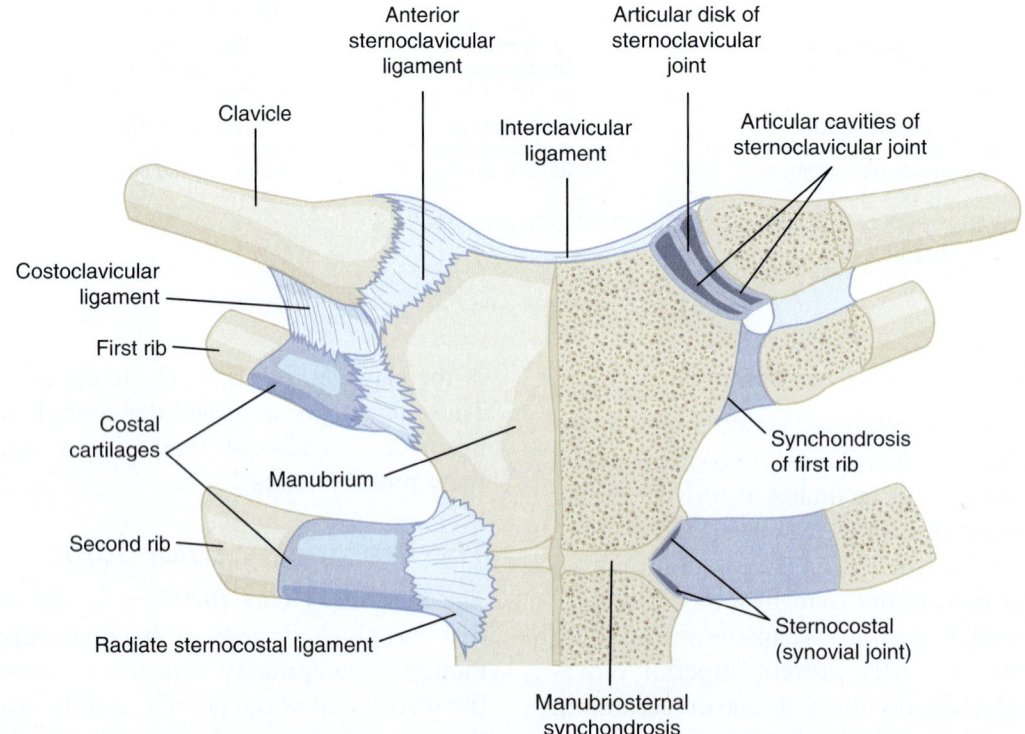

Figure 10.7 Drawing showing the sternoclavicular joint and its ligaments.

© Jones & Bartlett Learning

Table 10.1 Shoulder Muscles

Muscle	Origin	Insertion	Action	Innervation (Nerve Root)	Palpation	Manual Muscle Test
Supraspinatus	Supraspinatus fossa of scapula	Greater tubercle of humerus	Initiation of abduction up to 15° until the deltoid muscle takes over greater control. Also stabilizes head of humerus in glenoid cavity.	Suprascapular (C5, C6)	Find the acromion process and fall off the lateral edge moving toward the greater tuberosity.	Seated with the patient's shoulder abducted between 5° and 10° with the elbow at 90°. Ask patient to hold his or her arm in that position against resistance while the examiner attempts to push the patient's elbow toward the patient's side.
Infraspinatus	Medial two-thirds of the infraspinous fossa of the scapula	Greater tubercle of humerus	External rotation of the humerus.	Suprascapular (C5, C6)	With the patient in a prone position, landmark the medial border and spine of the scapula to feel the boundaries and then palpate the infraspinatus that sits in the infraspinous fossa and its tendon as it traverses toward the greater tubercle.	In a seated or standing position, abduct the patient's shoulder between 5° and 10° so there is enough room for the examiner to stabilize the patient at the elbow joint while the examiner's other hand goes to the wrist and attempts to push the patient's fist toward his or her own stomach.

(continues)

Table 10.1 Shoulder Muscles *(continued)*

Muscle	Origin	Insertion	Action	Innervation (Nerve Root)	Palpation	Manual Muscle Test
Teres minor	Posterolateral surface of the scapula	Inferior facet of the greater tubercle of the humerus	External rotation of the humerus.	Axillary nerve (C5, C6)	Flex the shoulder to 90°, then horizontally adduct into 10° to 20° of external rotation. Using the other hand to palpate, move two fingers just inferior to the greater tubercle and follow inferiorly and posteriorly to the lateral border of the scapular wall to palpate the teres minor muscle belly. It will be important to attempt to move the posterior deltoid out of the way to get to the teres minor tendon.	With the patient in a prone position, move the shoulder into abduction and 90° of flexion at the elbow. Stabilize the medial side of the patient's elbow with one hand and place the testing hand on the lateral side of the forearm. Instruct the patient to hold his or her arm steady while the testing hand attempts to push the forearm into internal rotation.

Subscapularis	Anterior surface on the medial two-thirds of the scapular fossa	Lesser tubercle of the humerus	Internal rotation of the humerus	Upper and lower subscapular nerves (C5–C7)	With the patient in a supine position, find the lesser tubercle or the humerus. The deltoid and pectoralis major muscles are more superficial; therefore, push through those muscles or try to push them aside to attempt to palpate the subscapularis. Alternatively, if the patient is side-lying, the examiner can attempt to find the subscapularis through the posterior axillary region by finding the lateral border of the scapula and then scooping the fingertips around the scapula to the anterior surface to feel the muscle belly. Once again, palpating in this manner forces the examiner to push through a number of other more superficial muscles, including the long head of the triceps, the latissimus dorsi, the teres major, and the teres minor.	Have the patient place his or her arm behind the back so the humerus is internally rotated and the posterior wrist is resting around the L5–S1 region. The patient can be seated or standing. Then, ask the patient to lift the wrist off his or her back and hold that position while the examiner resists the patient's lift-off motion (A). Alternatively, lay the patient supine with his or her shoulder slightly abducted, flexed with a 90° bent elbow. The examiner places his or her stabilizing hand on the lateral side of the elbow while the resisting hand is on the medial side of his or her wrist. The patient is asked to attempt to pull the wrist into internal rotation or toward the belly while the examiner resists (B).

(continues)

Table 10.1 Shoulder Muscles (continued)

Muscle	Origin	Insertion	Action	Innervation (Nerve Root)	Palpation	Manual Muscle Test
Deltoid	Inferior lip of the spine of the scapula, the lateral border of the acromion process, and the lateral one-third of the clavicle	Deltoid tuberosity of the humerus	Shoulder abduction beyond 15° of abduction (middle fibers). The posterior fibers assist in shoulder extension, while the anterior fibers assist in shoulder flexion.	Axillary nerve (C5, C6)	Stand beside the patient, facing the patient, and cup one hand on the anterior aspect of the deltoid and one hand on the posterior aspect of the deltoid. Both hands can move distally toward the deltoid tuberosity of the humerus. The middle deltoid lies between the anterior and posterior deltoid, with all combining distally to insert into the deltoid tuberosity of the humerus.	To test the middle deltoid, the patient should abduct the shoulder between 15° and 90° with the elbow bent to 90°. The examiner will place a stabilizing arm at the top of the shoulder on the AC joint. The examiner's testing hand will be just above the patient's elbow. The patient is instructed to hold the arm steady while the testing hand attempts to push the patient's arm toward his or her side (ie, caudad). The patient and examiner positioning for the posterior deltoid is similar except with the addition of the patient moving the shoulder into slight horizontal abduction (ie, posteriorly) (A). The anterior deltoid is often tested in a supine position with the shoulder placed into a minimum of 15° of abduction and a minimum of 15° of horizontal adduction with a flexed elbow (B). The examiner attempts to push the patient posteriorly or into horizontal abduction while the patient resists that motion.

Latissimus dorsi	Spinous processes of the lower six thoracic vertebrae and adjoining interspinous ligaments blending into the thoracolumbar fascia	Floor of the bicipital groove of the humerus	Extension, adduction, and internal rotation of the glenohumeral joint.	Thoracodorsal nerve (C6–C8)	In a prone position, identify the bony origins of the latissimus dorsi along the spinous processes of T6–T12 and into the iliac crest. The lateral border of the muscle can be palpated by following the lateral boundary of the back up toward the posterior axilla. To palpate the distal end of the latissimus dorsi, the patient should lie supine and the examiner should cradle the patient's flexed shoulder under his or her arm so the muscle is relaxed. Palpate the lateral boundary of the latissimus dorsi with the medial hand following the muscle belly into its tendon along the medial side of the humerus and into the bicipital groove.	The patient lies prone with the shoulder adducted, extended (10°), and medially rotated as much as he or she can with a fully extended elbow. With the testing hand at the patient's wrist, the patient is instructed to maintain this position while the examiner attempts to push the patient's arm into shoulder flexion or toward the table.
Teres major	Posterior-lateral and inferior surface of the scapula at the angle	Medial lip of the bicipital groove of the humerus	Glenohumeral adduction and medial rotation.	Lower subscapular nerve (C5, C6)	In a prone position, palpate the inferior angle of the scapula and follow the muscle belly along a similar pathway as the latissimus dorsi.	The patient should lie prone with the shoulder internally rotated and adducted with a flexed elbow (approximately 100°) with the posterior aspect of the wrist resting on the posterior aspect of the iliac crest. The examiner must place his or her hand against the patient's arm, just above the elbow. The patient will be asked to keep the wrist on the iliac crest and maintain that position while the examiner attempts to push the patient's arm into abduction and flexion.

(continues)

(continued)

Table 10.1 Shoulder Muscles

Muscle	Origin	Insertion	Action	Innervation (Nerve Root)	Palpation	Manual Muscle Test
Pectoralis minor	Anterior surfaces of ribs three to five	Coracoid process of the scapula	Protraction of the scapula and pulling the tip of the glenohumeral joint in an arc like fashion anteriorly and inferiorly.	Medial pectoral nerve (C5–T1)	Palpate the pectoralis minor muscle just inferior to the coracoid process.	The patient lies supine and attempts to roll his or her shoulder or glenohumeral joint anteriorly and inferiorly in an arc-like fashion. The examiner cups the glenohumeral joint and attempts to push it posteriorly while the patient resists this motion.
Pectoralis major	Clavicular head: Medial half of the clavicle. Sternocostal head: Boundary and anterior surface of the sternum down through the first through seventh costal cartilages	Lateral lip of the bicipital groove of the humerus	Flexion, adduction, and medial rotation of the humerus.	Clavicular head: Medial and lateral pectoral nerves (C5, C6) Clavicular head: C6, C7, T1	In a supine position with the shoulder slightly abducted and cradled by the examiner under his or her own arm, palpate the anterior axillary border and either extend to the insertion around the bicipital groove or to the origin side along the clavicle, sternum, and ribs.	In a supine position, test the clavicular head by flexing the patient's shoulder with an extended elbow to 90° and slight humeral medial rotation (thumb pointed toward the sky or head of patient). The patient is asked to hold this position while the examiner attempts to horizontally adduct the glenohumeral joint. To test the sternocostal head in a supine position, flex the patient's shoulder to approximately 75° of horizontal adduction and 10° of medial rotation. The patient is instructed to maintain this position while the examiner pulls the glenohumeral joint into abduction and extension.

Clinical Anatomy | **349**

Biceps brachii	Long head: Supraglenoid tubercle of the humerus and glenoid labrum Short head: Coracoid process of the scapula	Radial tuberosity of the radius	Shoulder flexion and elbow flexion.	Musculocutaneous nerve (C5–C7)	Identify the proximal attachments at the supraglenoid tubercle of the humerus pushing through the deltoid muscle or the coracoid process of the scapula. The examiner can trace the length of the biceps brachii along the anterior humerus to its insertion at the radial tuberosity.	The upper part of the biceps is tested using a special test called the speed test. The lower part of the biceps brachii muscle is tested by asking the patient to hold the elbow joint at a 90° angle while the examiner attempts to extend the elbow.
Coracobrachialis	Coracoid process of the scapula	Midshaft of the humerus on the medial side	Shoulder flexion and adduction.	Musculocutaneous nerve (C5–C7)	Palpate from the coracoid process and extend distally, pushing through the biceps brachii muscle to feel it.	In a seated position, the patient flexes his or her shoulder to 70° to 80° with a fully flexed elbow. The examiner asks the patient to hold that position while he or she attempts to push the shoulder into extension and slight abduction.

(continues)

350 **Chapter 10** Shoulder

Table 10.1 Shoulder Muscles

Muscle	Origin	Insertion	Action	Innervation (Nerve Root)	Palpation	Manual Muscle Test
Triceps brachii	Long head: Infraglenoid tubercle of the scapula Lateral head: Posterior surface of the humerus Medial head: Posterior surface of the humerus	Olecranon process of the ulna	Shoulder extension and elbow extension.	Radial nerve (C6–C8)	Palpate proximally just below the posterior deltoid for the shoulder attachment (long head). The muscle bulk of the three muscles is in the middle of the upper arm, and the rest of the muscle converges just proximally to the elbow, where it becomes more tendinous and ultimately passes across the posterior elbow to attach to the olecranon process.	The patient lies supine or is seated. All three heads of the triceps muscle (long head, lateral head, and medial head) are tested by flexing the patient's shoulder to 90° with the forearm supinated and elbow slightly flexed. The examiner's testing hand is situated at the wrist joint, and the stabilizing hand is just above the elbow joint. The examiner instructs the patient not to move while he or she attempts to flex the elbow.
Serratus anterior	Lateral surfaces of the first eight ribs	Anteromedial surface of the scapula	Scapular protraction. Also maintains the scapular position against the thoracic cage to prevent winging and rotates the angle of the scapula laterally with glenohumeral abduction and flexion.	Long thoracic nerve (C5–C7)	Begin at the lateral-inferior border of the scapula to the first eight ribs.	The patient lies supine with the shoulder flexed to 90° and elbow fully extended. The patient makes a fist and attempts to punch toward the sky. The patient holds this position while the examiner attempts to push the patient's fist back down toward the table.

(continued)

Muscle	Origin	Insertion	Action	Innervation	Identification	Testing
Rhomboids	Rhomboid minor: Ligamentum nuchae (lower end) and the spinous processes of C7 and T1. Rhomboid major: Spinous processes T2 to T5 inclusively as well as the interspinous ligament along that same path	Rhomboid minor: Medial border of the scapula from the spine of the scapula upward. Rhomboid major: Medial border of the scapula from the spine of the scapula distally to the apex	Rhomboid minor is primarily responsible for retraction while also having a minor role with elevation. Rhomboid major works with the middle trapezius muscle to retract the scapula.	Dorsal scapular nerve (C4, C5)	Identify the origin and insertion bony landmarks along the spine and the medial border of the scapula, respectively. The rhomboid muscles are deep to the trapezius, and, therefore, palpation must go through a layer of muscle to feel it.	In a prone position, the patient should abduct the shoulder to 90° and rotate the entire arm internally with an extended elbow so the thumb is pointed to the floor. The patient should be instructed to hold the arm in that position while attempting to move his or her hand toward the sky while also focusing on shoulder retraction.
Trapezius	Superior nuchal line, external occipital protuberance, medial margin of the ligamentum nuchae, C7 to T12 and the related supraspinous ligaments	Superior edge of the crest of the spine of the scapula, acromion, posterior border of the lateral one-third of the clavicle	Elevation, retraction, and depression of the scapula; scapular rotation during shoulder abduction; retraction of the scapula.	Cranial nerve XI (motor component). The sensation and proprioception of this muscle are innervated by the anterior rami of the third and fourth cervical nerves.	Outline the bony boundaries of the trapezius in a prone position with the head in a neutral position. The central boundary separates the right from the left trapezius muscles.	The upper trapezius muscle is best tested in a seated position with the examiner either in front of or behind the patient. The examiner places hands over both shoulders covering the acromioclavicular joints with the fingertips and palm of the hand cradling over the clavicle and the spine of the scapula. Because of the strength of the upper trapezius muscle, it is best to have the patient shrug his or her shoulders toward the sky and maintain the hold while the examiner tries to push the shoulders downward (or caudad) (A). The middle and lower trapezius muscles should be tested in a prone position. Similar to rhomboid manual muscle testing, the middle trapezius test is differentiated with the position of the thumb (ie, thumb up). The patient should lie prone on a table with the humerus abducted to 90° and elbow fully extended. The examiner will attempt to push the patient's arm toward the floor while the patient resists this motion (B).

(continues)

352 Chapter 10 Shoulder

Table 10.1 Shoulder Muscles *(continued)*

Muscle	Origin	Insertion	Action	Innervation (Nerve Root)	Palpation	Manual Muscle Test
Trapezius (continued)						Because of the wingspan of most patients, it is probably best to test right and left sides independently. The lower trapezius is also tested with the patient in a prone position similar to the middle trapezius muscle. However, the position of the humerus should be adjusted to approximately 120° of abduction or in line with the lower fibers of the trapezius muscle. Again, the examiner will attempt to push the patient's arm toward the floor while the patient resists this motion (C).

A

B

C

Clinical Anatomy

Muscle	Origin	Insertion	Action	Innervation	Palpation	Manual Muscle Test
Levator scapula	Transverse processes of C1–C4, inclusively; however, the muscle attachments on C3 and C4 attach to the posterior aspect of the transverse process	Posterior surface of the medial border of the scapula	Elevation of the scapula.	Anterior rami of C3 and C4 spinal nerves by the C5 branch of the dorsal scapular nerve.	Approach the patient from the side of the neck, just anterior to the upper fiber of the trapezius. Find the C1–C4 transverse processes both laterally and posteriorly to find the origin of the levator scapula and follow its pathway down to the medial border of the scapula.	With the patient lying prone and his or her head turned to the testing side, the patient should shrug the shoulder and tilt the head toward the testing side. The examiner will push the patient's shoulder down (caudad) while the patient resists that motion both at the shoulder and at the neck region. If necessary, the examiner should stabilize both the origin and insertion ends of the levator scapula by also cradling the patient's head around the occiput and mastoid process.

All figures in table © Jones & Bartlett Learning.

Reflex Testing. The closest reflex testing areas for the shoulder region are the biceps (C5–C6), the brachioradialis (C5–C6), and the triceps tendon (C7–C8) (**Figures 10.8** through **10.10**).

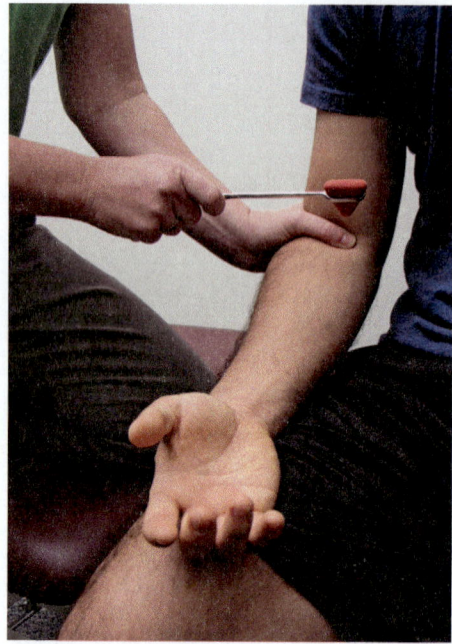

Figure 10.8 Photograph showing reflex testing of the biceps brachii.
© Jones & Bartlett Learning

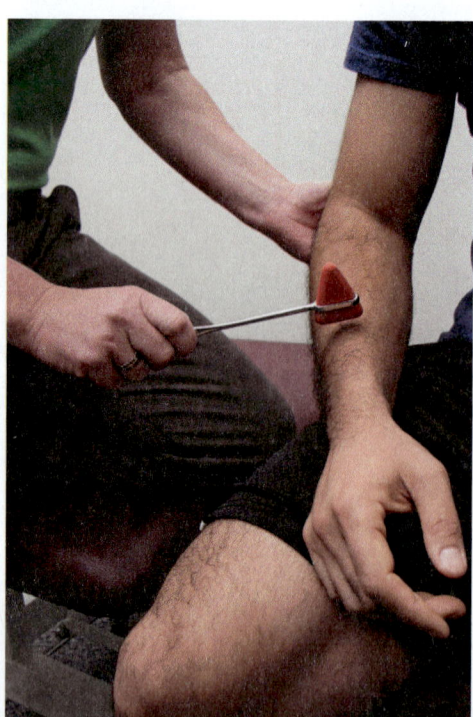

Figure 10.9 Photograph showing reflex testing of the brachioradialis.
© Jones & Bartlett Learning

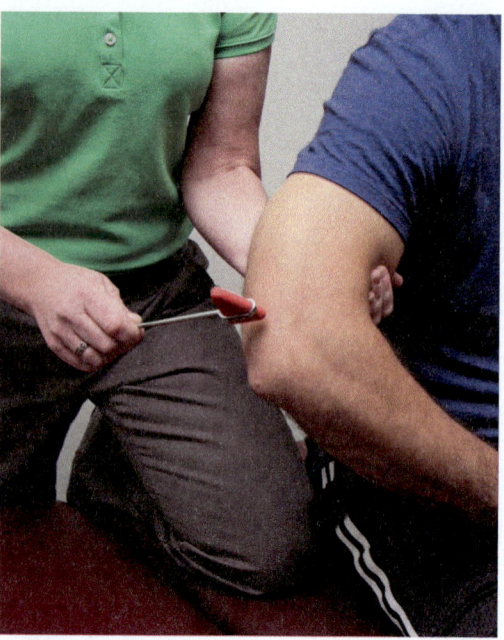

Figure 10.10 Photograph showing reflex testing of the brachioradialis.
© Jones & Bartlett Learning

Sensory Testing. The dermatomes that are most relevant to the shoulder include C4, C5, and C6 anteriorly and laterally. Posterior upper arm and shoulder dermatomes include the T1 and T2 dermatomes, whereas the scapular region dermatomes consist of mostly T2–T7.

The myotomes of most relevance to the shoulder region include C4 (scapular elevation), C5 (shoulder abduction), and, more peripherally, C6 (elbow flexion/wrist extension) and C7 (elbow extension/wrist flexion).

Vascular Anatomy

The axillary artery is a significant blood vessel that supplies the upper extremity with blood flow. Its proximity to bony and muscular structures leaves it susceptible to pathology. The first part of the axillary artery can be a complication with first rib or clavicular fractures, and, therefore, distal pulse checks with suspected fractures become an important screening for this complication. The second part of the axillary artery, where it passes deep to the pectoralis minor muscle, is a site for impingement leading to vascular signs or symptoms commonly associated with thoracic outlet syndrome (TOS). The third part of the axillary artery has two branches, called the anterior and posterior circumflex arteries. These two blood vessels can be involved in injury or pathology, particularly humeral head fractures. Both wrap around the head and neck of the head of the humerus and supply the GH joint and surrounding muscles with blood supply (**Figure 10.11**).

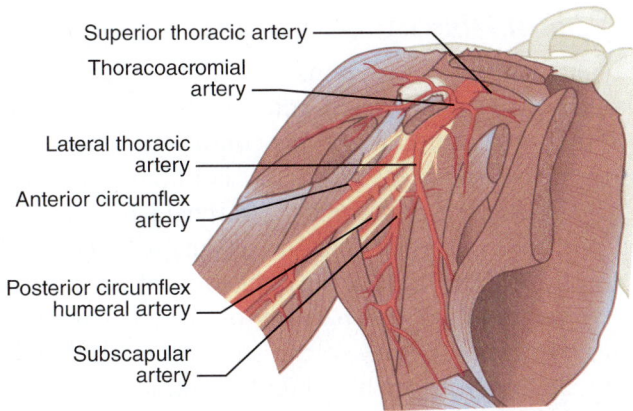

Figure 10.11 Drawing showing the anterior and posterior circumflex arteries.

© Jones & Bartlett Learning

Overview of Radiology and Imaging

Common Radiographic Views

AC joint sprains, anteroinferior glenohumeral dislocations, and posterior glenohumeral dislocation commonly present for imaging. These radiographic views are shown in **Figures 10.12** through **10.14**.

Common MRI Views and Injuries

Figure 10.15 and **Figure 10.16** show magnetic resonance images of a labral tear and Bankart lesion, respectively.

Other Imaging Options

Ultrasonography for Rotator Cuff Tear

Ultrasonography is the cost-effective method for diagnosing a rotator cuff tear.

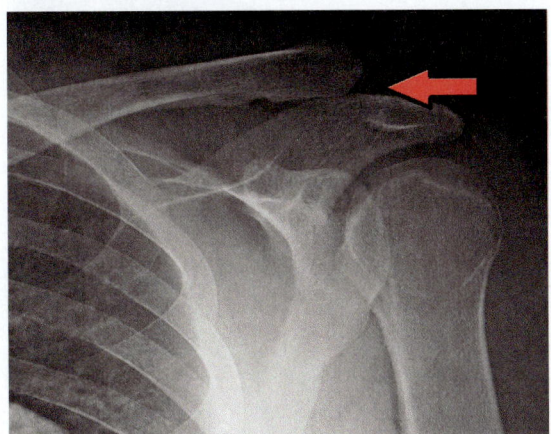

Figure 10.12 Radiograph of an acromioclavicular sprain (arrow).

Courtesy of James Heilman, MD.

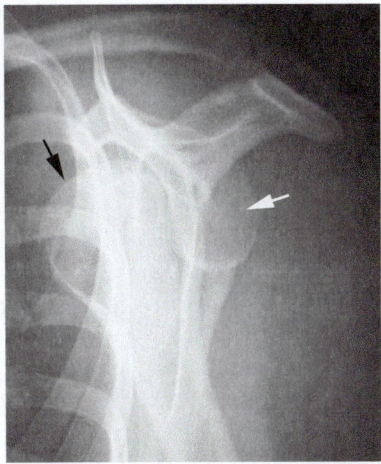

Figure 10.13 Radiograph of a glenohumeral anteroinferior dislocation (arrows).

Reproduced from Johnson TR, Steinbach LS. eds: *Essentials of Musculoskeletal Imaging*. Rosemont, IL, American Academy of Orthopaedic Surgeons, 2004.

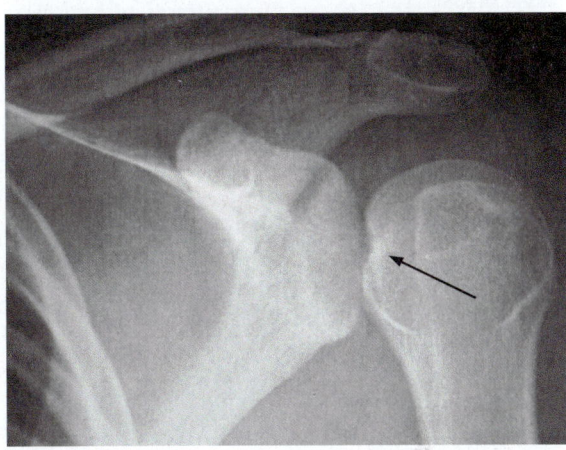

Figure 10.14 Radiograph of a glenohumeral posterior dislocation (arrow).

Reproduced from Armstrong AD, Hubbard MC. eds: *Essentials of Musculoskeletal Care*, ed 5. Burlington, MA, American Academy of Orthopaedic Surgeons, 2015.

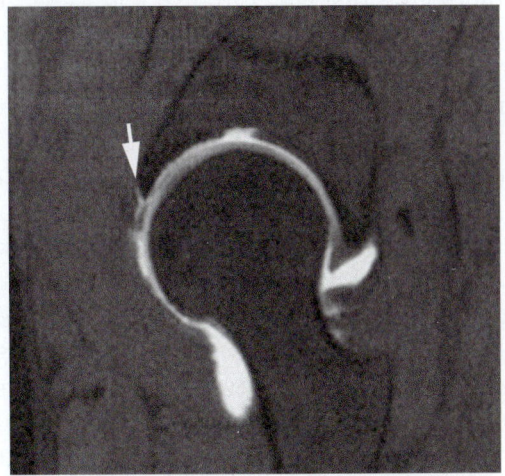

Figure 10.15 Magnetic resonance image showing a labral tear (arrow).

Reproduced from Johnson TR, Steinbach LS. eds: *Essentials of Musculoskeletal Imaging*. Rosemont, IL, American Academy of Orthopaedic Surgeons, 2004.

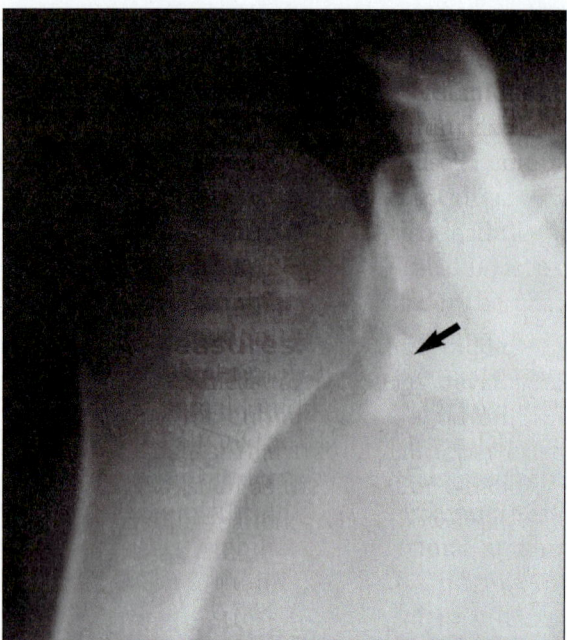

Figure 10.16 Radiograph of a bony Bankart lesion (arrow).

Reproduced from Johnson TR, Steinbach LS. eds: *Essentials of Musculoskeletal Imaging*. Rosemont, IL, American Academy of Orthopaedic Surgeons, 2004.

Evaluation of the Shoulder

A thorough evaluation of the shoulder includes performing history questions, an inspection, ROM assessment, palpation, and special tests.

History

Overview of Goal of History Taking

The goal of history taking in the shoulder region is to narrow the patient's complaint down to a very specific region or joint in the shoulder. Because of the complexity of the shoulder region and all of its joints, muscles, and innervations, primary and secondary sites can contribute to shoulder injury and pathology. Moreover, chronic conditions in the shoulder often result from poor posture and therefore contribute to poor biomechanics that underlie chronic conditions and pathologies. Therefore, shoulder evaluations can be quite challenging. Another challenging and unique aspect of the shoulder, relative to other joints in the upper extremity, is its proximity to the cervical and thoracic spine. Both the physical connection through musculature and the proximity to neurologic tissues should be considered in the history to ensure the primary injury site is actually in the shoulder and not being referred there by neurovascular structures.

Typical History Questions

Typical history questions for the shoulder are traditionally categorized into those for traumatic injuries and those for chronic conditions. Therefore, knowing the date of the injury is important. If the patient is able to pinpoint the mechanism of injury, it will more likely fit into the traumatic category of questions. The traumatic questions often involve investigating the mechanism of injury. Common mechanisms of injury of the shoulder include falling on an outstretched hand, commonly known as FOOSH. This type of mechanism of injury can result in anteroinferior GH dislocation or subluxation and complications that result from this type of injury including, but not limited to, Bankart lesions and Hill-Sachs lesions (an osteochondral lesion or fracture of the superior and/or posterior aspect of the head of the humerus). The FOOSH mechanism of injuries can be responsible for two other types of common injuries: traumatic subacromial bursitis and AC joint sprains. AC joint sprains can also be injured with the patient falling on the tip of his or her shoulder around the acromion process (**Figure 10.17**). This same mechanism is also responsible for clavicular fractures, SC sprains, and a lesser known first rib subluxation. Overall, knowing the mechanism of injury for traumatic conditions will help the examiner suspect the type of injury and appropriate testing that should follow.

If the patient has trouble identifying a specific date and the injury has gradually appeared over time (ie, insidious onset), it will likely fit into the chronic condition category of questions. Injuries or pathologies that are commonly associated with chronic or

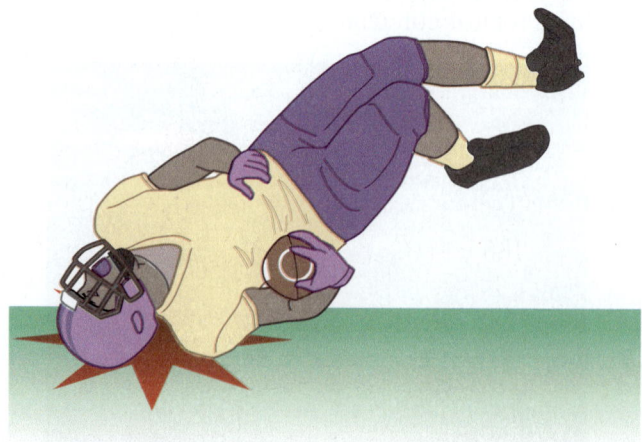

Figure 10.17 Illustration depicting an athlete falling on the tip of the shoulder around the acromion process.

© Jones & Bartlett Learning

overuse mechanisms of injury are more difficult to address with history taking. If the patient presents with no traumatic mechanism of injury, the examiner should attempt to drill deeper into chronic movements, postures, anthropometric changes, or changes to training and equipment that could contribute to the patient's injury, for example, overhead throwing sports, such as baseball or volleyball, are commonly associated with rotator cuff injuries, labral tears, bicipital impingement, and subacromial bursitis. Knowing about the intensity and volume of training, such as pitch count in baseball, is important to gain a full understanding of what may be contributing to the underlying condition.

Asking the patient whether there are certain positions, postures, or movements that are worse than others is useful in knowing more about chronic conditions. For example, people who sit for extended periods at work or school often have rounded shoulders (**Figure 10.18**) and excessive kyphosis in the thoracic spine. Both of these observations can lead to poor shoulder biomechanics and scapular dyskinesis. Scapular dyskinesis is poorly coordinated rhythm of scapular movement associated with GH movement (mostly flexion and abduction).[4] It is considered a secondary cause of shoulder impingement.[2]

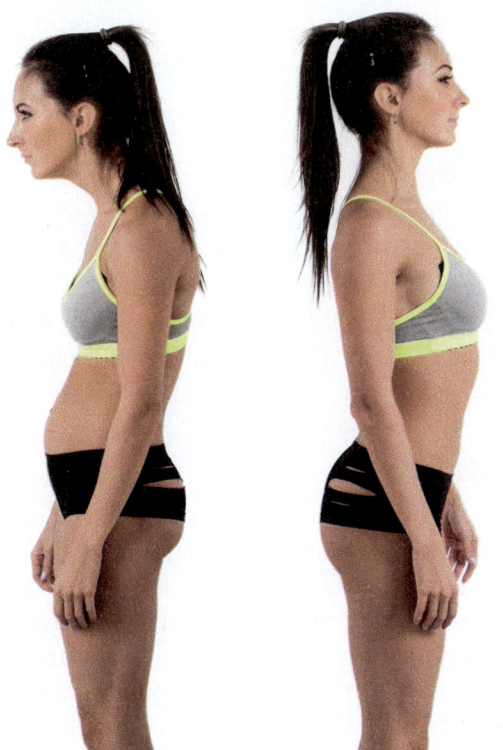

Figure 10.18 Clinical photographs showing rounded shoulders (left) and normal posture (right).
© Undrey/Shutterstock

Other secondary causes of shoulder impingement include abnormal GH arthrokinematics, poor posture (ie, excessive kyphosis), rotator cuff weakness or fatigue, poor muscle flexibility, GH capsular tightness, and inferior capsular adhesions.[2] Asking questions related to these secondary causes is important. However, if not possible, other components of the shoulder examination, such as observations and inspection, should be completed.

A common history question that should be asked for all injuries is related to the quality, quantity, and location of the pain. It may be important to have the patient point with one finger where the greatest amount of pain is located. Using a 0 to 10 pain scale may be helpful to determine the severity of the pain but may not be indicative of the volume of damage or pathology. For example, acute subacromial bursitis can be extremely painful, albeit not serious, and can be resolved in the long term. The quality and timing of the pain is also a useful question. For example, if the patient complains of pain at night when he or she sleeps, it could be indicative of subacromial bursitis, rotator cuff tears, or tumors. The role of the examiner is to screen for tumors, and, if the history suggests, it is important to refer back to a physician for an appropriate medical screening to confirm there are no underlying medical pathologies, such as cancer. Another example of deep, toothache-type pain, particularly when sleeping, is TOS. This may be due to the brachial plexus neuropathy associated with TOS. TOS can also involve vascular structures, and, in this case, the patient may complain about the upper limb "feeling heavy." It may also include tingling, numbness, or change in sensation in the upper extremity. Finally, another useful question is to ask the patient about circumstances that aggravate or relieve pain. This may help the athletic trainer to determine the mechanism or injury and also help in the development of treatment strategies later on for rehabilitation.

Another important question with all conditions may be asking the patient about abnormal sounds or sensations, such as clicking, catching, or locking. This may indicate a labral tear, for example. Labral tears (superior labrum anterior to posterior [SLAP] lesions, specifically) can be caused by chronic overhead activity and are associated with subacromial bursitis, rotator cuff impingement/pathology, or long head of biceps pathology. However, labral tears can also be associated with chronic GH dislocation or subluxations and, therefore, can also have associated sounds or sensations, such as clicking or catching.

Asking a patient about changes in sensation and weakness in the upper extremity is important to determine the involvement of other neurologic conditions. For example, if a patient has trouble lifting the arm up from the side (ie, abducting), it may be indicative of pathology of the suprascapular nerve or the axillary nerve. The suprascapular nerve can be damaged as it passes through the suprascapular notch, leading to paralysis of the supraspinatus and infraspinatus muscles. The supraspinatus muscle initiates abduction of the GH joint. The axillary nerve, the nerve supply for the deltoid muscle, is often damaged after anteroinferior GH dislocation or subluxation. Therefore, abduction of the GH joint may become difficult after the first 15° to 30° of abduction. A confirmatory sign of the axillary nerve pathology is the deltoid atrophy and rounding of the shoulder that would appear asymmetrical.

Other important history-taking questions include the presence of stiffness, instability, and previous injuries to the affected side. The examiner should also note sex, dominant hand, and occupation.

Inspection

The inspection of the shoulder complex is difficult because of the number of variables to consider with all the pathology that could occur. As a result, there are a number of specific inspection variables for each pathologic condition. General inspection of the shoulder complex should occur statically from the anterior-posterior perspectives first, followed by side/lateral views. From the anterior perspective, the following pathologic conditions should be considered: sulcus sign from a GH dislocation or subluxation; step deformity from an AC sprain; clavicular deformity that may be indicative of a clavicular fracture; bruising or a muscle divot around the pectoralis major muscle around the anterior axilla; bruising around the anterior shoulder, where the latissimus dorsi inserts, could be indicative of a tear of that muscle; and atrophy of the deltoid muscle on one side more than the other, which could be indicative of axillary nerve damage secondary to a GH dislocation. Posteriorly, inspection of the scapula is crucial to determine whether there is normal function. Abnormal scapular function with movement is a condition called scapular dyskinesis (covered in greater detail later in this chapter). From a lateral perspective, rounded shoulders relative to the head position, ears, and hips is often associated with poor scapular mechanics, which can lead to rotator cuff pathology and impingement. Rounded shoulders may also be accompanied by excessive thoracic spine kyphosis, which may also lead to secondary shoulder pathology.

ROM Assessment

The Cyriax method of evaluation calls for active ROM to determine the osteokinematic ROM in the shoulder, which is considered a stressing of both contractile and noncontractile tissues.[2,5] Passive ROM is intended to mostly isolate noncontractile tissues, such as bone, ligament, capsules, glenoid labrum, and bursae. Isometric resisted testing is intended to primarily test contractile tissue, including muscle, tendon, and tenosynovium, and may compress bursae. To summarize, active ROM tests both contractile and noncontractile tissues, which is why it is important to also perform passive ROM and isometric resisted testing to isolate tissues to know more about the structures involved in the pathology.

Active ROM

Magee[2] advocates for patients to be instructed to move through the entire active ROM to determine both the quality and quantity of motion. If active ROM is pain free, the examiner can stop at the patient's end range to apply an overpressure. The overpressure can act as a proxy to performing passive ROM if active ROM is pain free throughout the full ROM. A description of shoulder active ROM can be found in **Table 10.2**.

Passive ROM

Passive ROM is completed throughout a full ROM when overpressure during active ROM cannot be completed due to pain or restrictions. The quality of the passive ROM should be noted in addition to end feels. Passive ROM in the shoulder is described in **Table 10.3**.

Palpation

A good acronym to help focus palpation is SAM: skeletal, articular, and muscular. Focus on bony palpation first, including the clavicle, acromion process, spine of the scapula, head of the humerus, greater tubercle, bicipital groove, and lesser tubercle. The articular structures to palpate include, from medial to lateral, the SC joint, the AC joint, and the GH joint. Details of those bony and articular structures were covered in greater detail previously. Finally, muscular structure should be palpated relative to the bony and articular structures. Palpation of each muscle is outlined in greater detail in Table 10.1.

Table 10.2 Shoulder Range of Motion

Range of Motion	Degrees	Comments
Glenohumeral Joint		
Flexion	160–180	May need to stabilize the scapula to confirm where the motion comes from (ie, glenohumeral or scapulothoracic).
Extension	50–60	Examiner can stand beside the patient to see total range of motion for both arms.
Abduction	170–180	May need to stabilize the scapula to confirm where the motion comes from (ie, glenohumeral or scapulothoracic). A painful arc between 45° and 60° should be noted, as it is indicative of subacromial impingement. Ask the patient to slowly lower the arm to his or her side. If he or she is unable to do so under control, this could be a sign of a supraspinatus tear.
Adduction	50–75	Watch for controlled lowering of the arm from the abducted position.
Internal rotation (at 0° of abduction)	60–100	An alternative is to ask the patient to reach behind the back and then attempt to lift his or her wrist/hand off the back.
External rotation (at 0° of abduction)	80–90	The examiner should stand in front of the patient to observe the total ROM. The patient should tuck their bent elbows into their side, and move their forearms externally rotating the humerus.
Internal rotation (at 90° of abduction)	0–90	It may be important for the examiner to stabilize at the coracoid process if the patient's pectoralis minor is shortened.
External rotation (at 90° of abduction)	0–100	If an anteroinferior glenohumeral dislocation is suspected, this test should be approached carefully.
Horizontal adduction	130	It is important to note that this is also a special test for an AC sprain. Therefore, if this injury is suspected, caution should be taken.
Horizontal abduction		If a glenohumeral subluxation is suspected, caution should be taken at the extreme ROM.

Table 10.3 Passive Range of Motion in the Glenohumeral Joint

Range of Motion	End Feel	Comments
Flexion	Tissue stretch	Latissimus dorsi stretch or posterior capsule.
Extension	Tissue stretch	Biceps muscle or anterior capsule.
Abduction	Tissue stretch or bone to bone	Latissimus dorsi and pectoralis major stretch.
Adduction	Tissue approximation	
Internal rotation (at 0° of abduction)	Tissue stretch	
External rotation (at 0° of abduction)	Tissue stretch	
Internal rotation (at 90° of abduction)	Tissue stretch	This motion is similar to the Hawkins-Kennedy special test for shoulder impingement. Glenohumeral internal rotation deficit superior labrum anterior to posterior.
External rotation (at 90° of abduction)	Tissue stretch	This motion is similar to the apprehension special test for shoulder instability, so caution must be taken. Glenohumeral external rotation gain superior labrum anterior to posterior.
Horizontal adduction	Tissue stretch or approximation	If an acromioclavicular sprain is suspected, this is also a special test.
Horizontal abduction	Tissue stretch	Caution should be taken is a glenohumeral subluxation or laxity is suspected.

Special Tests

Special tests of the shoulder, as with other joints in the body, can be complicated to perform if there is a psychomotor component or skill required. In addition, the science of the testing can be questionable at times. The combination of developing skills with the questionable evidence of tests necessitates examiners to perform more than one test to improve the outcome and diagnostic accuracy.[6] Where possible, for each pathology discussed, the most scientifically valid tests will be covered first and confirmatory or other tests will also be listed to triangulate the diagnosis. A complete summary of special tests (ie, patient position, procedure, positive test, and implication) and associated evidence (ie, sensitivity, specificity, likelihood ratios, QUADAS scores [Quality Assessment of Diagnostic Accuracy Studies]) for the shoulder is presented in Table 10.18 and can be found at the end of this chapter.

Common Shoulder Pathologies

GH Dislocation/Subluxation

The incidence of acute, traumatic GH instability varies, depending on the source. The most common direction for the GH joint to dislocate is in an anteroinferior direction, with posterior dislocations occurring in only approximately 3% of dislocations.[7] Therefore, the focus of incidence is on anteroinferior dislocation and subluxations. Owens et al[8] reviewed data from the National Collegiate Athletic Association (NCAA) injury database and found an incidence of 0.2 per 1,000 athlete-exposures. In the general population, there are other estimates of an incidence of 8.2-51.0 per 100,000 athlete-exposures.[7,9-11] Males are more likely (between 70% and 75%) than females to experience an anteroinferior GH dislocation, except in older age groups (ie, 55 to 74 years).[7,11,12] The 15- to 19-year-old age group is the most common to redislocate, with up to a 90% chance.[7] **Table 10.4** presents quick tips for assessing dislocation and subluxations of the glenohumeral joint.

There are a number of complications and additional pathologies that often occur with an anteroinferior dislocation. In a study by Kraeutler et al,[13] 66% of patients had an anterior labral tear (also known as a Bankart lesion), and 41% had a Hill-Sachs lesion (an osteochondral lesion or fracture of the superior and/or posterior aspect of the head of the humerus). Atef et al.[14] found that 28% of patients had an additional rotator cuff tear, 21% had a Bankart lesion, 3% had axillary nerve pathology, and 13% had a combined Bankart lesion with axillary nerve pathology. Therefore, evaluation of a patient's primary shoulder dislocation should also involve testing for these complications, particularly with the labrum. Many of the special tests actually test both GH laxity and labral tears. Some labral tear testing is under the GH laxity, but some are also listed under the labral tear pathology.

Specific History Questions

The most common mechanisms of injury are falls, sports, and direct trauma.[7,14] Another common mechanism of injury is forced abduction and external

Table 10.4 Glenohumeral Dislocation/Subluxation Quick Tips

Pathology	Description	Presentation (HIPS)	Special Tests/Imaging	Differential Diagnosis	5-Min Sideline Assessment Tips
Glenohumeral dislocation/subluxation	The ball-and-socket joint is disrupted or dislocated, most often in an anterior-inferior direction.	Dislocation is typically traumatic with an abduction-external rotation. Mechanism of injury most common. There is a sulcus sign and the inability to move the shoulder.	Apprehension testing is useful in subluxation. Acute dislocation requires radiographs prior to reduction. Other tests include crank test, relocation test with surprise test, and load-and-shift test.	Acromioclavicular sprain. Pectoralis major tear. Long head of biceps muscle tear. Palpation to feel the integrity of the glenohumeral joint is important.	Palpation to determine the integrity of the glenohumeral joint is important. If it is dislocated, the head of the humerus can be palpated in the axilla. Vascular checks are important to determine severity.

HIPS, history, inspection, palpation, special tests.

rotation that happens in sports such as volleyball blocking, hockey goaltender glove handling, or combative positions in collision sports such as football or wrestling. Coincidentally, the abducted-externally rotated position is also used as a special test, the apprehension test, which is covered in more detail later in this chapter.

It is important to ask about tingling, numbness, and change of sensation or weakness because the axillary nerve is commonly damaged. Clicking or clunking is another sensation that should be questioned because the labrum is commonly damaged with a dislocation or subluxation. Because of recurrence rates for a younger population, it is important to ask the age of the patient and whether he or she has had this kind of injury in the past. It is common for someone with shoulder instability to experience pain and stiffness in the morning but for it to resolve with movement as the day goes on.

Inspection

If the shoulder is dislocated, the patient will complain of extreme pain and will often be grasping his or her arm at the elbow with it in slight abduction and internal rotation. The patient will likely be unable to move the shoulder. A classic sign of both shoulder dislocation and subluxation is the sulcus sign. The sulcus (also known as a divot) occurs around the middle or posterior deltoid muscle area just inferior to the acromion process (**Figure 10.19**). If the deltoid muscles are asymmetrical, it may be caused by arm dominance or if the patient had subluxated or dislocated their shoulder previously; this could also be a sign of axillary nerve (C5–C6) damage.

One of the first tests that should be performed if the examiner suspects an acutely dislocated shoulder is the distal pulse check because the head of the humerus can restrict blood flow at the axilla. It is important to compare the radial pulse bilaterally to evaluate for weakness. If the shoulder is dislocated, when the patient is asked to move the shoulder actively, he or she will likely refuse because of pain. If the shoulder was recently subluxated, active and passive ROM may be limited at the extreme ranges, particularly with abduction, external rotation, or a combination of those motions. In addition, weakness with shoulder abduction could be due to nerve involvement, which a full neurologic examination, including sensory testing, should help to discern. It may be important to refer the patient to a neurologist for

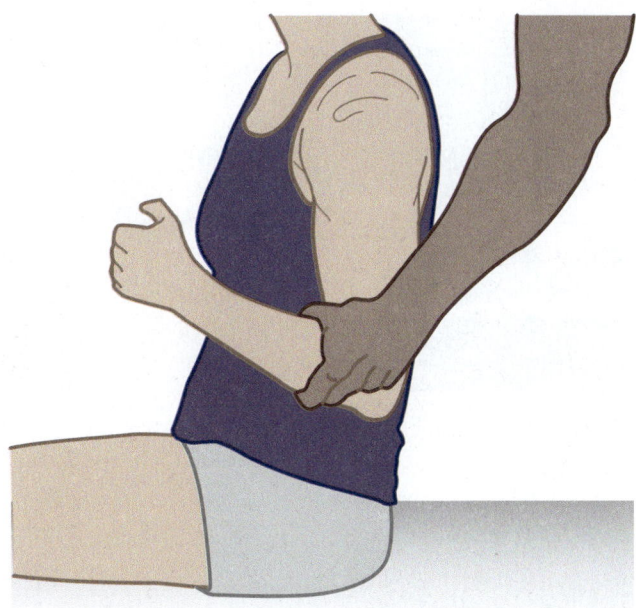

Figure 10.19 Illustration depicting the sulcus sign.
© Jones & Bartlett Learning

nerve conduction testing if there is concern about the axillary nerve involvement.

Palpations With Expected Outcomes

If the GH joint is dislocated, palpation should consist of only bony structures to confirm there is no displaced fracture and to apply a sling or support for the shoulder for transportation to further medical care so the joint can be reduced. If subluxation is suspected, it will be important to focus on all bone and muscle structures around the deltoid muscle. A common source of pain will present around the anterior GH ligaments, the bicipital groove, and the anteroinferior aspect of the axilla. Another bony protuberance that is involved with a subluxation is the coracoid process because the head of the humerus often subluxates just inferior to it. Differential diagnosis palpation should include the pectoralis minor, pectoralis major, latissimus dorsi, and all rotator cuff muscles.

Special Tests

The apprehension, crank, and relocation tests with a surprise test (**Figure 10.20**) are gross tests for instability and do not indicate severity or minute changes in laxity. Rather, they merely determine whether the patient shows apprehension during shoulder movement and therefore has an unstable GH joint. In order to assess severity or laxity, it is better to use the load-and-shift

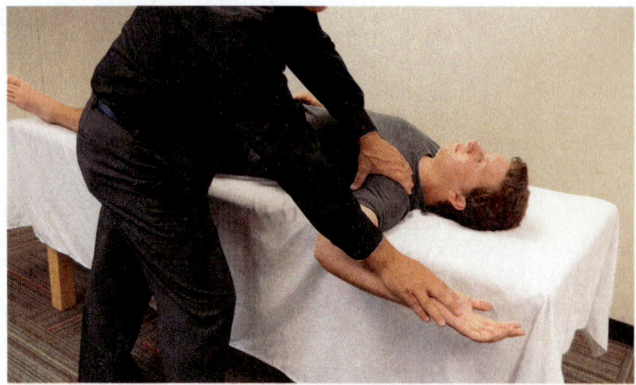

Figure 10.20 Clinical photograph demonstrating apprehension test, crank test, and relocation test with suprise test.
© Jones & Bartlett Learning

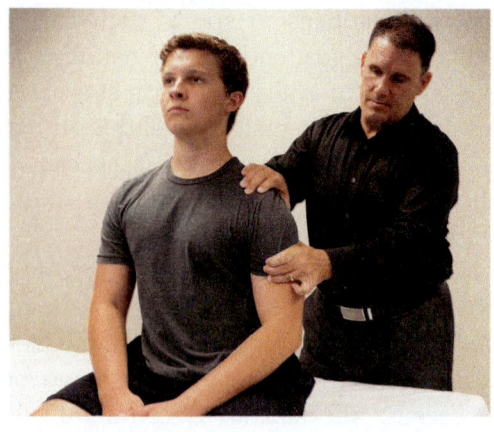

Figure 10.21 Clinical photograph demonstrating the load-and-shift test.
© Jones & Bartlett Learning

test (**Figure 10.21**). The implications of the crank test are that the glenoid labrum is likely damaged and this damage probably occurred when the patient experienced GH instability (dislocation or subluxation). In Figure 10.21, the examiner's left hand begins by compressing the humerus inwards or towards the patient, followed by shifting the humerus in an anterior and posterior gliding motion. See Table 10.18 for a complete description of these tests.

With the patient supine on the table, the patient should be far enough over that the humerus and forearm can be off the edge of the table. The patient's elbow should be bent to 90°.

The patient should be seated either on a low-backed chair or on the edge of the table with his or her arms hanging by the side. It is important for the patient to sit up straight and have proper posture because rounded shoulders could change the angle of the scapula and the angle of the glenoid fossa shifting the head of the humerus forward.

Functional Assessment/Outcome Measures

Functional assessment can include history questions related to activities of daily living (ADLs) such as combing hair, eating, tucking in the back of a shirt, wiping after going to the lavatory, or tying shoelaces. All of these movements require a variety of ROMs in the GH joint. Any or all of these are good questions to ask in the history if there is no clear mechanism of injury. Functional assessments, such as doing a push-up or being in a push-up position on a stool and hopping off onto the floor can also be performed.

Alternatively, there are a number of outcome measures that have been tested for the shoulder that may be useful in determining function and quality of life. Some of these outcome measures are specific to the shoulder (ie, region specific) and some are disease specific.[15-20] Examples of these outcome measures are listed in **Table 10.5**. Schmidt et al.[21] applied

Table 10.5 Shoulder and Disease-Specific Outcome Measures for Glenohumeral Dislocation/Subluxation

Outcome Measure Name	Target or Purpose	Reference
Simple Shoulder Test questionnaire form	General shoulder	Lippitt et al. 1993[15]
The 12-Item Shoulder Instability Questionnaire	Glenohumeral instability	Dawson et al. 1998[16]
Disabilities of the Arm, Shoulder and Hand (DASH)	General shoulder	Hudak et al. 1996[17]
Shoulder Pain and Disability Index (SPADI)	General shoulder	Roy et al. 2009[18]
American Shoulder and Elbow Surgeons' Shoulder Evaluation Form	General shoulder	Slobogean and Slobogean 2011[19]
Rotator Cuff Quality of Life Index	Rotator cuff disorders	Hollinshead et al. 2000[20]

Data from Hollinshead RM, Mohtadi NG, Vande Guchte RA, Wadey VM: Two 6-year follow-up studies of large and massive rotator cuff tears: comparison of outcome measures. *J Shoulder Elbow Surg* 2000; 9(5):373-381.

the Evaluating Measures of Patient Reported Outcomes tool to compare 11 shoulder instruments. The American Shoulder and Elbow Surgeons, Shoulder Evaluation Form, the Simple Shoulder Test, and the Oxford Shoulder Score were noted to be the strongest for shoulder outcome measures.

Clinical Diagnosis (Differential Diagnosis)

As noted previously, in traumatic GH instability, where a patient's dislocated joint has been relocated by a physician at a hospital, the diagnosis is likely known; the testing merely confirms the diagnosis. However, challenging cases occur when the patient does not have one traumatic incident but rather a number of smaller incidents whereby the GH joint is likely subluxating. These cases are much more subtle when it comes to determining the diagnosis. In addition, if there was either a dislocation or subluxation present, the labrum is likely to be damaged. Some of the anterior instability laxity tests listed previously will also test the labrum in addition to feelings of apprehension or laxity and if patients also feel pain. There are other tests discussed later that are specific to labral tears and, therefore, should also be included as part of the differential diagnosis. Other differential diagnoses include biceps brachii muscle strain or rupture, AC joint sprain, and cervical radiculopathy.

AC Joint Sprain

AC joint sprains make up 12% of sprains[22] and males are more than five times more likely to experience this injury than females.[23,24] In a longitudinal study of NCAA athletes, in more than 25 sports between 2009 and 2015, Hibberd et al found an injury rate of 1.7 per 10,000 athlete-exposures. Football accounted for just over one-half (50.4%) of all AC joint sprains.[24] The primary mechanism of injury tends to be player-on-player contact (~55%), followed by contact with the ground (~30%).[24] Most AC joint sprains (99%) are managed without surgery.[24,25] **Table 10.6** presents quick tips for assessing AC sprains.

Sprains of the AC joint (**Figure 10.22**) can involve a number of structures. The most common way to diagnose AC joint sprains is using the Rockwood

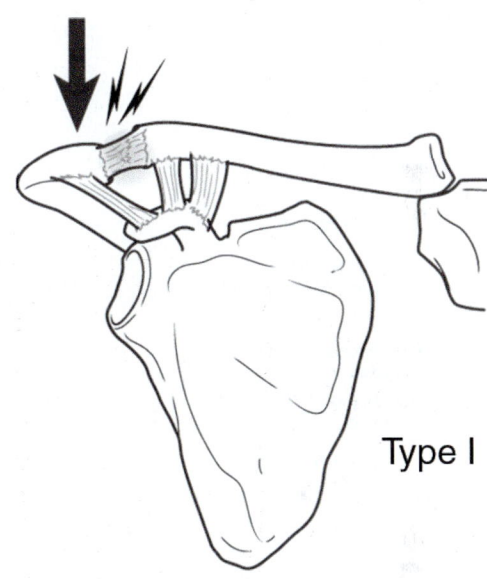

Figure 10.22 Drawing depicting type I acromioclavicular joint sprain.

Reproduced from Armstrong AD, Hubbard MC, eds: *Essentials of Musculoskeletal Care*, ed 5. Burlington, MA, American Academy of Orthopaedic Surgeons, 2015.

Table 10.6 Acromioclavicular Joint Sprain Quick Tips

Pathology	Description	Presentation (HIPS)	Special Tests/ Imaging	Differential Diagnosis	5-Min Sideline Assessment Tips
Acromioclavicular joint sprain	The clavicle is separate from the acromion process, often causing the distal end of the clavicle to stick up superiorly if severe enough.	There are two common mechanisms of injury: falling on an outstretched arm or direct contact with the tip of the shoulder and the ground, boards, or another athlete. A step deformity is the most common sign. There is an inability to perform horizontal adduction.	Horizontal adduction test, Paxinos test, or simple palpation of the AC joint is useful. Radiographs (weighted) will confirm the severity.	Glenohumeral subluxation, rotator cuff pathology, and clavicular fractures.	Palpation of the AC joint is usually a good indicator of the structures involved. This can be performed through equipment if necessary.

AC, acromioclavicular; HIPS, history, inspection, palpation, special tests.

classification system (**Figure 10.23**). There are six types of sprains, with the most discerning factor between types 2 and 3 being the disruption of the coracoclavicular (CC) ligaments in addition to the AC joint capsule. The best way to diagnose this condition and the severity is with a radiograph. Therefore, clinical evaluation must be supplemented by physician consultation and radiographs (see specifics in the next paragraphs).

Specific History

Asking the patient if he or she can reproduce the mechanism of injury is often an excellent start to understanding this diagnosis. Furthermore, asking about the pain location and whether the patient can place one finger (only) on the site of pain is also a clear sign of the problem. Most patients are able to pinpoint their pain to the very distal tip of the clavicle, where it articulates with the acromion process. In fact, this

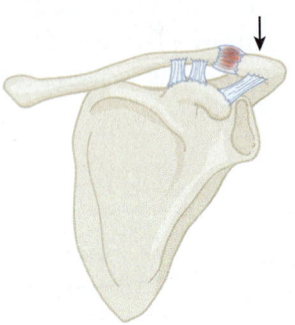

Type I

Pathology
Sprained AC ligaments; normal CC ligaments

Examination
Pain and swelling over the AC joint without a visible deformity

Radiography
Normal

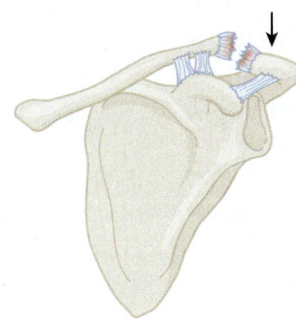

Type II

Pathology
Disruption of the AC ligaments; sprained CC ligaments

Examination
Distal clavicle is unstable to horizontal stress; pain over the CC interspace

Radiography
Widened AC joint and slight elevation of the clavicle (<25%)

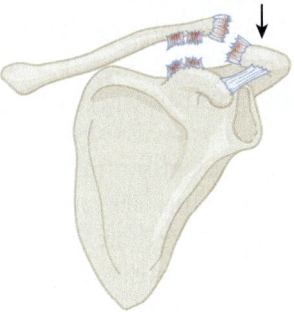

Type III

Pathology
Disruption of the AC and CC ligaments

Examination
Distal clavicle is unstable to horizontal and vertical stress; reducible

Radiography
Moderate elevation of the clavicle (25% to 100%)

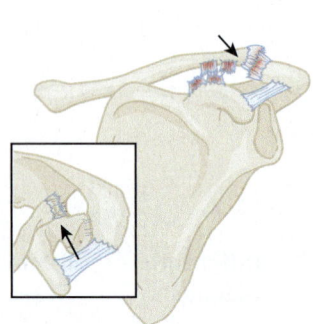

Type IV

Pathology
Posterior displacement into or through the trapezius muscle

Examination
Not reducible

Radiography
Axillary view shows posterior displacement

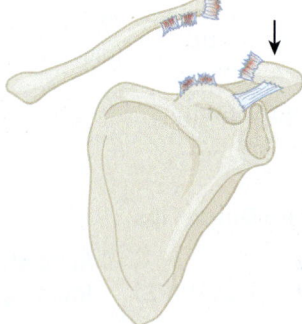

Type V

Pathology
Rupture of the deltotrapezial fascia

Examination
Clavicle palpable subcutaneously; not reducible

Radiography
Distal clavicle is elevated (>100% to 300%)

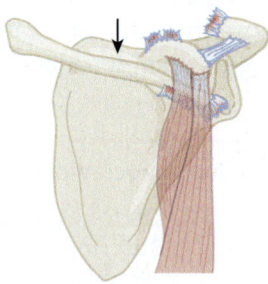

Type VI

Pathology
Inferior displacement of the distal clavicle under the conjoined tendon

Examination
Associated with rib fractures and neurovascular injury

Radiography
Clavicle is in a subacromial or subcoracoid position

Figure 10.23 Drawings showing the Rockwood classification.
AC, acromioclavicular; CC, coracoclavicular.
© Jones & Bartlett Learning

is also considered a special test with excellent sensitivity (96%).[26] ADLs are also a good indicator of the injury because most overhead movements, particularly those that involve some level of horizontal adduction, are very painful, if not impossible to do, for an acutely sprained AC joint. Hand dominance is important for context about ADLs. Knowing the patient's age is also important because most AC joint sprains occur in the third decade of life.[27]

Inspection

The most common observation that is made with AC joint sprains is the step deformity whereby the distal end of the clavicle is elevated. The height of elevation of the clavicle is usually a good indicator of severity of the condition.[23]

Generally, most active and passive ROMs, particularly at the extreme ranges, are painful. By far, the most painful range will be horizontal adduction, which is also considered a special test. However, there are a number of other conditions where this motion is also painful, including most patients presenting with subacromial impingement. Therefore, other special testing should be used to triangulate findings.

Palpations With Expected Outcomes

Palpation of the entire clavicle and scapula, particularly the acromion process, is essential. Palpation of the AC joint (ie, distal clavicle) is important and perhaps one of the best indicators of an AC sprain, with 96% sensitivity.[26] Soft tissues that support the AC joint may also be affected. For example, the pectoralis minor attaches to the coracoid process, and, if the coracoclavicular ligaments are involved, there may be considerable pain around this region. Palpation of the upper trapezius and levator scapula muscles may be important to understand collateral issues associated with AC joint sprains. The body's natural response is to protect a body region where there is a tendency for patients to hold the arm tight to the body with the shoulder shrugged. This may lead to spasm in those muscles that are responsible for the shrugging motion and, therefore, should be a focus when relieving the patient's pain in the first 7 to 10 days following the injury.

Special Tests

The Paxinos, O'Brien, and horizontal adduction tests (**Figures 10.24** through **10.26**) are used to assess AC joint instability. When performed in series or in parallel, these three tests can increase the probability of screening or confirming AC joint pathology. See Table 10.18 for a complete description of these tests.

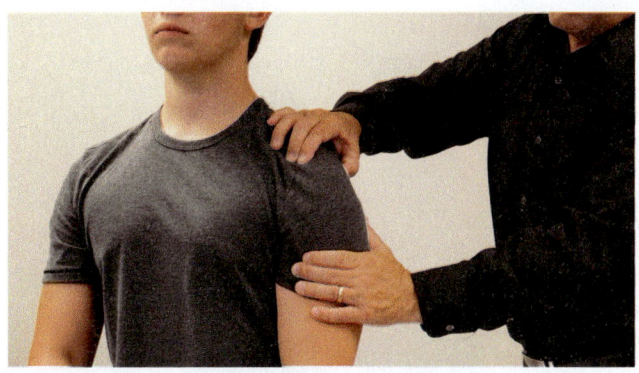

Figure 10.24 Clinical photograph demonstrating the Paxinos test.
© Jones & Bartlett Learning

- **Paxinos test:** The patient sits in a chair with the arm hanging by his or her side.
- **O'Brien test:** The patient stands and is asked to flex the glenohumeral joint to 90°, then horizontally adduct 10° with the humerus maximally internally rotated.
- **Horizontal adduction test:** The patient is usually standing, and this is typically completed as part of active and passive ROM testing of the shoulder. The patient is asked to abduct the glenohumeral joint to 90°, then horizontally adduct the shoulder with an extended elbow.

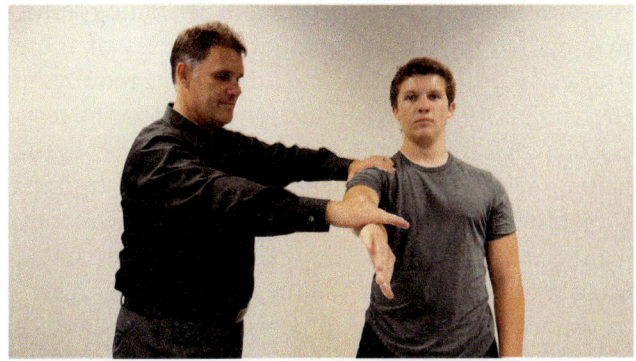

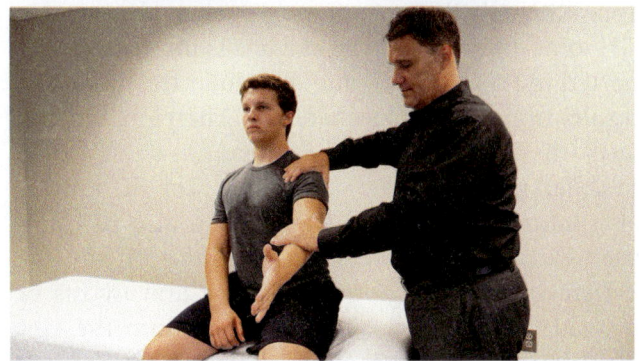

Figure 10.25 Clinical photographs demonstrating the O'Brien test.
© Jones & Bartlett Learning

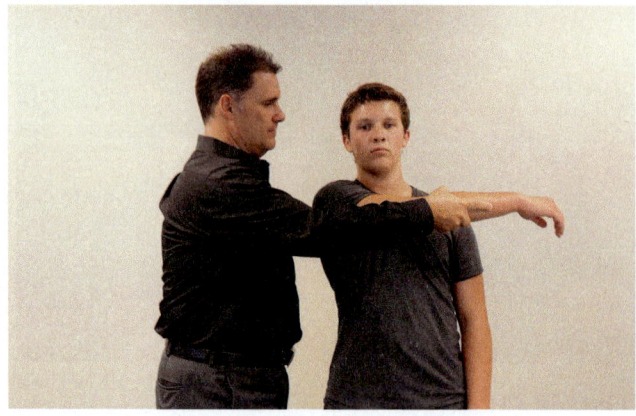

Figure 10.26 Clinical photograph demonstrating the horizontal adduction text.
© Jones & Bartlett Learning

Functional Assessment/Outcome Measures

Functional testing can be very similar to those tests listed for the GH joint. There are no outcome measures that are disease specific to AC joint sprains, but any of the other general shoulder outcome measures listed for the GH joint can be used.

Clinical Diagnosis (Differential Diagnosis)

AC joint sprains are confirmed with radiographic imaging. The list of differential diagnoses of these injuries is quite lengthy and, therefore, requires a careful history and triangulation with special tests to isolate AC joint sprains. Special tests, such as the Paxinos test, help to differentiate AC joint sprains from other conditions, such as labral injury, long head of biceps muscle impingement, subacromial bursa impingement, or rotator cuff impingement.[26] Furthermore, it may be important to also use tests associated with GH instability or labral tears because approximately 30% of AC joint sprains also involve GH joint pathology.[29] The clavicle is intimately connected to the AC joint, and clavicular fracture often results from similar mechanisms. Therefore, special tests (discussed later) and radiographs should help to differentiate the two conditions. The SC joint is also intimately connected and could also be damaged with similar mechanisms of injury. Finally, the patient hitting the ground with the arm by his or her side, whereby the arm is driven into the ribs (ie, from lateral to medial), often has an elevated first rib. Concomitant injury of the AC joint and first rib under rare conditions is discussed later in this chapter.

Glenohumeral Impingement

Whiting and Zernicke[28] define impingement syndrome as an increase in pressure within a confined anatomic space that has negative effects on tissue that occupies that space. Impingement is classified in two spaces: subacromial and internal.[28] Subacromial impingement syndrome is the most common source of shoulder pain, accounting for between 44% and 64% of all shoulder disorders.[30] Regarding subacromial impingement, it has been further classified as either primary or secondary.[2,31] Primary impingement occurs as the result of degeneration of the rotator cuff muscles, the acromion process shape, the coracoid process shape, and excessive stress. Primary impingement is most likely to occur after the fourth decade of life, whereas secondary impingement occurs in a younger population (15 to 35 years old) when there are abnormal force couples between the rotator cuff, the deltoid muscle, and scapular stabilizers.[30,32] Abnormal force couples are caused by abnormal GH mechanics, and when combined with overhead activities, results in impingement. The other contributing factor of secondary impingement could be hypermobility or hypomobility of the GH joint. Because of the complexity of all potential causes and effects, special tests are separated into muscle-related testing (strength and length), glenohumeral joint arthrokinematics and osteokinematics testing, and tests that re-create impingement or closure of the subacromial space. Muscle-related testing and glenohumeral joint osteokinematics will be discussed later in this chapter. **Table 10.7** presents quick tips for assessing glenohumeral impingement.

Glenohumeral arthrokinematics are challenging because problems are often associated with excessive laxity. In fact, inferior GH laxity and multidirectional instability are correlated and both can lead to abnormal arthrokinematics and subsequent impingement.[2] Traditional impingement special tests that reduce the subacromial space will be discussed with impingement or closure of the subacromial space.

Cools et al[31] proposed an algorithm to assist practitioners in organizing the various contributors to GH impingement, whether it is subacromial (external impingement) or internal impingement (**Figure 10.27**). This algorithm acts as an excellent conceptual guide to understanding the relationship between the cluster of symptoms that occur with all the structures that can be involved while also directing the examiner to use various special tests.

Internal impingement is the last type of impingement that is covered in this chapter and is the fourth type of special test covered later. It has been postulated that this impingement occurs in overhead

Common Shoulder Pathologies

Table 10.7 Glenohumeral Impingement Quick Tips

Pathology	Description	Presentation (HIPS)	Special Tests/ Imaging	Differential Diagnosis	5-Min Sideline Assessment Tips
Glenohumeral impingement	Entrapment of the supraspinatus muscle in the subacromial arch that causes inflammation of the tendon and/or bursa.	Most common sign is a painful arc in the midrange of active abduction. It is often difficult to pinpoint one structure.	A painful arc sign is positive. Empty can test is often positive. Weakness with abduction and external rotation is common.	Rotator cuff pathology, long head of biceps brachii pathology, or AC joint pathology.	Acutely, if the subacromial bursa is inflamed through direct contact or trauma, it may appear similar to AC joint pathology. Palpation of the AC joint helps differentiate the two.

AC, acromioclavicular; HIPS, history, inspection, palpation, special tests.

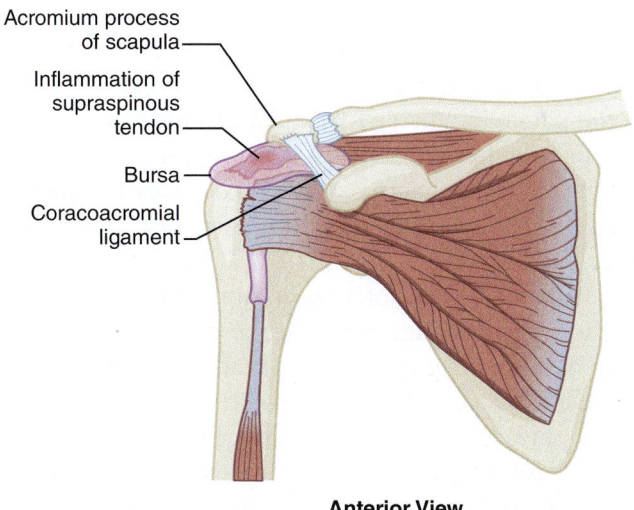

Figure 10.27 Drawing depicting glenohumeral impingement.
© Jones & Bartlett Learning

throwing–type sports. Repetitive impingement is thought to occur when the humerus is abducted and externally rotated or late in the cocking phase in throwing. In this position, the supraspinatus and infraspinatus tendons are impinged at the posterosuperior aspect of the GH joint.[31] Internal impingement is characterized by a reduced ROM, particularly with internal rotation, also known as glenohumeral internal rotation deficit.[33]

Specific History Questions

Some key history questions have been identified previously. Identifying a mechanism of injury is difficult in this case, particularly because injury onset is insidious in nature and often multifactorial. Therefore, asking history questions about the factors that typically contribute to the condition is critical. Knowing if the patient participates in overhead activity is not enough; the total amount of training in practices, competition, and other training is very important. The volume and intensity of those workouts will help both in the diagnosis and in the treatment plan afterward. Asking questions regarding the specific type of weight training and stretching that are done is also important because this may also help with the treatment plan. Overall, asking when the problem first began will help to understand chronicity.

As mentioned previously, age is a factor that will help to classify the type of impingement (ie, primary or secondary). It is important to ask about ADLs because knowing the exact position of the shoulder during an activity can tell the examiner about the condition. For example, reaching to the top shelf in the kitchen may outline a common symptom called painful arc. Painful arc (**Figure 10.28**) occurs when the patient abducts or flexes the GH joint between 45° and 120° because the subacromial space is most encroached due to the greater tuberosity passing under the acromion process.[2] Age is an important factor because various forms of impingement and rotator cuff pathology typically affect certain age groups. Primary subacromial impingement is associated with degeneration and older age. Litaker et al[34] demonstrated that patients older than 65 years who experience night pain and have weakness on external rotation often have confirmed tear of the supraspinatus or infraspinatus muscle. Secondary impingement is associated with a younger age group (15 to 35 years old), repetitive overhead activity, potential GH joint laxity, and scapular dyskinesis. Therefore, knowing the age group may help predict the type of special testing to use.

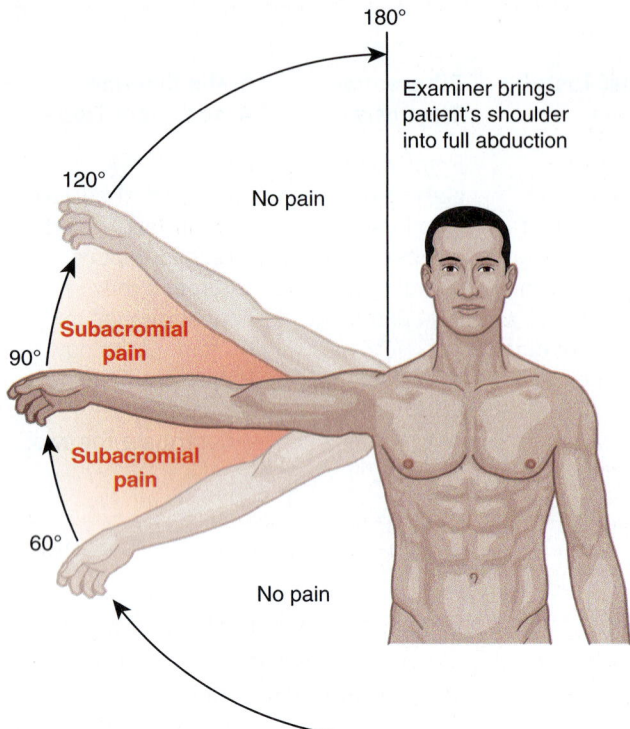

Positive test result: shoulder pain between 60° and 120° indicates subacromial or rotator cuff disorder.

Figure 10.28 Drawing depicting painful arc.

© Jones & Bartlett Learning

Inspection

Because of the multifactorial cause, some observations are more commonly linked than others. For example, observing the patient's posture from all angles will tell the examiner whether the patient has kyphosis or forward head posture and rounded shoulders. In this case, all of these signs can contribute to scapular dyskinesis and muscle imbalances, which can lead to impingement over time. A sulcus sign (discussed previously with GH instability) may be the result of a multidirectional instability of lax GH ligaments due to excessive overhead activity. This typically happens in sports such as baseball (ie, pitching) and swimming. Overall, muscle symmetry between the dominant hand and nondominant hand is useful. Observation of large muscle group hypertrophy may tell the examiner more about abnormal force coupling between the rotator cuff muscles and other larger muscles such as the latissimus dorsi, deltoid, and pectoralis major muscles. Scapular position should be tested both statically and dynamically. There is more information about scapular testing under the scapular dyskinesis section later in this chapter.

Active GH abduction is an important motion to observe. The supraspinatus muscle initiates abduction. If the supraspinatus muscle is involved due to weakness or a tear, the patient will often use the upper trapezius muscle to initiate abduction until the deltoid muscle can take over after the first 15°. The patient tends to shrug the shoulder and almost pull the humerus into abduction at the start of movement. This movement can be subtle but should be observed from in front of the patient and compared bilaterally. The most obvious sign of subacromial impingement occurs with abduction or flexion, painful arc (Figure 10.28).

Another sign of impingement, which often involves the long head of the biceps brachii muscle, is when the patient has pain with full flexion at the very top (ie, approximately 180°) of their ROM. When the examiner applies overpressure at the end ROM, the patient will have pain if impingement is present. This is also considered a special test called Neer impingement (discussed later in this chapter).

The examiner should also ask the patient to slowly lower the arm from full abduction to the side. If the patient is unable to control this motion straight through the full range to his or her side, it may also be a sign of supraspinatus involvement. This is considered a special test called the drop arm test (discussed later in this chapter).

Pain with active or passive horizontal adduction at the extreme range may also be indicative of subacromial impingement or long head of biceps brachii muscle impingement (Figure 10.26).

Reduced internal rotation is common with both active and passive internal impingement and may occur if the examiner asks the patient to put his or her arm behind the back around the belt line and asks him or her to lift the hand off the back (Gerber lift-off sign). If the patient is unable to complete this lift-off component of the motion, it could indicate tightness of the external rotators (ie, infraspinatus and teres minor) or the posterior capsule. It could also indicate weakness in the subscapularis. Rotation should also be tested with the GH joint abducted to 90°; this is often where a reduction of internal rotation (glenohumeral internal rotation deficit) is observed along with an increase in external rotation (glenohumeral external rotation gain)[2] (**Figure 10.29**).

There are a number of scapular motion observations that should be made with active, passive, and resisted ROM, discussed later with scapular dyskinesis.

Palpations With Expected Outcomes

Because of the complexity of GH impingement, painful palpation is dependent on the factors that are associated with that particular patient. The

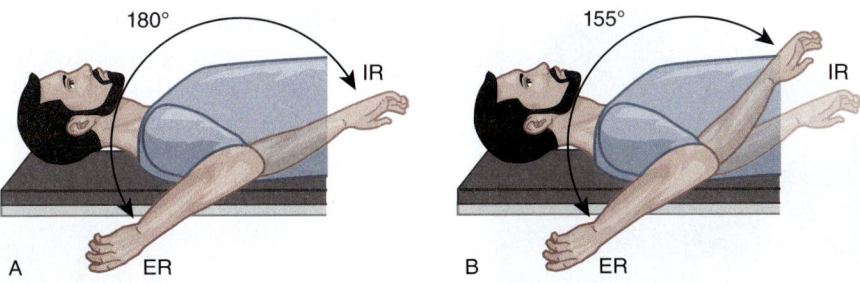

Figure 10.29 Drawings demonstrating total arc of motion **(A)** and glenohumeral internal rotation deficit **(B)**. ER, external rotation; IR, internal rotation.

© Jones & Bartlett Learning

subacromial bursa is a difficult structure to palpate because it is hidden under the deltoid muscle and acromion process/arch. If the bursa is inflamed or swollen, palpation may be possible by placing the patient's humerus into internal rotation, finding the edges of the acromion process, and dropping it off laterally and anteriorly. Again, if the patient has large deltoid muscles, this palpation is not feasible. Other sources of impingement are the supraspinatus and infraspinatus muscles. Therefore, palpation of these two muscle bellies (ie, their origin on the scapula) and their entire tendinous pathway is very important. The examiner should observe for hypertrophy (or atrophy), spasm (or not), and if there are any defects or breaks in the continuity of the muscle–tendon unit.

Special Test

Muscle-Related Special Tests. There are a number of muscle-related special tests that test the integrity of the muscle–tendon unit. These tests include the drop arm test, empty can test, full can test, rent test, hornblower sign, lift-off sign, belly press/Napoleon test, bear hug test, and internal rotation lag sign (**Figures 10.30** through **10.38**). See Table 10.18 for a complete description of these tests.

- **Drop arm test:** The patient should be standing with the arms at his or her side to start.
- **Empty can test:** The patient should be standing with the arms at his or her side. The examiner will provide instructions to the patient.
- **Full can test:** Similar to the empty can test, the patient should be standing with the arms at his or her side, and the examiner will provide instructions to the patient.
- **Rent test:** The patient is typically seated on the table with the arms by his or her side.
- **Hornblower sign:** The patient is seated and asked to abduct the glenohumeral joint to 90°.
- **Lift-off sign:** The patient performs active ROM while standing with the arm behind the back and is asked to actively lift the arm off the back.

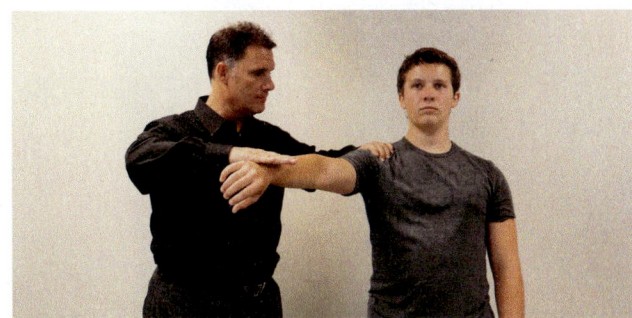

Figure 10.31 Photograph demonstrating the empty can test.

© Jones & Bartlett Learning

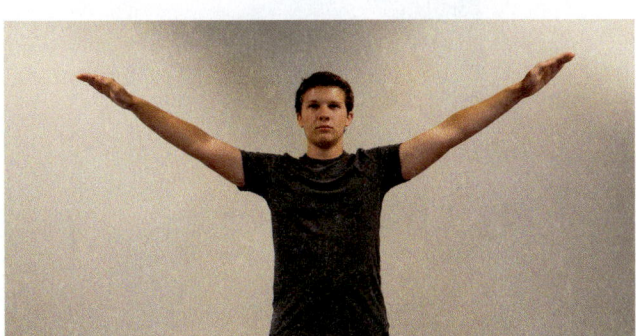

Figure 10.30 Photograph demonstrating the drop arm test.

© Jones & Bartlett Learning

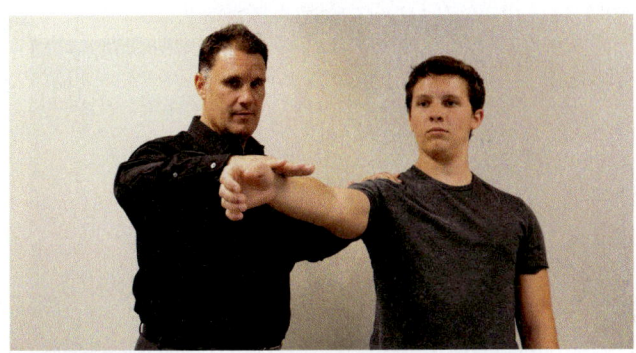

Figure 10.32 Photograph demonstrating the full can test.

© Jones & Bartlett Learning

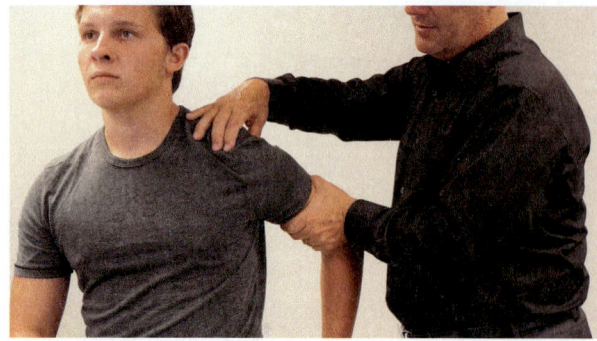

Figure 10.33 Photograph demonstrating the rent test.
© Jones & Bartlett Learning

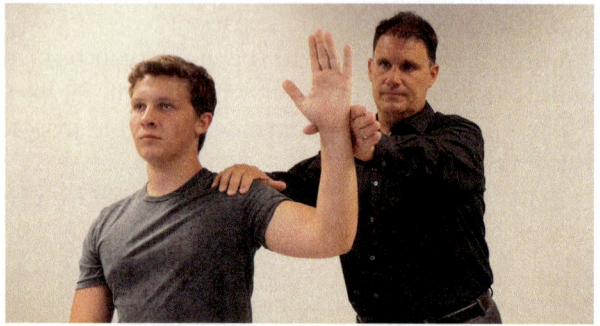

Figure 10.34 Photograph demonstrating the hornblower sign.
© Jones & Bartlett Learning

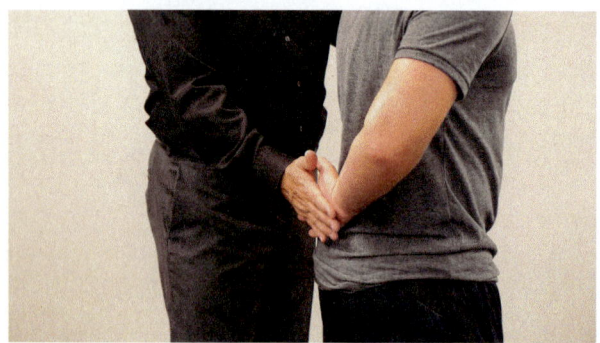

Figure 10.35 Photograph demonstrating the lift-off sign.
© Jones & Bartlett Learning

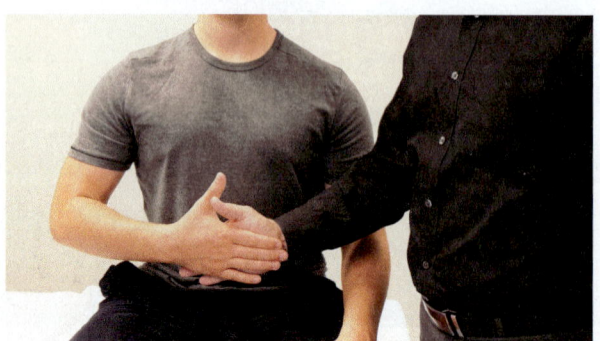

Figure 10.36 Photograph demonstrating the belly press test/Napoleon test.
© Jones & Bartlett Learning

- **Belly press test/Napoleon test:** The patient can be standing or seated with the elbow flexed to 90°, with the humerus internally rotated touching the stomach in a chicken wing–like position.

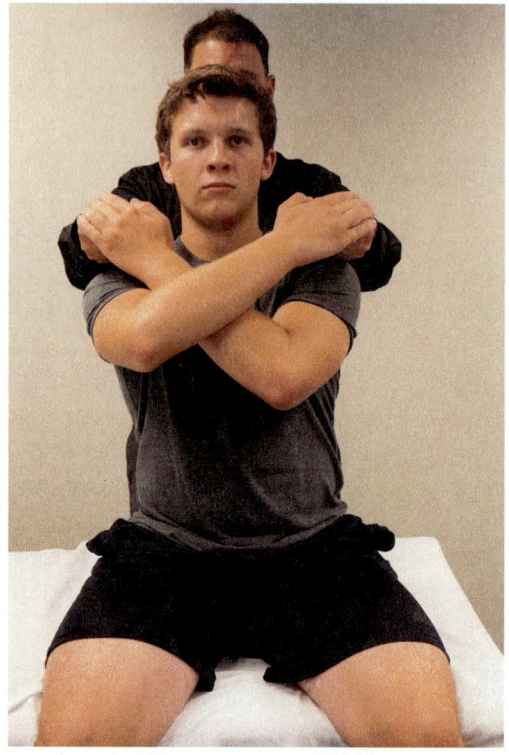

Figure 10.37 Photograph demonstrating the bear hug test.
© Jones & Bartlett Learning

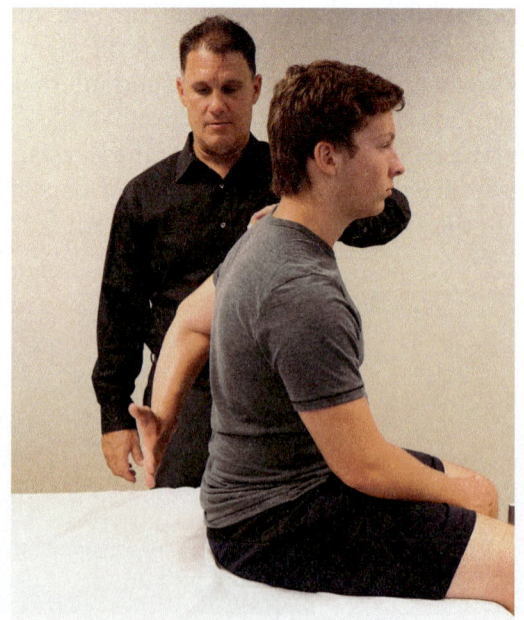

Figure 10.38 Photograph demonstrating the internal rotation lag sign (negative test).
© Jones & Bartlett Learning

Common Shoulder Pathologies

- **Bear hug test:** The patient can be seated or standing with the arm in horizontal adduction. The examiner can also ask the patient to scratch the back of his or her opposite shoulder.
- **Internal rotation lag sign:** The patient can either be standing or seated on a table relaxed with the arm by his or her side.

Glenohumeral Joint Testing. There are a number of glenohumeral joint–related special tests that test the integrity of the articular structures that support the glenohumeral joint, including the joint capsule, articular surface, and glenoid labrum. These tests include the sulcus sign, anterior drawer test, and the load-and-shift test (**Figures 10.39 and 10.40**). See Table 10.18 for a complete description of these tests.

- **Sulcus sign and test:** The patient can be seated or standing provided he or she is able to relax the shoulders completely.
- **Anterior drawer test:** The patient is supine with the shoulder abducted between 80° and 120°, forward flexed between 0° and 20°, and externally rotated between 0° and 30°. The patient rests his or her hand in the examiner's axilla. The anterior drawer test is multifunctional in that it will test GH instability and, when combined with an inferior superior capsule test, such as the sulcus sign, may be indicative of multidirectional instability. Multidirectional instability has been linked to secondary impingement with coupled with overhead throwing-type activities.
- **Load-and-shift test:** The patient should be seated either on a low-back chair or on the edge of the table with his or her arms hanging by the side. It is important for the patient to sit up straight and have proper posture because rounded shoulders could change the angle of the scapula and the angle of the glenoid fossa, shifting the head of the humerus forward (Figure 10.21).

Re-creation of Subacromial Space Impingement

There are two special tests that re-create subacromial space impingement. These tests include the Neer impingement test and the Hawkins-Kennedy test (**Figures 10.41 and 10.42**). See Table 10.18 for a complete description of these tests.

- **Neer impingement test:** The patient can be seated or standing depending on his or her comfort, his or her ability to relax the shoulder as the examiner moves him or her, and his or her height relative to the examiner's height.
- **Hawkins-Kennedy test:** The patient can be seated or standing with the shoulder completely relaxed while the examiner moves it.

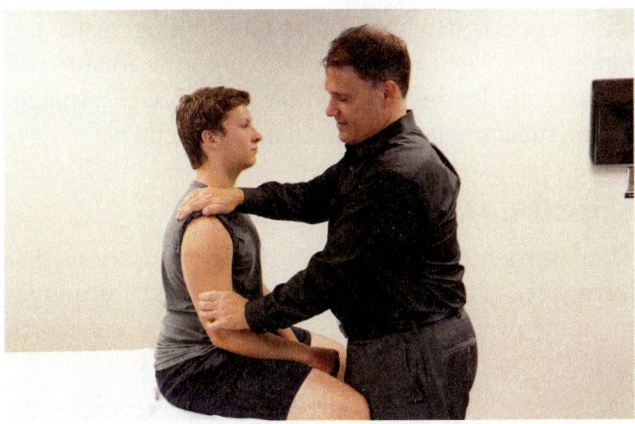

Figure 10.39 Photograph demonstrating the sulcus sign and test.

© Jones & Bartlett Learning

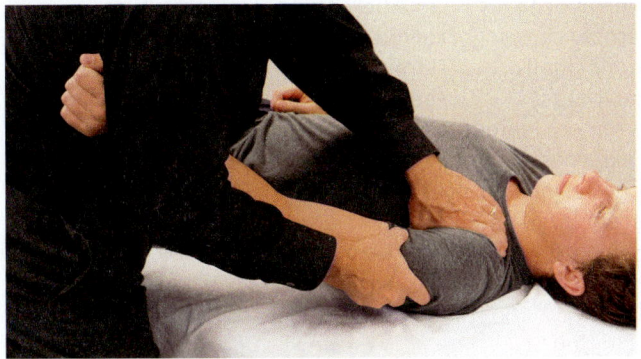

Figure 10.40 Photograph demonstrating the anterior drawer test.

© Jones & Bartlett Learning

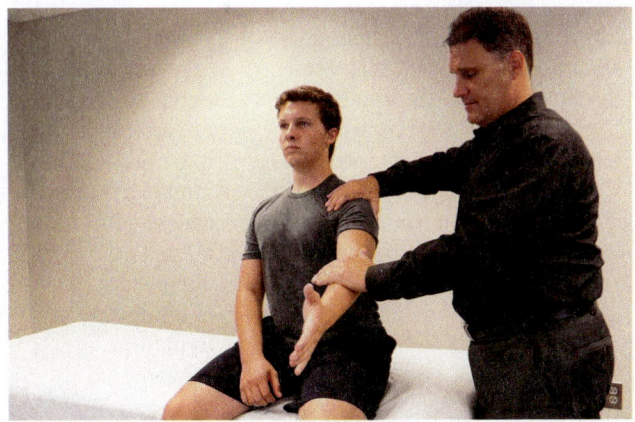

Figure 10.41 Photograph demonstrating the Neer impingement test.

© Jones & Bartlett Learning

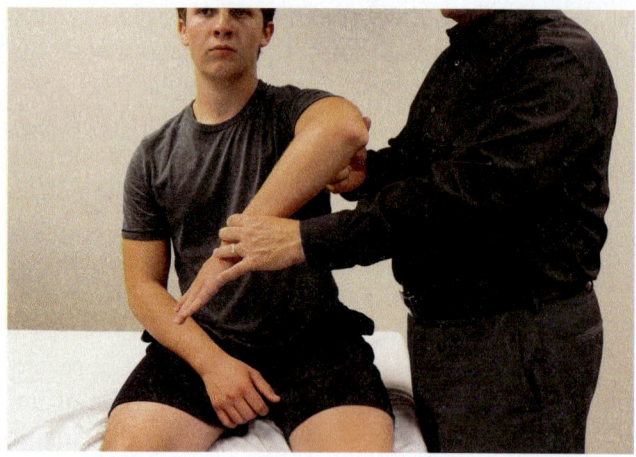

Figure 10.42 Photograph demonstrating the Hawkins-Kennedy test.
© Jones & Bartlett Learning

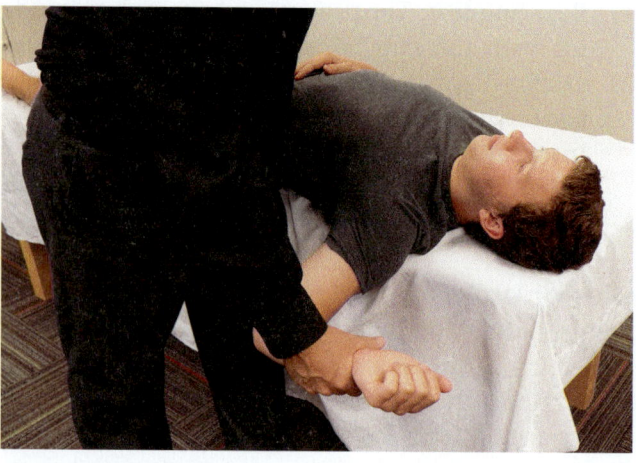

Figure 10.43 Photograph demonstrating the posterior impingement test.
© Jones & Bartlett Learning

Internal Impingement. There is only one test for internal impingement: the posterior impingement test (**Figure 10.43**). See Table 10.18 for a complete description of this test.

- **The posterior impingement test:** The patient should be lying down and actively move the glenohumeral joint in the following sequence: abducted to 90° to 110°, slight glenohumeral extension to 10° to 15°, and maximal external rotation.

Rotator Cuff Strain/Tear

Table 10.8 presents quick tips for assessing rotator cuff strains.

Supraspinatus

The rotator cuff muscle group comprises the supraspinatus, infraspinatus, teres minor, and subscapularis muscles (**Figure 10.44**). Tears, strains, tendinopathy, or any pathology is often part of a larger cluster of symptoms associated with subacromial impingement and rarely an isolated problem.[31,35] Often, the rotator cuff muscles are involved in some way with GH impingement (subacromial and internal impingement).

Specific History Questions

There are a number of specific history questions that have been identified previously for GH impingement. However, three history questions are worth

Table 10.8 Rotator Cuff Strain Quick Tips

Pathology	Description	Presentation (HIPS)	Special Tests/ Imaging	Differential Diagnosis	5-Min Sideline Assessment Tips
Rotator cuff strain/tear/ tendinopathy	If it is acute, there is often an excessive eccentric or concentric force followed by immediate pain. Strain and tendinopathy have a longer history of repetitive overhead motion.	Acutely, if there is a tear, there is initial pain and/ or weakness. If it is chronic, the longer history of overhead motion leads to a point where function is limited due to painful movement.	Supraspinatus: Drop arm for tears and empty can for tendinopathy. Infraspinatus/ teres minor: Tested with external rotation resistance. Subscapular: Lift-off sign. Ultrasonography or MRI can often confirm the diagnosis.	It is important to differentiate between muscle strains. Can be any rotator cuff or biceps brachii strain. Subacromial bursa involvement can be primary or secondary to the problem.	Quick muscle testing is important to differentiate between specific structures involved. If subacromial bursa is involved, a painful arc occurs with abduction.

HIPS, history, inspection, palpation, special tests.

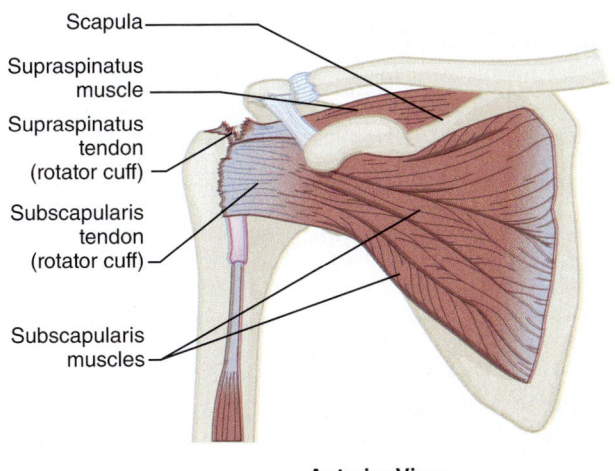

Figure 10.44 Drawing demonstrating rotator cuff strain.
© Jones & Bartlett Learning

highlighting again: (1) age, (2) activity type, and (3) activity level. The older the population, the more likely the presence of primary impingement and rotator cuff tear.[34] If the patient is younger, questions about the activity type, level, and intensity are important because rotator cuff pathology is often the result of overused overhead activities, such as baseball pitching, volleyball hitting, or swimming.

Inspection

Most observations have been outlined previously. The most important observation for rotator cuff pathology will be assessing scapulothoracic rhythm during active abduction and flexion of the GH joint.

As discussed previously, there is tremendous overlap between active, passive, and isometric resisted movements and all the special tests. The special tests that mimic these movements are discussed in detail later in this chapter.

Palpations With Expected Outcomes

Palpation of the rotator cuff was discussed previously; however, one special test can also be considered palpation: the rent test. The patient is typically seated on the table with the arms by his or her side during the rent test. The examiner passively extends the patient's shoulder while feeling just off the acromion process, just proximal to the greater tuberosity. The examiner will be feeling through the deltoid muscle, but that is also the pathway and attachment of the supraspinatus and infraspinatus muscles. If the examiner feels a "rent," or small sulcus, where the supraspinatus or infraspinatus muscles insert or travel to the greater tuberosity, the test is considered positive.

Special Tests

There are a number of special tests that assess supraspinatus pathology. These tests include the drop arm, empty can, full can, and rent tests. See Table 10.18 for a complete description of these tests.

- **Drop arm test:** The patient should be standing with the arms at his or her side to start (Figure 10.30).
- **Empty can test:** The patient should be standing with the arms at his or her side. The examiner will provide instructions to the patient to abduct the glenohumeral joint to 90°, then horizontally flex the glenohumeral joint to the plane of the scapula (approximately 30°) and internally rotate the humerus fully until the thumb is pointed toward the floor. This final motion is supposed to simulate a patient holding a can or drink in his or her hand and then pouring the drink out by tipping it over completely (Figure 10.31).
- **Full can test:** The patient should be standing with the arms at his or her side. The examiner will provide instructions to the patient to abduct the glenohumeral joint to 90° and then horizontally flex the glenohumeral joint to the plane of the scapula (approximately 30°) (Figure 10.32).
- **Rent test:** The patient is typically seated on the table with the arms by his or her side (Figure 10.33).

Radiographic Orders

Conventional radiography is often used as a diagnostic tool for chronic rotator cuff pathology. If rotator cuff pathology is suspected, the following radiographic views should be ordered at the initial visit: true anteroposterior (Grashey view), axillary, and transscapular lateral.[36] Studies have suggested that ultrasonography be the primary investigative tool for diagnosing rotator cuff pathology because it is accurate (>90%), fast, and cost effective.[37,38]

Functional Assessment/Outcome Measures

There have been four disease-specific outcome measures designed specifically for patients with rotator cuff pathology: The Rotator Cuff Quality of Life Index (RC-QOL), the Western Ontario Rotator Cuff Index (WORC), the Korean Shoulder Scoring System, and the Functional Shoulder Score (Table 10.9). Only the RC-QOL and WORC have been assessed for validity

Table 10.9 Disease-Specific Outcome Measures for Rotator Cuff Strain/Tear

Outcome Measure Name	Target or Purpose	Reference
Rotator Cuff Quality of Life Index	Rotator cuff disorders	Hollinshead et al. 2000[20]
Western Ontario Rotator Cuff Index	Rotator cuff disorders	Kirkley et al. 2003[40]
Korean Shoulder Scoring System	Rotator cuff disorders	Tae et al. 2009[42]
Functional Shoulder Score	Rotator cuff disorders	Iossifidis et al. 2015[43]

and reliability in accordance with the Consensus-Based Standards for the Selection of Health Measurements Instruments guidelines.[36,39] Both the RC-QOL and WORC are comparable across all categories.

Clinical Diagnosis (Differential Diagnosis)

The clinical diagnosis of supraspinatus pathology, strain, or tear is appropriate, depending on the outcomes of the specific tests. If there is complete weakness with the empty can test, for example, it is likely there is a complete tear, and this should be confirmed with ultrasonography. The differential diagnosis is much more challenging due to the multifactorial issues involved with the supraspinatus muscle and subacromial impingement pathologies.[31] Other conditions that are not part of that same model outlined by Cool et al.[31] may include red flags, such as cancer, particularly for patients who complain of night pain. The throbbing-type pain can also be indicative of neurologic involvement, so clearing the neck, nerve roots, and upper motor neuron lesions is also important.

Infraspinatus and Teres Minor Muscle Pathology

Of all the rotator cuff muscles, the infraspinatus and, in particular, teres minor seem to be least reported in the literature. However, there are no solid statistics comparing these muscle conditions.

Specific History Questions

Relative to the supraspinatus muscle, there are no unique history questions.

Inspection

Relative to the supraspinatus muscle, there are no unique observations. However, active external rotation may be weak, passive internal rotation may be tight, and isometric resisted external rotation both at 0° and 90° of abduction may be weak. Incidentally, many of the special tests mimic many of these motions and should also be positive.

Palpations With Expected Outcomes

Palpation of the rotator cuff was discussed previously. However, the rent test can also be performed during palpation as well.

Special Tests

There are a number of special tests that assess infraspinatus and teres minor pathology. These tests include external rotation lag and hornblower sign. See Table 10.18 for a complete description of these tests.

- **External rotation lag sign:** The patient is seated with the arms relaxed by his or her side and elbow bent to approximately 90° (**Figure 10.45**).
- **Hornblower sign:** The patient is seated and asked to abduct the glenohumeral joint to 90° (Figure 10.34).

Subscapularis Muscle Pathology

The subscapularis is a unique rotator cuff muscle because it is the only one that internally rotates the humerus. It works in unison with the other rotator

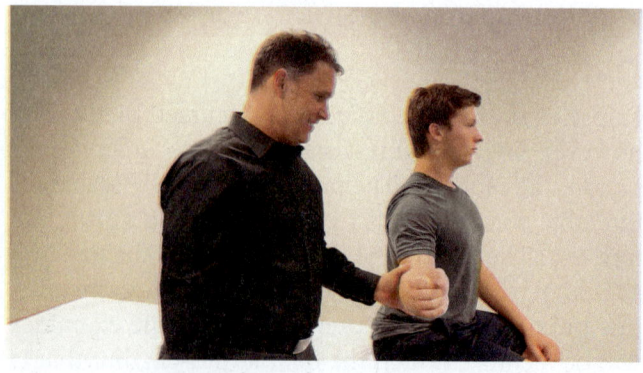

Figure 10.45 Photograph demonstrating the external rotation lag sign.

© Jones & Bartlett Learning

cuff muscles to stabilize the GH joint. There are powerful internal rotators of the shoulder (pectoralis major and latissimus dorsi), so the primary function of the subscapularis is stabilization, particularly in throwing motions.

Specific History Questions

The subscapularis muscle is grouped into all rotator cuff pathology and, thus, should use similar history questions. Perhaps the only unique history question may be inquiries about ADLs. Certain activities, such as tucking in the shirt at the back of the pants, may be helpful in directing the examiner to test or suspect the subscapularis muscle.

Inspection

There are no unique observations for the subscapularis muscle outside the other rotator cuff observations already mentioned.

Active internal rotation may be weak or difficult if the subscapularis is torn. Isometric resisted testing can be confusing because there are other, more powerful internal rotators that make it difficult to know if the subscapularis is involved. Therefore, special tests that isolate the subscapularis muscle become very important.

Palpations With Expected Outcomes

The subscapularis muscle is very difficult to palpate. The patient should be supine, and the examiner would need to go into the patient's armpit through the posterior part of the axilla. Some patients are uncomfortable with this means of palpation, so it is important to outline steps well in advance before attempting palpation.

Special Tests

There are a number of special tests that assess subscapularis pathology. Some of these tests were also used to assess glenohumeral impingement and include the lift-off sign and internal rotation lag, belly-press/Napoleon, and bear hug tests. See Table 10.18 for a complete description of these tests.

- **Lift-off sign:** This can be done when the patient is performing active ROM while standing. He or she is asked to tuck the arm behind the back, then lift the arm off the back (Figure 10.35).
- **Internal rotation lag test:** The patient can either be standing or seated on a table relaxed with the arm by his or her side (Figure 10.38).
- **Belly press test/Napoleon test:** The patient can be standing or seated with the elbow flexed to 90°, with the humerus internally rotated touching the stomach in a chicken wing–like position (Figure 10.36).
- **Bear hug test:** The patient can be seated or standing with the arm in horizontal adduction. The examiner can also ask the patient to scratch the back of his or her opposite shoulder (Figure 10.37).

Radiographic Orders

Radiographic imaging has previously been covered under the supraspinatus pathology section of this chapter.

Functional Assessment/Outcome Measures

Functional assessment and outcome measures have been covered previously.

Clinical Diagnosis (Differential Diagnosis)

The clinical diagnosis of subscapularis muscle strains or tears is difficult because there are more powerful muscles that are responsible for internal rotation of the GH joint, such as the latissimus dorsi and pectoralis major. Manual muscle testing of these two large muscles is helpful to differentiate from a subscapularis muscle strain or tear. Other differential diagnoses include labral tears and long head of biceps brachii impingement or tears.

Long Head of Biceps Brachii Strain/Tear/Impingement

The long head of the biceps brachii originates on the superior labrum and the supraglenoid tubercle.[44] The tendon has an intimate attachment and function with the superior GH ligament, the coracohumeral ligament, and the deep fibers of the subscapularis and supraspinatus tendons.[44] These intricate connections make the long head of the biceps brachii tendon susceptible to pathology when those structures are injured, such as GH instability, rotator cuff pathology, subacromial impingement,[45] and labral pathology.[46,47] As a result, when evaluating a patient's shoulder and any of those injuries are suspected, all special testing for all these conditions should be used to rule them out. In other words, GH instability, rotator cuff pathology, subacromial impingement, and labral pathology are also differential diagnoses for long head of biceps brachii muscle and tendon pathology, and also concurrent injuries. **Table 10.10** presents quick tips for assessing such pathology.

Table 10.10 Long Head of Biceps Brachii Tear, Strain, or Impingement Quick Tips

Pathology	Description	Presentation (HIPS)	Special Tests/Imaging	Differential Diagnosis	5-Min Sideline Assessment Tips
Long head of biceps brachii tear, strain, or impingement	A tear or strain often involves overhead motion and repetition. Acute tears can occur with eccentric clothesline motion.	Painful to flex glenohumeral joint. Pain at the extreme flexed state is indicative of impingement, particularly when coupled with repetitive overhead activity. Pain in the bicipital groove confirms involvement.	Neer impingement or speed test. If torn, radiography or ultrasonography may be useful.	Rotator cuff pathology or subacromial bursitis if it is chronic. If acute, pectoralis major or latissimus dorsi tears should be considered. Glenohumeral subluxation may also be present.	Palpation in the bicipital groove and speed test are quick assessment techniques on the sideline.

HIPS, history, inspection, palpation, special tests.

Specific History Questions

Long head of biceps brachii strains, tears, and impingement are often associated with other injuries, and, therefore, similar history questions to those injuries are important. Perhaps only three history questions may be helpful to differentiate biceps involvement from other injuries: pain location, ADLs, and abnormal sounds and sensations. The patient should be asked to point to the site of greatest pain, using one finger if possible. Pain in the bicipital groove is a good indicator of the long head of biceps brachii involvement. ADLs, such as brushing one's hair at the back, particularly if the dominant hand is responsible for brushing, can be painful in the same pain region pointed out earlier. Asking the patient if he or she has any abnormal sounds or sensations is useful if the examiner suspects either a SLAP lesion or a subluxating long head of biceps brachii from the bicipital groove. In the case of the subluxating biceps tendon, the examiner should suspect a torn transverse humeral ligament that holds the tendon in the bicipital groove. This can be confirmed with the Yergason test.

Inspection

There are no observations that would make the long head of the biceps brachii unique to other conditions previously mentioned.

Active ROM with forward flexion and overpressure or passive ROM at the extreme end of flexion are often painful. It should be noted that this is very similar to the Neer special test. Sometimes, passive extension at the very end range can also be painful. Isometric resisted forward flexion is often painful and can be weak if a significant tear is involved.

Palpations With Expected Outcomes

Palpation and assessing tenderness in the bicipital groove are useful in determining pathology.[46,48] Gill et al.[46] recommended palpating the tendon in the groove 3 to 6 cm below the acromion process with approximately 10° of internal rotation and the elbow at 90°. Table 10.18 provides the research evidence associated with those palpations.

Special Tests

There are a number of special tests that assess long head of biceps brachii muscle and tendon pathology and also concurrent injuries. These tests include the Speed, Yergason, and upper cut tests (**Figures 10.46** through **10.48**). See Table 10.18 for a complete description of these tests.

- **Speed test:** The patient should be standing with both arms out in front, flexed to approximately 60° with the palms up.
- **Yergason test:** The patient is seated with the elbow flexed to 90° and forearm fully pronated.
- **Uppercut test:** The patient can be seated or standing, depending on his or her height relative to the examiner's height. The patient should flex the shoulder to approximately 20° to 30° and keep a 90° bend in the elbow while making a full fist (ie, reproduce the uppercut motion from boxing).

Common Shoulder Pathologies

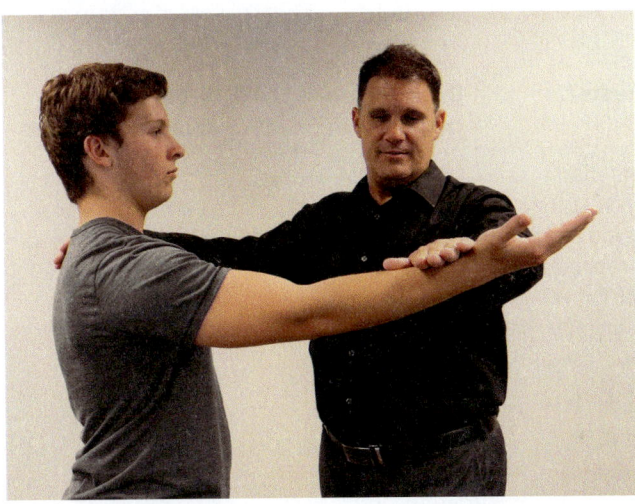

Figure 10.46 Photograph demonstrating the Speed test.
© Jones & Bartlett Learning

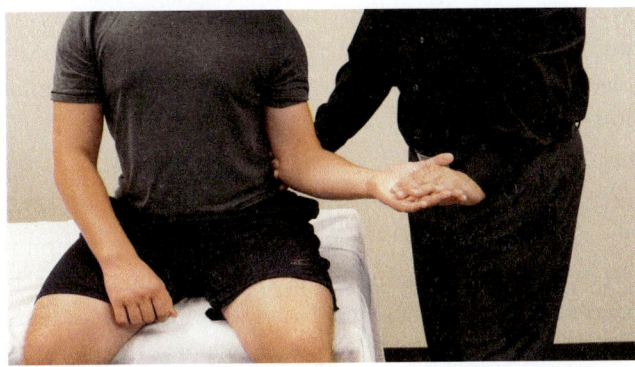

Figure 10.47 Photograph demonstrating the Yergason test.
© Jones & Bartlett Learning

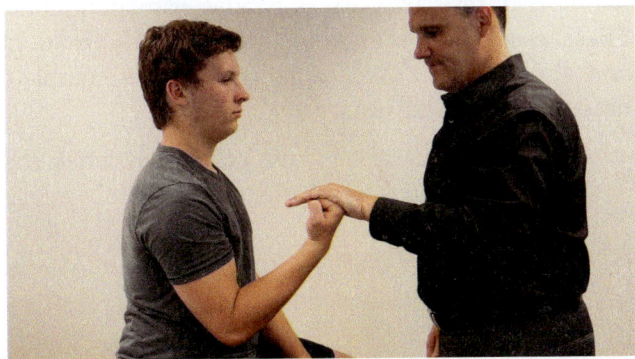

Figure 10.48 Photograph demonstrating the uppercut test.
© Jones & Bartlett Learning

Radiographic Orders

Ultrasonography is considered superior to arthrography for detecting tendon damage.[49] A more complete account of imaging was presented previously in the discussion of the rotator cuff. Ultrasonography was presented previously in the discussion of the rotator cuff.

Functional Assessment/Outcome Measures

There are no specific outcome measures associated with this specific condition. Functional assessment can be similar to the functional evaluation outlined previously.

Clinical Diagnosis (Differential Diagnosis)

The clinical diagnosis may include the tendon in the bicipital groove and microdamage to the tendon, tenosynovitis, or a subluxating tendon from the bicipital groove. There may also be damage to the proximal attachment of the long head of the biceps on the superior labrum. Type of diagnosis and differential diagnosis is outlined in the discussion on labral tears in the following paragraphs. As mentioned previously, GH instability, subacromial impingement, and rotator cuff pathology are not only considered differential diagnoses but also concomitant conditions with the long head of biceps brachii pathologies.

Labral Tears

One of the best analogies to understand labral pathology in the shoulder is to envision the glenoid labrum like a clock face. A Bankart lesion occurs when there is a labral tear between 3 o'clock and 6 o'clock, a reverse Bankart lesion occurs between 6 o'clock and 9 o'clock, and a SLAP lesion occurs between 9 o'clock and 3 o'clock. Bankart and reverse Bankart lesions are usually secondary to traumatic, acute anteroinferior, and posterior GH dislocations, respectively. SLAP lesions are commonly associated with chronic GH instability or laxity (or subluxation), subacromial impingement, rotator cuff pathology, and most commonly long head biceps brachii tendon pathology. Therefore, the testing that occurs with these other injuries should also include labrum testing when suspected. **Table 10.11** presents quick tips for assessing such pathology.

SLAP lesions were originally classified by Snyder et al.[50] into four types: (I) fraying and degeneration of the superior labrum, common with aging and wearing; (II) detachment of the superior labrum at the supraglenoid tubercle; (III) a bucket-handle tear of the labrum with an intact long head biceps brachii tendon, with the labrum commonly stuck in the joint; and (IV) similar to type III, but the long head biceps brachii tendon is involved with the tear. Testing for these four

Table 10.11 Labral Tear Quick Tips

Pathology	Description	Presentation (HIPS)	Special Tests/Imaging	Differential Diagnosis	5-Min Sideline Assessment Tips
Labral tear	Can accompany glenohumeral dislocation acutely. Chronically, often associated with repetitive overhead activity.	The patient often complains of clicking or popping sensation.	The biceps load test II, O'Brien test, or compression-rotation test may reproduce clicking or grinding. CT arthrography may be a useful imaging technique.	Often associated with rotator cuff pathology, long head of biceps brachii muscle pathology is secondary to a glenohumeral dislocation.	If the glenohumeral joint feels locked, an acute labral tear may be present.

HIPS, history, inspection, palpation, special tests.

different labral pathologies is separated by their classification, discussed in the following paragraphs.

Specific History Questions

The mechanism of injury for labral tears can typically be separated into traumatic or microtraumatic in nature. The traumatic causes of GH anteroinferior instability include FOOSH or extreme abduction with external rotation. These typically result in Bankart lesions. Reverse Bankart lesions can result from a traumatic blow with person-to-person or person-to-object (ground, building, etc) contact on the anterior aspect of the GH joint, pushing the head of the humerus posteriorly. However, SLAP lesions are often caused by repetitive microtrauma that occurs with overhead motions, such as throwing, hitting in volleyball, or swimming. Calcei et al[51] suggested that contributing factors may also be a tight posterior capsule and change in scapular mechanics (ie, scapular dyskinesis). Therefore, history questions that decipher some of the subtle microtrauma that contribute to SLAP lesions are important.

Perhaps one factor that may help to differentiate SLAP lesions from other conditions that occur with SLAP lesions is the question of abnormal sounds or sensations. Patients with SLAP lesions typically have clicking, grabbing, catching, locking, or clunking sensations.

Inspection

There are no unique observations with SLAP lesions. However, the scapular function (or dysfunction) is an important contributor to the cause, so information and testing of scapular dyskinesisis is helpful.

Active and passive ROM that mimics some of the special tests provides some evidence of labral tears. For example, extreme abduction and flexion may result in pain or abnormal sensations. If the patient's internal and external rotation is tested at 90° of abduction, pain or abnormal sensation may be indicative of labral tears. Resisted testing for shoulder flexion, internal rotation, or external rotation may be painful or weak, particularly if there are other conditions, such as rotator cuff involvement or subacromial impingement pathologies, present.

Palpations With Expected Outcomes

There is some evidence that palpation of the bicipital groove into its attachment at the superior labrum is indicative of SLAP lesions. However, other labral tears are difficult to palpate because they are deep in the GH joint.

Special Tests

Reverse Bankart Lesion Testing. There are two special tests that assess reverse Bankart lesions. These tests are the Kim test and jerk test (**Figure 10.49** and **Figure 10.50**). See Table 10.18 for a complete description of these tests.

- **Kim test:** This test is best performed when the patient is seated with the shoulder relaxed so

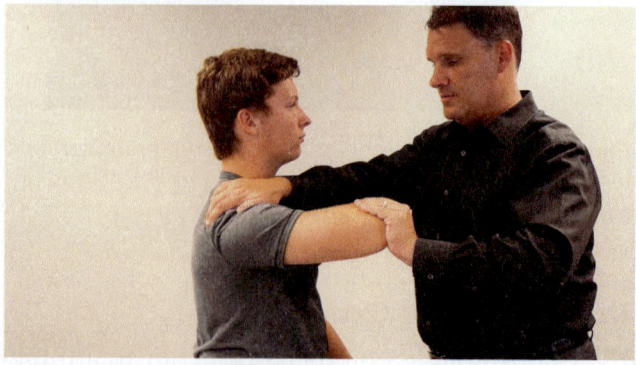

Figure 10.49 Photograph demonstrating the Kim test.
© Jones & Bartlett Learning

Common Shoulder Pathologies **379**

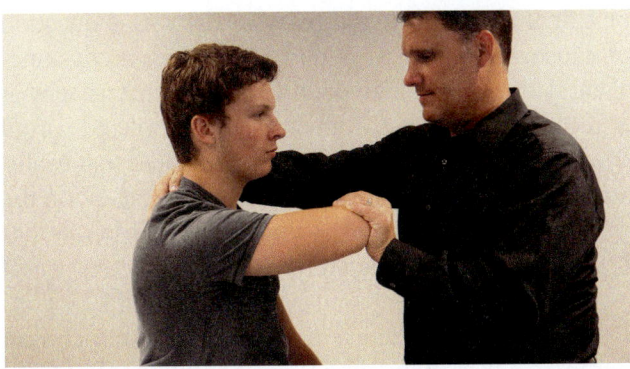

Figure 10.50 Photograph demonstrating the jerk test.
© Jones & Bartlett Learning

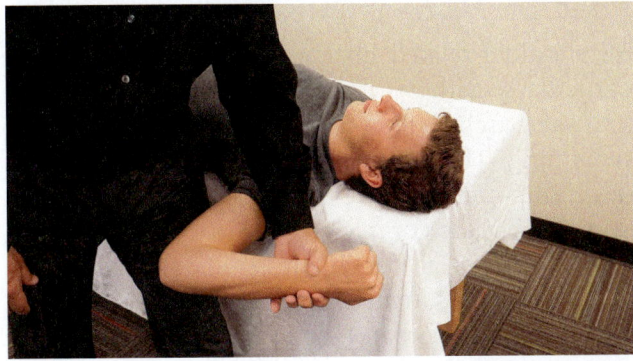

Figure 10.51 Photograph demonstrating the biceps load test II.
© Jones & Bartlett Learning

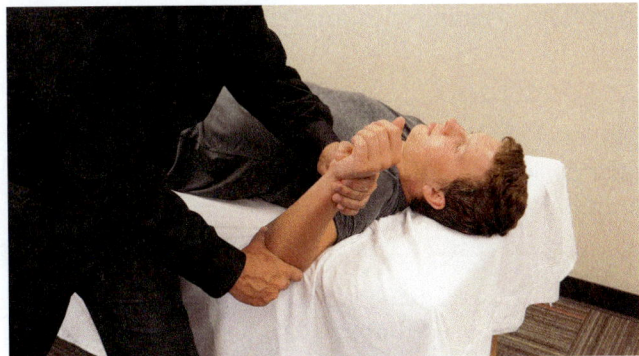

Figure 10.52 Photograph demonstrating the compression-rotation test.
© Jones & Bartlett Learning

the examiner can move it, but it can also be performed with the patient standing.
- **Jerk test:** The patient is seated with the arm/shoulder completely relaxed so the examiner can execute the test and shoulder motion.

SLAP Lesions. There are two special tests that assess SLAP lesions. These tests are the biceps load test II and compression-rotation test. (**Figure 10.51** and **Figure 10.52**). See Table 10.18 for a complete description of these tests.

- **Biceps load test II:** The patient lies on a table with the arm relaxed so the examiner can move it for testing purposes.
- **Compression-rotation test:** The patient lies supine on the table with the shoulder relaxed while the examiner moves the glenohumeral joint.

Radiographic Orders

Table 10.12 presents quick tips for assessing such pathology.

Functional Assessment/Outcome Measures

There are no specific or unique outcome measures or functional testing for SLAP lesions. Please refer to the outcome measures listed at the beginning of this chapter.

Clinical Diagnosis (Differential Diagnosis)

The clinical diagnosis is a SLAP lesion. There are a number of differential diagnoses related to SLAP lesions, including GH instability, GH impingement, AC sprain, and long head biceps tendon pathology. It is important to cross-reference with a number of special tests and be very specific about what a positive test should be with SLAP lesion versus other differential diagnoses.

Table 10.12 Evidence of Imaging in Diagnosis of SLAP Lesions

Study	Focus	Sensitivity	Specificity	LR+	LR-	QUADAS
Symanski et al 2017[52]	SLAP lesion: MRA	0.80	0.91	8.9	0.2	NR
Symanski et al 2017[52]	SLAP lesion: MRI	0.63	0.87	4.8	0.4	NR

LR+, positive likelihood ratio; LR–, negative likelihood ratio; MRA, magnetic resonance arthrography; NR, not reported; QUADAS, Quality Assessment of Diagnostic Accuracy Studies; SLAP, superior labrum anterior to posterior.

Scapular Dyskinesis

Scapular dyskinesis (**Figure 10.53**) has been defined simply as altered scapular motion and position.[4] Most of the literature focuses on the previous diagnoses in this chapter, and most studies likely involve some type of scapular dyskinesis as a contributing factor. As a result, there has been a call to test scapular function on all patients with shoulder pain because much of the dysfunction is a modifiable risk factor for most patients.[53] Hickey et al[53] have estimated that 43% of athletes have some form of scapular dyskinesis. Correcting scapular dyskinesis could prevent many of the shoulder conditions previously discussed. There are a number of causes of scapular dyskinesis, including bony (thoracic kyphosis and clavicular fracture), joint (AC joint instability, GH instability, or labral tear), and neurologic (cervical radiculopathy, long thoracic, or spinal accessory nerve palsy).[4] There is a question of cause and effect as it relates to scapular dyskinesis and other shoulder pathologies; so that is why it is recommended that evaluation be completed for all shoulder conditions. It should also be noted that evaluation of scapular dyskinesis is in its early stages and the evidence supporting the evaluations listed below has been questioned.[54] Despite the poor predictive validity and reliability, scapular evaluation should be considered with a critical eye and added to other clinical findings with specific pathologic conditions discussed previously. **Table 10.13** presents quick tips for assessing scapular dyskinesis.

Specific History Questions

All shoulder-related history questions are relevant, particularly with overhead throwing–type activities, such as baseball pitching, hitting in volleyball, or swimming. The volume of training for these activities is important relative to the other types of weight training that are completed. Certain weight-training activities, such as bench press, lateral pull-downs, and lateral raises, tend to work larger muscle groups, which can exacerbate scapular dyskinesis in the absence of balancing an athlete's weight-training program with other scapular stabilizers.

Knowing which arm is dominant may be helpful, particularly if there is significant hypertrophy (observation) on one side creating a muscle imbalance and, therefore, asymmetrical movement patterns.

Inspection

Kibler et al,[4] in their consensus article related to scapular dyskinesis, identified visual observation to be the number one factor when diagnosing this condition.

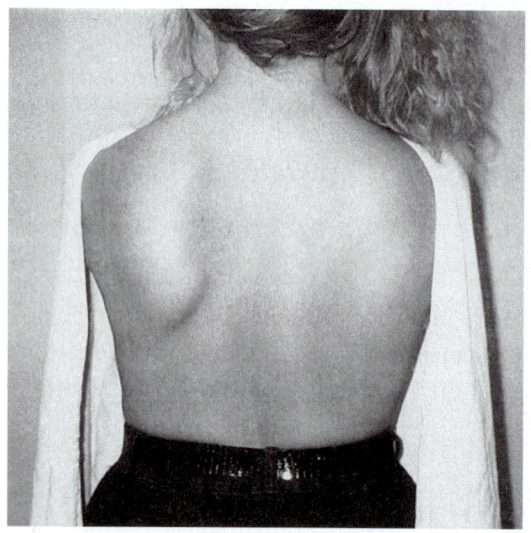

Figure 10.53 Photograph showing scapular dyskinesis.
© Jones & Bartlett Learning

Table 10.13 Scapular Dyskinesis Quick Tips

Pathology	Description	Presentation (HIPS)	Special Tests/Imaging	Differential Diagnosis	5-Min Sideline Assessment Tips
Scapular dyskinesis	This condition is characterized by biomechanical dysfunction and poor coordination of the scapulothoracic rhythm with the glenohumeral joint.	It is rare that this condition is painful or the primary site for an injury. Rather, it is more commonly associated with chronic, overhead repetitive activities and pathologies, such as glenohumeral impingement and rotator cuff pathology.	The best testing is observation of the scapulothoracic rhythm while performing active abduction and flexion. Symmetry with the opposite side and scapular winging are two positive signs. No imaging is useful.	This condition contributes to many conditions and, therefore, should be evaluated in a number of other chronic pathologies.	None.

HIPS, history, inspection, palpation, special tests.

Observation is central to many of the tests and, therefore, will be covered in greater detail in the following special tests.

Traditional active ROM should be tested, and abduction is usually the most useful. The lateral scapular slide test[55] is described later and can be considered in the special testing or active ROM component of the examiner's evaluation.

Palpations With Expected Outcomes

The primary palpation that is relevant to scapular dyskinesis is landmarking the borders of the scapula relative to the thoracic spine.

Special Tests

There is one special test that best assesses scapular dyskinesis, the lateral scapular slide test (**Figure 10.54**). See Table 10.18 for a complete description of this test.

- **Lateral scapular slide test:** The patient is asked to stand and abduct the glenohumeral joint to varying degrees.

Radiographic Orders

Imaging is not relevant to scapular dyskinesis because it is not a pathologic condition but rather merely considered a contributor to other conditions.

Functional Assessment/Outcome Measures

There are no functional assessments or outcome measures specific to scapular dyskinesis currently.

Clinical Diagnosis (Differential Diagnosis)

Technically, scapular dyskinesis is not a clinical diagnosis but rather considered a contributor to other conditions. However, the scientific evidence on the predictive validity to these other conditions is still controversial.[53,56]

Clavicular Fracture

Clavicular fractures (**Figure 10.55**) account for 5% of all fractures seen in emergency rooms and 44% of fractures in the shoulder region.[57] The most commonly fractured part of the clavicle is the middle third (69% to 81%) (**Figure 10.56**) because the clavicle changes shape at this exact point and also lacks muscular attachments that would provide additional support.[57]

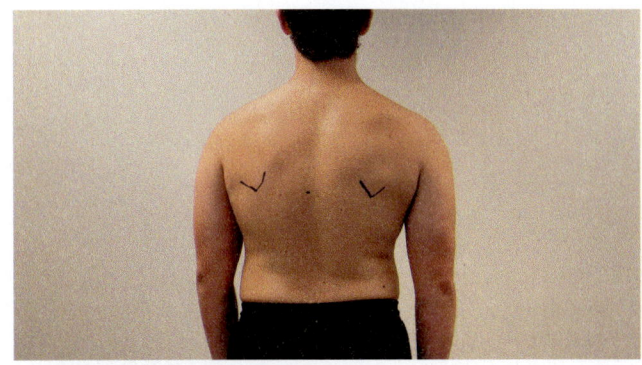
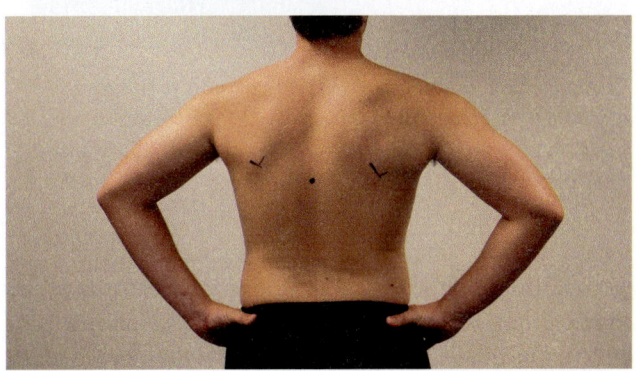
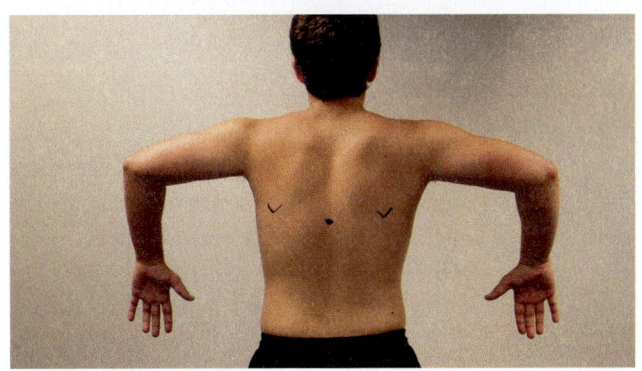

Figure 10.54 Photographs demonstrating the lateral scapula slide test.

© Jones & Bartlett Learning

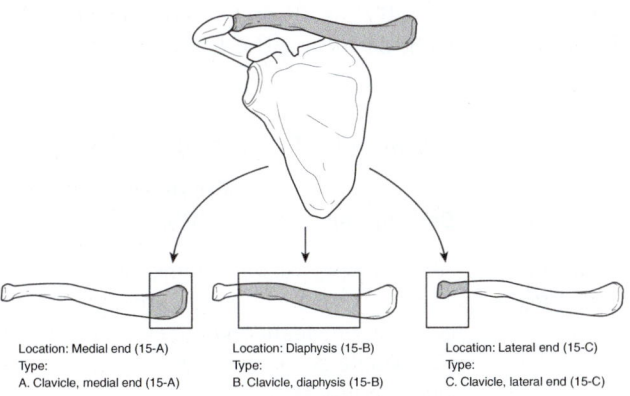

Figure 10.55 Drawing depicting types of clavicular fractures.

Reproduced from Armstrong AD, Hubbard MC, eds: Essentials of Musculoskeletal Care, ed 5. Burlington, MA, American Academy of Orthopaedic Surgeons, 2015.

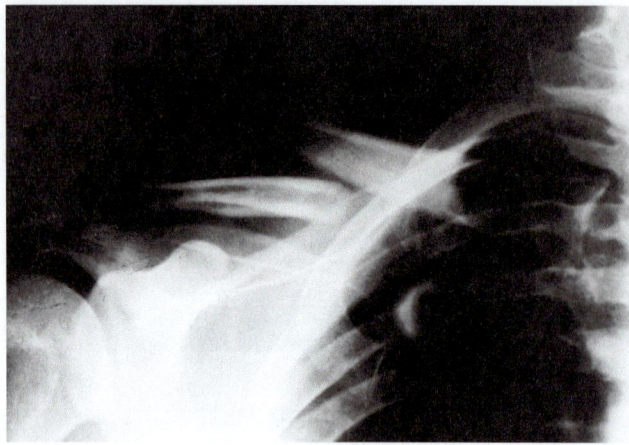

Figure 10.56 Radiograph showing middle-third clavicular fracture.

Reproduced from Armstrong AD, Hubbard MC, eds: *Essentials of Musculoskeletal Care*, ed 5. Burlington, MA, American Academy of Orthopaedic Surgeons, 2015.

Evaluation is typically done in the field during sports events, and clavicular fractures are managed as a traumatic condition that may require transportation. **Table 10.14** presents quick tips for assessing clavicular fractures.

Specific History Questions

Age is an important question because clavicular fractures tend to occur prior to age 40 years or after age 70 years. They are the most common fracture in the pediatric population. The mechanism of injury for these two populations is likely different as well, so knowing the events that preceded the injury is important. Adults older than 70 years tend to fall because of changes in balance with age, but it is important to determine the differential diagnosis for the fall because those conditions could be more serious than a fractured clavicle (upper motor neuron lesions, such as a stroke, for example). Other than FOOSH, other mechanisms of injury are similar to AC joint and SC joint sprains, such as hitting the top of the shoulder into another person (ie, collision sports), the ground, or boards (ice hockey).

Inspection

Observation of these injuries is usually quite useful because many of these fractures present with a deformity in the continuity of the clavicle, again mostly around the middle third.

The clavicle is required for motion in most directions and, therefore, most active and passive ROM is severely limited in the acute stage. Isometric resisted testing will be weak with any muscles that attach in or around the clavicle, primarily flexion, abduction, and horizontal adduction. Because of the proximity of the clavicle to the subclavian artery and the brachial plexus, distal pulse and sensation should be tested. A lack of pulse indicates a serious emergency and immediate medical care is required.

Palpations With Expected Outcomes

Palpation along the entire clavicle will be painful, but the site of the fracture will be most painful and should be approached very carefully to avoid undue pain and distress in the patient. Commencing palpation both distal and/or proximal to the suspected injury site is important. Differential diagnosis palpation includes both the AC and SC joints.

Special Tests

There are no special tests that are exclusive to clavicular fractures, and, most often, observation, inspection, and palpation are sufficient for diagnosis of a clavicular fracture. However, if the fracture is more subtle, the olecranon manubrium test is useful for all upper extremity fractures (**Figure 10.57**).

Radiographic Orders

Radiographs are the most common means of confirming the diagnosis of a clavicular fracture.

Table 10.14 Clavicular Fracture Quick Tips

Pathology	Description	Presentation (HIPS)	Special Tests/ Imaging	Differential Diagnosis	5-Min Sideline Assessment Tips
Clavicular fracture	Often results from a traumatic collision between two people or with the ground/ playing surface.	A deformity is often present when comparing sides.	Palpation is the best test in these cases. Radiographs are confirmatory.	AC sprain, SC sprain, rib fractures, or brachial plexus conditions.	Immediate and gentle palpation starting at the SC joint and moving laterally, feeling for bony continuity to the AC joint.

HIPS, history, inspection, palpation, and special tests; AC, acromioclavicular; SC, sternoclavicular.

Common Shoulder Pathologies

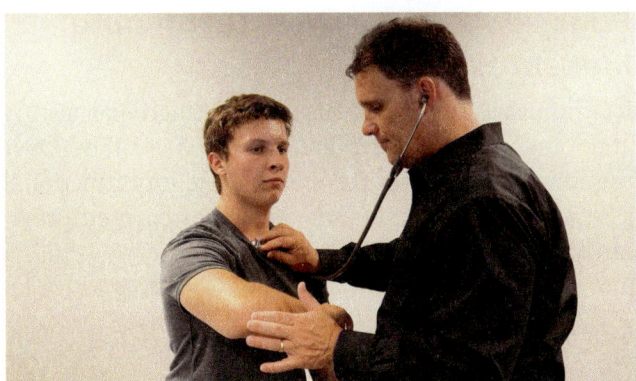

Figure 10.57 Photograph demonstrating the olecranon manubrium percussion test.

© Jones & Bartlett Learning

Functional Assessment/Outcome Measures

None.

Clinical Diagnosis (Differential Diagnosis)

The clinical diagnosis of a clavicular fracture requires referral to a physician to confirm the diagnosis with a radiograph. The differential diagnosis includes both AC and SC joint sprains.

Humeral Fracture

Humeral fractures (**Figure 10.58**) are more common in elderly patients, typically older than 60 years, in whom osteoporosis has been diagnosed.[58] The fractures account for approximately 5% of all fractures.[58] A FOOSH mechanism of injury is the most common for humeral fractures, but only in the older age group because other injuries covered previously in this chapter tend to be seen more in younger populations

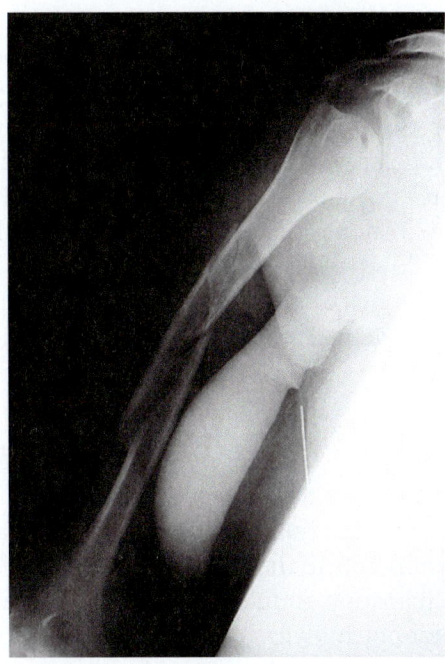

Figure 10.58 Radiograph showing humeral fracture.

Reproduced from Armstrong AD, Hubbard MC, eds: *Essentials of Musculoskeletal Care*, ed 5. Burlington, MA, American Academy of Orthopaedic Surgeons, 2015.

who have stronger bones. **Table 10.15** presents quick tips for assessing clavicular fractures.

Specific History Questions

The most important questions for this condition are age, the mechanism of injury, and previously diagnosed medical conditions, such as osteoporosis, because these are the main risks for this condition.

Inspection

The patient will likely be holding the arm in a position and unwilling to move it. Angulation and deformity may be present. Both of these signs, combined with

Table 10.15 Humeral Fracture Quick Tips

Pathology	Description	Presentation (HIPS)	Special Tests/ Imaging	Differential Diagnosis	5-Min Sideline Assessment Tips
Humeral fracture	This injury occurs as a result of significant upper body force or trauma.	A significant force is required to break this bone, so the sport or activity is important to note. Angulated fractures are relatively easy to discern, but stress fractures are less obvious. Aching and throbbing in the upper arm.	A percussion test at the distal end of the humerus may be useful clinically. Radiographs are confirmatory.	Glenohumeral impingement, rotator cuff pathology, long head of biceps brachii pathology, or triceps strain.	Feeling the continuity of the bony shaft compared to the opposite side can be useful.

HIPS, history, inspection, palpation, special tests.

the mental status of the patient, may necessitate emergency transportation for additional medical care.

It is unlikely the patient will be able to perform active or passive shoulder movement in any direction, particularly if the fracture is unstable. Isometric resisted testing should also cease if active and passive ROM are unsuccessful. An important test is checking for blood flow distally with assessment of either radial pulse or capillary refill. Compromised circulation is a medical emergency that would require emergency transportation.

Palpations With Expected Outcomes

Humeral fractures tend to occur around the midshaft or the neck of the humerus. During history taking, if the patient points to these sites as the greatest amount of pain, palpation should start distally at the medial and lateral epicondyles and slowly move proximally along the shaft of the humerus. As the examiner gets closer to the fracture site, the amount of palpation pressure should decrease according to the pain tolerance of the patient.

Special Tests

There are no specific special tests for humeral fractures. It may not be necessary to perform tests if there are any obvious signs in the observation, inspection, or palpation, discussed previously. However, if the fracture is more subtle, the olecranon manubrium percussion test (Figure 10.57) may prove useful in the diagnosis.

Radiographic Orders

Whenever a fracture is suspected, it is important to send the patient for follow-up care urgently or nonurgently for radiographs to confirm.

Functional Assessment/Outcome Measures

If a humeral fracture is suspected, functional testing and outcome measures are not used acutely. Over the long term, any of the upper extremity functional assessment tests or outcome measures covered previously may be useful.

Clinical Diagnosis (Differential Diagnosis)

The clinical diagnosis must be confirmed with a radiograph. The differential diagnosis may include triceps muscle strain, GH dislocation/subluxation, subacromial impingement, or labral tear, particularly if the fracture is around the head or neck of the humerus.

Frozen Shoulder (Adhesive Capsulitis)

Frozen shoulder, or adhesive capsulitis, has been classified as either primary or secondary.[57] Primary frozen shoulder has an insidious onset and therefore can be confusing to the examiner because there is little or no trauma in the patient's history. Secondary frozen shoulder occurs after a primary injury, such as GH dislocation/subluxation, AC sprain, or rotator cuff pathology. Table 10.16 presents quick tips for assessing frozen shoulder.

Specific History Questions

Age is an important question because frozen shoulder most often occurs during the fourth or fifth decade of life. Knowing the sex of the patient is important because women tend to be more susceptible to frozen shoulder. History questions about medical conditions are important because there is some correlation with

Table 10.16 Frozen Shoulder Quick Tips

Pathology	Description	Presentation (HIPS)	Special Tests/Imaging	Differential Diagnosis	5-Min Sideline Assessment Tips
Frozen shoulder	This condition is characterized by a chronic, slow-developing shrinkage of the glenohumeral capsule, often after some type of trauma, such as a glenohumeral dislocation/subluxation.	The most obvious sign is the inability of the patient to abduct or flex the shoulder. The patient often complains of an achy pain, particularly when sleeping.	Glenohumeral joint play and passive range of motion are significantly restricted.	Subacromial bursitis, glenohumeral impingement, rotator cuff tears, or glenohumeral instability.	None.

HIPS, history, inspection, palpation, special tests.

frozen shoulder and type 1 diabetes, type 2 diabetes, and hyperthyroidism.[57]

Inspection

There are no obvious deformities or other traditional observations that may help to diagnose this condition until the patient is asked to move. An inability to perform active or passive movement of the GH joint in multiple directions is the most obvious symptom to confirm the diagnosis. Passive ROM or overpressure at the end ranges occurs long before normal ROM and typically elicits pain because of tightness around the capsule. Otherwise, there is no pain with active or passive ROM. Isometric resisted testing usually results in no deficits in strength provided the patient is tested with the arm at the side.

Palpations With Expected Outcomes

It is difficult or impossible to find any particular body part in or around the shoulder that is painful upon palpation. A tight upper trapezius muscle may be present because of overrecruitment in shoulder motion (shrug sign).

Special Tests

There is one special test that best assesses frozen shoulder, the shrug sign. The patient is standing and asked to elevate or abduct the glenohumeral joint. (**Figure 10.59**). See Table 10.18 for a complete description of this test.

Radiographic Orders

There is no imaging modality that can help in the diagnosis of frozen shoulder. But ruling out other conditions is part of the diagnosis, so radiographs may be warranted for that reason.

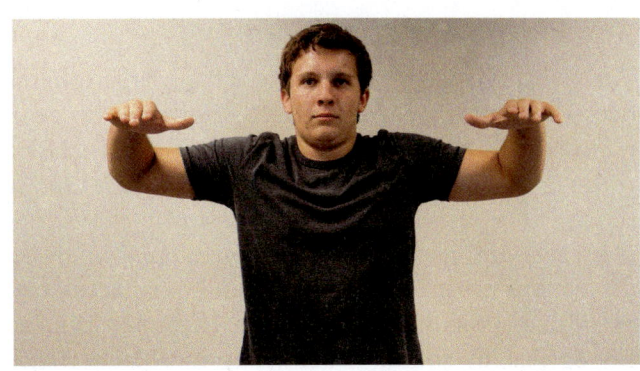

Figure 10.59 Photograph demonstrating the shrug sign.
© Jones & Bartlett Learning

Functional Assessment/Outcome Measures

The patient is unlikely to be able to complete many functional tests. However, some of the upper extremity outcome measures may be useful in the diagnosis and treatment plan.

Clinical Diagnosis (Differential Diagnosis)

The diagnosis is challenging and often a process of elimination of many other conditions covered previously in this chapter. Perhaps the most telling and differentiating sign from all other conditions is the lack of pain because the patient typically complains of a lack of function, rather than pain, as his or her most pressing complaint.

Peripheral Nerve Pathology

The most common peripheral nerve conditions of the shoulder include injuries to the spinal accessory, axillary, long thoracic, suprascapular and musculocutaneous nerves. **Table 10.17** presents quick tips for assessing peripheral nerve pathology.

Table 10.17 Peripheral Nerve Pathology Quick Tips

Pathology	Description	Presentation (HIPS)	Special Tests/ Imaging	Differential Diagnosis	5-Min Sideline Assessment Tips
Peripheral nerve pathology	Most nerve injuries have an immediate, acute, traumatic event that precedes the nerve damage. The nerve damage may become more obvious only later on due to muscle involvement.	Active range of motion or manual muscle testing is often compromised, depending on the specific nerve involved.	The special testing is a manual muscle test related to the nerves: shoulder elevation, shoulder abduction, scapular winging, or external humeral rotation.	Tears in any of the muscles that are innervated by these nerves are the primary differential diagnosis. However, upper motor neuron lesions should be ruled out.	Immediate weakness in various motions listed previously.

HIPS, history, inspection, palpation, special tests.

Spinal Accessory Nerve

The spinal accessory nerve is not actually a peripheral nerve but rather cranial nerve XI. However, because it innervates the trapezius muscle, it is discussed with nerve injuries here. Injury to this nerve is rare in sports.[59] The trapezius muscle is responsible for scapular elevation, retraction, and depression. Therefore, if a patient has scapular dyskinesis, spinal accessory nerve damage should be ruled out. The injury is most susceptible in sports, where it is most superficial around the posterior cervical triangle of the neck.[59] Blows to this region with a hockey or lacrosse stick make this nerve susceptible because it is a region where there is little padding or protective equipment.

Specific History Questions

A patient may complain of an inability to lift the arm, and, therefore, the main complaint is often function. This is similar to frozen shoulder, but, unlike frozen shoulder, the patient may have pain and a mechanism of injury where there is a direct blow to the base of the neck and shoulder. Another mechanism of injury may be traction or separation of the neck and shoulder similar to mechanisms resulting in brachial plexus injuries.

Inspection

Depending on the length of time the patient has had this condition, atrophy may have occurred, and, therefore, the shoulder height may appear different. The patient may also present with scapular winging (see scapular dyskinesis discussion).

Active ROM with abduction and flexion of the shoulder, particularly at the end ROM, is often affected. The examiner will be able to move the patient passively into this ROM. Any muscle testing involving the actions of the trapezius muscle will appear weak, or the patient may try to compensate with other muscles. Comparison bilaterally is critical to comparing the quality of strength in addition to the quantity.

Palpations With Expected Outcomes

Palpations rarely provide useful information other than that the trapezius muscle may appear to have less muscle bulk (ie, muscle atrophy).

Special Tests

There are two tests for the spinal accessory nerve; the lateral scapular slide test, outlined previously under scapular dyskinesis, can be useful in identifying scapular winging and the active elevation lag sign outlined below (**Figure 10.60**). Furthermore, manual muscle testing for the three trapezius muscle bellies can be useful.

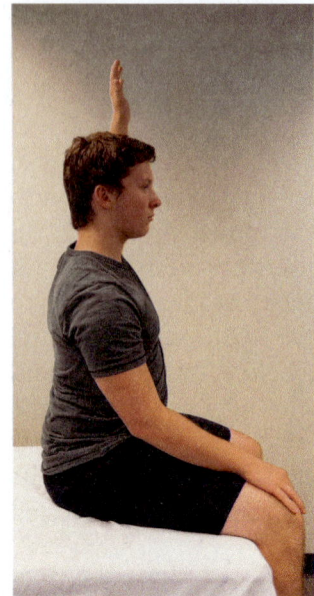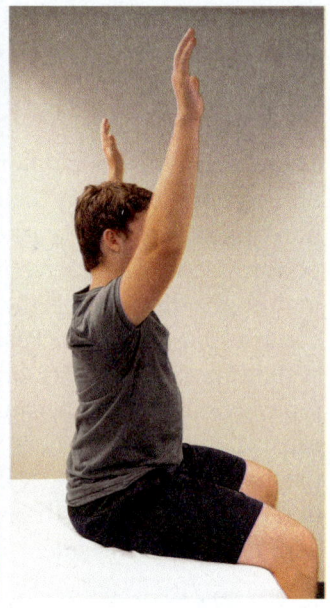

Figure 10.60 Photographs demonstrating the active elevation lag sign.
© Jones & Bartlett Learning

- **Active elevation lag sign:** Before the active elevation lag sign can be tested, the examiner must passively flex the affected shoulder fully to ensure there is no capsular or other restrictions preventing the patient from actively flexing his or her shoulder in the next steps. The patient is then asked to actively flex his or her shoulder until the patient's lumbar spine begins to extend. A decrease in flexion motion can be indicative of a spinal accessory nerve palsy.

Radiographic Orders

There is no imaging modality that helps with the diagnosis of this condition. Nerve conduction and electromyography (EMG) testing can be helpful in both the diagnosis of this condition and monitoring patient progress over time.

Functional Assessment/Outcome Measures

General functional assessment and outcome measures for the shoulder may be useful to identify both weaknesses and complaints from the patient.

Clinical Diagnosis (Differential Diagnosis)

The clinical diagnosis of spinal accessory nerve pathology or neuropathy is evident with positive tests listed previously. However, the differential diagnoses may be closely linked and difficult to rule out without confirmatory nerve conduction and EMG testing. These differential diagnoses include scapular dyskinesis due to unilateral or nondominant arm weakness, frozen shoulder, and rotator cuff pathology.

Axillary Nerve

Axillary nerve injuries are rare and account for fewer than 1% of all nerve injuries.[59] The axillary nerve (**Figure 10.61**) is responsible for teres minor and deltoid muscle innervation. It is uncommon for the axillary nerve to be injured in sport. One mechanism of injury is secondary to a traction injury that occurs with brachial plexus injuries or after a GH dislocation.[59] Another mechanism of injury in sport that has been reported is a direct blow to the anterior-lateral GH region with a hard implement or helmet.[60]

Specific History Questions

Asking about previous injuries is probably the most important question because nerve injuries tend to take time to show up clinically or for the patient to know. In addition, as mentioned previously, these injuries typically are secondary to another injury, such as a GH dislocation.

Inspection

Atrophy of the deltoid muscle relative to the other shoulder is the most obvious sign of this injury. Atrophy of the teres minor muscle may be more subtle and hard to discern.

The patient will have trouble actively abducting or externally rotating his or her shoulder. Shoulder flexion and extension is weaker but compensated by other synergistic muscles. Passive ROM is unremarkable. The patient's shoulder is usually weak with abduction, particularly if tested at 90° of abduction. The other motions that may be weak are GH external rotation, flexion, and extension. However, these motions may be compensated by other synergistic muscles as well.

Palpations With Expected Outcomes

There are usually no areas that are particularly painful with palpation. Atrophy will be present in the deltoid and teres minor muscles relative to the other shoulder.

Special Tests

There are no special tests for the axillary nerve. Hertel et al[61] introduced a test, called the deltoid extension lag sign, for which five male patients who had axillary nerve damage after an anteroinferior GH dislocation were tracked. However, this test does not have any other evidence in the literature other than a description. Therefore, C5–C6 dermatome and myotome testing is likely to be the best indicator of this condition.

Radiographic Orders

There is no imaging modality that helps with the diagnosis of this condition. Nerve conduction and EMG testing can be helpful in diagnosing this condition as well as monitoring patient progress over time.

Functional Assessment/Outcome Measures

General functional assessment and outcome measures for the shoulder may be useful to identify weaknesses and complaints from the patient.

Clinical Diagnosis (Differential Diagnosis)

The clinical diagnosis of an axillary nerve injury is usually secondary to other previous conditions. The most common differential diagnosis would be other muscles that perform a function similar to that of the affected muscles, such as supraspinatus and infraspinatus muscle pathology.

Long Thoracic Nerve

The long thoracic nerve is not commonly injured in the general public, but it is more common during sports participation. The long thoracic nerve (**Figure 10.62**) is susceptible to injury along its pathway. The two

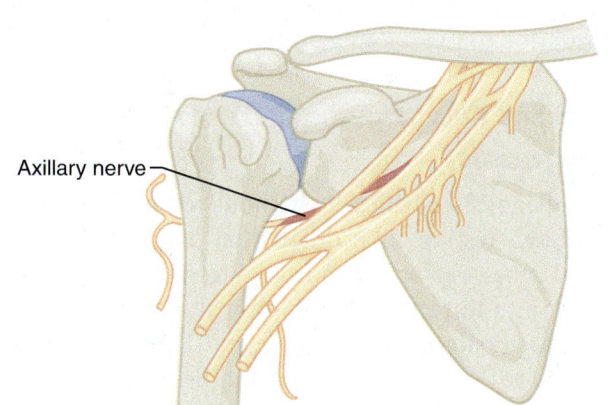

Figure 10.61 Drawing showing the axillary nerve.
© Jones & Bartlett Learning

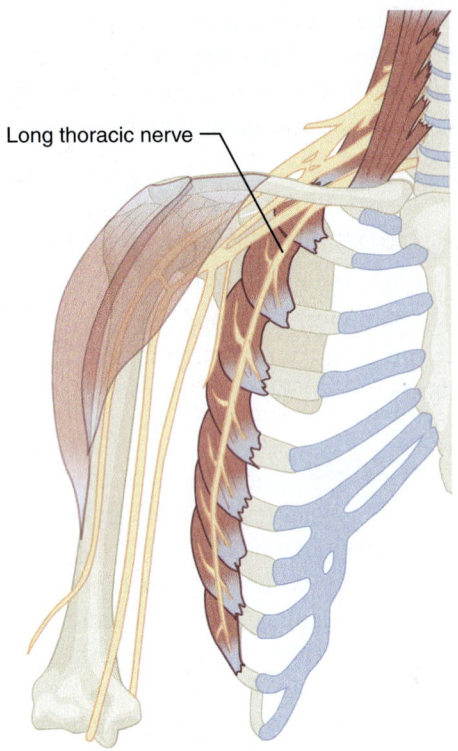

Figure 10.62 Drawing showing the long thoracic nerve.
© Jones & Bartlett Learning

common areas where it can be injured during sports participation are as it exits the neck region around the scalene muscles or in the axilla. The two mechanisms of injury tend to be either traction or compression related in the axilla.[62] The traction mechanism is typical with sports that require long, sustained, and repetitive overhead motions, such as volleyball, baseball, tennis, or gymnastics. Compression in the axilla is generally a secondary injury for athletes who use crutches inappropriately, pushing the top of the crutch into their armpit rather than using their ribcage wall. The long thoracic nerve is responsible for innervating the serratus anterior muscle. As covered previously at the beginning of this chapter, the serratus anterior muscle is responsible for stabilizing the scapula against the thoracic cavity, thus preventing winging during abduction and elevation of the GH joint.

Specific History Questions

History questions should attempt to discern between more common overhead activity shoulder conditions and long thoracic nerve pathology. Therefore, neurologic questions such as change of sensation or radicular type of pain are important and not common, with some of the other shoulder pathologies covered previously. Questions about difficulty with shoulder motion can be asked. Knowing the mechanisms stated previously is also helpful.

Inspection

Scapular dyskinesis is a common observation. Therefore, the lateral scapular slide test covered previously may be helpful.

Any active motions that require movement of the scapula may be limited or difficult, particularly at end ranges of motion (ie, flexion, extension, adduction, abduction, horizontal adduction, and horizontal abduction). Passive movement is not painful or helpful. Isometric resisted testing of the serratus anterior muscle would be weak.

Palpations With Expected Outcomes

Palpation would not reveal much pain in most places.

Special Tests

As mentioned previously, there are no special tests specific to the long thoracic nerve. However, dermatome and myotome testing should be completed to rule out other injuries. In addition, scapular dyskinesis testing is appropriate if it has not already been completed.

Radiographic Orders

There is no imaging modality that helps with the diagnosis of this condition. Nerve conduction and EMG testing can be helpful in both diagnosis of this condition and monitoring patient progress over time.

Functional Assessment/Outcome Measures

General functional assessment and outcome measures for the shoulder may be useful to identify both weaknesses and complaints from the patient. A push-up activity may reveal a great deal about this particular injury due to the scapular winging.

Clinical Diagnosis (Differential Diagnosis)

This diagnosis is difficult without nerve conduction and EMG testing. The differential diagnosis may be spinal accessory nerve pathology, rotator cuff pathology, or multidirectional instability of the GH joint that leads to subacromial impingement. However, special testing for those conditions would be negative; therefore, long thoracic nerve pathology is often diagnosed through a process of elimination.

Suprascapular Nerve

The suprascapular nerve (**Figure 10.63**) originates from the C5–C6 nerve root (sometimes with the addition of C4) and has both a sensory and motor component, so testing both is important. The nerve innervates the supraspinatus and infraspinatus muscles and therefore is responsible for initiation of abduction and external rotation of the GH joint. Injury to this nerve occurs where the nerve exits the suprascapular notch.[59] The mechanism of injury is similar to rotator cuff pathology and subacromial impingement: repeated overhead movement. However, the reason the mechanism of injury creates problems with this nerve is because of excessive tension on the nerve.

Specific History Questions

The mechanism of injury is similar to rotator cuff pathology and subacromial impingement, so this type of question may not help differentiate from suprascapular nerve pathology. Nerve involvement may involve neuropathy pain that is represented by toothache-type pain, throbbing-type pain, or radicular pain.

Inspection

Examiners should look for atrophy around the supraspinatus and infraspinatus muscles relative to the unaffected side.

The patient may present with shoulder shrug sign with active and resisted GH abduction. The patient's shoulder will also be weak with external rotation of the humerus. However, the patient does not have any pain with passive motion. The patient may present with numbness or change of sensation around the C4–C6 dermatome or cutaneous nerve distribution.

Palpations With Expected Outcomes

There may be pain around the suprascapular notch. The patient will also have significant atrophy of the supraspinatus and infraspinatus relative to the unaffected side.

Special Tests

Any special tests that require active or isometric resisted testing for the supraspinatus muscle and infraspinatus muscle should be applied.

Radiographic Orders

There is no imaging modality that helps with the diagnosis of this condition. Nerve conduction and EMG testing can be helpful in diagnosing this condition as well as monitoring patient progress over time.

Functional Assessment/Outcome Measures

There are no functional assessment or outcome measures specific to this condition. The general shoulder functional assessment and outcome measures can be applied.

Clinical Diagnosis (Differential Diagnosis)

The clinical diagnosis of suprascapular nerve palsy is extremely difficult, if not impossible, to differentiate from rotator cuff pathology clinically. Therefore, reliance on the nerve conduction and EMG testing is critical to the diagnosis.

Musculocutaneous Nerve

Injury to the musculocutaneous nerve (**Figure 10.64**) is more common as a result of another injury, such as GH dislocation or humeral fracture. It is a rare injury.[2]

Specific History Questions

The most important history questions are related to previous injuries because musculocutaneous nerve pathology is often secondary to those injuries. It is

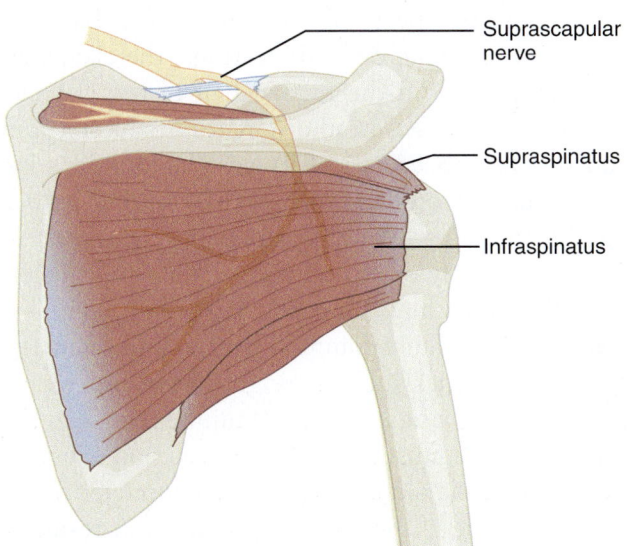

Figure 10.63 Drawing showing the suprascapular nerve.
© Jones & Bartlett Learning

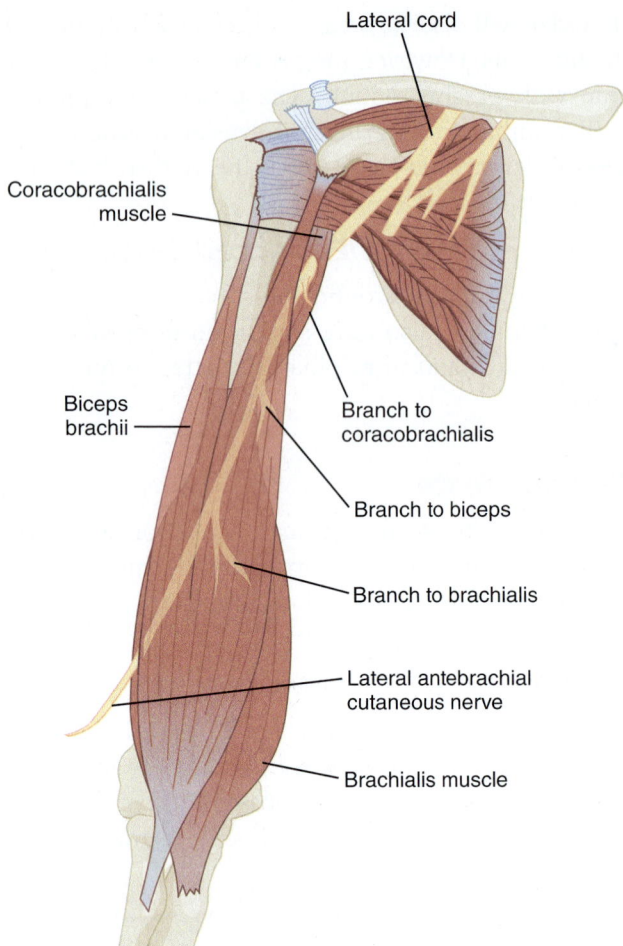

Figure 10.64 Drawing showing the musculocutaneous nerve

© Jones & Bartlett Learning

important to ask if the patient has any trouble with ADLs. It is likely he or she will notice a lack of normal function with elbow flexion.

Inspection
A unique observation, particularly if time has passed since the primary injury, is biceps brachii atrophy.

It is not normal to test elbow motion, but the history should lead the examiner to perform active, passive, and resisted testing in the elbow joint. The patient will present with weak active and resisted elbow flexion, but passive ROM is normal.

Palpations With Expected Outcomes
There is typically no pain with palpation, and the examiner may notice atrophy of only the anterior humerus (biceps brachii and brachialis) relative to the unaffected side.

Special Tests
There are no special tests for this specific condition.

Radiographic Orders
There is no imaging modality that helps with the diagnosis of this condition. Nerve conduction and EMG testing can be helpful in diagnosing this condition and monitoring patient progress over time.

Functional Assessment/Outcome Measures
There are no functional assessment or outcome measures specific to this condition. The general shoulder and arm functional assessment and outcome measures can be applied.

Clinical Diagnosis (Differential Diagnosis)
The clinical diagnosis of this condition is straightforward if the history matches the physical examination (ie, elbow flexion weakness). Failure to connect the primary injury with the secondary injury may leave the examiner confused. There are very few other injuries that lead to elbow flexion weakness.

Large Muscle Strains and Tears

Pectoralis Major Rupture
Proximally, the pectoralis major muscle has two parts that originate on two locations: the clavicular head originates on the medial half of the clavicle, and the sternocostal head originates on the sternum and superior six costal cartilages. The muscle is fan shaped and inserts distally on the bicipital groove on the humerus. Sprains and tears can occur to the muscle belly or at the musculotendinous insertion. Pectoralis major muscle strains and complete tears are moderately common in accidental injuries, sporting activities such as weight lifting and rodeo, and in elderly patients. FOOSH injuries can result in ruptures at the musculotendinous junction, whereas excessive tension on a maximally contracted muscle (ie, weight lifting, steer wrestling) can result in avulsion tears from its humeral attachment. Ruptures of the pectoralis major muscle are becoming more common.[63]

Specific History Questions

Most patients recall the specific mechanism of injury and report feeling a tearing or popping sensation. The patient should be asked to point with one finger, if possible, to his or her greatest site of pain or where the tearing/popping sensation was felt. Pain in the bicipital groove is a good indicator of a complete tear.

Inspection

Significant discoloration and swelling can appear over the anterior chest wall, with proximal strains and tears, and in the arm, with strains or tears with distal strains and tears. The muscle is fan shaped, inserts on the humerus, and appears in the upper arm or axilla with a distal tear. If the muscle has torn off its humeral attachment, look for a deformity and loss of contour of the anterior chest wall over the axilla, as the muscle has retracted.

Active ROM with adduction and internal rotation will be affected. The examiner will be able to perform passive movement of the patient's shoulder in all ROMs. Any muscle testing involving the actions of the pectoralis major muscle will appear weak, or the patient may try to compensate with other muscles. Comparison bilaterally is critical to comparing the quality of strength in addition to the quantity.

Palpations With Expected Outcomes

A palpable defect may be felt at the site of the tear; however, it might also be masked by swelling.

Special Tests

There is one special test that best assesses pectoralis major ruptures (**Figure 10.65**).

- **Pectoralis major muscle strength test:** Three strength tests can be performed when a pectoralis major muscle strain or tear is suspected. One test can test sternal fibers, one can test clavicular fibers, and one can be used for both sternal and clavicular fibers. The entire pectoralis major can be tested (ie, both heads) with the patient seated and the glenohumeral joint abducted to 90°. The clinician places one hand around the elbow of the patient and the other hand braces the patient around the scapula. The clinician asks the patient to try to pull his or her arm across the chest (ie, horizontal adduction). The clavicular head can be tested by placing the patient in a seated position; the glenohumeral joint is flexed to approximately 70° to 90° with an extended elbow. The clinician

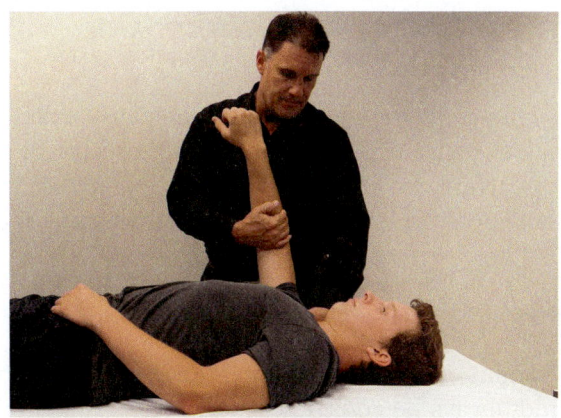

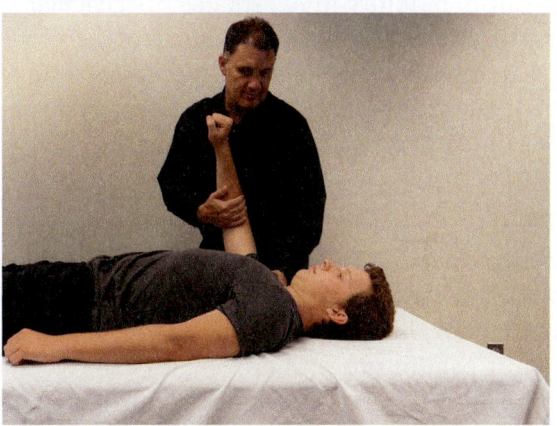

Figure 10.65 Photographs demonstrating the pectoralis major muscle strength test.
© Jones & Bartlett Learning

will apply a downward pressure while the patient applies an upward resistance. The sternal head can be tested in the same seated position, glenohumeral joint flexed to approximately 120°. The clinician places his or her hand around the posterior aspect of the elbow to apply an upward movement force while the patient applies extension resistance (ie, pushes toward the floor).

Radiographic Orders

It is important to refer to a physician for radiographs to rule out bony avulsions or humeral fractures with distal tears. Ultrasonography and MRI can be used to confirm grade; site; and, for complete tears, the amount of retraction of the muscle.[64]

Functional Assessment/Outcome Measures

There are no outcome measures associated with this specific condition. The general shoulder and arm functional assessment and outcome measures can be applied.

Clinical Diagnosis (Differential Diagnosis)

The clinical diagnosis is rather easy to make for complete distal tears because the asymmetry of the affected chest wall will be obvious. In rare cases, a patient could present with a congenital absence of the sternal head of the muscle.

SC Sprain

SC sprains are less common than AC sprains but should always be considered when there is a similar mechanism of injury to AC sprains or clavicular fractures. In particular, falling onto the tip of the shoulder (ie, acromion process) laterally and compressing the clavicle toward the midline of the body could result in SC joint sprains.

Specific History Questions

The mechanism of injury may be similar to AC joint sprains and clavicular fractures, but the painful location is quite different. Ask the patient to point to the most painful site with one finger. The only other structures that could be confused with this location are pectoralis major muscle strains/tears and first/second rib sprains. One unique history question to ask is whether the patient feels any abnormal sounds or sensations, such as clicking around the medial end of the clavicle.

Inspection

The patient should expose the clavicle and its attachment at both the AC and SC joints. If the SC joint is sprained, it will often result in an anterior deformity.

All the same motions that are painful with AC joint sprains and clavicular fractures are also painful with SC joint sprains. However, the pain is more diffuse and less specific to pinpoint for patients with SC joint sprains. Specifically, horizontal adduction will be most painful.

Palpations With Expected Outcomes

There will be pain on palpation on the SC joint and all around the proximal end of the clavicle and manubrium.

Special Tests

There are no special tests for SC joint sprains. However, joint play in a superior-inferior and anterior-posterior direction will result in greater laxity and pain if the SC joint is sprained.

Radiographic Orders

Radiographs to rule out AC sprains, rib fractures, and clavicular fractures are important. However, there is no specific technique for SC joint sprains unless there is a significant displacement of the clavicle medially.

Clinical Diagnosis (Differential Diagnosis)

The clinical diagnosis is easy to make because the painful site is unique. The other structures that are in the same region are the pectoralis major muscle and first two ribs. If the pectoralis major is strained or torn, it will likely result in bruising, whereas the SC joint sprain does not have this sign associated with it. Ribs are not as easy to differentiate from this condition. However, testing rib springing and thoracic spine passive accessory intervertebral motion may help to differentiate rib injuries from SC joint sprains.

Quick Tips for Evaluations for Pathology

In a sideline assessment, knowing and seeing the mechanism of injury can often direct the examiner to be more specific and focus his or her attention to the correct areas. In addition, the way an athlete is holding his or her arm/shoulder can also be useful. If there is equipment, such as in football or hockey, the examiner should be prepared to reach under the shirt and shoulder pads to feel for deformities. A useful acronym for a quick field evaluation is SAM, which stands for skeletal, articular, and muscular. In order of priority evaluation in a secondary survey, the examiner should feel bony structures (ie, skeletal) first to rule out any obvious fractures, such as clavicular or humeral. Then, feel the joints most commonly injured first, such as the GH and AC joints. The AC joint sprain will present with a step deformity and therefore is an easy place to start. If that is clear, move onto the GH joint. Feeling the roundness of the shoulder and in the athlete's armpit is a good quick test to determine if the GH joint is in place. It should be noted that the examiner should be asking the patient to direct him or her to the most painful site while using this SAM process. The final quick test should focus on the various muscles (Table 10.18 provides a summary of special tests). Obvious deformity in muscles that are

Quick Tips for Evaluations for Pathology

Table 10.18 Special Tests and Associated Evidence for the Shoulder

Test	Patient Position	Procedure	Positive Test	Implication
Apprehension test, crank test, and relocation test with a surprise test	Patient supine on the table. Table should support the patient's scapula, but the patient should be far enough over that the humerus and forearm can be off the edge of the table. The patient's elbow should be bent to 90°.	The examiner will slowly take the patient's arm from the side into abduction with the humerus internally rotated. Once the examiner gets the patient's shoulder to 90° of abduction, he or she should begin to slowly externally rotate the glenohumeral joint. It is important to tell the patient that if he or she feels any pain or discomfort to ask the examiner to stop. The examiner should also look for an "apprehensive" look in the patient's face. This can be difficult to assess for novices and may take many forms for different patients, so relying entirely on nonverbal cues of apprehension is not recommended.	Apprehension and pain are the main indicators of a test being positive. Essentially, the patient feels as if his or her shoulder may dislocate or subluxate when the external rotation or the surprise portions of the test are introduced. The patient will likely feel relief with the relocation aspect of the test. A positive crank test is when the patient complains of pain either with or without a clicking sensation.	The apprehension test is a gross test for instability and does not indicate severity or minute changes in laxity. Rather, it merely determines if the patient is apprehensive and therefore has an unstable glenohumeral joint.

Evidence for apprehension test, crank test, and relocation test with a surprise test	Study Author(s)	Special Test	Sensitivity	Specificity	LR+	LR−	QUADAS[a]
	Jia et al, 2009[65]	Apprehension test	0.72	0.96	18.0	0.3	7
	Fowler et al, 2010[66]	Apprehension test—Bankart lesion	0.79	0.82	4.3	0.3	NR
	Fowler et al, 2010[66]	Apprehension test—Hill-Sachs lesion	0.81	0.81	4.2	0.2	NR
	Lo et al, 2004[67]	Surprise test	0.64	0.99	64.0	0.4	
		Apprehension test	0.53	0.99	53.0	0.5	
		Relocation test	0.46	0.54	1.0	1.0	7
	Walsworth et al, 2008[68]	Crank test—Bankart lesion	0.61	0.55	1.4	0.7	11
	Liu et al, 1996[69]	Crank test—Bankart lesion	0.91	0.93	13.0	0.1	9

(continues)

Table 10.18 Special Tests and Associated Evidence for the Shoulder (continued)

Test	Patient Position	Procedure	Positive Test	Implication
Load-and-shift test	The patient should be seated either on a low-back chair or on the edge of the table with his or her arms hanging by the side. It is important for the patient to sit up straight and have proper posture because rounded shoulders could change the angle of the scapula and the angle of the glenoid fossa, shifting the head of the humerus forward.	The first part of the procedure is to evaluate the position of the head of the humerus. It may be more anterior (more common) or more posterior. Again, if the patient is in a slouched position with the scapulae more protracted, it is likely the head is sitting more anteriorly in the glenoid fossa. This is important to note because the "load" part of the test is to center the head of the humerus in the glenoid fossa. From this neutral position of the patient's glenohumeral joint, the "shift" portion of the test measures translation and end feels in both an anterior and posterior direction. The examiner pushes mostly with the thumb to test anterior instability and with the fingers to test posterior instability.	The laxity or translation of the glenohumeral joint should be measured using a grading system that has three grades.	The implications of a positive test are related to how long the problem has existed. If the patient has experienced this problem for a long period of time, the course of treatment may change. Generally, surgical consultation is important when there are positive laxity findings considering the reinjury rate, particularly with athletes younger than 25 years. The more laxity, the more important it may be to seek surgical advice, rather than tightening the shoulder with exercise.

Evidence for load-and-shift test	Study Author(s)	Special Test	Sensitivity	Specificity	LR+	LR−	QUADAS[a]
	McFarland et al, 2009[70]	Anterior instability	0.53	0.85	3.6	0.6	NR

Test	Patient Position	Procedure	Positive Test	Implication
Paxinos test and acromioclavicular palpation	The patient sits in a chair with the arm hanging by his or her side.	The examiner pushes the acromion process anterosuperiorly with the thumb while maintaining counterpressure with the fingers over the clavicle.	A positive test is pain in the acromioclavicular joint. Palpation of the acromioclavicular joint alone also elicits pain if it is sprained.	The amount of pain or movement will be one indicator of severity.

Evidence for Paxinos test	Study Author(s)	Special Test	Sensitivity	Specificity	LR+	LR−	QUADAS[a]
	Walton et al, 2004[26]	Paxinos test	0.79	0.50	1.6	0.4	13
	Walton et al, 2004[26]	AC sprain palpation	0.96	0.10	1.1	0.4	13

Quick Tips for Evaluations for Pathology **395**

Test	Patient Position	Procedure	Positive Test	Implication
O'Brien test	The patient stands and is asked to flex the glenohumeral joint to 90°, then horizontally adduct 10° with the humerus maximally internally rotated.	The examiner asks the patient to push toward the sky while he or she resists this motion (ie, isometric resistance). If there is pain in this position, the patient is asked to externally rotate and resist the flexion movement. If the pain or clicking disappears, this is also considered a positive test.	A positive test is when there is pain with the isometric resistance with the humerus internally rotated. The pain should be located at the acromioclavicular joint, not the anterior aspect of the shoulder, because that is indicative of a potential SLAP lesion. Another differentiating factor to the SLAP lesion is the presence of clicking or a similar sensation at the glenohumeral joint. Again, if the pain disappears or lessens when the arm is externally rotated and flexion resistance is applied, this is also considered a positive sign.	The acromioclavicular joint may be sprained, but, because this test is used for SLAP lesions as well, it is important to perform other acromioclavicular joint sprain tests and SLAP lesion tests to isolate the acromioclavicular sprain diagnosis.

Evidence for O'Brien test	Study Author(s)	Special Test	Sensitivity	Specificity	LR+	LR−	QUADAS[a]
	O'Brien et al, 1998[71]	AC sprain and labral tear	1	0.97	NA	NA	3
	Walton et al, 2004[26]	AC sprain and labral tear	0.16	0.90	1.6	0.9	13

Test	Patient Position	Procedure	Positive Test	Implication
Horizontal adduction test	The patient is usually standing, and this is typically completed as part of active and passive range of motion testing of the shoulder. The patient is asked to abduct the glenohumeral joint to 90°, then horizontally adduct the shoulder with an extended elbow.	Once the patient is unable to horizontally adduct any farther, the patient is asked to relax while the examiner grasps the patient's arm at the elbow joint with one hand and stabilizes the scapula with the other hand. The examiner applies an overpressure into horizontal adduction if the patient can handle the pain.	A positive test is pain in the acromioclavicular joint.	The acromioclavicular joint is stressed or compressed with this motion; pain in the acromioclavicular joint indicates a sprain of the joint. It is important for the patient to point out the painful site because this test is also used to test impingement of various structures in the glenohumeral joint.

(continues)

Table 10.18 Special Tests and Associated Evidence for the Shoulder *(continued)*

Evidence for horizontal adduction test	Study Author(s)	Special Test	Sensitivity	Specificity	LR+	LR−	QUADAS[a]
	Chronopoulos et al, 2004[72]	AC sprain	0.77	0.79	3.7	0.3	NR
	Jia et al, 2009[65]	AC sprain	0.77	0.79	3.7	0.3	6

Test	Patient Position	Procedure	Positive Test			Implication	
Drop arm test	The patient should be standing with the arms at his or her side to start.	This test can be performed during active range of motion testing in the glenohumeral joint for both abduction and adduction. The patient should be instructed to slowly abduct the shoulder, pause at the top, and then slowly lower the arm to his or her side, in a controlled fashion if possible.	A positive test is when the examiner observes the patient's inability to lower the arm to the side in a slow, controlled fashion. In other words, the arm drops without control, usually just after 90° of abduction.			If the patient is unable to control the lowering motion, it is probable he or she has supraspinatus pathology and possibly a tear.	

Evidence for drop arm test	Study Author(s)	Special Test	Sensitivity	Specificity	LR+	LR−	QUADAS[a]
	Nakagawa et al, 2005[73]	Glenohumeral laxity and superior labral tear	0.17	0.93	2.4	0.9	10

Test	Patient Position	Procedure	Positive Test			Implication	
Empty can test	The patient should be standing with the arms at his or her side. The examiner will provide instructions to the patient to abduct the glenohumeral joint to 90°, then horizontally flex the glenohumeral joint to the plane of the scapula (approximately 30°) and internally rotate the humerus fully until the thumb is pointed toward the floor. This final motion is supposed to simulate a patient holding a can or drink in his or her hand and then pouring the drink out by tipping it over completely.	Once the patient is in the empty can position, the examiner asks the patient to hold steady as the examiner pushes the hands toward the ground.	A test is considered positive if there is pain and/or weakness. For more information on how to interpret this test, particularly in relation to the full can test, please refer to what constitutes a positive test under the full can test.			A positive test is indicative of subacromial bursitis, supraspinatus pathology, or both (see notes under the full can test).	

Test	Patient Position	Procedure	Positive Test	Implication
Full can test	The patient should be standing with the arms at his or her side. The examiner will provide instructions to the patient to abduct the glenohumeral joint to 90° and then horizontally flex the glenohumeral joint to the plane of the scapula (approximately 30°).	Once the patient is in the full can position, the examiner asks the patient to hold steady while the examiner pushes the hands toward the ground. The full can position is supposed to simulate the patient holding a can or drink upright, thus not permitting it to spill.	Itoi et al[74] separated a positive test into pain, weakness, or both pain and weakness. Weakness is usually indicative of supraspinatus pathology at varying degrees of tearing with either a positive empty can or full can test. Alqunaee et al[35] suggested that, if the empty can test is positive for pain and the full can test is negative, impingement of the subacromial bursa is likely. However, if both tests are positive, both the subacromial bursa and supraspinatus pathology are suspected.	As highlighted previously, the patient will either have subacromial bursitis, supraspinatus pathology, or both. It is important to cross-reference with other tests to confirm.

Evidence for empty and full can tests	Study Author(s)	Special Test	Sensitivity	Specificity	LR+	LR−	QUADAS[a]
	Alqunaee et al, 2012[35]	Supraspinatus pathology	0.69	0.62	1.8	0.5	NR
	Calis et al, 2000[45]	Supraspinatus pathology	0.15	1	NA	NA	8
	Park et al, 2005[75]	Supraspinatus pathology	0.44	0.90	4.2	0.6	10
	Itoi et al, 1999[74]	Supraspinatus pathology	0.86	0.57	2.0	0.3	9
	Wolf and Agrawal, 2001[76]	Supraspinatus pathology	0.96	0.97	32	0.04	9

(continues)

Table 10.18 Special Tests and Associated Evidence for the Shoulder

(continued)

Test	Patient Position	Procedure	Positive Test	Implication
Rent test	The patient is typically seated on the table with the arms by his or her side.	The examiner passively extends the patient's shoulder while feeling just off the acromion process, just proximal to the greater tuberosity. The examiner will be feeling through the deltoid muscle, but that is also the pathway and attachment of the supraspinatus and infraspinatus muscles.	If the examiner feels a "rent," or small sulcus, where the supraspinatus or infraspinatus muscles insert or travel to the greater tuberosity, the test is considered positive.	A positive test indicates a torn supraspinatus and/or infraspinatus. Due to the proximity of the supraspinatus and infraspinatus ends to each other, further testing would be required to identify the specific muscle/tendon that is impacted.

Evidence for rent test	Study Author(s)	Special Test	Sensitivity	Specificity	LR+	LR−	QUADAS[a]
	Hertel et al, 1996[77]	Infraspinatus	0.70	1	NA	NA	8

Test	Patient Position	Procedure	Positive Test	Implication
External rotation lag sign	The patient is seated with the arms relaxed by his or her side and elbow bent to approximately 90°.	The examiner releases or lets the humerus go from the externally rotated position and asks the patient to hold the position steady.	A positive test is when the patient is unable to hold the arm in the externally rotated position—in other words, it lags.	The implication of a positive test indicates a varying degree of strain or tear of the infraspinatus and/or teres minor muscles.
Hornblower sign	The patient is seated and asked to abduct the glenohumeral joint to 90°.	The patient is asked to actively, in an isometric fashion, push the wrist backward or externally rotate the humerus.	If the patient is unable to provide external rotation resistance, he or she is thought to have either infraspinatus or teres minor pathology.	This may be a partial or full tear, depending on the grade of muscle resistance the patient is able (or unable) to apply.

Evidence for external rotation lag and hornblower signs	Study Author(s)	Special Test	Sensitivity	Specificity	LR+	LR−	QUADAS[a]
	Walch et al, 1998[78]	Infraspinatus and teres minor	1	0.93	NA	NA	3

Quick Tips for Evaluations for Pathology **399**

Test	Patient Position	Procedure	Positive Test	Implication
Lift-off sign	This can be done when the patient is performing active range of motion while standing. He or she is asked to tuck the arm behind the back, then lift the arm off the back.	The patient places his or her arm behind the back, reproducing the motion of tucking one's shirt into the back of the pants. Then, he or she is asked to lift the back of the wrist off his or her own back and hold that position if possible.	A positive test is when the patient cannot put the arm behind the back or he or she is unable to lift the arm off his or her back once it has been tucked behind him or her. Regarding the modification of the test, if the patient is strong but just has trouble getting into the position, it may be more indicative of external rotator or posterior capsule tightness as opposed to weakness in the subscapularis muscle.	If the patient is unable to lift the arm off the back, it may be that the subscapularis muscle is torn or partially torn. The modification described is useful because it helps with the differential diagnosis of a tight posterior capsule or external rotators.
Belly press/ Napoleon test	The patient can be standing or seated with the elbow flexed to 90°, with the humerus internally rotated touching the stomach in a chicken wing–like position.	The patient attempts to maintain the wrist/hand on his or her stomach.	A positive belly-off sign is when the patient is unable to maintain the arm on his or her stomach in the chicken-wing position as the examiner pulls his or her hand away. In the Napoleon test modification, if the patient moves to this chicken-wing position and compensates with wrist flexion, it is considered a positive test.	A partial or complete tear of the subscapularis.
Bear hug test	The patient can be seated or standing with the arm in horizontal adduction. The examiner can also ask the patient to scratch the back of his or her opposite shoulder.	The examiner grabs the patient's arm that is attempting to scratch the back and pulls it off the patient's shoulder slightly. Then, the patient is instructed to hold the arm in that position while the examiner attempts to move the arm back down to a resting position. In other words, the patient attempts to internally rotate from that position while the examiner attempts to externally rotate the humerus. This test should be performed isometrically.	A positive test is when the patient is weak.	Depending on the amount of weakness, the subscapularis muscle could be strained or torn.

(continues)

Table 10.18 Special Tests and Associated Evidence for the Shoulder (continued)

Test	Patient Position	Procedure	Positive Test	Implication
Internal rotation lag sign	The patient can either be standing or seated on a table relaxed with the arm by his or her side.	The patient is asked to relax while the examiner grasps the arms and attempts to pull them behind the back (adduction and internally rotated). It is a similar position to the lift-off position described above, but it is a passive test for the patient. The examiner pulls the patient into maximal internal rotation and asks the patient to maintain this position while the examiner takes away support.	If the patient is unable to maintain the arm in the internally rotated position that the examiner brought him or her to, it is considered a positive test.	The patient could have a torn subscapularis muscle of varying degrees, depending on the patient's strength.

Evidence for Lift-off sign, Belly press/Napoleon test, Bear hug test, Internal rotation lag sign

Study Author(s)	Special Test	Sensitivity	Specificity	LR+	LR−	QUADAS[a]
Hertel et al, 1996[77]	Subscapularis pathology	0.62	1	NA	NA	8
Barth et al, 2006[79]	Subscapularis pathology	0.25	0.98	12.5	0.8	11
Bartsch et al, 2010[80]	Subscapularis pathology	0.86	0.91	9.6	0.2	NR

Test	Patient Position	Procedure	Positive Test	Implication
Sulcus sign	The patient can be seated or standing provided he or she is able to relax the shoulders completely.	The sulcus sign is passive and, therefore, only requires the examiner to view the patient's shoulder/deltoid region. The sulcus test requires the examiner to pull on the humerus distally, away from the glenohumeral joint, and straight down toward the floor (caudad).	A positive test is the sulcus sign or a divot that is created just distal to the acromion process because the head of the humerus slides out of the joint inferiorly. The positive test is the same for both the sign that is completed in the observation phase of the evaluation and the test that is typically completed in the inspection phase of the evaluation.	If there is a positive sulcus sign, it indicates glenohumeral laxity. It is important to compare bilaterally.
Anterior drawer test	The patient is supine with the shoulder abducted between 80° and 120°, forward flexed between 0° and 20°, and externally rotated between 0° and 30°. The patient rests his or her hand in the examiner's axilla.	The examiner grasps the proximal end of the humerus around the humeral neck and pulls it anteriorly, or toward the ceiling.	If the examiner feels excessive anterior translation, it is a positive test. If the patient feels pain, it is also considered positive.	Excessive anterior translation indicates there is glenohumeral laxity that may be contributing to the subacromial impingement. Pain may indicate both laxity and a labral pathology.

Quick Tips for Evaluations for Pathology

	Evidence for anterior drawer test		Sensitivity	Specificity	LR+	LR−	QUADAS[a]
	Study Author(s)	Special Test	0.58	0.92	7.95	0.45	NR
	Van Kampen et al, 2006[81]	Anterior drawer					
Test	Patient Position	Procedure	Positive Test		Implication		
Neer impingement	The patient can be seated or standing, depending on his or her comfort, his or her ability to relax the shoulder as the examiner moves him or her, and his or her height relative to the examiner's height.	The examiner brings the patient's glenohumeral joint from the side into full flexion.	A positive test occurs when there is pain around the subacromial bursa. It is important to have the patient differentiate the site of pain between the subacromial bursa and the long head of the biceps brachii.		A positive test could indicate subacromial impingement of the bursa. However, it may also indicate a superior labral tear, long head of biceps brachii impingement, supraspinatus impingement, or infraspinatus impingement.		
Hawkins-Kennedy test	The patient can be seated or standing with the shoulder completely relaxed while the examiner moves it.	The examiner passively abducts the shoulder, then horizontally adducts the shoulder and internally rotates the humerus.	There is pain in the shoulder that is similar to the type of pain and location the patient normally feels.		It is possible there is impingement of the subacromial bursa, the supraspinatus tendon, or the infraspinatus tendon. A labral tear may also be present.		
Painful arc	This is typically tested with the patient standing during active range of motion testing.	The patient is asked to actively abduct the glenohumeral joint starting with the arm at his or her side and slowly moving to 180° of abduction.	A positive test occurs with pain in the arc of 60° to 120° of abduction. If this is positive and the patient is asked to externally rotate the humerus and he or she feels better, this is also a positive sign.		A positive test could indicate subacromial bursa impingement, supraspinatus impingement, or infraspinatus impingement.		
Horizontal adduction test	The patient can be seated or standing.	The patient is asked to actively horizontally adduct the glenohumeral joint. An overpressure at the end range of motion may be applied gently to provide additional provocation.	A positive test is associated with the location of the pain. With impingement, the pain presents around the subacromial bursa, the long head of biceps brachii, or the superior labrum where the long head of the biceps brachii attaches.		A positive test indicates impingement and subacromial bursitis.		
Posterior impingement test	The patient should be lying down and actively move the glenohumeral joint in the following sequence: abducted to 90° to 110°, slight glenohumeral extension to 10° to 15°, and maximal external rotation.	The patient actively moves the glenohumeral joint in the sequence described above.	A positive test is when the patient experiences deep pain in the posterior part of his or her shoulder.		The deep pain is indicative of internal impingement.		

(continues)

Table 10.18 Special Tests and Associated Evidence for the Shoulder *(continued)*

Evidence for impingement tests	Study Author(s)	Special Test	Sensitivity	Specificity	LR+	LR−	QUADAS[a]
	Alqunaee et al, 2012[35]	Impingement	0.78	0.58	1.9	0.4	NR
	Park et al, 2005[75]	Impingement	0.68	0.69	2.2	0.5	10
	Silva et al, 2008[82]	Impingement	0.68	0.30	1.0	1.1	11
	Alqunaee et al, 2012[35]	Impingement	0.74	0.57	1.7	0.5	NR
	Park et al, 2005[75]	Impingement	0.72	0.66	2.1	0.4	10
	Park et al, 2005[75]	Impingement	0.74	0.81	3.9	0.3	10
	Bassett et al, 2010[83]	Impingement	0.30	0.50	0.6	1.4	11
	Calis et al, 2000[45]	Impingement	0.33	0.81	1.7	0.8	8

Test	Patient Position	Procedure	Positive Test	Implication
Speed test	The patient should be standing with both arms out in front, flexed to approximately 60° with the palms up.	The patient is asked to lift the palms toward the sky while the examiner resists that motion (ie, isometric resisted).	If the patient has pain in the bicipital groove, the test is positive.	It is important for the patient to differentiate, if possible, pain in the bicipital groove from pain at the biceps attachment at the labrum.
Yergason test	The patient is seated with the elbow flexed to 90° and forearm fully pronated.	The patient is asked to supinate the wrist while the examiner resists that motion (ie, isometric testing).	A positive test results in pain in the bicipital groove. The patient may also experience a popping sensation in the bicipital groove.	If the patient is able to differentiate the site of pain between the bicipital groove and the superior labrum, it would be helpful in knowing all the structures involved with this pathology. If there is a popping sensation, the transverse humeral ligament may be torn.
Upper cut test	The patient can be seated or standing, depending on his or her height relative to the examiner's height. The patient should flex the shoulder to approximately 20° to 30° and keep a 90° bend in the elbow, while making a full fist (ie, reproduce the upper cut motion from boxing).	The examiner asks the patient to push up into his or her hand while resisting the upper cut motion.	This may elicit pain in the bicipital groove or a popping sensation in that same spot.	Pain in the bicipital groove indicates biceps pathology, and the popping sensation may indicate a torn transverse humeral ligament.

Evidence for biceps tendon pathology	Study Author(s)	Special Test	Sensitivity	Specificity	LR+	LR−	QUADAS[a]
	Gill et al, 2007[46]	Long head of biceps partial tear	0.50	0.67	1.5	0.75	12
	Oh et al, 2008[41]	Long head of biceps pathology	0.32	0.66	0.9	1.0	11
	Uhl et al, 2009[84]	Long head of biceps pathology	0.54	0.81	2.8	0.6	9
	Jia et al, 2009[65]	Biceps disease	0.50	0.67	1.5	0.8	6
	Uhl et al, 2009[84]	Biceps injury	0.41	0.79	1.9	0.7	9
	Uhl et al, 2009[84]	Biceps injury	0.73	0.78	3.4	0.3	9

Test	Patient Position	Procedure	Positive Test	Implication
Kim test	The patient can be seated (better) or standing with the shoulder relaxed so the examiner can move it.	While one of the examiner's hands is at the elbow (described previously), the other hand cups the head/neck of the humerus just below the glenohumeral joint to apply a downward (inferior) pressure toward the floor, along with a posterior pressure in the direction between six o'clock and nine o'clock, where the labral tear may exist.	A positive test is when the patient feels a clunking sensation or pain in his or her glenohumeral joint.	If there is a positive sign, particularly a clunking sensation, it is likely the posterior inferior labrum was torn when the patient dislocated the shoulder posteriorly.

Evidence for Kim test	Study Author(s)	Special Test	Sensitivity	Specificity	LR+	LR−	QUADAS[a]
	Kim et al, 2005[85]	Posterior inferior labral tear	0.80	0.94	13.3	0.2	9
	Kim et al, 2005[85]	Posterior inferior labral tear	0.73	0.98	36.5	0.3	9

Test	Patient Position	Procedure	Positive Test	Implication
Jerk test	The patient is seated with the arm/shoulder completely relaxed so the examiner can execute the test and shoulder motion.	The examiner applies an axial compression through the elbow toward the glenohumeral joint. Axial compression is maintained while the examiner horizontally adducts the glenohumeral joint.	A positive test is either a clunking sensation or pain in the glenohumeral joint around the six o'clock to nine o'clock position where posterior labral tears occur.	If there is pain alone, it may be possible to have other conditions, such as a tight posterior capsule. However, if there is both pain and a clunk (or click), the patient is likely to have a posterior inferior labral tear.

Evidence for Jerk test	Study Author(s)	Special Test	Sensitivity	Specificity	LR+	LR−	QUADAS[a]
	Nakagawa et al, 2005[73]	Posterior inferior labral tear	0.25	0.80	1.3	0.94	10

(continues)

Table 10.18 Special Tests and Associated Evidence for the Shoulder (continued)

Test	Patient Position	Procedure	Positive Test	Implication
Biceps load test II	The patient lies on a table with the arm relaxed so the examiner can move it for testing purposes.	The examiner passively abducts the patient's shoulder to 120° of abduction, 90° bend in the elbow, and the glenohumeral joint maximally external rotated. The patient is asked to flex the elbow at this stage, and the examiner resists this motion isometrically.	A positive test elicits pain in the superior labrum region where the long head of the biceps brachii tendon attaches. The differential diagnosis for anteroinferior instability is apprehension, so it is important to ask the patient what he or she is feeling and where he or she is feeling it.	Pain usually indicates a SLAP and/or an LHBT pathology.
Compression-rotation test	The patient lies supine on the table with the shoulder relaxed while the examiner moves the glenohumeral joint.	The examiner abducts the patient's glenohumeral joint to 90° with a bent elbow and neutral rotation of the humerus. Then, the examiner applies an axial load to the glenohumeral joint through the elbow and moves the humerus between internal and external rotation trying to catch the torn labrum in the process.	If the patient experiences pain, clicking, grabbing, or a clunking sensation, the test is considered positive.	If there is an abnormal sensation, there is likely a type 2 SLAP lesion.

Evidence for SLAP lesion tests	Study Author(s)	Special Test	Sensitivity	Specificity	LR+	LR−	QUADAS[a]
	Kim et al, 2001[86]	SLAP	0.90	0.97	26.4	0.1	10
	Oh et al, 2008[41]	SLAP	0.30	0.78	1.4	0.9	11
	Cook et al, 2012[90]	SLAP	0.67	0.51	1.4	0.7	NR
	McFarland et al, 2002[70]	SLAP	0.24	0.76	1.0	1.0	11
	Joo et al, 2008[48]	SLAP	0.61	0.54	1.3	0.7	11

Test	Patient Position	Procedure	Positive Test	Implication
Lateral scapular slide test	The patient is asked to stand and abduct the glenohumeral joint to varying degrees.	The examiner measures the distance between the inferior angle of the scapula and the thoracic spine for both right and left shoulders for comparison. This measurement is taken with the patient's shoulder at 0°, 45°, and 90° of abduction.	A positive test is present when there is a difference from side to side greater than 1 to 1.5 cm.	Scapular dyskinesis may be present if there is a bilateral difference in measurements.

Quick Tips for Evaluations for Pathology

	Study Author(s)	Special Test	Sensitivity	Specificity	LR+	LR−	QUADAS[a]
Evidence for scapular lateral slide test	Odom et al, 2001[87] 0° abduction 45° abduction 90° abduction	Interrater ICC[b] = .79 ICC = .45 ICC = .57	0.35 0.41 0.43	0.48 0.54 0.56	0.67 0.89 0.98	1.35 1.09 1.02	11
	Shadmehr et al, 2010[88] 0° abduction 45° abduction 90° abduction	Interrater ICC = .79 ICC = .70 ICC = .63	0.93–1 0.90–0.93 0.86–0.96	0.08–0.23 0.04–0.23 0.04–0.15	1.01 0.97 0.98	0 0.43 0.27	6

Test	Patient Position	Procedure	Positive Test	Implication
Olecranon manubrium percussion test	The patient is seated with his or her arms crossed.	The examiner taps on the olecranon process and listens to the sound through the stethoscope for both right and left sides.	If the examiner experiences different sounds between the affected and unaffected sides, a fracture should be suspected.	If a fracture is suspected, it is important to refer the patient to a physician so radiographs can be ordered.

	Study Author(s)	Special Test	Sensitivity	Specificity	LR+	LR−	QUADAS[a]
Evidence for olecranon manubrium percussion test	Adams et al, 1988[89]	Upper body fractures	0.84	0.99	84.0	0.27	13

Test	Patient Position	Procedure	Positive Test	Implication
Shrug sign	The patient is standing and asked to elevate or abduct the glenohumeral joint.	The patient is asked to elevate or abduct the shoulder actively.	A positive test occurs when the patient tries to abduct the glenohumeral joint but struggles to get full range of motion and, as a result, shrugs his or her shoulder, elevating his or her scapula and engaging his or her upper trapezius and levator scapula muscle in an attempt to gain more range of motion.	A positive test could be frozen shoulder if the patient is also lacking active and passive range of motion, as described previously. However, if the patient has good range otherwise, it may be indicative of rotator cuff pathology.

(continues)

Table 10.18 Special Tests and Associated Evidence for the Shoulder

Evidence for shrug sign	Study Author(s)	Special Test	Sensitivity	Specificity	LR+	LR−	QUADAS[a]
	Jia et al, 2008[65]	Frozen shoulder	0.95	0.50	1.9	0.1	10
Test	**Patient Position**	**Procedure**	**Positive Test**		**Implication**		
Active elevation lag test	The patient is either seated or standing. The patient relaxes while the examiner moves the arm and follows further instructions.	The patient is instructed to sit and move into full extension actively. Right and left sides are done separately for comparison.	A positive test is when the affected side cannot get into as much extension actively compared with the unaffected side.		Spinal accessory nerve pathology may be suspected if the patient is not able to actively move the arm through the full range of motion compared with the good side.		
Evidence for active elevation lag test	Study Author(s)	Special Test	Sensitivity	Specificity	LR+	LR−	QUADAS[a]
	Jia et al, 2008[65]	Rotator cuff pathology	0.96	0.53	2.0	0.1	10

(continued)

[a] QUADAS scores in this chapter are taken from Cook and Hegedus, 2013.[90]
[b] ICC = intraclass correlation coefficient

AC, acromioclavicular; LHBT, long head of biceps tendon; LR−, negative likelihood ratio; NA, not applicable; NR, not reported; QUADAS, Quality Assessment of Diagnostic Accuracy Studies; SLAP, superior labrum anterior to posterior.

completely torn may appear in the pectoralis major, long head of the biceps, or the rotator cuff muscle attachments around the greater tuberosity. This quick testing method is useful to get the examiner more quickly into complete testing, which has been covered in more detail previously.

CASE STUDY

This is a case presented by Butterwick et al.[91] related to a latissimus dorsi rupture. During the steer wrestling event at a rodeo performance, a professional steer wrestler reported to a member of the Canadian Professional Rodeo Sports Medicine Team with an injury to his right arm. In steer wrestling, the cowboy chases a steer while mounted on a horse, reaches down to grab its horns, drops down to the steer, and twists the steer to the ground. The mechanism of injury is similar to pectoralis major muscle strain in which the right shoulder was forced into abduction, external rotation, and horizontal abduction. During the twisting phase, the cowboy reported feeling a pop. He reported experiencing a burning sensation occurring at the superior aspect of the upper arm (ie, triceps brachii). Upon observation, the athletic therapist notices discoloration and swelling appearing over the back of the upper arm. An asymmetry was also noted over the posterolateral thorax. Active range of motion was full, but isometric testing was slightly limited in adduction and internal rotation. MRI was used to confirm the site and size of tear. The patient was successfully treated without surgery.

1. Are large muscles or muscle groups more or less susceptible to muscle tears?
2. What kinds of sports or activities have a large enough force to rupture large muscle groups?
3. What is a key history question the examiner should ask when he or she suspect a muscle rupture?
4. What does a defect in a muscle or tendon feel like and how would the examiner ensure he or she can find it?
5. Does a complete muscle rupture always have extreme pain associated with it?

ONE-IN-A-MILLION CASE STUDY

This is a case study presented by Lafave et al.[92] related to an AC joint sprain and concomitant first rib subluxation. The mechanism of injury is related to a cowboy falling off his horse and landing on the tip of his shoulder (**Figure 10.66**). This is the same mechanism of injury as an AC joint sprain, and, in fact, the patient suffered a definitive AC joint sprain, based on his pain location. However, the unique aspect of this case had to do with the change in sensation or transient neurologic symptoms the patient complained about immediately. In addition to pain in the tip of his shoulder (ie, AC joint), he also complained of a jolt into his "pinky." Due to the fall from a height and the presence of neurologic symptoms, neck evaluation was important to rule out other conditions. Neck motion resulted in somewhat stiff range of motion around the first rib, particularly with side-bending and rotation. Two special tests were completed. The first was rib cephalad to caudad springing. It was hypomobile and sitting more cephalad than the unaffected side. The cervical lateral flexion and rotation test was completed and was also positive. The patient was sent to a physician for follow-up radiographs to confirm the AC joint sprain. He also had a first rib sprain that was in an elevated position. Traditional AC joint sprain treatment was implemented as well as first rib mobilization. The first rib mobilization resulted in almost immediate relief for the patient, taking pressure off the AC joint because it had been pushing upward on the clavicle.

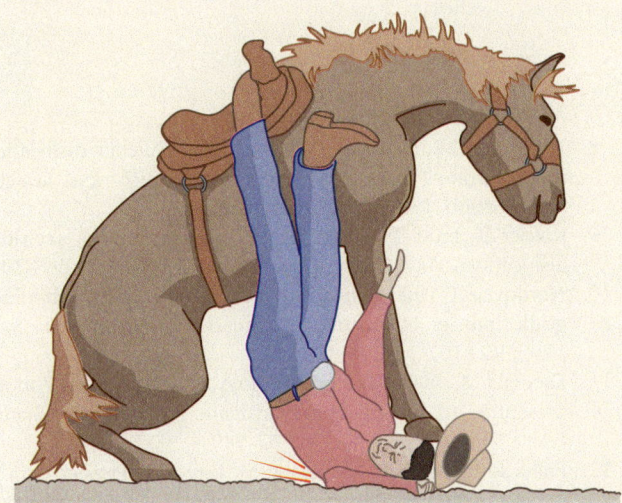

Figure 10.66 The mechanism of injury related to a rider falling off his horse and landing on the tip of his shoulder.

© Jones & Bartlett Learning

WRAP-UP

Critical Thinking Questions

1. The shoulder complex is a complicated body region due to several joint, muscle, and ligament injuries that can occur. Is there a way to simplify evaluation of the shoulder complex and identify diagnoses?
2. What are the common mechanisms of injury for shoulder conditions?
3. What shoulder conditions are more commonly associated with chronic mechanisms of injury as compared to acute or traumatic mechanisms of injury?
4. When are conditions serious enough to require immediate care from a physician or hospital? What are the signs and symptoms that would help make this determination?
5. When working through the evaluation process for the shoulder, what are some of the key history questions that help to determine the types of special tests that will be required to confirm a diagnosis?

Pearls and Pitfalls

- The shoulder complex is complicated and should be broken into various components.
- The FOOSH mechanism of injury is common but is not always associated with a single shoulder condition. Therefore, it is important to know all the conditions that could be associated with this mechanism of injury and have an arsenal of special tests that can help identify or eliminate those shoulder conditions. It is important not to jump to conclusions before the examiner has all the information.
- It is possible to have more than one condition; therefore, if an examiner finds a positive special test, it is important to continue to test other structures.
- When working in a sports or activity setting, knowing a shortened version of evaluation is important because the patient may need to be transported for additional care and observation. Therefore, it is important to identify some of those "yellow flags" early in the evaluation process to avoid further injury or damage.
- In the initial stages of developing evaluation skills for the shoulder, it may be important to keep good notes as the examiner goes through various components of the evaluation. There are a number of joints in the shoulder complex with more ROM to track than any other joint.

References

1. Oatis C: *Kinesiology: The Mechanics & Pathomechanics of Human Movement.* Philadelphia, PA, Lippincott Williams & Wilkins, 2004.
2. Magee DJ: *Orthopedic Physical Assessment*, vol 5. Toronto, Saunders, 2008.
3. Moore KL, Dalley AF: *Clinically Oriented Anatomy*, vol 5. Philadelphia: Lippincott, Williams and Wilkins, 2006.
4. Kibler WB, Ludewig PM, McClure PW, Michener LA, Bak K, Sciascia AD: Clinical implications of scapular dyskinesis in shoulder injury: the 2013 consensus statement from the "scapular summit." *Br J Sports Med* 2013;47(14):877-885.
5. Cyriax J: *Textbook of Orthopedic Medicine.* London: Bailliere Tindall, 1982.
6. Hegedus EJ, Cook C, Lewis J, Wright A, Park JY: Combining orthopedic special tests to improve diagnosis of shoulder pathology. *Phys Ther Sport* 2015;16(2):87-92.
7. Shields DW, Jefferies JG, Brooksbank AJ, Millar N, Jenkins PJ: Epidemiology of glenohumeral dislocation and subsequent instability in an urban population. *J Shoulder Elb Surg* 2018;27(2):189-195.
8. Waterman BR, Belmont PJ, Owens BD: Patellar dislocation in the United States: role of sex, age, race, and athletic participation. *J Knee Surg* 2012;1(212):51-58.
9. Krøner K, Lind T, Jensen J: The epidemiology of shoulder dislocations. *Arch Orthop Trauma Surg* 1989;108(5):288-290.
10. Nordqvist A, Petersson CJ: Incidence and causes of shoulder girdle injuries in an urban population. *J Shoulder Elb Surg* 1995;4(2):107-112.
11. Zacchilli M, Owens B: Epidemiology of shoulder dislocations presenting to emergency departments in the United States. *J Bone Joint Surg* 2010;92(3):542-549.
12. Frank RM, Chalmers PN, Moric M, Leroux T, Provencher MT, Romeo AA: Incidence and changing trends of shoulder stabilization in the United States. *Arthroscopy* 2018;34(3):784-792.
13. Kraeutler MJ, McCarty EC, Belk JW, et al: Descriptive epidemiology of the MOON shoulder instability cohort. *Am J Sports Med* 2018;46(5):1064-1069.
14. Atef A, El-Tantawy A, Gad H, Hefeda M: Prevalence of associated injuries after anterior shoulder dislocation: a prospective study. *Int Orthop* 2016;40(3):519-524.

15. Lippitt S, Harryman D, Matsen F: A practical tool for evaluating function: the Simple Shoulder Test, in *The Shoulder: A Balance of Mobility and Stability*. Rosemont, IL: American Academy of Orthopaedic Surgeons, 1993, pp 501-518.
16. Dawson J, Fitzpatrick R, Murray D, Carr A: Questionnaire on the perceptions of patients about total knee replacement. *J Bone Joint Surg Br* 1998;80(1):63-69.
17. Hudak PL, Amadio PC, Bombardier C: Development of an upper extremity outcome measure: the DASH (disabilities of the arm, shoulder, and head). *Am J Ind Med* 1996;29(6):602-608.
18. Roy JS, Macdermid JC, Woodhouse LJ: Measuring shoulder function: a systematic review of four questionnaires. *Arthritis Care Res* 2009;61(5):623-632.
19. Slobogean GP, Slobogean BL: Measuring shoulder injury function: common scales and checklists. *Injury* 2011;42(3):248-252.
20. Hollinshead RM, Mohtadi NGH, Vande Guchte RA, Wadey VMR: Two 6-year follow-up studies of large and massive rotator cuff tears: comparison of outcome measures. *J Shoulder Elb Surg* 2000;9(5):373-379.
21. Schmidt S, Ferrer M, González M, et al: Evaluation of shoulder-specific patient-reported outcome measures: A systematic and standardized comparison of available evidence. *J Shoulder Elb Surg* 2014;23(3):434-444.
22. Ringenberg JD, Foughty Z, Hall AD, Aldridge JM 3rd, Wilson JB, Kuremsky MA. Interobserver and intraobserver reliability of radiographic classification of acromioclavicular joint dislocations. *J Shoulder Elbow Surg*. 2018 Mar;27(3):538-544. Epub 2017 Nov 22.
23. Rockwood C, Matsen F: *The Shoulder*, ed 4. Philadelphia, PA, Saunders Elsevier, 2009.
24. Hibberd EE, Kerr ZY, Roos KG, Djoko A, Dompier TP: Epidemiology of acromioclavicular joint sprains in 25 National Collegiate Athletic Association Sports: 2009-2010 to 2014-2015 academic years. *Am J Sports Med* 2016;44(10):2667-2674.
25. Starkey C, Brown SD, Ryan J: *Examination of Orthopedic and Athletic Injuries*, vol 3. Philadelphia, FA Davis, 2010.
26. Walton J, Mahajan S, Paxinos A, et al: Diagnostic values of tests for acromioclavicular joint pain. *J Bone Joint Surgery Am* 2004;86(4):807-812.
27. Pallis M, Cameron KL, Svoboda SJ, Owens BD: Epidemiology of acromioclavicular joint injury in young athletes. *Am J Sports Med* 2012;40(9):2072-2077.
28. Whiting W, Zernicke R: *Biomechanics of Musculoskeletal Injury*, ed 2. Champaign, IL, Human Kinetics, 2008.
29. Pauly S, Kraus N, Greiner S, Scheibel M. Prevalence and pattern of glenohumeral injuries among acute high-grade acromioclavicular joint instabilities. *J Shoulder Elbow Surg*. 2013 Jun;22(6):760-766. Epub September 28, 2012.
30. Michener LA, Sharma S, Cools AM, Timmons MK: Relative scapular muscle activity ratios are altered in subacromial pain syndrome. *J Shoulder Elb Surg* 2016;25(11):1861-1867.
31. Cools AM, Cambier D, Witvrouw EE: Screening the athlete's shoulder for impingement symptoms: A clinical reasoning algorithm for early detection of shoulder pathology. *Br J Sports Med* 2008;42(8):628-635.
32. de Oliveira FCL, Bouyer LJ, Ager AL, Roy JS: Electromyographic analysis of rotator cuff muscles in patients with rotator cuff tendinopathy: a systematic review. *J Electromyogr Kinesiol* 2017;35:100-114.
33. Myers JB, Laudner KG, Pasquale MR, Bradley JP, Lephart SM: Glenohumeral range of motion deficits and posterior shoulder tightness in throwers with pathologic internal impingement. *Am J Sports Med* 2006;34(3):385-391.
34. Litaker D, Pioro M, El Bilbeisi H, Brems J: Returning to the bedside: using the history and physical examination to identify rotator cuff tears. *J Am Geriatr Soc* 2000;48(12):1633-1637.
35. Alqunaee M, Galvin R, Fahey T: Diagnostic accuracy of clinical tests for subacromial impingement syndrome: a systematic review and meta-analysis. *Arch Phys Med Rehabil* 2012;93(2):229-236.
36. Eubank BH, Mohtadi NG, Lafave MR, et al: Using the modified Delphi method to establish clinical consensus for the diagnosis and treatment of patients with rotator cuff pathology. *BMC Med Res Methodol* 2016;16(1).
37. Bachmann GF, Melzer C, Heinrichs CM, Möhring B, Rominger MB: Diagnosis of rotator cuff lesions: comparison of US and MRI on 38 joint specimens. *Eur Radiol* 1997;7(2):192-197.
38. De Jesus JO, Parker L, Frangos AJ, Nazarian LN: Accuracy of MRI, MR arthrography, and ultrasound in the diagnosis of rotator cuff tears: a meta-analysis. *Am J Roentgenol* 2009;192(6):1701-1707.
39. Longo U, Franceschi F, Berton A, Maffulli N, Denaro V: Conservative treatment and rotator cuff tear progression. *Med Sport Sci* 2012;57:90-99.
40. Kirkley A, Alvarez C, Griffin S: The development and evaluation of a disease-specific quality of life questionnaire for disorders of the rotator cuff: the Western Ontario Rotator Cuff Index. *Clin J Sport Med* 2003;13:84-92.
41. Oh JH1, Kim SH, Lee HK, Jo KH, Bae KJ. Transrotator cuff portal is safe for arthroscopic superior labral anterior and posterior lesion repair: clinical and radiological analysis of 58 SLAP lesions. *Am J Sports Med*. 2008 Oct;36(10):1913-21. Epub 2008 May 21.
42. Tae SK, Rhee YG, Park TS, et al: The development and validation of an appraisal method for rotator cuff disorders: the Korean Shoulder Scoring System. *J Shoulder Elb Surg* 2009;18(5):689-696.
43. Iossifidis A, Ibrahim EF, Petrou C, Galanos A: The development and validation of a questionnaire for rotator cuff disorders: the Functional Shoulder Score. *Shoulder Elb* 2015;7(4):256-267.
44. Khazzam M, George MS, Churchill RS, Kuhn JE: Disorders of the long head of biceps tendon. *J Shoulder Elb Surg* 2012;21(1):136-145.
45. Çalis M, Akgün K, Birtane M, Karacan I, Çalis H, Tüzün F: Diagnostic values of clinical diagnostic tests in subacromial impingement syndrome. *Ann Rheum Dis* 2000;59(1):44-47.
46. Gill HS, El Rassi G, Bahk MS, Castillo RC, McFarland EG: Physical examination for partial tears of the biceps tendon. *Am J Sports Med* 2007;35(8):1334-1340.
47. Virk M, Cole B: Proximal biceps tendon and rotator cuff tears. *Clin Sport Med* 2016;35:153-161.
48. Joo HO, Jae YK, Woo SK, Hyun SG, Ji HL: The evaluation of various physical examinations for the diagnosis of type II superior labrum anterior and posterior lesion. *Am J Sports Med* 2008;36(2):353-359.
49. Taylor SA, Newman AM, Nguyen J, et al: Magnetic resonance imaging currently fails to fully evaluate the biceps-labrum complex and bicipital tunnel. *Arthroscopy* 2016;32(2):238-244.
50. Snyder S, Karzel R, Del Pizzo W, Ferkel R, Friedman M: SLAP lesions of the shoulder. *Arthroscopy* 1990;6(4):274-279.
51. Calcei JG, Boddapati V, Altchek DW, Camp CL, Dines JS: Diagnosis and treatment of injuries to the biceps and superior

labral complex in overhead athletes. *Curr Rev Musculoskelet Med* 2018;11(1):63-71.

52. Symanski J, Subhas N, Babb J, Nicholson J, Gyftopoulos S: Diagnosis of superior labrum anterior-to-posterior tears by using MR imaging and MR arthrography. *Radiology* 2017;285(1):101-113.

53. Hickey D, Solvig V, Cavalheri V, Harrold M, Mckenna L: Scapular dyskinesis increases the risk of future shoulder pain by 43% in asymptomatic athletes: a systematic review and meta-analysis. *Br J Sports Med* 2018;52(2):102-110.

54. Lange T, Struyf F, Schmitt J, Lützner J, Kopkow C: The reliability of physical examination tests for the clinical assessment of scapular dyskinesis in subjects with shoulder complaints: a systematic review. *Phys Ther Sport* 2017;26:64-89.

55. Kibler WB: The role of the scapula in athletic shoulder function. *Am J Sports Med* 1998;26(2):325-337.

56. Wright AA, Wassinger CA, Frank M, Michener LA, Hegedus EJ: Diagnostic accuracy of scapular physical examination tests for shoulder disorders: a systematic review. *Br J Sports Med* 2013;47(14):886-892.

57. Suecki D, Brechter J: *Orthopedic Rehabilitation Clinical Advisor*. Maryland Heights, MO, Mosby Elsevier, 2010.

58. Kannus P, Palvanen M, Niemi S: Osteoporotic fractures of the proximal humeral in elderly Finnish persons: sharp increase in 1970-1998 and alarming projections for the new millennium. *Acta Orthop Scand* 2000;71(5):465-470.

59. Safran MR: Nerve injury about the shoulder in athletes, part 1: suprascapular nerve and axillary nerve. *Am J Sports Med* 2004;32(3):803-819.

60. Perlmutter GS, Apruzzese W: Axillary nerve injuries in contact sports: recommendations for treatment and rehabilitation. *Sport Med* 1998;26(5):351-361.

61. Hertel R, Lambert M, Ballmer F: The deltoid extension lag sign for diagnosis of axillary nerve palsy. *J Shoulder Elb Surg* 1998;7(2):5-7.

62. Safran MR: Nerve injury about the shoulder in athletes, part 2: long thoracic nerve, spinal accessory nerve, burners/stingers, thoracic outlet syndrome. *Am J Sports Med* 2004;32(4):1063-1076.

63. de Castro Pochini A, Ejnisman B, Andreoli C V, et al: Pectoralis major muscle rupture in athletes: a prospective study. *Am J Sports Med* 2010;38(1):92-98.

64. Petilon J, Carr DR, Sekiya JK, Unger DV: Pectoralis major muscle injuries: evaluation and management. *J Am Acad Orthop Surg* 2005;13(1):59-68.

65. Jia X, Petersen SA, Khosravi AH, Almareddi V, Pannirselvam V, McFarland EG: Examination of the shoulder: the past, the present, and the future. *J Bone Joint Surg* 2009;91(Suppl 6):10-18.

66. Fowler EM, Horsley IG, Rolf CG: Clinical and arthroscopic findings in recreationally active patients. *Sport Med Arthrosc Rehabil Ther Technol* 2010;2(1).

67. Lo IKY, Nonweiler B, Woolfrey M, Litchfield R, Kirkley A: An evaluation of the apprehension, relocation, and surprise tests for anterior shoulder instability. *Am J Sports Med* 2004;32(2):301-307.

68. Walsworth MK, Doukas WC, Murphy KP, Mielcarek BJ, Michener LA: Reliability and diagnostic accuracy of history and physical examination for diagnosing glenoid labral tears. *Am J Sports Med* 2008;36(1):162-168.

69. Liu SH, Henry MH, Nuccion SL: A prospective evaluation of a new physical examination in predicting glenoid labral tears. *Am J Sports Med* 1996;24(6):721-725.

70. McFarland EG, Garzon-Muvdi J, Jia X, Desai P, Petersen SA: Clinical and diagnostic tests for shoulder disorders: a critical review. *Br J Sports Med* 2010;44(5):328-332.

71. O'Brien SJ, Pagnani MJ, Fealy S, McGlynn SR, Wilson JB: The active compression test: a new and effective test for diagnosing labral tears and acromioclavicular joint abnormality. *Am J Sports Med* 1998;26(5):610-613.

72. Chronopoulos E, Kim TK, Park HB, Ashenbrenner D, McFarland EG: Diagnostic value of physical tests for isolated chronic acromioclavicular lesions. *AJSM:* 2004;32(3):665.

73. Nakagawa S, Yoneda M, Hayashida K, Obata M, Fukushima S, Miyazaki Y: Forced shoulder abduction and elbow flexion test: a new simple clinical test to detect superior labral injury in the throwing shoulder. *Arthroscopy* 2005;21(11):1290-1295.

74. Itoi E, Kido T, Sano A, Urayama M, Sato K: Which is more useful, the "full can test" or the "empty can test," in detecting the torn supraspinatus tendon? *Am J Sports Med* 1999;27(1):65-68.

75. Park HB, Yokota A, Gill HS, El Rassi G, McFarland EG: Diagnostic accuracy of clinical tests for the different degrees of subacromial impingement syndrome. *J Bone Joint Surg* 2005;87(7):1446-1455.

76. Wolf EM, Agrawal V: Transdeltoid palpation (the rent test) in the diagnosis of rotator cuff tears. *J Shoulder Elb Surg* 2001;10(5):470-473.

77. Hertel J, Lambert M, Gerber C: Lag signs in the diagnosis of rotator cuff rupture. *J Shoulder Elbow Surg* 1996;5(4):307-313.

78. Walch G, Boulahia A, Calderone S, Robinson A: The "dropping" and "hornblower's" signs in evaluation of rotator cuff tears. *J Bone Joint Surg Br* 1998;80(4):624-628.

79. Barth JRH, Burkhart SS, De Beer JF: The bear-hug test: a new and sensitive test for diagnosing a subscapularis tear. *Arthroscopy* 2006;22(10):1076-1084.

80. Bartsch M, Greiner S, Haas NP, Scheibel M: Diagnostic values of clinical tests for subscapularis lesions. *Knee Surg Sport Traumatol Arthrosc* 2010;18(12):1712-1717.

81. Van Kampen DA, Lovell MR, Pardini JE, Collins MW, Fu FH: The "value added" of neurocognitive testing after sports-related concussion. *Am J Sports Med* 2006;34(10):1630.

82. Silva L, Andréu JL, Muñoz P, et al: Accuracy of physical examination in subacromial impingement syndrome. *Rheumatology* 2008;47(5):679-683.

83. Bassett K, Lingman, Ellis R: The use and treatment efficacy of kinaesthetic taping for musculoskeletal conditions: a systematic review. *New Zeal J Physiother* 2010;38(2):56-62.

84. Uhl TL, Kibler WB, Gecewich B, Tripp BL: Evaluation of clinical assessment methods for scapular dyskinesis. *Arthroscopy* 2009;25(11):1240-1248.

85. Kim SH, Park JS, Jeong WK, Shin SK: The Kim test: a novel test for posteroinferior labral lesion of the shoulder: a comparison to the Jerk test. *Am J Sports Med* 2005;33(8):1188-1192.

86. Kim SH, Ha KI, Ahn JH, Kim SH, Choi HJ: Biceps load test II: a clinical test for SLAP lesions of the shoulder. *Arthroscopy* 2001;17(2):160-164.

87. Odom CJ, Taylor AB, Hurd CE, Denegar CR: Measurement of scapular asymmetry and assessment of shoulder dysfunction using the lateral scapular slide test: a reliability and validity study. *Phys Ther* 2001;81(2):799-809.

88. Shadmehr A, Bagheri H, Ansari NN, Sarafraz H: The reliability measurements of lateral scapular slide test at three

different degrees of shoulder joint abduction. *Br J Sports Med* 2010;44(4):289-293.
89. Adams S, Yarnold P: Clinical use of the olecranon-manubrium percussion sign in shoulder trauma. *Ann Emerg Med* 1988;17(5):484-487.
90. Cook C, Hegedus E: *Orthopedic Physical Examination Tests*. ed 2. Boston, Pearson, 2013.
91. Butterwick DJ, Mohtadi NG, Meeuwisse WH, Frizzell JB: Rupture of latissimus dorsi in an athlete. *Clin J Sport Med* 2003;13(3):189-191.
92. Lafave MR, Butterwick DJ, Bugg B, Roberts D: 1st degree acromioclavicular sprain, elevated 1st rib, or both: a case study of a rodeo cowboy. *Open J Ther Rehabil* 2014;2014.

CHAPTER 11

Abdomen and Thorax

Mikaela Boham, EdD, LAT, ATC

OVERVIEW

Injuries to the thoracic and abdominal cavities have a decreased incidence compared to injuries to the extremities. However, injuries to the heart, lungs, and visceral organs can be serious and may even be life threatening. Early identification of injuries to the thorax and abdomen is important for treatment and the best patient outcomes.

LEARNING OBJECTIVES

After completing this chapter, the reader will be able to do the following:

1. Understand and identify the anatomy associated with the thorax and abdomen.
2. Be familiar with techniques associated with assessing thoracic and abdominal injuries.
3. Recognize common injuries in the thorax and abdominal regions.
4. Identify medical emergencies associated with the thorax and abdomen.
5. Explain measures used to prevent injuries to the thorax and abdomen.

FUN FACTS ABOUT THE ABDOMEN AND THORAX

- The heart lies in the thoracic cavity; it is slightly larger than a patient's clenched fist.
- The ribs move like a bucket handle, swinging upward during each breath, allowing the thoracic cavity to expand, and then swinging downward as a person exhales and breathes out, compressing the thoracic cavity.
- It has been said women have more ribs than men. Sex plays no part in the number of ribs a person has: everyone has 12 ribs. However, regardless of sex, approximately 20% of individuals do have an "extra" rib called a cervical rib.
- Although the ribs are resilient, a rib fracture can occur during sneezing or coughing. Forceful vomiting can also result in a rib fracture.
- When a person blushes, the lining of the stomach also turns red.
- The longest attack of constant hiccups lasted 68 years.
- The liver weighs about the same as a Chihuahua (often as much as 3 lb).

Introduction

The thoracic cavity houses the heart and lungs, which are responsible for maintaining body homeostasis and signs of life.[1] The heart and lungs are protected by the ribs in the thoracic cavity. Muscles surround and protect the internal organs of the abdomen and are less protected because they are not covered by the bony structure of the rib cage. The organs of the abdomen include the liver; the spleen; and the organs of the digestive, urinary, and reproductive systems.[2] The thoracic and abdominal cavities protect these internal structures well; however, blunt-force trauma or subtle abnormalities can result in damage to the organs and may result in life-threatening injuries. The abdominal organs are resilient to trauma because they are not attached to the skeletal system, which increases their ability to absorb shock and distribute forces during trauma. The internal organs, not including the liver, are largely hollow, providing additional shock-absorbing capabilities.

Injuries to the visceral organs in the abdominal cavity and thoracic cavity can range from minor to severe to catastrophic.[1,2] Understanding the signs and symptoms, mechanisms of injury, and body systems is imperative for the proper management and recognition of these conditions. In many instances, injuries to the abdominal and thoracic cavities are progressive in nature, so early intervention and follow-up examinations and evaluations of the involved structures are important to the quality of care required to treat these injuries.

In the past, conditions affecting the heart, lungs, or visceral organs may have resulted in elimination of physical activity for an individual. Advancements in knowledge, treatment, and care have allowed more individuals to participate in exercise activities, even following organ transplant. Exercise is a vital component to overall physical and mental health and well-being, so safe participation is important for all individuals.

Unique/Special History Questions

Pain in the thoracoabdominal region may be the result of trauma or a new or chronic medical condition. For example, low back pain may be the result of an infection in the kidney or trauma to the low back.

Injuries to the internal organs and ribs commonly are a result of high-velocity trauma to the affected area, resulting in trauma to the area directly below the point(s) of impact.[2] Individuals may also have a contrecoup injury, in which organs on the opposite side of the point of impact may be injured when they rebound off bony structures following the impact. These conditions may not present immediately after the impact but can progress quickly into life-threatening conditions for the patient.[2]

Past Medical History

Some conditions that once eliminated individuals from participation in physical activity now may be managed with the use of medications and other medical treatments. Strenuous physical activity is no longer precluded for conditions such as cystic fibrosis, asthma, HIV infection, spastic colitis, Crohn disease, renal disease, hypertension, and undescended testicles. Identifying preexisting medical conditions can provide patients with thorough medical care and allow for safe participation in exercise and physical activity.

General Medical History

An individual's medical history is important to document. In cases such as exercise-induced asthma, the patient may have a history of asthmatic conditions, or this may be a new complaint. Patients may have other illnesses that may predispose the internal organs to acute or chronic injuries; for example, mononucleosis can enlarge the spleen and expose the organ to an increased incidence of injury.

Cardiac events may go unrecognized or unreported in individuals who are physically active.[1] Asking patients about their history of previous symptoms and any family history of cardiovascular disease may help identify potential future issues.[3]

Family Medical History

A thorough family history may help to identify individuals potentially at high risk for cardiopulmonary distress.[3] A family history of cardiac abnormalities, disorders, and conditions as well as cardiac-related sudden death may predispose a patient to cardiac disability because many of these conditions have a hereditary component.[3-5] Conditions such as hypertrophic cardiomyopathy, myocardial infarctions, and other heart-related conditions may increase the risk of a cardiac event resulting in sudden death.[1,3-5] The preparticipation medical history questionnaire may help to identify any family history of cardiac-related sudden death and any identifiers should warrant a full examination by a cardiologist.[3]

Medication and Drug Use

Clinicians should be sure to ask questions regarding recent use of prescription medications, drugs, alcohol, and tobacco because these substances may alter a patient's normal cardiovascular or respiratory function.[3]

Mechanism of Injury

The questions the clinician should ask to evaluate thoracic and abdominal injuries are somewhat different from questions commonly used to evaluate musculoskeletal injuries of the extremities. The primary mechanism of injury should be assessed first.

- What happened?
- What activity were you doing when you started having pain or discomfort?
- Was there direct contact or a direct blow?
- What position were you in during the trauma?
- What type of pain are you experiencing? (Is the pain sharp, shooting, dull, localized, etc.?)

- Do you feel any pain other than in the area where the injury occurred?
- Do you have any radiating pain away from the source of pain?
  - Is there any burning, numbness, or tingling (paresthesia) of hands, arms, neck, back, legs, or feet following the injury?
  - Is there any decrease in sensation in hands, arms, neck, back, legs, or feet?
  - Can you move your hands and/or feet?
  - Is there any weakness in legs or feet? (Please instruct your patients to toe-walk and heel-walk to look for a normal gait.)
- Are certain positions more comfortable than others?
- Did you notice any unusual sounds, such as a pop, snap, or crack, during the episode?
  - Did you hear or feel a pop, snap, or crack in your chest?
- Are you experiencing any catching, slipping, or locking sensations?
- Have you had any muscle spasms?
- Do you have a headache, dizziness, nausea, tinnitus, etc.?
- Have you experienced any vomiting or vomiting of blood?
- Have you had any difficulty or pain during urination?
  - Was your bladder full or empty during impact?
- Have you experienced any blood in the urine? Have you experienced any changes in bowel or bladder signs?
  - How long has it been since you have eaten?
  - Is there a personal or family history of any heart problems, abdominal issues, or other diseases involving the thorax and abdomen that you are aware of?

Onset of the Injury/Illness

Determining when the injury occurred is very important because many abdominal and thoracic injuries do not present immediately after trauma.

- Was this a sudden episode, or did the condition become painful or make you ill over time?
- Did the symptoms have an acute or chronic/insidious onset?

Breathing Evaluation

Maintaining airway and breathing is essential to sustain life; altered breathing mechanics may cause issues with respiratory function resulting in altered respiratory chemistry, which induces muscle contraction due to changes in pH levels, electrolyte imbalance, and decreased tissue oxygenation.[6] Although severe breathing issues are rare, a clinician should continuously monitor an injured patient for changes in respiration and respiratory patterns.

- Is the patient breathing?
- Have you had any difficulty breathing or trying to catch your breath?
- Are you experiencing any breathing pain?
- Is the patient refusing to take a deep breath or is breathing shallow?
- Is there symmetry in movement of the ribs and chest during breathing?
- If the patient had the "wind knocked out of them," did normal breathing returning rapidly, or is there prolonged difficulty?

Table 11.1 includes an overview of clinical deductions based on responses.

Table 11.1 Possible Clinical Deductions

Mechanism of Injury	
What happened? What activity were you doing when you started having pain or discomfort?	Please note that the patient may not know or remember the onset of the activity because some conditions are cumulative or chronic rather than acute.
Was there direct contact or a direct blow?	A contusion to the abdomen may injure an internal organ, either on the same or opposite side of the direct trauma. It is important for the clinician to note it may take hours for pain from an injury to be noticed by a patient, such as in the case of internal bleeding and the accumulation of blood within an organ or the abdominal cavity.
Do you have any radiating pain away from the source of pain?	Pain radiating into the buttocks or down into one leg or both legs may indicate neurologic involvement. Pain radiating into the left upper quadrant or left shoulder, also known as Kehr sign, may indicate a ruptured spleen, which is then irritating the diaphragm.

(continues)

Table 11.1 Possible Clinical Deductions (continued)

Mechanism of Injury

	Referred pain may also occur in musculoskeletal areas, such as the ribs, cartilage, or abdominal area. Patients will usually report pain or tenderness at the site of pain.
	Referred pain from internal organs may result in diffuse pain, referred pain, or pain at rest.
Do you have a headache, dizziness, nausea, tinnitus, etc.?	These signs and symptoms may indicate the presence of a head injury, such as a sports concussion, mild traumatic injury of the head, or traumatic brain injury. Concussions may result from a direct blow to the head or a force on the chest or back that results in a whipping motion ("whiplash") of the head. Nausea and vomiting can also indicate abdominal injury.
Have you experienced any vomiting or vomiting of blood?	Vomiting or vomiting of blood may indicate an internal organ injury, a genital injury, or a possible ulcer.
Have you experienced any blood in the urine?	Hematuria, or blood in the urine, may indicate an internal organ injury, a genital injury, a urinary tract infection, or a sexually transmitted infection.
Have you experienced any changes in bowel or bladder signs?	A condition known as cauda equina syndrome, which is the result of a lower nerve root lesion, may alter a patient's ability to control his or her bowel or bladder.

Onset of Injury

Did the symptoms have an acute or chronic/insidious onset?	If the clinician suspects the mechanism of injury was the result of axial loading, the patient should be evaluated and referred to an emergency department immediately.
	A spinal fracture may be a medical emergency and needs to be treated conservatively and as rapidly as possible.
	Ultrasonography or radiographs may be necessary to help evaluate possible spinal, sternum, or rib injuries.

Breathing Evaluation

Is the patient breathing?	If the patient is not breathing, assess pulse.
	If the patient has a pulse but is not breathing, then initiate rescue breathing.
	If the patient does not have a pulse and is not breathing, then initiate cardiopulmonary resuscitation.
Have you had any difficulty breathing or trying to catch your breath?	Hyperventilation, asthma, rib injury, or lung injury should be suspected. Attempt to help the patient slow his or her breathing.
	Mirror breathing, or having the individual mimic your breathing; pursing the lips as if blowing a kiss; or plugging one nostril can aid to slow down rapid breathing.
Are you experiencing any breathing pain?	Difficulty breathing may be associated with rib trauma or fracture, costal cartilage injury, asthma, muscle spasm, or the incidence of shock.
Is the patient refusing to take a deep breath or breathing shallowly?	Difficulty breathing may be associated with rib trauma or fracture, costal cartilage injury, asthma, muscle spasm, or the incidence of shock.
Is there symmetry in the movement of the ribs and chest during breathing?	A costochondral or lung injury may not allow the rib cage to be symmetrical during inspiration and expiration.
If the patient had the "wind knocked out of them," is normal breathing returning rapidly or is there prolonged difficulty?	Prolonged difficulty may indicate a more serious or severe internal thoracic injury.

Observation

Functional Inspection

A clinician should observe the patient's overall posture. Leaning of the thorax to the affected side may indicate the patient is trying to protect an injury on that side, is experiencing cramps, or is having difficulty breathing. Leaning of the thorax to the side opposite the injury may result from the patient trying to stretch a cramped muscle. If the individual is grasping the torso or abdomen, he or she may be attempting to splint the painful area. Being unwilling to move, curling up into a fetal position, or a preference to lie supine with the knees flexed may indicate that the patient has an internal organ injury. Additional inspection by the clinician should include the following:

- Sweating: Profuse sweating is a common sign of cardiac arrest. This sign may be difficult to observe in an individual who has been participating in vigorous physical activity, as sweating is commonly associated with physical activity.
- Throat: Observe the trachea and larynx in their normal positions along the midline of the cervical spine. Deviation from the midline position may indicate trauma to these structures or the presence of a pneumothorax.
- Muscle tone: The contour of muscle tone in the abdomen should be monitored over time. As an internal organ injury progresses, the injured area may become distended because of blood accumulating in the abdominal cavity.
- Skin features: Document the location of the primary injury (ie, the location of the direct trauma). Look for any contusions, wounds, or abrasions in the direct area of injury. Discolorations may serve to warn of possible injury to or bleeding of underlying internal organs.
- Kyphosis: Kyphosis is a condition in which the thoracic spine is exaggerated and the curvature of the spine is more pronounced than normal. A slight kyphotic (or posterior) curvature of the thoracic spine is to be expected.
- Scoliosis: Scoliosis is a spinal deformity characterized by lateral curvature of the spine. Scoliosis may occur as an isolated incident in the thoracic spine, in the thoracolumbar area, or in the lumbar spine. Scoliosis may occur in multiple spinal segments as the severity of the condition increases.
- Chest deformities: Different deformities occur at the thoracic cavity affecting the chest, such as pectus excavatum, pectus carinatum, barrel chest, Poland syndrome, Jeune syndrome, and defects of the ribs and sternum.[7,8]
- Pigeon chest (pectus carinatum) is a deformity in which the sternum projects forward and downward, narrowing the anterior portion of the chest at the sternum (**Figure 11.1**). This congenital deformity gives the chest a birdlike appearance and affects breathing, as the change in chest shape restricts the volume of air allowed in the chest. Additionally, this condition may be associated with heart disease, scoliosis, kyphosis, and musculoskeletal defects.[7]
- Funnel chest (pectus excavatum) is a congenital deformity in which the sternum is pushed posteriorly by an overgrowth of the ribs.[6] Because of the displacement of the sternum, the heart may be displaced as well (**Figure 11.2**). The anteroposterior dimension of the chest is diminished, which affects the patient's ability to take a full, deep breath. Kyphosis, scoliosis, or Marfan syndrome may also be present with this deformity.[7,9]
- Barrel chest: The sternum projects upward and forward, increasing the diameter of the chest. The chest appears to be partially inflated all the time, as if the patient is in the middle of taking a deep breath (**Figure 11.3**). This condition is common in patients suffering from emphysema, osteoarthritis, chronic obstructive pulmonary disorder, cystic fibrosis, or chronic asthma.[8]
- Less common types of chest wall abnormalities include Poland syndrome (underdeveloped chest muscles), Jeune syndrome (breathing difficulties resulting from restricted rib growth and a small chest restricting expansion of the lungs), and other defects of the ribs and sternum.[7]

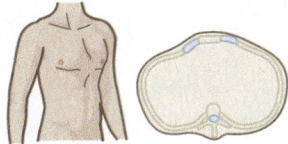

Figure 11.1 Drawing showing pigeon chest.
© Jones & Bartlett Learning

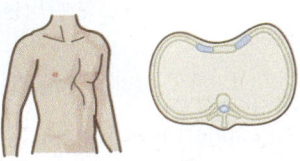

Figure 11.2 Drawing showing funnel chest.
© Jones & Bartlett Learning

Chapter 11 Abdomen and Thorax

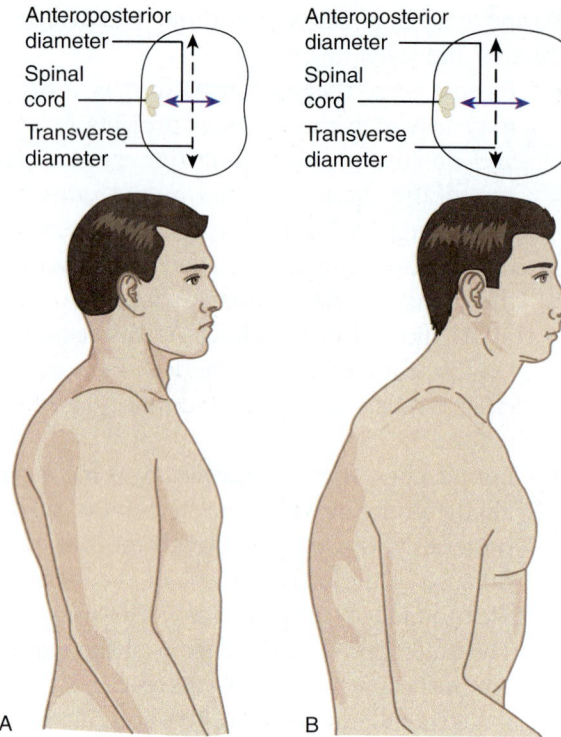

Figure 11.3 Drawing showing a normal chest **(A)** compared to a barrel chest **(B)**.

© Jones & Bartlett Learning

Anatomic Inspection

Clinicians are recommended to develop a protocol for inspecting the thorax and abdomen. Some individuals choose to start superior and move inferior; other clinicians start on one side and move to the other side (ie, left to right or right to left); and another approach is to inspect from superficial to deep (**Figure 11.4**). By developing an inspection protocol, clinicians are less likely to miss anatomic inspections. Each individual has to decide what system works best for them. The anatomic inspection sites have been broken down into anterior, posterior, and lateral locations.

- Anterior
    - Height of the shoulders (one shoulder, usually the dominant one, may be slightly lower)
    - Sternum
    - Clavicle
    - Ribs
    - Normal breathing: Symmetrical rise of the rib cage, or expansion of the abdominal cavity, or both
    - Nipple line in males should be approximately at the fourth rib (or slightly below). In women, the level varies greatly.

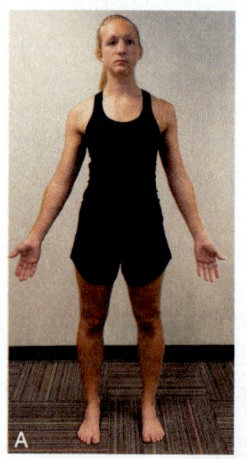 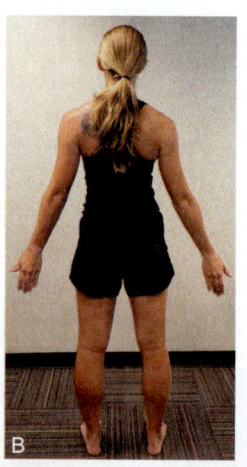 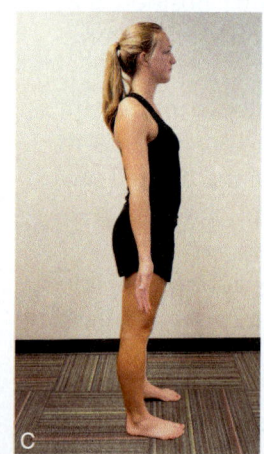 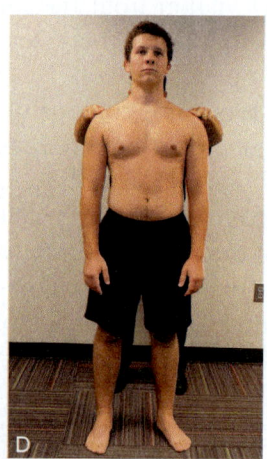

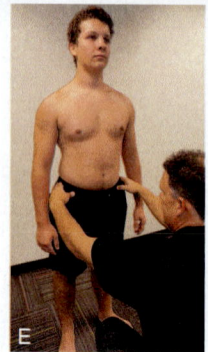 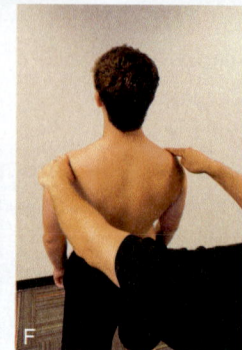 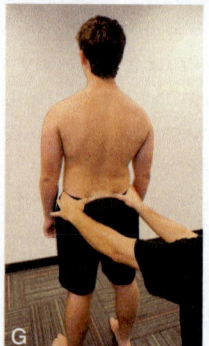

Figure 11.4 Clinical photographs depicting anatomic views and inspection. **A.** Anterior view. **B.** Posterior view. **C.** Lateral view. **D.** Shoulder height. **E.** Anterior superior iliac crest. **F.** Acromion process. **G.** Posterior superior iliac crest.

© Jones & Bartlett Learning

- Skin coloring (look for ecchymosis, erythema, or pallor)
- Skin temperature
• Posterior
  - Height of the shoulders (one shoulder, usually the dominant one, may be slightly lower)
  - Ribs
  - Spinous process of the vertebrae (look for alignment)
  - Normal breathing: Symmetrical rise of the rib cage, or expansion of the abdominal cavity, or both
  - Skin coloring (look for ecchymosis, erythema, or pallor)
  - Skin temperature
• Lateral
  - Ribs
  - Normal breathing: Symmetrical rise of the rib cage, or expansion of the abdominal cavity, or both
  - Skin coloring (look for ecchymosis, erythema, or pallor)
  - Skin temperature

Palpation

Skeletal Anatomy

The chest, or thoracic cavity, lies between the base of the neck and the diaphragm. Posteriorly there are 12 thoracic vertebrae.[7] Wrapping around from posterior to anterior, there are 12 pairs of ribs with associated costal cartilage and the sternum. The primary function of the thoracic cavity is to protect the organs responsible for respiration (lungs) and the circulatory (heart) system from injury.[5] The ribs assist with respiration: both inhalation and expiration during the breathing process. The thymus[10,11] lies within the thoracic cavity (anterior and superior to the heart) and stores mature lymphocytes known as T cells.[11,12] The T cells migrate to lymphatic tissue to respond to foreign substances in the body.[10-12]

The clavicle should be palpated along the length of the bone for abnormal bumps (history of fracture or callus formation) or tenderness (**Figure 11.5**).

The "breastbone ridge" includes the sternum and its associated landmarks.[13] The sternum includes bony landmarks, such as the jugular notch, manubrium, body of the sternum, and xiphoid process (**Figure 11.6**). All of these structures are fused together, but muscles and cartilage insert on different parts of the sternum. Understanding the different anatomic palpations can be important.[13]

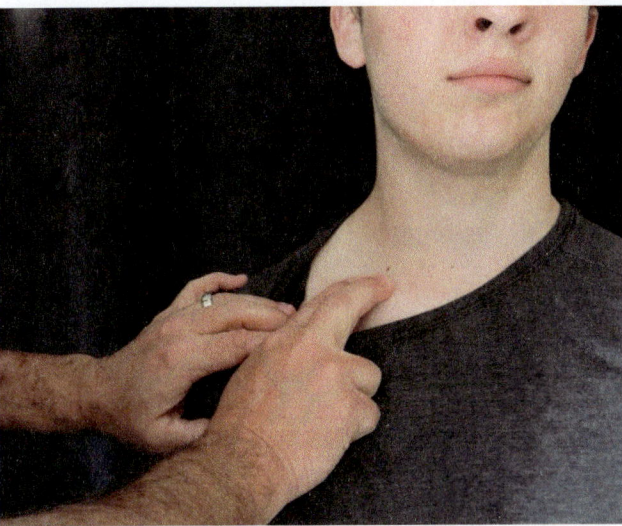

Figure 11.5 Clinical photograph showing palpation of the clavicle.
Courtesy of Matt Kutz.

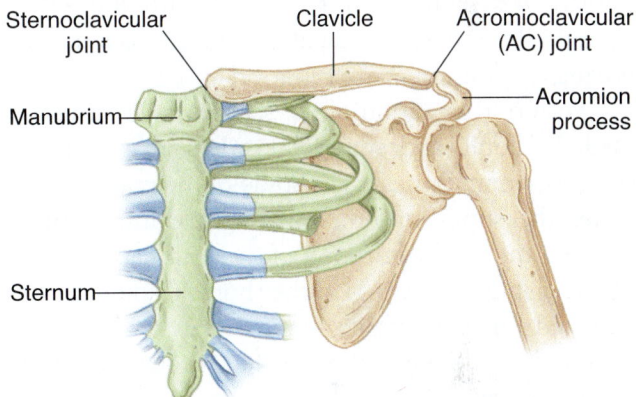

Figure 11.6 Drawing showing palpation landmarks of the sternum and ribs.
© Jones & Bartlett Learning

The ribs are flat bones found in or around the thoracic cavity, surrounding the soft tissue of the lungs. The ribs articulate posterior to the thoracic vertebrae and anteriorly with the sternum via costal cartilage. The upper seven ribs are referred to as true ribs or sternal ribs, as each of the ribs articulate with the sternum by a separate costal cartilage. The 8th to 10th ribs are commonly referred to as false ribs and have a common costal cartilage articulating to the 7th rib before articulating to the sternum. The 11th and 12th ribs are referred to as floating ribs because they do not attach to the sternum; they do, however, have muscular attachments and are therefore still important for function (**Figure 11.7**). Each individual rib articulation produces a slight gliding action.

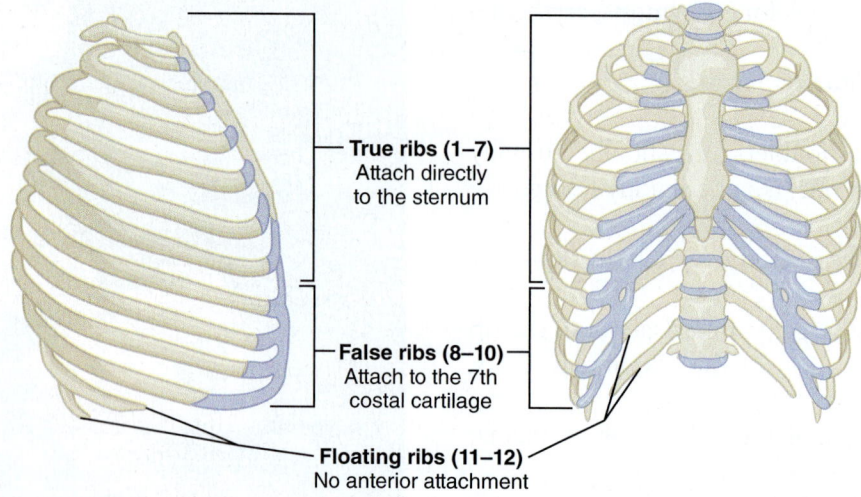

Figure 11.7 Drawing showing true ribs, false ribs, and floating ribs.
© Jones & Bartlett Learning

The inside of the thoracic cavity is lined with a thin, double-layered membrane called a pleura[6] (**Figure 11.8**). The pleura is filled with fluid that permits the lungs to slide along the thoracic cavity during inspiration and expiration.[6,13]

Posterior palpation of the scapula, including the medial, lateral, and superior borders, may indicate swelling or tenderness. The spine of the scapula separates the supraspinous fossa and the infraspinous fossa on the posterior aspect of the scapula.

The spinous process of the thoracic spine can be palpated for abnormality. Approximately 2 to 3 cm (0.8 to 1.2 in.) laterally from the spinous processes, a clinician can palpate the facet joints of each vertebrae. Overlying musculature makes palpation of the facet joints difficult unless there is some pathology (**Figure 11.9**).

Fibrocartilaginous disks provide cushioning between the bodies of articulating vertebrae. The disks consist of a thick outer ring (annulus fibrosus) surrounding an inner gelatinous substance (nucleus pulposus).[13] The disks serve to reduce and distribute shock and allow movement at the spine.

Specific bony landmarks can help orient a clinician during palpation:[13]

- Spinous process of C7: sits at the base of the neck (this is usually a large protuberance compared to other spinous processes)
- Spinous process of T2: sits at the superior angle of the scapula

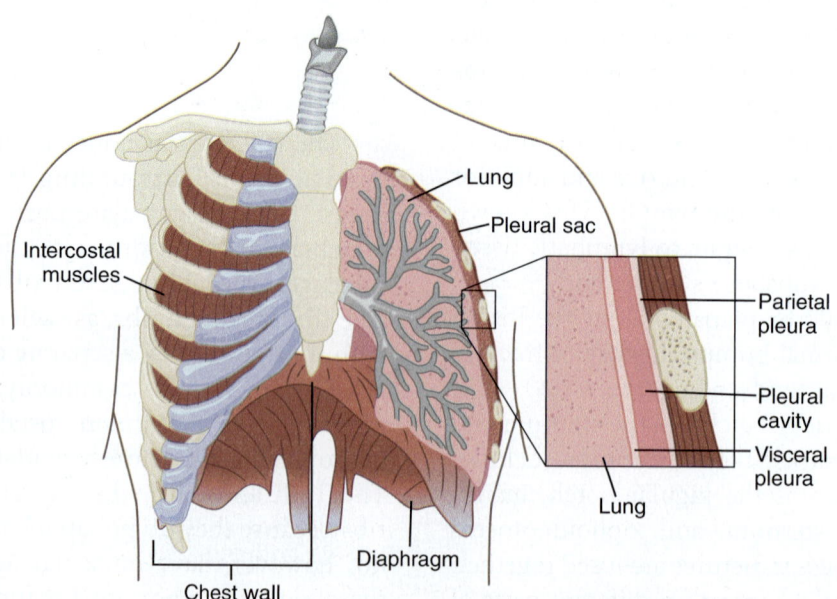

Figure 11.8 Drawing showing the pleural cavity.
© Jones & Bartlett Learning

- Spinous process of T7: sits at the inferior angle of the scapula
- Spinous process of T12: sits at the level of the 12th rib
- Spinous process of L4: sits at the top of the iliac crest

Articulations and Ligamentous Support

Costovertebral, Costotransverse, Costochondral, and Sternocostal Joints

The costovertebral joints are synovial joints located between the ribs and vertebral bodies of the spine. There are 24 costovertebral joints in the human body. Ribs 1, 10, 11, and 12 articulate with a single vertebra. Ribs 2 through 9 articulate with two adjacent vertebrae and the intervening intervertebral disk.

The costotransverse joints are synovial joints located between the ribs and transverse processes of the vertebra of the same level for ribs 1 through 10. Ribs 11 and 12 do not articulate with the transverse processes.

The costochondral joints articulate the ribs and costal cartilage. The sternocostal joints are the articulation for the costal cartilage and the sternum (**Table 11.2**).

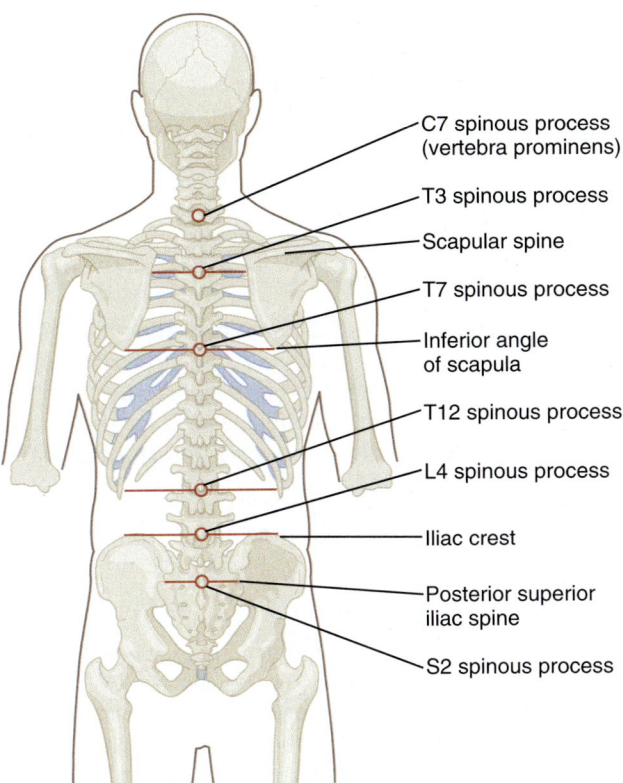

Figure 11.9 Drawing showing spinous process landmarks.

© Jones & Bartlett Learning

Table 11.2 Soft-Tissue Anatomy

Ligament	Origin	Insertion	Palpation
Radiate ligament	The radiate ligament consists of three flat fasciculi (bundle of skeletal muscles) that attach on the anterior part of the head of the rib	The superior fasciculus ascends and inserts on the body of the vertebra above The inferior fasciculus descends and inserts on the body of the vertebra below The middle fasciculus inserts horizontally to the intervertebral fibrocartilage	Not palpable, deep
Intra-articular ligament of the head of the rib (first through ninth ribs)	Crest separating the two costal facets on the head of the rib	Intervertebral disk between the two vertebrae (this ligament divides the joint into two cavities)	Deep palpation between the superior costal facet and the inferior costal facet
Superior costotransverse ligament (may be absent for the first rib)	The anterior fibers originate on the crest of the superior border of the neck of each rib The posterior fibers originate on the crest of the superior border of the neck of the rib	The anterior fibers insert on the anterior surface of the transverse process of the vertebra immediately superior The posterior fibers insert on the inferior border of the transverse process of the vertebra immediately superior	Deep palpation between the superior costal facet and the inferior costal facet

(continues)

Table 11.2 Soft-Tissue Anatomy (continued)

Ligament	Origin	Insertion	Palpation
Costotransverse ligament	Neck of the first rib	Transverse process at the same level	Transverse process
Lateral costotransverse ligament	Posterior surface of the tip of the transverse process of the vertebra	Tubercle of the corresponding rib	Transverse process
Anterior longitudinal ligament	Upper edge of the vertebral body	Lower edge of the vertebral body	The ligament runs the entire length of the spine from the base of the skull to the sacrum. It is not palpable, as it is located on the anterior portion of the spine
Posterior longitudinal ligament	Upper edge of the vertebral body	Lower edge of the vertebral body	The ligament runs the entire length of the spine from the base of the skull to the sacrum. It is deep and difficult to palpate
Supraspinous ligament	Above the seventh cervical vertebrae, the supraspinous ligament is continuous with the nuchal ligament. Spinous process of the seventh cervical vertebrae to the sacrum	Between the spinous processes the supraspinous ligament is continuous	Palpated deep between the spinous processes of the vertebrae. The most superficial fibers of this ligament extend over three or four vertebrae; fibers more deeply seated pass between two or three vertebrae, while the deepest connect the spinous processes of neighboring vertebrae
Ligamentum flavum	Pedicles of the vertebrae	Pedicle of the adjacent vertebrae	Vertebral pedicles

Facet Joints of the Spine

The facet joints of the spine are synovial joints articulating two adjacent vertebrae in the spine. There are two facet joints in each spinal motion segment, and each facet joint is innervated by the recurrent meningeal nerves.

Blood Supply of the Lungs

Two separate circulatory systems, the bronchial and pulmonary, supply blood to the lungs. Bronchial circulation comes from the aorta and intercostal arteries and provides oxygenated blood to the bronchi, large blood vessels, hilar lymph nodes, and visceral pleura. The bronchial circulation ends at the terminal bronchioles, joining with the pulmonary capillaries and venules.

The pulmonary artery (originating from the right ventricle) starts the pulmonary circulation. Pulmonary circulation moves poorly oxygenated blood from the right side of the heart to the alveoli, where oxygen is added and carbon dioxide is removed from the blood. Blood from the lungs is returned to the heart through the pulmonary vein and then is pumped out to the rest of the body, supplying the entire body with oxygenated blood.

Blood Supply to the Heart

The blood supply to the heart occurs via the coronary arteries branching from the aorta (**Figure 11.10**). The cardiac veins empty into the right atrium.

Aorta

The aorta is the largest and main artery of the body; it supplies oxygenated blood to the circulatory system. The aorta begins at the left ventricle and passes over the heart. Three leaflets (on the aortic valve) open and close with each ventricular contraction to allow one-way flow of blood. The heart pumps blood from left ventricle into the aorta through the aortic valve. The aorta continues down to the lower body through the abdomen anterior to the spine. In the abdomen, the aorta is approximately one foot long and approximately one inch in diameter. A deep palpation of the aorta is shown in **Figure 11.11** and discussed[14] in **Table 11.3**. The aorta is divided into four sections:

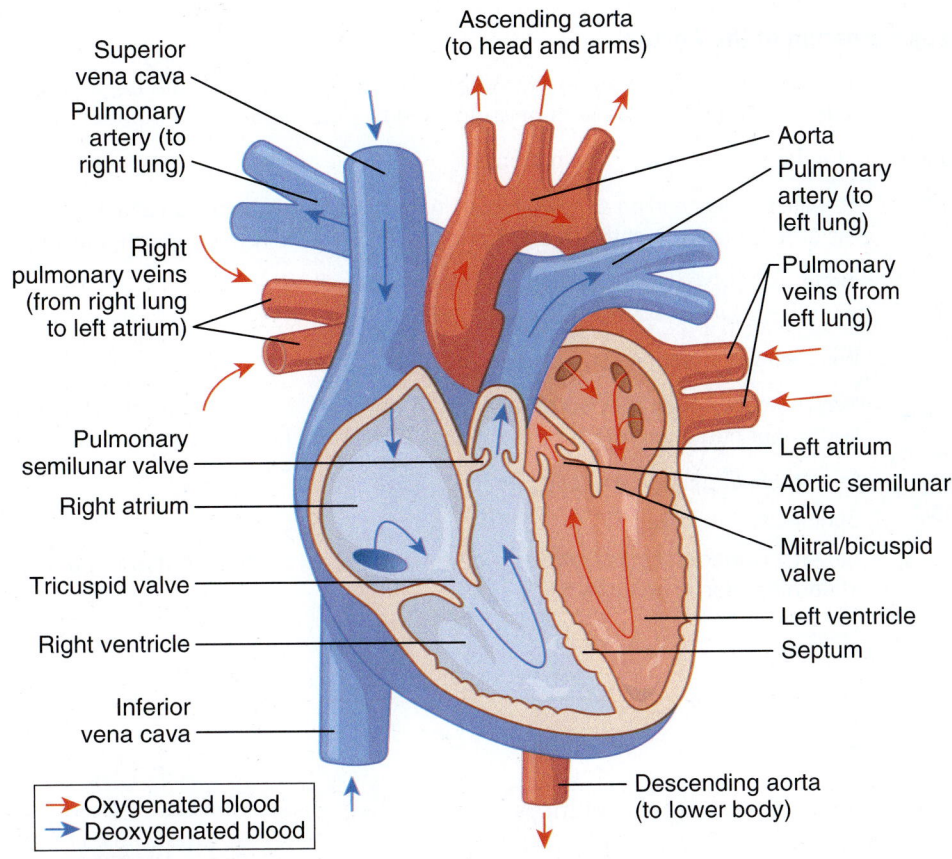

Figure 11.10 Drawing showing the blood flow pathway to the heart.

© Jones & Bartlett Learning

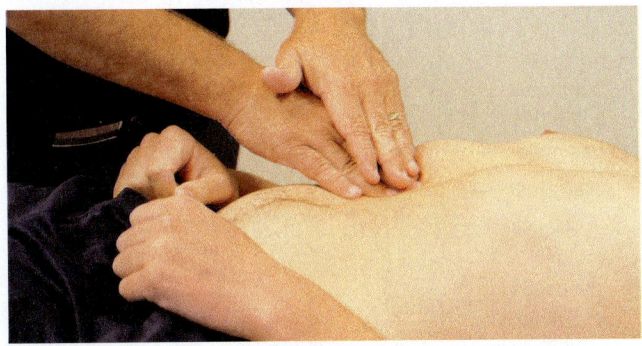

Figure 11.11 Clinical photograph showing deep palpation of the aorta.

© Jones & Bartlett Learning

1. The ascending aorta is approximately two inches long and connects directly to the heart (left ventricle). The coronary arteries branch off of the ascending aorta to supply the heart with oxygenated blood.
2. The aortic arch is the section of the artery curving over the heart. Branches come off the aortic arch supplying blood to the head, neck, and upper extremities.
3. The descending thoracic aorta continues down through the thoracic cavity. The small branches of the descending thoracic aorta supply blood to the ribs and some of the thoracic anatomy.
4. The abdominal aorta begins at the level of the diaphragm. The abdominal aorta splits to become the paired iliac arteries in the lower abdomen. Many major organs in the abdominal cavity receive blood from the branches of the abdominal aorta.

Superior Vena Cava

The superior vena cava is a large vein receiving deoxygenated blood from the head, neck, upper extremities, and thorax. The superior vena cava delivers blood to the right atrium of the heart.

Inferior Vena Cava

The inferior vena cava is a large vein receiving deoxygenated blood from the lower extremities and abdomen. The inferior vena cava delivers blood to the right atrium of the heart.

Renal Arteries

The renal arteries are a pair of large blood vessels branching off of the abdominal aorta that supply oxygenated blood to each kidney. In a normal person at rest, the renal arteries deliver approximately 1.2 L of blood per minute to the kidneys. At this delivery rate, the entire volume of blood found in the body circulates to the kidneys once every 4 to 5 minutes.

Table 11.3 Deep Palpation of the Aorta

Patient positioning	The patient is supine on an examination table. The head should be on a pillow, arms at the side. The knees can be bent or supported by pillows to help the patient relax the abdomen.
Examiner positioning	Standing at the side of the patient.
Procedure	Palpate the descending aorta with both index fingers. The palpation should be performed just above the umbilicus and slightly left of the midline. Press down firmly to locate the pulse of the aorta.
Modifications (if available)	None.
Positive test	Wide aortic pulsations (> 4 cm) or lateral pulsations.
Implications	May indicate abdominal aortic aneurysm; the patient should be referred for evaluation. Width, not pulsation intensity, is the significant finding.
Research-based evidence to support test	Sensitivity of palpation = 0.68 Specificity = 0.75 Sensitivity increases with the size of the abdominal aortic aneurysm, up to 0.82 for an abdominal aortic aneurysm > 5 cm.
Notes/record-keeping tips	None.

Renal Veins

The renal veins carry blood filtered by the kidneys back to the inferior vena cava.

Muscles of the Vertebral Column

Multiple muscles work on the vertebral column to support the chest, torso, and abdomen during activities of daily living. Without these muscles working together, the body would have a difficult time maintaining an upright posture, especially for an extended length of time.[13] **Table 11.4** and **Figures 11.12** through **11.14** discuss some of these muscles.

Vertebral Column Flexion

The spine's bending forward is known as vertebral flexion. Multiple muscles are activated during vertebral flexion, which allows activities such as bending over to tie a shoe or performing an abdominal crunch[12,13,15] (**Table 11.5**).

Vertebral Column Extension

Muscles help hold the spine upright and allow for a small amount of backward bending, also known as extension. Most of these muscles are used as postural stabilizing muscles, rather than large movers of the body[13,15] (**Table 11.6**).

Vertebral Column Rotation

The spine is unique, as it allows for rotation as well as flexion and extension. This rotation allows for individuals to twist, such as looking for a ball

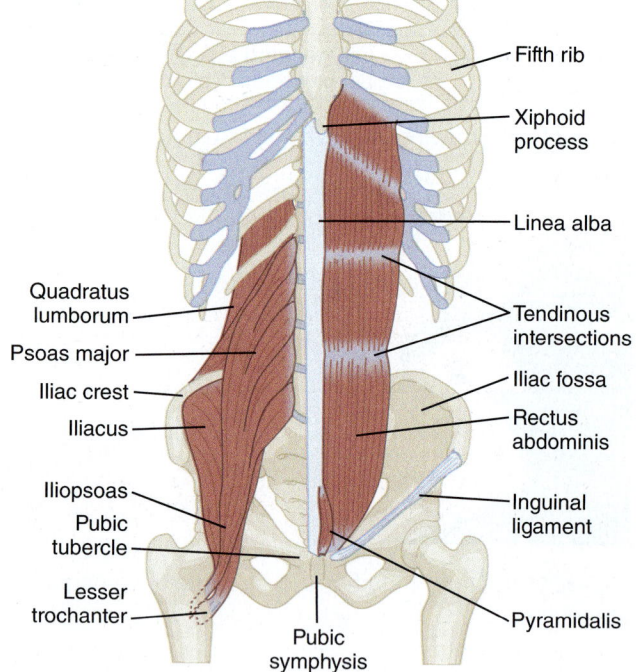

Figure 11.12 Drawing showing deep abdominal muscles.
© Jones & Bartlett Learning

or opponent during athletic participation or looking over your shoulder while driving. In addition to moving the spine, many of these muscles also help compress the abdominal contents to provide support to the torso[13,15] (**Table 11.7**).

Vertebral Column Lateral Flexion

The muscles around the abdomen and thorax can cause lateral flexion of the spine, meaning that the torso (shoulder) can move toward the hip. An example

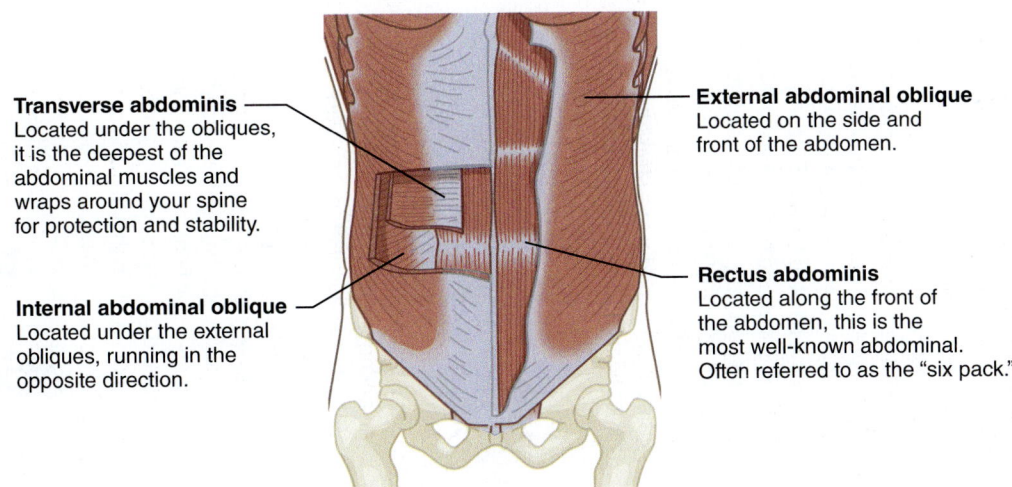

Figure 11.13 Drawing showing superficial abdominal muscles.

© Jones & Bartlett Learning

Table 11.4	Synergist Muscles Working Together on the Vertebral Column
Vertebral column flexion (antagonist on extension)	Rectus abdominis External oblique (bilaterally) Internal oblique (bilaterally) Psoas major (with the origin fixed) Iliacus (with the origin fixed)
Vertebral column extension (antagonist on flexion)	Longissimus (bilaterally) Iliocostalis (bilaterally) Multifidi (bilaterally) Rotatores (bilaterally) Semispinalis capitis Spinalis (bilaterally) Quadratus lumborum (assists) Interspinalis Intertransversarii (bilaterally) Latissimus dorsi (assists when arm is fixed)
Vertebral column rotation (all unilaterally)	External oblique (to the opposite side) Internal oblique (to the opposite side) Multifidi (to the opposite side) Rotatores (to the opposite side)
Vertebral column lateral flexion (unilaterally to the same side)	Iliocostalis External oblique Internal oblique Longissimus Quadratus lumborum Psoas major (assists) Intertransversarii Spinalis Latissimus dorsi (assists)
Vertebral column stabilization	Transverse abdominis

Data from Biel A: Trail Guide to the Body, ed rev 5. Boulder, CO, Books of Discovery, 2014.

of lateral spinal flexion would be when a person stands with the hands at his or her sides touching the thigh. As the hand slides down the thigh toward the knee, the spine laterally bends or flexes, resulting in the desired movement. This movement is important because occasionally a person drops things, and this movement allows a person to bend. These muscles exist on either side of the abdomen and thorax but act unilaterally to perform lateral flexion[13,15] (**Table 11.8**).

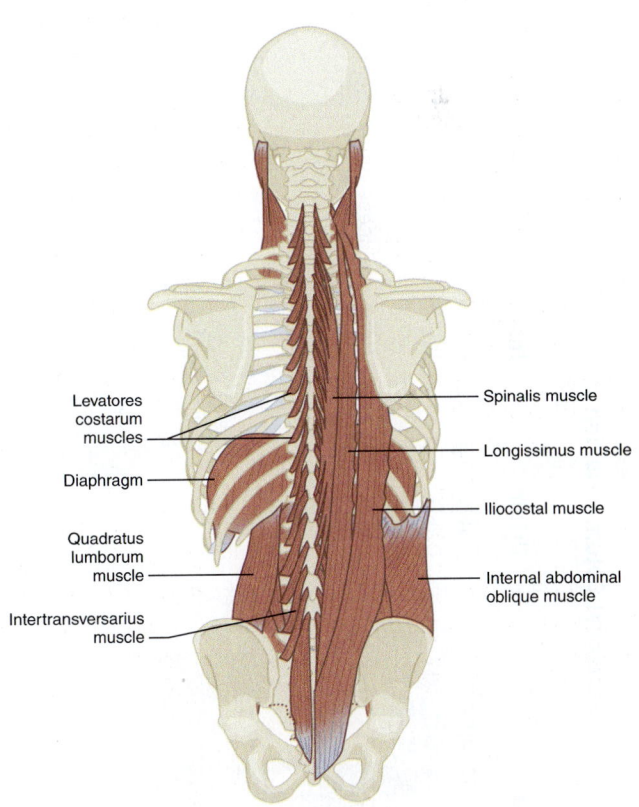

Figure 11.14 Drawing showing posterior abdominal muscles.

© Jones & Bartlett Learning

Table 11.5 Vertebral Column Flexion

Muscle	Origin	Insertion	Action	Innervation (Nerve Root)	Palpation	Manual Muscle Test
Rectus abdominis	Pubic crest Pubic symphysis	Cartilage of the fifth, sixth, and seventh ribs Xiphoid process	Flex the vertebral column Tilt pelvis posteriorly	T5–T12, ventral rami	Most superficial abdominal muscle ("six-pack abs"). Palpate the rectus abdominis while the patient lies supine but flexes the trunk (abdominal curl or crunch).	To test the upper abdominal muscles, the patient is supine with the legs extended. If the hip flexor muscles are short and prevent posterior pelvic tilt with flattening of the lumbar spine, place a roll under the knees to passively flex the hips enough to allow the back to flatten. Stabilize the patient's feet and have the patient do a trunk curl very slowly, completing spine flexion (A). Have the patient continue to the hip flexion phase (ie, the sit-up) to perform a strength test of the abdominal muscle group (B). Many individuals can perform trunk flexion with the arms placed behind the head; however, some patients will struggle. The patient may begin by reaching the arms forward, then folding the arms across the chest, and then placing arms behind the head if performing an abdominal crunch is difficult (C). When the abdominal muscles are too weak to perform the curl, the hip flexors will tilt the pelvis anteriorly, and hyperextension of the lumbar spine may occur until the trunk is raised to a seated position. If the examiner must hold the feet of the patient to do a trunk curl, then this also indicates significant abdominal weakness.

Rectus abdominis *(continued)*

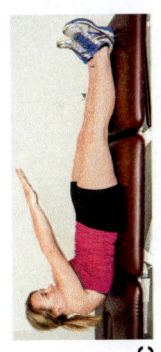

C

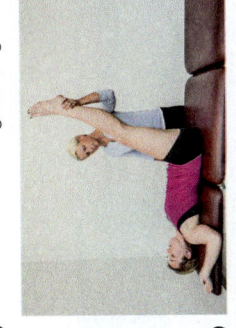

D

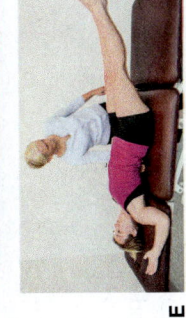

E

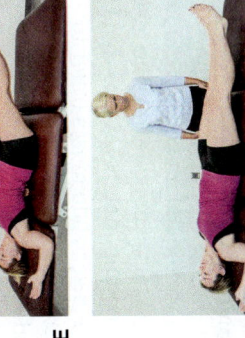

F

To test the lower abdominal muscles, the patient lies supine with the legs extended. The patient crosses the arms across the chest. The examiner will assist the patient in raising the legs to a vertical position while keeping the knees straight (D). Have the patient flatten the lumbar spine by performing a posterior pelvic tilt while contracting the abdominal muscles (E). Have the patient hold the lower back flat against the table while slowly lowering the legs to the table, keeping the knees straight (F). The head and shoulders should stay on the table during testing.

(continues)

Table 11.5 Vertebral Column Flexion *(continued)*

Muscle	Origin	Insertion	Action	Innervation (Nerve Root)	Palpation	Manual Muscle Test
External oblique	External surface of the 5th to 12th ribs	Anterior portion of iliac crest Abdominal aponeurosis to linea alba	Laterally flex vertebral column to same side (unilaterally) Rotate vertebral column to opposite side (unilaterally) Flex vertebral column (bilaterally) Compress abdominal contents (bilaterally)	T5–T12	Hands on hips: If you place your hands on your own hips, this is the direction of fiber orientation for the external oblique muscle. Have the patient rotate the trunk toward the opposite side, and palpate just below the rib cage.	The abdominal muscles, including the external oblique, may be tested as a group together as the upper and lower abdominals (refer to manual muscle test for the rectus abdominis).
Internal oblique	Lateral inguinal ligament Iliac crest Thoracolumbar fascia	Internal surface of lower three ribs Abdominal aponeurosis to linea alba	Laterally flex vertebral column to same side (unilaterally) Rotate vertebral column to the same side (unilaterally) Flex the vertebral column (bilaterally) Compress abdominal contents (bilaterally)	T7–L1 Iliohypogastric and ilioinguinal Ventral rami	The internal obliques are deep to the external obliques and are therefore difficult to palpate.	The abdominal muscles, including the internal oblique, may be tested as a group together as the upper and lower abdominals (refer to manual muscle test for the rectus abdominis).

Psoas major	Bodies and transverse processes of the lumbar vertebrae	Lesser trochanter	Flex the hip (coxal joint [with the origin fixed]) May laterally rotate the hip (coxal joint [with the origin fixed]) Flex the trunk toward the thigh (with the insertion fixed) Tilt the pelvis anteriorly (with the insertion fixed) Assist to laterally flex the lumbar spine (unilaterally)	Anterior rami off of the lumbar plexus L1–L4	Have the patient side lying with the hips flexed. The examiner's fingers should be curled into the abdomen. If the patient is supine during palpation, have the patient flex the hip to help palpate the psoas major muscle. Palpate the muscle by pressing into the inner surface of the pelvis right by the anterior superior iliac spine.	The psoas major and iliacus are commonly tested together. To test the iliopsoas muscle with emphasis on the psoas major, the patient is supine. Stabilize the opposite iliac crest and have the patient use the quadriceps to stabilize the knee into extension. The hip is flexed with slight abduction and slight lateral rotation (external rotation). Apply pressure against the anteromedial leg in the direction of extension and slight abduction.

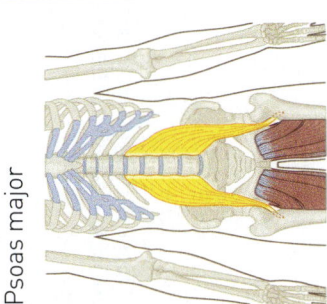

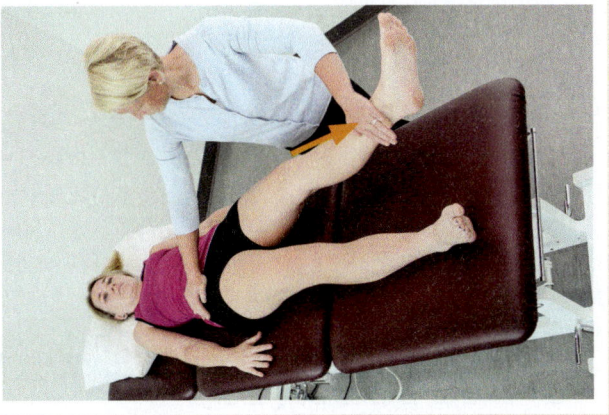

(continues)

Table 11.5 Vertebral Column Flexion

Muscle	Origin	Insertion	Action	Innervation (Nerve Root)	Palpation	Manual Muscle Test
Iliacus	Iliac fossa	Lesser trochanter	Flex the hip (coxal joint) (with the origin fixed) May laterally rotate the hip (coxal joint) (with the origin fixed) Flex the trunk toward the thigh (with the insertion fixed) Tilt the pelvis anteriorly (with the insertion fixed)	Femoral, L2–L4	Have the patient side lying with the hips flexed. The examiner's fingers should be curled into the abdomen. The examiner may also stand in front of a side-lying patient, using the thumbs to palpate the iliacus muscle on the medial surface of the pelvis just round from the iliac crest.	The psoas major and iliacus are commonly tested together. To test for common hip flexors as a group, have the patient short-sit on a table. Resist hip flexion with the knee flexed, raising the thigh off the table by a few inches (A). To test the iliopsoas muscle group, have the patient short-sitting on the table and then perform full hip flexion with the knee flexed (B).

(continued)

All figures in table © Jones & Bartlett Learning.
Data from Biel A: *Trail Guide to the Body*, ed rev 5. Boulder, CO, Books of Discovery, 2014; and Kendall FP, McCreary EK, Provance PG, Rodgers MM, Romani WA: *Muscles: Testing and Function with Posture and Pain*, ed 5. Baltimore, MD, Lippincott Williams & Wilkins, 2005.

Table 11.6 Vertebral Column Extension

Muscle	Origin	Insertion	Action	Innervation (Nerve Root)	Palpation	Manual Muscle Test
Longissimus	Common tendon (thoracis) Transverse process of the upper five thoracic vertebrae (cervicis and capitis)	Lower nine ribs and transverse process of the thoracic vertebrae (thoracis) Transverse process of the cervical vertebrae (cervicis) Mastoid process of the temporal bone (capitis)	Laterally flex the vertebral column to the same side (unilaterally) Extend the vertebral column (bilaterally) Primary mover for spinal extension, assists in lateral bending and spinal rotation on the same side	Spinal	Palpated as a group with the spinalis, longissimus, and iliocostalis. Have the patient lie on his or her stomach and raise the arms above the head. Have the patient actively extend the upper body off the table and palpate the muscle mass next to the spine.	There is no specific manual muscle test for the longissimus muscle.
Iliocostalis	Common tendon (lumborum) Posterior surface of ribs 1–12 (thoracis and cervicis)	Transverse process of L1–L3 and posterior surface of ribs 6–12 (lumborum) Posterior surface of ribs 1–6 (thoracis) Transverse process of lower cervicals (cervicis)	Laterally flex the vertebral column to the same side (unilaterally) Extend the vertebral column (bilaterally) Primary mover for spinal extension, assists in lateral bending and spinal rotation on the same side	Spinal	Easily palpated the entire length of back and neck close to spine. The examiner is positioned behind the patient. The patient extends the head to relax fascia. Knead the muscles looking for tenderness, spasm, defects, and bilateral size.	There is no specific manual muscle test for the iliocostalis muscle.
Multifidi	Sacrum and transverse processes of lumbar through cervical vertebrae	Spinous processes of lumbar vertebrae through second cervical vertebrae The multifidi span two to four vertebrae	Rotate the vertebral column to the opposite side (unilaterally) Spinal extension (bilaterally) The multifidi play an important role in the dynamic, segmental stabilization of the lumbar spine	Spinal	Palpation is deep to erector spinae. Have the patient lie prone; palpate the multifidi by finding the lamina groove on the opposite side of the body with the thumbs sliding away from the vertebrae.	There is no specific manual muscle test for the multifidi muscle.

(continues)

Table 11.6 Vertebral Column Extension *(continued)*

Muscle	Origin	Insertion	Action	Innervation (Nerve Root)	Palpation	Manual Muscle Test
Multifidi *(continued)*			These muscles rotate the spinal column, especially above the lumbar level, slight contribution to spinal extension and lateral bending			
Rotatores	Transverse processes of lumbar through cervical vertebrae	Spinous processes of lumbar vertebrae through second cervical vertebra. The rotatores span one to two vertebrae	Rotate the vertebral column to the opposite side (unilaterally) Spinal extension (bilaterally) The rotatores play important role in the dynamic, segmental stabilization of the lumbar spine These muscles rotate the spinal column, especially above the lumbar level; slight contribution to spinal extension and lateral bending	Spinal	Palpation is deep to erector spinae. Have the patient lie prone. Palpate the rotatores by moving the fingers toward the vertebrae.	There is no specific manual muscle test for the rotatores muscle.
Semispinalis capitis	Transverse processes of C4–T5	Between the superior and inferior nuchal lines of the occiput	Extend the vertebral column and head	Cervical	Have the patient lie prone; palpate the muscle between the spinous process and transverse processes of the vertebrae. Deep along the thoracic and cervical vertebrae.	There is no specific manual muscle test for the semispinalis capitis muscle. The muscle may be tested with the posterolateral neck extensor muscle group (splenius capitis, splenius cervicis, semispinalis capitis, semispinalis cervicis, and cervical erector spinae). Have the patient lie prone on the table with the shoulders abducted, elbows bent, and the hands resting overhead on the table. Have the patient extend the neck with the face turned toward the side being tested.

Spinalis	Spinous process of the upper lumbar and lower thoracic vertebrae (thoracis) Ligamentum nuchae, spinous process of C7 (cervicis)	Spinous process of the upper thoracic (thoracis) Spinous processes of cervicals, except C1 (cervicis)	Laterally flex the vertebral column to the same side (unilaterally) Extend the vertebral column (bilaterally) Primary mover for spinal extension, assists in lateral bending and spinal rotation on the same side	Spinal	Easily palpated entire length of back and neck close to spine. The examiner is positioned behind the patient. The patient extends the head to relax fascia. Knead the muscles looking for tenderness, spasm, defects, and bilateral size.	There is no specific manual muscle test for the spinalis muscle.
Quadratus lumborum	Posterior iliac crest	Last rib and transverse process of first through fourth lumbar vertebrae	Lateral pelvic tilt (unilaterally) Lateral spinal flexion (unilaterally) Assist to extend vertebral column (unilaterally) Fix the last rib during forced inhalation and exhalation (bilaterally)	Lumbar plexus (T12–L3)	The quadratus lumborum is palpated deep beneath thoracolumbar aponeurosis and erector spinae muscle. Have the patient lie prone; palpate from the transverse process of the lumbar spine out. The quadratus lumborum may also be palpated with the patient side lying with the hips flexed; palpate superior to the iliac crest on the patient's side.	Place the patient prone on the table. The leg to be tested should be abducted away from the midline and should be slightly off the table. Resistance is provided in the form of traction on the extremity with slight extension and abduction. Grading the strength of the quadratus lumborum muscle numerically is not recommended; rather, the test is performed to determine whether the muscle is weak or strong.

(continues)

Table 11.6 Vertebral Column Extension (continued)

Muscle	Origin	Insertion	Action	Innervation (Nerve Root)	Palpation	Manual Muscle Test
Interspinalis	Spanning the spinous process of C2–T3 (cervical) Spanning the spinous process of T12–L5 (lumbar)	Spanning the spinous process of C2–T3 (cervical) Spanning the spinous process of T12–L5 (lumbar)	Extend the vertebral column	Spinal	This is a very deep muscle; palpate between the spinous processes of adjacent vertebrae with the patient lying prone.	There is no specific manual muscle test for the interspinalis muscle.
Intertransversarii	Spanning the transverse process of C2–C7 (cervical) Spanning the transverse process of L1–L5 (lumbar)	Spanning the transverse process of C2–C7 (cervical) Spanning the transverse process of L1–L5 (lumbar)	Laterally flex the vertebral column to the same side (unilaterally) Extend the vertebral column (bilaterally)	Spinal	Palpate deep between the transverse processes of adjacent vertebrae.	There is no specific manual muscle test for the intertransversarii muscle.
Latissimus dorsi	Inferior angle of the scapula Spinous process T6–T12 Last three or four ribs Thoracolumbar aponeurosis Posterior iliac crest	Intertubercular groove of the humerus	Extend the shoulder (glenohumeral joint) Adduct the shoulder (glenohumeral joint) Medially rotate (internal rotation) of the shoulder (glenohumeral joint)	Thoracodorsal (C6–C8)	The latissimus dorsi is a relatively large muscle with a large palpation site toward the lower thoracic spine. Have the patient lie prone with the shoulder off the table. Internally rotate the shoulder to feel the fibers of the latissimus dorsi muscle. The latissimus dorsi muscle can be palpated by having the patient lie supine, raise the shoulder to 90° and then have the patient press the elbow toward the hip against resistance. The latissimus dorsi may be palpated close to the rib cage.	Place the patient in a prone position with the head facing the arm being tested. Have the patient adduct the arm with extension in the medially rotated (internally rotated) position. The examiner provides pressure against the forearm in the direction of abduction and slight flexion of the arm.

All figures in table © Jones & Bartlett Learning.
Data from Kendall FP, McCreary EK, Provance PG, Rodgers MM, Romani WA: *Muscles: Testing and Function with Posture and Pain*, ed 5. Baltimore, MD, Lippincott Williams & Wilkins, 2005.

Table 11.7 Vertebral Column Rotation

Muscle	Origin	Insertion	Action	Innervation (Nerve Root)	Palpation	Manual Muscle Test
External oblique	External surface of the 5th to 12th ribs	Anterior portion of iliac crest; Abdominal aponeurosis to linea alba	Laterally flex vertebral column to same side (unilaterally); Rotate vertebral column to opposite side (unilaterally); Flex vertebral column (bilaterally); Compress abdominal contents (bilaterally)	(T5–T6), T7–T12	Hands on hips: When the hands are placed on the hips, this is the direction of fiber orientation for the external oblique muscle. Have the patient rotate the trunk toward the opposite side, palpate just below the rib cage.	There is no specific muscle test for the external oblique muscle. The abdominal muscles may be tested as a group together as the upper and lower abdominals (refer to manual muscle test for the rectus abdominis).
Internal oblique	Lateral inguinal ligament; Iliac crest; Thoracolumbar fascia	Internal surface of lower three ribs; Abdominal aponeurosis to linea alba	Laterally flex vertebral column to same side (unilaterally); Rotate vertebral column to the same side (unilaterally); Flex the vertebral column (bilaterally); Compress abdominal contents (bilaterally)	T7–L1; Iliohypogastric and ilioinguinal; Ventral rami	The internal obliques are deep to the external obliques and therefore are difficult to palpate.	There is no specific muscle test for the external oblique muscle. The abdominal muscles may be tested as a group together as the upper and lower abdominals (refer to manual muscle test for the rectus abdominis).
Multifidi	Sacrum and transverse processes of lumbar through cervical vertebrae	Spinous processes of lumbar vertebrae through second cervical vertebrae; The multifidi span two to four vertebrae	Rotate the vertebral column to the opposite side (unilaterally); Spinal extension (bilaterally); The multifidi play an important role in the dynamic, segmental stabilization of the lumbar spine; These muscles rotate the spinal column, especially above the lumbar level; slight contribution to spinal extension and lateral bending	Spinal	Palpation is deep to erector spinae. Have the patient lie prone and palpate the multifidi by finding the lamina groove on the opposite side of the body with the thumbs sliding away from the vertebrae.	There is no specific manual muscle test for the multifidi muscle.
Rotatores	Transverse processes of lumbar through cervical vertebrae	Spinous processes of lumbar vertebrae through second cervical vertebra; The rotatores span one to two vertebrae	Rotate the vertebral column to the opposite side (unilaterally); Spinal extension (bilaterally); The rotatores play important role in the dynamic, segmental stabilization of the lumbar spine; These muscles rotate the spinal column, especially above the lumbar level; slight contribution to spinal extension and lateral bending	Spinal	Palpation is deep to erector spinae. Have the patient lie prone. Palpate the rotatores by moving the fingers toward the vertebrae.	There is no specific manual muscle test for the rotatores muscles.

Data from Biel A: *Trail Guide to the Body*, rev ed 5. Boulder, CO, Books of Discovery, 2014; and Kendall FP, McCreary EK, Provance PG, Rodgers MM, Romani WA: *Muscles: Testing and Function with Posture and Pain*, ed 5. Baltimore, MD, Lippincott Williams & Wilkins, 2005.

Table 11.8 Vertebral Column Lateral Flexion

Muscle	Origin	Insertion	Action	Innervation (Nerve Root)	Palpation	Manual Muscle Test
Iliocostalis	Common tendon (lumborum) Posterior surface of ribs 1–12 (thoracis and cervicis)	Transverse process of L1–L3 and posterior surface of ribs 6–12 (lumborum) Posterior surface of ribs 1–6 (thoracis) Transverse process of lower cervicals (cervicis)	Laterally flex the vertebral column to the same side (unilaterally) Extend the vertebral column (bilaterally) Primary mover for spinal extension, assists in lateral bending and spinal rotation on the same side	Spinal	Easily palpated entire length of back and neck close to spine. The examiner is positioned behind the patient. The patient extends the head to relax fascia. Knead the muscles looking for tenderness, spasm, defects, and bilateral size.	There is no specific manual muscle test for the iliocostalis muscle.
External oblique	External surface of the 5th to 12th ribs	Anterior portion of iliac crest Abdominal aponeurosis to linea alba	Laterally flex vertebral column to same side (unilaterally) Rotate vertebral column to opposite side (unilaterally) Flex vertebral column (bilaterally) Compress abdominal contents (bilaterally)	(T5–T6), T7–T12	Hands on hips: When the hands are placed on the hips, this is the direction of fiber orientation for the external oblique muscle. Have the patient rotate the trunk toward the opposite side, palpate just below the rib cage.	There is no specific muscle test for the external oblique muscle. The abdominal muscles may be tested as a group together as the upper and lower abdominals (refer to manual muscle test for the rectus abdominis).
Internal oblique	Lateral inguinal ligament Iliac crest Thoracolumbar fascia	Internal surface of lower three ribs Abdominal aponeurosis to linea alba	Laterally flex vertebral column to same side (unilaterally) Rotate vertebral column to the same side (unilaterally) Flex the vertebral column (bilaterally) Compress abdominal contents (bilaterally)	T7–L1 Iliohypogastric and ilioinguinal Ventral rami	The internal obliques are deep to the external obliques and therefore are difficult to palpate.	There is no specific muscle test for the external oblique muscle. The abdominal muscles may be tested as a group together as the upper and lower abdominals (refer to manual muscle test for the rectus abdominis).

Quadratus lumborum	Posterior iliac crest	Last rib and transverse process of first through fourth lumbar vertebrae	Lateral pelvic tilt (unilaterally) Lateral spinal flexion (unilaterally) Assist to extend vertebral column (unilaterally) Fix the last rib during forced inhalation and exhalation (bilaterally)	Lumbar plexus (T12–L3)	The quadratus lumborum is palpated deep beneath thoracolumbar aponeurosis and erector spinae muscle. Have the patient lie prone, palpate from the transverse process of the lumbar spine out. The quadratus lumborum can be palpated with the patient side lying with the hips flexed, palpating just superior to the iliac crest on the patient's side.	Place the patient prone on the table. The leg to be tested should be abducted away from the midline and should be slightly off the table. Resistance is proved in the form of traction on the extremity with slight extension and abduction. Grading the strength of the quadratus lumborum muscle numerically is not recommended; rather, the test is performed to determine whether the muscle is weak or strong.
Psoas major	Bodies and transverse processes of the lumbar vertebrae	Lesser trochanter	Flex the hip (coxal joint [with the origin fixed]) May laterally rotate the hip (coxal joint [with the origin fixed]) Flex the trunk toward the thigh (with the insertion fixed) Tilt the pelvis anteriorly (with the insertion fixed) Assist to laterally flex the lumbar spine (unilaterally)	Anterior rami off of the lumbar plexus L1–L4	Have the patient side lying with the hips flexed. The examiner's fingers should be curled into the abdomen. If the patient is supine during palpation, have the patient flex the hip to help palpate the psoas major muscle group. Palpate the muscle group by pressing into the inner surface of the pelvis right by the anterior superior iliac spine.	The psoas major and iliacus are commonly tested together. To test the iliopsoas muscle with emphasis on the psoas major, the patient is supine. Stabilize the opposite iliac crest and have the patient use the quadriceps to stabilize the knee into extension. The hip is flexed with slight abduction and slight lateral rotation (external rotation). Apply pressure against the anteromedial leg in the direction of extension and slight abduction.

(continues)

Table 11.8 Vertebral Column Lateral Flexion (continued)

Muscle	Origin	Insertion	Action	Innervation (Nerve Root)	Palpation	Manual Muscle Test
Intertransversarii	Spanning the transverse process of C2–C7 (cervical) Spanning the transverse process of L1–L5 (lumbar)	Spanning the transverse process of C2–C7 (cervical) Spanning the transverse process of L1–L5 (lumbar)	Laterally flex the vertebral column to the same side (unilaterally) Extend the vertebral column (bilaterally)	Spinal	Palpate deep between the transverse processes of adjacent vertebrae.	There is no specific manual muscle test for the intertransversarii muscle.
Spinalis	Spinous process of the upper lumbar and lower thoracic vertebrae (thoracis) Ligamentum nuchae, spinous process of C7 (cervicis)	Spinous process of the upper thoracic (thoracis) Spinous processes of cervicals, except C1 (cervicis)	Laterally flex the vertebral column to the same side (unilaterally) Extend the vertebral column (bilaterally) Primary mover for spinal extension, assists in lateral bending and spinal rotation on the same side	Spinal	Easily palpated entire length of back and neck close to spine. The examiner should be positioned behind the patient and have him or her extend the head to relax fascia. Knead the muscles looking for tenderness, spasm, defects, and bilateral size.	There is no specific manual muscle test for the spinalis muscle.

Latissimus dorsi	Inferior angle of the scapula Spinous process T6–T12 Last three or four ribs Thoracolumbar aponeurosis Posterior iliac crest	Intertubercular groove of the humerus	Extend the shoulder (glenohumeral joint) Adduct the shoulder (glenohumeral joint) Medially rotate (internal rotation) of the shoulder (glenohumeral joint)	Thoracodorsal (C6–C8)	The latissimus dorsi is a relatively large muscle with a large palpation site toward the lower thoracic spine. Have the patient lie prone with the shoulder off the table. Internally rotate the shoulder to feel the fibers of the latissimus dorsi muscle. The latissimus dorsi muscle can be palpated by having the patient lie supine; raise the shoulder to 90° and have the patient press the elbow toward the hip against resistance. The latissimus dorsi may be palpated close to the rib cage.	Place the patient in a prone position with the head facing the arm being tested. Have the patient adduct the arm with extension in the medially rotated (internally rotated) position. The examiner provides pressure against the forearm in the direction of abduction and slight flexion of the arm.
Longissimus	Common tendon (thoracis) Transverse process of the upper five thoracic vertebrae (cervicis and capitis)	Lower nine ribs and transverse process of the thoracic vertebrae (thoracis) Transverse processes of cervical vertebrae (cervicis) Mastoid process of the temporal bone (capitis)	Laterally flex the vertebral column to the same side (unilaterally) Extend the vertebral column (bilaterally)	Spinal	Have the patient lie prone, palpate the longissimus along the spine while the patient extends the spine or raises the feet to activate the muscle.	There is no specific manual muscle test for the longissimus muscle.

Data from Biel A: *Trail Guide to the Body*, rev ed 5. Boulder, CO, Books of Discovery, 2014; and Kendall FP, McCreary EK, Provance PG, Rodgers MM, Romani WA: *Muscles: Testing and Function with Posture and Pain*, ed 5. Baltimore, MD, Lippincott Williams & Wilkins, 2005.

Table 11.9 Vertebral Column Stabilization

Muscle	Origin	Insertion	Action	Innervation (Nerve Root)	Palpation	Manual Muscle Test
Transverse abdominis	Lateral inguinal ligament Iliac crest Thoracolumbar fascia Internal surface of lower six ribs	Abdominal aponeurosis to linea alba	Compress abdominal contents	T7–L1 Iliohypogastric and ilioinguinal Ventral divisions	The transverse abdominis is the innermost muscular layer of the abdomen. The transverse abdominis forces expiration by pulling the abdominal wall in and stabilizing the lumbar spine. Because of the muscle's depth, palpation of the transverse abdominis is extremely difficult.	There is no specific muscle test for the transverse abdominis muscle. The abdominal muscles may be tested as a group together as the upper and lower abdominals (refer to manual muscle test for the rectus abdominis).

Data from Biel A: *Trail Guide to the Body*, rev ed 5. Boulder, CO, Books of Discovery, 2014; and Kendall FP, McCreary EK, Provance PG, Rodgers MM, Romani WA: *Muscles: Testing and Function with Posture and Pain*, ed 5. Baltimore, MD, Lippincott Williams & Wilkins, 2005.

Vertebral Column Stabilization

The muscles of the vertebral column often work together to help stabilize the abdomen and thorax. Particiularly, the transverse abdominis acts much like a girdle to compress the abdominal contents and provides stabilization to the entire lower back and core muscles. Activation of the transverse abdominis helps compress and support the internal organs and expel air during forced exhalation. Weakness in the transverse abdominis is often the most common reason people experience lower back pain. If the transverse abdominis is weak, the abdominal wall will often bulge forward, and the pelvis may rotate forward as well, resulting in increased lordosis. The transverse abdominis is the deepest layer of all the abdominal muscles and one of the most difficult muscles to train[13,15] (Table 11.9).

Muscles Used for Breathing

During quiet breathing, the diaphragm is the predominant muscle used during respiration[13] (Table 11.10). During inspiration, the diaphragm contracts, and the pleural pressure drops, which decreases the alveolar pressure and draws the air down and in from the pressure gradient from the mouth to the alveoli[15] (Table 11.11). Expiration is a relatively passive process—respiratory muscles relax, and the elastic lung and chest wall return passively to their resting volume[15] (Table 11.12).

During exercise or bouts of breathing emergencies, such as asthma, other muscles may become more important and involved in respiration. During inspiration, the external intercostals help to raise the lower ribs up and out, which increases the lateral and anteroposterior dimension of the thorax (Table 11.11). Additionally, the scalene muscles and sternocleidomastoid also become involved and help raise and push out the upper ribs and sternum. During active expiration, the most important muscles are those of the abdominal wall, which increase the intraabdominal pressure when they contract and thus pushes up the diaphragm, raising the pleural pressure and alveolar pressure driving out the air (Table 11.12). The internal intercoastal muscles also activate in active expiration by pulling the ribs down and in, decreasing the thoracic volume.

The muscles of the thorax and abdomen are essential to basic functions of nearly all movements. Without core control, an individual cannot move their arms or legs; therefore, when evaluating or rehabilitating injuries, the clinician should always consider including core conditioning in the rehabilitation protocols.

Table 11.10 Muscles Used for Breathing

Accessory respiratory muscles (inhalation)
- Sternocleidomastoid muscle
- Pectoralis minor muscle
- Serratus anterior muscle

Primary respiratory muscles (inhalation)
- External intercostal muscles
- Diaphragm

Accessory respiratory muscles (exhalation)
- Internal intercostal muscles
- Transversus thoracis muscle
- External oblique muscle
- Internal oblique muscle
- Rectus abdominis

Ribs and thorax elevation/expansion (involved in inhalation; antagonists on depression)	Diaphragm Anterior scalene (bilaterally) Middle scalene (bilaterally) Posterior scalene (bilaterally) Sternocleidomastoid (assists) External intercostals (assists) Serratus posterior superior Pectoralis major (all fibers may assist if the arm is fixed) Pectoralis minor (if scapula is fixed) Serratus anterior (if scapula is fixed) Subclavius (first rib)
Ribs and thorax depression/collapse (involved with exhalation; antagonist on elevation)	Internal intercostals (assists) Serratus posterior inferior

Data from Biel A: *Trail Guide to the Body*, rev ed 5. Boulder, CO, Books of Discovery, 2014.

Injury Conditions to the Thorax and Abdomen

Many injuries can occur to the thorax and abdomen. Some conditions explored in this chapter may be life threatening, while others are relatively minor. All clinicians should maintain their cardiopulmonary resuscitation training in the event an emergency occurs in their presence. Many of these injuries are often extremely painful and can be debilitating to the athletic and physically active population. Injury conditions to the thorax and abdomen[16-70] will be explored in **Tables 11.13** through **11.33**.

Table 11.11 Ribs and Thorax Elevation/Expansion for Inhalation

Muscle	Origin	Insertion	Action	Innervation (Nerve Root)	Palpation	Manual Muscle Test
Diaphragm	Costal attachment: Inner surface of the lower six ribs Lumbar attachment: Upper two or three lumbar vertebrae Sternal attachment: Inner part of the xiphoid process	Central tendon of the diaphragm	Draw down the central tendon of the diaphragm Increase the volume of the thoracic cavity during inhalation	Phrenic nerve C3–C5	Have the patient lie prone to palpate the diaphragm. Hook the thumb or fingers under the rib cage and encourage the patient to relax and feel for breathing. The diaphragm can be palpated with the patient side lying and the examiner's fingers curled around the ribs to access the diaphragm.	There is no specific manual muscle test for the diaphragm muscle.
Anterior scalene	Transverse process of the third through sixth cervical vertebrae (anterior tubercles)	First rib	With the ribs fixed, laterally flex the head and neck to the same side (anterior, middle, and posterior scalene muscles [unilaterally]) Rotate head and neck to the opposite side (anterior, middle, and posterior scalene muscles [unilaterally]) Elevate the ribs during inhalation (anterior, middle, and posterior scalene muscles [bilaterally])	C3–C8	The scalene muscles are typically palpated together as a group. Have the patient lie supine and palpate the muscle group between the sternocleidomastoid and anterior flap of trapezius; contraction of the muscles can be felt as the patient inhales. The anterior fibers are associated with the anterior scalene, middle fibers are associated with the middle scalene, and posterior fibers are associated with the posterior scalene.	There is no specific manual muscle test for the anterior scalene muscle. The muscle may be tested by testing the anterior neck flexor group (longus capitis, longus colli, rectus capitis anterior, sternocleidomastoid, anterior scalene, suprahyoid, and infrahyoid muscles). To test the anterior neck flexor group, have the patient lie supine with the shoulders abducted and flexed, the elbows bent, and the hands overhead resting on the table. Have the patient flex the neck while keeping the chin depressed and approximated toward the sternum against resistance. In addition, the anterior scalene muscle may be tested as a group with the anterolateral neck flexors (sternocleidomastoid, anterior scalene, middle scalene, and posterior

Injury Conditions to the Thorax and Abdomen

Muscle	Attachment	Attachment	Action	Innervation	Palpation	Manual Muscle Test
			Flex the head and neck (anterior, middle, and posterior scalene muscles [bilaterally])		The brachial plexus runs between the anterior and the middle scalene muscles, so caution should be exercised with palpation in this area.	scalene). To test the anterolateral neck flexors, the patient is supine with the shoulders abducted and flexed, the elbows bent, and the hands overhead resting on the table. Have the patient flex the head with rotation toward the same side being tested.
Middle scalene	Transverse process of the second through seventh cervical vertebrae (posterior tubercle)	First rib	With the ribs fixed, laterally flex the head and neck to the same side (anterior, middle, and posterior scalene muscles [unilaterally]) Rotate head and neck to the opposite side (anterior, middle, and posterior scalene muscles [unilaterally]) Elevate the ribs during inhalation (anterior, middle, and posterior scalene muscles [bilaterally]) Flex the head and neck (anterior, middle, and posterior scalene muscles [bilaterally])	C3–C8	The scalene muscles are typically palpated together as a group. Have the patient lie supine and palpate the muscle group between the sternocleidomastoid and anterior flap of trapezius; contraction of the muscles can be felt as the patient inhales. The anterior fibers are associated with the anterior scalene, middle fibers are associated with the middle scalene, and posterior fibers are associated with the posterior scalene. The brachial plexus runs between the anterior and the middle scalene muscles, so caution should be exercised with palpation in this area.	There is no specific manual muscle test for the middle scalene muscle. The middle scalene muscle may be tested as a group with the anterolateral neck flexors (sternocleidomastoid, anterior scalene, middle scalene, and posterior scalene). To test the anterolateral neck flexors, the patient is supine with the shoulders abducted and flexed, the elbows bent, and the hands are overhead resting on the table. Have the patient flex the head with rotation toward the same side being tested.

(continues)

Table 11.11 Ribs and Thorax Elevation/Expansion for Inhalation (continued)

Muscle	Origin	Insertion	Action	Innervation (Nerve Root)	Palpation	Manual Muscle Test
Posterior scalene	Transverse process of the sixth and seventh cervical vertebrae (posterior tubercles)	First rib	With the ribs fixed, laterally flex the head and neck to the same side (anterior, middle, and posterior scalene muscles [unilaterally]) Rotate head and neck to the opposite side (anterior, middle, and posterior scalene muscles [unilaterally]) Elevate the ribs during inhalation (anterior, middle, and posterior scalene muscles [bilaterally]) Flex the head and neck (anterior, middle, and posterior scalene muscles [bilaterally])	C3–C8	The three scalene muscles are typically palpated together as a group. Have the patient lie supine and palpate the muscle group between the sternocleidomastoid and anterior flap of trapezius; contraction of the muscles can be felt as the patient inhales. The anterior fibers are associated with the anterior scalene, middle fibers are associated with the middle scalene, and posterior fibers are associated with the posterior scalene.	There is no specific manual muscle test for the posterior scalene muscle. The posterior scalene muscle may be tested as a group with the anterolateral neck flexors (sternocleidomastoid, anterior scalene, middle scalene, and posterior scalene). To test the anterolateral neck flexors, the patient is supine with the shoulders abducted and flexed, the elbows bent, and the hands overhead resting on the table. Have the patient flex the head with rotation toward the same side being tested.
Sternocleidomastoid	Top of manubrium (sternal head) Medial one-third clavicle (clavicular head)	Mastoid process of temporal bone Lateral portion of superior nuchal line of occiput	Rotation skull to opposite side (unilaterally) Laterally flex cervical spine (unilaterally) Neck flexion (bilaterally) Assist to elevate rib cage during inhalation	C1–C3	Have the patient lie supine to palpate the sternocleidomastoid muscle. Ask the patient to turn the head to the contralateral (opposite) side of palpated muscle. The sternocleidomastoid will stick out, and the belly of the muscle can be grasped. The patient can flex the head/neck to engage the sternocleidomastoid muscle.	There is no specific manual muscle test for the sternocleidomastoid muscle. The sternocleidomastoid muscle may be tested as a group with the anterolateral neck flexors (sternocleidomastoid, anterior scalene, middle scalene, and posterior scalene). To test the anterolateral neck flexors, the patient is supine with the shoulders abducted and flexed, the elbows bent, and the hands overhead resting on the table. Have the patient flex the head with rotation towards the same side being tested.

External intercostals	Inferior border of the rib above	Superior border of the rib below	Draw the ribs superiorly (increasing the space of the thoracic cavity) to assist with inhalation	Thoracic	Have the patient lie supine, palpate the external intercostals between the ribs. The examiner will feel the muscle activate during inhalation.	There is no specific manual muscle test for the external intercostal muscles.
Serratus posterior superior	Spinous process of C7 to T3	Posterior surface of the second through fifth ribs	Elevate the ribs during inhalation	T1–T4	Have the patient lie prone and palpate the serratus posterior superior close to the transverse process between C7 and T3.	There is no specific manual muscle test for the serratus posterior superior muscle.
Pectoralis major	Medial half of the clavicle, sternum and cartilage of the first through sixth ribs	Crest of the greater tubercle of the humerus	Adduct the shoulder (glenohumeral joint [all fibers]) Medially rotate the shoulder (glenohumeral joint [all fibers]) Assist in elevation of the thorax during forced inhalation (with the arm fixed [all fibers]) Flex the shoulder (glenohumeral joint [upper fibers]) Horizontally adduct the shoulder (glenohumeral joint [upper fibers])	Lateral pectoral C5–C7 (upper fibers) Lateral and medial pectoral C6–T1 (lower fibers)	Have the patient lie supine, palpate the pectoralis major by medially rotating the patient's shoulder against resistance. With the patient's arm raised (abducted and flexed), contraction of the lower fibers can be palpated. The pectoralis major can be palpated by having the patient side lying and palpating the muscle belly.	There are two tests for the pectoralis major: a manual muscle test for the upper fibers and a manual muscle test for the lower fibers. To test the upper fibers of the pectoralis major, place the patient supine and have the patient flex the shoulder to 90° with slight medial rotation (internal rotation) while keeping the elbow straight. The humerus is horizontally adducted toward the sternal end of the clavicle with the examiner providing resistance. To test the lower fibers of the pectoralis major, place the patient supine, have the patient flex the shoulder (approximately 45°) with slight medial rotation (internal rotation), the elbow remains straight. The humerus is adducted toward the opposite iliac crest with the examiner providing resistance.

Injury Conditions to the Thorax and Abdomen

(continues)

Table 11.11 Ribs and Thorax Elevation/Expansion for Inhalation (continued)

Muscle	Origin	Insertion	Action	Innervation (Nerve Root)	Palpation	Manual Muscle Test
Pectoralis major (continued)			Extend the shoulder (glenohumeral joint) [lower fibers]			
Pectoralis minor	Third, fourth, and fifth ribs	Medial surface of the coracoid process of the scapula	Depress the scapula (scapulothoracic joint) Abduct the scapula (scapulothoracic joint) Downwardly rotate the scapula (scapulothoracic joint) Assist to elevate the thorax during forced inhalation (with the scapula fixed)	Medial pectoral, with fibers from a communicating branch of the lateral pectoral C6–T1	The pectoralis minor is palpated underneath the pectoralis major. Have the patient lie supine and slide the fingers under the pectoralis major to access the pectoralis minor. The pectoralis minor can also be palpated in a side-lying position with the patient's arm flexed while palpating along the ribs.	Place the patient in a supine position with the arm being tested by the patient's side. Have the patient thrust the shoulder forward while the arm remains by the patient's side. The examiner will apply a downward pressure on the head of the humerus. The patient should not be pressing down on the table during the test. If necessary, have the patient raise the hand or elbow off the table to test.

Injury Conditions to the Thorax and Abdomen

Serratus anterior	External surfaces of the upper eight or nine ribs	Anterior surface of the medial border of the scapula	Abduct the scapula (scapulothoracic joint [with the origin fixed]) Upwardly rotate the scapula (scapulothoracic joint [with the origin fixed]) Depress the scapula (scapulothoracic joint [with the origin fixed]) Hold the medial border of the scapula against the rib cage (scapulothoracic joint [with the origin fixed]) May act to elevate the thorax during forced inhalation (with the scapula fixed)	Long thoracic (C5–C8)	The serratus anterior can be isolated by having the patient lie supine with the shoulder elevated. The patient will reach the hand toward the ceiling, and the serratus anterior can be palpated along the ribs. The serratus anterior can also be palpated with the patient side lying; the examiner's fingers can be curled under the medial border of the scapula to palpate the insertion point of the muscle.	There are three tests that have been suggested for the serratus anterior muscle.

The preferred serratus anterior manual muscle test occurs with the patient sitting. The patient attempts to stabilize the scapula while the arm is in a position of approximately 120° to 130° shoulder flexion. The examiner applies resistance against the dorsal surface of the humerus (between the shoulder and elbow) in a downward direction toward extension with slight pressure against the lateral border of the scapula in the direction of rotating the inferior angle medially. This test emphasizes the upward rotation action of the serratus in the shoulder abducted position (A).

The supine serratus anterior manual muscle test is performed with the patient lying supine. The patient flexes the shoulder to 90°. The patient performs abduction of the scapula by projecting the upper extremity anteriorly (upward from the table, as if punching in the air). The examiner provides resistance to the patient's hand by transmitting pressure down the upper extremity to the scapula in the direction of adducting the scapula. Slight pressure may be applied to the lateral border of the scapula or against the fist. The muscles from the pectoralis minor, levator scapula, and rhomboids may assist with this motion; therefore, examiners may misrepresent the strength available to the patient from the serratus anterior muscle (B).

The standing serratus anterior manual muscle test is performed with the patient standing and facing a wall |

(continues)

Table 11.11 Ribs and Thorax Elevation/Expansion for Inhalation *(continued)*

Muscle	Origin	Insertion	Action	Innervation (Nerve Root)	Palpation	Manual Muscle Test
Serratus anterior *(continued)*						with the elbows straight. The patient places both hands against the wall at shoulder level (or slightly above). The patient allows the thorax to sag forward so the scapula is in a position of adduction. The patient pushes hard against the wall, displacing the thorax backward. This is a strenuous test due to the weight of the thorax, and therefore muscle grading should not be used. This test is only used to determine strong and weak muscles.
Subclavius	First rib and cartilage	Inferior surface of the middle third of the clavicle	Depress the clavicle and draw it anteriorly Elevate the first rib (to assist during inhalation) Stabilize the sternoclavicular joint	Subclavian C5–C6	Palpate the subclavius muscle by having the patient side lying with the arm flexed and palpating just inferior to the clavicle. Use the thumb or finger to pin the muscle belly to the clavicle during palpation.	There is no specific manual muscle test for the subclavius muscle.

All figures in table © Jones & Bartlett Learning.
Data from Kendall FP, McCreary EK, Provance PG, Rodgers MM, Romani WA: *Muscles: Testing and Function with Posture and Pain*, ed 5. Baltimore, MD, Lippincott Williams & Wilkins, 2005.

Table 11.12 Ribs and Thorax Depression/Collapse for Exhalation

Muscle	Origin	Insertion	Action	Innervation (Nerve Root)	Palpation	Manual Muscle Test
Internal intercostals	Inferior border of the rib above	Superior border of the rib below	Draws ribs inferiorly (decreasing the space of the thoracic cavity) to assist with exhalation	Thoracic	Have the patient lie supine, palpate the internal intercostals between the ribs. Muscle activation can be felt during exhalation.	There is no specific manual muscle test for the internal intercostal muscles.
Serratus posterior inferior	Spinous processes of T12–L3	Posterior surface of the 9th through 12th ribs	Depress the ribs during exhalation	T9–12	Have the patient lie prone and palpate the serratus posterior inferior close to the transverse process of T12 to L3.	There is no specific manual muscle test for the serratus posterior inferior muscle.

Data from Kendall FP, McCreary EK, Provance PG, Rodgers MM, Romani WA: *Muscles: Testing and Function with Posture and Pain*, ed 5. Baltimore, MD, Lippincott Williams & Wilkins, 2005.

Table 11.13 Rib Contusion Quick Tips

Pathology	Description	Presentation (HIPS)	Special Test/Imaging	Differential Diagnosis	5-Min Sideline Assessment Tips
Rib contusions	A blow to the rib cage can bruise the intercostal muscles or, if severe enough, produce a fracture. Because the intercostal muscles are essential for breathing, both expiration and inspiration can become very painful when the intercostal muscles are bruised.	*Unique/directed history questions for the identified pathology* • Did you sustain a direct blow to the ribs? • Are you having any difficulty breathing? • Have you been coughing up any frothy or bloody sputum? *Common observations unique to specific pathology* • Pain with breathing. • Sharp pain during coughing and sneezing. • Bruising and ecchymosis may be present over the affected rib. *Common observation findings* • Contusion or laceration over the area of trauma. *Palpations with expected outcomes* • Point tenderness over the specific rib. • Pain during breathing. • Pain with rib cage compression.	No specific special tests clinically diagnose a rib contusion. The clinical diagnosis is made from the history and palpation. *Review of body systems* • Cardiovascular: Rapid, thready pulse if in shock. • Respiratory: Shallow breaths, increased frequency if in shock. • Gastrointestinal: Within normal limits. • Genitourinary: Within normal limits. • Neurologic: Within normal limits. *Imaging* • Radiographic examination should be routine if a rib contusion occurs to rule out possible fracture. *Functional assessment/ outcome measures* • General unwillingness to move. • Pain aggravated by movement.	Rib fracture Rib stress fracture Abdominal muscle strain Lung injury Pneumothorax	Nonsurgical management and anti-inflammatory agents are both commonly used for treatment of rib contusions. Contusions are self-limiting.

HIPS, history, inspection, palpation, special tests.

Table 11.14 Rib Fractures Quick Tips

Pathology	Description	Presentation (HIPS)	Special Test/Imaging	Differential Diagnosis	5-Min Sideline Assessment Tips
Rib fractures A radiograph of a rib fracture. Reproduced from Armstrong AD, Hubbard MC, eds: *Essentials of Musculoskeletal Care*, ed 5. Burlington, MA, American Academy of Orthopaedic Surgeons. 2015.	Rib fractures are the most common serious injury of the chest occurring in sports participation. Rib fractures are extremely common in sports as the result of direct trauma. Collision sports, such as football, lacrosse, rugby, and wrestling, are frequently associated with rib fractures following a blow to the thoracic cavity. Direct impact causes the most serious damage, as the external force frequently displaces the rib inwardly toward the delicate lungs. The jagged edges from the fracture may cut, tear, or perforate the tissue of the pleurae, causing a hemothorax, or they may even collapse one lung (called a pneumothorax). Fractures can be the result of either direct or indirect trauma. Occasionally, albeit infrequently, rib fractures can be the result of violent muscular contractions. An indirect force is generally the result of compression of the rib cage as may occur in football or wrestling when a participant falls or someone falls on top of someone else. Ribs may also fracture from high-velocity forces during coughing and sneezing. An indirect fracture will cause the rib to spring outward away from the thoracic cavity, which will	*Unique/directed history questions for the identified pathology* • Did you sustain a direct blow to the ribs? • Did anyone fall on you or run into you? • Are you having any difficulty breathing? • Have you been coughing up any frothy or bloody sputum? • Are you feeling or hearing any unusual sounds (ie, crepitus in a rib) during breathing? • Wheezing: Asthma may potentially complicate a potential rib fracture. *Common observations unique to specific pathology* • Pain with breathing. • Difficulty breathing. • Bruising and ecchymosis may be present over the affected rib. • Swelling may be present over the affected rib. *Common observation findings* • Severe, sharp pain during inspiration. • Contusion or discoloration over site of impact. • Pain with rib cage compression. • Rule out open fracture of the ribs (sucking chest wound).	*Special tests* • Mobility of the first rib. • Compression test for rib fracture. 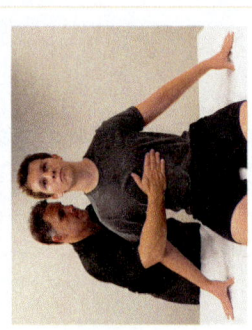 © Jones & Bartlett Learning *Imaging* • Ultrasonography should be routine if a rib contusion occurs to rule out possible fracture (radiographs are a less desirable method of evaluation, but may still be able to assess rib fractures).	Severe rib contusion Costochondral separations Muscle strains (erector spinae injury) Stress fracture Pneumothorax Hemothorax	Injuries to the pectoral muscles may mask the signs and symptoms of a rib fracture. An uncomplicated fracture can be difficult to diagnose on radiograph; therefore, the most common treatment is to treat the symptoms of the rib fracture and make the patient as comfortable as possible. A rib brace can offer some support, stabilization, and comfort to the patient. Rib supports may predispose a patient to the development of hypostatic pneumonia, which can occur when a patient cannot take full inspirations because of pain and/or has a mechanical restriction.

Injury Conditions to the Thorax and Abdomen 451

result in an oblique or transverse fracture.

Stress fractures of the ribs can also occur and are becoming more common in sports. Stress fractures can occur from repetitive arm movements, such as those occurring in overhead athletes. Stress fractures may also occur from repetitive coughing or laughing.

Ribs five through nine are the most commonly fractured. Multiple rib fractures are considered a severe injury and may be extremely painful for the patient. A flail chest involves three or more fractures of consecutive ribs on the same side.

- Possible splinting posture, or the patient holding the affected area.
- Patient may be leaning toward the affected side.

Palpations with expected outcomes

- Severe, sharp pain during palpation over the affected rib.
- Point tenderness over the area of impact.
- Sharp pain during coughing and sneezing.
- Crepitus during palpation.
- Possible deformity.
- Possible indentation at the fracture site.

- MRI or CT may be used to rule out concurrent injury to the lungs or other tissues.

Functional assessment/outcome measures

- Movement of the torso produces pain along the fracture site.
- Torso movement may be limited.
- Active motion, deep respiration, coughing, or sneezing may induce pain.

HIPS, history, inspection, palpation, special tests.
Data from Connolly LP, Connolly SA: Rib stress fractures. *Clin l Nucl Med* 2004;29(10):614-616; Dodds S: Injuries to the pectoralis major. *Sports Med* 2002;32(14):945; Du Preez G: Fractured ribs may result in serious complications. *Nursing Times* 2003;99(20):27.; Marasco S, Davies AR, Cooper J, et al: Prospective randomized controlled trial of operative rib fixation in traumatic flail chest. *J Am Coll Surg* 2013;216l5:924-932; McGown A: Blunt abdominal and chest trauma. *Athl Ther Today* 2004;9(1):40; Miles JW, Barrett GR: Rib fractures in athletes. *Sports Med* 1991;12(1):66-69; Pishbin E, Ahmadi K, Foogardi M, Salehi M, Toosi FS, Rahimi-Movaghar V: Comparison of ultrasonography and radiography in diagnosis of rib fractures. *Clin J Traumatol* 2017;20(4):226-228; and Ryan J: Abdominal injuries and sport. *Br J Sports Med* 1999;33(3):155.

Table 11.15 Costochondral Separation and Dislocation Quick Tips

Pathology	Description	Presentation (HIPS)	Special Test/Imaging	Differential Diagnosis	5-Min Sideline Assessment Tips
Costochondral separation and dislocation	Costochondral separation and dislocation has an extremely high incidence in sports, even higher than rib fractures. This injury occurs from a direct blow to the anterolateral thorax or can occur indirectly from a sudden twist or a fall on some object, compressing the rib cage.	*Unique/directed history questions for the identified pathology* • Did you sustain a direct blow to the ribs? • Did anyone fall on you or run into you? • Are you having any difficulty breathing? • Have you been coughing up any frothy or bloody sputum? *Common observations unique to specific pathology* • Difficulty breathing deeply; the patient may be breathing very shallowly. • Sharp pain during sudden movement of the trunk. • Sharp pain during coughing and sneezing. • Possible contusion or discoloration at site of injury. *Common observation findings* • Point tenderness with swelling at the site of injury. • Possible rib deformity. • Possible crepitus as the rib moves in and out of place. *Palpations with expected outcomes* • Pain localized in the junction of the rib cartilage and rib.	*Special tests* • Compression test for rib fractures. *Imaging* • Radiograph examination should be routine if a rib contusion occurs to rule out possible fracture. *Functional assessment/outcome measures* • Movement of the torso produces pain. • Torso movement may be limited. • Active motion, deep respiration, coughing, or sneezing may induce pain.	Severe rib contusion Rib fracture Muscle strains of the thorax Stress fracture Pneumothorax Hemothorax	Costochondral separation is managed by rest and immobilization with a rib brace. Complete healing takes several months. Any strenuous activity should be eliminated until the patient is symptom free.

HIPS, history, inspection, palpation, special tests.
Data from Du Preez G: Fractured ribs may result in serious complications. *Nursing Times* 2003;99(20):27.; Pishbin E, Ahmadi K, Foogardi M, Salehi M, Toosi FS, Rahimi-Movaghar V: Comparison of ultrasonography and radiography in diagnosis of rib fractures. *Clin J Traumatol* 2017;20(4):226-228.; and Prentice WE: *Principles of Athletic Training: A Guide to Evidence-Based Clinical Practice*, ed 16. New York, NY, McGraw-Hill Education, 2017.

Table 11.16 Rib Tip Syndrome Quick Tips

Pathology	Description	Presentation (HIPS)	Special Test/Imaging	Differential Diagnosis	5-Min Sideline Assessment Tips
Rib tip syndrome	Rib tip syndrome involves ribs 8, 9, and 10 and the cartilage attached to each rib. The connections of ribs 8, 9, or 10 are damaged due to trauma; the ribs can dislocate and impinge on the intercostal nerve, which results in pain. This injury is most common in contact sports.	*Unique/directed history questions for the identified pathology* • Did you sustain a direct blow to the ribs? • Did anyone fall on you or run into you? • Are you having any difficulty breathing? *Common observations unique to specific pathology* • No unusual observations of the rib cage are typically noted. *Common observation findings* • Pain with lateral flexion and hyperextension toward the opposite side. • Slight possibility of discoloration or contusion at the site of injury. *Palpations with expected outcomes* • Pain can be reproduced by hooking the fingers under the inferior rib and pulling the rib anteriorly. A positive test produces a click sound either heard or felt. • Pain in the upper abdomen or inferior costal area (frequently sharp, shooting, or stabbing pain).	*Special tests* • No specific special tests clinically diagnose rib tip syndrome. The clinical diagnosis is made from the history and palpation. *Review of body systems* • Cardiovascular: Rapid, thready pulse if in shock. • Respiratory: Shallow breaths, increased frequency. • Gastrointestinal: Within normal limits. • Genitourinary: Within normal limits. • Neurologic: Intercostal nerve pain. *Imaging* • Radiographs are not recommended for this type of injury. *Functional assessment/outcome measures* • Pain in ribs 8, 9, and/or 10. • General unwillingness to move. • The patient may be holding the abdomen or ribs in the area of trauma.	Costochondral separation Rib contusion Rib fracture Muscle strains of the thorax Stress fracture	It is uncommon for the patient to report a popping sensation or slipping movement of the ribs with this condition. The ribs will be extremely sore and may need support if possible.

HIPS, history, inspection, palpation, special tests.
Data from Prentice WE: *Principles of Athletic Training: A Guide to Evidence-Based Clinical Practice*, ed 16. New York, NY, McGraw-Hill Education, 2017.

Table 11.17 Sternum Fracture Quick Tips

Pathology	Description	Presentation (HIPS)	Special Test/Imaging	Differential Diagnosis	5-Min Sideline Assessment Tips
Sternum fracture	Fracture of the sternum results from a high-velocity blow to the center of the chest. Sternum fractures are more frequently the result of injury from an automobile accident than from sports. An impact strong enough to cause fracture of the sternum may also cause trauma to the underlying cardiac muscle, which is a significant concern.	*Unique/directed history questions for the identified pathology* • Have you recently sustained a blow to the center of the chest? • Are you having any difficulty breathing? • Are you having difficulty catching your breath? *Common observations unique to specific pathology* • Difficulty breathing, especially with deep inspiration and forceful expiration. • Signs of shock may be present in the patient. • Weak, rapid pulse may indicate a more severe internal injury. • If the patient is not breathing, activate the emergency action plan. *Common observation findings* • Bruising around the sternum and associated ribs. • Possible crepitus with breathing. *Palpations with expected outcomes* • Point tenderness over the sternum at the site of the fracture.	*Special tests* • No specific special tests clinically diagnose a sternum fracture. The clinical diagnosis is made from the history and palpation. *Review of body systems* • Cardiovascular: Rapid, thready pulse if in shock. • Respiratory: Shallow breaths, increased frequency if in shock. • Gastrointestinal: Within normal limits. • Genitourinary: Within normal limits. • Neurologic: Within normal limits. *Radiographic orders if appropriate* • The patient should be sent for radiographs and be closely monitored for signs of shock and signs of trauma to the heart. *Functional assessment/outcome measures* • Pain in the chest. • General unwillingness to move. • Difficulty breathing, difficulty catching breath or regulating breathing.	Rib fracture Costochondral separation Pericarditis Pneumothorax	A sternum fracture is going to result in a significant amount of pain. Because of the force required to fracture the sternum, cardiac involvement should be suspected.

HIPS, history, inspection, palpation, special tests.
Data from Du Preez G: Fractured ribs may result in serious complications. *Nursing Times* 2003;99(20):27; and Prentice WE: *Principles of Athletic Training: A Guide to Evidence-Based Clinical Practice*, ed 16. New York, NY, McGraw-Hill Education, 2017.

Table 11.18 Disk Herniation Quick Tips

Pathology	Description	Presentation (HIPS)	Special Test/Imaging	Differential Diagnosis	5-Min Sideline Assessment Tips
Disk herniation	A herniated disk is also called a bulged, slipped, or ruptured disk. A fragment of the disk, the nucleus pulposus, is pushed out of the annulus fibrosus and into the spinal canal through a tear or rupture in the annulus fibrosus. Disk herniations are extremely common with more than 3 million cases per year in the United States.	*Unique/directed history questions for the identified pathology* • Have you recently lifted anything heavy? • Are you having any back pain? • Are there any positions that make the pain better or worse? *Common observations unique to specific pathology* • Most patients are asymptomatic. • Some people may be unwilling to move or leaning to one side. • Possible numbness or tingling into the upper extremities. *Common observation findings* • None *Palpations with expected outcomes* • None	*Special tests* • For the thoracic spine, no specific special tests clinically diagnose a disk herniation. The clinical diagnosis is made from the history and palpation. *Review of body systems* • Cardiovascular: Within normal limits. • Respiratory: Within normal limits. • Gastrointestinal: Within normal limits. • Genitourinary: Within normal limits. • Neurologic: Likely within normal limits. Possible numbness or tingling into the upper extremities. *Radiographic orders if appropriate* • The patient should be sent for radiographs. • MRI can identify and assess disk herniations. MRI should only be used to confirm a clinical diagnosis and reported pain. Disk herniation has been identified in asymptomatic individuals and does not necessarily indicate a pathologic injury in the absence of pain. • CT can be used to evaluate bony tissue, the spinal contents, and the surrounding soft tissues. *Functional assessment/outcome measures* • General unwillingness to move.	Muscle spasm Spinal fracture Neuropathy	Some disk herniations cause no symptoms. Others can irritate nearby nerves, which restuls in pain, numbness, neuropathy, or weakness in an extremity.

HIPS, history, inspection, palpation, special tests.
Data from Wood KB, Blair JM, Aeppie DM, et al: The natural history of asymptomatic thoracic disc herniations. *Spine* 1997;22:525-530; and Wood KB, Garvey TA, Gundry C, Heithoff KB: Magnetic resonance imaging of the thoracic spine. *J Bone Joint Surg Am* 1995;77:1631-1638.

Table 11.19 Thoracic Outlet Syndrome Quick Tips

Pathology	Description	Presentation (HIPS)	Special Test/Imaging	Differential Diagnosis	5-Min Sideline Assessment Tips
Thoracic outlet syndrome	TOS involves the brachial plexus, the subclavian artery, or the subclavian vein (collectively known as the neurovascular bundle) being compressed between muscles within the interscalene triangle, the costoclavicular space, and the subcoracoid space. TOS is classified as either vascular or neurologic. The neurovascular bundle passes between the clavicle and the first rib and is susceptible to pressure. The neurovascular bundle may also be impinged between the clavicle and the first rib. The neurovascular bundle can be compressed between the pectoralis minor and the rib cage or between the anterior and middle scalene muscles.	*Unique/directed history questions for the identified pathology* • Do your symptoms change with activity? Do they increase with overhead activity? • Do certain activities appear to increase your symptoms? • Does carrying a purse or backpack on your shoulder increase your symptoms? • Do you feel like your arms fall asleep? • Do you have any shoulder or arm pain? • Is there a specific time of the day that your symptoms are the most severe? • Do you have any numbness or paresthesia? • Have you had any recent neck injury? • Can you describe your symptoms? • Do you feel like your extremity gets cold during episodes? *Common observations unique to specific pathology* • Poor posture. • The patient may be supporting the affected arm.	*Special tests* • Allen test • Costoclavicular syndrome test (military brace position test) • Cyriax release test • Hyperabduction test • Morley sign • Roos test (EAST) • Supraclavicular pressure test • Tinels sign • Wright test *Imaging* • Radiographs can confirm (or rule out) the presence of a cervical rib. • Ultrasonography to identify arterial or venous insufficiency. • Angiography can confirm arterial TOS. • MRI can identify the presence of causative factors for TOS. *Functional assessment/outcome measures* • Active ROM: Cervical rotation combined with lateral cervical flexion may reveal muscle tightness in the scalenes. • Neurogenic: Cervical rotation to the opposite side and overhead movement may increase symptoms. • MMT: Neurogenic: weakness of the muscles of the hand. • Passive ROM: Neurogenic: Symptoms may be exacerbated during overhead motion.	Cervical disk herniation Carpal tunnel syndrome Cubital tunnel syndrome Vascular occlusive disease Malignant tumor Multiple sclerosis Fibromyalgia Raynaud disease Complex regional pain syndrome Angina	Nerve conduction studies and electromyography are used to diagnose TOS. Patients who have vascular symptoms should be immediately referred to a physician for further testing.

© Jones & Bartlett Learning

Vascular TOS is less common (arterial TOS less than 1%; venous TOS between 3% and 5%) than neurogenic TOS. TOS may be linked to the presence of a cervical rib (an extra rib present in approximately 1% of the population), which is more commonly found in women than men.	*Common observation findings* • Rounded shoulders and/or forward head posture. • Pallor and/or cyanosis in the involved arm. • Pooling edema. • Distended veins in the shoulder and chest. • Atrophy of the thenar eminence (Gilliatt-Sumner hand). *Palpations with expected outcomes* • Pooling edema may be palpated in the extremity. • Tenderness and spasm of the scalene muscles may be palpated. • Decreased skin temperature. • Point tenderness at Erb point (located at the third intercostal space and the left lower sternal border).

EAST, elevated arm stress test; HIPS, history, inspection, palpation, special tests; MMT, manual muscle test; ROM, range of motion; TOS, thoracic outlet syndrome.

Data from Demirbag D, Unlu E, Ozdemir F, et al: The relationship between magnetic resonance imaging findings and postural maneuver and physical examination tests in patients with thoracic outlet syndrome: results of a double-blind, controlled study. *Arch Phys Med Rehabil* 2007;88(7):844-851; Ferrante MAL: The thoracic outlet syndrome. *Muscle Nerve* 2012;45:780; Hooper TL, Denton J, McGalliard MK, Brismee JM, Sizer PS Jr: Thoracic outlet syndrome: a controversial clinical condition, part I: anatomy and clinical examination/diagnosis. *J Man Manip Ther* 2010;18(2):74-84.[27] Klaassen Z, Sorenson E, Tubbs RS, et al: Thoracic outlet syndrome: a neurological and vascular disorder. *Clin Anat* 2014;27(5):724-732; Prentice WE: *Principles of Athletic Training: A Guide to Evidence-Based Clinical Practice*, ed 16. New York, NY, McGraw-Hill Education, 2017; Sanders RJ, Hammond SL, Rao NM: Diagnosis of thoracic outlet syndrome. *J Vasc Surg* 2007;46:601; and Tender GC, Thomas AJ, Thomas N, Kline DG: Gilliat-Sumner hand revisited: a 25-year experience. *Neurosurgery* 2004;55(1):883-890.

Table 11.20 Muscle Injuries Quick Tips

Pathology	Description	Presentation (HIPS)	Special Test/Imaging	Differential Diagnosis	5-Min Sideline Assessment Tips
Muscle injuries	The muscles of the thorax and abdomen are subjected to trauma (contusions and strains) as a result of athletic participation. The intercostal muscles are especially vulnerable. Traumatic injuries can occur from direct blows or sudden torsion of the athlete's trunk.	*Unique/directed history questions for the identified pathology* • Are you experiencing any pain? • Where is the pain? • What is the type of pain? • Does pain increase with movement? • Do you recall any recent trauma? • Are you having any difficulty breathing or catching your breath? *Common observations unique to specific pathology* • Pain with active movement. • Pain during inspiration and expiration. • Pain with laughing, coughing, and/or sneezing. *Common observation findings* • Possible discoloration or contusion around the trauma site. *Palpations with expected outcomes* • Tenderness to palpation at the affected muscle site.	*Special tests* • No specific special tests clinically diagnose a sternum fracture. The clinical diagnosis is made from the history and palpation. • Manual muscle tests for specific muscles may help to identify the muscle injury. *Review of body systems* • Cardiovascular: Within normal limits. • Respiratory: Possible shallow breaths, increased frequency. • Gastrointestinal: Within normal limits. • Genitourinary: Within normal limits. • Neurologic: Within normal limits. *Imaging* • No radiographs are indicated for muscular injuries. • CT scans may help diagnose abdominal or thoracic muscular injuries. *Functional assessment/outcome measures* • Pain in the affected muscle. • General unwillingness to move. • Muscle splinting and guarding. • Leaning toward the affected side.	Rib fracture Costochondral separation Angina	Conservative care following trauma can assist with muscular injuries of the thorax and abdomen. Making the patient comfortable with rest and support can assist with the injury recovery process.

HIPS, history, inspection, palpation, special tests.

Injury Conditions to the Thorax and Abdomen **459**

Table 11.21 Injuries to the Lungs Quick Tips

Pathology	Description	Presentation (HIPS)	Special Test/Imaging	Differential Diagnosis	5-Min Sideline Assessment Tips

Injuries to the lungs	Sports trauma resulting in lung injuries is rare. Early recognition of signs and symptoms of lung injuries is important for allied health care providers. The most serious lung conditions are pneumothorax, tension pneumothorax, hemothorax (hemorrhaging into the lungs), and traumatic asphyxia.	*Unique/directed history questions for the identified pathology*
		• Have you received a direct blow to the chest?
		• Are you having difficulty breathing?
		• Have you been coughing up blood or bloody sputum?
		• Are you having pain when breathing?
		Common observations unique to specific pathology
		• Pain with active movement.
		• Pain during inspiration and expiration.
		• Pain with laughing, coughing, or sneezing.
		• Resting respiratory rate greater than 22 breaths per minute.
		• Cyanosis.
		• Hemoptysis (coughing up blood or blood-stained mucus from the bronchi, larynx, trachea, or lungs).
		• Hematemesis (vomiting of blood).
		Common observation findings
		• Pneumothorax: Pleural cavity becomes filled with air that has entered through an opening in the chest wall.
		  • As the plural cavity fills with air (due to the negative pressure), the lung on the affected side collapses.
			No specific special tests clinically diagnose lung injuries. The clinical diagnosis is made from the history and palpation.
			Review of body systems
			• Cardiovascular: Rapid, thready pulse if in shock.
			• Respiratory: Increased respiratory rate if in shock.
			• Gastrointestinal: Within normal limits.
			• Genitourinary: Within normal limits.
			• Neurologic: Within normal limits.
			Auscultations of the lungs
			• Assess breath sounds with a stethoscope, comparing side to side over the different lobes of the lung.
			• Listen for normal breath sounds, and note any abnormal breath sounds (ie., egophony or bronchophony).
			• Three sounds are assessed in normal individuals, depending on the position of the stethoscope.
			  • Bronchial breath sounds.
			  • Bronchovesicular breath sounds
			  • Vesicular breath sounds.
				Rib fracture
				Costochondral separation
				Abdominal or thoracic muscle strain
				Sternal fracture
				Rib stress fracture
					Lung injuries should be treated as a medical emergency; patients should be transported to an emergency department immediately for evaluation, care, and treatment.

(continues)

Table 11.21 Injuries to the Lungs Quick Tips *(continued)*

Pathology	Description	Presentation (HIPS)	Special Test/Imaging	Differential Diagnosis	5-Min Sideline Assessment Tips
Injuries to the lungs *(continued)*		• The collapse of one lung may produce pain, difficulty breathing, and anoxia (lack of oxygen). • Tension pneumothorax: The pleural sac on one size fills with air and displaces the lung and heart toward the opposite side, resulting in compression of the opposite lung. • Shortness of breath and chest pain are noted on the side of the injury. • Absence of breath sounds. • Cyanosis. • Distention of neck veins. • Tracheal shift toward the compressed lung (away from the side of the injury). • A total collapse of the opposite lung is possible (medical emergency). • Hemothorax: The presence of blood within the pleural cavity. • This injury occurs because of tearing or puncturing of the lung or the pleural tissue, involving damage to the blood vessels in the area. • Pain with breathing. • Difficulty breathing. • Cyanosis. • A forceful blow or compression of the chest without fracture to the rib may cause the lung to hemorrhage.	*Percussion of the lungs* • Tapping generates sounds transmitted through the organs and cavities of the body. • Percuss over the lobes of the lungs listening for tympany, resonance, hyperresonance, and dull and flat sounds. *Imaging* • Radiograph can rule out rib fractures. • CT or MRI can be used to evaluate lung injury. *Functional assessment/outcome measures* • Pain in the thoracic cavity. • General unwillingness to move. • Difficulty catching a breath. • Difficulty breathing.		

- Severe pain during breathing.
- Coughing up frothy blood.
- Signs and symptoms of shock.
- This injury warrants an immediate referral to an emergency department (medical emergency).
- Traumatic asphyxia: The result of a violent blow or compression of the rib cage, resulting in an arrest of breathing.
  - Cyanosis or a purple discoloration of the upper trunk and head.
  - Bright red coloring of the conjunctivae.
  - This condition is a medical emergency and should be treated with mouth-to-mouth cardiopulmonary resuscitation if the patient is not breathing along with immediate activation of advanced medical services.

Palpations with expected outcomes
- There are no specific palpations associated with lung injuries. Be sure to rule out rib fracture.

HIPS, history, inspection, palpation, special tests.
Data from Curtin S: Pneumothorax in sports: issues in recognition and follow-up care. *Physician Sports-Med* 2000;28(8):23; Kersey R: Primary spontaneous pneumothorax in a collegiate soccer player. *Ath Ther Today* 2000;5(2):48; Lively M: Pulmonary contusion in football players. *Clin J Sports Med* 2006;16(2):177; Smith D: Chest injuries, what the sports physical therapist should know. *Int J Sports Phys Ther* 2011;6(4):257-260; Walsh KM, Cuppett M: *General Medical Conditions in the Athlete*, ed 3. St. Louis, MO, Elsevier Mosby, 2017; and Weder M: Pulmonary disorders in athletes. *Clin Sports Med* 2011;30(3):525-536.

Table 11.22 Hyperventilation Quick Tips

Pathology	Description	Presentation (HIPS)	Special Test/Imaging	Differential Diagnosis	5-Min Sideline Assessment Tips
Hyperventilation	Excessive rapid ventilation, which may be due to anxiety-induced stress or asthma. This condition may develop in a patient during athletic participation. The rapid ventilation will result in the development of decreased amounts of carbon dioxide in the blood, a condition called hyocapnia.	*Unique/directed history questions for the identified pathology* • Are you having difficulty breathing? • Are you having difficulty catching your breath? • Do you have a history of asthma? • Have you ever been diagnosed with anxiety? *Common observations unique to specific pathology* • Difficulty with breathing, struggling to breathe. • Shallow, rapid breathing. • Patient appears to be in a panicked state. • Gasping or wheezing. *Common observation findings* • None *Palpations with expected outcomes* • None	*Special tests* • No specific special tests clinically diagnose hyperventilation. The clinical diagnosis is made from the history and palpation. *Review of body systems* • Cardiovascular: Within normal limits. • Respiratory: Increased respiratory rate. • Gastrointestinal: Within normal limits. • Genitourinary: Within normal limits. • Neurologic: Within normal limits. *Imaging* • None *Functional assessment/outcome measures* • General anxiety and possible panic.	Anxiety Lung injury Rib contusion	Although the patient is concerned about feeling as if he or she is not getting enough oxygen, the primary concern and issue is the patient's level of carbon dioxide is too low relative to the amount of oxygen in the blood. If hyperventilation continues, eventually the patient may pass out (experience syncope). The clinician needs to be prepared to act. The immediate treatment for hyperventilation is to decrease the rate of carbon dioxide loss by slowing breathing. Try to have the patient focus on his or her breathing to slow the rate of respiration. Ask the patient to focus on his or her breathing while breathing in through the nose and exhaling through the mouth. Another technique is to have the patient inhale and exhale through one nostril, with the other pinched closed and the mouth closed. The technique of having a patient breathe into a paper or plastic bag was recommended in the past but is not used as often because other breathing techniques are more effective. The breathing techniques should help to increase the level of carbon dioxide within a few minutes, and breathing should return to a normal level. After acute hyperventilation has been addressed, determining the underlying cause and recommending appropriate treatment is important for the patient's future. There is a possibility of recurrence, so teaching patients breathing strategies is encouraged.

HIPS, history, inspection, palpation, special tests.
Data from Prentice WE: *Principles of Athletic Training: A Guide to Evidence-Based Clinical Practice*, ed 16. New York, NY, McGraw-Hill Education, 2017 and Suman O: Airway obstruction during exercise and isocapnic hyperventilation in asthmatic subjects. *J App Physiol* 1999;87(3):1107.

Injury Conditions to the Thorax and Abdomen 463

Table 11.23 Sudden Cardiac Death Syndrome in Athletes Quick Tips

Pathology	Description	Presentation (HIPS)	Special Test/Imaging	Differential Diagnosis	5-Min Sideline Assessment Tips
Sudden cardiac death syndrome in athletes **Marfan syndrome.** © Jones & Bartlett Learning	Although rare, it is extremely catastrophic when a young athlete dies while participating in athletic activity for no apparent reason. Annually, an estimated 1 in 280,000 males younger than 30 years will experience sudden death. In individuals younger than 35 years, the most common cause of exercise-associated sudden cardiac death is due to a congenital cardiovascular abnormality. Three of the most common cardiac conditions affecting athletic populations are hypertrophic cardiomyopathy, anomalous origin of the coronary artery, and Marfan syndrome. Hypertrophic cardiomyopathy occurs when there is a thickening of the cardiac muscle, which decreases the size of the chamber of the ventricle because of extensive myocardial scarring. It is a relatively common genetic cardiac disease with a prevalence of 1 in 500 in the general population. Hypertrophic cardiomyopathy is associated with an increased frequency of ventricular arrhythmias. Anomalous origin of the coronary arteries is a condition in which one of the two coronary vessels originates in a site other than normal, which obstructs or compromises the artery. These	*Unique/directed history questions for the identified pathology* • Early identification of cardiac conditions in athletes is important. Counseling, screening, and early identification of preventable causes of sudden death may help to avoid future emergencies. • The use of diagnostic tests to screen for cardiovascular abnormalities in an athletic population have been largely ineffective and are extremely costly. • Utilization of the Physical Activity Readiness Questionnaire during preparticipation physical examinations may be beneficial and could help to identify athletes who have cardiac abnormalities. *Common observations unique to specific pathology* • Chest pain or discomfort with exertion • Heart palpitations or flutters • Syncope • Nausea • Profuse sweating • Heart murmurs • Shortness of breath • General malaise • Fever	*Special tests* • No specific special tests clinically diagnose cardiac predisposition for sudden death in sports. The Physical Activity Readiness Questionnaire should be used to identify patients at an increased risk. A cardiologist should perform follow-up testing. *Imaging* • Electrocardiography can be performed on high-risk athletes to determine heart rhythm abnormalities. • Diagnostic ultrasonography can measure the size and shape of the vessels and chambers of the heart to examine for abnormalities. *Functional assessment/outcome measures* • None	Heart contusion Lung injuries Angina Heart attack (myocardial infarction) Sternal fracture Rib fracture	Be prepared for a cardiac emergency. Activate the emergency action plan as soon as possible; recognition of cardiac symptoms, early access to an automated external defibrillator, and advanced medical care can help care for athletes experiencing cardiac emergencies.

(continues)

Table 11.23 Sudden Cardiac Death Syndrome in Athletes Quick Tips *(continued)*

Pathology	Description	Presentation (HIPS)	Special Test/Imaging	Differential Diagnosis	5-Min Sideline Assessment Tips
Sudden cardiac death syndrome in athletes *(continued)*	congenital malformations of the coronary arteries are detectable with the utilization of imaging modalities. The prevalence of occurrence ranges from 0.21% to 5.79% of the general population. Marfan syndrome is characterized by an abnormality within the connective tissue. The weakening of the connective tissue, especially the aorta and cardiac valves, can lead to sudden death in athletes. Mitral valve prolapse has been linked to both hypertrophic cardiomyopathy and Marfan syndrome. The prevalence of Marfan syndrome has been approximated to be 2 in 10,000 individuals in the general population; however, Marfan syndrome may be underdiagnosed and could affect as many as 1 in 3,000. Other conditions may result in sudden cardiac death as well. Coronary artery disease is a condition resulting from a narrowing of the coronary arteries (arteriosclerosis). Peripheral artery disease results from large plaques (containing red blood cells, fibrin aggregates, and cholesterol) dislodging from arteries in the extremities, which then migrate as an embolus (with sufficient size to occlude a major coronary artery).	• Be prepared to perform cardiopulmonary resuscitation. *Common observation findings* • Most patients are asymptomatic prior to the life-threatening or catastrophic event. *Palpations with expected outcomes* • None			

Right ventricular dysplasia is a condition characterized by enlargement of the right ventricle, resulting in a potentially lethal disturbance in the heartbeat.

Cardiac conduction system abnormalities may result from a disturbance in the electrical signals of the sinus or atrioventricular nodes.

Aortic stenosis is a narrowing of the artery or the valve. The narrowing prevents the valve from opening fully, which restricts blood flow from the heart into the main artery and out to the body. When the blood flow through the aortic valve is reduced or blocked, the heart needs to work harder to pump blood to the body.

Wolff-Parkinson-White syndrome is a cardiac rhythm abnormality resulting in ventricular tachycardia.

Myocarditis is an inflammation of the heart associated with a viral condition.

HIPS, history, inspection, palpation, special tests.

Data from Casa DJ, Guskiewicz KM, Anderson SA, et al: National Athletic Trainers' Association position statement: preventing sudden death in sports. *J Ath Train* 2012;47(1):96-118; Hipp A: Hypertrophic cardiomyopathy – sports-related aspects of diagnosis, therapy, and sports eligibility. *Int J Sports Med* 2004;25(1):20; Judge DP, Dietz HC: Marfan's syndrome. *Lancet* 2005;366(9501):1965-1976; Koester M: A review of sudden cardiac death in young athletes and strategies for preparticipation cardiovascular screening. *J Athl Train* 2001;36(2):197; Lufukuja GJ: Anomalous origin of the coronary arteries. *Ital J Anat Embryol* 2016;121(3):253-257; Maron BJ: Hypertrophic cardiomyopathy: a systematic review. *JAMA* 2002;287(10):1308-1320; McGrew C: Sudden cardiac death in competitive athletes. *J Orthop Sports Phys Ther* 2003;33(10):589; Merrick M: Cardiovascular pathologies: to screen or not to screen? *Ath Ther Today* 2001;6(4):28; National Academy of Sports Medicine (NASM): Physical Activity Readiness Questionnaire. https://www.nasm.org/docs/default-source/PDF/nasm_par-q-(pdf-21k).pdf. Accessed 12, 2018; Pérez-Pomares JM, Luis de la Pompa J, Franco D, et al: Congenital coronary artery anomalies: a bridge from embryology to anatomy and pathophysiology: a position statement of the development, anatomy and pathology ESC Working Group. *Cardiovasc Res* 2016;109:204-216; Perron A: Chest pain in athletes. *Clin Sports Med* 2003;22(1):37; Toresdahl B, Courson R, Börjesson M, et al: Emergency cardiac care in the athletic setting: from schools to the Olympics. *Br J Sports Med* 2012;46:i85-i89; and Turk E: Natural and traumatic sports-related fatalities: a 10-year retrospective study. *Brit J Sports Med* 2008;42:604-608.

Table 11.24 Pericardial Tamponade Quick Tips

Pathology	Description	Presentation (HIPS)	Special Test/Imaging	Differential Diagnosis	5-Min Sideline Assessment Tips
Pericardial tamponade	The heart has a sac, the pericardium, containing a thin layer of fluid. The fluid in the pericardium surrounds the heart and prevents friction between the layers when the heart moves during contractions. If too much fluid accumulates in the pericardial space around the heart, it may become difficult for the heart to expand normally and restrict the ability for the ventricles to fill with blood. This is known as reduced ventricular filling. This results in a hemodynamic compromise (less blood entering the body from the heart, reducing the amount of oxygen-rich blood going out to the body). Fluid can build up in the pericardium either quickly or slowly. If the fluid builds up quickly, it can lead to acute (short-term) cardiac tamponade, which is life threatening if not treated immediately. Subacute tamponade can happen when the fluid builds up more slowly. Chest pain occurs among athletes and the general population, accounting for approximately 20% to 30% of all hospital visits. Cardiac tamponade is not common, but this health problem can develop in anyone.	*Unique/directed history questions for the identified pathology* • Do you feel like your heart is heavy? • Do you feel like it is hard to breathe? • Do you feel a loss of energy? • Have you had a direct blow to the left side of the chest (over the heart)? *Common observations unique to specific pathology* • Chest pain or discomfort. • Shortness of breath. • Fast breathing. • Increased heart rate. • Enlargement of the veins of the neck. • Fainting. • Swelling in the arms and legs. • Pain in the right upper quadrant of the abdomen. • Upset stomach. • Fever, if infection is involved. *Common observation findings* • Dyspnea. • Tachycardia. • Tachypnea. • Low blood pressure. *Palpations with expected outcomes* • None	*Special tests* • No specific special tests clinically diagnose pericardial tamponade. *Imaging* • Several imaging modalities can help diagnose pericardial tamponade: • Echocardiogram examines and measures the fluid around the heart and heart motion • Electrocardiography to evaluate the heart's electrical rhythm • Chest radiograph to view the heart's anatomy • CT or MRI to view the heart's anatomy and surrounding soft-tissue structures • If the patient has symptoms of shock, additional tests may be needed, including: • Blood tests to evaluate infection • Blood tests to diagnose autoimmune disease(s) • Analysis of fluid removed from around the heart to check for cancer or infection • Blood tests to evaluate metabolic issues *Functional assessment/outcome measures* • None	Heart contusion Lung injuries Angina Heart attack (myocardial infarction) Sternal fracture Rib fracture	Be prepared for a cardiac emergency. Activate the emergency action plan as soon as possible; recognition of cardiac symptoms, early access to an automated external defibrillator, and advanced medical care can help care for athletes suffering from cardiac emergencies.

HIPS, history, inspection, palpation, special tests.

Data from Maron BJ, Gohman TE, Kyle SB, Estes NAM, Link M: Clinical profile and spectrum of commotio cordis in the athlete. *J Am Med Assoc* 2002;287(9):1142-1146; Singh AM, McGregor RS: Differential diagnosis of chest symptoms in the athlete. *Clin Rev Allergy Immunol* 2005; 29(2):87-96; and Spodick DH: Acute cardiac tamponade. *N Engl J Med* 2003;349:684.

Injury Conditions to the Thorax and Abdomen **467**

Table 11.25 Commotio Cordis Quick Tips

Pathology	Description	Presentation (HIPS)	Special Test/Imaging	Differential Diagnosis	5-Min Sideline Assessment Tips
Commotio cordis	Commotio cordis occurs because of a low to mild blow to the chest wall causing a sudden arrhythmic death. Commotio cordis is most prevalent in young individuals between the ages of 8 and 18 years, most commonly in sports involving projectiles (baseballs, hockey pucks, or lacrosse balls). Projectiles can strike the athlete in the heart during practice or competition. If the projectile strike occurs in the middle of the chest with a low to moderate impact, it can cause the heart to enter an arrhythmia. Martial arts, in which another individual's foot or hand could strike the chest, may change the rhythm of the heart with a specific strike. Without immediate CPR and defibrillation, the prognosis for commotio cordis is bleak. Unfortunately, many individuals do not survive the resulting arrhythmia caused by the blow to the chest.	*Unique/directed history questions for the identified pathology* The patient may not be conscious. You may have to ask bystanders: • Did the patient get hit in the chest? • When did the patient lose consciousness? *Common observations unique to specific pathology* • Unconscious following blow to chest. *Common observation findings* • Most patients are asymptomatic prior to the cardiac event. Once they are struck in the chest, the patient will rapidly decline and will likely lose consciousness. • Possible bruising to the chest. *Palpations with expected outcomes* • None	*Special tests* • No specific special tests clinically diagnose commotio cordis. *Imaging* • A number of imaging modalities can help diagnose pericardial tamponade and the effects of commotio cordis: • Echocardiography to examine heart and heart motion • Electrocardiography to evaluate the heart's electrical rhythm • Chest radiograph to view the heart's anatomy • CT or MRI to view the heart's anatomy and surrounding soft-tissue structures *Functional assessment/outcome measures* • None	Heart attack (myocardial infarction) Sternal fracture Rib fracture	Be prepared for a cardiac emergency. Activate the emergency action plan as soon as possible; recognition of cardiac symptoms, early access to an automated external defibrillator, and advanced medical care can help care for athletes suffering from cardiac emergencies.

HIPS, history, inspection, palpation, special tests.
Data from Casa DJ, Guskiewicz KM, Anderson SA, et al: National Athletic Trainers' Association position statement: preventing sudden death in sports. *J Ath Train* 2012;47(1):96-118; and Maron BJ, Gohman TE, Kyle SB, Estes NAM, Link M: Clinical profile and spectrum of commotio cordis. *J Am Med Assoc* 2002;287(9):1142-1146.

Table 11.26 Athletic Heart Syndrome Quick Tips

Pathology	Description	Presentation (HIPS)	Special Test/Imaging	Differential Diagnosis	5-Min Sideline Assessment Tips
Athletic heart syndrome	Athletic heart syndrome results in structural and functional changes often seen in individuals who train athletically for more than 1 hour per day, most days of the week. The left ventricle enlarges in mass due to left ventricle diastolic activity. As an athlete trains, both maximal stroke volume and cardiac output increase, which results in a lower resting heart rate and an increase in the function of the heart (longer diastolic filling time). Changes in the cardiac muscle can be observed by using echocardiography. Differences between athlete and nonathlete populations are generally minimal. Athletic heart syndrome tends to occur less often in women than in men.	*Unique/directed history questions for the identified pathology* • There are no specific history questions for athletic heart syndrome. Athletic heart syndrome is largely asymptomatic. *Common observations unique to specific pathology* • None *Common observation findings* • Bradycardia (decreased heart rate). • Systolic murmur. • Extra heart sounds. *Palpations with expected outcomes* • None	*Special tests* • No specific special tests clinically diagnose athletic heart syndrome. The PAR-Q should be utilized to identify patients at an increased risk, and a cardiologist should perform follow-up testing. *Review of body systems* • Cardiovascular: Possible abnormal rhythm. • Respiratory: Within normal limits. • Gastrointestinal: Within normal limits. • Genitourinary: Within normal limits. • Neurologic: Within normal limits. *Imaging* • Electrocardiogram abnormalities are common. *Functional assessment/outcome measures* • After other serious cardiac abnormalities have been ruled out and a diagnosis of athletic heart syndrome has been made, no treatment is necessary.	Heart contusion Lung injuries Angina Heart attack (myocardial infarction) Sternal fracture Rib fracture	Be prepared for a cardiac emergency. It may be necessary to activate the emergency action plan. Recognition of cardiac symptoms and early access to an automated external defibrillator and advanced medical care can help care for athletes suffering from cardiac emergencies.

HIPS, history, inspection, palpation, special tests.

Data from Maron BJ, Gohman TE, Kyle SB, Estes NAM, Link M: Clinical profile and spectrum of commotio cordis. *J Am Med Assoc* 2002;287(9):1142-1146; National Academy of Sports Medicine (NASM): Physical Activity Readiness Questionnare. https://www.nasm.org/docs/default-source/PDF/nasm_par-q-1pdf-21kl.pdf. Accessed September 12, 2018; and Puffer JC, Thompson PD: The athletic heart syndrome. *Physician Sports-Med* 2002;7:41-47.

Table 11.27 Heart Contusion Quick Tips

Pathology	Description	Presentation (HIPS)	Special Test/Imaging	Differential Diagnosis	5-Min Sideline Assessment Tips
Heart contusion	A heart contusion can occur if a patient sustains a high-velocity blow to the chest or the heart is compressed between the sternum and the spine by a strong force. The most severe consequence of a violent impact to the heart may result in a ruptured aorta, which is considered a life-threatening condition.	*Unique/directed history questions for the identified pathology* • Did you recently receive a blow to the chest? • Has anyone fallen on your chest recently? • Are you having any difficulty breathing? • Are you having any chest pains? • Do you feel like your heart is fluttering? *Common observations unique to specific pathology* • The patient may be highly anxious or may appear scared. *Common observation findings* • Severe heart pain. • Shock. • Cardiac arrhythmia. • Possible contusion or bruising at the trauma site. • Possible rib fracture. *Palpations with expected outcomes* • None	*Special tests* • No specific special tests clinically diagnose heart contusions. The clinical diagnosis is made from the history. *Review of body systems* • Cardiovascular: Rapid, thready pulse if in shock. Possible altered rhythm. • Respiratory: Increased respiratory rate if in shock. • Gastrointestinal: Within normal limits. • Genitourinary: Within normal limits. • Neurologic: Within normal limits. • Auscultations of the heart. • A stethoscope is used to listen to cardiac sounds of the heart. Four sites are used to determine cardiac sounds: aortic, located at the second intercostal space at the right sternal border; pulmonic, located at the second intercostal space at the left sternal border; tricuspid, located at the left lower sternal border; and mitral, located at the cardiac apex. *Imaging* • An electrocardiogram can be performed to determine heart rhythm abnormalities. • Diagnostic ultrasonography can measure the size and shape of the vessels and chambers of the heart to examine for abnormalities. *Functional assessment/outcome measures* • The heart may exhibit an arrhythmia, which may decrease the patient's cardiac output. If the cardiac arrhythmia is not addressed quickly, then death may follow.	Lung injuries Angina Heart attack (myocardial infarction) Sternal fracture Rib fracture	This is considered a medical emergency, and the patient should be transported to the emergency department as quickly as possible. Any allied health care professional treating a patient with a suspected heart contusion should be prepared to administer cardiopulmonary resuscitation and to treat the athlete for shock.

HIPS, history, inspection, palpation, special tests.
Data from Holanda MS, Dominguez MJ, Lopez-Espadas F, Lopez M, Diaz-Reganon J, Rodriguez-Borregan JC: Cardiac contusion following blunt chest trauma. *Eur J Emerg Med* 2006;13(6):373-376; and Walsh KM, Cuppett M: *General Medical Conditions in the Athlete*, ed 3. St. Louis, MO, Elsevier Mosby, 2017.

Table 11.28 Kidney Contusion or Laceration Quick Tips

Pathology	Description	Presentation (HIPS)	Special Test/Imaging	Differential Diagnosis	5-Min Sideline Assessment Tips
Kidney contusion or laceration	Even though the kidneys are relatively well protected by the muscles of the abdomen and the ribs, injuries can happen, such as contusions, lacerations, or ruptures. The kidneys may be predisposed to injury, as they are normally distended with blood. Direct trauma, usually to the back of the patient, can cause extension of an engorged kidney, which results in injury. The degree of injury is largely dependent on the extent of kidney distension and the angle and force of the trauma.	*Unique/directed history questions for the identified pathology* • Have you recently had a blow to the back? • Have you fallen recently? • Have you had anyone fall on top of you? • Do you have any lower back pain? • Are you nauseated? • Have you been vomiting? • Have you noticed any blood in your urine? *Common observations unique to specific pathology* • Signs and symptoms of shock. • Nausea. • Vomiting. *Common observation findings* • Contusion or laceration at the site of trauma may be present. • Hematuria (blood in the urine). This is a medical emergency, and patients should be referred to an emergency department immediately. • Referred pain (pain in the costovertebral angle radiating forward around the trunk into the lower abdominal region). *Palpations with expected outcomes* • Rigidity of the back muscles. • Rigidity of the abdominal muscles. • Tenderness over the impact site.	*Special tests* • No specific tests are available to indicate a kidney contusion and/or laceration. • Abdominal observation. • Urine test for hematuria. *Review of body systems* • Cardiovascular: Hypotension. • Respiratory: Breathing may become rapid. • Gastrointestinal: Nausea and vomiting are possible; abdominal rigidity. • Genitourinary: Macroscopic or microscopic traces of blood may be present in the urine. Possible pain with urination. • Neurologic: Within normal limits. *Imaging* • CT with contrast can be used to diagnose a kidney contusion or laceration. *Functional assessment/outcome measures* • General unwillingness to move.	Urinary tract infection Abdominal contusion Rib fracture Kidney stone Kidney infection Muscle strain Muscle contusion	Kidney injuries can hemorrhage and result in shock. Therefore, the condition should be treated as a medical emergency. Early intervention is extremely important.

HIPS, history, inspection, palpation, special tests.
Data from McAleer IM, Kaplan GW, LoSasso BE: Renal and testis injuries in team sports. *J Urol* 2002;168(4 suppl),1805-1807; and Walsh KM, Cuppett M: *General Medical Conditions in the Athlete*, ed 3. St. Louis, MO, Elsevier Mosby, 2017.

Table 11.29 Liver Contusion Quick Tips

Pathology	Description	Presentation (HIPS)	Special Test/Imaging	Differential Diagnosis	5-Min Sideline Assessment Tips
Liver contusion	Injuries to the liver are the second most common of the internal organ injuries, although they happen infrequently during athletic participation. Direct trauma to the right side of the rib cage and upper right abdominal quadrant may result in a contusion or laceration of the liver. The liver is especially susceptible if the liver is enlarged due to disease, such as hepatitis. Hepatitis is a disease characterized by inflammation of the liver. Large amounts of alcohol consumption may also damage the liver. The cells of the liver will die if the viral infection (hepatitis) or alcohol consumption is not addressed. The dead cells are replaced with scar tissue and may lead to cirrhosis or impaired liver function. Cirrhosis is a disease of the liver, progressive in nature, resulting in significant scarring, fibrosis, and disruption of the hepatic blood flow, eventually resulting in liver failure. Cirrhosis is most often a complication of chronic alcoholism.	*Unique/directed history questions for the identified pathology* • Have you been hit in the abdomen or back recently? • Have you fallen or had anyone fall on top of you? • Are you having any stomach pain? • Are you nauseated? • Do you have any pain in your back or chest area? • Do you have any chest pain? *Common observations unique to specific pathology* • Signs and symptoms of shock. • Nausea. • Vomiting. *Common observation findings* • Bruising in the upper right quadrant of the abdomen. • Referred pain just below the right scapula, right shoulder, and substernal area. • Referred pain in the anterior left side of the chest. *Palpations with expected outcomes* • Rigidity in the upper right quadrant of the abdomen.	*Special tests* • No specific tests are available to indicate a liver contusion and/or laceration *Review of body systems* • Cardiovascular: Rapid, thready pulse if in shock. • Respiratory: Increased respiratory rate if in shock. • Gastrointestinal: Nausea and vomiting are possible. Abdominal rigidity. • Genitourinary: Within normal limits. • Neurologic: Referred pain to the right scapula, right shoulder, substernal area, or left side of the chest. *Imaging* • Diagnostic ultrasonography can be used to examine liver injury. *Functional assessment/outcome measures* • Pain below the right scapula, right shoulder, and substernal area. • Pain in the anterior left side of the chest. • Pain aggravated by movement. • General unwillingness to move.	Rib fracture Abdominal or thoracic muscle injury Kidney injury Gallbladder injury	Liver injuries can cause significant hemorrhage and result in shock. This condition should be treated as a medical emergency. Early surgical intervention is extremely important.

HIPS, history, inspection, palpation, special tests.
Data from Mileski W: Injuries to the liver, in Flint L, ed: *Trauma: Contemporary Principles and Therapy*. Philadelphia, PA, Lippincott Williams & Wilkins, 2007, pp 433-442; and Parks NA, Davis JW, Forman D, Lemaster D: Observation for nonoperative management of blunt liver injuries: how long is long enough? *J Trauma* 2011;70(3):626-629.

Table 11.30 Splenic Injury Quick Tips

Pathology	Description	Presentation (HIPS)	Special Test/Imaging	Differential Diagnosis	5-Min Sideline Assessment Tips
Splenic injury	The spleen is a solid, rather fragile organ located on the left side of the abdomen. The spleen is supported by ligaments attached to the kidney, colon, stomach, and diaphragm. The function of the spleen is to produce and destroy blood cells when the body experiences systemic infection (such as during an illness). Specific diseases, such as mononucleosis, pneumonia, or other systemic infections, can cause the spleen to become enlarged and engorged with blood, allowing the spleen to protrude below the ribs and leaving the organ susceptible to injury. If the spleen is injured, surgical removal may be required. In the case of spleen removal, the organ function is replaced by the liver and bone marrow. When determining readiness for contact-sport play following illness, such as mononucleosis, general consensus indicates that the athlete must be asymptomatic from all symptoms, including fever, fatigue, and pharyngitis, before any return to activity protocol is initiated. Resolution of abnormalities evaluated via laboratory tests (such as elevated white blood cell counts or abnormal liver function tests) does not play a role in assisting return-to-play decisions. There seems to be little consensus regarding the optimal time to wait before returning an athlete to activity. The highest risk for splenic injury occurs within the first 21 days following the illness. Splenomegaly is palpable in only about 20% of people who have the condition.	*Unique/directed history questions for the identified pathology* • Have you been hit in the abdomen recently? • Have you fallen or had anyone fall on top of you? • Are you having any abdominal pain (particularly in the upper left quadrant)? • Do you have any pain in your shoulder (particularly the left shoulder)? • Are you nauseated? • Have you recently been ill? • Have you been diagnosed with mononucleosis? *Common observations unique to specific pathology* • Signs and symptoms of shock. • Nausea. • Vomiting (undigested food, red from blood, or greenish from bile). • Holding the abdominal area. *Common observation findings* • Bruising in the upper left quadrant of the abdomen. • Pain in the upper left quadrant of the abdomen. • Referred pain in the left shoulder (Kehr sign). • Referred pain in the anterior left side of the chest. • Site of impact may show signs of a rib contusion or rib fracture. *Palpations with expected outcomes* • Rigidity in the upper left quadrant of the abdomen. • Tenderness over impact site. • Cold and clammy skin with the onset of shock.	*Special tests* • No specific special tests indicate a splenic injury. *Review of body systems* • Cardiovascular: Rapid, thready pulse if in shock. • Respiratory: Increased respiratory rate if in shock. • Gastrointestinal: Nausea and vomiting are possible. Abdominal rigidity. • Genitourinary: Within normal limits. • Neurologic: Kehr sign. *Imaging* • MRI can be used to identify splenic trauma. • Diagnostic ultrasonography. *Functional assessment/outcome measures* • Pain in the upper left quadrant of the abdomen and shoulder are aggravated by any movement of the patient. • General unwillingness to move.	Liver trauma Kidney injury Rib fracture	Patients with suspected splenic trauma should be referred to the emergency department for immediate evaluation, observation, and treatment.

Research does not indicate any increased risk of injury with early return to light activity; however, there is a lack of evidence-based return-to-play protocols. Increased intra-abdominal pressure and contact sports may place the chest or abdomen at risk for trauma for athletes participating in activity following mononucleosis. Splenic rupture is extremely rare (< 0.5%) in those with a diagnosis of mononucleosis; however, if it does happen, the consequences may be severe. Research suggests athletes with a diagnosis of mononucleosis should rest for a minimum of 3 weeks and then begin with light activity.

HIPS, history, inspection, palpation, special tests.

Data from Mileski W: Injuries to the liver, in Flint L: *Trauma: Contemporary Principles and Therapy.* Philadelphia, PA, Lippincott Williams & Wilkins, 2007; Noffsinger J: Physical activity considerations in children and adolescents with viral infections. *Pediatr Ann* 1996;25:585-589;[59] Putukian M, O'Connor FG, Stricker PR, et al: Mononucleosis and athletic participation: an evidence-based subject review. *Clin J Sport Med* 2008;18:309-315; Rea TD, Russo JE, Katon W, Ashley RL, Buchwald DS: Prospective study of the natural history of infectious mononucleosis caused by Epstein-Barr virus. *J Am Board Fam Pract* 2001;14:234-242; Rinderknecht AS, Pomerantz WJ: Spontaneous splenic rupture in infectious mononucleosis: case report and review of the literature. *Pediatr Emerg Care* 2012;28,1377; Turner J, Gard M: Splenomegaly and sports. *Curr Sports Med Rep* 2008;7:113-116; Walsh KM, Cuppett M: *General Medical Conditions in the Athlete,* ed 3. St. Louis, MO, Elsevier Mosby, 2017; and Waninger KN, Harcke HT: Determination of safe return to play for athletes recovering from infectious mononucleosis. *Clin J Sport Med* 2005;15:410.

Table 11.31 Gallbladder Conditions Quick Tips

Pathology	Description	Presentation (HIPS)	Special Test/Imaging	Differential Diagnosis	5-Min Sideline Assessment Tips
Gallbladder conditions *Murphy sign.* © Jones & Bartlett Learning	The gallbladder fills with bile produced by the liver, and after eating, bile empties into the small intestine to help digest food consumed. The gallbladder functions like a balloon, filling and emptying during the day. Injury to the gallbladder (usually because of direct trauma) is most likely to occur when the gallbladder is full of bile. The gallbladder may develop complications (stones or inflammation). Inflammation of the gallbladder is known as cholecystitis. Gallstones can be formed by cholesterol, which is secreted by the liver, and the stones may block the pancreatic duct, leading to pancreatitis.	*Unique/directed history questions for the identified pathology* • Do you have any pain in the upper right quadrant of the abdomen? • Do you feel nauseated? • Do you feel anxious? *Common observations unique to specific pathology* Cholecystitis • Pain. • Fever. • Tenderness in the upper right quadrant of the abdomen. Gallstones • May be asymptomatic. • Jaundice. • Nausea. • Severe pain in the upper right quadrant of the abdomen. *Common observation findings* • Possible bruising in the upper right quadrant of the abdomen. *Palpations with expected outcomes* • Possible rigidity in the upper right quadrant of the abdomen.	*Special tests* • Murphy sign *Review of body systems* • Cardiovascular: Rapid, thready pulse if in shock. • Respiratory: Increased respiratory rate if in shock. • Gastrointestinal: Nausea and vomiting are possible. Abdominal rigidity. • Genitourinary: Within normal limits. • Neurologic: Kehr sign. *Imaging* • Radiographs can spot gas or gallstones containing calcium in the gallbladder. • Diagnostic ultrasonography can be used to diagnose cholecystitis and gallstones. • CT can help diagnose gallstones. • Cholescintigraphy or hepatobiliary scintigraphy (HIDA scan) is a test where a small amount of radioactive dye is administered and tracked as it moves into the gallbladder. This test can detect a blocked duct or acute inflammation but does not evaluate chronic gallbladder inflammation or gallstones. *Functional assessment/outcome measures* • Pain in the upper right quadrant. • Pain aggravated by movement. • General unwillingness to move.	Irritable bowel syndrome Gastroesophageal reflux disease Crohn disease or ulcerative colitis Inflammation of the pancreas Kidney stones Urinary tract infection Viral hepatitis Appendicitis	Rest and antibiotics are the typical treatment for cholecystitis. Diagnostic ultrasonography of the upper right abdominal quadrant can be used to determine whether there are gallstones. Gallstones, depending on the size, are usually managed by waiting and letting the stones pass naturally. If stones are too large or patients have recurrent gallstones, surgical intervention to remove the gallbladder may be required. The gallbladder is considered a nonessential organ, and removal does not cause any complications with digestion or to a patient's overall health.

HIDA, hepatobiliary iminodiacetic acid; HIPS, history, inspection, palpation, special tests.
Data from Jarvis C: *Physical Examination and Health Assessment*, ed 5. St. Louis, MO, Saunders-Elsevier, 2008; Urbano FL, Carroll MB: Murphy's sign of cholecystitis. *Hospital Physician* 2000;11:51-51,70;66 and Walsh KM, Cuppett M: *General Medical Conditions in the Athlete*, ed 3. St. Louis, MO, Elsevier Mosby, 2017.

Table 11.32 Gastroesophageal Reflux Disease Quick Tips

Pathology	Description	Presentation (HIPS)	Special Test/Imaging	Differential Diagnosis	5-Min Sideline Assessment Tips
Gastroesophageal reflux disease	GERD occurs when there is a backward flow (reflux) of the acidic gastric contents into the esophagus. This can occur because of a malfunctioning lower esophageal sphincter or a hiatal hernia. Typically, the occurrence of GERD increases with exercise. If GERD continues to happen, the lower esophagus may become inflamed (esophagitis).	*Unique/directed history questions for the identified pathology* • Do you have heartburn after exercise? • Do you have heartburn when you lie down at night? • Do you have any pain in your chest? • Do you feel like you burp up food after eating? • Do you wake up with a sour taste in your mouth? • Do you feel as if you have difficulty swallowing? *Common observations unique to specific pathology* • No unique observations. *Common observation findings* • Heartburn pain that can progress to a gripping chest pain, which may mimic angina pectoris. • Burning feeling with a sour liquid taste in the throat. • Difficulty swallowing. *Palpations with expected outcomes* • None	*Special tests* • No specific special tests indicate GERD. *Review of body systems* • Cardiovascular: Within normal limits. • Respiratory: Within normal limits. • Gastrointestinal: Sour taste in the mouth, acid reflux. Nausea and vomiting are possible. • Genitourinary: Within normal limits. • Neurologic: Within normal limits. *Imaging* • A barium swallow radiograph can rule out any structural problem with the esophagus. • An endoscopy (small tube with camera inserted into the esophagus) is a procedure to investigate the esophagus and stomach to examine the lining. *Functional assessment/outcome measures* • Pain in the stomach and upper abdomen. • Pain lying down with reflux.	Crohn disease or ulcerative colitis Inflammation of the pancreas Kidney stones Cholecystitis Urinary tract infection Viral hepatitis Appendicitis	GERD can be controlled effectively by medication. If medication does not stop the reflux, then surgery may be needed.

GERD, gastroesophageal reflux disease; HIPS, history, inspection, palpation, special tests.

Table 11.33 Appendicitis Quick Tips

Pathology	Description	Presentation (HIPS)	Special Test/Imaging	Differential Diagnosis	5-Min Sideline Assessment Tips
Appendicitis **McBurney point.** © Jones & Bartlett Learning	Inflammation of the appendix can be either acute or chronic and may be caused by a variety of conditions, such as fecal obstruction, lymph swelling, or even a carcinoid tumor. Appendicitis is most likely to occur in males between the ages of 15 and 25 years. The symptoms of acute appendicitis can be mistaken for other gastric disorders. In the early stage of acute appendicitis, the appendix becomes red and swollen. As the condition progresses, the appendix becomes gangrenous and eventually ruptures, spilling its contents into the intestines and peritoneal cavity, which causes peritonitis. A bacterial infection is a serious complication when the appendix ruptures.	*Unique/directed history questions for the identified pathology* • Do you have pain in the lower right quadrant? • Have you been nauseated? • Have you been vomiting? • Have you had a fever? *Common observations unique to specific pathology* • The patient may appear pale (pallor). *Common observation findings* Early acute appendicitis: • Mild-to-severe pain in the lower abdomen. • Nausea. • Vomiting. • Low-grade fever ranging from 99°F to 100°F (37°C to 38°C). Late acute appendicitis: • Cramps in the lower abdomen. • Pain in the lower right quadrant. *Palpations with expected outcomes* • Pain and tenderness at McBurney point during palpation. • McBurney point can be located between the anterior superior iliac crest and the umbilicus, about 1 to 2 inches (2.5 to 5 cm) above the umbilicus. • Rigidity of the abdomen, particularly in the lower right quadrant.	*Special tests* • Blumberg sign (rebound tenderness) for appendicitis. • Iliopsoas muscle test for appendicitis. • Obturator muscle test for appendicitis. *Imaging* • Diagnostic ultrasonography. • MRI or CT can be used to identify appendicitis. *Functional assessment/outcome measures* • Pain in the lower right quadrant of the abdomen. • Pain aggravated by movement. • General unwillingness to move.	Irritable bowel syndrome Crohn disease or ulcerative colitis Inflammation of the pancreas Kidney stones Cholecystitis Urinary tract infection Viral hepatitis	Appendicitis should be treated as an emergency, and a patient with suspected appendicitis should be referred to an emergency department immediately. Antibiotic therapy for uncomplicated appendicitis has proven effective in many cases. Surgical removal of the appendix may be necessary. If the appendix does rupture, it is a life-threatening condition requiring medical attention immediately. Strains of the iliopsoas muscle group or an abscess in the sheath of the psoas or iliacus may be mistaken for appendicitis.

HIPS, history, inspection, palpation, special tests.

Data from Cook, CE: *Orthopedic Manual Therapy: An Evidence-Based Approach*, ed 2. Upper Saddle River, NJ, Pearson Education, 2012; Kreis ME, Edler V, Koch F, Jauch KW, Friese K: The differential diagnosis of right lower quadrant pain. *Dtsch Arztebl* 2007;104(45):A3114–3121; Salminen P, Paajanen H, Rautio T: Antibiotic therapy vs. appendectomy for treatment of uncomplicated acute appendicitis. *JAMA* 2015;313(23):2340-2348; Venes D: *Taber's Cyclopedic Medical Dictionary*. Philadelphia, PA, FA Davis Co, 2013; and Walsh KM, Cuppett M: *General Medical Conditions in the Athlete*, ed 3. St. Louis, MO, Elsevier Mosby, 2017.

Physical Activity Readiness Questionnaire (PAR-Q)

The Physical Activity Readiness Questionnaire (PAR-Q) is a self-screening tool that can be used by someone who is starting an exercise or athletic activity program. The questions are designed to identify individuals who are at an increased health risk associated with exercise participation. Physical activity is safe for most individuals. Answering yes to the questions on this questionnaire should result in the individual being referred to a doctor or qualified exercise professional before engaging in physical acitivty.

Special Tests

Osteokinematic Assessment

Thoracic Spine Flexion and Extension

Have the patient seated with hands interlaced behind the neck. Have the patient move through active flexion while ensuring the patient keeps the elbows in. For extension, instruct the patient to lift the elbows to the sky while extending the thoracic spine (**Figure 11.15**).

Restrictions in thoracic spine mobility may be a result of pain in the thoracic, shoulder, or cervical regions.[67]

Thoracic Spine Rotation

Have the patient seated (stabilizing the pelvis and lower extremity). The patient is instructed to raise the shoulders and spinal column (as if they are looking backward over the shoulder). Trunk rotation occurs primarily at the thoracic spine (**Figure 11.16**). The amount of rotation should be approximately equal in each direction. Overpressure can be applied to the patient's shoulders to assess the end feels for spinal rotation.[67]

Reflex Testing

Deep tendon reflexes occur when the threshold response following a quick stretch of the muscle tendon occurs, causing a reflexive muscle contraction.[12] To induce a reflexive muscle contraction, the clinician must tap on the tendon with a reflex hammer with enough force to elicit the desired response. The reflex can be graded on a four-point scale (**Table 11.34**).

The reflexes in the extremity being tested should be assessed and compared to the bilateral reflex. The clinician must determine whether the elicited response is normal or abnormal. It is important to

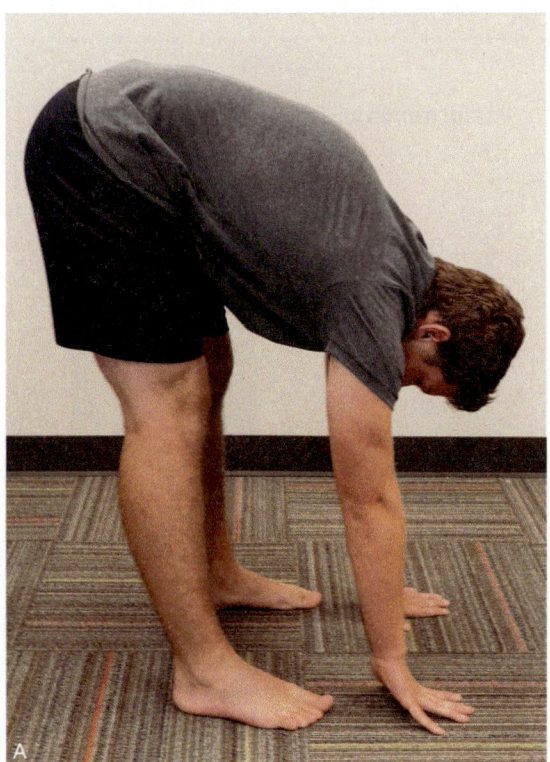
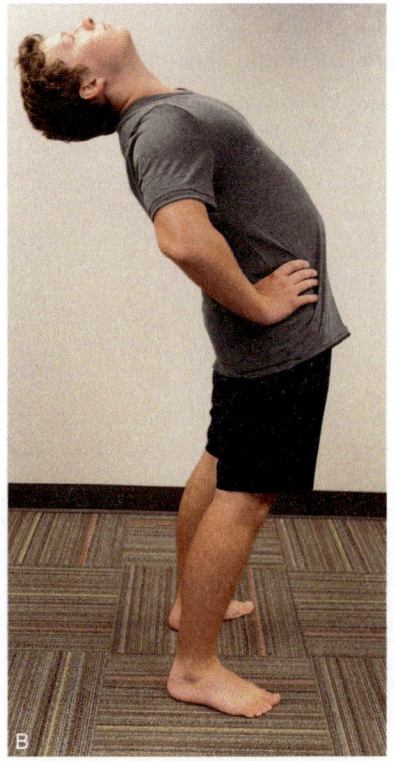

Figure 11.15 Clinical photographs showing thoracic spine flexion **(A)** and extension test **(B)**.
© Jones & Bartlett Learning

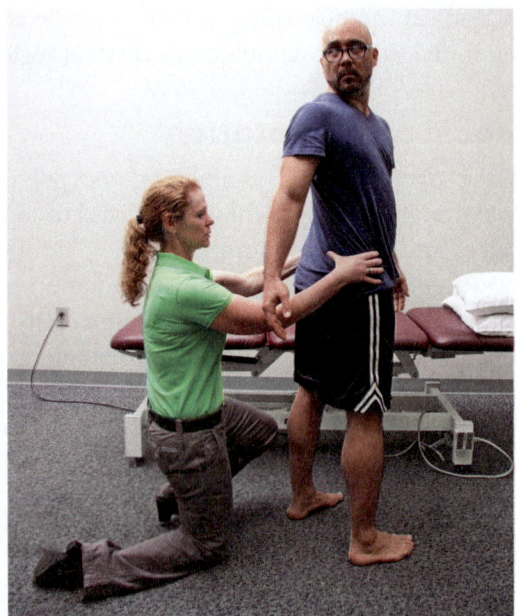

Figure 11.16 Clinical photograph demonstrating the thoracic spine rotation test.

© Jones & Bartlett Learning

Table 11.34	Graded Reflex Response
Grade	Response
0	No reflex elicited
1+	Hyporeflexia: Reflex elicited with reinforcement (precontracting the muscle)
2+	Normal response
3+	Hyperreflexia (brisk)
4+	Hyperactive with clonus

injury. Superficial reflexes disappear with both upper and lower motor neuron disease and may also be impaired during thoracic or abdominal injuries. It is important to remember that superficial reflexes are absent in approximately 20% of individuals, more so in elderly populations. The observation of an asymmetric reflex pattern is commonly associated with neurologic disease (**Table 11.35**).

Dermatome Testing

Dermatomes are areas of the skin that are innervated by a single dorsal root of spinal nerves. Dorsal roots are organized into segments in the body, and, as such, dermatomees are as well. Neighboring dorsal roots often overlap, as the sensory fibers have

note that a reflex that must be elicited with reinforcement could be considered abnormal; however, future assessment may also indicate other reflexes are also a grade 1, which would then become the baseline for the individual.

A neurologic screening should be done on any individual who has suffered an abdominal or thoracic

Table 11.35	Neurologic Screening	
Nerve Root Level	Reflex Testing	Performing the Test
C1–C4	None	
C5	Biceps brachii reflex test (musculocutaneous nerve)	The clinician's thumb is tapped with the reflex hammer.
C6	Brachioradialis reflex test (radial nerve)	The distal portion of the brachioradialis tendon is tapped with the reflex hammer. The proximal tendon may also be used.

Nerve Root Level	Reflex Testing	Performing the Test
C7	Triceps brachii reflex test (radial nerve)	The distal triceps brachii tendon is tapped with the reflex hammer.
C8	None	
T1	None	
L1	None	
L2	Femoral nerve (partial)	N/A
L3	Femoral nerve (partial)	N/A
L4	Patellar tendon (quadriceps femoris) reflex test (femoral nerve [partial])	The patellar tendon is tapped with the reflex hammer.
L5	Tibialis posterior reflex test	The tibialis posterior tendon is tapped with the reflex hammer posteriorly and just proximal to the medial malleolus.
L5 (cont.)	Semitendinosus and medial hamstring reflex (tibial nerve)	The medial hamstring tendon is tapped via the finger with the reflex hammer.
S1	Achilles tendon (triceps surae muscle group) reflex test (tibial nerve)	The Achilles tendon is tapped with the reflex hammer.
S2	Biceps femoris reflex test (tibial nerve)	The biceps femoris tendon is tapped with the reflex hammer.

All figures in table © Jones & Bartlett Learning.

multiple branches in the spinal cord. This overlap means that if a single spinal nerve is affected, there is likely still an innvervation to that section of skin. If a dermatome is completely numb, usually at least three neighboring dorsal roots are also affected. Assessing dermatomes is important to total body evaluation, including injuries to the thorax and abdomen (**Table 11.36**).

Table 11.36 Dermatome Testing

Nerve Root Segment	Nerve	Sensory Testing
C1		No dermatome distribution
C2		Forehead, temporal and occipital region of the head
C3		Neck and posterior cheek
C4	Supraclavicular nerve	Upper trapezius and clavicle
C5	Proximal lateral branch of the cutaneous nerve	Upper lateral arm
C6	Lateral antebrachial cutaneous nerve	Lateral forearm, thumb, and index finger
C7	Radial nerve	Middle finger
C8	Ulnar nerve (mixed)	Ring and little finger, medial forearm
T1	Medial branch of the cutaneous nerve	Medial arm
L1	Femoral cutaneous nerve	Oblique band across upper anterior thigh (gluteal region and around to anterior hip above hip crease line)
L2	Femoral cutaneous nerve	Oblique band across anterior portion of the upper thigh
L3	Femoral cutaneous nerve	Oblique band across the anterior midthigh
L4	Saphenous nerve	Oblique band across the anterior thigh above the knee, down the medial side of the foot and leg
L5	Superficial peroneal nerve	Lateral side of the leg starting at the midthigh, lateral side of the crest of the tibia and medial dorsum of the foot
S1	Superficial peroneal nerve	Lateral calf (about halfway up) and lateral plantar surface of the foot
S2	Tibial nerve and common peroneal nerve	Medial surface of the foot, posterior midcalf, posterior thigh

Myotome Testing

A myotome is a group of muscles that are innervated by a single spinal nerve root. Clinically, myotome testing may help to determine whether damage has occurred to the spinal cord and at which level (**Table 11.37**). Myotomes are tested in terms of power and graded 0 through 5. A grade of 0 indicates total paralysis; grade 1 is a palpable or visible contraction; grade 2 is an active movement with full range of motion with gravity eliminated; grade 3 is active movement with full range of motion against gravity; grade 4 is active movement with full range of motion against gravity with moderate resistance against gravity; and grade 5 is active movement with full range of motion against gravity and full resistance against gravity.

Range of Motion

Active Range of Motion

The ROM at each vertebra can be difficult to measure. One technique is to use a soft tape measure to measure the length of the spine from the spinous process at C7 to the spinous process at T12 with the patient standing in anatomic position. Then, ask the patient to bend forward at the spine and measure again. A 2.7-cm (1.1-inch) difference in tape measure length is a normal finding (**Table 11.38**). The spine can also be measured from the spinous process at C7 to the spinous process at S1 with the patient standing in the anatomic position. The patient is then asked to bend forward at the spine and measurements are taken (**Figure 11.17**). A 10-cm (4-inch) difference in measured length is considered within normal limits.

Table 11.37 Myotome Testing

Nerve Root Segment	Action Tested
C1–C2	Neck flexion
C3 and cranial nerve XI	Lateral neck flexion
C4 and cranial nerve XI	Shoulder elevation
C5	Shoulder abduction
C6	Elbow flexion and/or wrist extension
C7	Elbow extension and/or wrist flexion
C8	Thumb extension and/or ulnar deviation
T1	Finger abduction and adduction
L1	Short sitting hip flexion with knee flexed to 90°
L2	Short sitting hip flexion with knee flexed to 90°
L3	Short sitting knee extension
L4	Long sitting, dorsiflexion
L5	Long sitting, extension of the first metatarsophalangeal joint (big toe)
S1	Long sitting, ankle eversion
S2	Prone knee flexion

Table 11.38 Active Range of Motion Norms for the Thoracic Spine

Movement	Goniometer Measurement
Forward spine flexion	20° to 45°
Spine extension	25° to 45°
Spine side flexion (left and right)	20° to 40°
Spinal rotation (left and right)	35° to 50°
Movement	**Centimeters**
Costovertebral expansion	3–7.5

These measures evaluate movement of the thoracic and lumbar spine, the greatest amount of movement (approximately 7.5 cm [3 inches]) occurring between T12 and S1.[67]

Another measure for spinal flexion is to have the patient bend forward at the hips (keeping the knees straight) and try to touch the toes (**Figure 11.18**). A tape measure can be used to measure from the fingertips to the floor. This measure is somewhat functional in nature, as it does not isolate the thoracic spine but rather includes the lumbar spine and hip range of motion in the movement as well.[67]

As with flexion, extension can be measured using a soft tape measure between the spinous process at C7 and the spinous process at T12. A 2.5-cm (1-inch) difference in tape measure length between standing and extension is within normal limits.[67]

Passive Range of Motion

Capsular Patterns.
- Facet joints of the thoracic spine:[71]
  - Resting position: Midway between flexion and extension
  - Close packed position: Extension
  - Capsular pattern: Side flexion and rotation equally limited, then extension

End Feels.
- Passive movements of the thoracic spine and normal end feels:[71]
  - Forward flexion: Tissue stretch
  - Extension: Tissue stretch
  - Side flexion (left and right): Tissue stretch
  - Rotation (left and right): Tissue stretch

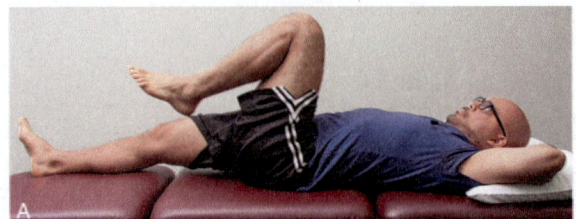
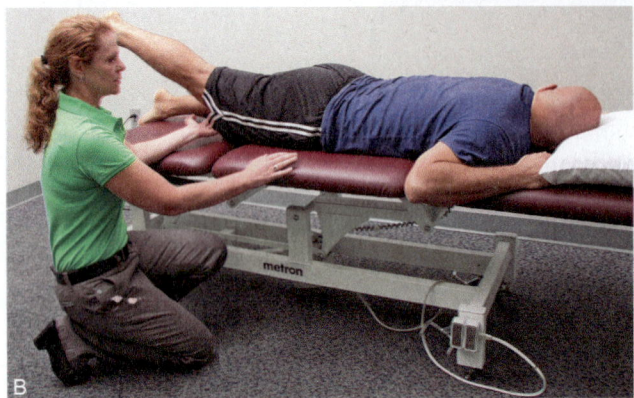
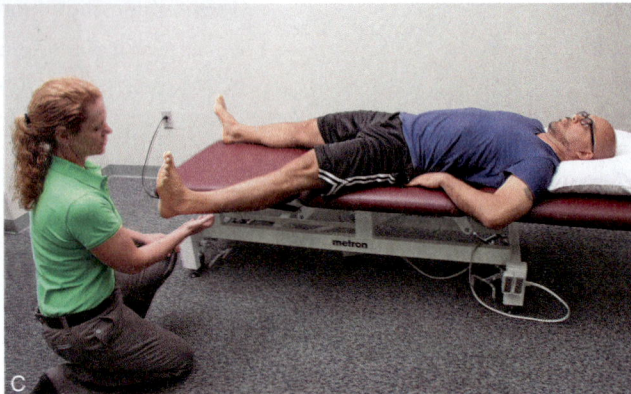
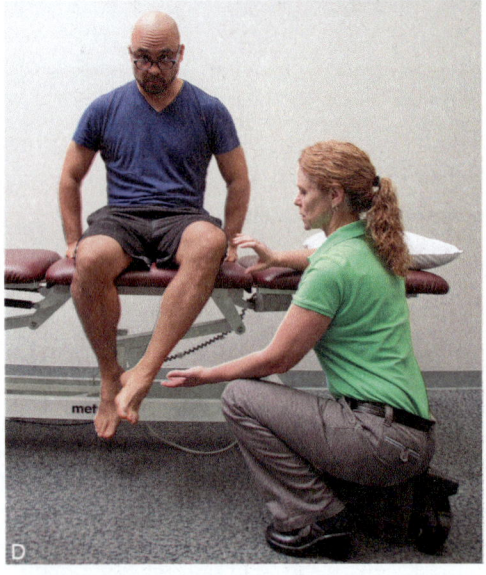
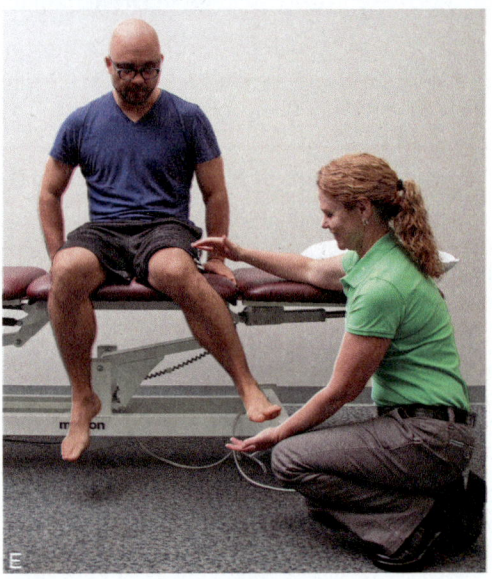

Figure 11.17 Clinical photographs showing assessment of active range of motion. **A.** Hip flexion. **B.** Hip extension. **C.** Hip abduction. **D.** Hip external rotation. **E.** Hip internal rotation.

© Jones & Bartlett Learning

Joint Orientation: Thoracic Spine.

T1–T11[71]

- Superior articular facets:
  - Convex
  - Face posteriorly, slightly superiorly and laterally
- Inferior articular facets:
  - Concave
  - Face anteriorly, slightly inferiorly and medially

T12[66]

- Superior articular facets:
  - Thoracic-like
  - Convex
  - Face posteriorly, slightly superiorly and laterally
- Inferior articular facets:
  - Lumbar-like
  - Convex
  - Face laterally and anteriorly

Cobb Method to Measure Spinal Curvature Associated With Scoliosis

The Cobb method has been described as a system to evaluate scoliosis by measuring angles calculated after obtaining AP radiographs[72-74] (**Figure 11.19**). Based on

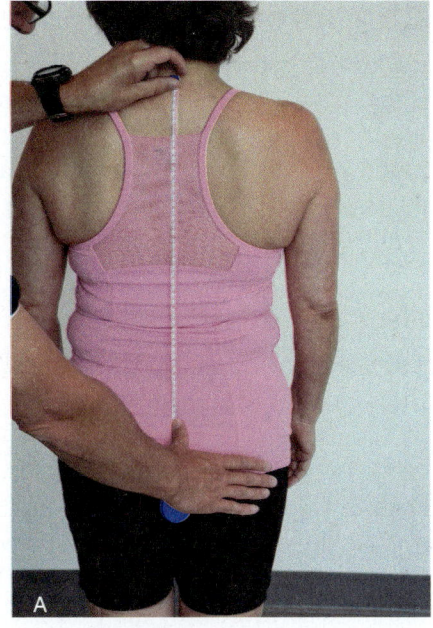
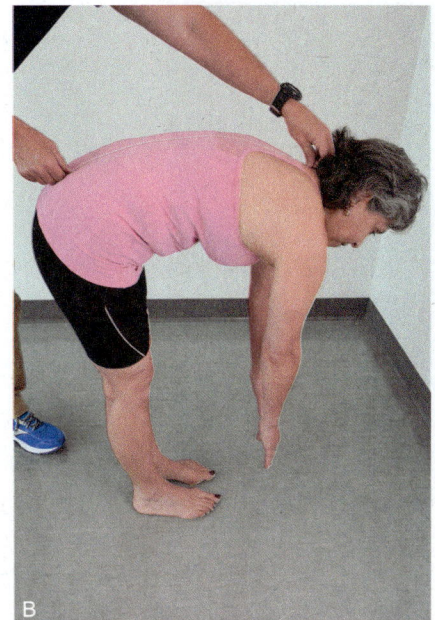
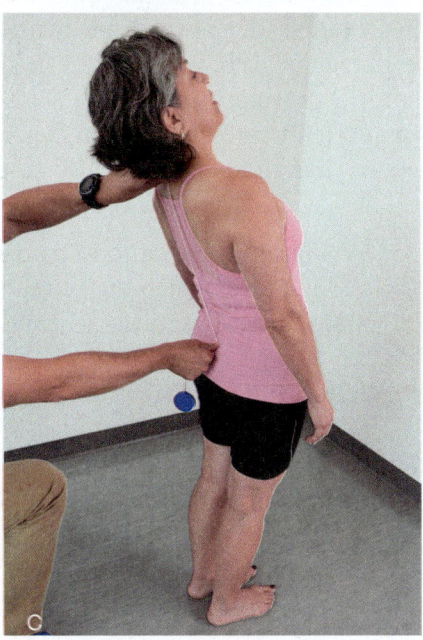
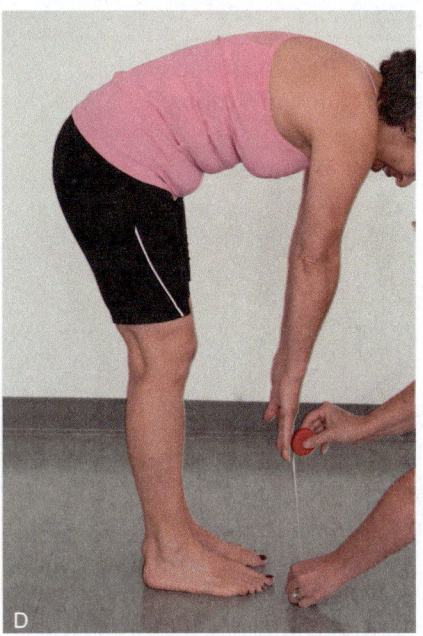

Figure 11.18 Clinical photographs showing alternative methods to assess spinal range of motion. **A.** Measurement of the spine along the spinous process from C7 and T12 is assessed using a soft tape measure. **B.** Clinician has the patient perform spinal flexion and measures the spine. **C.** Clinician has the patient perform spinal extension and measures the spine. **D.** Clinician has the patient perform spinal flexion and measures from the patient's fingertips to the floor (if the patient cannot touch the floor).

© Jones & Bartlett Learning

the angle calculated via the Cobb method, the severity of clinical scoliosis can be diagnosed in an individual.[74] From an AP radiograph view, a line is drawn parallel to the superior cortical plate of the proximal end of the vertebra.[72,74] A second line is drawn from the inferior cortical plate of the distal end vertebra.[72,74] A perpendicular line connects each of these two lines, and the angle resulting represents the spinal curvature resulting from scoliosis.[72] The Scoliosis Research Society has classified the degree of scoliosis according to the degree of curvature[73] (**Table 11.39**).

Common Radiographic Views
AP View

In an AP radiograph view, look for the following features:

- Normal symmetry of the ribs (bilateral comparison)
- Normal disk spaces between vertebrae

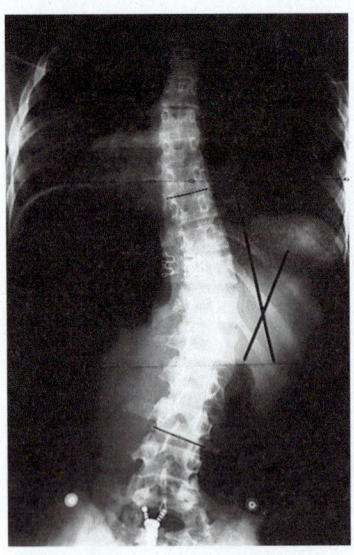

Figure 11.19 Radiograph showing the Cobb method.

Reproduced from Armstrong AD, Hubbard MC, eds: *Essentials of Musculoskeletal Care*, ed 5. Burlington, MA, American Academy of Orthopaedic Surgeons, 2015.

Table 11.39 Scoliosis Research Society Classification of Scoliosis

Classification	Cobb Score
Group 1	0° to 20°
Group 2	21° to 30°
Group 3	31° to 50°
Group 4	51° to 75°
Group 5	76° to 100°
Group 6	101° to 125°
Group 7	126° or greater

Reproduced from Keim HA: Scoliosis. *Clin Symposia* 1973;25:1-25.

- Wedging of the vertebrae
- Scoliosis (lateral bending) of the vertebrae
- Possible osteophytes

Lateral View

In a lateral radiograph view, look for the following features:

- Normal mild kyphosis of the thoracic spine
- Normal angle of the ribs
- Normal disk spaces between the vertebrae
- Wedging of the vertebrae
- Possible osteophytes

Neurologic Assessment

Check the neurologic status if thoracic nerve root involvement is suspected.

Cardiorespiratory Assessment

Cardiorespiratory status should be monitored for signs of shock and internal hemorrhage. Record and monitor vital signs, such as heart rate and pulse, blood pressure, and respiration quantity and quality. Assessing skin color, moisture, and temperature also can be helpful.

Heart Rate and Pulse

The strength and rate of the surge of blood circulating through the blood vessels is indicated with each beat of the heart.

Rate. Gently place the flat pad of the index or middle finger over the patient's superficial arteries to palpate and count the number of beats per minute (bpm), also known as the pulse. Count the number of beats over 15 seconds and then multiply by 4. A heart rate under normal, resting conditions is strong and regular, typically beating 60 to 80 bpm in an adult.[75] Normal pulse rate in a child is 80 to 100 bpm. Heart rates may be higher in untrained, sedentary individuals (80 to 100 bpm) than in highly trained athletes (40 to 60 bpm).[75]

- Do not use the thumb to palpate because it has a strong pulse, which may confuse the assessment.
- Bradycardia describes a heart rate falling below the normal range.
- Tachycardia describes a rapid heart rate.

Rhythm and Strength. The rhythm of the pulse should be steady, and the pulse strength should be consistent. Changes in pumping quality or demands on the heart may alter the rhythm and strength of the pulse.

Blood Pressure

The blood must be circulated throughout the body to survive, and, therefore, adequate blood pressure must be maintained to help facilitate that movement. Blood pressure is measured with a stethoscope and sphygmomanometer (blood pressure cuff) and is recorded in millimeters of mercury (mmHg). Blood pressure is reported as a fraction—the systolic over the diastolic (eg, 120/80 mm Hg). The systolic pressure measures the pressure against the artery walls when the heart pumps.[76-78] The diastolic pressure measures the pressure exerted against the artery walls when the heart is relaxed.[77, 78]

Have the patient relax and sit in a chair with the feet on the floor (ask him or her to uncross the feet if they are crossed). The patient should rest for at least 5 minutes prior to evaluation.[78] Position the sphygmomanometer (be sure to choose the right size based on the patient such that the bladder encircles 80% of the patient's arm) just above the patient's elbow, aligning the arrow (center of the bladder) with the brachial artery.[76,78] An uninflated cuff should be snug around the arm but not too tight. The patient's arm should be relaxed with the elbow and forearm level with the heart.[78] Place the stethoscope over the brachial artery, just under the cuff, in the antecubital fossa and hold firmly with the nondominant hand.[76,78] Make sure the bladder is closed, and then squeeze the hand pump to inflate the bladder of the cuff until the pressure gauge reads 200 mm Hg. Listen for a pulse, while inflating the cuff. Increase pressure until the pulse sound is absent.[77] Gradually open the bladder valve to release air slowly from the cuff and gradually drop the pressure (at a rate of 3–5 mm Hg per second).[78] Listen for the first strong thump of the pulse also known as Korotkoff sounds.[78] Mentally note the number of the first thump heard and continue to listen as the pressure falls until the pulse can no longer be heard. The diastolic pressure is the value at which the last audible pulse is heard.[76-78] After the diastolic pressure is identified, open the valve completely to release the rest of the pressure and restore blood flow to the extremity. Normal blood pressure in adults ranges between 90/60 and 130/85 mm Hg. The American College of Cardiology and the American Heart Association have new recommendations for normal blood pressure[76,78] (**Table 11.40**).

Although it is not uncommon for athletes and highly trained individuals to have blood pressures at or below the normal limit, a systolic pressure below 80 mm Hg for adults (and 70 mm Hg for children) should be considered critically low.[77] A critically low systolic blood pressure may indicate injury or illness. Low systolic blood pressure is a sign that the body is not sufficiently compensating for changes in the circulatory system and is unable to maintain adequate blood perfusion.[78]

Respiration

Rate. Record the rate of respiration in breaths per minute by counting the number of breaths the patient takes in a 30-second time interval and multiplying by two.[79] Count the breaths by watching the chest or abdomen rise and fall, placing a hand on the patient's back to feel the rise and fall of the chest, or listening to the breaths with a stethoscope. Normal respiration rates under resting conditions are 12 to 20 breaths per minute for adults and 20 to 30 breaths per minute for children.[79]

Quality. The quality of respiration is somewhat subjective in nature. It can be difficult to identify abnormal breathing, especially during exercise or athletic activity.[79] Watch and listen to the patient's breathing. Labored breathing may occur if an individual has difficulty speaking or appears to exert unusual effort to inhale.[12,79] Activation of accessory muscles of the neck, abdomen, and thorax during breathing or leaning over (hands on the knees in a tripod position) may indicate the increased effort to pull more air into the lungs by an individual.[12] Noisy breathing may indicate an airway obstruction (audible wheezing or stridor). Fluid in the lungs may make a gurgling or bubbling sound during breathing.[79]

Rhythm and Depth. Watch the patient's chest rise and fall or listen to the breaths. Determine whether the patient is breathing at a regular interval or breathing seems to speed up or slow down without reason. If the patient appears to be having difficulty drawing a deep breath (shallow breathing), minimal oxygen delivery may be occurring. Deeper breathing may suggest

Table 11.40 Blood Pressure Categories

Blood Pressure Category	Systolic mm Hg (Upper Number)		Diastolic mm Hg (Lower Number)
Normal	Less than 120	and	Less than 80
Elevated	120–129	and	Less than 80
High blood pressure (hypertension) stage 1	130–139	or	80–89
High blood pressure (hypertension) stage 2	140 or higher	or	90 or higher
Hypertensive crisis (consult your doctor immediately)	Higher than 180	and/or	Higher than 120

Reprinted with permission © American Heart Association, Inc.

Table 11.41 Abnormal Breathing Patterns

Term	Description	Location of Possible Neurologic Lesion
Hyperpnea	Abnormal increase in the depth and rate of respiration	
Apnea	Periods of no breathing	Pons
Ataxic breathing (Biot respiration)	Irregular breathing pattern; random periods of deep and shallow breathing	Medulla
Hyperventilation	Prolonged, rapid hyperpnea. Results in decreased carbon dioxide blood levels	Midbrain, pons
Cheyne-Stokes respirations	Periods of hyperpnea regularly alternating with periods of apnea (no breathing). Regular acceleration and deceleration in depth of breathing	Cerebrum, cerebellum, midbrain, pons
Cluster breathing	Disordered sequence of breaths with irregular pauses between	Pons, medulla

Reproduced from Hickey JV: *The Clinical Practice of Neurological and Neurosurgical Nursing*, ed 7. Philadelphia, PA, Lippincott Williams & Wilkins, 2013.

oxygen deprivation.[12] Abnormal findings may indicate that the patient has suffered a head injury or is in respiratory distress or arrest. Cheyne-Stokes respirations, characterized by a rhythmic fluctuation between rapid, deep breathing (hyperpnea) and slow or absent breathing (apnea), are an abnormal rhythm and depth sometimes found with head injury[80,81] (**Table 11.41**).

Skin Assessment

The skin can provide valuable information to the clinician regarding the amount of oxygen perfusion throughout the body, the amount of peripheral circulation, and body temperature.[12,79] The skin should be assessed for color, temperature, and moisture.[79] Various clinical conditions may affect these skin characteristics in different ways.

Skin Coloring. Ashen, pale (pallor), or grayish skin may indicate poor blood perfusion in conditions such as heat exhaustion, hypothermia, and/or shock. A reddish tint to the skin can be found in athletes who are exercising but may also be a sign of a pathologic condition, such as hypertension, heatstroke, or carbon dioxide poisoning. Blueish (cyanotic) skin may suggest hypoxia, a lack of oxygen to the tissues[79] (**Figure 11.20** and **Table 11.42**). Yellowish skin may signify a liver issue. It may be more difficult to determine color changes in patients with darker skin pigmentation, so a clinician should examine the nail beds, mucosa of the mouth, the lips, and the palms or soles of the feet.

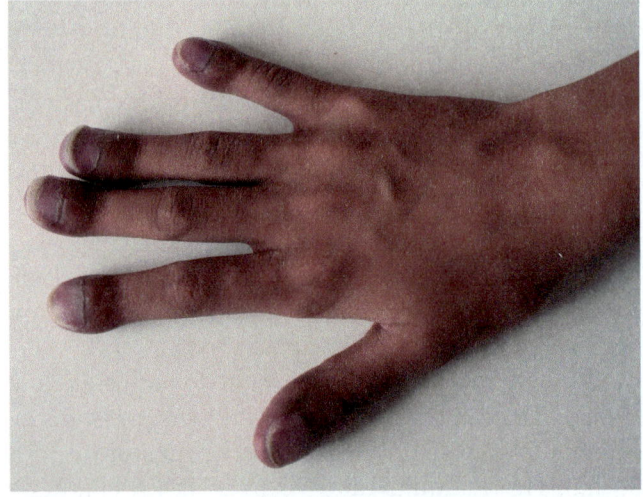

Figure 11.20 Photograph showing cyanotic skin color in the fingertips.
© kris4to/Shutterstock.

Skin Temperature. Skin temperature can be evaluated by the clinician using a handheld surface thermometer. Normal skin temperature is approximately 98.6°F (37°C). The skin is normally warm and dry to the touch. If a patient is exercising, the skin may be moist and warm (or hot). In conditions such as hypothermia, the skin may be very cold to the touch. Cool, clammy skin is found in patients suffering from heat exhaustion. The skin will feel hot with conditions such as fever and burns. The skin will likely be hot and dry with a patient suffering from heatstroke, as the body has lost the ability to cool itself via sweating.

Table 11.42 Skin Coloring Evaluation to Determine Circulatory Status

Color	Indication	Likely Condition
Pink	Good tissue perfusion	Normal
Pale, ashen	Poor tissue perfusion	Heat exhaustion, hypothermia, shock
Red	Increased tissue perfusion	Normal exercise, hypertension, heatstroke, carbon dioxide poisoning
Blue	Cyanotic (lack of oxygen to tissues)	Hypoxia

Reproduced from Shultz SJ, Houglum PA, Perrin DH: *Examination of Musculoskeletal Injuries*, ed 4. Champaign, IL, Human Kinetics, 2016.

Vascular Assessment

Carotid Pulse. The carotid artery is palpated between the thyroid cartilage and sternocleidomastoid. The carotid artery is used to determine the frequency, quality, and rhythm of the pulse.

Orthopaedic Special Tests

Special tests are used to rule in and rule out abdominal and thoracic injuries. Spinal pathology should be ruled out prior to performing any special tests. If a spinal injury is suspected, refer the patient to an emergency department as soon as possible while maintaining spinal stabilization.

Additionally, any difficulty breathing may be a rib or lung injury and should be closely monitored. If a patient has sustained difficulty breathing, refer the patient to an emergency department for further evaluation. Patients may exhibit signs, such as coughing up blood (hemoptysis) or vomiting blood (hematemesis).

Abdominal rigidity could indicate a medical emergency with injury (specifically rupture) to the spleen, which requires activation of an emergency action plan. The next section will examine common pathologies and special tests to identify other thoracic and abdominal pathologies when available. Special tests are used to rule in and rule out pathologies. It is important that clinicians are trained to perform these special tests before they conduct an evaluation. Special tests often lead health care professionals to other medical referrals for treatment.

Mobility of the First Rib

The ribs should be slightly mobile to allow for regular respiration. Occasionally a rib can become stuck, so assessing the mobility of the ribs, particularly the first rib is important (**Table 11.43**).

Compression Test for Rib Fracture

The compression test can assess possible rib fractures. Clinicians need to be cautious when performing this special test because, if the rib is fractured, it possibly has sharp ends that could be pressed into the thorax or underlying blood vessels (**Table 11.44**).

Table 11.43 Mobility of the First Rib

Test	Patient Position	Procedure	Positive Test	Implication	Evidence
Mobility of the first rib	Prone.	Palpate the posterior aspect of the first rib (anterior to the upper trapezius and above the medial [vertebral] border of the scapula). Provide an inferior glide to the first rib.	Hypomobility and/or pain.	Restricted mobility of the first costovertebral joint.	Absent or inconclusive in the literature.

Table 11.44 Compression Test for Rib Fractures

Test	Patient Position	Procedure	Positive Test	Implication	Evidence
Compression test for rib fractures	Seated or standing.	The examiner compresses the rib cage in an anteroposterior direction and quickly releases the pressure. The rib cage is then compressed from the patient's sides, and the pressure is quickly released.	Pain in the rib cage isolated to the fracture site.	Damage to the rib cage (may indicate possible rib fracture, rib contusion, or costochondral separation).	Absent or inconclusive in the literature.

Table 11.45 Adson Test for Thoracic Outlet Syndrome

Test	Patient Position	Procedure	Positive Test	Implication	Evidence
Adson test for TOS	The patient is sitting; the shoulder is abducted to 30°. The elbow is extended with the thumb pointed upward, and the humerus is externally rotated.	Find the radial pulse, externally rotate and extend the patient's shoulder while the patient's face is rotated toward the involved side, and then the patient extends the neck. The patient should be instructed to inhale deeply and hold his or her breath.	The radial pulse disappears and/or is markedly diminished compared with the opposite side or a reproduction of the symptoms.	The subclavian artery and/or brachial plexus is occluded between the anterior and middle scalene muscle and the pectoralis minor.	Sensitivity: 50 79 Specificity: Vascular changes 87 89 Paresthesia: 74 89 Pain: 100 Nonspecific: 76 16–20 + Likelihood ratio: 3.3 − Likelihood ratio: 0.27

TOS, thoracic outlet syndrome.
Data from Gillard J, Perez-Cousin M, Hachulla E, et al: Diagnosing thoracic outlet syndrome: contribution of provocative tests, ultrasonography, electrophysiology, and helical computed tomography in 48 patients. *Joint Bone Spine*. 2001;68:416-424; Lee AD, Agawal S, Sadhu D. Doppler Adson's test: predictors of outcome of surgery in non-specific thoracic outlet syndrome. *World J Surg* 2006;30:291-292; Nord KM, Kapoor P, Fisher J, et al: False positive rate of thoracic outlet syndrome diagnostic maneuvers in healthy patients. *Electromyog Clin Neurophysiol*. 2008;48:67-74; Plewa MC, Delinger M: The false-positive rate of thoracic outlet syndrome shoulder maneuvers in healthy patients. *Acad Emerg Med* 1998;5:337-342; and Rayan GM, Jensen C: Thoracic outlet syndrome provocative examination maneuvers in a typical population. *J Shoulder Elbow Surg* 1995;4:113-117.

Thoracic Outlet Syndrome

Thoracic outlet syndrome (TOS) is a condition in which the blood vessels and/or the nerves become trapped between the clavicle (collarbone) and the first rib. This condition causes pain in the shoulders and neck and numbness into the fingers. TOS can result from physical trauma, such as a car accident; sporting incident; repetitive injuries; or anatomic defects, such as being born with an extra rib. There are multiple causes of TOS. Clinicans can use several special tests to identify TOS[82-95] and evaluate the possible structures involved with the condition (**Tables 11.45** through **11.54**).

Auscultations of the Lungs

Breath sounds are the noises produced by the movement of the lungs during respiration. A stethoscope, most often the bell of the stethoscope, can be used

Table 11.46 Allen Test for Thoracic Outlet Syndrome

Test	Patient Position	Procedure	Positive Test	Implication	Evidence
Allen test for TOS	The patient is sitting with the head facing forward.	The elbow is flexed to 90° while the clinician abducts the shoulder to 90°. The shoulder is passively horizontally abducted and placed into external rotation. The patient is then instructed to rotate the head toward the opposite shoulder.	The radial pulse disappears and/or neurologic symptoms are reproduced.	The pectoralis minor muscle is compressing the neurovascular bundle.	Absent or inconclusive in the literature.

TOS, thoracic outlet syndrome.
Data from Brismee JM, Gilbert K, Isom K, et al: Rate of false positive using the Cyriax release test for thoracic outlet syndrome in an asymptomatic population. *J Man Manipulative Ther* 2004;12:73-81.

Table 11.47 Costoclavicular Syndrome Tests for Thoracic Outlet Syndrome

Test	Patient Position	Procedure	Positive Test	Implication	Evidence
Costoclavicular syndrome test (military brace position test) for TOS	The patient is standing with the shoulders in a relaxed position and the head is looking forward.	The patient retracts and depresses the shoulder (as if coming to military attention). The humerus is extended (50° to 60°) and abducted to 30°. The neck and head are hyperextended during the test.	The radial pulse disappears, and/or neurologic symptoms are reproduced.	The subclavian artery and/or lower trunks of the brachial plexus are impinged by the costoclavicular structures of the shoulder.	Sensitivity: Absent or inconclusive in the literature. Specificity: Vascular changes 53 79 Paresthesia: 98 85 Pain: 100 + Likelihood ratio: Absent or inconclusive in the literature − Likelihood ratio: Absent or inconclusive in the literature

TOS, thoracic outlet syndrome.
Data from Plewa MC, Delinger M: The false-positive rate of thoracic outlet syndrome shoulder maneuvers in healthy patients. *Acad Emerg Med.* 1998;5:337-342; and Rayan GM, Jensen C: Thoracic outlet syndrome provocative examination maneuvers in a typical population. *J Shoulder Elbow Surg* 1995;4:113-117.

Table 11.48 Cyriax Release Test for Thoracic Outlet Syndrome

Test	Patient Position	Procedure	Positive Test	Implication	Evidence
Cyriax release test for TOS	The patient is sitting or standing.	The examiner grabs under the forearms, holding the elbows at approximately 80° to 90° elbow flexion while maintaining the forearms, wrists, and hands in a neutral position. The examiner then leans into the patient's trunk posteriorly, approximately 15° from vertical, and elevates the patient's shoulder girdle close to the end range (in a lifted position). This position is held for up to 3 minutes.	Replication of sensory and/or motor symptoms in the extremity.	Vascular and/or neurologic TOS.	Sensitivity: Inconclusive or absent in the literature Specificity: 97 + Likelihood ratio: Inconclusive or absent in the literature − Likelihood ratio: Inconclusive or absent in the literature

TOS, thoracic outlet syndrome.
Data from Brismee JM, Gilbert K, Isom K, et al: Rate of false positive using the Cyriax release test for thoracic outlet syndrome in an asymptomatic population. *J Man Manipulative Ther* 2004;12:73-81.

Table 11.49 Hyperabduction Test for Thoracic Outlet Syndrome

Test	Patient Position	Procedure	Positive Test	Implication	Evidence
Hyperabduction test for TOS	The patient is sitting with the back straight.	Both arms are placed at the side of the patient. The examiner takes the radial pulse. The patient is instructed to place the arms above 90° abduction and in full shoulder external rotation. The arms are held in this position 1 to 2 minutes. The examiner palpates the radial pulse in the hyperabducted and externally rotated position.	The radial pulse disappears and/or neurologic symptoms are reproduced.	The subclavian artery and/or lower trunks of the brachial plexus are impinged by the costoclavicular structures of the shoulder.	Sensitivity: Pulse abolition 52 Symptom reproduction 84 Specificity: Vascular changes 43 38 Paresthesia: 90 64 Pain: 79 Pulse abolition 90 Symptom reproduction 40 + Likelihood ratio: Pulse abolition 5.2 Symptom reproduction 1.4 − Likelihood ratio: Pulse abolition 0.53 Symptom reproduction 0.4

TOS, thoracic outlet syndrome.
Data from Gillard J, Perez-Cousin M, Hachulla E, et al: Diagnosing thoracic outlet syndrome: contribution of provocative tests, ultrasonography, electrophysiology, and helical computed tomography in 48 patients. *Joint Bone Spine* 2001;68:416-424; Plewa MC, Delinger M: The false-positive rate of thoracic outlet syndrome shoulder maneuvers in healthy patients. *Acad Emerg Med* 1998;5:337-342; and Rayan GM, Jensen C: Thoracic outlet syndrome provocative examination maneuvers in a typical population. *J Shoulder Elbow Surg* 1995;4:113-117.

to listen to the sounds of the lungs, also known as auscultations of the lungs (Table 11.55). It is extremely common for health care professionals to listen and assess lung sounds. During auscultions of the lungs, the patient breaths deeply with the mouth open, and the clinican listens to assess for normal breathing sounds, decreased or absent breath sounds, and abnormal breath sounds (Table 11.56).

Table 11.50 Morley Sign for Thoracic Outlet Syndrome

Test	Patient Position	Procedure	Positive Test	Implication	Evidence
Morley sign for TOS	The patient is sitting with the arms at his or her side.	The examiner palpates the supraclavicular fossa with his or her thumb.	Tenderness in the supraclavicular fossa. This test will also likely be painful for a patient with cervical radiculopathy.	Vascular and/or neurologic TOS	Absent or inconclusive in the literature.

TOS, thoracic outlet syndrome.
Data from Plewa MC, Delinger M: The false-positive rate of thoracic outlet syndrome shoulder maneuvers in healthy patients. *Acad Emerg Med* 1998;5:337-342; Nord KM, Kapoor P, Fisher J, et al: False positive rate of thoracic outlet syndrome diagnostic maneuvers in healthy patients. *Electromyog Clin Neurophysiol* 2008;48:67-74.

Table 11.51 Roos Test for Thoracic Outlet Syndrome

Test	Patient Position	Procedure	Positive Test	Implication	Evidence
Roos test (EAST) for TOS	The patient is sitting or standing; the shoulders are abducted to 90°, and the humerus is externally rotated. The elbows are flexed to 90° during the test.	The patient rapidly opens and closes both hands for 3 minutes.	Inability to maintain the testing position. Replication of sensory and/or motor symptoms in the extremity.	Vascular and/or neurologic TOS.	Sensitivity: 82 84 Specificity: 100 47 30 + Likelihood ratio: 1.2 − Likelihood ratio: 0.53

EAST, elevated arm stress test; TOS, thoracic outlet syndrome.
Data from Gillard J, Perez-Cousin M, Hachulla E, et al: Diagnosing thoracic outlet syndrome: contribution of provocative tests, ultrasonography, electrophysiology, and helical computed tomography in 48 patients. *Joint Bone Spine* 2001;68:416–424; Howard M, Lee C, Dellon AL: Documentation of brachial plexus compression (in the thoracic inlet) utilizing provocative neurosensory and muscular testing. *J Reconstr Microsurg* 2003;19:303-312; and Nord KM, Kapoor P, Fisher J, et al: False positive rate of thoracic outlet syndrome diagnostic maneuvers in healthy patients. *Electromyog Clin Neurophysiol* 2008;48:67-74.

Table 11.52 Supraclavicular Pressure Test for Thoracic Outlet Syndrome

Test	Patient Position	Procedure	Positive Test	Implication	Evidence
Supraclavicular pressure test for TOS	The patient is sitting with the arms by the side.	The examiner places his or her fingers on the upper trapezius and the thumbs on the lowest portion of the anterior scalene near the first rib. The examiner then squeezes the fingers and thumb together for 30 seconds.	Changes in paresthesia or reproduction of TOS symptoms.	Vascular and/or neurologic TOS.	Sensitivity: Absent or inconclusive in the literature. Specificity: Vascular changes 79 Pain: 98 Paresthesia: 85 General symptoms: 56 + Likelihood ratio: Absent or inconclusive in the literature − Likelihood ratio: Absent or inconclusive in the literature

TOS, thoracic outlet syndrome.
Data from Nord KM, Kapoor P, Fisher J, et al: False positive rate of thoracic outlet syndrome diagnostic maneuvers in healthy patients. *Electromyog Clin Neurophysiol* 2008;48:67-74; and Plewa MC, Delinger M: The false-positive rate of thoracic outlet syndrome shoulder maneuvers in healthy patients. *Acad Emerg Med* 1998;5:337-342.

Table 11.53 Tinel Sign for Thoracic Outlet Syndrome

Test	Patient Position	Procedure	Positive Test	Implication	Evidence
Tinel sign for TOS	The patient is sitting with the arms at the side.	The examiner taps the supraclavicular fossa with a reflex hammer.	Tenderness in the supraclavicular fossa.	Vascular and/or neurologic TOS. Additional testing should be performed to confirm the TOS clinical diagnosis.	Sensitivity: 46 Specificity: 56 + Likelihood ratio: 1.04 − Likelihood ratio: 0.96

TOS, thoracic outlet syndrome.
Data from Gillard J, Perez-Cousin M, Hachulla E, et al: Diagnosing thoracic outlet syndrome: contribution of provocative tests, ultrasonography, electrophysiology, and helical computed tomography in 48 patients. *Joint Bone Spine* 2001;68:416-424.

Table 11.54 Wright Test for Thoracic Outlet Syndrome

Test	Patient Position	Procedure	Positive Test	Implication	Evidence

Wright test for TOS	The patient is sitting with the shoulders hyperabducted and the elbow flexed to 90° during the test. The head is turned toward the unaffected side.	The patient holds this position for 1 to 2 minutes while the examiner palpates the radial artery.	Replication of sensory and/or motor symptoms in the extremity.	Vascular and/or neurologic TOS. Pectoralis minor syndrome.	Sensitivity:
					  Pulse abolition: 70
					  Symptom reproduction: 90
					Specificity:
					  Pulse abolition: 53
					  Symptom reproduction: 29
					+ Likelihood ratio:
					  Pulse abolition: 1.5
					  Symptom reproduction: 1.3
					− Likelihood ratio:
					  Pulse abolition: 0.56
					  Symptom reproduction: 0.34

TOS, thoracic outlet syndrome.
Data from Gillard J, Perez-Cousin M, Hachulla E, et al: Diagnosing thoracic outlet syndrome: contribution of provocative tests, ultrasonography, electrophysiology, and helical computed tomography in 48 patients. *Joint Bone Spine* 2001;68:416-424.

Table 11.55 Auscultations of the Lungs

Test	Patient Position	Procedure	Positive Test	Implication	Evidence
Auscultations of the lungs	Patients are instructed to breathe deeply through an open mouth.	A stethoscope is used to listen to the lungs to evaluate breath sounds. Move from one side to the other, comparing the symmetry of the lung sounds. The clinician should listen for at least one full breath at each site (six sites starting at the clavicle and moving down toward the ribs in a J shape in the anterior portion of the chest and seven sites starting at the upper apex of the scapula and working down in a J shape from the back).	Crackles Fine crackles Coarse crackles Wheezes Rhonchi Stridor Pleural rub Mediastinal crunch Absence of sounds	No specific implications; however, possible upper respiratory tract infection, pneumonia, chronic heart failure, airway obstruction, or asthma.	Absent or inconclusive in the literature.

Data from JoVE Science Education Database: *Physical Examinations I. Respiratory Exam II: Percussion and Auscultation*. JoVE, Cambridge, MA, 2019.

Table 11.56 Abnormal Breath Sounds

Sound	Characteristic
Crackles	May result from abnormalities of the lungs (eg, pneumonia, fibrosis, or early congestive heart failure) or the airways (eg, bronchitis or bronchiectasis).
Fine crackles	Soft, high-pitched popping and very brief (5–10 msec).
Coarse crackles	Somewhat louder than fine crackles, lower in pitch, and not quite so brief (20–30 msec).
Wheezes	Relatively high pitched (~400 MHz or higher) with a hissing or shrill quality. Wheezing indicates a narrowing of the airway (eg, asthma, bronchitis, chronic obstructive pulmonary disease, and congestive heart failure).
Rhonchi	Relatively low-pitched (~200 MHz or lower) with a rumbling, gurgling, rattle-like or snoring quality. The thickened mucus inhibiting the passage of air through the bronchi usually causes rhonchi.
Stridor	Stridor is a high pitched, whistle-like sound and is predominantly inspiratory. Often louder in the neck than over the chest wall. Indicates partial obstruction of the larynx or trachea.
Pleural rub	Inflamed or roughened pleural surfaces grate against each other producing a creaking sound.
Mediastinal crunch	A series of precordial crackles synchronous with heartbeats not respirations. These sounds are best heard in the left lateral position (Hamman sign) and are caused by mediastinal emphysema.
Absence of sounds	May be caused by pleural effusion, pneumothorax, tension pneumothorax, hemothorax, or traumatic asphyxia.

Data from JoVE Science Education Database: *Physical Examinations I. Respiratory Exam II: Percussion and Auscultation.* JoVE, Cambridge, MA, 2019; Walker HK, Hall WD, Hurst JW, eds: *Clinical Methods: The History, Physical, and Laboratory Examinations,* ed 3. London, Butterworths, 1990; Scifers J: *Special Tests for Neurological Examination.* Thorofare, NJ, Slack Incorporated, 2008.

Percussion of the Lungs

Percussion is an assessment technique in which the clinician taps on the patient's chest wall to produce sounds. Tapping on the chest wall produces different sound resonances based on the amount of air in the lungs (Table 11.57).

Abdominal Observations

An observation of the abdomen can provide the clinician with information following an injury. The clinician must expose the abdomen to evaluate and observe. It is extremely important to communicate with the patient prior to conducting an evaluation and to be sensitive to cultural differences in comfort levels in exposing the abdomen. The clinician should be sure to drape and cover the lower half of the patient (below the hips) and the upper chest; a clinician should expose only what he or she needs to see. The clinician should note the general shape, contour, symmetry, and color and any scars seen on the abdomen (Table 11.58). The internal organs are located in the abdomen and may become enlarged and swollen when injured. Additionally, bruising may occur over the site of the injuries, so it is important to be able to portion the abdomen into quadrants to evaluate it. Depending on the organ injured, pain may present differently for each patient. It's important to understand which organs are hollow and which ones are solid. Pain in the abdomen can give the clinician insight into the cause of the condition. Additionally, pain from injuried or diseased organs can be referred to other areas of the body.

Urine Test for Hematuria

When blood is present in the urine, it is known as hematuria. The blood present in urine does not have to be visible to the naked eye (gross hematuria); in fact, often it occurs in such small quantities that individuals do not know that it is there, yet it

Chapter 11 Abdomen and Thorax

Table 11.57 Percussion of the Lungs

Test	Patient Position	Procedure	Positive Test	Implication	Evidence
Percussion of the lungs	Make sure the patient is undressed down to the waist if possible. Percuss both the posterior and anterior aspect of the thorax.	Have the patient lean forward while sitting on the edge of the treatment table. To start the percussion, place the nondominant hand against the patient's right or left midback area (evaluates the lower levels of the lungs). Tap the opposite fingers against the hand placed on the back to perform the percussion and listen for the sound. A normal sound would be hollow, representing an air-filled lung. A dull sound may represent fluid in the plural cavity. Repeat the percussion up the back in the intercostal spaces. The best position to perform an anterior respirator examination and lung percussions is with the patient lying on table reclined about 30°–45° and the examiner standing at the right side of the patient. Percuss the chest all around, particularly in the intercostal spaces.	Absence of hollow sound.	Pneumothorax Tension pneumothorax Hemothorax Lung injury	Absent or inconclusive in the literature.

Reproduced from JoVE Science Education Database: *Physical Examinations I. Respiratory Exam II: Percussion and Auscultation*. JoVE, Cambridge, MA, 2019; and Walsh KM, Cuppett M: *General Medical Conditions in the Athlete*, ed 3. St. Louis, MO, Elsevier Mosby, 2017.

---

can be seen under a microscope or via a urine test (microscopic hematuria). An individual could have blood in his or her urine from a variety of injuries or conditions, including infection of the urinary tract system, trauma, vigorous exercise, hepatitis, sexually transmitted infection, or menstruation. More serious conditions associated with hematuria include cancer, kidney stones, bacterial or viral infections, or kidney disease. The most common evaluation for hematuria is testing the urine (**Table 11.59**).

Murphy Sign

The gallbladder is a small pouch that is located just under the liver and is responsible for storing bile that is produced by the liver, which is used to help digest fats. After meals, the gallbladder is empty and flat, resembiling a deflated balloon. Before a meal, the gallbladder is commonly full of bile and swells to the size of a small pear. The gallbladder may become injured or inflamed and has a significant impact on a patient's quality of life. The gallbladder is often called an accessory digestive organ, as it is helps with digestion but is not part of the digestive tract. When the gallbladder becomes inflamed or has stones, the patient will likely have a positive Murphy sign[66] (**Table 11.60**).

Rebound Sign for Appendicitis

The appendix is another pouch-like sac of tissue found in the abdomen. It is located in the first part of the colon (the cecum) in the lower right abdomen. Like the gallbladder, the appendix is also considered an accessory digestive organ. Inflammation of the appendix is known as an appendicitis; this is often a medical emergency and should be taken seriously. Common signs and symptoms of appendicitis include pain in the lower right abdomen, loss of appetite, nausea and vomiting, swollen abdomen, fever, and an inability to pass gas.[62,87,88] Several special tests[91-95] should be utilized by a clinician if a patient is complaining of pain in the lower right quadrant (**Tables 11.61** through **11.63**).

Orthopaedic Special Tests 495

Table 11.58 Abdominal Observation

Test	Patient Position	Procedure	Positive Test	Implication	Evidence

Abdominal observation	Supine on an examination table with head on a pillow, arms at the side, and knees bent to 90° or supported by pillows (allowing for abdominal relaxation).	Visual observation for contour, symmetry, umbilicus, skin integrity, and pulsation or movement.	Contour: Protuberance or distention of the abdomen may indicate ascites (the accumulation of fluid in the peritoneal cavity resulting in abdominal swelling) or obesity; sunken may indicate emaciation.
			Symmetry: Localized bulging, masses, or hernias.
			Umbilicus: Protruding, discolored, or inflamed.
			Skin: Redness, jaundice, tautness, striae, rashes, angiomas, scars, poor turgor, or dilated veins.
			Bulging along the inguinal canal when the patient is asked to cough suggests an inguinal hernia.
			Pulsation or movement: Marked pulsation of the aorta or distended abdomen with marked peristalsis.
			Cullen sign: Ecchymosis around the umbilicus due to retroperitoneal hemorrhage.
			Grey Turner sign: Ecchymosis around the flanks due to retroperitoneal hemorrhage.
			Notes/record-keeping tips:
			• Normal findings:
			  • Contour: Flat or rounded
			  • Symmetry: Equal bilaterally. Umbilicus: Midline, inverted.
			  • Skin: Smooth, similar color overall
			  • Pulsation or movement: Pulsation from the aorta, peristalsis, or respiration. The abdomen should rise and fall rhythmically with respirations.
			• Special considerations: Use a warm room, warm stethoscope, and warm hands during the abdominal inspection. Consider the normal anatomy.
				No specific implications; general evaluation for abdominal deviations.	Absent or inconclusive in the literature.

Abdominal quadrants.

© Jones & Bartlett Learning

Data from Jarvis C: *Physical Examination and Health Assessment*, ed 5. St. Louis, MO, Saunders-Elsevier, 2008; Scifers J: *Special Tests for Neurological Examination*. Thorofare, NJ, Slack Incorporated, 2008; Walker HK, Hall WD, Hurst JW, eds: *Clinical Methods: The History, Physical, and Laboratory Examinations*, ed 3. London, Butterworths, 1990; and White MJ, Counselman FL: Troubleshooting acute abdominal pain. Part 1. *Emerg Med* 2002;20;34–42.

Table 11.59 Urine Test for Hematuria

Test	Patient Position	Procedure	Positive Test	Implication	Evidence
Urine test for hematuria	None	The patient will provide a urine sample in a clean (designated) container. A urine test strip is immersed in the patient's urine no longer than 2 seconds, and any access urine is removed. Once the test strip is removed, the results should be analyzed and read after 60–120 seconds. Do not read the results after 2 minutes, as this may produce a false positive.	Hold the urine strip to evaluate the reagent strips. The examiner will compare color changes to the chromatic scale provided by the manufacturer. The examiner should utilize personal protective equipment (ie, gloves) while handling body fluids.	Evaluation for the presence of blood in the urine is important for the assessment of kidney injury, sexually transmitted infections, or exercise-induced hematuria.	Absent or inconclusive in the literature.

Table 11.60 Murphy Sign

Test	Patient Position	Procedure	Positive Test	Implication	Evidence
Murphy sign	Supine on an exam table with the head on a pillow, arms at the side, and knees bent to 90° or supported by pillows (allowing for abdominal relaxation)	Have the patient take a deep breath in; as the patient exhales, the examiner hooks his or her fingers under the costal margin of the right upper abdominal quadrant to feel for the liver. Have the patient inhale again deeply.	Sharp pain with inspiration, with the patient frequently unable to complete a deep inspiration.	Test may indicate inflammation of the gall bladder.	Sensitivity 97.2% Specificity 48.3% + Likelihood ratio = 70% – Predictive value 93.3%

Data from Urbano FL, Carroll MB: Muphy's sign of cholecystitis. *Hospital Physician* 2000;11:51-52, 70.

Table 11.61 Rebound Sign for Appendicitis

Test	Patient Position	Procedure	Positive Test	Implication	Evidence
Rebound sign for appendicitis	Supine on an exam table. The patient should relax with his or her knees bent or supported by a pillow.	Palpate the right lower abdominal quadrant over McBurney point. Slowly and firmly press down deeply on the abdomen. Hold for a second or two and then release quickly but smoothly.	Pain decreases with abdominal compression, and pain increases when compression is released.	Potential appendicitis.	Absent or inconclusive in the literature.

Data from White MJ, Counselman FL: Troubleshooting acute abdominal pain. Part 1. *Emerg Med* 2002:20;34-42.

Table 11.62 Iliopsoas Muscle Test for Appendicitis

Test	Patient Position	Procedure	Positive Test	Implication	Evidence
Iliopsoas muscle test for appendicitis	Supine on an exam table with the head on a pillow and the arms at the side.	Flex the right hip to 90° against light resistance. The patient then turns to a left lateral decubitus position (patient lying on the left side) to extend the right leg.	Pain in the lower right abdominal quadrant with right knee flexion or extension.	Potential appendicitis.	Specificity .95 Sensitivity .16

Data from Jarvis C: *Physical Examination and Health Assessment*, ed 5. St. Louis, MO, Saunders-Elsevier, 2008; and Wagner JM, McKinney WP, Carpenter JL: Does this patient have appendicitis? *JAMA* 1996;276:1589-1594.

Table 11.63 Obturator Muscle Test for Appendicitis

Test	Patient Position	Procedure	Positive Test	Implication	Evidence
Obturator muscle test for appendicitis	Supine on an exam table with the head on a pillow and the arms at the side.	Passively abduct the right hip to 45° and the knee to 90° while internally rotating the patient's hip.	Pain in the lower right abdominal quadrant but not the lower left abdominal quadrant.	Potential appendicitis.	Absent or inconclusive in the literature. May accompany other signs and symptoms of appendicitis, such as lower right abdominal quadrant pain, rigidity, and migration of pain from umbilicus.

Data from Jarvis C: *Physical Examination and Health Assessment*, ed 5. St. Louis, MO, Saunders-Elsevier, 2008; Orient JM: *Sapria's Art & Science of Bedside Diagnosis*, ed 3. Philadelphia, PA, Lippincott Williams & Wilkins, 2005; and Wagner JM, McKinney WP, Carpenter JL: Does this patient have appendicitis? *JAMA* 1996;276:1589-1594.

Summary

Injuries to the thorax and abdomen may be prevented using appropriate protective equipment, especially in high-impact collision sports. For example, football pads are designed and should be fitted to extend at least below the level of the sternum to protect the thoracic cavity both anteriorly and posteriorly. Additional padding, such as rib protectors, may also be worn to cover the entire thoracic cage if wanted or as necessary.

Additionally, ensuring hollow organs, such as the stomach and bladder, are not full prior to athletic participation may help reduce the risk of injury. Meals should be eaten 3 to 4 hours prior to athletic participation to allow foods to be digested and cleared from the stomach. Urinating immediately prior to participation in athletic activity can help protect the bladder from injury.

Strengthening of the core musculature (muscles of the abdomen) can help support the underlying viscera and improve posture.

Quick Tips for Abdominal and Thoracic Injuries

The most important aspect to assess during an on-the-field evaluation is the involvement of the thoracic spine. If a thoracic spine injury is suspected, immediately perform spinal stabilization and activate emergency medical services.

Red flags warranting immediate referral or immobilization:

- Pain, point tenderness, or deformity along the thoracic spine
- Pain radiating into the extremities
- Trunk or abdominal pain (referred from visceral organs)
- Loss or changes in sensation
- Paralysis or inability to move a body part
- Diminished or absent reflexes
- Diminished or absent pulse
- Muscle weakness in a myotome
- Prolonged vomiting or vomiting blood
- Coughing up blood
- Passing blood in the urine or feces

CASE STUDY 1

A 22-year-old man who plays hockey was checked into the boards with an opponent's stick hitting him right under the rib cage on the left side of his body. He reports to you as the athletic trainer, and he is having difficulty breathing. His breaths are rapid and shallow, refusing to take a deep breath. He is leaning toward the left side. When you raise the athlete's shirt and remove his pads, you notice a linear bruise (in the shape of the stick) along the back of the rib cage on the left side in the thoracic region. The patient has a rapid pulse and appears agitated.

1. What conditions might you include in a differential diagnosis?
2. What are the signs and symptoms of shock?
3. What emergency conditions might you consider? How could you test for these emergency conditions?

CASE STUDY 2

A 14-year-old girl who is a wrestler is competing in a wrestling match. Her opponent slams her to the mat, landing on her chest. The female wrestler immediately calls for help and appears to be having difficulty breathing. Upon inspection, you notice a bump forming around the sternum, and the patient tells you that she felt a pop in her chest when she was slammed to the mat and fallen on. She is grabbing her rib cage and chest and complains of pain. The patient is tender to palpation in the costochondral joint at ribs 7–12. There is crepitus and a crunchy feeling when you palpate the costochondral cartilage at the same levels. You notice an indentation where the costochondral cartilage should articulate with the sternum. The patient is having trouble catching her breath and is having a hard time answering your questions due to pain.

1. While activating emergency medical services to transport the athlete, what instructions or positions would you place the patient in to help ease breathing?
2. What are some special tests that could be used to evaluate the ribs for fracture?
3. What associated lung injuries would you be concerned about based on the mechanism of injury?

ONE-IN-A-MILLION CASE STUDY

Rodeo is an extreme sport with a high risk of injury. This case involved an 18-year-old man injured while riding bareback during a rodeo competition. The athlete was competing in a remote rural site, far from medical attention. Livestock were loaded into a metal chute, and the rider climbed on the horse to start the ride. The horse was agitated in the chute, and, as the rider nodded his head to start the ride, the horse slammed the rider into the back of the metal chute, forcing the rider's legs into his chest. The rider felt a "pop" in his lower back followed by excruciating pain; he attempted to free his hand from the rigging on the horse and struggled to dismount the animal. During the dismount, the rider was kicked by the horse. He immediately motioned for medical assistance and walked out of the arena and then collapsed behind the chutes. The rider immediately reported to the medical staff that he had broken his back. Medical professionals noted few physical symptoms other than tenderness to palpation at the midline of the thoracolumbar junction. He had full muscle strength in the lower extremity. The patient was transported to a level 1 trauma center where CT scans of the cervical, thoracic, and lumbar spine were obtained. The CT scans revealed a compression fracture of the T12 vertebra, indicating an unstable chance fracture, with only approximately 30% of the anterior vertebral body height maintained. The patient also had a 20° kyphotic angulation in the T12 vertebral body and a transverse fracture through the bilateral pedicle lamina and spinous process at T12. Surgical fixation was required, including bilateral pedicle screws and Harrington rod fixation. The patient was discouraged from returning to rodeo competition, but, after a year of functional training and rehabilitation, he returned to riding wearing a protective flak jacket. It is extremely rare for an athlete to sustain a thoracolumbar fracture. Most chance fractures are associated with intra-abdominal injuries, as the most frequent occurrence of chance fractures are associated with seat belt injuries during car accidents. Understanding the mechanism of a chance fracture can assist with the thoracic spine injury evaluation and diagnosis. Spinal hyperflexion and distraction injury causing a split in the spinous process of the vertebrae, fracture of the pedicles, and ruptures in the posterior ligaments result in significant damage and distruction to the spinal segment and are a very serious injury. Any suspected spinal fracture should be treated with care and referred to an emergency department for further evaluation.[95]

WRAP-UP

Critical Thinking Questions

1. After assessing level of consciousness, airway, breathing, and circulation, what vital signs should be assessed during the primary assessment?

2. What are some mechanisms that could cause a fracture to the chest wall? What are some potential complications that could arise with a fracture to the chest wall?

Are any of these conditions emergency conditions?
3. What are the differences among the signs and symptoms of abdominal organ injuries (appendix, gallbladder, kidney, liver, spleen)? What are the pain referral patterns for each injury?
4. What structures are located in each of the four quadrants of the abdomen?
5. What are some techniques that could be utilized with someone who is suffering from hyperventilation? Why is it important to help the patient slow down his or her breathing?

Pearls and Pitfalls

- Injuries to the heart, lungs, and abdominal organs can be serious or even life threatening if not addressed and managed appropriately.
- The primary survey by a clinician evaluating injury to the abdomen or thorax should focus on signs and symptoms associated with life-threatening conditions. Asking complete and detailed history questions, observing body positioning and posture, and completing palpation of structures are critical to identifying injuries.
- Rib fractures and contusions, costochondral separations, sternum fractures, and muscle strains are common injuries to the thoracic cavity.
- Injuries involving the lungs include pneumothorax, tension pneumothorax, hemothorax, and traumatic asphyxia.
- Sudden cardiac death is traumatic and rare in an athletic population. It is most often the result of a congenital cardiovascular abnormality. Identifying participants at risk for cardiac emergencies is key during preparticipation physical examinations.
- A number of conditions may develop over time. Therefore, it is important to educate an injured patient to recognize the signs and symptoms associated with emergency conditions (such as liver contusion, kidney contusion, gallbladder trauma, or appendix injury).
- The abdominal cavity lies between the diaphragm and the bones of the pelvis. The organs within the abdominal cavity include both hollow and solid organs, which may be damaged with direct trauma to the abdomen or thoracic and lumbar spine.

References

1. Leski M: Sudden cardiac death in athletes. *South Med J* 2004;97:861.
2. Ryan J: Abdominal injuries and sport. *Br J Sports Med* 1999; 33(3):155.
3. Lyznicki JM, Nielsen NH, Schneider, JF: Cardiovascular screening of student athletes. *Am Fam Phys* 2000;62:765.
4. O'Brien LD, Rogers IR: Athlete's heart syndrome: a diagnostic dilemma in the emergency department. *Emerg Med* 1999;11:277.
5. Sen-Chowdhry S, McKenna WJ: Sudden cardiac death in the young: a strategy for prevention by targeted evaluation. *Cardiology* 2006;105:196.
6. McLaughlin L, Goldsmith CH, Coleman K: Breathing evaluation and retraining as an adjunct to manual therapy. *Man Ther* 2011; 16(1):51-52.
7. University of California San Francisco. *Chest wall deformities*: https://surgery.ucsf.edu/conditions--procedures/chest-wall-deformities.aspx. Published unknown date 2019. Accessed Dec 17, 2019.
8. Pierce JA: The barrel deformity of the chest, the senile lung and obstructive pulmonary emphysema. *Am J Med* 1958;25(1):13.
9. Sutherland ID: Funnel chest. *J Bone Joint Surg Br* 1958;40: 244-251.
10. Miller JFAP, Osoba D: Current concepts of the immunological function of the thymus. *Physiol* 1967;7:437-520.
11. Dirckx JH, ed: *Stedman's Concise Medical Dictionary for the Health Professions*. Baltimore, MD, Lippincott Williams & Wilkins, 2001.
12. Prentice WE: *Principles of Athletic Training: A Guide to Evidence-Based Clinical Practice*, ed 16. New York, NY, McGraw-Hill Education, 2017.
13. Biel A: *Trail Guide to the Body*, rev ed 5. Boulder, CO, Books of Discovery, 2014.
14. Fink HA, Lederle FA, Roth CS, Bowles CA, Nelson DB, Haas MA The accuracy of physical examination to detect abdominal aortic aneurysm. *Arch Intern Med* 2000;160: 833-836.
15. Kendall FP, McCreary EK, Provance PG, Rodgers MM, Romani WA: *Muscles: Testing and Function with Posture and Pain*, ed 5. Baltimore, MD, Lippincott Williams & Wilkins, 2005.
16. Connolly LP, Connolly SA: Rib stress fractures. *Clinl Nucl Med* 2004;29(10):614-616.
17. Dodds S: Injuries to the pectoralis major. *Sports Med* 2002;32(14):945.
18. Du Preez G: Fractured ribs may result in serious complications. *Nursing Times* 2003;99(20):27.
19. Marasco S, Davies AR, Cooper J, et al: Prospective randomized controlled trial of operative rib fixation in traumatic flail chest. *J Am Coll Surg* 2013;(216)5:924-932.
20. McGown A: Blunt abdominal and chest trauma. *Athl Ther Today* 2004;9(1):40.
21. Miles JW, Barrett GR: Rib fractures in athletes. *Sports Med* 1991;12(1):66-69.
22. Pishbin E, Ahmadi K, Foogardi M, Salehi M, Toosi FS, Rahimi-Movaghar V: Comparison of ultrasonography and

radiography in diagnosis of rib fractures. *Chin J Traumatol* 2017;20(4):226-228.
23. Wood KB, Blair JM, Aepple DM, et al: The natural history of asymptomatic thoracic disc herniations. *Spine* 1997;22:525-530.
24. Wood KB, Garvey TA, Gundry C, Heithoff KB: Magnetic resonance imaging of the thoracic spine. *J Bone Joint Surg Am* 1995;77:1631-1638.
25. Demirbag D, Unlu E, Ozdemir F, et al: The relationship between magnetic resonance imaging findings and postural maneuver and physical examination tests in patients with thoracic outlet syndrome: results of a double-blind, controlled study. *Arch Phys Med Rehabil* 2007;88(7):844-851.
26. Ferrante MAL: The thoracic outlet syndrome. *Muscle Nerve* 2012;45:780.
27. Hooper TL, Denton J, McGalliard MK, Brismee JM, Sizer PS Jr: Thoracic outlet syndrome: a controversial clinical condition, part I: anatomy and clinical examination/diagnosis. *J Man Manip Ther* 2010;18(2):74-84.
28. Klaassen Z, Sorenson E, Tubbs RS, et al: Thoracic outlet syndrome: a neurological and vascular disorder. *Clin Anat* 2014;27(5):724-732.
29. Sanders RJ, Hammond SL, Rao NM: Diagnosis of thoracic outlet syndrome. *J Vasc Surg* 2007;46:601.
30. Tender GC, Thomas AJ, Thomas N, Kline DG: Gilliat-Sumner hand revisited: a 25-year experience. *Neurosurgery* 2004;55(1):883-890.
31. Curtin S: Pneumothorax in sports: issues in recognition and follow-up care. *Physician Sports-Med* 2000;28(8):23.
32. Kersey R. Primary spontaneous pneumothorax in a collegiate soccer player. *Ath Ther Today* 2000;5(2):48.
33. Lively M. Pulmonary contusion in football players. *Cl J Sports Med* 2006;16(2):177.
34. Smith D. Chest injuries, what the sports physical therapist should know. *Int J Sports Phys Ther* 2011;6(4):257-260.
35. Walsh KM, Cuppett M: *General Medical Conditions in the Athlete*, ed 3. St Louis, MO, Elsevier Mosby, 2017.
36. Weder M: Pulmonary disorders in athletes. *Clin Sports Med* 2011;30(3):525-536.
37. Suman O: Airway obstruction during exercise and isocapnic hyperventilation in asthmatic subjects. *J App Physiol* 1999;87(3):1107.
38. Casa DJ, Guskiewicz KM, Anderson SA, et al: National Athletic Trainers' Association position statement: preventing sudden death in sports. *J Ath Train* 2012;47(1):96-118.
39. Hipp A: Hypertrophic cardiomyopathy: sports-related aspects of diagnosis, therapy, and sports eligibility. *Int J Sports Med* 2004;25(1):20.
40. Judge DP, Dietz HC: Marfan's syndrome. *Lancet* 2005;366(9501):1965-1976.
41. Koester M: A review of sudden cardiac death in young athletes and strategies for preparticipation cardiovascular screening. *J Athl Train* 2001;36(2):197.
42. Lufukuja GJ: Anomalous origin of the coronary arteries. *Ital J Anat Embryol* 2016;121(3):253-257.
43. Maron BJ: Hypertrophic cardiomyopathy: a systematic review. *JAMA* 2002;287(10):1308-1320.
44. McGrew C: Sudden cardiac death in competitive athletes. *J Orthop Sports Phys Ther* 2003;33(10):589.
45. Merrick M: Cardiovascular pathologies: to screen or not to screen? *Ath Ther Today* 2001;6(4):28.
46. National Academy of Sports Medicine (NASM): Physical Activity Readiness Questionnare. https://www.nasm.org/docs/default-source/PDF/nasm_par-q-(pdf-21k).pdf. No Date. Accessed Sep 12, 2018.
47. Pérez-Pomares JM, Luis de la Pompa J, Franco D, et al: Congenital coronary artery anomalies: a bridge from embryology to anatomy and pathophysiology: a position statement of the development, anatomy and pathology ESC Working Group. *Cardiovasc Res* 2016;109:204-216.
48. Perron A: Chest pain in athletes. *Clin Sports Med* 2003;22(1):37.
49. Toresdahl B, Courson R, Börjesson M, et al: Emergency cardiac care in the athletic setting: from schools to the Olympics. *Br J Sports Med* 2012;46:i85-i89.
50. Turk E: Natural and traumatic sports-related fatalities: a 10-year retrospective study. *Brit J Sports Med* 2008;42:604-608.
51. Singh AM, McGregor RS: Differential diagnosis of chest symptoms in the athlete. *Clin Rev Allergy Immunol* 2005;29(2):87Y96.
52. Spodick DH: Acute cardiac tamponade. *N Engl J Med* 2003;349:684.
53. Maron BJ, Gohman TE, Kyle SB, Estes NAM, Link M: Clinical profile and spectrum of commotio cordis. *J Am Med Assoc* 2002;287(9):1142-1146.
54. Puffer JC, Thompson PD: The athletic heart syndrome. *Physician Sports-Med* 2002;7:41-47.
55. Holanda MS, Dominguez MJ, Lopez-Espadas F, Lopez M, Diaz-Reganon J, Rodriguez-Borregan JC: Cardiac contusion following blunt chest traumaa. *Eur J Emerg Med* 2006;13(6):373-376.
56. McAleer IM, Kaplan GW, LoSasso BE: Renal and testis injuries in team sports. *J Urol* 2002;168(suppl 4):1805-1807.
57. Mileski W: Injuries to the liver, in Flint L, ed *Trauma: Contemporary Principles and Therapy*. Philadelphia, PA, Lippincott Williams & Wilkins, 2007.
58. Parks NA, Davis JW, Forman D, Lemaster, D: Observation for nonoperative management of blunt liver injuries: how long is long enough? *J Trauma* 2011;70(3):626-629.
59. Noffsinger J: Physical activity considerations in children and adolescents with viral infections. *Pediatr Ann* 1996;25:585-589.
60. Putukian M, O'Connor FG, Stricker PR, et al: Mononucleosis and athletic participation: an evidence-based subject review. *Clin J Sport Med* 2008;18:309-315.
61. Rea TD, Russo JE, Katon W, Ashley RL, Buchwald DS: Prospective study of the natural history of infectious mononucleosis caused by Epstein-Barr virus. *J Am Board Fam Pract* 2001;14:234-242.
62. Rinderknect AS, Pomerantz WJ: Spontaneous splenic rupture in infectious mononucleosis: case report and review of the literature. *Pediatr Emerg Care* 2012;28:1377.
63. Turner J, Gard M. Splenomegaly and sports. *Curr Sports Med Rep* 2008;7:113-116.
64. Waninger KN, Harcke HT. Determination of safe return to play for athletes recovering from infectious mononucleosis: a review of the literature. *Clin J Sport Med* 2005;15:410-416.
65. Jarvis C. *Physical Examination and Health Assessment*, ed 5. St Louis, MO, Saunders-Elsevier, 2008.
66. Urbano FL, Carroll MB: Murphy's sign of cholecystitis. *Hospital Physician* 2000;11:51-51,70.
67. Cook, CE: *Orthopedic Manual Therapy: An Evidence-Based Approach*, ed 2. Upper Saddle River, NJ, Pearson Education, 2012.
68. Kreis ME, Edler V, Koch F, Jauch KW, Friese K: The differential diagnosis of right lower quadrant pain. *Dtsch Arztebl* 2007;104(45):A3114-3121.

69. Salminen P, Paajanen H, Rautio T: Antibiotic therapy vs. appendectomy for treatment of uncomplicated acute appendicitis. *JAMA* 2015;313(23):2340-2348.
70. Venes D: *Tabers' Cyclopedic Medical Dictionary*. Philadephia, PA, FA Davis Co, 2013.
71. Magee DJ: *Orthopedic Physical Assessment*, ed 5. St. Louis, MO, Elsevier, Inc., 2008.
72. Adam CJ, Izatt MT, Harvey JR, Askin GN: Variability in Cobb angle measurements using reformatted computerized tomography scans. *Spine* 2005;50:1664-1669.
73. Keim HA: Scoliosis. *Clin Symposia* 1973;25:1-25.
74. Loder RT, Spiegel D, Gutknecht S, et al: The assessment of intraobserver and interobserver error in measurement of noncongenital scoliosis in children = 10 years of age. *Spine* 2004;29:2548-2553.
75. Wilmore JH, Costill DL: *Physiology of Sport and Exercise*. Champaign, IL, Human Kinetics, 1994.
76. Centers for Disease Control and Prevention, National Center for Health Statistics. High Blood Pressure Fact Sheet. https://www.cdc.gov/dhdsp/data_statistics/fact_sheets/fs_bloodpressure.htm. Accessed Sept 11, 2018.
77. Nwankwo T, Yoon SS, Burt V, Gu Q: Hypertension among adults in the US: National Health and Nutrition Examination Survey, 2011-2012. NCHS Data Brief, No. 133. Hyattsville, MD, National Center for Health Statistics, Centers for Disease Control and Prevention, US Dept of Health and Human Services, 2013.
78. Whelton PK, et al: 2017 ACC/AHA/AAPA/ABC/ACPM/AGS/APhA/ASH/ASPC/NMA/PCNA Guideline for the prevention, detection, evaluation, and management of high blood pressure in adults. *Am Coll Cardiol* 2018;71(19):e127-248.
79. Shultz SJ, Houglum PA, Perrin DH: *Examination of Musculoskeletal Injuries*, ed. 4. Champaign, IL, Human Kinetics, 2016.
80. Meyer JS: Studies of cerebral circulation in brain injury. *Electroencephalogr Clin Neurophysiol* 1957;9(1):83-100.
81. Hickey JV: *The Clinical Practice of Neurological and Neurosurgical Nursing*, ed 7. Philadelphia, PA, Lippincott Williams & Wilkins 2013.
82. Gillard J, Perez-Cousin M, Hachulla E, et al: Diagnosing thoracic outlet syndrome: contribution of provocative tests, ultrasonography, electrophysiology, and helical computed tomography in 48 patients. *Joint Bone Spine* 2001;68:416-424.
83. Lee AD, Agawal S, Sadhu D: Doppler Adson's test: predictors of outcome of surgery in non-specific thoracic outlet syndrome. *World J Surg* 2006;30:291-292.
84. Nord KM, Kapoor P, Fisher J, et al: False positive rate of thoracic outlet syndrome diagnostic maneuvers in healthy patients. *Electromyog Clin Neurophysiol* 2008;48:67-74.
85. Plewa MC, Delinger M: The false-positive rate of thoracic outlet syndrome shoulder maneuvers in healthy patients. *Acad Emerg Med* 1998;5:337-342.
86. Rayan GM, Jensen C: Thoracic outlet syndrome provocative examination maneuvers in a typical population. *J Shoulder Elbow Surg* 1995;4:113-117.
87. Brismee JM, Gilbert K, Isom K, et al: Rate of false positive using the Cyrax Release test for thoracic outlet syndrome in an asymptomatic population. *J Man Manipulative Ther* 2004;12:73-81.
88. Howard M, Lee C, Dellon AL: Documentation of brachial plexus compression (in the thoracic inlet) utilizing provocative neurosensory and muscular testing. *J Reconstr Microsurg* 2003;19:303-12.
89. JoVE Science Education Database: *Physical Examinations I. Respiratory Exam II: Percussion and Auscultation*. JoVE, Cambridge, MA, 2019.
90. Walker HK, Hall WD, Hurst JW, eds: *Clinical Methods: The History, Physical, and Laboratory Examinations*, ed 3. London, Butterworths, 1990.
91. Scifers J: *Special Tests for Neurological Examination*. Thorofare, NJ; Slack Incorporated, 2008.
92. White MJ, Counselman FL: Troubleshooting acute abdominal pain. Part 1. *Emerg Med* 2002;20:34-42.
93. Wagner JM, McKinney WP, Carpenter JL: Does this patient have appendicitis? *JAMA* 1996;276:1589-1594.
94. Orient JM: *Sapria's Art & Science of Bedside Diagnosis*, ed 3. Philadelphia, PA, Lippincott Williams & Wilkins, 2005:451.
95. Boham M, O'Connell K: Unusual mechanism of injury resulting in a thoracic chance fracture in a rodeo athlete: a case report. *J Athl Train* 2014;49(2):274-279.

CHAPTER 12

Spine

Thomas G. Palmer, PhD, ATC, CSCS*D, TSAC
Andrea E. Cripps, PhD, ATC
Sara Stiltner, EdD, ATC

OVERVIEW

The spine plays a significant role as the primary mediator between the appendicular and axial skeleton and the environment. Center to all movements, the spine's architecture allows for varying mobility and stability at the proximal segments of the body while promoting distal extremity function. The individual characteristics of the cervical, thoracic, and lumbar spine serve to influence dynamic synergistic activities of several body regions. Such function results in the transfer and distribution of ground reaction forces and related interactions with environmental obstacles. An evaluation of the spine will entail a strong understanding of the spine posture, neuromuscular and musculoskeletal anatomy, function, and associated injury pathologies. This chapter will outline general orthopaedic properties of injury, evaluation, and treatment as they relate to the cervical, thoracic, and lumbar spine.

LEARNING OBJECTIVES

After completing this chapter, the reader will be able to do the following:

1. Outline general anatomic functions and specific soft and skeletal tissues of each spinal region.
2. Describe common injurious mechanics to the spine for chronic and traumatic pathologies specific to each region of the spine.
3. Describe techniques used to clinically evaluate each region of the spine, with emphasis on functional anatomy, palpation, postural observation, range of motion, and structural joint integrity as well as treatment plans for each region of the spine.

FUN FACTS ABOUT THE SPINE

- The spinal column is typically not fully developed until age 6 years.
- The spinal cord does not always need to receive signals from the brain to cause muscle actions.
- Although a person is born with 33 vertebral segments, the formation of the pelvis and sacrum results in having only 26 segments at adulthood.
- There are approximately 100 spinal joints, more than 120 muscles, and more than 220 ligaments supporting the three regions of the spine.
- People are taller in the morning than at night due to constant daily pressure from gravity on the intervertebral disk.
- Approximately 80% of all adults will experience a form of back pain that requires medical attention.
- Back pain and spinal pathologies are among the top reasons for physician visits and disability claims in the United States.
- Injury to the spinal cord at any level is generally irreversible for repair.

Introduction

The vital neurovascular properties of the brain, spinal cord, and associated structures are conveyed inferiorly through an excessively mobile cervical column to a moderately itinerant thoracic region and fairly static lumbar region. This design provides the ability to contort and maintain body function and structure throughout a variety of ballistic and/or static activities, such as standing or sitting for long periods of time. The mobility and structural integrity of the cervical spine make it vulnerable to injury yet provide an extensive range of motion and functional properties to allow the head, eyes, ears, and nose to interact with the environment. As a driver of direction and body position for nearly every activity, dynamic control of the cervical column is critical to function in daily life and sport. The thoracic spine provides an extensive amount of thorax and shoulder girdle support for scapular function and muscular support for many of the primary movers of the upper extremity and the proximal rib cage. The larger and less mobile lumbar spine segments provide added stability to the center of mass and play a primary role in absorbing and distributing forces to and from the upper spine, the extremities, and the environment.

The diverse demands on the spine, differences in vertebral body size, intricacy of the vertebral disks, and magnitude of muscular correspondence with the spine at each region of the body make it extremely impressionable for function and injury. The location and properties of the spine make it an essential component to consider when performing most orthopaedic evaluations. A magnitude of traumatic and chronic pathologies throughout the spinal column may result from overload stressors, such as habitual/chronic poor posture tasks or high-impact injuries resulting in a whiplash, or shear, compressive, and/or tensile injury mechanisms. Such pathologies are often associated with muscle spasm/strain, neurologic disruptions, joint sprains, and/or disk lesions. The common occurrence of spine pathologies necessitates a systematic understanding of the different spinal regions and the associated evaluation techniques.

Clinical Anatomy

Skeletal Anatomy

The spine consists of 31 stacked and 9 fused vertebrae; each spinal segment is identified by sequential differences in the skeletal anatomy. There are 5 spinal sections: 7 cervical, 12 thoracic, 5 lumbar, 5 fused sacral, and 4 fused coccygeal vertebrae[1] (**Figure 12.1**). The spine consists of four curves in the sagittal plane: anteriorly convex/lordosis at the cervical and lumbar regions and anteriorly concave/kyphotic at the thoracic and sacral regions. The thoracic and sacral curves are referred to as the primary curves because they maintain an erect frontal plane position

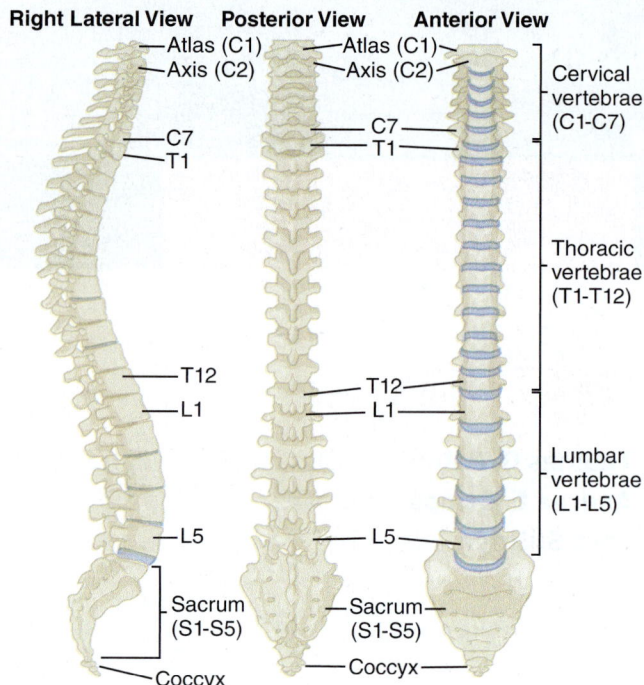

Figure 12.1 Drawings showing the spinal column.
© Jones & Bartlett Learning

with a kyphotic sagittal plane posture in development from infancy to adulthood. The cervical and lumbar lordotic curves develop secondarily, resisting gravity to raise the head and ambulate upright. Scoliotic or frontal plane curvatures are abnormal developmental curves that contort the normal function of the spine to absorb and transfer forces throughout different regions of the body and often become pathologic.[1-4]

The vertebrae in each region of the spine consist of an anterior vertebral body and a posterior neural track, collectively forming the vertebral canal, where the spinal cord is housed. The neural track forms a posterior arch and extends to a posterior projection called the spinous process. Flexion of the spine often makes the spinous process of all the spinal regions more prominent for distinctive palpation. Palpation to the structure serves as a landmark to identify spinal region and segment locations. Typically, the spinous process aligns with the spinal segment space below the actual vertebral body. The superficial prominence of these ridged projections and their serving as major muscle and ligament attachments make the spinous processes vulnerable to injury, especially in the C6-T1 cervical region. The lateral projections off the vertebral body, referred to as the transverse process, also serve as a primary site of ligament and muscle attachment.[5]

The transverse process is connected to the body of the vertebra via the pedicles. The laminae is a part

Clinical Anatomy

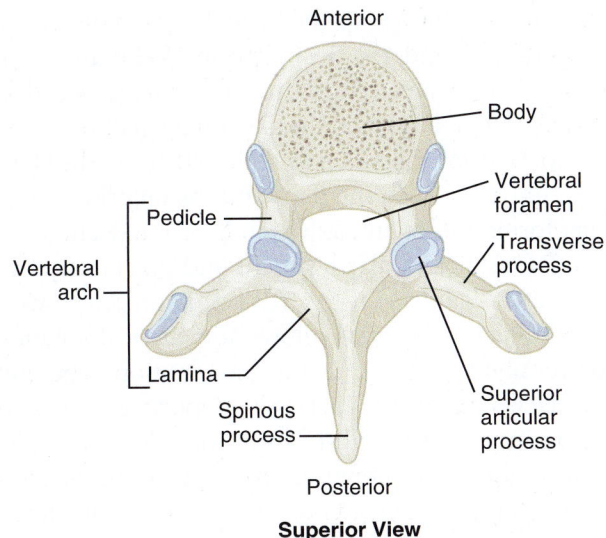

Figure 12.2 Drawing of a thoracic spinal vertebra.
© Jones & Bartlett Learning

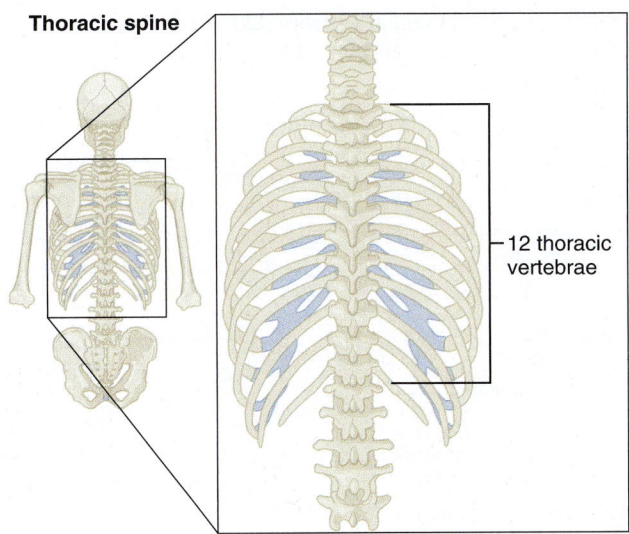

Figure 12.4 Drawings showing the thoracic spine.
© Jones & Bartlett Learning

of the vertebral arch and connects the two transverse processes. The superior and inferior unions of the laminae and pedicles form two superior and inferior synovial joint articular facets with the vertebral segments above and below. The pedicle of each vertebra is notched at its superior and inferior edges. The union of the vertebral segments forms an intervertebral foramen, or spacing, through which spinal cord nerve roots can pass to provide motor and sensory distributions for the musculoskeletal system, such as the cervical, brachial, lumbar, and sacral nerve plexuses[1,6-8] (**Figure 12.2** and **Figure 12.3**).

Inferior to the cervical spine is the thoracic spine. Developmentally, the thoracic vertebrae adopt some of the form of the cervical vertebrae above but gradually increase in size with vertical articular facets and thinner spinous processes. The lower thoracic segments continue to increase in body size, with the transverse and spinous processes increasing in thickness with slight lateral articular facets. Each thoracic vertebrae contains two pairs of articular facets for the ribs on the body and one on each corresponding transverse process (**Figure 12.4** and **Figure 12.5**). The ribs articulate with the inferior facet of the body and the transverse process and the superior facet of the vertebra below. The 11th and 12th thoracic vertebrae articulations are unique, because they lack a superior costal facet.[2,7,9]

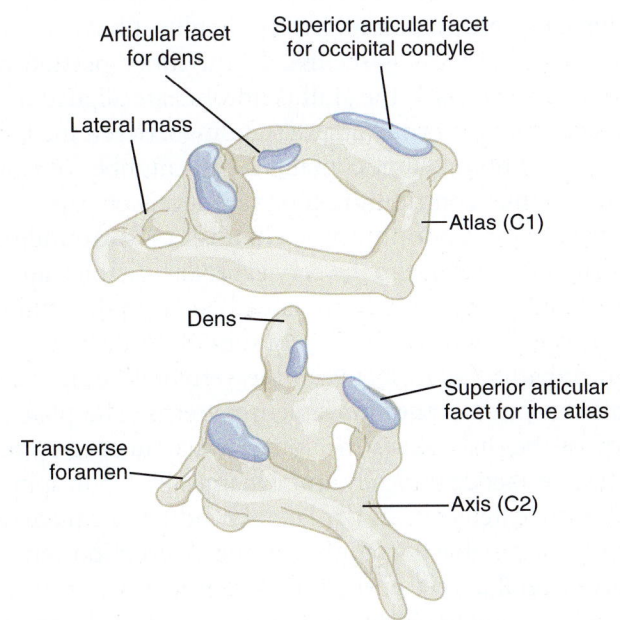

Figure 12.3 Drawings showing the atlas and axis.
© Jones & Bartlett Learning

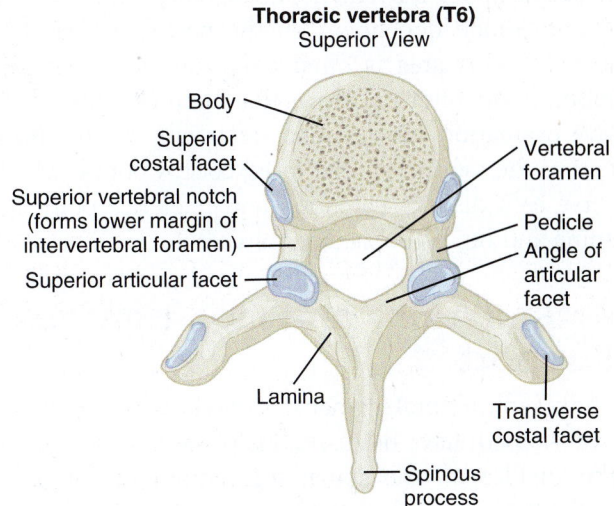

Figure 12.5 Drawing showing a thoracic vertebra.
© Jones & Bartlett Learning

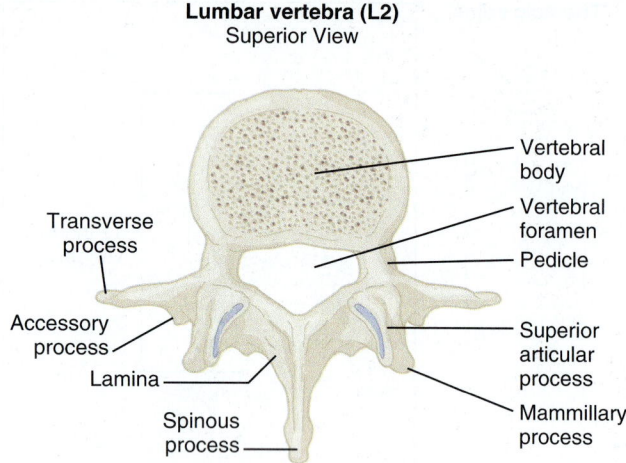

Figure 12.6 Drawing of a lumbar vertebra.
© Jones & Bartlett Learning

Lumbar spine vertebrae have the largest vertebral bodies, with thick spinous and transverse processes. The parasagittal facets allow for excessive sagittal trunk range of motion into flexion and extension but limited rotation. These vertebral bodies serve as a significant attachment for the proximal deep muscles of the spine and the lumbothoracic fascia. The high levels of muscle contour and force transmission at the lumbar spine make it vulnerable to high-intensity, shear, and compressive forces[1,10] (**Figure 12.6**).

Inferior to the lumbar spine and central and posterior to the iliac pelvic bones are the five fused sacral vertebrae. The sacrum is an extremely stable structure; it has anterior and posterior foramina housing rami for the sacral plexus. The common major sacral landmarks are the S1 (sacral promontory), the medial sacral crest (fused spinous process), and the lateral sacral crest (fused transverse process). The relationship for movement and stability at the sacrum is very much dependent on the posterior sacroiliac joint.[1,11] This area is often compromised by excess mobility or oblique postures that often warrant extensive evaluation prowess and treatment. At the distal end of the sacrum are the fused coccyx bones, which serve as a distinct palpation and reference point for spine and hip orthopaedic evaluations.

Articulations and Ligamentous Support

The seven vertebral segments of the cervical column are oval shaped, have bifid spinous processes, are among the smallest of the spinal segments, and are often difficult to see and distinctively palpate. The prominence of each cervical segment increases from C1-C7, with C7 being the most prominent. The union of the atlas and axis make up the synovial joins of cervical vertebrae C1 and C2, respectively[2,12] (Figure 12.3). These oddly shaped structures are characterized by the absence of a vertebral body and a small bony vertical protrusion on the axis, referred to as the dens. This union between the dens and the anterior arch of atlas forms the atlantoaxial joint. Secured anteriorly by a left and right alar ligament and posteriorly by a transverse ligament of the atlas, this union between the skull and the atlas allows for cervical rotation, commonly referred to as the "no" motion. The concave facets of the atlas act as a supportive mount for the occiput of the skull to form the atlanto-occipital joint, commonly known as the "yes" joint, as cervical flexion and extension are accessible at this union. Adjacent vertebral segments are joined by intervertebral articulations between the superior and inferior pars interarticularis zygapophyseal facet articulations. The C1-C2 facets lie in a horizontal position and lack stability. The remaining facets lie in a vertical fashion at approximately 45° from the horizontal and frontal planes of motion, which provides additional support throughout the segments of the spine.[2,12]

Intervertebral Disks and Articulations

The 23 intervertebral disks between the vertebrae serve to promote mobility and dexterity while providing a pressure gradient between the vertebrae. Each disk is designed to serve as a shock absorber. The vibrant nucleus pulposus is a gel-like substance that makes up the inner circle of the disk (**Figure 12.7**). Typically encompassed by the anulus fibrosus, the nucleus pulposus is secured to the inner portion of disk. The layers of the anulus fibrosus are aligned in a cross-helix pattern to assure stability between the layers. This fibrous unit contains a high number of pain fibers, thus contributing to severe levels of pain and dysfunction upon injury to the disk or surrounding structures. Unique to the cervical collar are thick anterior and posterior (but not lateral) areas of the anulus fibrosus (Figure 12.7). The contour of the disks assists in providing space between the vertebral bodies that allows for smoother movement patterns. The pliability of the disk assists the spine in maintaining structural resilience statically and dynamically. Upon spinal flexion, extension, and/or lateral bending, the nucleus pulposus is able to compress to the anterior, posterior, and lateral aspect of the intervertebral space, respectively. Simultaneously, the opposite end of the intervertebral space expands, allowing the compressed nucleus fluid to displace into the open spacing. The

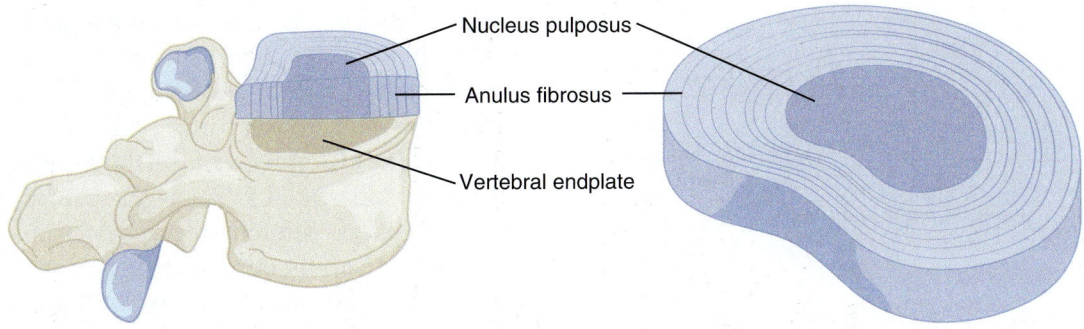

Figure 12.7 Drawings showing the nucleus pulposus.
© Jones & Bartlett Learning

balancing of space distribution allows for smooth multiplanar motions to occur incrementally about each spinal segment.[1,7] Distribution of pressure on the disk changes with different positions of the spine. The lumbar spine is often a location of injury due to the high amount of exorbitant fluctuation in force, pressure, and position change. Lying supine seems to produce the least amount of pressure on the lumbar disks, whereas standing can increase the pressure on the disks to approximately 100 kg. A slightly flexed position of leaning forward increases the pressure to approximately 150 to 220 kg while lifting from a flexed position of approximately 20° to 30° of spinal lumbar flexion. Seated in an upright position results in approximately 130 to 150 kg of pressure, whereas forward flexion from a seated position increases the pressures to well above 185 kg. The greatest amount of pressure on the lumbar spine, exceeding 250 to 275 kg, occurs while seated, flexed, and lifting an object. Therefore, it is critical to often maintain more erect positions of the spine and keeping the object close to the body to reduce the stress on the disks.[1,9,13,14]

Disk-space narrowing is often associated with back or nerve pain/pathology as the result of the vertebral disk losing fluid contour due to age, degenerative processes, or injury. A failure in the anulus fibrosus from an acute or chronic amount of pressure can result in a defect or herniation of the nucleus pulposus. Typically, the inner ring of the anulus fibrosus is disrupted or breached by the nucleus pulposus, thus offsetting the pressure gradient for the nucleus to evenly distribute pressures between vertebral segments. Damage to the nucleus pulposus and anulus fibrosus often augments and compromises the opening between the vertebral bodies and creates a stenosis at the level of the spinal nerve root. As a result, individuals experience nerve root signs and symptoms or nerve-oriented pain of numbness, tingling, and/or burning in the distal extremities; localized muscle spasm; pain; and altered biomechanics.[9,14,15]

Spinal Ligamentous Support

The shape of the skeletal anatomy and the anterior and posterior longitudinal ligaments at the spine reinforce the disk and vertebral unions for the length of the column[1] (**Figure 12.8**). The anterior longitudinal ligament maintains a strong and robust thickness throughout the length of the spine, whereas the posterior longitudinal ligament decreases in width and thickness as it progresses to the lumbar spinal segments. The loss of integrity and narrowing of the posterior longitudinal ligament results in most disk lesions occurring at the posterior lateral section of the lumbar region. Both the anterior and posterior longitudinal ligaments help to resist excessive cervical extension and flexion, respectively. The anterior atlantoaxial and atlanto-occipital ligaments are an extension of the anterior longitudinal ligament and help to support the diskless C1-C2 and C0-C1 unions.[1,9] The ligamentum nuchae, the interspinous ligament, and the ligamentum flavum add additional support in resisting terminal flexion and rotation

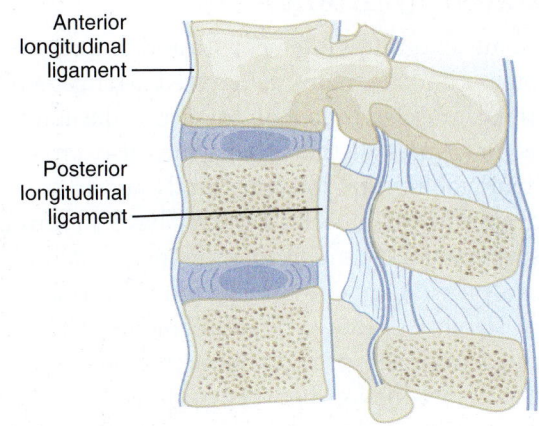

Figure 12.8 Drawing showing the anterior and posterior longitudinal ligaments.
© Jones & Bartlett Learning

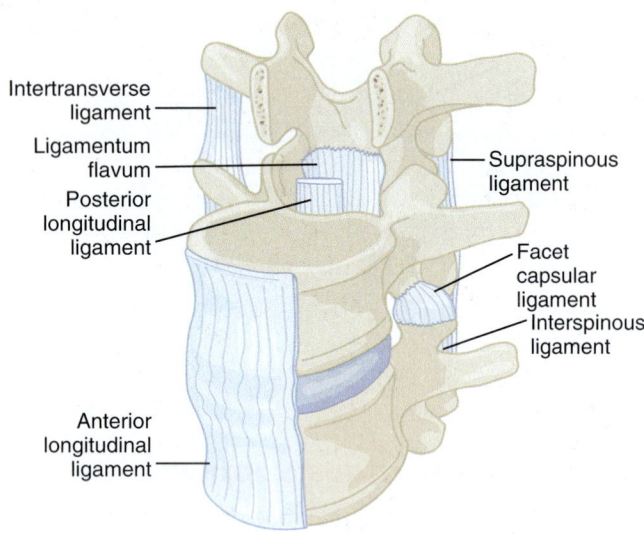

Figure 12.9 Drawing showing the additional spinal ligaments.
© Jones & Bartlett Learning

for the spine. The ligamentum flavum lies deep to the interspinous ligament and attaches to the preceding lamina of the cervical vertebra; it adds an elastic-resistive contact for a somewhat flexible end field.[1,2,12]

The small vertebral synovial joints formed by the union of the superior and inferior vertebral facets rely on small capsular ligaments. The supraspinous and interspinous ligaments secure the union between adjacent spinous processes at the distal and proximal process, respectively. Adjacent transverse processes are secured at the laminae and linked together via the intertransverse ligaments and the ligamentum flavum[1,2] (**Figure 12.9**).

Soft-Tissue Anatomy

Muscular Anatomy

Several muscle groups interact with and/or manipulate the spine. Fundamentally, the layered arrangement of the spinal muscles functions to secure the intersegmental properties of the spine while also providing proximal stability for forceful distal muscle actions. The deep intrinsic muscles typically have an intimate intersegmental attachment to vertebrae, which allow them to provide an anticipatory function and incremental stability of the vertebral segments. The larger superficial muscles provide more regional stability and power production between regions of the spine and the body/extremities.[1,16]

The back extensor muscles of the spine and trunk also contribute to trunk rotation and lateral flexion. The deep spine-supporting muscles are categorized into the erector spinae and the transversospinalis. The erector spinae or sacrospinalis muscles extend from the base of the skull to the pelvis and help to keep the body erect. The three layers of muscles consist of the iliocostalis (rib), longissimus, and spinalis. Each group of muscles has attachments at different regions of the spine. The longissimus capitis is unique in that it assists with rotation of the head. The interwoven presentation of these muscles from the cervical to the lumbar spine provides a vast pillar of slender, overlapping muscles. The iliocostalis lumborum and thoracic erector spinae muscles branch from the lumbar aponeurosis and into the lower thoracic spine, attaching to the lower ribs. An extension of these muscles to the cervical spine transverse process is the iliocostalis cervicis. The spinalis are the most medial part of the erector spinae, spanning from the lumbar aponeurosis to regions of the lumbar and thoracic spinous processes. The transversospinalis lie deeper and extend over several vertebral segments of the spinous and transverse process relative to the thoracic, cervical, and skull regions (thoracic, cervicis, and capitis). From superficial to deep, these muscles are composed of the semispinalis, multifidus, and rotatores. This orientation creates a closer relationship with the spinal segments. Among these are the rotatores longus and the multifidus. The multifidus extends from C2 to L5 and has been reported to influence precise control over the spine's position. Isolated to the deep lumbar musculature, the quadratus lumborum muscle connects to rib 12 and transverse processes L1–L5 and the posterior iliac crest. In conjunction with muscle stability of the spine, these deep muscles are interwoven into a thick, fibrous membrane referred to as the thoracolumbar fascia. This support of the spine consists of three layers (posterior, medial, and anterior) and transitions muscle-to-fibrous support in this area. Muscle atrophy, weakness, or poor motor control in these muscles has been associated with chronic low back pain, chronic dysfunction, and higher risk for lower extremity injuries[16,17] (**Figure 12.10**).

The abdominal muscles (superficial to deep: rectus abdominis, external oblique, internal oblique, and transverse abdominis) serve to manage muscular force and body position, as they relate to the trunk, pelvis, and spine via direct or indirect attachment to the vertebral segments. The rectus abdominis is primarily a sagittal plane trunk/pelvic flexor, whereas the remaining muscles assist with flexion. The oblique muscles primarily provide lateral flexion and rotation of the trunk. The transverse

Clinical Anatomy 509

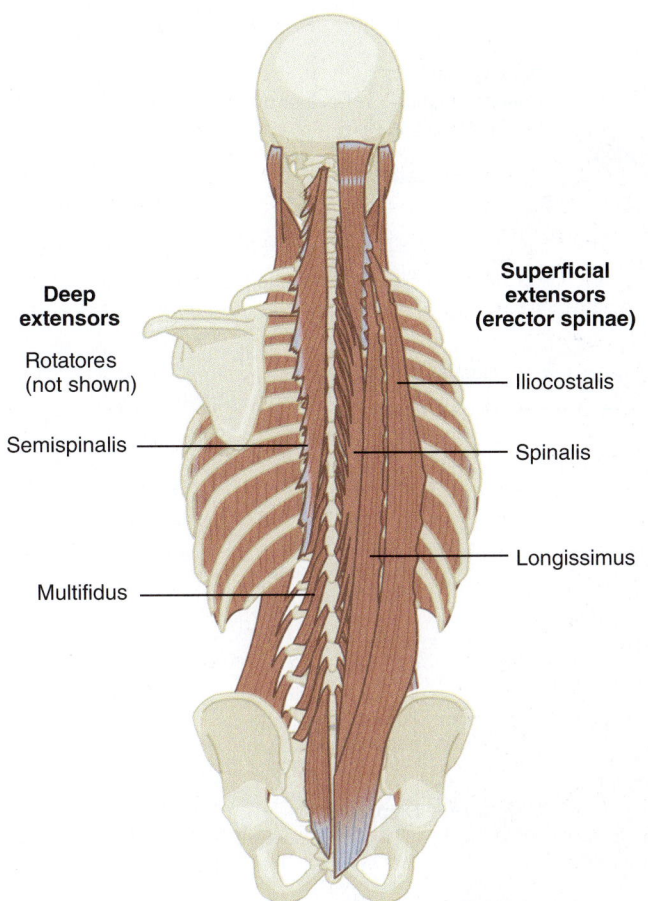

Figure 12.10 Drawing showing the back extensor muscles.
© Jones & Bartlett Learning

abdominis supports all motions by maintaining the intra-abdominal pressure[16,18-21] (**Figure 12.11**).

The pelvic floor consists of deep and superficial muscular layers known as the levator ani and the perineal, respectively.[22] The levator ani consists of the caudal vertebral flexors and abductors: ischiococcygeus, iliococcygeus, and pubococcygeus. Collectively, this mass spans from the pubic pectinate line and the obturator internus to the coccyx. The peroneal layer consists of the puborectalis and the pubovisceralis muscles, which originate at the inferior pubic rami.[22] The pubovisceralis muscle is made up of three parts: the pubococcygeus, puborectalis, and puboperineal, which support the deep visceral organs and sphincter function of the abdomen.[22] It has been reported the pelvic floor muscles cocontract with the deep spinal stabilizers of the spine in anticipation of global muscle activation of the pelvis and trunk[23-25] (**Figure 12.12**).

The diaphragm (**Figure 12.13**) is the roof of the spinal stability system that assists in maintaining intra-abdominal pressure and spinal stability through coactivation with the transverse abdominis.[26-28] In situations when respiration is under distress, the stability provided by the diaphragm has been reported to be compromised.[28] The diaphragm and the pelvic floor muscles act jointly with the abdominal musculature and skeletal structures of the spine to provide proximal stability.[23-25,27,28] It has been suggested that the layers of the thoracolumbar fascia and the adjacent aponeurosis of the latissimus dorsi assist in supporting the spine and the abdominal musculature similar to a weight-lifting belt.[29] The shared attachments to the transverse abdominis allow the fascia to serve as a link between the upper and lower extremities while providing proprioceptive feedback for trunk positioning.[5,29] This assists the entire lumbopelvic area to withstand forces from the global muscles and intra-abdominal pressures.[30,31]

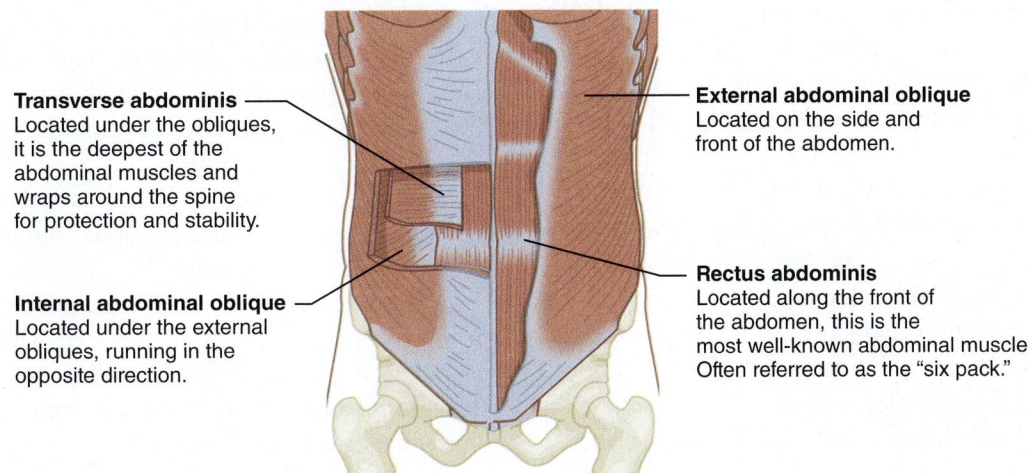

Figure 12.11 Drawing showing the abdominal muscles.
© Jones & Bartlett Learning

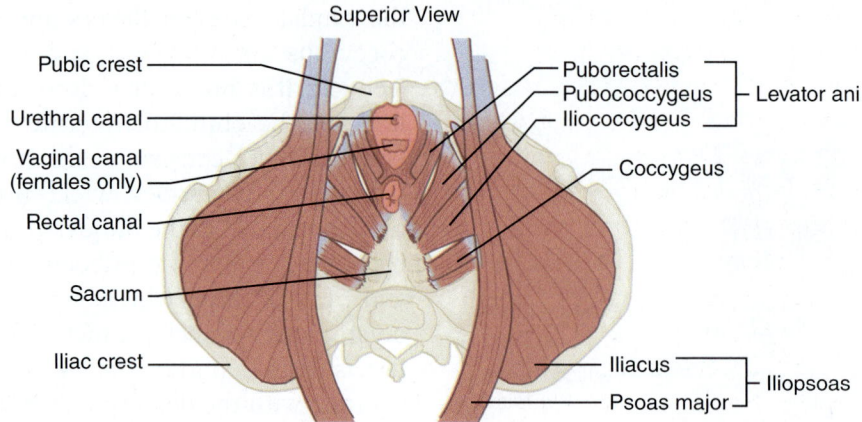

Figure 12.12 Drawing showing the pelvic floor muscles (superior view).
© Jones & Bartlett Learning

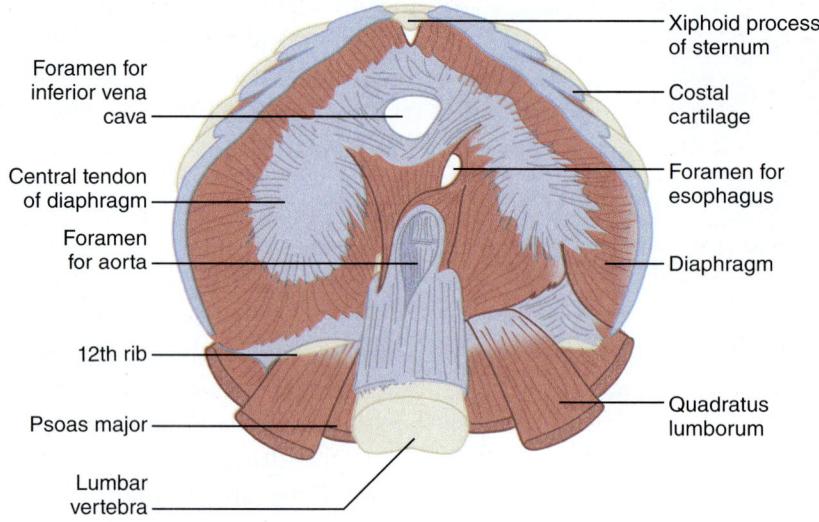

Figure 12.13 Drawing of the diaphragm (inferior view).
© Jones & Bartlett Learning

The Theoretical Model of Spinal Stability

The spinal stabilizing system, described by Bergmark,[30] Panjabi,[32] and earlier studies, has promoted the evolution of the proximal stabilization concept.[30,33-36] Spinal integrity or stiffness must be established to provide a proximal support for the distal body segments.[37] Skeletally, the pelvis and trunk are inherently rigid supports, whereas the lumbar spine is supple with five separate joined segments in the vertebrae.[30] The intervertebral segments of the spinal column receive forces from multiple directions, which must be controlled or redirected in order for body movement and function to be maintained and perform work.[30,32]

The spinal stabilizing system has been described as having three structural subsystems: passive, active, and neurologic.[30,32] The passive structures are predominantly the static or immovable bone and ligaments. The active structures consist of the deep and superficial muscles and tendons. The neurologic, or motor control, system encompasses the functions of the central nervous system, primarily anticipated and unanticipated neurologic feedback. Panjabi[32] stressed the importance of the interdependent nature of these subsystems to attain spinal stability. He stated that the subsystems must work synergistically to provide optimal and immediate proximal stiffness, or a "base of support" at the lumbar spine, which, in turn, allows the more distal segments of the pelvis and trunk to counter static and dynamic postural demands.[30,32]

As the spine encounters different postural demands, the intervertebral segments are stressed. The supporting passive ligaments/capsules maintain static alignment between the adjacent vertebrae and are often stretched to provide static blocks toward the end range of motion. In response, mechanoreceptors initiate afferent proprioceptive neurologic signals to the central nervous system. Immediate efferent feedback in the form of active muscle stiffness and/or relaxation is initiated to support the impending load(s).[30,32,38,39] McGill et al[40,41] describe the symmetrical alignment of the spinal muscles as supporting guy wires. The local (deep) and global (superficial) muscles are described to act on the proximal segments on three dimensions to accomplish intervertebral, pelvic, and trunk control.[39,40,42] The amplitude and timing of the muscle co-contractions around the spine must work in concert to achieve intervertebral stability consistent with the direction and magnitude of the load.[39,42-44] It has been reported that inappropriate contraction sequences can cause excess mobility of a single segment, resulting in compensatory loads to passive structures or other subsystems resulting in an instability.[40,45,46] Increases in instability accompanied with a perturbation or unexpected movement request put the spinal stability system in jeopardy of failing.[47-50] An example of this was reported by Cholewicki and McGill.[46] Lumbar spine instability of the L2 vertebra was observed in a weightlifter from a sagittal view using a video fluoroscope. The visual evidence of a spinal instability was accompanied by pain and a failure of the weightlifter to sustain the lift.

The feed forward and feedback neural processes communicate with the active subsystem to anticipate, implement, and alter the warranted spinal stiffness needs.[30,32,36] The spinal muscles work synergistically to balance their individual contributions of stability.[30,32,36] Local muscles provide a rigid spine, whereas the global muscles interact with the forces generated about the trunk and the more distal extremities.[30,32] It has been reported that the complexity of the neuromuscular system allows for immediate spinal stability prior to unexpected perturbations.[38,49] Cholewicki et al[38] reported an increased reflex response of trunk muscle activation and lumbar spine stability prior to the implementation of a sudden trunk load.[51-53]

The multiplanar motion of the spinal column is guided by a neutral zone.[36] When operating optimally, the coordinated efforts of the subsystems control spinal segment motion to ensure the column stays within a safe range of motion that places negligible stress on the intervertebral disks and capsular ligaments.[36] It has been reported that disruption to a subsystem can create intervertebral laxity that translates into an increased neutral zone, which may alter muscle stability schemes, causing an unstable spine and potential weakness.[42,45,54,55]

Spinal disruptions usually come in the form of pain, injury, degeneration, disease, and/or inappropriate motor control patterns.[37,42,44] Originally proposed to occur when a vertebra is beyond its end range of motion, recent literature has reported spinal degradation to occur at midrange of the neutral zone and without vertebral displacement.[37,45,54] Commonly associated with low back pain, instability in this area can impede the function of the spine and alter the effectiveness of force distribution at the spine.

Muscular Supports for the Spinal Segments

Naturally unstable, the spine depends greatly on the highly synchronized characteristics of the local and global musculature about the proximal segments.[30,32,34,40,54] **Table 12.1** describes the local and

Table 12.1 Quick Guide to Local Versus Global Muscles

	Local Muscles	Global Muscles
Description	Involved primarily with joint support or stabilization	Primarily responsible for functional movement
Location	Deeper muscles, located closer to skeletal system	More superficial, larger muscles
Example of Muscles	• Deep cervical flexors • Rotator cuff • Rhomboids • Mid and lower trapezius • Transverse abdominis • Multifidus • Diaphragm • Pelvic floor muscles • Gluteus medius • Gluteus minimus • Hip external rotators • Vastus medialis	• Sternocleidomastoid • Upper trapezius • Levator scapulae • Pectoralis major • Deltoid • Latissimus dorsi • Rectus abdominis • Internal obliques • External obliques • Erector spinae • Gluteus maximus • Hamstring group • Rectus femoris • Iliopsoas • Hip adductors

global muscles and movement schemes. The transverse abdominis, multifidus, erector spinae, internal oblique, posterior fibers of internal oblique, quadratus lumborum, diaphragm, and pelvic floor muscles have been classified as local muscles supporting the lumbar spine curvature and proximal cavity of the pelvis. These smaller and relatively single-jointed muscles provide intervertebral stability by means of their deep origin and insertional attachments.[30,35,55] The local muscles anticipate the loads at individual spinal segments and adjacent structures, which provide localized mechanical stiffness to the spine.[30,52] The interaction of the local muscles provides a stable column responsible for maintaining the curvature and posture of the spine.[30,35,56] As mentioned previously, the pelvic floor and the diaphragm work synergistically with the deep and superficial musculature of the spine to secure functional capacity about the spine.

The global muscles, which include portions of the internal oblique, external oblique, latissimus dorsi, gluteus maximus, iliopsoas, and rectus abdominis, are the larger superficial muscles spanning over several body segments of the pelvis and trunk.[30,32,35] They are responsible for creating, transferring, and reducing loads between the thoracic cage and the pelvis.[30,34] The global muscles provide mobility and stability about the proximal segments, depending on the given task.[39] Mobility can occur at high forces, whereas stability tends to be incrementally based on intensity of the activity.[35]

The muscular complex of the hip has been suggested by some as a primary component of the proximal spinal stabilizers,[57,58] whereas others have described the hip involvement as a support structure of the kinetic chain.[44,59-61] The close proximity of the hip complex is ideal for force production relative to the pelvis but not for implementing intersegmental support to the spinal vertebrae or related structures.[36,39,62-65] McGill et al[39] and Naito et al[64] reported variations in peak electromyographic muscle activation between the deep transverse abdominis muscle and the distal biceps femoris and gluteus muscles of the hip. These authors concluded that the activation patterns demonstrated an interaction between the proximal and distal segments necessary for the distribution of ground reaction forces. Although the local muscles stabilize the spine, the forces from the hip assist to overcome rotational inertias about the ground, lower extremity, and trunk and throughout the kinetic chain. Therefore, the primary role of the hip has been referred to as a generator and mediator of forces transmitted from the ground, rather than a stabilizer of the lumbar spine or core.[44,60,64]

Counterrotation between the trunk and pelvis, which normally occurs in acts of walking or throwing, contributes to the body's ability to perform diagonal movements necessary for activities of daily living and sports participation.[55] Expressed as the serape effect,[66] it has been hypothesized that the contralateral pelvis/hip and trunk work in tandem to absorb and distribute loads to and from the extremities through a stable spine.[55,67] The term is coined from the way a Mexican serape or poncho aligns from contralateral upper to lower extremities. The contralateral connection incorporates activation of the rhomboids, serratus anterior, external oblique, and internal oblique muscles.[66] These muscles are commonly active in overhead athletics and the inclusion of diagonal movements and act as a direct link between the local and global muscles of the lumbopelvic area.[63,66,68]

Distinct Roles of the Local and Global Muscles. There are distinct responsibilities for the local and global muscles that contribute to proximal stability.[59] Kiefer et al[6] used two spinal geometric muscle models to evaluate the distinct stabilizing mechanisms of the local and global activation patterns. Asymmetrical co-contractions of the global muscles were noted, whereas co-contractions of the multifidus muscle were symmetrical during a variety of trunk and arm positions. Others have reported the symmetrical action of the multifidus, transverse abdominis, and quadratus lumborum provides stability similar to guy wires of a bridge. It is commonly thought that the local and global muscles work collectively but have distinctive roles in providing proximal stabilization. Electromyographic analysis supports the exclusive roles of the global muscles and intra-abdominal pressure to provide stability and mobility predicated upon the intensity and type of task being performed.[39,44,69,70] Hodges et al[51] and others[71,72] have described the different functional responsibilities of the local and global muscles. For example, the transverse abdominis and the multifidus muscles have been reported to be active prior to rapid arm movement and the more global muscles of the trunk (ie, external oblique).[51] The multifidus also acts concurrently with the erector spinae to assist in providing an outlet for force distribution from the deep and proximal muscles to the superficial global muscles.[71] Regardless of arm direction or intensity of movement, the deep spinal stabilizing muscles appear to be primarily responsible for providing a stiff lumbar spinal segment.[51] This natural progression of co-contraction provides intervertebral stabilization, enabling the global muscles to position and orient the spine and adjacent segments.[51,73] The data from these studies highlight the anticipatory nature of the proximal stabilizers and offer important insight regarding motor control strategies and training implications.

The extremities rely on the dynamic and static stabilizing capabilities of the proximal kinetic chain to support distal function. Activation of the deep spinal stabilizer muscles has not demonstrated adaptability to task but has consistently been reported to maintain a predominant role of intersegmental stability in anticipation of movement.[70,74-77] The distinct relationship between the local and global muscles provides a nice blueprint for training and assessment practices. It appears that healthy individuals would need to maintain adequate function of this relationship in order to perform movement tasks efficiently. Thus, monitoring functional performance of the local and global muscles is likely a critical piece for training and assessment practices.

Neurologic Anatomy

The spinal cord lies within the vertebral canal from the foramen magnum of the skull to the L1-L2 intervertebral segments, where it forms a cone shape at the terminal end known as the conus medullaris. All of the spinal nerves from L2 to the coccygeal nerves pass caudally through the conus medullaris. Though protected by three fibrous meninges layers—the dura mater, arachnoid mater, and pia mater—the spinal cord remains vulnerable to both injury and infection.[1,29,78] The dura mater is a tough, fibrous sheath that covers the spinal nerves leaving the spinal canal and forming a protective layer dorsal root ganglion. The arachnoid, or arachnoid mater, has a spider-web appearance and lies on the inferior surface of the dura mater; the subdural space between these structures is a common location for fluid displacement from infection and/or injury. The pia mater is deep to the arachnoid mater and protects the spinal cord to the L2 vertebra caudal end. Here, the filum terminale attaches the end of the spinal cord to the caudal end of the dura mater. Further, the denticulate ligaments branch off the pia mater to connect the spinal cord to the dura mater. The subarachnoid space between the arachnoid mater and pia mater is synonymous with the cerebrospinal fluid and spinal cord[1,78] (**Figure 12.14**).

Plexuses. The sensory and motor distributions for the spine's cervical, brachial, lumbar, and sacral plexuses serve as great contributors to joint stability and function throughout the axial and appendicular skeleton. The cervical nerve supply of C2-C8 travels through the intervertebral foramen formed by the posterior lateral spacing of the vertebrae. The foramen spacing is often a cause of injury due to a spacing stenosis caused by joint inflammation, degeneration, and cervical hyperextension. On the contrary, cervical flexion and/or traction will increase the posterior lateral pathway, thus resulting in less stress on the nerve roots and/or the facet joints. The cervical nerve roots branch off the spinal cord into anterior/ventral and posterior/dorsal roots, providing the arm and trunk with sensory and motor supply. In addition, the horizontal foramen in the transverse process serves as a passage through the cervical column for the cervical arteries and veins. The anterior branches of the nerve roots serve C1-C4 sensory input and are referred to as the cervical plexus (**Figure 12.15**). The C4-C8 make up the brachial plexus (**Figure 12.16**) and serve as the motor distribution of the upper extremity. The distribution of the brachial plexus progresses from the proximal nerve root to nerve trunks, divisions, cords, and terminal branches of the musculocutaneous, axial, radial, median, and ulnar nerves.

The lumbar plexus and sacral plexus consist of nerve networks form T12-L5 and L4-S1, respectively. The L4 and L5 and a portion of the lumbosacral trunk project downward to form the beginning of the

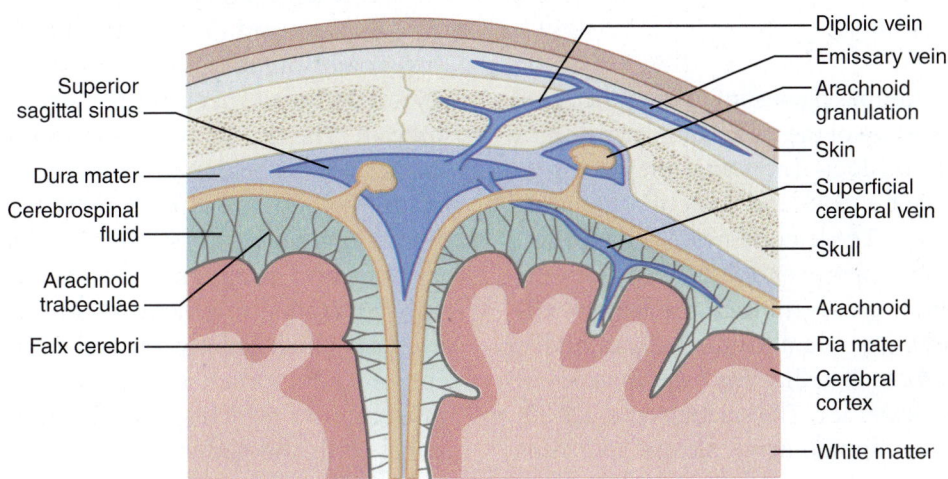

Figure 12.14 Drawing of the subarachnoid space.
© Jones & Bartlett Learning

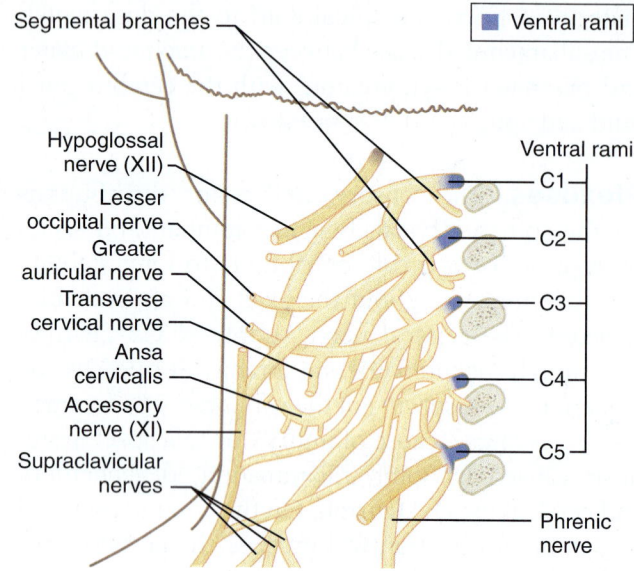

Figure 12.15 Drawing of the cervical plexus.
© Jones & Bartlett Learning

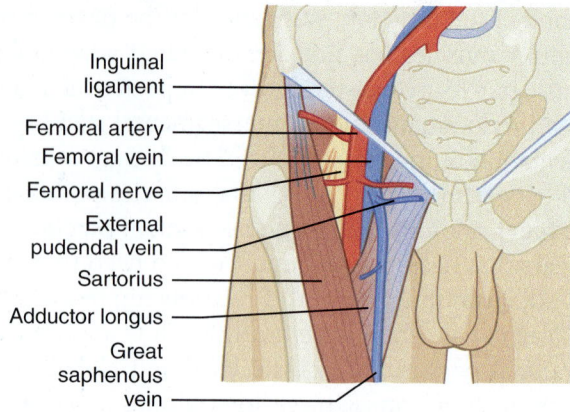

Figure 12.17 Drawing of the femoral triangle.
© Jones & Bartlett Learning

in the popliteal fossa, the sciatic nerve divides into the common peroneal nerve and the tibial nerve to innervate the anterior, lateral, and posterior compartments of the lower leg and foot. Damage to the common peroneal nerve or more proximally at the sciatic nerve can result in a muscle weakness/dysfunction resulting in a foot drop symptom.

Vascular Anatomy

Vascular anatomy of the spine is rarely discussed in the athletic training profession, but it is important to understand the fundamentals of the spinal vascular anatomy to prevent oversight of any potential pathologies. Functional blood supply to the spinal anatomy occurs through a variety of vessels. Although there are numerous arteries that could be discussed in this chapter, only the main sources of vascular blood supply will be covered. The aorta and its associated aortic arch are the main sources of arterial blood supply for the entire body. The aortic arch and its corresponding major branches, listed right to left, are (1) the brachiocephalic trunk, (2) the left common carotid artery, and (3) the left subclavian artery. These three major branches provide the arterial blood supply to the head, neck, upper extremities, and thorax wall. The descending aorta projects to numerous smaller vessels before it pierces the diaphragm. Once inside the abdominal cavity, the vessel, now called the abdominal aorta, supplies the abdominal walls and viscera. The abdominal aorta ends at the L4 level and then splits into the right and left common iliac arteries, which supply the pelvis and lower limbs. The other important vessels are the posterior intercostal arteries, which supply the deep spinal muscles, spinal cord, and vertebrae.

Table 12.2 provides a summary of the muscle groups as they relate to the spine.

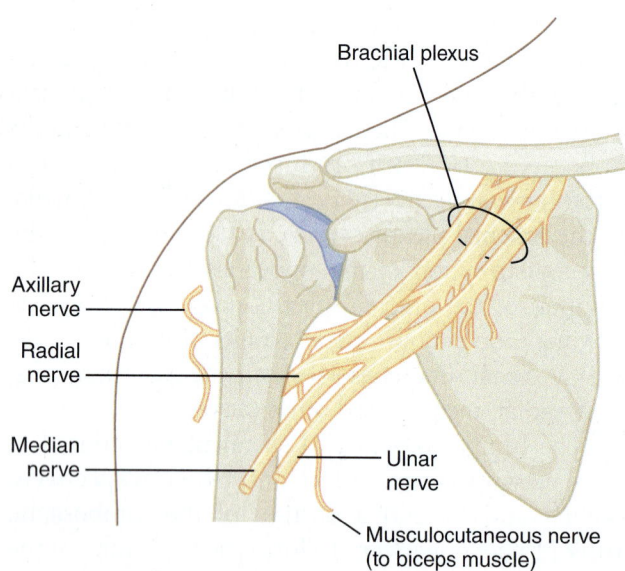

Figure 12.16 Drawing of the brachial plexus.
© Jones & Bartlett Learning

sacral plexus. The lumbar plexus innervates the anterior and medial muscles of the thigh and dermatomes of the medial leg and foot. The sacral plexus innervates muscles of the buttocks and posterior upper leg (via the sciatic nerve). The femoral nerve is the largest branch of the lumbar plexus and is derived from the L2-L4 nerve roots. It passes through the femoral triangle (**Figure 12.17**), just lateral to the femoral artery, and has articular branches that feed the muscles of the hip, knee, and lower leg. The sciatic nerve, L4-S3, is derived from the lumbosacral plexus and runs beneath the piriformis muscle of the pelvis to the posterior thigh via the greater sciatic foramen. Distally,

Table 12.2 Muscle Groups Related to the Spine

Muscle	Origin	Insertion	Action	Nerve Root Innervation	Palpation
Erector Spinae Group					
Spinalis (formed by the thoracis, cervicis, and capitis)	Spinous processes of the upper lumbar and lower thoracic vertebrae (thoracis); Ligamentum nuchae, spinous process of C7 (cervicis)	Spinous processes of upper thoracic (thoracis); Spinous processes of cervical vertebrae, except C1 (cervicis)	**Unilaterally:** Lateral flexion of vertebral column to same side **Bilaterally:** Extend vertebral column	Spinal	Easily palpated entire length of trunk and neck proximal to spine
Iliocostalis (formed by the lumborum, thoracis, and cervicis)	Common tendon (lumborum); Posterior surface of ribs 1-12 (thoracis and cervicis)	Transverse processes of L1-L3 and posterior surface of ribs 6-12 (lumborum); Posterior surface of ribs 1-6 (thoracis); Transverse processes of lower cervical vertebrae (cervicis)			
Longissimus (formed by the thoracis, cervicis, and capitis)	Common tendon (thoracis); Transverse processes of upper five thoracic vertebrae (cervicis and capitis)	Lower nine ribs and transverse processes of thoracic vertebrae (thoracis); Transverse processes of cervical vertebrae (cervicis); Mastoid process of temporal bone (capitis)			

(continues)

Table 12.2 Muscle Groups Related to the Spine (continued)

Muscle	Origin	Insertion	Action	Nerve Root Innervation	Palpation
Intrinsic Spinal Muscles					
Transversospinalis muscle group					
Multifidi and rotatores	Sacrum and transverse processes of lumbar through cervical vertebrae (multifidi) Transverse processes of lumbar through cervical vertebrae (rotatores)	Spinous processes of lumbar vertebrae through second cervical vertebrae (multifidi span 2-4 vertebrae; rotatores span 1-2 vertebrae)	**Unilaterally:** Rotate the vertebral column to the opposite side **Bilaterally:** Spinal extension	Spinal	Deep to erector spinae
Semispinalis capitis	Transverse processes of C4-T5	Between the superior and inferior nuchal lines of the occiput	Extend the vertebral column and head	Cervical	Deep along the thoracic and cervical vertebrae
Intertransversarii	Cervical: Spanning the transverse processes of vertebrae C2-C7 Lumbar: Spanning the transverse processes of vertebrae L1-L5		**Unilaterally:** Laterally flex the vertebral column to the same side **Bilaterally:** Extend the vertebral column	Spinal	Deep, nonpalpable
Interspinalis	Cervical: Spanning the spinous processes of C2-T3 Lumbar: Spanning the spinous processes of T12-L5		Extend the vertebral column	Spinal	Deep, nonpalpable
Splenius Muscles					
Splenius capitis	Inferior half of ligamentum nuchae and spinous processes of C7-T4	Mastoid process and lateral superior nuchal line	**Unilaterally:** Neck and head rotation same side	Cervical	Upper back and posterior neck
Splenius cervicis	Spinous processes of T3-T6 vertebrae	Transverse processes of C1-C3 vertebrae	**Unilaterally:** Head and neck lateral flexion **Bilaterally:** Extend head and neck		

Muscles of the Neck

Muscle		Origin	Insertion	Action	Innervation	Palpation
Sternocleidomastoid		Top of manubrium (sternal head); Medial one-third of the clavicle (clavicular head)	Mastoid process of temporal bone; Lateral portion of superior nuchal line of occiput	**Unilaterally:** Head and neck lateral flexion same side; head and neck rotation to opposite side **Bilaterally:** Flexion neck; assist to elevate rib cage during inhalation	Spinal accessory (XI)	Ask athlete to turn head to the opposite side of muscle to be palpated
Scalenes	Anterior	Transverse process of C3-C6 (anterior tubercles)	First rib	Laterally flex head to same side (with ribs fixed); Rotate head and neck to opposite side (all)	C3, C4-C8	Between sternocleidomastoid and anterior flap of trapezius
	Middle	Transverse process of C2-C7 (posterior tubercles)				
	Posterior	Transverse process of C6-C7 (posterior tubercles)				
Longus capitis		Transverse processes of C3 through C6	Inferior surface of occiput	**Unilaterally:** Laterally flex the head and neck to the same side; rotate head and neck to the same side **Bilaterally:** Flex the head and neck	C1-C3	Base of the occiput
Longus colli		Bodies of C5 through T3, transverse processes of C3 through C5	Tubercle on anterior arch of the atlas; bodies of the axis, C3, and C4; transverse processes of C5 and C6	**Unilaterally:** Laterally flex the head and neck to the same side; rotate the head and neck to the same side **Bilaterally:** Flex the head and neck	C2-C7	Base of occiput
Platysma		Fascia covering superior part of pectoralis major	Base of mandible, skin of lower part of face	Assists to depress the mandible; Tighten the fascia of the neck; Draw down the corner of the mouth	Facial	Anterior lateral tissue of neck when patient juts jaw forward

(continues)

Table 12.2 Muscle Groups Related to the Spine

Muscle	Origin	Insertion	Action	Nerve Root Innervation	Palpation
Suboccipital Muscles					
Rectus capitis posterior major	Spinous processes of the axis (C2)	Inferior nuchal line of the occiput	Rock and tilt the head back into extension; Rotate the head to the same side	Suboccipital	Curling the fingers under the occiput
Rectus capitis posterior minor	Tubercle of the posterior arch of the atlas (C1)	Inferior nuchal line of the occiput	Rock and tilt the head back into extension		
Obliquus capitis superior	Transverse process of the atlas (C1)	Between the nuchal lines of the occiput	Rock and tilt the head back into extension; Laterally flex the head to the same side		
Obliquus capitis inferior	Spinous process of the axis (C2)	Transverse process of the atlas (C1)	Rotate the head to the same side		
Muscles of the Abdominal Wall					
Quadratus lumborum	Posterior iliac crest	Last rib and transverse process of L1-L4	**Unilaterally:** Lateral pelvic tilt; lateral flexion vertebral column to same side; assist to extend vertebral column **Bilaterally:** Fix the last rib during forced inhalation and exhalation	Lumbar plexus	Deep beneath thoracolumbar aponeurosis and erector spinae

(continued)

		Origin	Insertion	Action	Innervation	Notes
Rectus abdominis		Pubic symphysis Pubic crest	Costal cartilage of ribs 5–7 Xiphoid process	Flex the vertebral column Tilt pelvis posteriorly	T5–T12, ventral rami	Most superficial abs ("6 pack")
External oblique		External surface of ribs 5–12	Anterior superior iliac spine and anterior portion of iliac crest Abdominal aponeurosis to linea alba	**Unilaterally:** Laterally flex vertebral column to same side; rotate vertebral column to opposite side **Bilaterally:** Flex vertebral column; compress abdominal contents	T5–T12	Done in "hands on hips" position; just above iliac crest
Internal oblique		Lateral inguinal ligament Iliac crest Thoracolumbar fascia	Internal surface of lower three ribs Abdominal aponeurosis to linea alba	**Unilaterally:** Laterally flex vertebral column to same side; rotate vertebral column to same side **Bilaterally:** Flex the vertebral column; compress abdominal contents (bilaterally)	T7–T12, L1, Iliohypogastric and ilioinguinal Ventral rami	Deep under external obliques

(continues)

Table 12.2 Muscle Groups Related to the Spine

Muscle	Origin	Insertion	Action	Nerve Root Innervation	Palpation
Transverse abdominis	Lateral inguinal ligament Iliac crest Thoracolumbar fascia Internal surface of lower 6 ribs	Abdominal aponeurosis to linea alba	Compress abdominal contents	T7–T12, L1 Iliohypogastric and ilioinguinal Ventral divisions	Deep; nonpalpable
Muscles of the Thorax					
Diaphragm	Costal attachment: Inner surface of lower six ribs Lumbar attachment: Upper two or three lumbar vertebrae Sternal attachment: Inner part of xiphoid process	Central tendon	Draw down the central tendon of the diaphragm	Phrenic C3–C5	Curled around ribs to access the diaphragm during exhalation
Intercostals	Inferior border of the rib above	Superior border of the rib below	External intercostals: Draw the ribs superiorly (increasing the space of the thoracic cavity) to assist with inhalation Internal intercostals: Draw the ribs inferiorly (decreasing the space of the thoracic cavity) to assist with exhalation	Thoracic	Between each rib

(continued)

All figures in table © Jones & Bartlett Learning.

Overview of Radiology and Imaging

Imaging of the spine is accomplished using a variety of modalities, such as radiographs, CT, and MRI. Radiographs and CT are used to identify bone or more detailed information regarding the fracture of or stress reactions to the bone.[79-82] CT offers higher resonance than a radiograph regarding bone and soft tissue, whereas MRI offers more detailed information for multiple sections of the structures being evaluated, especially with soft tissue. Therefore, MRI is, many times, the choice when the differential diagnosis is need for soft tissue, such as the spinal cord, nerve roots, ligaments, muscles, tendons, and disks.[83-85] Radiography is generally very dependable for noting stress reactions and often does not require higher levels of detection; however, if radicular pain is present, CT or MRI is generally the modality of choice[85] (**Figure 12.18**).

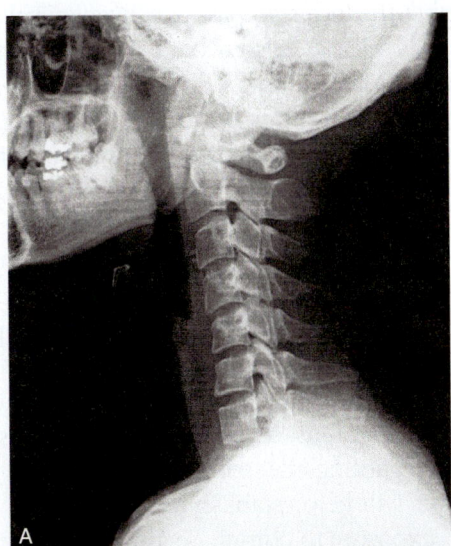

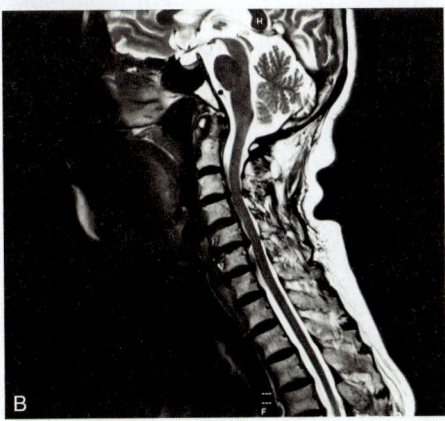

Figure 12.18 Imaging of the spine. **A.** Cervical spine radiograph. **B.** T2-weighted magnetic resonance image showing cervical myelopathy.

A. © mapo_japan/Shutterstock; **B.** © Yok_onepiece/Shutterstock.

Evaluation of the Spine

A typical evaluation of the spine consists of an evaluation of the cervical, thoracic, and/or lumbar regions. Generally, because of their close proximity, it is important to consider all spinal regions during evaluation to determine all potential mechanistic contributions to the current pathology. The evaluation should be systematic and focused on the spinal region bearing the primary complaint; however, if possible, information regarding the history, inspection, palpation, and functional testing should include factors related to the axial and appendicular skeleton.

History

Gathering a history during a spinal evaluation will necessitate some general questions regarding chief complaint, mechanism of injury, previous injury, and location and onset of pain. However, specific history questions concerning neurologic and postural implications regarding the signs and symptoms will be critical to all spinal evaluations. Determining the pain status in the history as localized, radiating, or referred will assist in plotting out a systematic algorithm for injuries that are related to a bone, disk, or nerve, respectively. Pain from inflammation about the spine or nerve roots typically remains unchanged unless the inflammation is reduced, whereas mechanical forces (compressions, distraction) can often elevate or alleviate pain. Determining the mechanical direction of force will also be very similar in all spinal regions. For example, hyperflexion of the spine will compress the anterior structures of the spine while transmitting forces on the vertebral disk in a posterior direction, potentially compromising the integrity of the disk or the nerve roots. Conversely, hyperextension imposes the opposite implication with compression forces to posterior facets, nerve foramen, and bony structures. However, axial loads or the whiplash mechanism are typically more common among patients undergoing cervical evaluation.

Onset of a pathology, acute or chronic, typically is similar throughout the spinal regions. However, acute injuries noted with a primary mechanism and location of pain help to isolate the primary injury structures.[85,86] Muscle strain and spasm often are associated with acute injuries but tend to have insidious onsets that typically indicate muscle fatigue/imbalance, poor fitness/biomechanics, delayed onset of soreness or inflammation, and/or chronic degenerative properties of the spine.[3,13,39] The history for any spinal evaluation should include occupational questions regarding the types of body postures used during employment (seated, standing, overhead activity) and the intensity and duration of these activities. Prolonged occupational postures tend to foster muscle imbalances and poor biomechanics, resulting in both chronic and acute pathologies.[86-90]

Objective patient feedback can be quantified through self-reporting outcome scales specific to the thoracic spine. Quantifiable measures of spinal disabilities can be used to gain subjective patient perspectives regarding pain, function, and activities of daily living. General numeric pain rating scales from 1 to 10 can be an easy way to quantify patient perspective, as these ratings generally match well with severity of injury and functional capacity. The following are common objective and validation measures for spinal assessment: Oswestry Disability Index, Neck Disability Index, Patient-Specific Functional Scale, and Roland-Morris Low Back Pain and Disability Questionnaire.[91,92] These forms and questionnaires can be found in **Appendix 12.A** through **12.D**.

Cervical Spine History

The nature of any spinal pathology necessitates routine history questions that target the mechanism of injury and the primary complaint. The primary concern while evaluating the cervical collar is to rule out any traumatic spinal cord or head injury. Therefore, it is necessary to ask memory- and cognitive-related history questions to establish the patient's level of consciousness. Whiplash and axial load mechanisms typically occur at the cervical spine, revealing a multitude of injuries related to potential fracture, sprain, muscle strain, and nerve pathologies. Determining whether the localized pain at a given spinal segment corresponds with a sensory or motor function will be critical in determining causation and the potential of nerve root involvement. Thus, questions related to the type of stress, neck position, point of contact or direct blows, and/or specific involvement of the brachial plexus nerve roots must be asked. Specific questions must also attempt to establish daily active and/or chronic posture throughout the day.[93,94]

Thoracic Spine History

The uniqueness of the thoracic spine is attributed to its being a mobile region that acts as a foundation for the scapula while also collaborating with the thoracic rib cage. The thoracic spine will experience traditional spinal pathologies. However, complications involving different postures, such as kyphosis or scoliosis, and/or rib cage variations necessitate history questions targeting congenital and/or developmental spine postures.[95-97] Further, the rib cage and potential costal, breathing, and internal organ injuries associated with the thoracic spine could complicate an orthopaedic evaluation and must be addressed during a medical history. Determining whether the localized pain at a given spinal segment corresponds with a sensory or motor function will be critical in defining causation and the potential of nerve root involvement. Thus, questions related to the type of stress; point of contact or direct blows; and/or specific involvement of a nerve root versus peripheral disorders, or both, need to be addressed. Specific questions must also attempt to establish daily active and/or chronic postures associated with activities of daily living.

Lumbar Spine History

The primary concern while evaluating the lumbar spine is to rule out isolated spine pathology versus pathologies that involve multiple spinal properties. Determining whether the localized pain at a given spinal segment corresponds with a sensory or motor function will be critical in defining causation and the potential of nerve root involvement.[98] Thus, questions related to the type of stress; point of contact or direct blows; and/or specific involvement of a nerve root versus peripheral disorders, or both, are important.[99-101] L4-S1 disk and nerve root levels are highly susceptible to injury, so questions for lumbar pathologies should address potential neurologic implications from these spinal segments. Many pathologies of the lumbar spine relate to lifting mechanics that often involve improper spine flexion and faulty hip and/or knee motions. Thus, specific questions should be asked regarding the patient's normal acts of daily living. This will help establish an understanding of the potential exposure to chronic seating/standing postures and/or lifting behaviors associated with daily activities and the current signs and symptoms.[102,103]

Inspection

Inspection of the spine should include routine posture assessments, but specific concern regarding the true characteristics of the spinal regions and the appendicular skeleton is critical. For example, the roles of mobility versus stability of the cervical collar are different from those of the thoracic and lumbar regions, or how unwarranted excess motion at the lumbar spine might be used to attain hip function/mobility, thus breaching the integrity of the lumbar structures. Regardless of the spinal segment being evaluated, both history and inspection should be used to determine whether total body functional assessments versus isolated, linear assessments can be performed. When possible, total body flexion, extension, rotation, and loading (nonweighted squat, lunge) should accompany all spine evaluations. Such motions will help attain additional potential etiologic contributions.

Clinical Presentation for Posture of the Spine

A postural assessment is a common aspect of any orthopaedic examination because curvature, muscle imbalance, or limitation at the spine often results in altered mechanics at a distal segment. Spinal posture should be examined from all planes and from a regional interdependence and intradependence perspective. Understanding the role of the spine as it relates to adjacent and regional body segments can assist in finding potential compensatory mechanics and related pathologies. Using common landmarks to assess static posture associated with or without a plumb line can assist in determining potential mechanisms of injury or related cause-and-effect relationships. Generally, visual screening of the axial skeleton and adjacent body regions in all planes should be performed from anatomic position prior to an extensive evaluation.

Posture: General Static Screen

The cervical spine serves as the primary mover and support of the head. The lordotic curve of cervical vertebra (**Figure 12.19**) serves as a primary observable

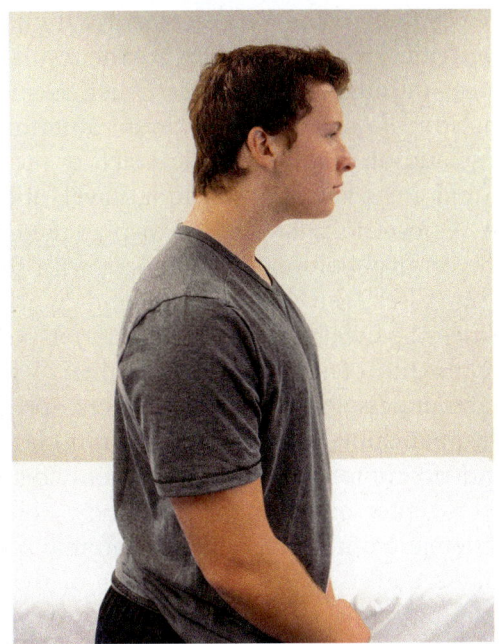

Figure 12.20 Photograph depicting a forward head.
© Jones & Bartlett Learning

postural landmark. From a lateral/sagittal view, the curve is anterior to the occiput and C7. The auricle and center of the ear align vertically with the center of the acromion. Loss of lordosis is noted with deformities, such as a forward or protracted head (**Figure 12.20**) in which the C1 and C2 are extended on flexed C3-C7 spinal segments. A backward or retracted head (**Figure 12.21**) is the result of excessive flexion at C1-C2 with an extended

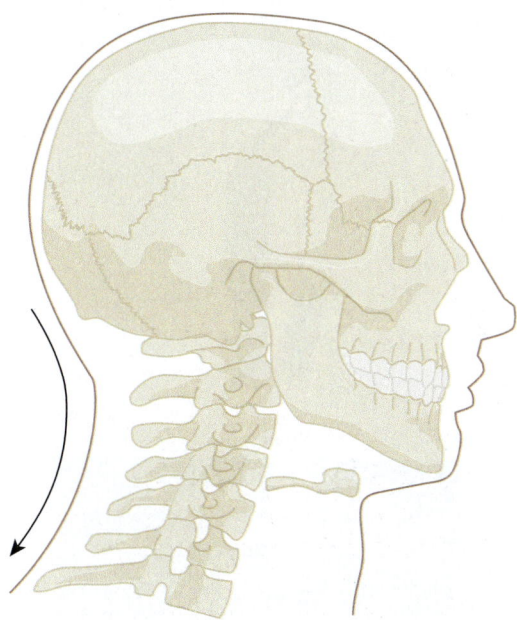

Figure 12.19 Drawing showing the lordotic curve of cervical vertebrae.
© Jones & Bartlett Learning

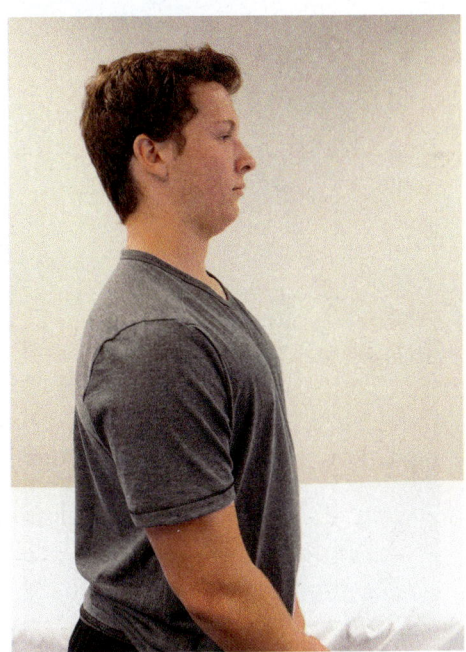

Figure 12.21 Photograph depicting a backward head.
© Jones & Bartlett Learning

C3-C7.[1,16,59] Often the result of poor habitual postural activities, these conditions are the result of disturbances in muscular properties, such as strength, length, and motor control. From an anterior view, the nose and philtrum or medical cleft of the upper lip should align with the sternum, navel, and mid-stance. A posterior view should display the occiput and the cervical column in alignment with the spinous processes, the sacrum, and mid-stance. The feet, knees, pelvis/hip (anterior/posterior superior iliac spine and crest), greater trochanter, leg muscles, acromioclavicular joint/shoulders, pectoralis muscles, paraspinal muscles, deltoid muscles, scapula, and rib contour should all be evenly displaced from the center of the spine and body. Following is a systematic outline of normal anatomic postural landmarks and associated alignments of the spine using a plumb line.

Plumb Line Checklist: Spine Posture Assessment

Anterior View. Disruptions noted in bolded text in the following list indicate areas that influence the normal characteristics of the spine and demonstrate abnormalities/asymmetries in the frontal and transverse planes (**Figure 12.22**).

- Feet, knees (patella), and hips facing anterior with equal distance from plumb line
- Tibial crest: slight external rotation
- Lateral malleoli, fibular head, and iliac crest should be bilaterally equal to the plumb line.
- **Anterior superior iliac spine (ASIS) height to floor and distance** to plumb line
  - **Chest musculature, umbilicus, sternum, and jugular notch** aligned and symmetrical with plumb line.
  - **Head: nasal bridge, cleft of chin, and upper lip** bisected equally by the plumb line.
- **Shoulder musculature/acromion processes** height/evenly spaced from the plumb line.

Lateral View. Disruptions noted in bolded text in the following list indicate areas that influence the normal characteristics of the spine and demonstrate abnormalities/asymmetries in the sagittal and transverse planes (**Figure 12.23**).

- **Lateral malleolus:** Slightly posterior to plumb line with tibia parallel.
- **Lateral femoral condyle:** Slightly anterior to the plumb line.
- **Lordosis at cervical and lumbar spine**
- Plumb line bisects **greater trochanter, midthoracic region, acromion process, and auditory meatus.**

Posterior View. Disruptions noted in bolded text in the following list indicate areas that influence the normal characteristics of the spine and demonstrate

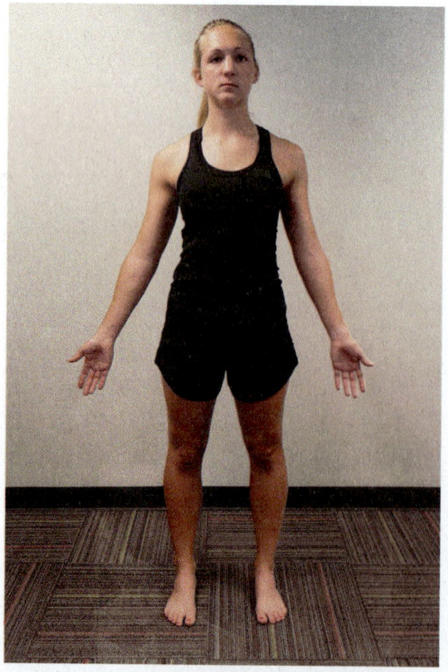

Figure 12.22 Photograph showing the anterior anatomic view.

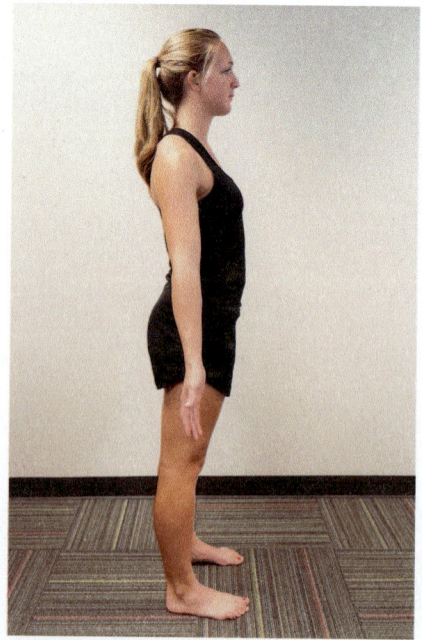

Figure 12.23 Photograph showing the lateral anatomic view.

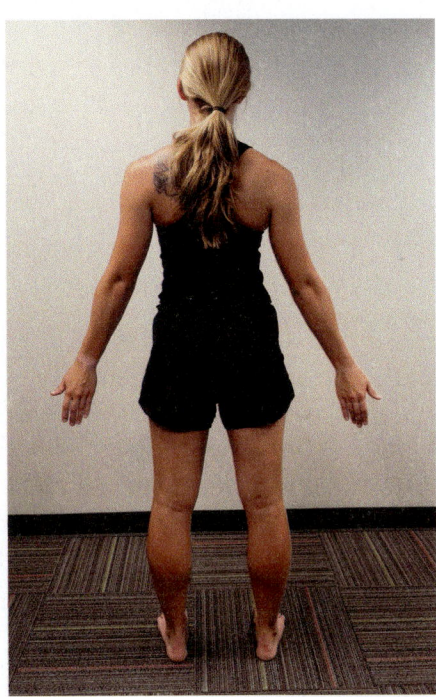

Figure 12.24 Photograph showing the posterior anatomic view.
© Jones & Bartlett Learning

abnormalities/asymmetries in the frontal and transverse planes (**Figure 12.24**).

- Feet, knees, and hips are evenly spaced, slight lateral rotation, and lateral two toes are visible
- Plumb line equally bisects **sacrum, spinous processes, paraspinal musculature, scapular borders, occipital protuberance, and skull**
- Calf, thigh, **gluteal/pelvic, paraspinal, deltoid, and neck posterior musculature bilaterally symmetrical** heights and distance from plumb line
- **Shoulder heights equal** or dominant side slightly lower

Common Spine Postural Deficits

Muscle imbalances or skeletal asymmetries at the spine often cause irregular muscle tightness/shortening resulting in hypomobility and hypermobility at adjacent and/or spinal segments. As a result, muscle synergy in adjacent muscle regions is lost. The propagation of muscle weakness or hypertonic dysfunction promotes potential faulty mechanics, pain, and injury. Common postural abnormalities noted at or associated with the spine are scoliosis (C and S curves), forward head, flat back, swayback, excessive lumbar lordosis, and thoracic kyphosis.[17,59,104,105]

Congenital and/or habitually formed sclerotic deviations are some of the common spinal misalignments noted visually (**Figure 12.25**). Scoliosis generally

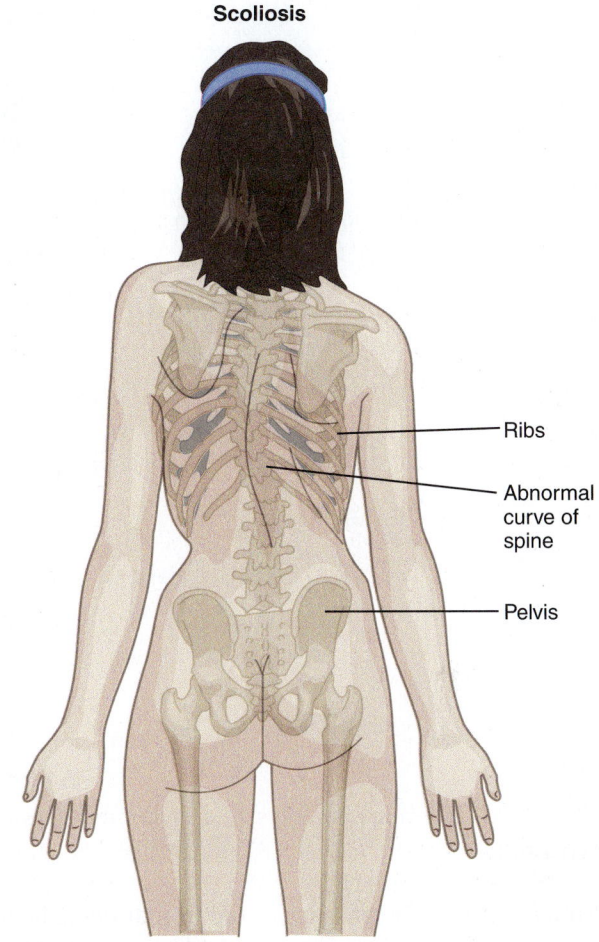

Figure 12.25 Drawing showing scoliosis.
© Jones & Bartlett Learning

occurs in prepubescent patients and is associated with a rapid growth spurt. C and S curves are commonly noted as a frontal and transverse plane abnormality but are often associated with multiplanar deviations (**Figure 12.26**). These structural deviations in the spine often cause mechanical alterations to joint function, resulting in inappropriate degenerative stress and damage. A left or right C curve is best noted posteriorly, whereas an S curve is more commonly seen from all planar views. Often, both conditions can place additional strain on the rib cage alignment and disrupt thoracic pressure gradients against the lungs and heart, making it more difficult to breathe and compromising the rhythm of the heart to pump blood. An observable ipsilateral rib cage convexity/hump is notable in patients with sclerosis during standing trunk flexion (**Figure 12.27**). A forward head is a frontal plane malalignment commonly associated with several other mechanical dysfunctions at the spine. Specifically, the head protracts anteriorly due to shortened levator scapulae, sternocleidomastoid, upper trapezius, and posterior cervical suboccipital spine muscles. Flatback is

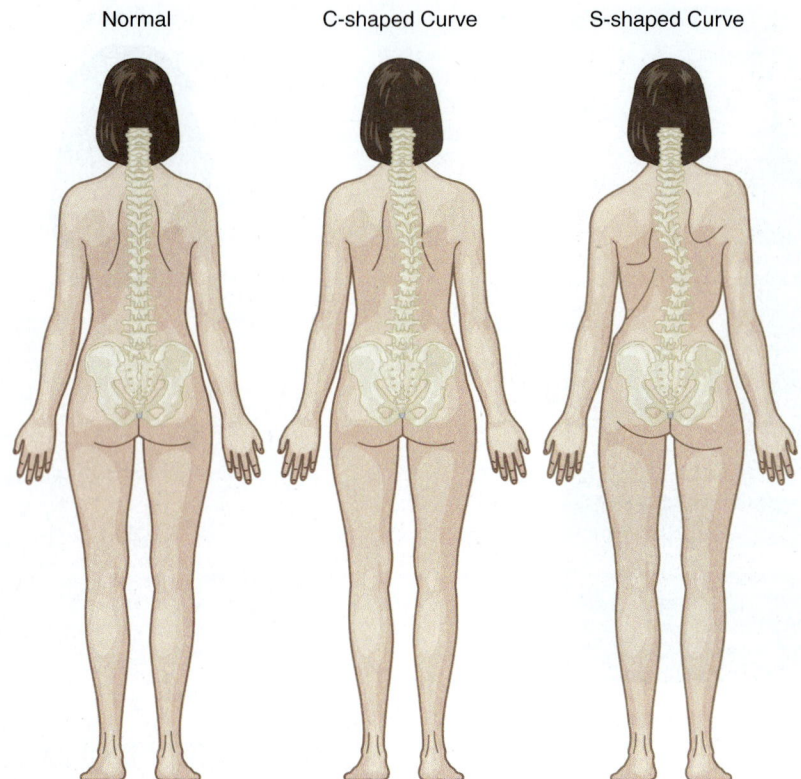

Figure 12.26 Drawing showing scoliosis: C curve versus S curve.

© Jones & Bartlett Learning

characterized by the absence of the frontal plane lumbar lordosis, a flat thoracic spine with a slight kyphosis in the upper thoracic spinal segments, extension at the terminal segments of the cervical column, and a forward head (**Figure 12.28**). Similarly, a swayback posture is hallmarked by a forward head and slight cervical extension but a more remarkable and lengthy

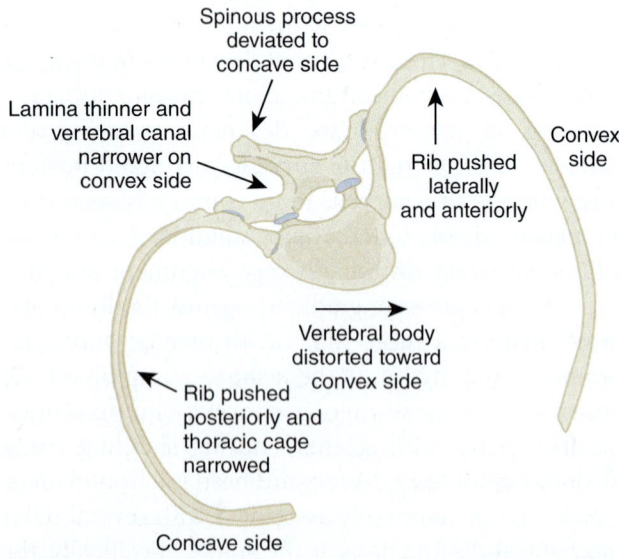

Figure 12.27 Drawing showing the ipsilateral rib cage hump.

© Jones & Bartlett Learning

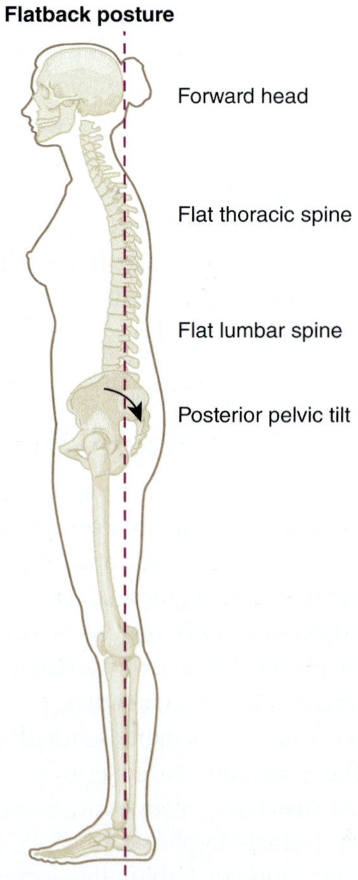

Figure 12.28 Drawing showing flatback posture.

© Jones & Bartlett Learning

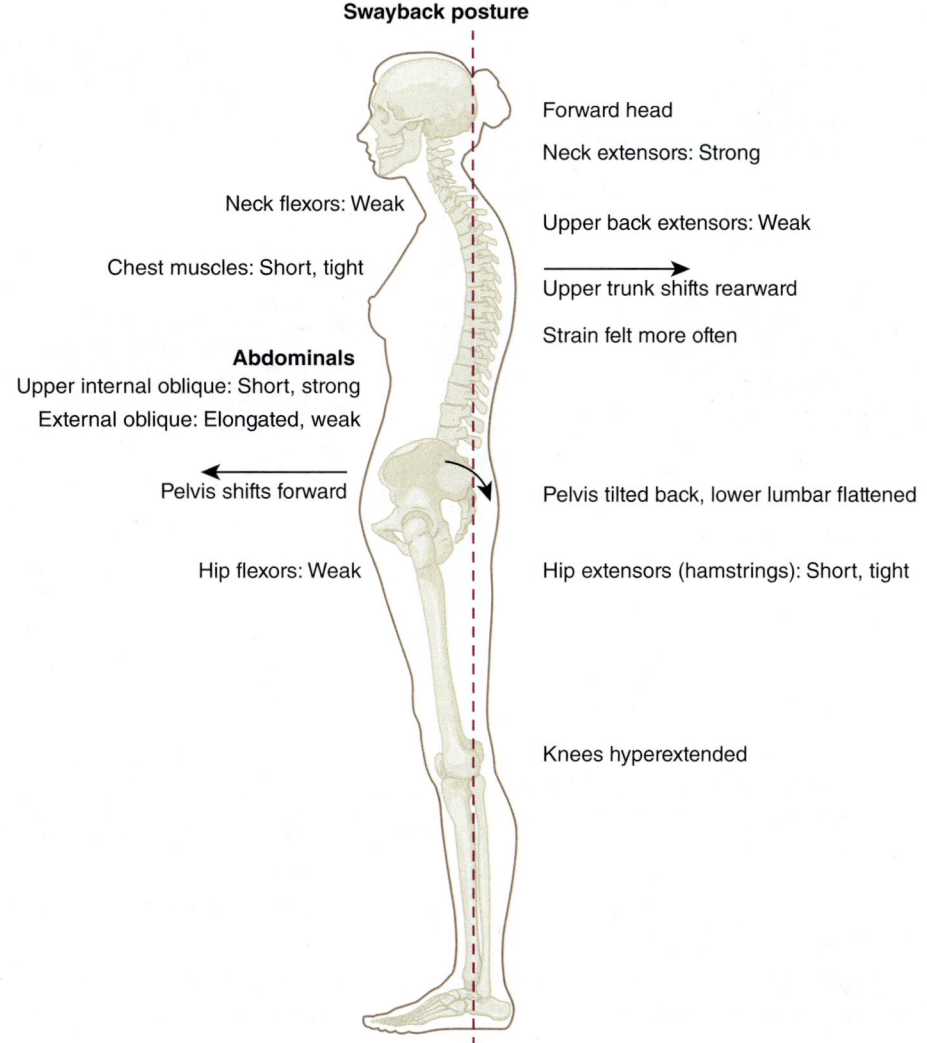

Figure 12.29 Drawing showing swayback posture.
© Jones & Bartlett Learning

swayed/flexed kyphotic thoracic spine, flat lumbar spine, and posterior tilted pelvis. Typically, this results in the hips and knees being hyperextended to balance the center of mass (**Figure 12.29**). An excessive lumbar lordosis, or anterior curve, in the spine often is the result of an anteriorly rotated pelvis. Elongation and weakness in the abdominal muscles combined with tight hip flexors and back erector spinae extensors compromises the level state of the pelvis, creating a sagittal postural defect. Thoracic kyphosis, or an extreme posterior curve to the thoracic spine, is commonly the result of congenital factors, such as Scheuermann disease, or compensatory habitual factors. This sagittal malalignment is often associated with shoulder girdle dysfunction and cervical column adaptations, such as cervical hyperextension and a forward head.[17,32,106,107]

Often, a combination of postural defects between the spine and the extremities and adjacent regions results in upper-cross and lower-cross syndromes (**Figure 12.30**). The upper- and lower-cross syndromes are theorized to be habitual neuromuscular defects, rather than structural in nature. Isolated muscle tightness/lengthening and hypotonic or hypertonic activity in the muscles about the upper and lower spine and extremities create dysfunctional motor patterns, resulting in systematic musculoskeletal compensation and postural disruptions. Upper cross syndrome is the result of muscular weakness and lengthening of the rhomboids, serratus anterior, and lower trapezius muscles associated with hypertonic/tight upper trapezius, levator scapula, and pectoralis muscle activation. It is characterized by a forward head, excessive cervical lordosis, thoracic kyphosis, elevated and protracted scapula/shoulder girdle, and winging of the scapula. In lower cross syndrome, the thoracolumbar extensors and hip flexors become tight/hypertonic, while the abdominals and gluteus maximus lengthen and become weak. The combination of tight muscles and weak muscles, from a side view, is seen as an X (or cross). In both conditions the

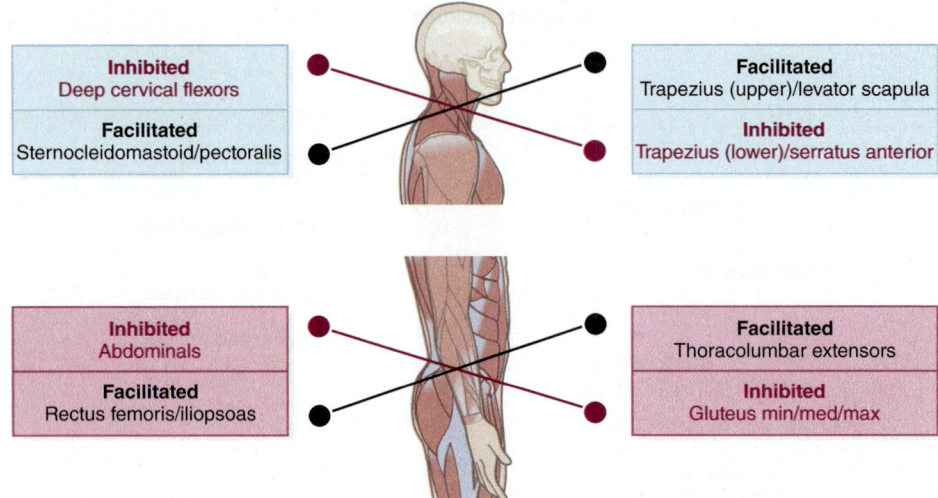

Figure 12.30 Drawing explaining upper and lower cross syndromes.
© Jones & Bartlett Learning

lengthened muscles become neurologically inhibited as the tight hypertonic muscles become mechanically dysfunctional.[16,19,108,109] The imbalance creates joint dysfunction, particularly at the atlanto-occipital joint, C4–C5 segment, cervicothoracic joint, glenohumeral joint, and T4–T5 segment.

Cervical Spine Inspection

Evaluation of the cervical spine should begin with inspection of any postural abnormalities or structural asymmetries. The anterior prominence of the hyoid bone and thyroid cartilage as well as the orientation of the head to the cervical vertebrae help to establish a basis for anatomic orientation. Being able to identify the skull's occipital inion; superior nuchal line; mastoid process; mental region/chin with the erect lordotic cervical curve; C7 spinous process; thyroid cartilage; and corresponding contour of the trapezius, deep paraspinal muscles, sternocleidomastoid, and supporting musculature of the shoulder girdle is a critical foundation for a cervical spine orthopaedic assessment.[1,2,9,11]

Thoracic Spine Inspection

Normal spinal posture and function should be evaluated, noting symmetry and observable abnormalities. Common postural thoracic abnormalities, such as kyphosis, scoliosis, and rib-augmented variations, are standard foundational influences for injury.[110,111] General posture and gait analysis, noting asymmetries or inappropriate movement sequences, should be performed to monitor skeletal contributors to injury rooted to the thoracic spine or outriggers of the thoracic cage[112,113] (**Figure 12.31**).

Lumbar Spine Inspection

Normal spinal posture and function should be evaluated, noting symmetry and observable abnormalities. Common postural thoracic and lumbar abnormalities such as kyphosis, scoliosis, and lordosis are standard foundational influences for injury.[114-116] Noted asymmetries in muscle tone or atrophy in the gluteal muscles or leg/thigh could be indicative of a deficit in nerve root transfer. General posture and gait analysis, noting asymmetries or inappropriate movement sequences, should be made to monitor skeletal contributors to injury.[99,100,102,117-119] Often, individuals with disk or nerve root pain avoid loading the spine or a given pathological leg. Upon standing up from a seated position, these individuals will use their upper body strength to lift themselves out of a chair and generally offload a pathological leg.

Palpation

Cervical Spine Palpation

The prominences of musculoskeletal structures serve as landmarks for primary palpation and postural references.[94] The inion serves as a center point for palpation of the center of the spine. At approximately one fingerbreadth inferior lies the area of the C2–C7 spinous process. Lateral to the spinous processes, left and right, are the facet joints and paraspinal muscles. The anterior hyoid bone, thyroid cartilage, and the first cricoid ring serve sequentially as primary landmarks for the approximate location of the posterior C3–C6 facet joints.[2,6,9,11] Pathology is often detected by palpable defect, pain, asymmetry, muscle spasm, and/or localized

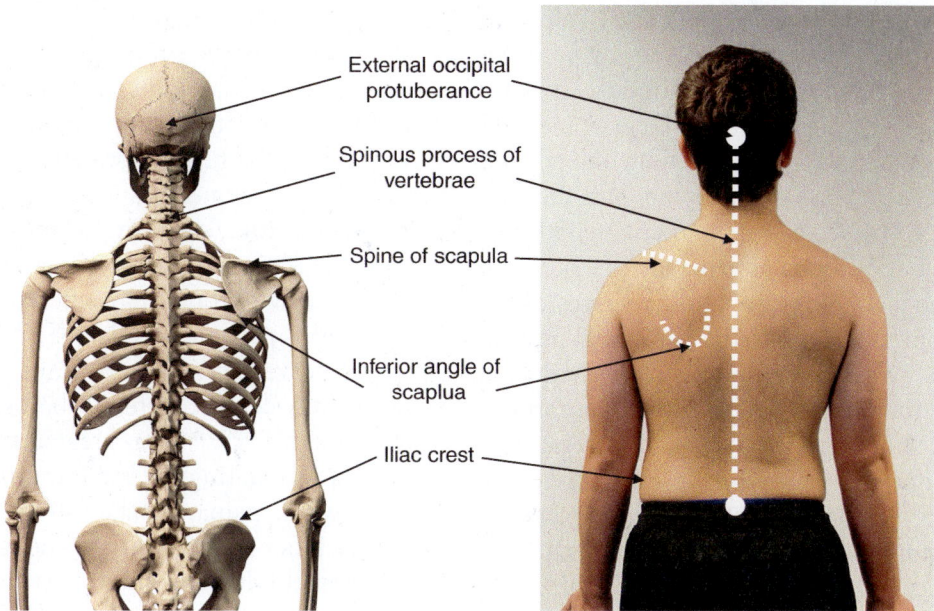

Figure 12.31 Illustration of the palpation and bony landmarks for thoracic and lumbar spine.
(Left) © iStockphoto/Thinkstock; (Right) © Jones & Bartlett Learning

pain. Although nerve root, disk, and facet pathologies are common in the areas between C5 and C7, dexterity in palpation is often required to determine these pathologies.[11,120] Distal neurologic symptoms (C5-C8) may be exasperated by palpation or movement, resulting in a stenosis or pressure on the spinal facets.[86,120-122]

The posterior muscles, such as the trapezius, the levator scapulae, and the paraspinal muscles, cover a portion of the spinal segments; thus, palpation may require the patient to lie down to relax and reduce the muscle tone. The trapezius muscle shares a common proximal attachment at the base of the skull with the anterior lateral sternocleidomastoid muscle and is extremely active, as its broad origin spans from the inion to T12.[2] The levator scapulae has a broad attachment from the transverse process of C1-C4 to the superior angle and medial border of the scapula. The upper one-third of the trapezius extends the spine and elevates the shoulder girdle, whereas the levator scapulae elevates the superior angle of the scapula, which laterally rotates the scapula, bringing the inferior angle of the scapula closer to the spine. All three of these muscles work bilaterally and unilaterally to laterally flex the cervical spine. Assisting these muscles are the anterolateral anterior/medial/posterior scalenus muscles.[2,10] The close orientation of the scalenus muscles and related structures with the neurovascular bundles (plexuses) of the neck often contributes to injury or complications of the cervical and brachial plexus from compressive or distraction mechanisms, such as burners/stingers[2,10,123] (**Figure 12.32**).

Thoracic Spine Palpation

The traditional orientation of the thoracic spine between the cervical and lumbar spines makes it easy to palpate. Further, the large reference landmarks of the skull and the scapula provide additional assurance

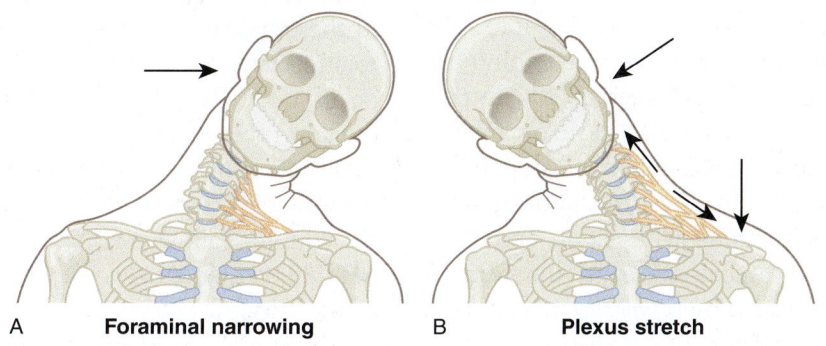

A **Foraminal narrowing**   B **Plexus stretch**

Figure 12.32 Drawings showing brachial plexus neurapraxia.
© Jones & Bartlett Learning

in identifying specific thoracic landmarks. Palpation of the C7 spinous process serves as a starting point for the prominence of the proceeding thoracic spinous processes T1-T12.[98,124] The superior angle, spine, and inferior angle of the scapula align with the second rib, third spinous process of the spine, and the seventh rib of the thoracic cage. The intervertebral disk space and nerve root foramen generally are lateral to and at the same level of the spinous processes of the superior vertebrae and deep to the paraspinal musculature.[125] These areas are commonly associated with palpable pain from a nerve root, disk, facet, and/or muscle strain. Thoracic spine pain and visceral pain can mimic symptoms that originate from T1 to the lumbar spine.[126] Segments T4-T7 have the potential to cause chest pain as well as symptoms generated by a cough, sneeze, rapid breathing, forceful palpation, and/or compression of the thoracic cage.[98,124,127] Palpation and light pressure along the corresponding ribs and vertebral transverse processes help to establish thoracic cage stability and spinal joint integrity.

Lumbar Spine Palpation

Specialized palpation should include landmarks of the specific spinous processes and corresponding disk spaces from T12-L1 to the spine of the sacrum and the coccyx bone. The prominence of the skeletal anatomy is often hindered by the lumbosacral fascia, the supraspinous and interspinous ligaments, paraspinal muscles, and multifidi and quadratus lumborum muscles. If possible, placing the patient in slight spinal flexion, seated or lying prone with a pillow under the abdominal area, will help to increase the exposure of the lumbar skeletal anatomy. When performing palpation, it is important to understand that, in many cases, it may be difficult to isolate specific muscle, fascia, and skeletal anatomy, and so understanding the location of specific landmarks and regions of the lumbar spine will assist in identifying pathologic tissues.[99,103,128]

A good place to start palpation is the apex of the iliac crest. The vertebral space between spinous processes L4 and L5 can be palpated at the same level as the iliac crest and serve as a primary reference for the remaining skeletal anatomy.[5,7,11,80] Palpating inferiorly from the iliac crest to the posterior superior iliac spine will line up with the S2 spinous process. The intervertebral disk space and transverse process for L4 can be located by palpating in a lateral and deep fashion the inferior aspect of the L4 spinous process. The inferior and superior transverse processes, nerve root disk segments, and area of the vertebral bodies can be palpated superior and inferior along the spinous process. Inability to locate a spinous process may indicate spina bifida, a congenital defect, or a skeletal disruption, such as a spondylolysis, warranting further investigation.[79-81,129] Palpation of the lumbar segments should serve to identify specific nerve root, disk, or facet pathology. Therefore, palpable pain at the spine associated with distal radicular symptoms may offer insight to a disk or nerve root pathology.[11,15,118,130,131] The branch of the sciatic nerve can be found in the sciatic notch of the pelvis between the ischial tuberosity and the greater trochanter.[118,130,131] The greater trochanter is easily located by rotating the hip joint internally and externally while palpating the lateral hip. Knee flexion will facilitate accessibility of the ischial tuberosity in the gluteal fold. The anterior structures of the spine are difficult to access due to the depth of soft tissue in the abdominal region. The L5-S1 articulation may be accessible inferior and lateral to the umbilicus in a supine, knees-flexed position. Palpable pain in this area usually indicates potential sacroiliac joint and/or L5-S1 disk pathology, abdominal herniation, or muscle tightness/strain.

Table 12.3 discusses manual muscle testing of the spine.

Special Tests

Range of Motion Assessment

Cervical Range of Motion Assessment. Active and passive range of motion (ROM) should be assessed in all three planes, monitoring for function and compensation tendencies. The skeletal orientation of C1-C7 requires the spinal segments to work synergistically to achieve spinal flexion, extension, rotation, and lateral flexion. General mechanical stress for flexion and extension requires spinal segments to slide on preceding segments in the sagittal plane, adding compressive and distractive stressors anteriorly and posteriorly, respectively, for flexion; extension would result in the opposite motions[10,86,132] (**Figure 12.33**). Cervical rotation requires the first 35° to 45° of axial rotation to occur at the C1-C2 joint. Additional rotation in either direction requires the lower segments to displace and rotate anterior and posterior at each preceding segment. Lateral bending requires coupling motions. Spinal coupling allows segments to work independently in multiple planes to accomplish single planar motions of the cervical column. C2-C7 coupling motions for lateral bending require the inferior segments to translate inferior and posterior to the bending side while the opposite facet joints slide superior and anterior

Table 12.3 Spine Manual Muscle Testing

Muscle	Manual Muscle Test	Figure of Manual Muscle Test
Spinal extensors	Patient is prone on table with hands interlocked behind head. Examiner stabilizes patient's lower legs. Full strength is ability to perform movement off table. If needed, examiner can assist patient to lift chest off table and then patient should be instructed to hold position.	
Quadratus lumborum	Patient prone. Patient abducts and extends leg. Examiner provides traction on the extremity, opposite to the line of pull of the muscle.	
Upper abdominal muscles	Patient supine with legs extended. The patient is instructed to perform a trunk flexion sit-up. Grading is accomplished by the hand position during the sit-up. Normal: Hand clasped behind head, patient is able to complete full sit-up (A). Good: Arms are folded across chest, patient is able to complete full sit-up (B). Fair: With arms extended forward, patient is able to complete full sit-up (C).	

(continues)

Chapter 12 Spine

Table 12.3 Spine Manual Muscle Testing (continued)

Muscle	Manual Muscle Test	Figure of Manual Muscle Test
Lower abdominal muscles	Patient supine with hips flexed to 90° and knees extended; forearms should be folded across chest. Patient is instructed to posterior tilt pelvis so low back is flat against table. Patient is then instructed to slowly lower legs to table while maintaining the low back position against table. Examiner may place one hand beside low back to help determine point to grade. Grading is based on the ability to keep the low back flat against the table. The grade is assigned at the time the low back comes off the table. Normal: Patient is able to maintain position while lowering legs to the table (complete range of motion) (A). Good: Patient is able to keep low back against surface until legs less than 30° from table (B). Fair: Patient is able to keep low back against surface until legs are less than 60° from table (C).	*Courtesy of Andrea Cripps.*
Anterolateral neck flexors	Patient supine. Examiner puts pressure on the temporal region of the head.	© Jones & Bartlett Learning
Posterolateral neck extensors	Patient prone and instructed to extend and rotate head. Examiner puts pressure on posterior lateral portion of head and pushes into an anterolateral direction.	© Jones & Bartlett Learning

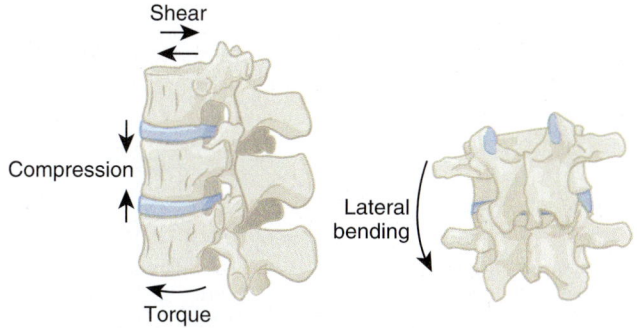

Figure 12.33 Drawing showing compressive and shear forces on vertebrae.

© Jones & Bartlett Learning

(**Figure 12.34**). Isolated manual muscle testing for the sternocleidomastoid, upper trapezius, scalene, and levator scapulae muscles is often associated with establishing specific functional capacities for the cervical column. Ancillary motions for the glenohumeral, scapular, thoracic, abdominal, and pelvic regions may also provide insight into the mechanical capacities of the cervical spine.[86,133,134]

Lumbar Spine ROM Assessment. Active and passive ROM should be assessed in all three planes, monitoring function and compensation tendencies.[116,135] The skeletal orientation of the T1–T12 and L1–L5 vertebrae requires the spinal segments to work synergistically to achieve spinal flexion, extension, rotation, and lateral flexion. The thoracic spine is classified as a mobility region of the spine, whereas the lumbar spine is classified as retaining stability. Thus, isolated and combined ROM assessments should be performed for flexion, extension, and rotation. General thoracic and lumbar flexion and extension are 55°/45° and 75°/30°, respectively.[101,136] Lateral flexion and rotation for the thoracic and lumbar regions are roughly 45°/40° and 25°/20°, respectively.[101,124,127,137] Often, pathologies arise when the thoracic and/or the hip region lacks mobility, which forces the lumbar spine to attain injurious increases in motion. Thus, assessing motion with a tape measure and/or a goniometer will obtain a baseline measure of mobility. Holding or locking the hips and/or lumbar spine in place will allow for an isolated mobility assessment for the flexion, extension, and rotation of the thoracic and lumbar spine.

Neurologic Testing

The prevalence of nerve injury or complications suggests sensory and motor neurologic assessments should accompany not only an orthopaedic spine evaluation but all orthopaedic evaluations. Neurologic evaluations should include the assessment of myotomes, dermatomes, and reflexes.

Peripheral nerve assessment for the cervical upper extremity branches will include the radial, ulnar, median, axillary, and musculocutaneous nerves. Neurologic assessments of the lumbar and sacral regions are often common practice for lower extremity screenings, as they relate to orthopaedic evaluations and/or vertebral disk or nerve pathologies. Common deficits in both motor and sensory output are often the result of a vertebrae, disk, or degenerative disruption, such as spondylolisthesis, spondylolysis, compression fracture, disk lesion, and/or a nerve root stenosis. This relationship between the peripheral nerve roots in the plexuses and the upper and lower extremities prompts evaluators to consider dermatome and myotome assessments of the nerve root branches as a regular practice for all orthopaedic upper extremity and/or cervical spine evaluations.[117]

Dermatome and Myotome Testing. A dermatome is an area of skin innervated by cutaneous neurons of a spinal or cranial nerve. Myotomes are a muscle or group of muscles innervated by a spinal or cranial nerve. The dermatomal pattern for the body is shown in **Figure 12.35**. **Table 12.4** summarizes the specific spinal nerve functions and how to functionally examine them.

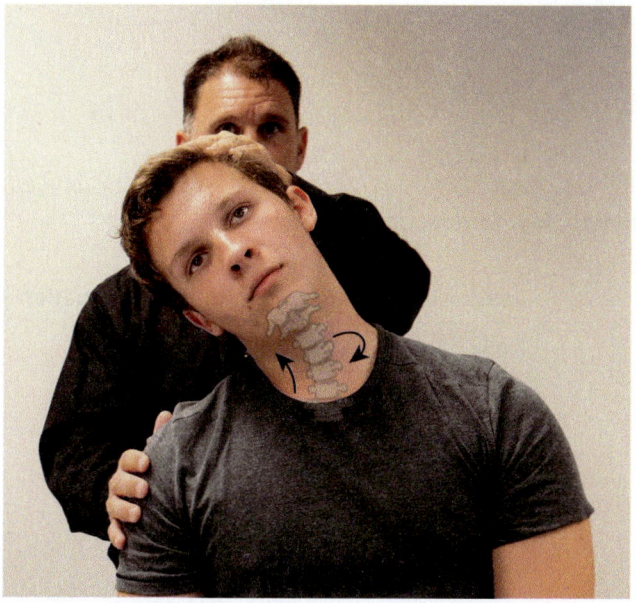

Figure 12.34 Photograph showing lateral bending coupling.

© Jones & Bartlett Learning

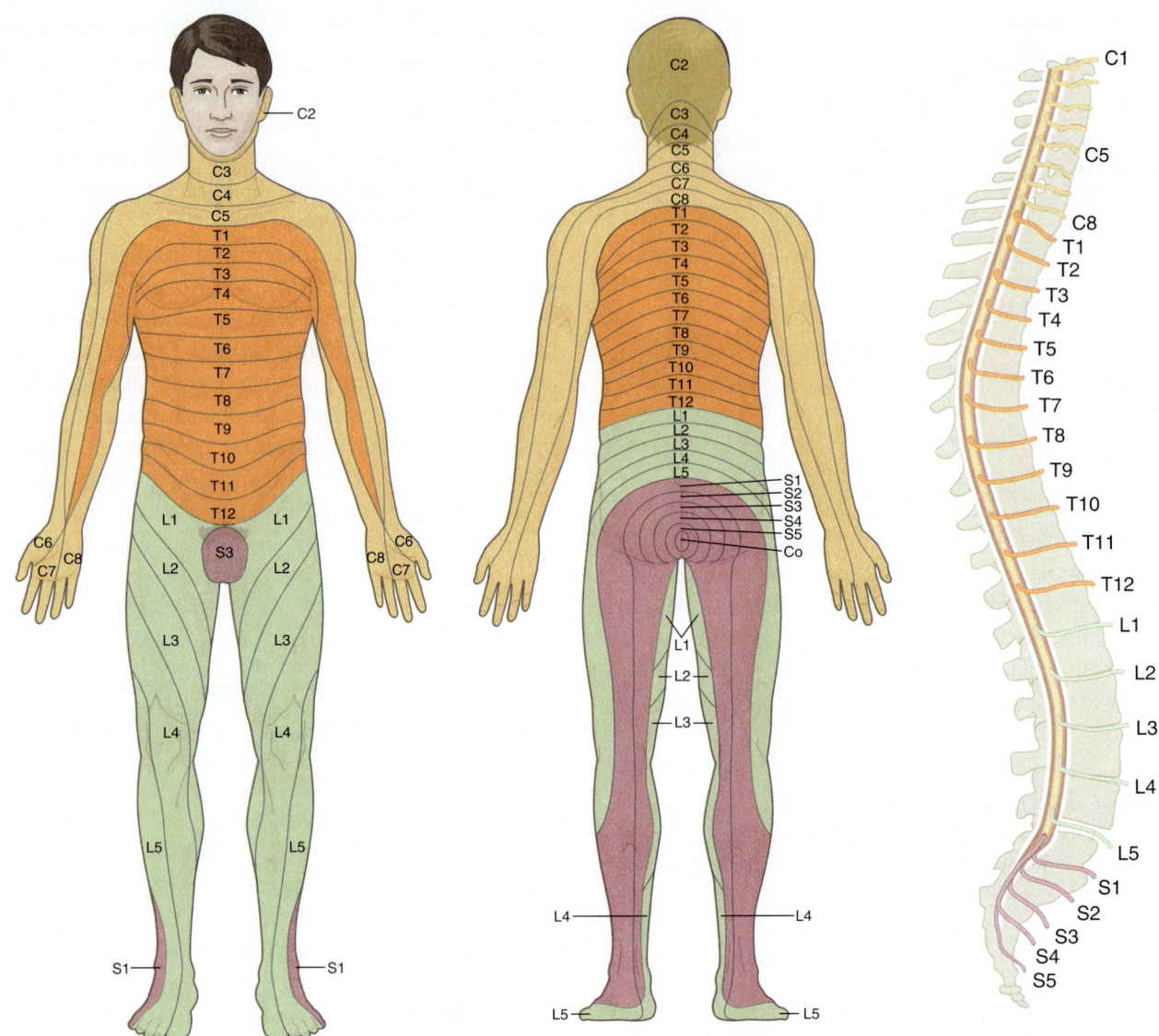

Figure 12.35 Drawings showing the dermatomal chart.
© Jones & Bartlett Learning

Table 12.4 Spinal Nerve Roots and Associated Dermatomes, Myotomes, and Reflexes

Nerve Root	Dermatome (Sensory)	Myotome (Motor)	Associated Reflex	Functional Examination
C1	Vertex of skull	Upper neck muscle	None	Upper cervical flexion
C2	Temple, forehead, occiput	Upper neck muscle	None	Upper cervical extension/neck rotation
C3	Entire neck, posterior cheek, temporal area	Upper trapezius, splenius capitis	None	Cervical lateral flexion
C4	Top of shoulder, clavicular area	Upper trapezius, levator scapulae	None	Shoulder shrug
C5	Deltoid insertion, anterior aspect of arm to base of first digit	Supraspinatus, infraspinatus, deltoid, biceps brachii	Biceps brachii	Shoulder abduction and external rotation

Nerve Root	Dermatome (Sensory)	Myotome (Motor)	Associated Reflex	Functional Examination
C6	Anterior arm, radial side of hand to first and second digits	Biceps brachii, supinator, wrist extensors	Biceps brachii, brachioradialis	Elbow flexion and wrist extension
C7	Lateral arm and forearm to fourth and fifth digits	Triceps brachii, wrist flexors	Triceps brachii	Elbow extension and wrist flexion
C8	Medial side of forearm to fourth and fifth digits	Ulnar deviators, extensors and adductors of thumb	None	Thumb extension and ulnar deviation
T1	Medial arm and forearm to wrist	Intrinsic muscles of the hands (except opponens pollicis and abductor pollicis brevis)	None	Finger adduction and abduction
T2	Medial side of upper arm to medial elbow, pectoral, and midscapular area	Intercostal muscles	None	Proper breathing technique
T3-T12	Circumferential rings at level of nerve root	Intercostal muscles and abdominal muscles	None	None
L1	Lower abdomen, groin, L2-L4, upper and outer aspect of buttocks	Quadratus lumborum	None	Hip flexion
L2	Lower lumber region, upper buttocks, anterior thigh	Iliopsoas, quadriceps	None	Hip flexion (adduction and medial rotation)
L3	Medial aspect of thigh to knee, anterior aspect of lower thigh to just below patella	Psoas, quadriceps	Patella	Leg/knee extension
L4	Medial aspect of lower leg and foot, great toe	Tibialis anterior, extensor hallucis, extensor digitorum longus, peroneals	Patella	Dorsiflexion
L5	Lateral border of leg, anterior surface of lower leg, dorsum of foot, second to fourth toes	Extensor hallucis longus, extensor digitorum longus, peroneal, gluteus maximus, gluteus medius, dorsiflexors	None	First toe extension
S1	Posterior aspect of lower leg, foot (including heel), lateral border of foot and sole	Gastrocnemius, soleus, gluteus maximus, gluteus medius, hamstrings, peroneals	Achilles	Ankle plantarflexion and eversion
S2	Posterior middle of leg from three-quarters way down leg to gluteal fold	Gastrocnemius, soleus, gluteus maximus, hamstring group	None	Knee flexion
S3	Groin, medial thigh to knee	Intrinsic foot muscles	None	None
S4	Perineum, genitals, lower sacrum	Bladder, rectum	None	Bladder and rectum function
S5	Perianal	Coccygeus muscle	None	Bladder and rectum function
Co	Skin of back of coccyx	None	None	Bladder and rectum function

Testing Considerations for Dermatome and Myotome Status

Dermatome Testing

- Test for abnormalities in sensitivity by using a filament, pinwheel, paper clip, or fingernail.
- Superficial sensation: Touch dermatomes with cotton.
- Superficial pain: Touch dermatomes with sharp, rather than dull, object.
- Deep pressure pain: Squeeze a muscle.
- Sensitivity of temperature: Touch dermatomes with ice cube.
- Sensitivity of vibration: Touch dermatomes with tuning fork.
- Position sense: Move fingers, toes, and extremities passively and ask patient to indicate body position.
- With eyes closed, the patient gives feedback with regard to various stimuli.
- All tests should be compared bilaterally (**Figure 12.36**).

Myotome Testing

- Functional movements against gravity with and without resistance
- Full range of motion with isometric, isotonic, and/or functional tasks
- All tests should be compared bilaterally.

Reflex Testing

Deep tendon reflexes include C5 (biceps tendon), C6 (brachioradialis tendon), C7 (triceps tendon), L4 (patellar tendon), L5 (hamstrings), and S1 (Achilles tendon). **Table 12.5** outlines how reflexes are graded.

There are four pathologic reflexes. A positive test indicates a lesion in the descending upper motor neurons (**Figure 12.37**).

- Babinski: Slide a smooth, pointed object along the lateral plantar surface and metatarsal heads of the foot; positive test produces extension and splaying of toes.
- Chaddock rub: Glide a smooth, pointed object along peroneals distal to the lateral malleolus; positive test produces extension and splaying of toes.

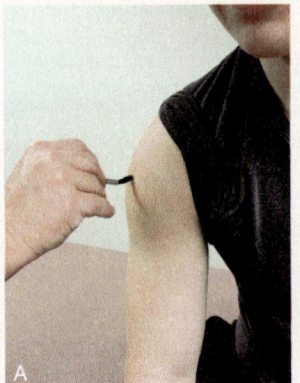
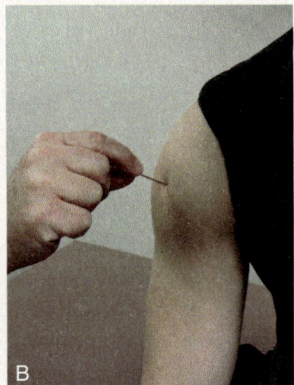
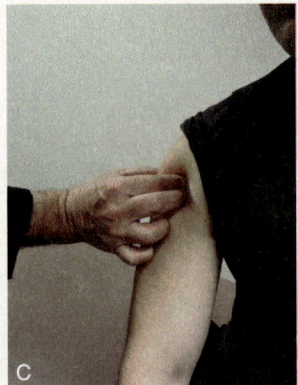
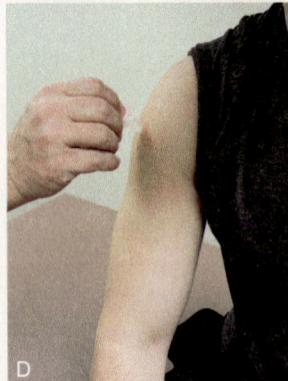
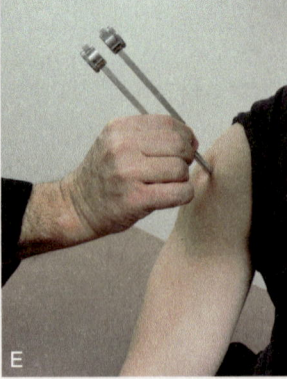

Figure 12.36 Photographs of dermatome testing. **A.** Superficial sensation. **B.** Superficial pain. **C.** Deep pressure pain. **D.** Sensitivity of temperature. **E.** Sensitivity of vibration.

Courtesy of Andrea Cripps.

Table 12.5 Reflex Grading

Result	Grade	Definition
Absence of reflex	0	Areflexia
Diminished reflex	1	Hyporeflexia
Average/normal reflex	2	Against gravity/resistance
Exaggerated reflex	3	Hyperreflexia (increased but not pathologic)
Markedly hyperactive	4	Often associated with clonus, but clonus is not required for grade 4

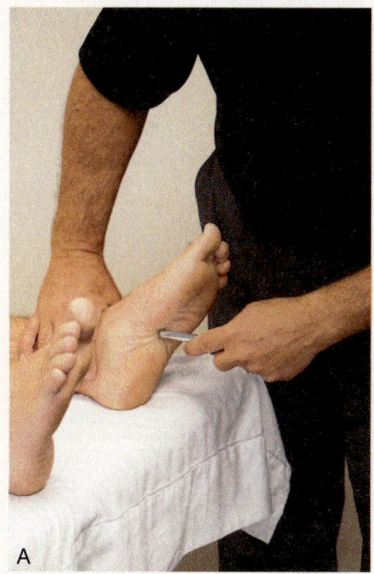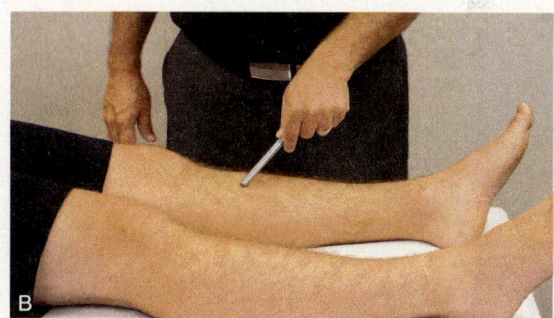

Figure 12.37 Photographs of two of the four pathologic reflexes. **A.** Babinski test. **B.** Oppenheim test.
© Jones & Bartlett Learning

- Oppenheim test: Glide a smooth, pointed object proximal to distal along the crest of the tibia; positive test produces extension and splaying of toes.
- Clonus test: Forcefully and quickly dorsiflex the foot from a relaxed position; positive test produces a rhythmic plantar flexion to dorsiflexion "beating" of the foot in the hand.

Superficial reflexes are those elicited by stimulation of the skin for a reflex muscle contraction:

- Upper abdominal (T7-T9), lower abdominal (T11-T12), cremasteric (T12-L1), plantar (S1-S2), and gluteal (L4-S3)
- Absence of superficial reflexes is indicative of a lesion in the descending corticospinal tract.

A summary of special tests[138-166] can be found in **Table 12.6**.

Common Spine Pathologies

Spinal Body Fracture

Fracture to spinal vertebrae often results from traumatic episodes of compressive or shear mechanisms and can be experienced at all segments of the spinal column (Figure 12.33). Osteoporotic conditions or weakening of the bone as a result of age or poor nutrition will compromise the integrity of the bone and increase the occurrence of fractures about the spinal column. Often resulting from high-velocity direct blows, traumatic falls from heights, and/or repetitive traumatic compressive forces, these fractures can be associated with spinal cord injury or damage to adjacent structures. In addition, fracture to the transverse process can result from severe rotational and/or lateral bending mechanisms. Common signs and symptoms for traumatic episodes include severe, localized, palpable, and descriptive pain at the site of the fracture with an antalgic trunk

538 Chapter 12 Spine

Table 12.6 Orthopaedic Special Tests

Special Test	Patient Positioning	Test Procedure	Positive Test	Indications	Evidence
Cervical distraction test	Supine or seated	Secure the base of the skull from a neutral spine position and apply a steady traction/distraction force	Relief of localized or radicular pain	Nerve root compression/stenosis, disk compression, facet pathology/compression	Interrater reliability = 0.50 Sensitivity = 0.43 Specificity = 0.985
Cervical foramina compression test	Seated or standing with cervical collar in a neutral position	Apply downward compression to cervical spine from the top of the head for 10 seconds	Increase in pain and signs/symptoms related to facet or nerve	Nerve root stenosis causing a compression/impingement, facet joint irritation	Interrater reliability = 0.61 Sensitivity = 0.83 Specificity = 0.34
Jackson cervical foramina rotation compression test	Seated or standing with cervical collar rotated to one side	Apply downward compression to the cervical spine from the top of the head for 10 seconds	Increase in pain and signs/symptoms related to facet or nerve to the rotated side	Nerve root compression of cervical spine while rotated to involved side. Nerve root compression from disk, osteophyte, or tumor	

© Jones & Bartlett Learning

Common Spine Pathologies

Test	Position	Action	Positive Finding	Implication	Statistics
Spurling cervical foramina compression test	Seated or standing with cervical collar rotated, laterally flexed, and extended to one side	Apply downward compression to the cervical spine from the top of the head for 10 seconds	Increase in pain and signs/symptoms related to facet or nerve to the rotated side	Nerve root compression of cervical spine while rotated/extended to involved side. Nerve root compression from disk, osteophyte, or tumor	Interrater reliability = 0.46; Sensitivity = 0.55; Specificity = 0.92
Valsalva test	Seated or standing with cervical collar in a neutral position	Hold breath and bear down	Increase in pain and signs/symptoms related to nerve pathology	Intrathecal (spinal cord) pressure from space occupying lesion, tumor, disk, or osteophyte	Interrater reliability = 0.63; Sensitivity = 0.73; Specificity = 0.95
Swallow test	Seated or standing with cervical collar in a neutral position	Perform a forceful and exaggerated swallow	Increase in pain and signs/symptoms while swallowing	Bony impingement, osteophyte, or soft-tissue swelling in anterior portion of canal	
Lhermitte sign	Long sit	Perform a simultaneous neck and hip flexion with knees fully extended	Pain and/or signs/symptoms along a spinal nerve into upper/lower extremities	Irritation of cervical spine dural/meningeal areas	

(continues)

Table 12.6 Orthopaedic Special Tests (continued)

Special Test	Patient Positioning	Test Procedure	Positive Test	Indications	Evidence
Shoulder abduction test (Bakody sign)	Seated or standing	Abduct shoulder, flex elbow, and rest hand at the top of the head	Decrease in pain or diminished signs and symptoms	Potential vascular problem, disk lesion, or nerve root compression to C4-C5 or C5-C6 level	Interrater reliability = 0.20-0.21 Sensitivity = 0.43 Specificity = 0.90
Shoulder traction-depression test	Seated, standing, or supine	Simultaneously perform passive or active lateral flexion of cervical spine away from involved side while placing downward pressure on shoulder of involved side	Increase in neurologic symptoms and/or pain indicates brachial plexus	Increases in symptoms could indicate potential thoracic outlet syndrome Brachial plexus for affected side, cervical spine foramina encroachment, or osteophyte for opposite side	Preliminary data
Vertebral artery test	Supine with head off end of table	Examiner passively extends cervical spine, and the head is then passively rotated and held to one side for 30 seconds. Repeat procedure on opposite side. Note: Examiner must watch patient's pupillary response during test.	Dizziness, nystagmus, pupil changes (unilaterally), nausea, confusion	Vertebral artery occlusion (cervical)	Sensitivity = 0.67 Specificity = 0.86

Common Spine Pathologies **541**

Disk test		Seated, standing, or supine	Active or passive hyperflexion and lateral flexion of cervical spine away from involved side	Increase in neurologic symptoms and/or pain at the posterior-lateral disk space	Disk lesion, vertebral fracture, or ligament sprain	
Brachial plexus Tinel test		Seated, standing, or supine	Tapping over brachial plexus superior to the middle third of the scapula	Increase in radiating symptoms and/or pain	Brachial plexus nerve lesion	Limited data available
Brachial plexus squeeze test		Seated or standing	Examiner squeezes clavicle and brachial plexus into upper trapezius and scapula	Increase in radiating symptoms and/or pain	Brachial plexus nerve lesion	Sensitivity = 0.63 Specificity = 0.67

(continues)

Table 12.6 Orthopaedic Special Tests

Special Test	Patient Positioning	Test Procedure	Positive Test	Indications	Evidence
Median nerve test (Elvey test #1)	Shoulder abduction to 110°, maintain posture noted previously, extend wrist and fingers with forearm supination, extend elbow last Modification of this test (Evans test): Active abduction to 90° with elbow flexed. Patient then extends shoulder with head laterally flexed to the opposite side, followed by elbow extension	Perform shoulder position first, followed by other joints, saving the elbow position for last	Increase in radiating symptoms and/or pain	Nerve lesion or related nerve stenosis	Sensitivity = 0.3 Specificity = 0.8
Median, musculocutaneous, and axillary nerve test (Elvey test #2)	Abduct shoulder to minus 10° and externally rotate while maintaining posture noted previously, followed by same joint positions as Elvey test #1	Perform shoulder position first, followed by other joints, saving the elbow position for last	Increase in radiating symptoms and/or pain	Nerve lesion or related nerve stenosis	Sensitivity = 0.3 Specificity = 0.8

(continued)

Courtesy of Andrea Cripps.

Common Spine Pathologies **543**

Radial nerve test (Elvey test #3)	Abduct shoulder to 10° with internal rotation while maintaining posture noted previously, wrist and finger flexion with ulnar deviation and pronation, elbow extension last	Perform shoulder position first, followed by other joints, saving the elbow position for last	Increase in radiating symptoms and/or pain	Nerve lesion or related nerve stenosis	Limited data available
Ulnar nerve test (Elvey test #4)	Abduct shoulder to 90° with external rotation while maintaining posture noted previously, wrist and finger extension with radial deviation and supination, elbow flexed toward head last Modification of the test (Evans test): Active abduction to point of discomfort, then externally rotate to point of symptoms; clinician holds the position for the patient while the patient actively flexes the elbow to place hands behind head (brachial plexus tension test)	Perform shoulder position first, followed by other joints, saving the elbow position for last	Increase in radiating symptoms and/or pain	Nerve lesion or related nerve stenosis	Sensitivity = 0.45 Specificity = 0.71

Courtesy of Andrea Cripps.

(continues)

Table 12.6 Orthopaedic Special Tests (continued)

Special Test	Patient Positioning	Test Procedure	Positive Test	Indications	Evidence
Straight leg raise (SLR) test (Laseque test)	Supine	Assist patient into straight leg hip flexion to a point of pain, then reduce hip flexion slightly and dorsiflex foot/ankle (Bragard test)	Pain during SLR and reproduced with dorsiflexion in lumbar spine (disk or sciatic nerve) Pain in posterior thigh during SLR and not reproduced with dorsiflexion (muscle tightness) *If the patient reports no pain and is able to get to 80° of hip flexion, any reported symptoms are likely from another pathology.	Indications: Nerve root compression, disk pathology, or muscle tightness *Note: Should be performed in tandem with tests for piriformis syndrome or hip	Interrater reliability = 0.68 Sensitivity = 0.68 Specificity = 0.56
Well straight leg raise test	Supine	Passively lift the uninvolved leg into a straight leg position	Pain or re-creation of neurologic symptoms to the opposite/affected side and or lumbar spine	Nerve root/disk space-occupying lesion	Sensitivity = 0.25 Specificity = 0.93
Slump test	Patient sitting in a slumped cervical and thoracic flexed position	Actively extend knee while examiner holds dorsiflexion of ankle	Increase in spine pain, radicular symptoms, or radicular pain in the leg	Suggests tension on sciatic nerve; many times, patient will extend neck or back to relieve pain, which then allows more knee extension	Interrater reliability = 0.95 Sensitivity = 0.42 Specificity = 0.73

Common Spine Pathologies **545**

Kernig test		Supine	Active straight leg raise with extended knee, knee is flexed actively upon the occurrence of pain	Pain reduction or relief of radicular symptoms	Nerve root impingement, disk-occupying lesion/bulge	Limited data available
Brudzinski/Kernig test		Supine	Passive cervical flexion combined with active/passive straight leg raise	Pain in lumbar, thoracic, and/or cervical spine, reproduction of spine pain or radicular symptoms	Nerve root impingement, disk-occupying lesion/bulge	Sensitivity = 0.47 Specificity = 0.68
Forward flexion test		Seated or standing	Perform forward spinal flexion	Pain at lumbar spine or posterior thigh, radicular symptoms localized to the spine and/or lower leg	Disk-occupying lesion, ligament; pain coming out of flexion may indicate muscular pathology ***Note:** Watch knee on affected side for bending to relieve sciatic tension	Sensitivity = 0.55 Specificity = 0.73

(continues)

Table 12.6 Orthopaedic Special Tests

Special Test	Patient Positioning	Test Procedure	Positive Test	Indications	Evidence
Hyperextension test	Seated or standing	With hands on hips, patient actively extends spine to maximum level	Localized lumbar pain, radicular symptoms	Spondylolisthesis/spondylolysis, sacroiliac joint pain, facet impingement	Limited data available
Stork stand (single leg hyperextension test)	Standing on single leg	With hands on hips, patient actively extends spine while balancing on a single leg to maximum level	Localized lumbar pain, radicular symptoms	Spondylolisthesis/spondylolysis, sacroiliac joint pain, facet impingement	Interrater reliability = 0.88–1.0 Sensitivity = 0.50–0.55 Specificity = 0.46–0.68

(continued)

Common Spine Pathologies **547**

Test	Position	Procedure	Positive findings	Pathology	Data
Quadrant test (Kemps sign)	Standing	Unilateral spine rotation and hyperextension	Localized lumbar pain, radicular symptoms to the side rotating	Sacroiliac joint pain, facet impingement, spinal stenosis	Limited data available
Bowstring test (cram or popliteal pressure sign)	Supine	Straight leg raise to pain, flex knee to 20° while thigh remains at the same level, apply pressure to the popliteal fossa *Variation: Sitting erect, passive knee extension to point of pain, lower slightly, finger pressure in popliteal fossa; increase in pain suggests sciatic nerve irritation	Localized lumbar pain, radicular symptoms	Increase in pain or radicular symptoms suggests the sciatic nerve is irritated or a potential disk or nerve root stenosis	Preliminary data Sensitivity = 0.42 Specificity = 0.77
Percussion test	Seated or prone	Clinician applies the thumb or the palm of his or her hand to a spinous process, then applies a percussion force with a reflex hammer, tuning fork, or the palm of a hand	Radicular and/or localized pain	Fracture, unstable spinal segment	Limited data available

(continues)

Table 12.6 Orthopaedic Special Tests *(continued)*

Special Test	Patient Positioning	Test Procedure	Positive Test	Indications	Evidence
Milgram test	Supine	Two-inch active bilateral leg raise for 30 seconds	Lowering of leg, pain or reproduction of radicular symptoms	Intrathecal lesion, disk- or space-occupying lesion	Limited data available
Spring test (anterior-posterior glide)	Prone	Place thumb or finger on spinous process, apply posterior to anterior pressure	Pain, displacement, radicular symptoms	Facet joint dysfunction, spondylolisthesis/spondylolysis, nerve root irritation	Limited data available
Hip motion test (piriformis test)	Supine	Passive internal/external rotation of the hip	Increased pain on internal rotation and decreased pain on external rotation	Piriformis muscle *Note:* If both internal and external result in pain, likely the sciatic nerve is the primary complaint	Interrater reliability = 0.28–0.37 Interrater reliability = 0.60 Sensitivity = 0.52 Specificity = 0.73

Common Spine Pathologies **549**

				Preliminary data
Ely test	Prone	Passive extension of hip with knee at 90°; flexion-stabilize pelvis	L2-L4 nerve root impingement (pain along femoral nerve distribution) or sacroiliac joint (pain over joint) ***Note:** Nachlas prone bending test: Knee flexed as far as possible to buttocks, positive for femoral nerve root/tight rectus femoris muscle	Femoral nerve, hip flexor tightness, sacroiliac joint pathology
Femoral nerve traction test	Lying on unaffected side	Passive hip extension (15°) with knee straight, then passive knee flexion; increased pain down anterior thigh: traction on L2-L4 nerve roots	Localized pain, radicular symptoms	Femoral nerve pathology Sensitivity = 0.52 Specificity = 0.76
Spinal segmental motion tests thoracic and lumbar pathology	Patient sitting with arms crossed in front of chest, hands on shoulders; flexion/extension	Clinician places one arm around elbows to use for passive leverage, fingers of other hand over and between spinous processes feeling for opening and closing, patient sitting with hands clasped behind head; lateral flexion/rotation: Clinician places one arm over elbows for passive leverage, fingers of other hand along spinous processes feeling for movement	Laxity and pain/radicular symptoms	Vertebral spine instability Limited data available

(continues)

Table 12.6 Orthopaedic Special Tests *(continued)*

Special Test	Patient Positioning	Test Procedure	Positive Test	Indications	Evidence
Hoover test	Supine	Clinician places hands beneath the patient's heel while the patient performs an active straight leg raise to each side individually	No noted unilateral pressure in the heel of the opposite foot lifted	Cause is most likely psychogenic	Limited data available
Neri bowstring sign	Standing	Patient flexes forward as to touch toes	Unilateral knee flexion associated with a report of decreased symptomatic or radicular pain	Nerve root, disk lesion, tight posterior musculature	Preliminary data Sensitivity = 0.42 Specificity = 0.77
Lewin standing sign	Standing	Patient flexes forward to touch toes, add knee flexion	Knee flexion reduces leg/lumbar pain	Neural tension, disk lesion, nerve root pathology	Limited data available

Test	Position	Procedure	Purpose	Statistics
Scoliosis testing (Adams forward bending test)	Standing	Patient flexes forward to touch toes	Observable hump and spinal flexion/rotation	Establishes existence of scoliosis	Interrater reliability = 0.61 Sensitivity = 0.73 Specificity = 0.64
Scoliosis testing (Hanging test)	Standing	Visual observation reveals notable scoliosis; have patient hang from bar and observe spine position and angles	Notable reduction in scoliosis upon hanging: functional scoliosis	Establishes functional versus structural scoliosis; if no change in spinal curves during hanging position, the scoliosis is said to be congenital or related to leg length	Limited data available
Babinski test	Supine	Using a blunt device (eg, end of reflex hammer, pen, etc.) examiner runs the device up the plantar aspect of the foot, making an arc from the calcaneus medially to the ball of the great toe	The great toe extends, the other toes splay Note: In newborns the Babinski reflex occurs normally and will spontaneously go away soon after birth.	Upper motor neuron lesion	Interrater reliability = 0.30 Sensitivity = 0.34 Specificity = 0.95

(continues)

Table 12.6 Orthopaedic Special Tests

Special Test	Patient Positioning	Test Procedure	Positive Test	Indications	Evidence
Oppenheim test	Supine	Examiner stands at patient's side and uses a blunt object or examiners fingernail along the crest of the anteromedial tibia	The great toe extends, and other toes splay	Upper motor neuron lesion caused by pathology in brain or spinal cord	Limited data available
Beevor sign	Supine	Examiner stands at the side of the patient as the patient performs a partial sit-up	The umbilicus moves. Movement can be up, down, left, right, or diagonally.	Nerve pathology of rectus abdominis innervations (T5-T12)	Limited data available

(continued)

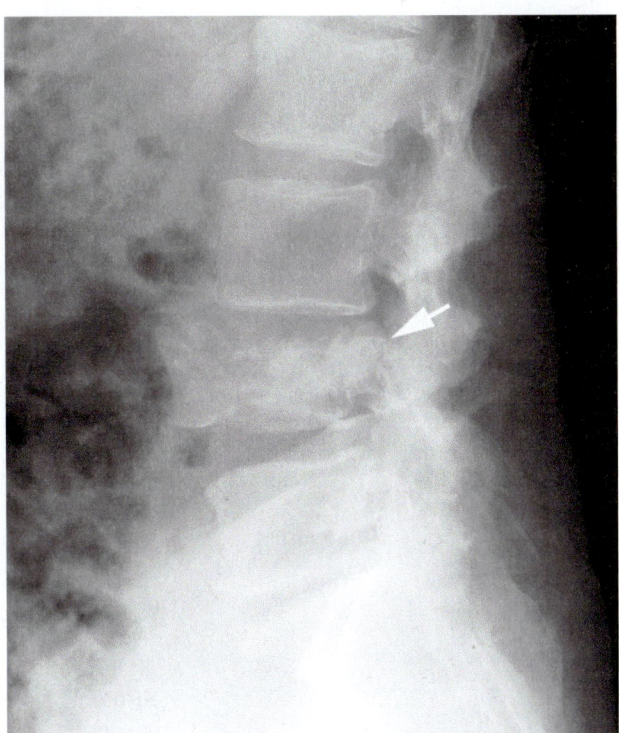 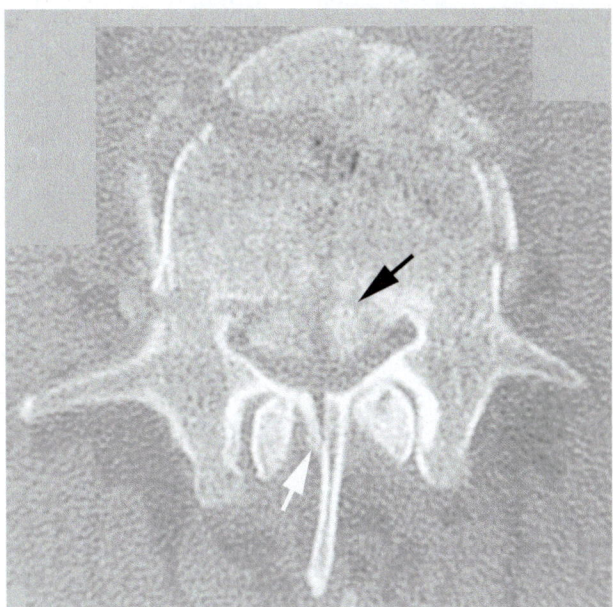

Figure 12.38 Radiograph (left) and axial CT scan (right) showing a spinal burst fracture (arrows).

Reproduced from Johnson TR, Steinbach LS, eds: *Essentials of Musculoskeletal Imaging*. Rosemont, IL, American Academy of Orthopaedic Surgeons, 2004.

posture, significant loss of mobility, difficulty with deep breaths, loss of bowel or bladder control, and distal extremity numbness and tingling. If a transverse or spinous process is fractured, a noted asymmetric abnormality may be visually observed or palpated. Insidious or chronic onsets may mimic these symptoms, with more classifications of dull chronic pain increasing in severity over time. Diagnosis and treatment parameters require radiography, CT, and/or MRI to ensure exact location(s) of the damaged bone and appropriate treatment. Such fractures are generally categorized as rotational, flexion, or extension injuries.[7,8] Compression and axial-loaded fractures are often the result of loaded vertebral segments from compressive flexion and extension moments, respectively. These fractures often remain nondisplaced, with limited damage to the spinal cord and nerve roots. In severe cases, the vertebral body may fracture in multiple places, resulting in a crushed segment or burst fracture[3,7,11,13,36] (**Figure 12.38**). A collapse in the vertebral body from any compression fracture may result in a mechanical spinal defect and an exaggerated flexion or kyphotic posture. Often, these injures do not require surgery but do require extensive bracing, rest, and therapeutic guidance. In severe cases, with mechanical deficits, surgery may be needed to reestablish nerve root canals or spinal column integrity (**Table 12.7**).

Spondylolysis and Spondylolisthesis

Chronic compressive spinal extension mechanisms, such as those seen in gymnastics, football, and Olympic lifting, may result in a bone stress reaction resulting in a fracture. A spondylolysis is a stress fracture to the pars interarticularis or isthmus of the lamina of the vertebral segments. Commonly referred to as a "Scotty-dog neck" fracture, the radiograph of the fracture line mimics that of a collar on a Scottish Terrier[33,167] (**Figure 12.39**). Common in the lumbar spine, these injuries often present with chronic localized pain and muscle spasm along the corresponding segments with no neurologic implications. Over time, these injuries can progress into an open fracture of the pars interarticularis, resulting in an anterior translation of the corresponding vertebral body, known as a spondylolisthesis.[79-81] Here, patients generally have increased sensitivity to palpation, spinal extension, and standing upright and may complain of radicular irritation about the posterior pelvis, gluteal muscles, and lateral hip. Radiography or MRI are traditionally used to diagnose the incidence and severity of these injuries. Grades of severity of anterior translations are classified as first to fourth equal to 25%, 50%, 75%, and 100%, respectively. A fifth-degree translation is identified

Table 12.7 Spinal Body Fracture Quick Tips

Pathology	Description	Presentation (HIPS)	Special Tests/ Imaging	Differential Diagnosis	5-Min Sideline Assessment Tips
Spinal body fracture	A traumatic, high-velocity force applied to the spinal vertebrae resulting in fracture Spinal body fractures can also occur in an atraumatic manner	H: Patient reports a traumatic compressive or shear force or one is observed. Report of nonradiating, stabbing, or aching back pain. Report of urinary retention. I: Weakness or decreased sensation at vertebral level of injury. Presence of abrasions, point tenderness, or local kyphosis. P: Palpable gap between spinous processes may be present.	• Percussion test • Spinal segment motion tests (thoracic and lumbar pathologies) • Radiograph, MRI, and CT scan	Traumatic: • Hyperflexion or hyperextension injury • Nonspecific low back pain • Spondylolysis/ spondylolisthesis Atraumatic: • Degenerative disk disease • Osteoporosis	• Approach patient as a life-threatening injury is expected • Activate EAP immediately • Immediate stabilization • All injury evaluation efforts must ensure immobilization of injury • Dependent on location of spinal fracture, neurologic signs may not be present

EAP, emergency action plan; HIPS, history, inspection, palpation, special tests.

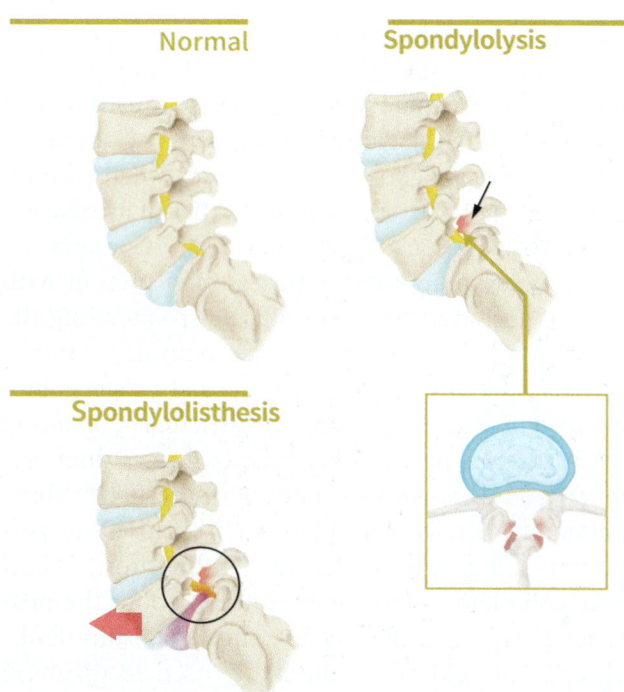

Figure 12.39 Drawing showing spondylolysis and spondylolisthesis.
© Chu KyungMin/Shutterstock

as movement of the complete vertebral body length and is referred to as a spondyloptosis.[79-81] Most commonly seen in the lumbar and sacral spine (L4-S1), development of these injuries is often exacerbated or influenced by degenerative spine disease associated with age or excessive overuse of spinal hyperextension movement patterns. Periods of rest, modified activity, basic spinal strengthening, flexibility and equilibrium therapy, and limiting spinal extension movements usually result in full recovery. More severe cases may require surgery to alleviate spinal nerve root impingements and/or provide mechanical spinal stability (**Table 12.8**).

Facet Joint Pathology

The superior and inferior spinal facets of the vertebral bodies are commonly subjected to a great deal of multiplanar compressive and shear movements, resulting in periosteal and articular irritations. Commonly associated with other pathologies, such as disk and skeletal degeneration, nerve root impingements, sprains, and hyperextension movements, facet arthropathologies can occur throughout all spinal regions. Facet articulations play a

Table 12.8 Spondylolysis and Spondylolisthesis Quick Tips

Pathology	Description	Presentation (HIPS)	Special Tests/Imaging	Differential Diagnosis	5-Min Sideline Assessment Tips
Spondylolysis	Stress fracture within the vertebrae Occurs unilaterally	H: Patient will likely report sudden trauma of hyperextension I: Chronic, localized pain and spasm along corresponding segments. Mild to moderate aching, stiffness, and fatigue across low back. Movement will assess as normal until position is held for extended period of time. Patient may also be asymptomatic P: Localized tenderness	• Hyperextension test • Stork stand • Radiograph for diagnostic imaging • Spondylolisthesis will require MRI	• Disk herniation • Vertebral injury • Muscle strain	• Assess for spasm of the erector spinae musculature • Patient may appear with antalgic gait • Hypersensitive to palpation (spondylolisthesis) • Dermatome/myotome acute and subacute assessment • Referral and diagnostic imaging
Spondylolisthesis	A spondylolysis that has spread bilaterally, potentially creating an open fracture of the pars interarticularis	H: Patient will likely report a direct blow, a sudden twist, or a chronic low back strain I: Increased sensitivity to prior palpations of spondylolysis. Radicular irritation. Patient may appear asymptomatic P: Localized tenderness, segmental hypermobility		• Spondylolysis • Muscle strain	

HIPS, history, inspection, palpation, special tests.

critical part in the numerous synovial joints about the spinal segments. The general role of the facets is to maintain spinal alignment and integrity among adjacent segments, which explains why they are subject to a variety of mechanical-related stressors.[1,29,86,121] Compressive, rotational, and distraction movements, such as those seen in contact sports, can irritate these particular properties, resulting in counterirritations from swelling, muscle spasm, and ligament damage—similar to other synovial joints throughout the body, just at a lower magnitude. In addition, chronic overuse/repetitive movement patterns or static postures can load and irritate the facets. In some cases, muscle fatigue can result in less dynamic muscle control, placing additional accessory stressors on the facets in an attempt to maintain spinal integrity.[10,13,14] Facet injury is characterized by localized joint facet palpable tenderness and increased pain with compressive or rotational movements toward the affected facet, which usually includes standing erect, localized spinal extension, lateral bending, and/or rotation. Radiography and MRI may be used to determine the severity of arthritic integrity and damage, but conservative treatment often relieves signs and symptoms prior to a precise diagnosis.[83] Rest and avoiding compressive rotational movements or chronic postures generally results in a reduction of symptoms and/or full recovery. Biomechanical analysis and preventive movement techniques, such as mobility, flexibility, and strengthening, may be necessary to avoid reoccurrence[168] (**Table 12.9**).

Facet Articulation Dislocation and Subluxation

Dislocation and subluxation of the articulating facets are common at the C4-C6 regions of the cervical spine. Severe spinal flexion and rotation movements result in the inferior facet becoming disassociated and overlapping the superior vertebral facet. The patient will have an extreme limitation in movement and appear to be stuck in cervical rotation and flexion facing away from the affected side.[86,121] Patients may additionally report a "buckling" mechanism of injury in high-impact events. To create this buckling movement, significant compressive forces result in flexion at the lower vertebrae spine and extension of the upper vertebrae.[169] These disassociations are noted with palpable and visual malalignment of the spine associated with limited mobility and localized to radicular signs and symptoms. Such moments can result in bilateral dislocations and/or facet fractures. Radiography and CT are generally used to confirm diagnosis and management. A lateral radiograph will reveal a bow-tie sign of the vertebral segments. Treatment varies, depending on the diagnosed damage[121] (**Table 12.10**).

Scheuermann Kyphosis

Scheuermann kyphosis is a diagnostic disorder defined as a degenerative thoracic kyphosis with an anterior wedge fracture.[170] Radiographically, Scheuermann kyphosis presents with three or more contiguous vertebrae wedged at a minimum of 5° anteriorly. As a

Table 12.9 Facet Joint Pathology Quick Tips

Pathology	Description	Presentation (HIPS)	Special Tests/Imaging	Differential Diagnosis	5-Min Sideline Assessment Tips
Facet joint pathology	Chronic or general inflammatory condition of the superior and/or inferior facets of the vertebral bodies	H: Patient reports a history of repetitive trauma, overloading extension, and occurrence secondary to disk degeneration I: Increased pain with compressive or rotational movements toward affected facet P: Localized joint facet tenderness	• Cervical distraction test • Cervical foramina compression test • Hyperextension test • Stork stand • Quadrant test (Kemp sign) • Spring test • Radiography and MRI	• Disk degeneration • Skeletal degeneration • Nerve root impingements • Sprains	• Often associated with paraspinal muscle spasm • Rule out major spinal neurologic or osteologic damage

HIPS, history, inspection, palpation, special tests.

Table 12.10 Facet Articulation Dislocation and Subluxation Quick Tips

Pathology	Description	Presentation (HIPS)	Special Tests/Imaging	Differential Diagnosis	5-Min Sideline Assessment Tips
Facet articulation, dislocation, and subluxation	Anterior translation of one vertebral body onto another without fracture	H: Patient reports severe spinal flexion and rotation mechanism, or a "buckling" mechanism I: Weakness and tingling in C5, C6, and C7. Possible vertebral protuberance P: Anterior translation and possible vertebral protuberance. Point tenderness over involved vertebral bodies. Trigger points over back musculature	• Compression and distraction test • Spring test • Radiograph, MRI, and CT scan	• Disk herniation • Posterior spinal ligament injury • Incomplete spinal cord injury • Nerve root injury	• Rule out major spinal neurologic or osteologic damage • Complete neurologic assessment • Palpate for vertebral protuberance or possible anterior translation • Patient may appear with head tilted toward affected side • Do not move patient until neurologic assessment is unremarkable and palpation reveals no translation or protuberance

HIPS, history, inspection, palpation, special tests.

result, the nucleus pulposus is at risk and prolapses, resulting in further damage to the vertebral body. In approximately 0.4% to 8.0% of adolescents ages 10 to 12 years, the condition is more common among those participating in activities that require increased demands on the thoracic or thoracolumbar segments of the spine, such as gymnastics, extreme weighted squats, or the butterfly stroke in swimming. Often, patients will present with impaired circulation, thoracic kyphosis, and lordosis of the lumbar spine. Pain is secondary to the deformation. Patients can typically be treated with conservative interventions targeting pain modulation with mobility and anti-inflammatory medication when the thoracic curvature is less than 70° to 75°[171] (**Table 12.11**). To diagnose Scheuermann kyphosis, it is essential to consult an orthopaedic specialist for appropriate diagnosis and treatment protocol.

Muscle Strain

Muscle strains are common throughout the spine. The overlapping and interwoven nature of the musculoskeletal anatomy adds to the complexity of these injuries. The common mechanisms of injury are generally related to muscular capacity overloads, fatigue, or high-velocity impacts to the body or head. Injury to the cervical muscles usually occurs from a high-impact injury, such as seen in football when a ball carrier receives a blow to the trunk and the cervical muscles supporting the head are forced to stabilize at high velocities.[16,112,172] Repetitive or chronic lifting movement patterns combined with poor posture (referring to posture of the spine), limited ROM, and/or poor musculoskeletal fitness can lead to muscle and joint mismechanics, resulting in both muscle and joint failure in all areas of the spine (**Table 12.12**). Submaximal efforts that require sustained loads on the spine (prolonged sitting or standing) and/or continuous repetitive movement patterns often have a cumulative effect of musculoskeletal failure at the spine. Excessive eccentric loads and/or a lack of anticipatory stability at the spine can result in muscle, ligament, and bone/facet injuries. Such injuries often result in localized pain and swelling over the specific joint spaces and muscle lengths.[32,86] Due to the close approximation and intimate relationship between the spinal segments, facets, nerve roots, and spinal muscles, it is often difficult to differentiate which structures are symptomatic versus being truly damaged.[86,121] For example, a disk lesion may result in pressure on a given nerve root, which results in muscle pain or spasm. Facet or isolated muscle spasm can often result in very similar signs and symptoms. Muscle guarding or contractile spasms

Table 12.11 Kyphosis Quick Tips

Pathology	Description	Presentation (HIPS)	Special Tests/Imaging	Differential Diagnosis	5-Min Sideline Assessment Tips
Scheuermann kyphosis	Structural deformity of the thoracic or lumbothoracic spine. Diagnostically defined as thoracic kyphosis	H: Patient will not necessarily report a specific mechanism; rather the signs and symptoms and obvious deformity will identify the disease I: Assess the thoracic and lumbar curvature. Patient may report pain and diminished circulation. Pain may intensify with increased activity. Muscular tightness P: Point tenderness over spinous process	• Radiography, MRI, and CT scan	• Postural kyphosis • Poorly healed compression fracture	• This is rarely a condition that is evaluated on the sideline • Identify any impairment in circulation, sensory, and motor sensations • Gather thorough history of activity biomechanics • Muscular tightness and point tenderness may indicate later stages of Scheuermann kyphosis

HIPS, history, inspection, palpation, special tests.

---

are also a common sign of nerve root and/or facet irritation rather than an isolated muscle strain. On occasion, palpation may indicate pain and spasm, but further testing, such as muscle tests and/or special tests, are necessary to rule out other skeletal versus soft-tissue abnormalities. Isolated muscle testing can help locate specific muscle damage or irritation, but should be used in combination with all aspects of the orthopaedic evaluation. Thus, it is important to have a thorough assessment using a multitude of tests that target specific pathologies.

Vertebral Disk Injury

Vertebral disk injuries are common among all spinal regions, with the highest occurrence of disk pathologies at the C5-C7 and L3-S1.[3,13-15] Many disruptions to the disk or disk pathologies are associated

Table 12.12 Muscle Strain Pathology Quick Tips

Pathology	Description	Presentation (HIPS)	Special Tests/Imaging	Differential Diagnosis	5-Min Sideline Assessment Tips
Muscle strain	Deformation of muscle in response to a force	H: Patient reports a force of tension or shearing was applied through hyperextension, flexion, or a twisting motion I: Spasm, decreased ROM, neurologic testing P: Point tenderness	• Spinal segment motion tests • Neri bowstring sign • Clinical palpation test • MMT of suspected involved musculature • ROM testing in forward and lateral flexion • MRI for diagnostic imaging	• Spinal bony injury • Herniated disk or disk rupture	• Rule out major spinal neurologic or osteologic damage • Facilitate patient's comfort • Assess ROM and MMT • Determine any muscle guarding and spasm • Rule out any nerve involvement

HIPS, history, inspection, palpation, special tests; MMT, manual muscle test; ROM, range of motion.

with a high degree of repetitive movement patterns and improper spine stability and/or biomechanics. Degenerative disk changes are often the result of age or excessive repetitions. Deterioration of the spinal segments, facet surfaces, joint foramen, and nerve properties often accompanies changes in the disk. A decrease in fluid properties and disk pliability also contributes to the decrement of adjacent structures. A disk disruption of a minor classification is described as a disruption, or annular tear, while the nucleus stays intact.[10] However, more serious injuries, such as a disk prolapse and extrusion, often result in the nucleus fluid compressing the spinal nerve roots, resulting in pain and dysfunction at the spine/distal extremities. In severe cases, the disk will sequester or have a breach in the anulus fibrosus, resulting in the nucleus pulposus emptying into the spinal canal[13,53,127] (**Figure 12.40**). As a result, there is generally severe nerve root disruptions resulting in pain and/or sensory and motor dysfunction. The high frequency of movement transitions, such as those seen at C5-T1 and L3-S1, commonly subject these areas to disk herniation and associated peripheral nerve pathologies[27,32,117] (**Table 12.13**).

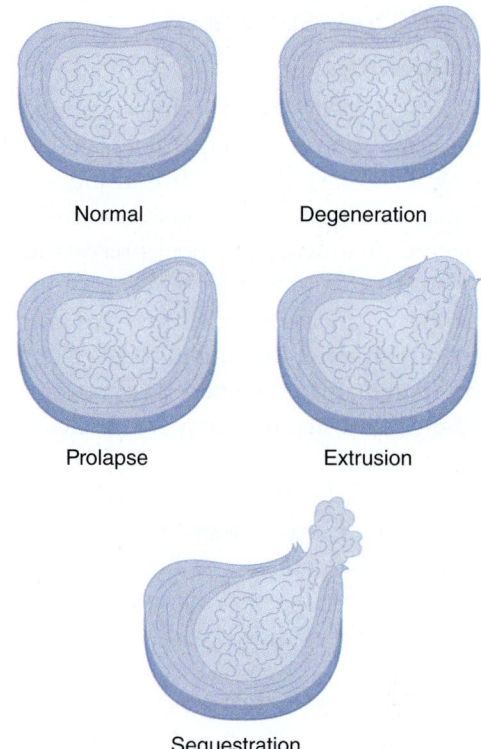

Figure 12.40 Drawing showing the stages of disk injury.
© Jones & Bartlett Learning

Table 12.13 Vertebral Disk Injury Quick Tips

Pathology	Description	Presentation (HIPS)	Special Tests/ Imaging	Differential Diagnosis	5-Min Sideline Assessment Tips
Vertebral disk injury	High degree of repetitive movement patterns, such as forward bending and twisting, resulting in pain, discomfort, and other associated neurologic signs and symptoms	H: Patient reports repetitive faulty body mechanics or an acute trauma. At times, both may be reported I: Pain, sensory loss, and motor dysfunction. Sharp pain that is centrally located. Pain may radiate to one side. Restriction in motion may be present P: Assess for cardinal signs of inflammation; palpate for point tenderness and pain patterns	• Valsalva test • Lewin forward standing sign • Forward flexion test • Kernig test • Well straight leg raise • Straight leg raise • Disk test • Brudzinski test • Bowstring test • Neri bowstring test • Milgram test • Radiography, MRI, CT scan	Due to the number of potential vertebral disk injuries, definitive diagnosis can be difficult. • Lumbosacral sprain • Herniated disk • Annular tear • Degenerative disk change • Vertebral fracture	• Gather as much history as possible • Do not recreate motion that initiated initial injury • Determine whether signs and symptoms are unilateral or bilateral • Rule out major spinal neurologic or osteologic damage • Identify type of pain and whether it has radiating characteristics • Immediate response should be to modulate pain

HIPS, history, inspection, palpation, special tests.

Vertebral Disk Stages of Herniation Injury

1. Disk degeneration results from a combination of physical and chemical changes associated with age, causing the disks to become brittle and weaken.
2. Prolapse is a minor disruption to the anulus fibrosus where the nucleus pulposus results in spinal canal pressure from a slight bulge or protrusion.
3. Extrusion of the disk is characterized by a more severe disruption in the spinal canal. The nucleus pulposus remains contained but breaks through the anulus fibrosus, resulting in significant spinal canal pressure.
4. Sequestered disks are characterized by a breach in the anulus fibrosus wall by the nucleus pulposus fluid, which encroaches into the spinal canal, resulting in a severe disruption of the spinal nerves and pain.

Spinal Cord and Nerve Root Injury

The spinal cord and corresponding nerve roots are commonly at risk for compression, traction, and tearing mechanisms. Axial loading, hyperflexion, hyperextension, and hyperrotation of the spine are among the most common mechanisms that can disrupt both sensory and motor capabilities of the spinal cord.[82,173,174] In addition, corresponding nerve roots are also at risk to be injured individually or collectively with the spinal cord. The structural integrity of skeletal anatomy is critical in protecting and maintaining neurologic distributions from the central nervous system to the peripheral system. A narrowing, or spinal stenosis, of the spinal canal is often a congenital defect, though it may be caused by skeletal variations, such as osteophytes. A stenosis puts the cord at risk for damage and potential lost function. Fairly common in the cervical region, the narrowing can be further compromised by poor biomechanics and/or injury to adjacent structures.[102] Repeated episodes of transient paralysis may occur from activities of daily living that involve a degree of axial loading, hyperflexion, or hyperextension. Signs and symptoms may be provoked with simple functional movements that require multiple body segments or proprioception, such as a nonweighted overhead squat, walking lunge, or touching the toes. Symptoms may be purely sensory or have a motor component. Signs of muscle fatigue and/or atrophy may indicate a spinal canal stenosis[121,174,175] (Table 12.14). These individuals warrant high levels of diagnostic tests and should be referred to an orthopaedic spine

Table 12.14 Spinal Cord and Nerve Root Injury Quick Tips

Pathology	Description	Presentation (HIPS)	Special Tests/ Imaging	Differential Diagnosis	5-Min Sideline Assessment Tips
Spinal cord and nerve root injury	An axial load, hyperflexion, hyperextension, or hyperrotation of the spine resulting in disruption to the sensory and/or motor capabilities of the spinal cord	H: Patient reports a compression, traction, or tearing mechanism resulting in diminished or absent sensory and/or motor capabilities I: Assess for any diminished and/or absent dermatomes and myotomes as well as deep tendon reflexes. Potential difficulty in coordinated limb movement P: Temperature difference, point tenderness	• Femoral nerve stretch test • Assess dermatomes for hypersensitivity or hyposensitivity • Assess myotomes for appropriate motor response • MRI and CT scan	• Spinal stenosis • Muscle strain • Facet joint inflammation • Disk degeneration • Arthritic change to spinal cord	• Determine mechanism immediately • Rule out major spinal neurologic or osteologic damage • Severity will be dependent upon vertebral level of signs and symptoms • Assess dermatome and myotome activation for appropriate removal from competition field • These injuries can require activation of the EAP or could require less invasive and immediate action

EAP, emergency action plan; HIPS, history, inspection, palpation, special tests.

specialist to determine the degree of severity of the stenosis. All sport participation should be discontinued until advanced diagnostic testing is performed.

Peripheral nerve damage can occur in many forms and often is associated with disruption at the spinal root in the form of a compression, distraction, or muscle fatigue/failure mechanism. Compression often comes from a stenosis within the vertebral foramen from a direct blow/impact, high-velocity movements (whiplash/axial load), disk degeneration, muscle spasm, joint facet inflammation, arthritic bony or soft-tissue changes due to age or injury, and/or a mechanical restriction from range of motion, such as cervical extension.[86,176,177] Distraction or stretching areas of the nerve or within the muscles/fascia supporting the nerves is often the result of high-velocity movements where one body segment is secured and a distal or proximal segment is rapidly displaced. A proximal disruption localized at the nerve root often accompanies a distal extremity dermatome and/or myotome complication along the branches of the nerve. Often, determining the location of the proximal disruption and associated distal deficits to the dermatome/myotome can provide insight into the injury mechanism and potential treatment options. All motor and sensory assessments should be performed bilaterally.[120,178] Myotome assessments should focus on determining muscle function and control, whereas dermatome assessments are geared toward determining hypersensitivity or hyposensitivity; two-point discrimination; and potential kinesthetic ailments regarding force, pressure, and position. More extensive muscle function grading can accompany any neurologic assessment to gain more insight into the current pathology.[1,16]

Peripheral Nerve Damage

There are three classifications of nerve damage: neurapraxia, axonotmesis, and neurotmesis (**Figure 12.41**). The neurotmesis has two subclassifications of complete nerve transections—endoneurium nerve fiber neurotmesis and perineurium nerve fiber neurotmesis. Neurapraxia is the least severe and results in a temporary loss of conduction properties about an injury site due to a physiologic nerve block. Conduction properties are intact above and below the injury, and the nerve fibers are fully intact. Nerve neurapraxia transient paralysis is commonly caused by a spinal stenosis from a disk, foramen, or muscle spasm.[123,133,179] Full nerve capacity is usually restored in hours to days. Axonotmesis results from damage to the axon and the myelin protective sheath. The connective tissue of the nerve remains intact and will generally recover back to normal within a few weeks of rest and general modalities (**Table 12.15**). On rare occasions, surgical interventions are warranted to débride scar

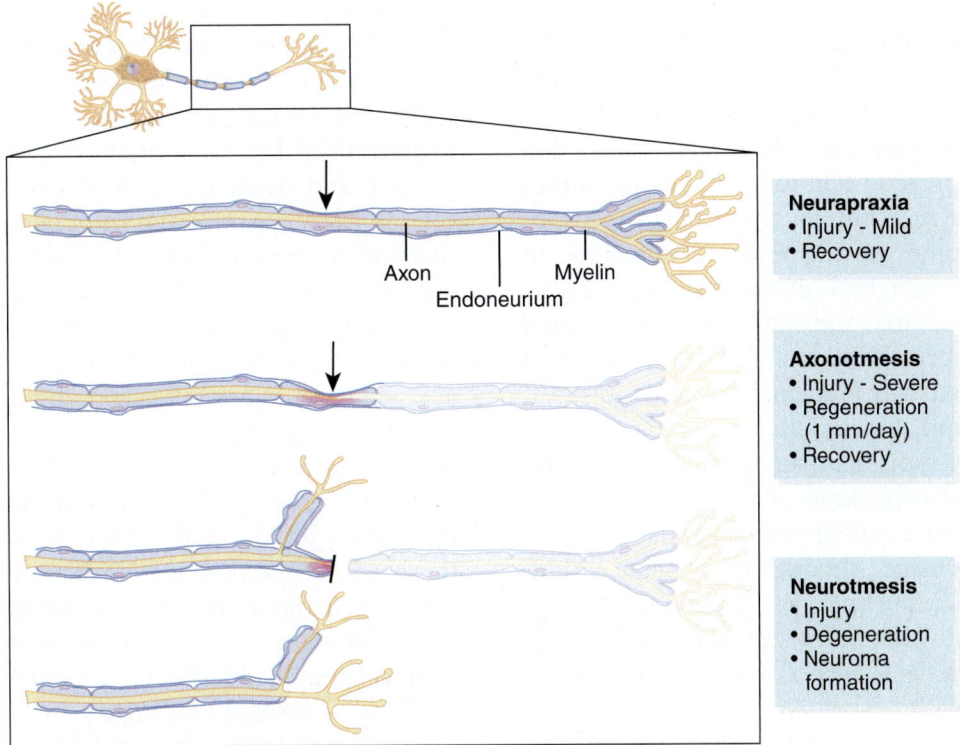

Figure 12.41 Drawing depicting the stages of nerve injury.

© Jones & Bartlett Learning

Table 12.15 Peripheral Nerve Damage Quick Tips

Pathology	Description	Presentation (HIPS)	Special Tests/Imaging	Differential Diagnosis	5-Min Sideline Assessment Tips
Peripheral nerve damage	A temporary, but in rare cases a permanent, loss of conduction properties to an injury site due to physiologic nerve block resulting from one of five classifications Generally, a secondary injury from a primary cause, such as forceful hyperextension, scar tissue formation, or muscle spasm	H: Dependent on classification of nerve damage. Patient may report severe traumatic incident or sensations of muscle spasm entrapping a nerve root I: General neurologic symptoms of numbness and tingling, may identify radiating pain to one or both sides, dependent on level of nerve root involvement and classification of nerve damage P: Secondary bony translation or protuberance	• MRI, electromyography, nerve conduction velocity test	• Facet joint pathology • Spinal fracture • Spinal cord and nerve root injury	• Early evaluation, diagnosis, and treatment are essential to noncomplicated recovery • Rule out major spinal neurologic or osteologic damage • Assess signs and symptoms prior to moving patient • Identify whether onset of symptoms was acute or insidious

HIPS, history, inspection, palpation, special tests.

tissue formation in the area. Neurotmesis is a total severing of the nerve fiber endoneurium, but the epineurium and perineurium are intact. In a perineurium nerve fiber neurotmesis, the endoneurium and the perineurium are severely damaged, hampering the nerve's capability to send messages distal to an injury. Neurotmesis and complete nerve transection require surgical intervention to repair the properties of the nerve but may not always result in recovery. A nerve laceration or tearing of the nerve may occur secondary to a vertebral dislocation or fracture, resulting in a potential paralysis below the injured site. Nerve hemorrhage develops from all vertebral trauma associated with vertebral fractures, dislocations, strains, and sprains. Nerve contusions may result from sudden displacement or rapid disruption of a vertebra that compresses the cord and/or nerve roots, resulting in swelling and potential paralysis and long-term damage. Although many nerve pathologies result from acute episodes, chronic nerve compressions or contusions will result in various degrees of discontinuity as well, such as those seen in the brachial plexus.[123,133,179]

In cases of violent or high-velocity movements, the spinal cord can experience an acute trauma referred to as a spinal cord shock.[180] As a result, there is an immediate loss of function below the level of the lesion; limbs are flaccid and potentially spastic with a total loss of associated deep tendon reflexes and hyperreflexia. Although the spinal cord cannot necessarily be damaged in the lumbar region, it is extremely vulnerable to damage in the cervical and thoracic regions. Cord lesions at or above C3 will impair respiration and result in death, whereas lesions below C4 will allow for some return of nerve root function. Incomplete lesions of the cord can result in a central cord syndrome, caused by hemorrhage or ischemia in the central portion of the cord. Often, these cases result in a quadriplegia with nonspecific sensory loss and sexual and bowel/bladder dysfunction. Brown-Séquard syndrome is caused by a unilateral spinal cord injury resulting in a loss of sensory and motor function, dexterity of touch, and proprioception on the damaged side of the body. If the anterior two-thirds and/or the posterior portion of the spinal cord is damaged, the result is an anterior and posterior spinal cord syndrome.[180-182] Here, there is a loss of motor, sensory, and bladder/bowel function. If the posterior cord is isolated with injury, motor function may remain intact. Spinal cord and nerve injuries require a tremendous degree of diligence and care requiring high levels of medical care and diagnostic precision.

Brachial Plexus Neurapraxia. Commonly referred to as a stinger or burner, the transient neurapraxia resulting from stretching or compression of the brachial plexus is the most common of all cervical neurologic injuries in athletes, occurring during sports such as football, rugby, and ice hockey.[123] The neurapraxia causes disruption in normal function of a peripheral nerve without any degenerative changes, unless there is chronic exposure to the mechanism. When the cervical collar and head are forced laterally to one side and pressure is placed on the apex of the shoulder girdle, the nerve roots on the opposite side of the lateral flexion of the head are subject to be stretched or tractioned.[123,179] The nerve roots on the same side of the head's lateral flexion are subject to compression.[123] Both potential mechanisms result in pain, numbness, and tingling radiating proximal to distal into the hand, generally aggravating nerve roots C6-C8. C5 involvement is indicated if there is weakness to the deltoid, upper trapezius, biceps brachii, and brachialis. Signs and symptoms may last for several minutes to hours with the potential for long-term weakness. Generally, treatment requires rest and modalities to control pain and swelling[133,179] (**Table 12.16**). Monitoring the neurologic peripheral properties, light mobility and strengthening about the neck musculature are usually implemented with a modification of protective padding about the shoulders and neck.

Neuropathic injury to the lumbar and sacral plexus can occur due to direct blows or falls to the ground. In many cases, these injuries are noted with a degree of lumbar pain that may or may not have radicular symptoms into the hip or leg.[179] Lumbar plexus lesion may cause symptoms about the iliohypogastric, genitofemoral, ilioinguinal, femoral, and obturator nerves. Often, weakness of hip flexion, knee extension, and thigh adduction results in antalgic gait. Sensory loss in the lower abdomen, inguinal region, and circumferential about the pelvis and thigh and distal to the lower leg is often noted following neuropathic injuries. Common neuropathies of L4 and L5 result in anterior thigh pain/numbness and dorsum of the foot pain of sensory loss, respectively.[103] The distribution of the sciatic nerve, located midway between the greater trochanter and ischial tuberosity in the greater sciatic foramen, is associated with posterior lateral hip and gluteal pain due to disk pathology or piriformis muscle impingement.[130,131] Such injuries generally require specialized therapy and/or advanced surgical interventions.

Table 12.16 Brachial Plexus Neurapraxia Quick Tips

Pathology	Description	Presentation (HIPS)	Special Tests/Imaging	Differential Diagnosis	5-Min Sideline Assessment Tips
Brachial plexus neurapraxia	A transient neurapraxia from a stretching or compressive force on the brachial plexus, resulting in disruption to peripheral nerves without degenerative changes	H: Patient reports a forced lateral motion to opposite side while shoulder is depressed or forced neck extension and rotation to the affected side I: Pain, tingling, and numbness radiating to hand from proximal to distal. Potential weakness of deltoids, biceps, and brachialis P: Tenderness over trapezius	• Brachial plexus traction test • Shoulder distraction/depression test • Brachial plexus Tinel sign • Brachial plexus squeeze test	• Nerve root compression • Brachial plexus lesion	• Rule out major spinal neurologic or osteologic damage • Determine pattern of numbness and tingling • If patient reports no weakness of deltoids, biceps, or brachialis, return to participation may be acceptable • Neck range of motion will generally assess as normal, while loss of function and sensation in shoulder and hand may be present

HIPS, history, inspection, palpation, special tests.

Summary

The multifaceted and complex nature of the spine contributes to the functional dexterity and intricate details associated with the potential for injury. As a primary mediator between the upper and lower extremities, both appendicular and axial musculoskeletal systems must be considered to have a causative effect on the spine. This allows the body to be highly interactive with the surrounding environment. As a result, spine function is rooted to the transfer and distribution of ground reaction forces and related interactions with environmental obstacles. Therefore, evaluation procedures should consider both whole-body and isolated limb assessments as they relate to posture, ROM, function, neuromuscular control, vascular properties, and biomechanics.

There are several general pathologies related to strains, sprains, and fractures; however, the intricate detail of the spinal nerve complexes make them challenging to treat and properly diagnose. These structures are of great importance and must be treated and evaluated with great caution to avoid life-threatening alterations, especially when dealing with acute, high-impact trauma. Muscle compensation and improper musculoskeletal function about the spine often result in destructive movement patterns that contribute to both acute and chronic pathologies.

Furthermore, the individual characteristics of the cervical, thoracic, and lumbar spine warrant a high degree of protection and precision when determining best practices for the evaluation and treatment process. An evaluation of the spine will entail a strong understanding of the spine posture, neuromuscular and musculoskeletal anatomy, function, and associated injury pathologies.

CASE STUDY 1

A football player reports to your athletic training room with unilateral right-side cervical collar pain. He reports one episode of numbness and tingling in his neck, shoulder, and elbow areas after making a hard tackle nearly 1 week prior to reporting to you. He states he has weakness in his right arm and difficulty sleeping and putting pressure on the shoulder and cannot hit hard without feeling a repeated episode of radicular pain. There is a C5 motor and sensory deficit.

1. What do you suspect?
2. What five history questions would you like to ask and why?
3. List five major areas of palpation you think will tell you more about the injury.
4. If he has pain and reproduces neurologic symptoms on lateral cervical flexion to the right, what do you suspect? And what special test might you perform to confirm your suspicions?

CASE STUDY 2

A right-handed softball pitcher reports to you with right-sided thoracic spine pain in the areas of the T5-T7 spinous process. She states she is having some stiffness and difficulty with rotation and side bending to the right. She has trouble pitching but less with overhead throwing. She reports pitching 14 innings on Saturday and 18 innings on Sunday but does not report any acute episodes that could have caused pain in that area. She states feeling slightly congested with difficulty breathing and pressure in her chest.

1. What do you suspect?
2. What five history questions would you like to ask and why?
3. List five major areas of palpation you think will tell you more about the injury.
4. If she has pain and reproduces neurologic symptoms with trunk flexion, what do you suspect? And what special test might you perform to confirm your suspicions?

ONE-IN-A-MILLION CASE STUDY

A 17-year-old gymnast reports to you with aching anterolateral right thigh pain following a practice 3 weeks before the national championship qualifying meet. The pain migrates no lower than her knee. She states that the discomfort has been there for about 2 weeks but comes and goes throughout the day. The irritation increases upon standing up after sitting for a period of time. She has full ROM and a slight increase in discomfort with trunk flexion and hyperextension. She does not remember an isolated episode that caused her trauma, but she does state increasing the volume on the balance beam and an increased number of falls. After receiving extensive rehabilitation for 1 week, there is little to no improvement in her signs and symptoms. A radiograph was obtained and MRI was performed.

Physical exam findings:

- Full range of motion in lumbar spine, but increase in pain >35° of flexion and >5° of extension
- All manual muscle tests are within normal limits
- Abnormal neurologic finding: L5 myotomes and L2-L3 dermatomes show bilateral deficits (reflexes all normal)

Imaging findings: AP and lateral standing lumbar radiographs reveal a grade III spondylolisthesis of L5 on S1 (**Figure 12.42**). Axial and sagittal T2-weighted MRI sequences reveal the following:

- Excessive lumbar lordosis
- Unicameral (noncancerous) bone cyst resulting in an L5-S1 spondylolisthesis
- L5-S1 spinal stenosis of spinal canal and neural foramina on the right side

If you were performing an examination on this individual, which special tests would you perform? Provide the rationale for your choices.

1. Based on the radiology findings of excessive lumbar lordosis and an L5-S1 spondylolisthesis, what postural deviations would you expect to find?
2. What signs or symptoms concern you most, and which would require an immediate referral?

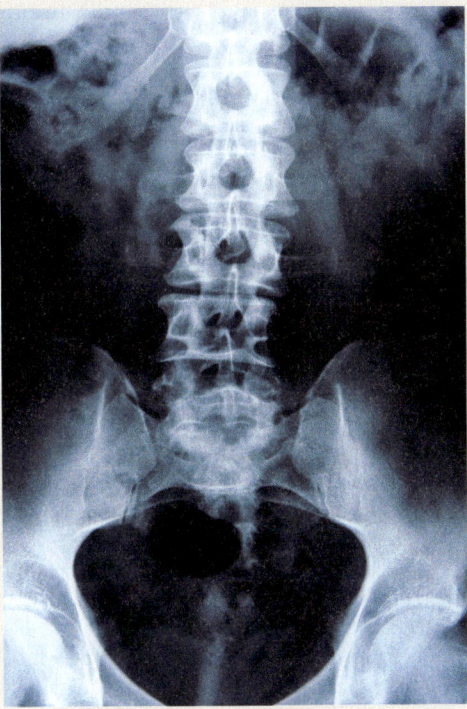

Figure 12.42 Grade III spondylolisthesis of L5 on S1.
© Fmajor/E+/Getty Images

WRAP-UP

Critical Thinking Questions

1. Describe the differences between a spondylolisthesis and a spondylosis. What clinical findings (eg, strength, ROM, special tests) would be expected for each? Which one is more serious?
2. What is the most reliable way to determine the health of the spine and spinal column?
3. A bone cyst will heal similarly to a normal spinal compression fracture. What precautions will you take in the rehabilitation strengthening components?
4. Provide three to five reasons a postural evaluation is important in determining spinal pathologies.
5. Complete a mock injury report using descriptive properties for history, inspection, palpation, ROM, special tests, and neurologic exam.
6. Identify spinal pathologies that would warrant immediate activation of the emergency action plan.

Pearls and Pitfalls

- The spine is central to all human movement, resulting in multifactorial properties, and therefore should be considered as a contributing factor in all pathologies.
- Understanding the anatomy and function of the spine is critical in maximizing sensitivity and specificity of diagnosis and treatment.
- Always consider the potential of a life-threatening situation until it has been ruled out.
- An assessment of neurologic function, the dermatomes and myotomes, and the potential pain distributions (referred and radicular) should always be considered for any spine-related pathology.
- Pain and muscle spasm are often common symptoms of spine pathologies, which require a diligent evaluation and constant follow-up evaluation and care.
- Sensory and motor function disruptions about the spine commonly result from improper compensatory muscle activations of local versus global muscles.
- Pain and muscle spasm can inhibit the evaluation process and may need to be treated prior to establishing a full diagnosis.
- Insidious onset of pain and dysfunction often is a result of pathologies associated with arthritic degeneration, improper compensatory muscle function, and increased overload or work volume. Treating pain prior to evaluation may allow for more in-depth evaluation results.

References

1. Drake R, Vogl AW, Mitchell, AWM: *Gray's Anatomy for Students*, ed 3. Amsterdam, Netherlands: Churchill Livingstone Publishing, Elsevier, 2015.
2. Hatcher J: Manual therapy student handbook: Assessment and treatment of the cervical spine—Part 11. *Co-Kinetic J* 2018;75(11):30-35.
3. Koreska J, Robertson D, Mills RH, Gibson DA, Albisser AM: Biomechanics of the lumbar spine and its clinical significance. *Orthop Clin North Am* 1977;8(1):121-133.
4. Petrides S: Clinical anatomy and management of thoracic spine pain. *Br J Sports Med* 2002;36(2):154-156.
5. Vleeming A, Pool-Goudzwaard AL, Stoeckart R, van Wingerden JP, Snijders CJ: The posterior layer of the thoracolumbar fascia: its function in load transfer from spine to legs. *Spine* 1995;20(7):753-758.
6. Kiefer A, Shirazi-Adl A, Parnianpour M: Stability of the human spine in neutral postures. *Eur Spine J* 1997;6(1):45-53.
7. Clark P, Letts M: Trauma to the thoracic and lumbar spine in the adolescent. *Can J Surg* 2001;44(5):337-345.
8. Patel AA, Vaccaro AR: Thorocolumbar spine trauma classification. *J Am Acad Orthop Surg* 2010;18(2):63-71.
9. Lee J, Lee Y, Hansoo K, Lee J: The effects of cervical mobilization combined with thoracic mobilization on forward head posture of neck pain patients. *J Phys Ther Sci* 2013;25:7-9.
10. Wu Q, Huang JH: Intervertebral disc aging, degeneration, and associated potential molecular mechanisms. *J Head Neck Spine Surg* 2017;1(4):1-5.
11. Garcia KM, Harrison MF, Sargsyan AE, Ebert D, Dulchavsky SA: Real-time ultrasound assessment of astronaut spinal anatomy and disorders on the International Space Station. *J Ultrasound Med* 2018;37(4):987-999.
12. Bodon G, Patonay L, Baksa G, Olerud C: Applied anatomy of a minimally invasive muscle-splitting approach to posterior C1-C2 fusion: an anatomical feasibility study. *Surg Radiol Anat* 2014;36(10):1063-1069.
13. Bostelmann R, Steiger H-J, Cornelius JF: Effect of annular defects on intradiscal pressures in the lumbar spine: an in vitro biomechanical study of diskectomy and annular repair. *J Neurol Surg A Cent Eur Neurosurg* 2017;78(1):46-52.
14. Vergroesen P-P, Veen A, Royen B, Kingma I, Smit T: Intradiscal pressure depends on recent loading and correlates with disc height and compressive stiffness. *Eur Spine J* 2014;23(11):2359-2368.
15. Kirkaldy-Willis WH, Farfan HF: Instability of the lumbar spine. *Clin Orthop Relat Res* 1982;165:110-123.
16. Kendall HO, Kendall FP, Wadsworth CE: *Muscles: Testing and Function*, ed 4. Baltimore, Williams & Willkins, 2003.
17. Kendall HO, Kendall FP: Developing and maintaining good posture. *Phys Ther* 1968;48(4):319-336.
18. Behm DG, Cappa D, Power GA: Trunk muscle activation during moderate- and high-intensity running. *Appl Physiol Nutr Metab* 2009;34(6):1008-1016.
19. Kohler JM, Flanagan SP, Whiting WC: Muscle activation patterns while lifting stable and unstable loads on stable and unstable surfaces. *J Strength Cond Res* 2010;24(2):313-321.
20. Lehman GJ, Hoda W, Oliver S: Trunk muscle activity during bridging exercises on and off a Swiss ball. *Chiropr Osteopat* 2005;13:14.
21. Mok NW, Yeung EW, Cho JC, Hui SC, Liu KC, Pang CH: Core muscle activity during suspension exercises. *J Sci Med Sport* 2015;18(2):189-194.
22. Raizada V, Mittal RK: Pelvic floor anatomy and applied physiology. *Gastroenterol Clin North Am* 2008;37(3):493.
23. Sapsford R: Rehabilitation of pelvic floor muscles utilizing trunk stabilization. *Man Ther* 2004;9(1):3-12.
24. Sapsford R: Explanation of medical terminology. *Neurourol Urodyn* 2000;19(5):633-634.
25. Sapsford RR, Hodges PW: Contraction of the pelvic floor muscles during abdominal maneuvers. *Arch Phys Med Rehabil* 2001;82(8):1081-1088.
26. Hodges PW, Cresswell AG, Thorstensson A: Perturbed upper limb movements cause short-latency postural responses in trunk muscles. *Exp Brain Res* 2001;138(2):243-250.
27. Hodges P, Kaigle Holm A, Holm S, et al: Intervertebral stiffness of the spine is increased by evoked contraction of transversus abdominis and the diaphragm: in vivo porcine studies. *Spine* 2003;28(23):2594-2601.
28. McGill SM, Sharratt MT, Seguin JP: Loads on spinal tissues during simultaneous lifting and ventilatory challenge. *Ergonomics* 1995;38(9):1772-1792.

29. Solomonow M, Zhou BH, Harris M, Lu Y, Baratta RV: The ligamento-muscular stabilizing system of the spine. *Spine* 1998;23(23):2552-2562.
30. Bergmark A. Stability of the lumbar spine: a study in mechanical engineering. *Acta Orthop Scand Suppl* 1989;230:1-54.
31. Cholewicki J, Juluru K, McGill SM: Intra-abdominal pressure mechanism for stabilizing the lumbar spine. *J Biomech* 1999;32(1):13-17.
32. Panjabi MM: The stabilizing system of the spine: part I: function, dysfunction, adaptation, and enhancement. *J Spinal Disord* 1992;5(4):383.
33. Knutssen F: The instability associated with disc degeneration in lumbar spine. *Acta Radiography* 1944;25:593-609.
34. Comerford MJ, Mottram SL: Functional stability re-training: principles and strategies for managing mechanical dysfunction. *Man Ther* 2001;6(1):3-14.
35. Comerford MJ, Mottram SL: Movement and stability dysfunction–contemporary developments. *Man Ther* 2001;6(1):15-26.
36. Panjabi MM: The stabilizing system of the spine: part II: neutral zone and instability hypothesis. *J Spinal Disord* 1992;5(4):390.
37. Steindler A, ed: *Kinesiology of the Human Body Under Normal and Pathological Conditions*. Springfield, IL, Charles C. Thomas, 1977.
38. Cholewicki J, Simons AP, Radebold A: Effects of external trunk loads on lumbar spine stability. *J Biomech* 2000;33(11):1377-1385.
39. McGill SM, Karpowicz A, Fenwick CMJ: Ballistic abdominal exercises: muscle activation patterns during three activities along the stability/mobility continuum. *J Strength Cond Res* 2009;23(3):898-905.
40. McGill SM, Cholewicki J: Biomechanical basis for stability: an explanation to enhance clinical utility. *J Orthop Sports Phys Ther* 2001;31(2):96-100.
41. McGill S, Grenier S, Bluhm M, Preuss R, Brown S, Russell C: Previous history of LBP with work loss is related to lingering deficits in biomechanical, physiological, personal, psychosocial and motor control characteristics. *Ergonomics* 2003;46(7):731.
42. McGill SM, Grenier S, Kavcic N, Cholewicki J: Coordination of muscle activity to assure stability of the lumbar spine. *J Electromyogr Kinesiol* 2003;13(4):353-359.
43. Cholewicki J, Van Vliet JJ: Relative contribution of trunk muscles to the stability of the lumbar spine during isometric exertions. *J Orthop Sports Phys Ther* 2002;17(2):99-105.
44. McGill SM, McDermott ART, Fenwick CMJ: Comparison of different strongman events: trunk muscle activation and lumbar spine motion, load, and stiffness. *J Strength Cond Res* 2009;23(4):1148-1161.
45. Janda V: Introduction to functional pathology of the motor system, in Howell ML, Bullock MI, eds: *Physiotherapy in Sport*. St. Lucia, Queensland, University of Queensland 1983; pp 39-42.
46. Cholewicki J, McGill SM: Lumbar posterior ligament involvement during extremely heavy lifts estimated from fluoroscopic measurements. *J Biomech* 1992;25(1):17-28.
47. Houck JR, Duncan A, De Haven KE: Comparison of frontal plane trunk kinematics and hip and knee moments during anticipated and unanticipated walking and side step cutting tasks. *Gait Posture* 2006;24(3):314-322.
48. Santana JC, Vera-Garcia FJ, McGill SM: A kinetic and electromagnetic comparison of the standing cable press and bench press. *J Strength Cond Res* 2007;21(4):1271-1277.
49. Faulkner JA, Claflin DR, McCully KK: Power output of fast and slow fibers from human skeletal muscles, in McCartney NL, McComas AJ, eds: *Human Muscle Power*. Champaign, IL, Human Kinetics, 1984.
50. Vera-Garcia FJ, Elvira JLL, Brown SHM, McGill SM: Effects of abdominal stabilization maneuvers on the control of spine motion and stability against sudden trunk perturbations. *J Electromyogr Kinesiol* 2007;17(5):556-567.
51. Hodges P, Cresswell A, Thorstensson A: Preparatory trunk motion accompanies rapid upper limb movement. *Exp Brain Res* 1999;124(1):69-79.
52. Hodges PW, Richardson CA: Contraction of the abdominal muscles associated with movement of the lower limb. *Phys Ther* 1997;77(2):132-142.
53. Cholewicki J, McGill SM: Mechanical stabilty of in vivo lumbar spine: implictions for injury and chronic low back pain. *Clin Biomech* 1996;11(1):1-15.
54. Kulas AS, Hortobágyi T, Devita P: The interaction of trunk-load and trunk-position adaptations on knee anterior shear and hamstrings muscle forces during landing. *J Athl Train* 2010;45(1):5-15.
55. Voss DE: Proprioceptive neuromuscular facilitation. *Am J Phys Med* 1967;46(1):838-899.
56. Meakin JR, Hukins DW, Aspden RM: Euler buckling as a model for the curvature and flexion of the human lumbar spine. *Proc Biol Sci* 1996;263(1375):1383-1387.
57. Kibler WB, Press J, Sciascia A: The role of core stability in athletic function. *Sports Med* 2006;36(3):189-198.
58. Leetun DT, Ireland ML, Willson JD, Ballantyne BT, Davis IM: Core stability measures as risk factors for lower extremity injury in athletes. *Med Sci Sports Exerc* 2004;36(6):926-934.
59. Borghuis J, Hof AL, Lemmink KAPM: The importance of sensory-motor control in providing core stability. *Sports Med* 2008;38(11):893-916.
60. Akuthota V, Nadler SF: Core strengthening. *Arch Phys Med Rehabil* 2004;85(3 Suppl 1):S86-S92.
61. Liemohn WP, Baumgartner TA, Gagnon LH: Measuring core stability. *J Strength Cond Res* 2005;19(3):583-586.
62. Elliott B, Marsh T, Overheu P: A biomechanical comparison of the multisegment and single unit topspin forehand drives in tennis. Comparaison biomecanique d'un topspin en coup droit multisegmentaire ou monosegmentaire en tennis. *Int J Sports Mech* 1989;5(3):350-364.
63. Hirashima M, Kadota H, Sakurai S, Kudo K, Ohtsuki T: Sequential muscle activity and its functional role in the upper extremity and trunk during overarm throwing. *J Sports Sci* 2002;20(4):301-310.
64. Naito K, Fukui Y, Maruyama T: Multijoint kinetic chain analysis of knee extension during the soccer instep kick. *Human Movement Sci* 2010;29(2):259-276.
65. Hibbs AE, Thompson KG, French D, Wrigley A, Spears I: Optimizing performance by improving core stability and core strength. *Sports Med* 2008;38(12):995-1008.
66. Northrip JW, Logan GA, McKinney WC: *Analysis of Sport Motion: Anatomic and Biomechanic Perspectives*, ed. 3. Dubuque, IA, W.C. Brown, 1983.
67. Konin JG, Beil N, Werner G: Facilitating the serape effect to enhance extremity force production. *Athl Ther Today* 2003;8(2):54-56.
68. Stodden DF, Langendorfer SJ, Fleisig GS, Andrews JR: Kinematic constraints associated with the acquisition of overarm throwing: part I: step and trunk actions. *Res Q Exerc Sport* 2006;77(4):417-427.

69. Cresswell AG, Grundström H, Thorstensson A: Observations on intra-abdominal pressure and patterns of abdominal intramuscular activity in man. *Acta Physiol Scand* 1992;144(4):409-418.
70. Hodges PW: Is there a role for transversus abdominis in lumbo-pelvic stability? *Man Ther* 1999;4(2):74-86.
71. Arokoski JP, Valta T, Airaksinen O, Kankaanpää M: Back and abdominal muscle function during stabilization exercises. *Arch Phys Med Rehabil* 2001;82(8):1089-1098.
72. Cresswell AG, Oddsson L, Thorstensson A: The influence of sudden perturbations on trunk muscle activity and intra-abdominal pressure while standing. *Exp Brain Res* 1994;98(2):336-341.
73. Hodges PW, Richardson CA: Feedforward contraction of transversus abdominis is not influenced by the direction of arm movement. *Exp Brain Res* 1997;114(2):362-370.
74. Hodges P, Richardson C, Jull G: Evaluation of the relationship between laboratory and clinical tests of transversus abdominis function. *Physiother Res Int* 1996;1(1):30-40.
75. Hodges PW: Core stability exercise in chronic low back pain. *Orthop Clin NA* 2003;34(2):245-254.
76. O'Sullivan P, Dankaerts W, Burnett A, et al: Lumbopelvic kinematics and trunk muscle activity during sitting on stable and unstable surfaces. *J Orthop Sports Phys Ther* 2006;36(1):19-25.
77. Richardson CA, Jull GA, Toppenberg RMK, Comerford MJ: New perspectives in lumbar spine stabilisation prior to exercise, in Sanders TL, ed: *Australian Sports Medicine Federation, Sports Performance Through the "Ages": Proceedings of the 27th National Annual Scientific Conference of ASMF.* Belconnen, ACT, Australian Sports Medicine Federation Ltd, 1990, pp 37-50.
78. Zazulak BT, Hewett TE, Reeves NP, Goldberg B, Cholweicki J: Deficits in neuromuscular control of the trunk predict knee injury risk: a prospective biomechanical-epidemiologic study. *Am J Sports Med* 2007;35(7):1123-1130.
79. Cecchinato R, Boriani S: Spondylolisthesis and tumors: a treatment algorithm. *Eur Spine J* 2018;27:206-212.
80. Foreman P, Griessenauer C, Watanabe K, et al: L5 spondylolysis/spondylolisthesis: a comprehensive review with an anatomic focus. *Childs Nerv Syst* 2013;29(2):209-216.
81. Lily B: Computed tomography evaluation of spondylolysis and spondylolisthesis in asymptomatic patients. *Spine* 2006;31(24):907-910.
82. Hale AT, Alvarado A, Bey AK, et al: X-ray vs. CT in identifying significant C-spine injuries in the pediatric population. *Childs Nerv Syst* 2017;33(11):1977-1983.
83. Xu C, Lin B, Ding Z, Xu Y: Cervical degenerative spondylolisthesis: analysis of facet orientation and the severity of cervical spondylolisthesis. *Spine J* 2016;16(1):10-15.
84. American College of Sports Medicine: American College of Sports Medicine position stand: progression models in resistance training for healthy adults. *Med Sci Sports Exerc* 2009;41(3):687-708.
85. Hides J, Stanton W, Freke M, Wilson S, McMahon S, Richardson C: MRI study of the size, symmetry and function of the trunk muscles among elite cricketers with and without low back pain. *Br J Sports Med* 2008;42(10):809-813.
86. Nadeau M, McLachlin SD, Bailey SI, Gurr KR, Dunning CE, Bailey CS: A biomechanical assessment of soft-tissue damage in the cervical spine following a unilateral facet injury. *J Bone Joint Surg* 2012;94(21):e156.
87. Biering-Sorensen F: Physical measurements as risk indicators for low-back trouble over a one-year period. *Spine* 1984;9(2):106-119.
88. Cholewicki J, McGill SM, Norman RW: Lumbar spine loads during the lifting of extremely heavy weights. *Med Sci Sports Exerc* 1991;23(10):1179-1186.
89. Bjerkefors A, Ekblom MM, Josefsson K, Thorstensson A: Deep and superficial abdominal muscle activation during trunk stabilization exercises with and without instruction to hollow. *Man Ther* 2010;15(5):502-507.
90. Willardson JM: A periodized approach for core training. *ACSM Health Fitness J* 2008;12(1):7-13.
91. Grönblad M, Järvinen E, Hurri H, Hupli M, Karaharju EO: Relationship of the Pain Disability Index (PDI) and the Oswestry Disability Questionnaire (ODQ) with three dynamic physical tests in a group of patients with chronic low-back and leg pain. *Clin J Pain* 1994;10(3):197-203.
92. Van Dillen LR, Maluf KS, Sahrmann SA: Further examination of modifying patient-preferred movement and alignment strategies in patients with low back pain during symptomatic tests. *Man Ther* 2009;14(1):52-60.
93. Steffen K, Pensgaard AM, Bahr R: Self-reported psychological characteristics as risk factors for injuries in female youth football. *Scand J Med Sci Sports* 2009;19(3):442-451.
94. Chia-Chi Y, Fong-Chin S, Lan-Yuen G: A new concept for quantifying the complicated kinematics of the cervical spine and its application in evaluating the impairment of clients with mechanical neck disorders. *Sensors (14248220).* 2012;12(12):17463-17475.
95. LaBan MM: An intercostal muscular hernia as a consequence of intercostal nerve root compromise after trauma to the thoracic spine. *Am J Phys Med Rehabil* 2017;96(4):e68-e69.
96. Edmondston SJ, Singer KP: Thoracic spine: anatomical and biomechanical considerations for manual therapy. *Man Ther* 1997;2(3):132-143.
97. Hein V: Postural alignment in different standing position and the trunk muscle strength among girls aged 8-16 years. *Biol Sport* 1999;16(2):125-138.
98. Ernst MJ, Rast FM, Bauer CM, Marcar VL, Kool J: Determination of thoracic and lumbar spinal processes by their percentage position between C7 and the PSIS level. *BMC Res Notes* 2013;6(1):1-6.
99. Ferreira APA, Póvoa LC, Zanier JFC, Machado DC, Ferreira AS: Sensitivity for palpating lumbopelvic soft tissues and bony landmarks and its associated factors: A single-blinded diagnostic accuracy study. *J Back Musculoskelet Rehabil* 2017;30(4):735-744.
100. Hides J, Scott Q, Jull G, Richardson C: A clinical palpation test to check the activation of the deep stabilizing muscles of the lumbar spine. *Int Sport Med J* 2000;1(4):1.
101. Troke M, Schuit D, Petersen CM: Reliability of lumbar spinal palpation, range of motion, and determination of position. *BMC Musculoskelet Disord* 2007;8:103-106.
102. Epstein NE: More nerve root injuries occur with minimally invasive lumbar surgery: let's tell someone. *Surg Neurol Int* 2016;7(Suppl 3):1-4.
103. Niemi-Nikkola V, Saijets N, Ylipoussu H, et al: Traumatic spinal injuries in northern Finland. *Spine* 2018;43(1):E45-E51.
104. Costa LOP, Maher CG, Latimer J, et al: Motor control exercise for chronic low back pain: a randomized placebo-controlled trial. *Phys Ther* 2009;89(12):1275-1286.
105. Mahdavie E, Rezasoltani A, Simorgh L: The comparison of the lumbar multifidus muscles function between gymnastic athletes with sway-back posture and normal posture. *Int J Sports Phys Ther* 2017;12(4):607-615.

106. Roy AL, Keller TS, Colloca CJ: Posture-dependent trunk extensor EMG activity during maximum isometrics exertions in normal male and female subjects. *J Electromygr Kinesiol* 2003;13(5):469-476.
107. Sahrmann S. Posture and muscle imbalances. *Phys Ther* 1987;67:1840-1844.
108. Izquierdo M, Häkkinen K, Gonzalez-Badillo JJ, Ibáñez J, Gorostiaga EM: Effects of long-term training specificity on maximal strength and power of the upper and lower extremities in athletes from different sports. *Eur J Appl Physiol* 2002;87(3):264-271.
109. Stodden DF, Campbell BM, Moyer TM: Comparison of trunk kinematics in trunk training exercises and throwing. *J Strength Cond Res* 2008;22(1):112-118.
110. Brasiliense LBC, Lazaro BCR, Reyes PM, Dogan S, Theodore N, Crawford NR: Biomechanical contribution of the rib cage to thoracic stability. *Spine* 2011;36(26):E1686-E1693.
111. Lee DG: Rotational instability of the mid-thoracic spine: assessment and management. *Man Ther* 1996;1(5):234-241.
112. Cholewicki J, Panjabi MM, Khachatryan A: Stabilizing function of trunk flexor-extensor muscles around a neutral spine posture. *Spine* 1997;22(19):2207-2212.
113. Wirth B, Amstalden M, Perk M, Boutellier U, Humphreys BK: Respiratory dysfunction in patients with chronic neck pain: influence of thoracic spine and chest mobility. *Man Ther* 2014;19(5):440-444.
114. Maluf KS, Sahrmann SA, Van Dillen LR: Use of a classification system to guide nonsurgical management of a patient with chronic low back pain. *Phys Ther* 2000;80(11):1097-1111.
115. Van Dillen LR, Sahrmann SA, Norton BJ, Caldwell CA, McDonnell MK, Bloom NJ: Movement system impairment-based categories for low back pain: stage 1 validation. *J Orthop Sports Ther* 2003;33(3):126-142.
116. Silfies SP, Bhattacharya A, Biely S, Smith SS, Giszter S: Trunk control during standing reach: a dynamical system analysis of movement strategies in patients with mechanical low back pain. *Gait Posture* 2009;29(3):370-376.
117. Hodges PW, Martin Eriksson AE, Shirley D, Gandevia SC: Intra-abdominal pressure increases stiffness of the lumbar spine. *J Biomech* 2005;38(9):1873-1880.
118. Eser F, Aktekin LA, Bodur H, Atan Ç: Etiological factors of traumatic peripheral nerve injuries. *Neurol India* 2009;57(4):434-437.
119. Sun J, Liu Y-C, Yan S-H, Wang S-S, Lester DK, Zeng J-Z, et al: Clinical gait evaluation of patients with lumbar spine stenosis. *Orthop Surg* 2018;10(1):32-39.
120. Epstein NE, Hollingsworth R: C5 nerve root palsies following cervical spine surgery: a review. *Surg Neurol Int* 2015;6:S154-S163.
121. Quarrington RD, Jones CF, Tcherveniakov P, Clark JM, Sandler SJI, Lee YC, et al: Traumatic subaxial cervical facet subluxation and dislocation: epidemiology, radiographic analyses, and risk factors for spinal cord injury. *Spine J* 2018;18(3):387-398.
122. Radcliff KE, Ben-Galim P, Dreiangel N, Martin SB, Reitman CA, Lin JN, et al: Comprehensive computed tomography assessment of the upper cervical anatomy: what is normal? *Spine J* 2010;10(3):219-229.
123. Dailey A, Harrop JS, France JC. High-energy contact sports and cervical spine neuropraxia injuries. *Spine* 2010;35(21S):S193-S194.
124. Walker BF, Koppenhaver SL, Stomski NJ, Hebert JJ: Interrater reliability of motion palpation in the thoracic spine. *eCAM* 2015:1-6.
125. Gkasdaris G, Tripsianis G, Kotopoulos K, Kapetanakis S: Clinical anatomy and significance of the thoracic intervertebral foramen: a cadaveric study and review of the literature. *J Craniovertebr Junction Spine* 2016;7(4):228-235.
126. Filippovaa LV, Nozdrachev AD: Modern concepts on the mechanisms of encoding visceral nociceptive stimuli. *Hum Physiol* 2010;36(1):107-117.
127. Menck JY, Requejo SM, Kulig K: Thoracic spine dysfunction in upper extremity complex regional pain syndrome type 1. *J Orthop Sports Phys Ther* 2000;30(7):401-409.
128. Behm DG, Drinkwater EJ, Willardson JM, Cowley PM: The use of instability to train the core musculature. *Appl Physiol Nutr Metab* 2010;35(1):91-108.
129. Fanfar HF: The pathological anatomy of a degenerative spondylolisthesis: cadaver study. *Spine* 1980;5(5):412-418.
130. Güngör I, Zinnuroğlu M, Taş A, Tezer T, Beyazova M: Femoral nerve injury following a lumbar plexus blockade. *Balkan Med J* 2014;31(2):184-186.
131. Hopayian K, Song F, Riera R, Sambandan S: The clinical features of the piriformis syndrome: a systematic review. *Eur Spine J* 2010;19(12):2095-2109.
132. Johnson KD, Grindstaff TL: Thoracic rotation measurement techniques: clinical commentary. *N Am J Sports Phys Ther* 2010;5(4):252-256.
133. Rihn JA, Anderson DT, Lamb K, Deluca PF, Bata A, Marchetton PA, et al: Cervical spine injuries in American football. *Sports Med* 2009;39(9):697-708.
134. Tsang SMH, Szeto GPY, Lee RYW: Movement coordination and differential kinematics of the cervical and thoracic spines in people with chronic neck pain. *Clin Biomech* 2013;28(6):610-617.
135. Beach TAC, Frost DM, Callaghan JP: FMS™ scores and low-back loading during lifting—whole-body movement screening as an ergonomic tool? *Appl Ergon* 2014;45(3):482-489.
136. Elvira JLL, Barbado D, Flores-Parodi B, Moreside JM, Vera-Garcia FJ. Effect of movement speed on trunk and hip exercise performance. *Eur J Sport Sci* 2014;14(6):547-555.
137. Cleland JA, Childs JD, Fritz JM, Whitman JM, Eberhart SL: Development of a clinical prediction rule for guiding treatment of a subgroup of patients with neck pain: use of thoracic spine manipulation, exercise, and patient education. *Phys Ther* 2007;87(1):9-23.
138. Bertilson BC, Grunnesjo M, Strender LE: Reliability of clinical tests in the assessment of patients with neck/shoulder problems: impact of history. *Spine* 2003:28(19):2222-2231.
139. Cook C, Brown C, Isaacs R, Roman M, Davis S, Richardson W: Clustered clinical findings for diagnosis of cervical spine myelopathy. *J Man Manip Ther* 2010;18:175-180.
140. Viikari-Juntura E, Porras M, Laasonen EM: Validity of clinical tests in the diagnosis of root compression in cervical disease. *Spine* 1989;4:253-257.
141. Wainner RS, Fritz JM, Irrgang JJ, Boninger ML, Delitto A, Allison S: Reliability and diagnostic accuracy of the clinical examination and patient self-report measures for cervical radiculopathy. *Spine* 2003:28:52-62.
142. Raney NH, Petersen EJ, Smith TA, Cowan JE, Rendiero DG, Deyle GD, et al: Development of a clinical prediction rule to identify patients with neck pain likely to benefit from cervical traction and exercise. *Eur Spine J* 2009;3:382-391.
143. Sandmark N, Nisell R: Validity of five common manual neck pain provoking tests. *Scand J Rehabil Med* 1995;27:131.

144. Latimer J, Maher CG, Refshauge K, Colaco I, et al: The reliability and validity of the Biering-Sorensen test in asymptomatic subjects and subjects reporting current or previous non-specific low back pain. *Spine (Phila Pa 1976)* 1999;24(20):2085-2089.

145. Malanga GA, Landes P, Nadler DF: Provocation tests in cervical spine examination: historical basis and scientific analysis. *Pain Physician* 2003;6:199.

146. Richter RR, Reinking MF: How does evidence on the diagnostic accuracy of the vertebral artery test influence teaching of the test in a professional physical therapist education program? *Phys Ther* 2005;85:589.

147. Albeck MJ: A critical assessment of clinical diagnosis of disc herniation in patients with monoradicular sciatica. *Acta Neurochir* 1996;138:40.

148. Capra F, Vanti C, Donati R, Tombetti S, O'Reilly C, Pillastrini P: Validity of the straight-leg raise test for patients with sciatic pain with or without lumbar pain using magnetic resonance imaging results as a reference standard. *J Manipulative Physiol Ther* 2011;34:231.

149. Deville WLJM, van der Windt DA, Dzaferagic A, Bezemer PD, Bouter LM: The test of Lesegue: systematic review of the accuracy in diagnosing herniated discs. *Spine* 2000:25(9):1140-1147.

150. Kerr RS, Cdoux-Hudson TA, Adams CB: The value of accurate clinical assessment in the surgical management of the lumbar disc protrusion. *J Neurol Neurosurg Psychiatry* 1988;51:169-173.

151. Majlesi J, Togay H, Unalan H, Toprak S: The sensitivity and specificity of the slump and straight-leg raising tests in patients with lumbar disc herniation. *J Clin Rheumatol* 2008;14:87-91.

152. Rose MJ: The statistical analysis of the intraobserver repeatability of four clinical measurement techniques. *Physiotherapy* 1991;77:89.

153. Strender L, Sjoblom A, Sundell K, Ludwig R, Taube A: Interexaminer reliability in physical examination of patients with low back pain. *Spine* 1997;22:814.

154. Jonsson B, Stomqvist B: The straight-leg raising test and the severity of symptoms in lumbar disc herniation: a preoperative evaluation. *Spine* 1995;20:27.

155. Paatelma M, Karvonen E, Heiskanen J: Clinical perspective: how do clinical test results differentiate between chronic and subacute pain patients from "nonpatients"? *J Man Manip Ther* 2009;17:11.

156. Tucker N, Reid D, McNair P: Reliability and measurement error of active knee extension range of motion in a modified slump test position: a pilot study. *J Man Manip Ther* 2007; 15:E85.

157. Masci L, Pike J, Malara F, Phillips B, Bennell K, Brukner P: Use of the one-legged hyperextension test and magnetic resonance imaging in the diagnosis of active spondylolysis. *Br J Sports Med* 2006;40:940-946.

158. Tidstrand J, Homeij E: Interrater reliability of three standardized functional tests in patients with low back pain. *BMC Musculoskelet Disord* 2009;2:10.

159. Dreyfuss P, Michaelsen M, Pauza K, McLarty J, Bogduk N: The value of medical history and physical examination in diagnosing sacroiliac joint pain. *Spine* 1996;21:2594.

160. Flynn T, Fritz J, Whitman J, et al: A clinical predication rule for classifying patients with low back pain who demonstrate short-term improvement with spinal manipulation. *Spine* 2002;27:2835.

161. Kokmeyer DJ, Van der Wurff P, Aufdemkampe G, Fickensher TC: The reliability of multitest regimens with sacroiliac pain provocation tests. *J Manipulative Physiol Ther* 2002;25:42.

162. Laslett M, Aprill CN, McDonald B, Young SB: Diagnosis of sacroiliac joint pain: validity of individual provocation tests and composites of tests. *Man Ther* 2005;10:207.

163. Cote P, Kreitz BG, Cassidey JD, Dzus AK, Martel J: A study of the diagnostic accuracy and reliability of the Scoliometer and Adam's forward bend test. *Spine* 1998;23:796.

164. Yawn BP, Yawn RA, Hodge D, et al: A population-based study of school scoliosis screening. *JAMA* 1999;282:1427.

165. Estanol B, Jimenez-Gil FJ, Cardenas E, Corona T: Babinski's sign: statistical validity of a classic sign in medicine. *Neurologica* 1995;10:307.

166. Miller TM, Johnston SC: Should the Babinski sign be part of the routine neurologic examination? *Neurology* 2005;25:1165.

167. O'Sullivan PB, Phyty GD, Twomey LT, Allison GT: Evaluation of specific stabilizing exercise in the treatment of chronic low back pain with radiologic diagnosis of spondylolysis or spondylolisthesis. *Spine* 1997;22(24):2959-2967.

168. McGill SM: Distribution of tissue loads in the low back during a variety of daily and rehabilitation tasks. *J Rehabil Res Dev* 1997;34(4):448.

169. O'Shaughnessy J, Grenier JM, Stern PJ: A delayed diagnosis of bilateral facet dislocation of the cervical spine: a case report. *J Can Chirop Assoc* 2014;58(1):45-51.

170. Wood KB, Melikian R, Villamil F: Adult Scheuermann kyphosis: evaluation, management, and new developments. *J Am Acad Orthop Surg* 2012;20(2):113-121.

171. Sardar ZM, Ames RJ, Lenke L: Scheuermann's kyphosis: diagnosis, management, and selecting fusion levels. *J Am Acad Orthop Surg* 2019;27(10):462-472.

172. Crisco JJ, Panjabi MM. Postural biomechanical stability and gross muscular architecture in the spine, in Winters JM, Woo S.L-Y, eds: *Multiple Muscle Systems: Biomechanics and Movement Organization*. New York, NY, Springer-Verlag, 1990, pp 438-450.

173. Boland RA, Lin CSY, Engel S, Kiernan MC: Adaptation of motor function after spinal cord injury: novel insights into spinal shock. *Brain* 2011;134(2):495-505.

174. Hagen EM, Eide GE, Rekand T, Gilhus NE, Gronning M: A 50-year follow-up of the incidence of traumatic spinal cord injuries in Western Norway. *Spinal Cord* 2010;48(4):313-318.

175. Hall L, Tsao H, MacDonald D, Coppieters M, Hodges PW: Immediate effects of co-contraction training on motor control of the trunk muscles in people with recurrent low back pain. *J Electromyogr Kinesiol* 2009;19(5):763-773.

176. Cone JR, Berry NT, Goldfarb AH, Henson RA, Schmitz RJ, Wideman L, Shultz SJ: Effects of an individualized soccer match simulation on vertical stiffness and impedance. *J Strength Cond Res* 2012;26(8):2027-2036.

177. Udermann BE, Mayer JM, Graves JE, Murray SR: Quantitative assessment of lumbar paraspinal muscle endurance. *J Athl Train* 2003;38(3):259-262.

178. Mihara A, Kanchiku T, Nishida N, Tagawa H, Ohgi J, Suzuki H, et al: Biomechanical analysis of brachial plexus injury:

availability of three-dimensional finite element model of the brachial plexus. *Exp Ther Med* 2018;15(2):1989-1993.
179. Gill SS, Boden BP: The epidemiology of catastrophic spine injuries in high school and college football. *Sports Med Arthrosc* 2008;16(1):2-6.
180. Chien-Chang L, Shie-Huei L, Chia-Hung Y, Wang-Tso L, Shyr-Chyr C: Complete recovery of spinal cord injury without radiographic abnormality and traumatic brachial plexopathy in a young infant falling from a 30-feet-high window. *Pediatr Neurosurg* 2006;42(2):113-115.
181. Deltombe T, Nisolle JF, Boutsen Y, Gustin T, Gilliard C, Hanson P: Cervical spinal cord injury in sapho syndrome. *Spinal Cord* 1999;37(4):301.
182. Fehlings MG, Wilson JR, Dvorak MF, Vaccaro A, Fisher CG: The challenges of managing spine and spinal cord injuries. *Spine* 2010;35(21S):S161-S165.

Appendix 12.A

Oswestry Low Back Pain Disability Questionnaire

The Oswestry Disability Index (also known as the Oswestry Low Back Pain Disability Questionnaire) is an extremely important tool that researchers and disability evaluators use to measure a patient's permanent functional disability. The test is considered the 'gold standard' of low back functional outcome tools.

Scoring Instructions

For each section the total possible score is 5: if the first statement is marked the section score = 0; if the last statement is marked, it = 5. If all 10 sections are completed the score is calculated as follows:

Example: 16 (total scored)
50 (total possible score) × 100 = 32%

If one section is missed or not applicable the score is calculated:

16 (total scored)
45 (total possible score) × 100 = 35.5%

Minimum detectable change (90% confidence): 10% points (change of less than this may be attributable to error in the measurement)

Interpretation of Scores

0–20%: minimal disability	The patient can cope with most living activities. Usually no treatment is indicated apart from advice on lifting sitting and exercise.
21–40%: moderate disability	The patient experiences more pain and difficulty with sitting, lifting and standing. Travel and social life are more difficult and they may be disabled from work. Personal care, sexual activity, and sleeping are not grossly affected and the patient can usually be managed by conservative means.
41–60%: severe disability	Pain remains the main problem in this group but activities of daily living are affected. These patients require a detailed investigation.
61–80%: crippled	Back pain impinges on all aspects of the patient's life. Positive intervention is required.
81–100%	These patients are either bedbound or exaggerating their symptoms.

Instructions

This questionnaire has been designed to give us information as to how your back or leg pain is affecting your ability to manage in everyday life. Please answer by checking ONE box in each section for the statement which best applies to you. We realize you may consider that two or more statements in any one section apply but please just shade out the spot that indicates the statement which most clearly describes your problem.

Section 1 – Pain Intensity
- ☐ I have no pain at the moment
- ☐ The pain is very mild at the moment
- ☐ The pain is moderate at the moment
- ☐ The pain is fairly severe at the moment
- ☐ The pain is very severe at the moment
- ☐ The pain is the worst imaginable at the moment

Section 2 – Personal Care (Washing, Dressing, etc)
- ☐ I can look after myself normally without causing extra pain
- ☐ I can look after myself normally but it causes extra pain
- ☐ It is painful to look after myself and I am slow and careful
- ☐ I need some help but manage most of my personal care
- ☐ I need help every day in most aspects of self-care
- ☐ I do not get dressed, I wash with difficulty and stay in bed

Section 3 – Lifting
- ☐ I can lift heavy weights without extra pain
- ☐ I can lift heavy weights but it gives extra pain
- ☐ Pain prevents me from lifting heavy weights off the floor, but I can manage if they are conveniently placed (eg. on a table)
- ☐ Pain prevents me from lifting heavy weights, but I can manage light to medium weights if they are conveniently positioned
- ☐ I can lift very light weights
- ☐ I cannot lift or carry anything at all

Section 4 – Walking
- ☐ Pain does not prevent me walking any distance
- ☐ Pain prevents me from walking more than 1 mile
- ☐ Pain prevents me from walking more than 1/2 mile
- ☐ Pain prevents me from walking more than 100 yards
- ☐ I can only walk using a stick or crutches
- ☐ I am in bed most of the time

Section 5 – Sitting
- ☐ I can sit in any chair as long as I like
- ☐ I can only sit in my favorite chair as long as I like
- ☐ Pain prevents me sitting more than 1 hour
- ☐ Pain prevents me from sitting more than 30 minutes
- ☐ Pain prevents me from sitting more than 10 minutes
- ☐ Pain prevents me from sitting at all

Section 6 – Standing
- ☐ I can stand as long as I want without extra pain
- ☐ I can stand as long as I want but it gives me extra pain
- ☐ Pain prevents me from standing for more than 1 hour
- ☐ Pain prevents me from standing for more than 30 minutes
- ☐ Pain prevents me from standing for more than 10 minutes
- ☐ Pain prevents me from standing at all

Section 7 – Sleeping
- ☐ My sleep is never disturbed by pain
- ☐ My sleep is occasionally disturbed by pain
- ☐ Because of pain I have less than 6 hours sleep
- ☐ Because of pain I have less than 4 hours sleep
- ☐ Because of pain I have less than 2 hours sleep
- ☐ Pain prevents me from sleeping at all

Section 8 – Sex Life (if applicable)
- ☐ My sex life is normal and causes no extra pain
- ☐ My sex life is normal but causes some extra pain
- ☐ My sex life is nearly normal but is very painful
- ☐ My sex life is severely restricted by pain
- ☐ My sex life is nearly absent because of pain
- ☐ Pain prevents any sex life at all

Section 9 – Social Life
- ☐ My social life is normal and gives me no extra pain
- ☐ My social life is normal but increases the degree of pain
- ☐ Pain has no significant effect on my social life apart from limiting my more energetic interests (eg, sport)
- ☐ Pain has restricted my social life and I do not go out as often
- ☐ Pain has restricted my social life to my home
- ☐ I have no social life because of pain

Section 10 – Travelling
- ☐ I can travel anywhere without pain
- ☐ I can travel anywhere but it gives me extra pain
- ☐ Pain is bad but I manage journeys over 2 hours
- ☐ Pain restricts me to journeys of less than 1 hour
- ☐ Pain restricts me to short necessary journeys under 30 minutes
- ☐ Pain prevents me from travelling except to receive treatment

Reference

Fairbank JC, Pynsent PB: The Oswestry Disability Index. *Spine* 2000;25(22):2940-2952; discussion 2952.

Appendix 12.B

Office Use Only

Name _____

Date _____

Neck Disability Index

This questionnaire has been designed to give us information as to how your neck pain has affected your ability to manage in everyday life. Please answer every section and **mark in each section only the one box that applies to you.** We realise you may consider that two or more statements in any one section relate to you, but please just mark the box that most closely describes your problem.

Section 1: Pain Intensity

☐ I have no pain at the moment
☐ The pain is very mild at the moment
☐ The pain is moderate at the moment
☐ The pain is fairly severe at the moment
☐ The pain is very severe at the moment
☐ The pain is the worst imaginable at the moment

Section 2: Personal Care (Washing, Dressing, etc.)

☐ I can look after myself normally without causing extra pain
☐ I can look after myself normally but it causes extra pain
☐ It is painful to look after myself and I am slow and careful
☐ I need some help but can manage most of my personal care
☐ I need help every day in most aspects of self care
☐ I do not get dressed, I wash with difficulty and stay in bed

Section 3: Lifting

☐ I can lift heavy weights without extra pain
☐ I can lift heavy weights but it gives extra pain
☐ Pain prevents me lifting heavy weights off the floor, but I can manage if they are conveniently placed, for example on a table
☐ Pain prevents me from lifting heavy weights but I can manage light to medium weights if they are conveniently positioned
☐ I can only lift very light weights
☐ I cannot lift or carry anything

Section 4: Reading

☐ I can read as much as I want to with no pain in my neck
☐ I can read as much as I want to with slight pain in my neck
☐ I can read as much as I want with moderate pain in my neck
☐ I can't read as much as I want because of moderate pain in my neck
☐ I can hardly read at all because of severe pain in my neck
☐ I cannot read at all

Section 5: Headaches

☐ I have no headaches at all
☐ I have slight headaches, which come infrequently
☐ I have moderate headaches, which come infrequently
☐ I have moderate headaches, which come frequently
☐ I have severe headaches, which come frequently
☐ I have headaches almost all the time

Section 6: Concentration

☐ I can concentrate fully when I want to with no difficulty
☐ I can concentrate fully when I want to with slight difficulty
☐ I have a fair degree of difficulty in concentrating when I want to
☐ I have a lot of difficulty in concentrating when I want to
☐ I have a great deal of difficulty in concentrating when I want to
☐ I cannot concentrate at all

Section 7: Work

☐ I can do as much work as I want to
☐ I can only do my usual work, but no more
☐ I can do most of my usual work, but no more
☐ I cannot do my usual work
☐ I can hardly do any work at all
☐ I can't do any work at all

Section 8: Driving

☐ I can drive my car without any neck pain
☐ I can drive my car as long as I want with slight pain in my neck
☐ I can drive my car as long as I want with moderate pain in my neck
☐ I can't drive my car as long as I want because of moderate pain in my neck
☐ I can hardly drive at all because of severe pain in my neck
☐ I can't drive my car at all

Section 9: Sleeping

☐ I have no trouble sleeping
☐ My sleep is slightly disturbed (less than 1 hr sleepless)
☐ My sleep is mildly disturbed (1-2 hrs sleepless)
☐ My sleep is moderately disturbed (2-3 hrs sleepless)
☐ My sleep is greatly disturbed (3-5 hrs sleepless)
☐ My sleep is completely disturbed (5-7 hrs sleepless)

Section 10: Recreation

☐ I am able to engage in all my recreation activities with no neck pain at all
☐ I am able to engage in all my recreation activities, with some pain in my neck
☐ I am able to engage in most, but not all of my usual recreation activities because of pain in my neck
☐ I am able to engage in a few of my usual recreation activities because of pain in my neck
☐ I can hardly do any recreation activities because of pain in my neck
☐ I can't do any recreation activities at all

Score: _____ /50   **Transform to percentage score x 100 =** _____ %points

Scoring: For each section the total possible score is 5: if the first statement is marked the section score = 0, if the last statement is marked it = 5. If all ten sections are completed the score is calculated as follows:

    Example: 16 (total scored)
    50 (total possible score) x 100 = 32%

If one section is missed or not applicable the score is calculated: 16 (total scored)
    45 (total possible score) x 100 = 35.5%

Minimum Detectable Change (90% confidence): 5 points or 10 %points

NDI developed by: Vernon, H. & Mior, S. (1991). The Neck Disability Index: A study of reliability and validity. Journal of Manipulative and Physiological Therapeutics. 14, 409-415

Appendix 12.C

Patient-Specific Functional Scale

Clinician to read and fill in: Complete at the end of the history and prior to physical

Read at Baseline Assessment

I'm going to ask you to identify up to five important activities that you are unable to do or have difficulty with as a result of your problem.

Today, are there any activities that you are unable to do or have difficulty with because of your problem? (show scale)

Read at Follow-up Visits

When I assessed you on (state previous assessment date), you told me that you had difficulty with (read 1, 2, 3, 4, 5 from list).

Today, do you still have difficulty with 1 (have patient score each activity); 2 (have patient score each activity); 3 (have patient score each activity); 4 (have patient score each activity); 5 (have patient score each activity).

Scoring scheme (show patient scale):

0	1	2	3	4	5	6	7	8	9	10
Unable to perform activity										Able to perform activity at preinjury level

Activity	Date/score				
1					
2					
3					
4					
5					
Additional					
Additional					

Reproduced from Stratford P, Gill C, Westaway M, Binkley, J: Assessing disability and change on individual patients: A report of a patient specific measure. *Physiother Can* 1995;47(4): 258-263.

Appendix 12.D

The Roland-Morris Disability Questionnaire

When your back hurts, you may find it difficult to do some of the things you normally do.

This list contains sentences that people have used to describe themselves when they have back pain. When you read them, you may find that some stand out because they describe you *today*.

As you read the list, think of yourself *today*. When you read a sentence that describes you today, put a tick against it. If the sentence does not describe you, then leave the space blank and go on to the next one. Remember, only tick the sentence if you are sure it describes you today.

1. I stay at home most of the time because of my back.
2. I change position frequently to try and get my back comfortable.
3. I walk more slowly than usual because of my back.
4. Because of my back I am not doing any of the jobs that I usually do around the house.
5. Because of my back, I use a handrail to get upstairs.
6. Because of my back, I lie down to rest more often.
7. Because of my back, I have to hold on to something to get out of an easy chair.
8. Because of my back, I try to get other people to do things for me.
9. I get dressed more slowly then usual because of my back.
10. I only stand for short periods of time because of my back.
11. Because of my back, I try not to bend or kneel down.
12. I find it difficult to get out of a chair because of my back.
13. My back is painful almost all the time.
14. I find it difficult to turn over in bed because of my back.
15. My appetite is not very good because of my back pain.
16. I have trouble putting on my socks (or stockings) because of the pain in my back.
17. I only walk short distances because of my back.
18. I sleep less well because of my back.
19. Because of my back pain, I get dressed with help from someone else.
20. I sit down for most of the day because of my back.
21. I avoid heavy jobs around the house because of my back.
22. Because of my back pain, I am more irritable and bad tempered with people than usual.
23. Because of my back, I go upstairs more slowly than usual.
24. I stay in bed most of the time because of my back.

Note to Users

This questionnaire is taken from: Roland MO, Morris RW. A study of the natural history of back pain. Part 1: Development of a reliable and sensitive measure of disability in low back pain. *Spine* 1983;8:141-144.

The score of the questionnaire is the total number of items checked (ie, from a minimum of 0 to a maximum of 24).

It is acceptable to add boxes to indicate where patients should tick each item.

Reproduced from Roland MO, Morris RW: A study of the natural history of back pain. Part 1: Development of a reliable and sensitive measure of disability in low back pain. *Spine* 1983;8:141-144.

CHAPTER 13

Head and Face

Johna K. Register-Mihalik, PhD, LAT, ATC, FACSM

OVERVIEW

The head and face are key areas of concern for evaluation because injuries to these areas may affect the brain. Additionally, due to emergent as well as cosmetic concerns, prompt evaluation and treatment are essential for optimal outcomes. This chapter will provide guidance for key aspects of evaluation and common injuries to the head and face, including case studies, critical thinking questions, and pearls and pitfalls for clinical consideration.

LEARNING OBJECTIVES

After completing this chapter, the reader will be able to do the following:

1. Identify the key anatomy of the head and face.
2. Describe the evaluation process for the head and face.
3. Describe common injuries of the head and face.
4. Compare and contrast differential diagnoses for the head and face.

FUN FACTS ABOUT THE HEAD AND FACE

- The skull contains a total of 22 primary bones (8 cranial and 14 facial).
- The sphenoid bone in the skull is shaped like a butterfly.
- The temporomandibular joint is the only freely moveable joint in the skull.
- The outer meningeal layer, the dura mater, means "tough mother" in Latin.
- The brain has four lobes, which may have some distinct functions; they also contain elaborate communication systems in which neural signals are transmitted.
- Concussions cannot be identified on standard medical imaging.
- Orbital fractures can impinge eye musculature and nerves and may impede eye movement.

Introduction

Injuries to the head and face receive significant attention from athletes, families, coaches, and medical professionals given that these injuries can have a serious effect on a patient's quality of life and may be catastrophic. Proper recognition, immediate and serial response, and proper treatment are essential. Because of improvements in care and equipment over the past 30 years, there have been significant decreases in the incidence of catastrophic injuries to the head and face.[1]

More recently, attention concerning traumatic brain injury in sport has risen to an all-time high. The evidence regarding the best ways to evaluate and treat these injuries is constantly being informed by new research. This chapter provides an overview of the clinical anatomy, evaluation components and strategies, and common pathologies of the head and face.

Clinical Anatomy

Skeletal Anatomy

The bones of the head and face make up the skull; there are 22 primary bones. Key bony structures of the head and face include the 8 cranial bones and the

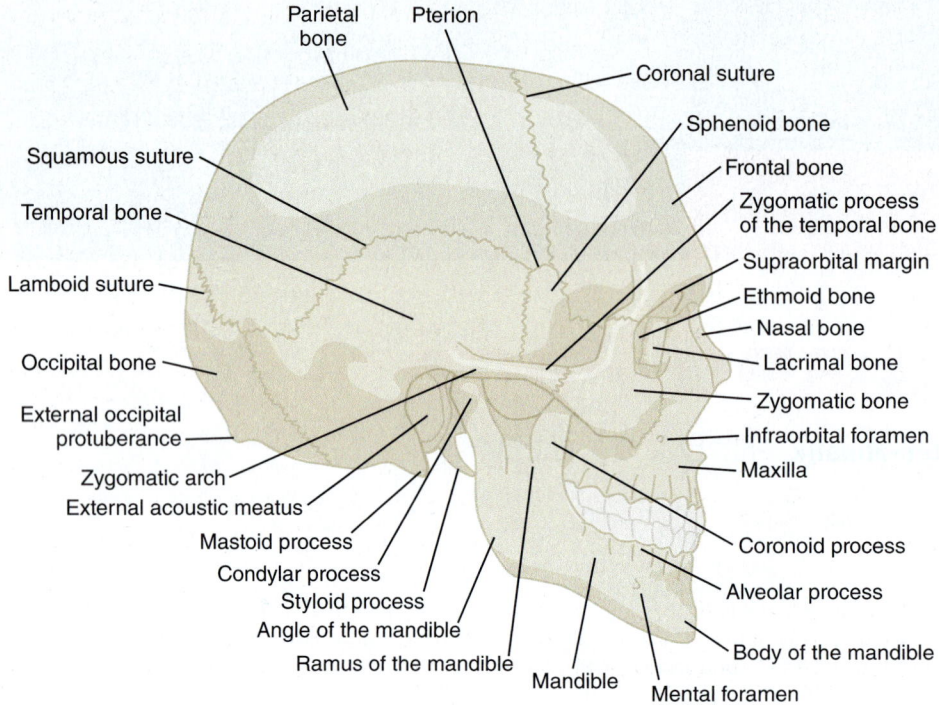

Figure 13.1 Drawing showing the bones of the head and face.
© Jones & Bartlett Learning

14 bones of the face (**Figure 13.1**). The eight cranial bones include the frontal, occipital, sphenoid, and ethmoid bones plus the temporal and parietal bones, of which there are two each. These cranial bones are fused together, creating the encased structure for the brain. The structure and shape of the cranium allow for protection of the key structures housed within. The frontal, parietal, temporal, and occipital bones align with the lobes of the brain and make up most of the cranium. The sphenoid bone (shaped like a butterfly) forms the floor of the cranium and has the space that houses the pituitary gland (sella turcica). The 14 bones of the face include two each of the nasal, maxillary, lacrimal, zygomatic, and palatine bones; two inferior nasal conchae; one mandible; and one vomer. These facial bones add to the protective structure of the head and face.

A key bony clinical region is the orbit. The orbit is formed by seven bones: the frontal, zygomatic, sphenoid, maxillary, palatine, lacrimal, and ethmoid bones. **Table 13.1** outlines where these bones are in relation to the orbit.

Additionally, the bones that make up the nasal region are clinically important. The ethmoid bone separates the nasal cavity from the brain. The nasal bones (one on each side) join the frontal bone superiorly and the maxillary bones laterally to form the nasal bridge. The nasal septum is formed posteriorly by the perpendicular plate for the ethmoid and vomer bones. Additionally, the septum is bordered anteriorly by the hard palate and posteriorly by the soft palate.

Table 13.1 Bones and Borders of the Orbit

Border	Bones
Superior (roof)	Frontal bone Lesser wing of the sphenoid bone
Inferior (floor)	Orbital surface of maxilla Orbital surface of zygomatic bone Orbital process of palatine bone
Medial	Orbital plate of ethmoid bone Frontal process of maxilla Lacrimal bone
Lateral	Frontal process of zygomatic bone Greater wing of the sphenoid bone

Articulations and Ligamentous Support

Key articulations of the head and face include the sutures that divide the cranial bones. These are immoveable articulations in adults that hold the cranial bones together. There are four sutures: coronal (unites frontal and both parietal bones), sagittal (unites the two parietal bones), lambdoid (unites the two parietal

Clinical Anatomy

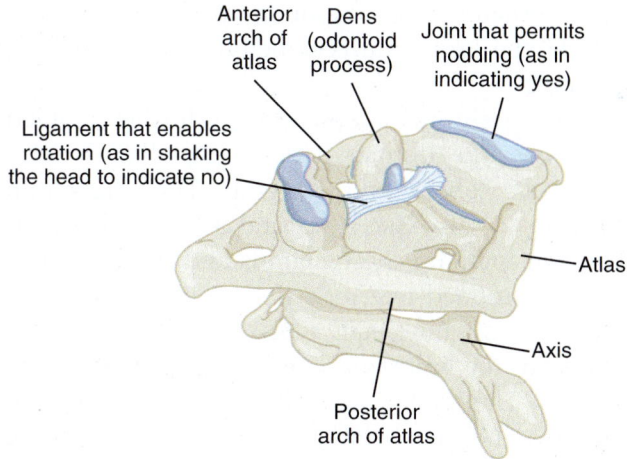

Figure 13.2 Drawing of C1: Atlas.
© Jones & Bartlett Learning

bones to the occipital bone), and squamous (unites the parietal and temporal bones). Additionally, the articulation where the cranium joins the atlas (C1) is also a key articulation when considering the evaluation of the head (**Figure 13.2**).

The temporomandibular joint (TMJ) is a key articulation in the face that is formed by the junction between the temporal bone and the mandible. Specifically, the TMJ is formed by the articulation of the condylar process of the mandible with the mandibular fossa and articular tubercle of the temporal bone. At the articulation point, there is an articular disk, much like the meniscus in the knee. Additionally, as with all synovial joints, there is a capsule surrounding the joint. The TMJ is a unique joint and is considered a combined hinge and planar (synovial) joint due to its ability to function with motions of both joint types: the joint slides above the disk and hinges below the disk. The primary motions of the TMJ are opening and closing (depression and elevation) and protracting and retracting of the jaw. It is the only freely moveable joint of all of the cranial and facial joints (**Figure 13.3**).

The articulation of the teeth with the alveolar bone is also of clinical importance. These joints are considered immovable, fibrous joints called gomphoses (**Figure 13.4**).

There are only a few ligaments of concern for the head and face. For the face, the clinically important ligaments are those surrounding the TMJ and those connecting the teeth to the jaw. Although there are other ligaments near the TMJ, the primary ligament is the temporomandibular ligament, which is the thickened lateral portion of the capsule surrounding the TMJ. The ligament has two parts: an outer oblique portion and an inner horizontal portion (Figure 13.3). The periodontal ligament connects the tooth to the

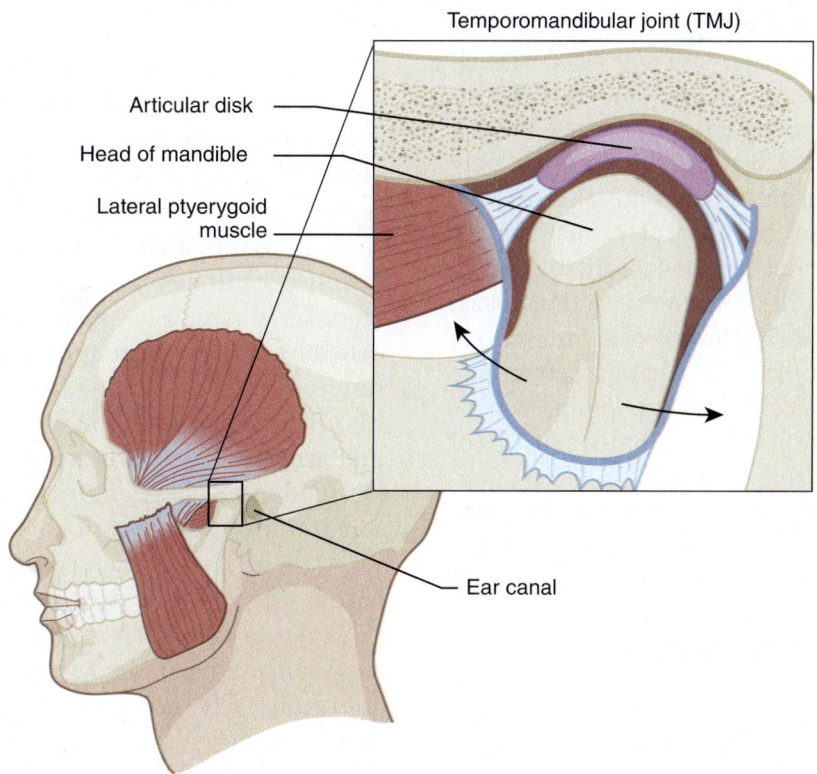

Figure 13.3 Drawing showing the temporomandibular joint.
© Jones & Bartlett Learning

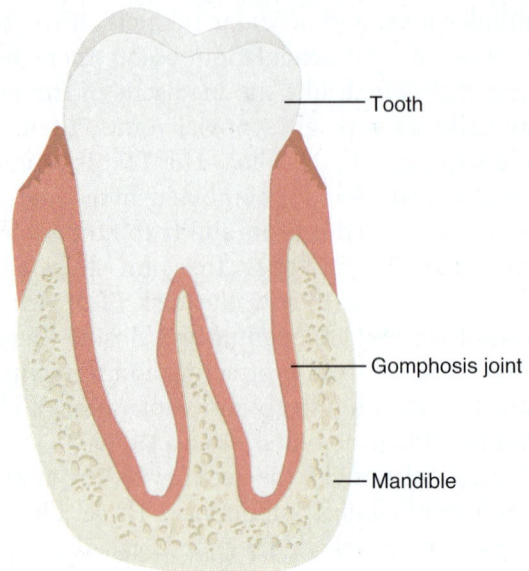

Figure 13.4 Drawing showing the gomphosis joint (tooth).
© Jones & Bartlett Learning

alveolar bone. It is fibrous connective tissue that has neurovascular components and connects the cementum covering the root of the tooth to the alveolar bone (Figure 13.4).

Soft-Tissue Anatomy

Muscular Anatomy

Key clinically important muscles of the head and face include the muscles of mastication and facial expression. Origins, insertions, actions, and innervations for selected muscles of mastication and expression can be found in **Table 13.2**. These muscles are not only important because of their function but also because they are innervated by branches of cranial nerves. Should these muscles not function properly, cranial nerve dysfunction of the trigeminal and/or facial nerves may be indicated. The testing of the muscles of mastication can be completed by having a patient bite down and open; this may include having the patient chew gum or some other soft food. For the muscles of expression, these same tests may provide information. Additionally, the clinician may have the patient smile, frown, purse the lips, and make funny faces. It can be difficult to isolate which muscle may be directly affected, but these types of tests can suggest a problem needing further follow-up and evaluation.

Neurologic Anatomy

Neurologic anatomy is a primary consideration in the evaluation of the head and face. The key neurologic anatomy includes the brain and cranial nerves. Anatomically important parts of the brain include the cerebrum, cerebellum, diencephalon, and pons.

The cerebrum (**Figure 13.5**) is further divided into lobes: the frontal, parietal (two lobes), temporal (two lobes), and occipital. The cerebellum (**Figure 13.6**) also has lobes and a body. The diencephalon includes the thalamus and the hypothalamus. Positioned inferiorly is the pons, which acts as the coordinating center between the two hemispheres of the brain and connects the cortex to the medulla. The medulla is part of the brainstem and sits above the spinal cord. The medulla serves as the major connection between the brain and the spinal cord (**Figure 13.7**). Surrounding all of the tissue in the central nervous system, including the brain, are meninges, layers of protection around the brain and other central nervous system structures that also circulate cerebrospinal fluid (CSF). The layers of the meninges, from the most superficial to the deepest, are the dura mater, the arachnoid mater, and the pia mater. The subarachnoid space between the arachnoid and pia maters is where CSF circulates.

Vascular Anatomy

The primary clinical vascular anatomy for the head and face includes the vessels that circulate blood in the brain. The blood flow within the brain is tightly regulated to meet the brain's metabolic demands.[2,3] The arteries carry oxygenated blood and glucose to the brain, and the veins carry deoxygenated blood back to the heart. The primary circulation center for blood flow in the brain is the cerebral circulation center, called the circle of Willis (**Figure 13.8**). The circle of Willis includes the arteries and veins that supply the primary blood flow to the brain. Cerebral blood flow is said to represent 12% to 15% of cardiac output, flowing at approximately 750 mL/min.[4] Anterior cerebral circulation includes the internal carotid arteries and the branches (anterior cerebral arteries and middle cerebral artery). The anterior communicating artery connects both anterior cerebral arteries. Posterior circulation includes the vertebral arteries, which come together to form the basilar artery. Off of the basilar artery are the anterior inferior cerebellar artery, pontine branches, the superior cerebellar artery, and the posterior cerebral artery on each side. The posterior communicating artery connects the anterior and posterior circulation centers. There are both deep and superficial venous drainage systems within the brain that return blood to the heart.

Table 13.2 Select Muscles of Mastication and Facial Expression

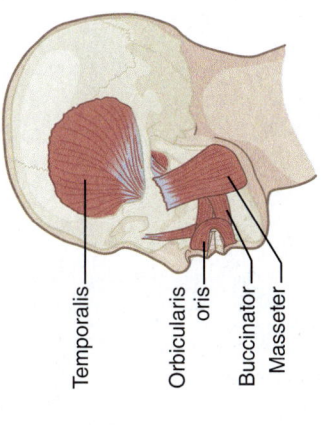

Temporalis
Orbicularis oris
Buccinator
Masseter

Muscle Name	Origin	Insertion	Action	Innervation	Palpation	Manual Muscle Test
Masseter	Zygomatic arch	Lateral surface of mandibular ramus	Elevates mandible and closes jaws	Mandibular branch of the trigeminal nerve		No standard manual muscle tests, but can ask patient to perform the primary action and observe
Temporalis	Along temporal lines of skull	Coronoid process of mandible	Elevates mandible			

(continues)

Table 13.2 Select Muscles of Mastication and Facial Expression (continued)

Muscle Name	Origin	Insertion	Action	Innervation	Palpation	Manual Muscle Test
Medial and lateral pterygoids	Lateral pterygoid plate	Medial surface of mandibular ramus	Medial: Elevates the mandible, closes the jaw, or performs lateral excursion. Lateral: Opens jaws, protrudes mandible, or performs lateral excursion			
Buccinator	Alveolar processes of maxillary bone and mandible	Blends into fibers of orbicularis oris	Compresses cheeks	Facial nerve		

Occipitofrontalis
Procerus
Levator labii superioris alaeque nasi
Temporalis
Orbicularis oculi
Levator labii superioris
Zygomaticus minor
Zygomaticus major
Levator anguli oris
Masseter
Buccinator
Orbicularis oris
Depressor anguli oris
Depressor labii inferioris
Mentalis
Platysma

Depressor labii inferioris	Mandible between the anterior midline and the mental foramen	Skin of lower lip	Depresses lower lip
Levator labii superioris	Inferior margin of orbit, superior to the infraorbital foramen	Orbicularis oris	Elevates upper lip
Mentalis	Incisive fossa of mandible	Skin of chin	Elevates and protrudes lower lip

(continues)

Table 13.2 Select Muscles of Mastication and Facial Expression *(continued)*

Muscle Name	Origin	Insertion	Action	Innervation	Palpation	Manual Muscle Test
Orbicularis oris	Maxillary bone of mandible	Lips	Compresses, purses lips			
Risorius	Fascia surrounding parotid salivary gland	Angle of mouth	Draws corner of mouth to the side			
Depressor anguli oris	Anterolateral surface of mandibular body	Skin at angle of mouth	Depresses corner of mouth			

Zygomaticus major	Zygomatic bone near zygomaticomaxillary suture	Angle of mouth	Retracts and elevates corner of mouth
Zygomaticus minor	Zygomatic bone posterior to zygomaticotemporal suture	Upper lip	Retracts and elevates upper lip

All figures in table © Jones & Bartlett Learning except where noted.

588 Chapter 13 Head and Face

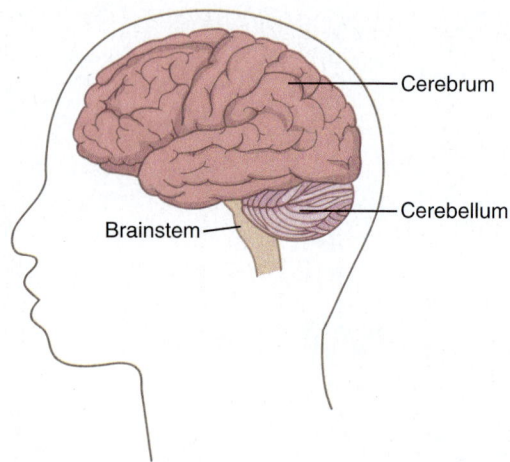

Figure 13.5 Drawing showing the cerebrum and cerebellum.
© Jones & Bartlett Learning

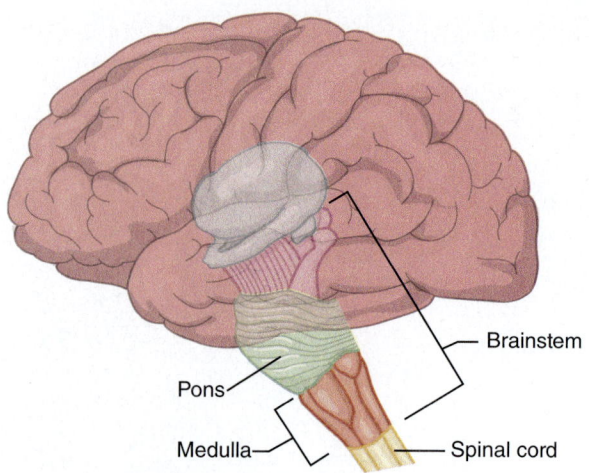

Figure 13.7 Drawing showing the spinal cord, pons, and medulla.
© Jones & Bartlett Learning

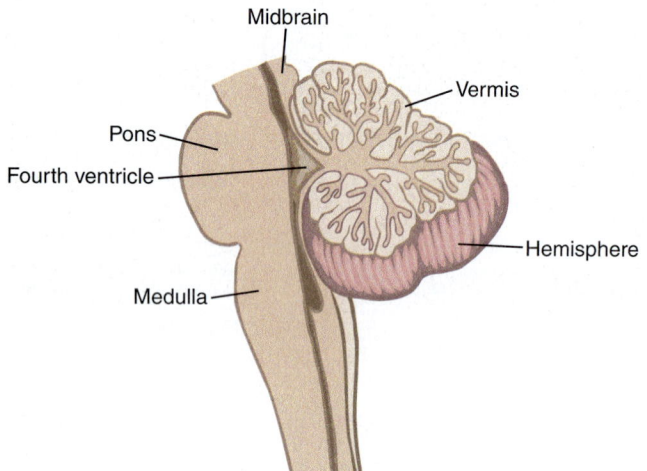

Figure 13.6 Drawing showing the cerebellum.
© Jones & Bartlett Learning

Overview of Radiology and Imaging

Common Radiographic Views

Common skull views include lateral, anterior, and posterior views; these views may be altered and the x-ray beam focused on specific areas of interest as well. **Figure 13.9** includes all of these views as normal and with an abnormal presentation of skull fracture. For the face, standard views include occipitomental at 30°. Specifically, for the mandible, common views include orthopantomogram and mandible views. For inspection of the mandible, both views are needed, as a fracture may be seen on only one of the views. For

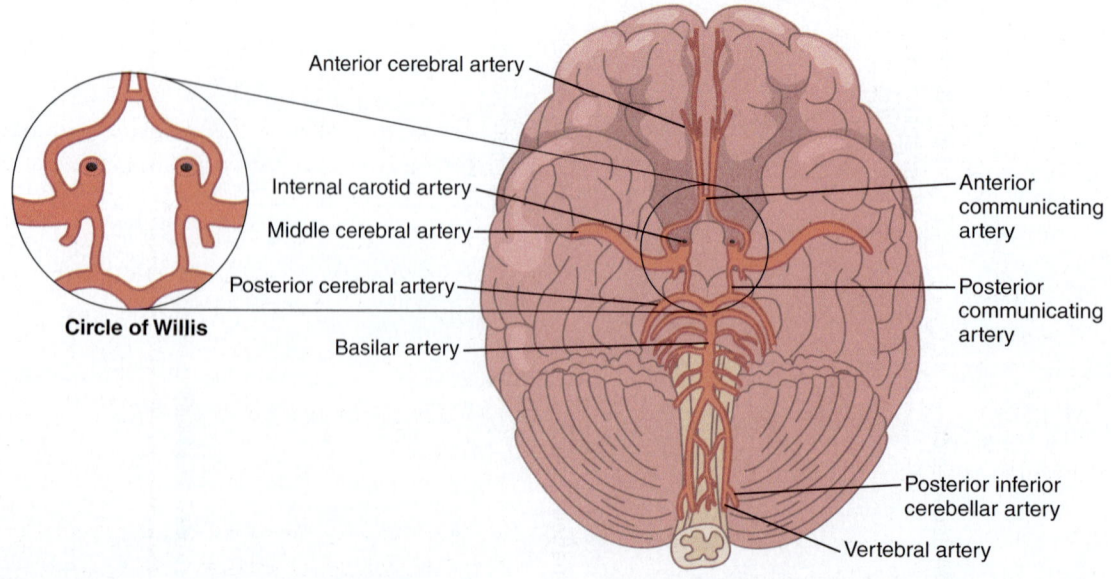

Figure 13.8 Drawing showing the circle of Willis.
© Jones & Bartlett Learning

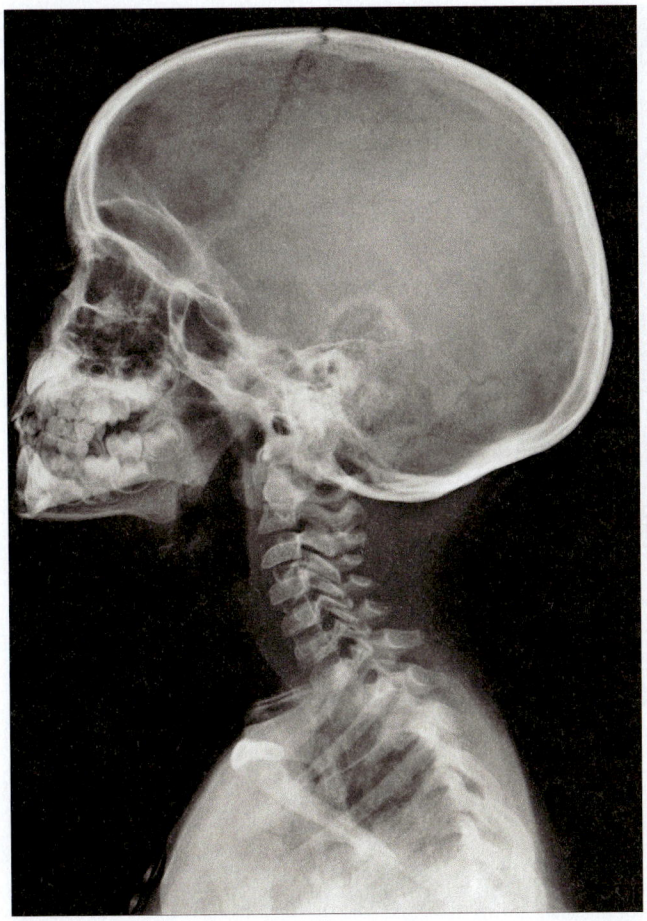
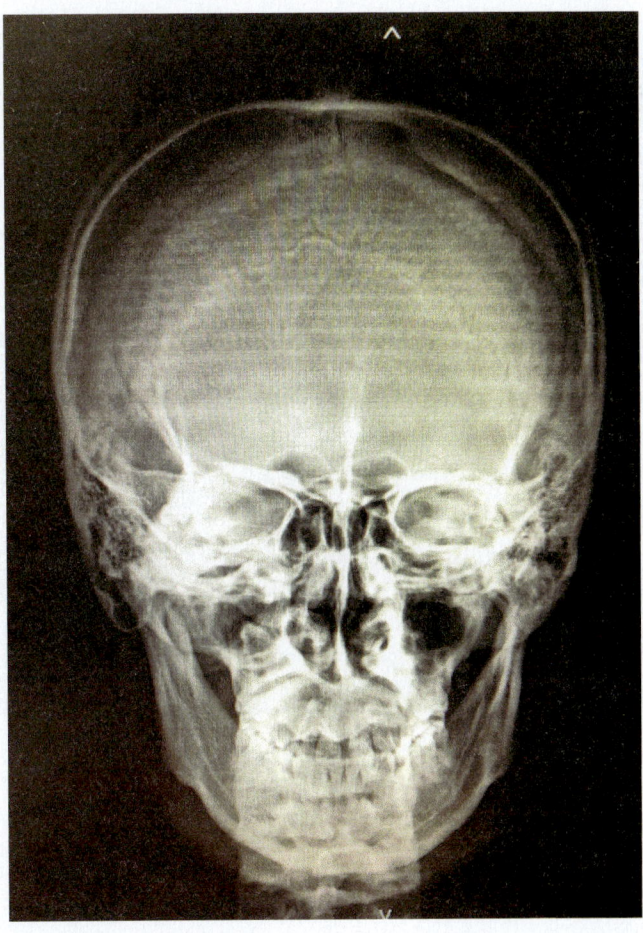

Figure 13.9 Common radiographic views of the skull. **A.** Lateral view. **B.** AP view.

A. © narcoz52/Shutterstock; **B.** © Chisanupong Chantapoon/Shutterstock

the head and face, radiographs are primarily used to identify and rule out fractures.

Common MRI Views

MRI is often used to assess soft-tissue damage. MRI provides a map of proton density within tissues. MRI of the entire head is most commonly used to assess the head and face. **Figure 13.10** provides examples of normal and pathologic views of brain tissue via MRI.

Different types of MRI sequences can be used to identify various pathologies, including T1- and T2-weighted images, which are the most basic types. In T1-weighted images, fat tissue is highlighted; in T2-weighted images, fat tissue and water are highlighted. There are other specific sequences that may be used to identify specific pathologies. With fluid-attenuated inversion recovery, the signal from free fluid in the ventricles is suppressed. These views are compared with T2-weighted images. Diffusion-weighted imaging is used in combination with apparent diffusion coefficient imaging. Areas with high diffusion-weighted imaging signal and low apparent diffusion coefficient imaging signal indicate cell death as seen through the districted diffusion.

Other Imaging Options

CT scans provide a three-dimensional map of the head based on density variations of anatomic structures. CT is often used in an emergency department setting to rule out suspected intracranial hemorrhage. It is important to note that concussion cannot be identified or diagnosed using imaging techniques.

Evaluation of the Head and Face

Evaluation of the head and face, as with other parts of the body, begins with the primary survey for airway, breathing, circulation, and other key life- or limb-threatening signs or symptoms. Determining

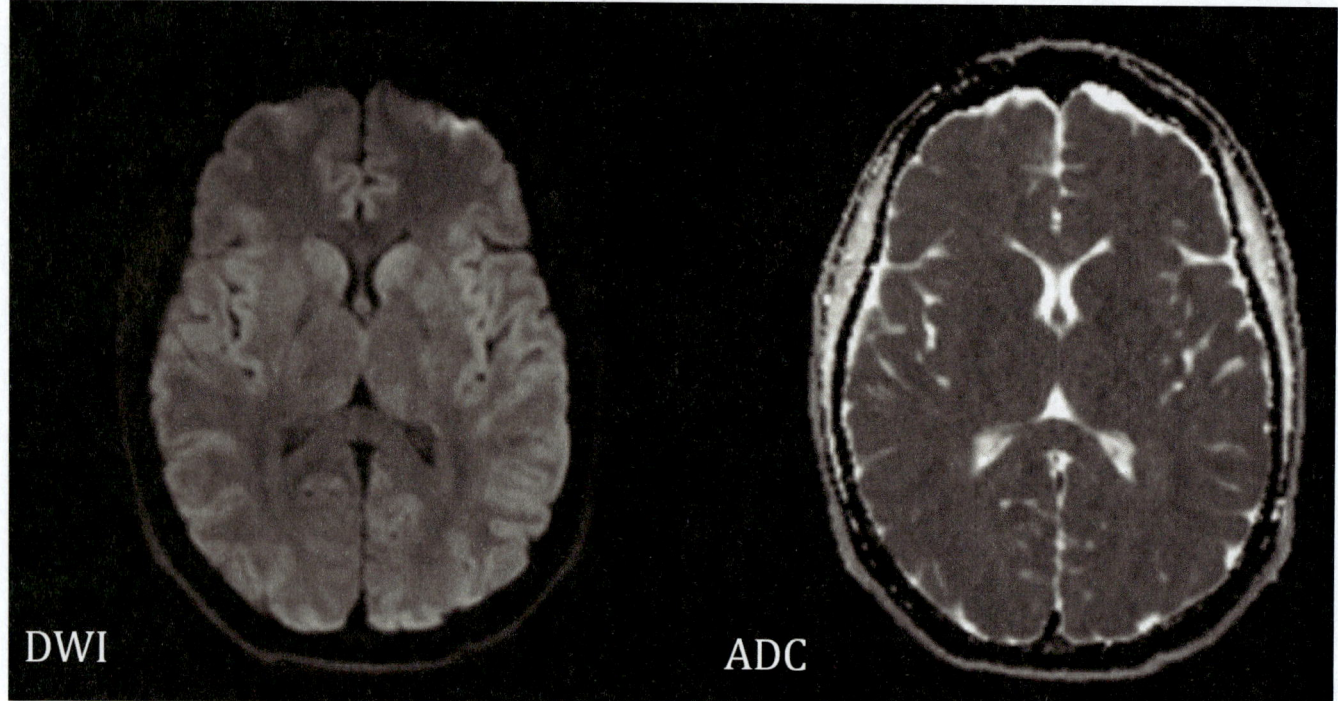

Figure 13.10 Examples of magnetic resonance images.
ADC, apparent diffusion coefficient; DWI, diffusion-weighted imaging.
© springsky/Shutterstock

level of consciousness for any head injury is key. Although the Glasgow Coma Scale (GCS) is not necessarily helpful for individuals with mild traumatic brain injury (TBI)/concussion, it can provide valuable information for patients with more severe injury, as it provides assessment of level of consciousness and ability to respond to commands. The GCS is embedded in the Sport Concussion Assessment Tool-5 (SCAT-5), which can be found in **Appendix 13.A**. This primary survey, including level of consciousness, is especially important for the head and face because these structures enclose the brain, so neurologic injuries should always be considered with any injuries to this region. The following paragraphs describe a detailed process for evaluation of injuries to the head and face.

History
Overview of Goals of History

Key aspects of history taking should include general personal and family history, with specific focus on preexisting conditions, especially those that are neurologic in origin. This is important because many preexisting conditions, such as headaches/migraines; learning disorders, such as attention deficit hyperactivity disorder; and psychological and psychiatric issues/illnesses may affect presentation and recovery. Additionally, considerations of previous injuries to the head, face, and neck are key because they may contribute to presentation and outcomes following subsequent injuries to the same structures (eg, for suspected concussions, it is important to know whether it was a single impact or the patient has received multiple impacts over time).[5,6] For injuries involving the TMJ, a history of teeth grinding is important to note.

The history should also include injury characteristics, including but not limited to mechanism of injury (especially if not observed), environment in which the injury occurred, equipment involvement, and patient response to the injury (such as whether he or she received any immediate care or continued to play postinjury). The common mechanisms for brain injury, including concussion, may include a coup (trauma on the side of impact) or contrecoup (trauma on the side opposite of the injury) injury. The forces that cause trauma may be linear, shear, or rotational and may come from a single impact or multiple impacts. More recently, a mechanistic concern is repeated subconcussive forces and the trauma these forces may cause over time.[7]

Pain location and intensity, as well as anything done to alleviate the pain, are key in the assessment of the head and face, as pain location can indicate areas of concern. If the TMJ is involved, pain may be present over the TMJ region, or the patient may report headache and ear pain. Key pain questions include the following:

- Rate your pain (1-10).
- When did the pain start and what started the pain?
- What makes the pain better/worse?
- Can you fully describe the pain and pinpoint areas of pain?
- Ask about all areas of pain to avoid overlooking anything, especially considering the many connections one injury to the head and face may have to another (eg, a force great enough to cause a facial fracture may also lead to a concussion).
- Specific to concussion/brain injury:
  - Describe the type of head pain (pressure, throbbing, etc).
  - Rate the head pain (mild, moderate, severe).
  - If severe, would the patient describe it as the worst headache of his or her life? (This indicates a red flag.)

Last, ask about symptoms the patient is experiencing, including onset, timing, and any changes in symptoms. Common symptoms of concussion range from headache to trouble sleeping. A symptom checklist (**Table 13.3**) is typically used to check for symptom presence and severity. For facial injuries, such as those involving the nose or bones of the face, pain and bleeding may be present. If the affected bones are part of the orbit, eye pain or visual symptoms may be reported. In addition, knowing whether the patient feels or hears anything unusual, particularly when moving the affected part, can provide useful information; for example, for the TMJ, it is important to know whether the patient reports popping and clicking as he or she opens and closes the mouth. There may also be difficulty with mastication and opening/closing the mouth.

Table 13.3 Postconcussion Symptom List

- Headache
- Feeling of pressure in the head
- Neck pain
- Nausea or vomiting
- Dizziness
- Blurred vision
- Balance problems
- Sensitivity to light
- Sensitivity to noise
- Feeling slowed down
- Feeling like "in a fog"
- Patient reports "not feeling right"
- Difficulty concentrating
- Difficulty remembering
- Fatigue or low energy
- Confusion
- Drowsiness
- More emotional
- Irritability
- Sadness
- Nervous or anxious
- Trouble falling asleep

Overview of Possible Clinical Deductions

- Personal history of headache, learning disorders, and/or attention deficit hyperactivity disorder may influence presentation, and the patient may be at higher risk for suffering a concussion and/or a prolonged recovery following concussion.[5,6]
- Previous history of concussion, especially if there are multiple previous injuries, may result in more severe presentation and higher risk for prolonged recovery.
- Patients with a high initial symptom burden following concussion may be at risk for prolonged recovery.[8,9]
- Patients with a history of previous facial injury may have a resulting palpable or visible deformity that may be mistaken as acute without the historical context.
- Patients reporting grinding of the teeth at night may be at risk for TMJ problems, and this can indicate a potential source of injury for the TMJ.

Inspection

For head and facial injuries, observe for overall demeanor; general coordination; emotional state; and any obvious deformity, hematoma, or bleeding in the head or facial region. Pupillary response to light should also be observed. With any evaluation of the head and face, you should also inspect for any signs of neck-related trauma.

Osteokinematic and Arthrokinetic Assessment

Because most of the joints in the head and face are immobile, the only range of motion to be assessed is the motion at the TMJ. Both active and passive motion of this joint, including depression and elevation (opening and closing the mouth) and protraction and retraction of the mandible, should be evaluated.

Neurologic Assessment

A neurologic assessment of the head and face is essential given the key neurologic structures in this anatomic region. This should include a cranial nerve assessment. **Table 13.4** outlines the cranial nerves, their functions, and example of assessment tasks. Additionally, a thorough review of dermatomes and myotomes is also warranted (**Figure 13.11**). Typically, these assessments will be normal with most injuries to the head and face; however, they may be abnormal with more severe injuries, such as subdural and epidural hematomas, and indicate immediate referral.

Table 13.4 Cranial Nerve Function and Assessment Example

Number	Name	Function	Assessment Example
I	Olfactory	• Smell	Smell an alcohol pad
II	Optic	• Vision	Read a sign
III	Oculomotor	• Pupillary response • Eye tracking	Pen light to check pupillary response
IV	Trochlear	• Upward eye movement	Look up
V	Trigeminal	• Facial sensation • Teeth sensation • Tongue sensation • Mastication	Chew gum
VI	Abducens	• Lateral eye movement	Look to each side
VII	Facial	• Movement of facial muscles • Taste • Salivary glands	Eat an orange and state its taste
VIII	Vestibular	• Hearing • Equilibrium	Stand on one leg Respond to clapping at ear
IX	Glossopharyngeal	• Taste • Swallowing • Tongue sensation	Swallow with examiner's hand on throat
X	Vagus	• Taste • Swallowing • Parasympathetic outflow to visceral organs	Blood pressure
XI	Spinal accessory	• Turning head • Shrugging	Shrug shoulders
XII	Hypoglossal	• Tongue movement	Speak

Cranial Nerve Sideline Assessment

Function	Cranial Nerves Tested	Assessment Method	
Visual Assessment	II, III, IV, VI	• Visual acuity	

Cranial Nerve Sideline Assessment

Function	Cranial Nerves Tested	Assessment Method
		• Pupillary reaction
		• Eye tracking
Balance	VIII	• Romberg • Balance error scoring system
Speaking/Hearing	VIII, IX, X, XII	• Patient speaking and responding to questions
Facial Movement	V, VII, XII	• Smile

(continues)

Table 13.4 Cranial Nerve Function and Assessment Example (continued)

Cranial Nerve Sideline Assessment

Function	Cranial Nerves Tested	Assessment Method
		• Frown 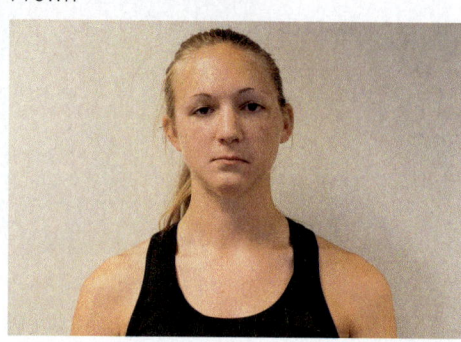
		• Stick out tongue 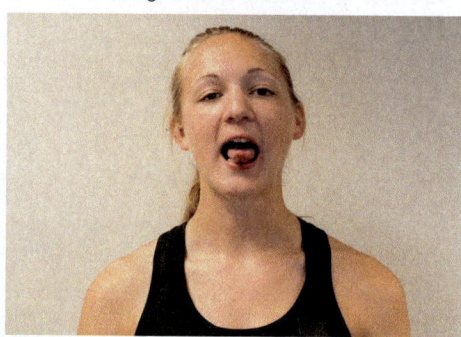
Smell	I	• Smelling salts 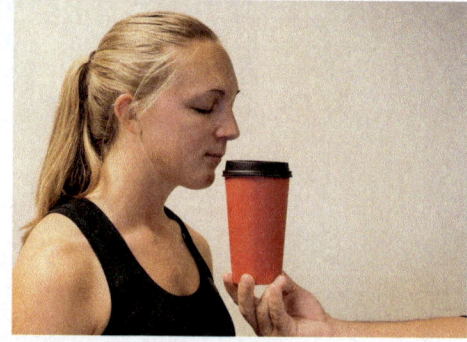 • Self-reported symptom
Shoulder Shrug	XI	• Resist shoulder shrug 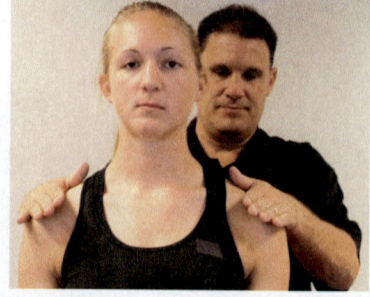 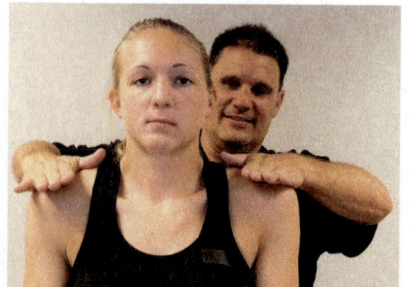 A B

All figures in table © Jones & Bartlett Learning.

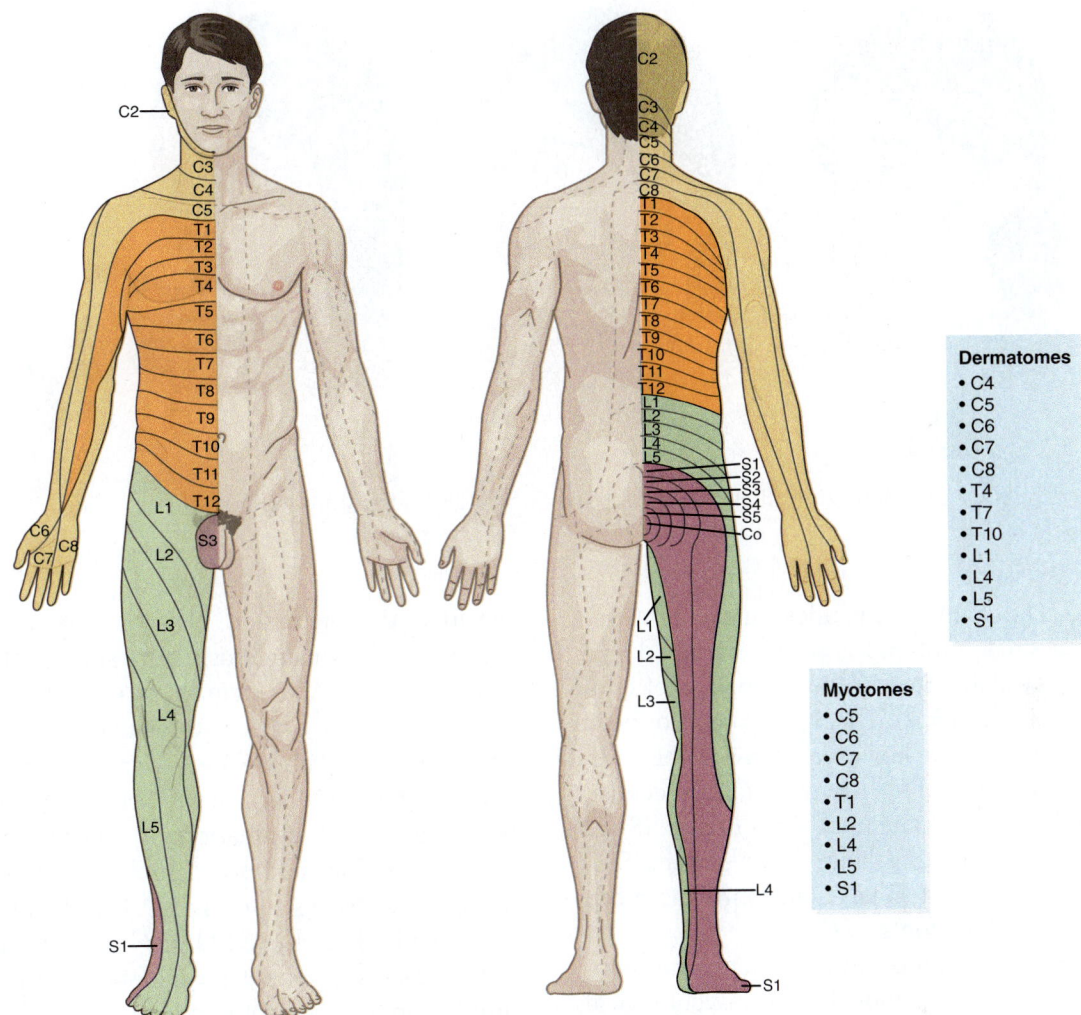

Figure 13.11 Drawing of the dermatome–myotome chart.
© Jones & Bartlett Learning

Vascular Assessment

Although there is no peripheral vascular assessment specific to the head and face, vital signs, which are indicative of overall vascular function, should be checked; these include respiration rate, blood pressure, pulse pressure, and pulse. Increases in intracranial pressure from hemorrhage, hematoma, or skull fracture can result in damage to brain tissue, which may lead to deterioration of these vital signs.

Palpation

Key areas of palpation include all areas around and near points of pain.

Bony

The entire skull should be palpated. This includes the base of the skull and all of the cranial bones, moving anteriorly toward the face and including the temporal bones (and mastoid process of each), parietal bones, frontal bones, sphenoid bones, and zygomatic bones (Table 13.2). Continuing along the face, the nasal bones, maxilla bones, and mandible should be palpated along their full length. For the face, this may also include palpation of the TMJ both internally and externally (**Figure 13.12**).

Soft Tissue

Considerations for soft-tissue palpation include the muscles of the face and scalp, specifically those of mastication and facial expression (Table 13.2).

Special Tests

The special tests for the head and face primarily consist of those that would be included in the evaluation of concussion and TBI. These special tests typically evaluate cognitive, motor, and visual-vestibular

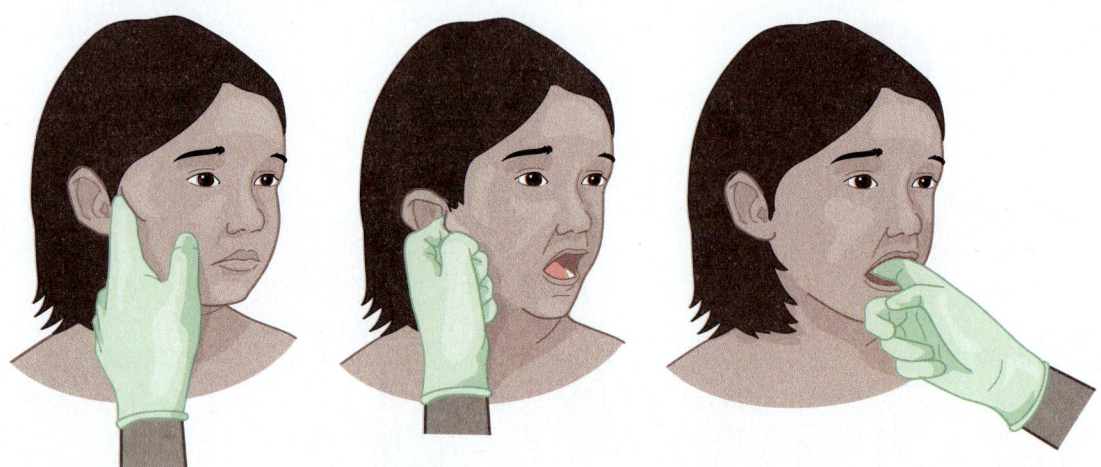

Figure 13.12 Drawings showing external and internal palpations of the temporomandibular joint.
© Jones & Bartlett Learning

capabilities. The SCAT-5 includes many of these domains in a single tool and is widely accepted as a useful, freely available tool in the evaluation of concussion[10] (Appendix 13.A). The SCAT-5 has not been validated in its entirety; however, many of the individual measures, including the symptom checklist, the Standardized Assessment of Concussion (SAC, described later), and the Balance Error Scoring System (BESS, described later) have, and thus those can be used as stand-alone tools.

Cognitive testing can be done via paper and pencil testing, such as traditional neuropsychological testing or mental status testing. Another common way cognition is tested is via computerized testing batteries. Both versions of these tests provide evaluation of thinking, memory, reaction time, and other key cognitive functions. **Table 13.5** outlines domains of cognitive assessment. The SAC, a mental status measure, can be used on the sideline or across the injury process. However, it is most sensitive in the first 48 hours after a concussion. The SAC includes questions of orientation, immediate memory, concentration, and delayed memory.[11,12] Motor assessments are typically conducted via assessments of balance, such as BESS (**Figure 13.13**), a clinical test that is cost-effective and sensitive to concussion. Additionally, coordination can be assessed using basic tests such as the tandem gait test. The SCAT-5 includes an example of this task.

More recently, visual-vestibular screening tasks, such as the Vestibular-Ocular Motor Screening (VOMS; **Figure 13.14**), have been suggested to be beneficial in the evaluation of concussion.[13] These tasks provide an additional tool to understand dysfunction following concussion. The Buffalo Concussion Treadmill Test (BCTT) has been introduced as a way to assess potential physiologic dysfunction and provide an additional functional marker of recovery. The BCTT includes measuring heart rate while gradually increasing intensity on a treadmill, with symptoms and exertion measured to produce a measure of exercise tolerance.[14-16] In addition, when returning a patient to activity following concussion or TBI, a stepwise progressive return to activity is necessary. This progression is outlined in the concussive injury section of this chapter.

For the face, functional testing of the TMJ includes observing deviations (with the lateral incisors as the reference point) as the mandible depresses and elevates (**Figure 13.15**).

Table 13.5 Potential Cognitive Deficits

- Attention/concentration
- Working memory
- Memory consolidation/retrieval
- Processing speed
- Reaction time
- Cognitive flexibility
- Executive
- Fatigue

Common Pathologies of the Head and Face

Concussion

There are an estimated 1.1 to 1.9 million sport-related concussions that occur each year.[17] Concussion causes a diffuse presentation of symptoms following a blow to the head or body that transmits forces through the brain (**Table 13.6**). The injury causes a neurometabolic

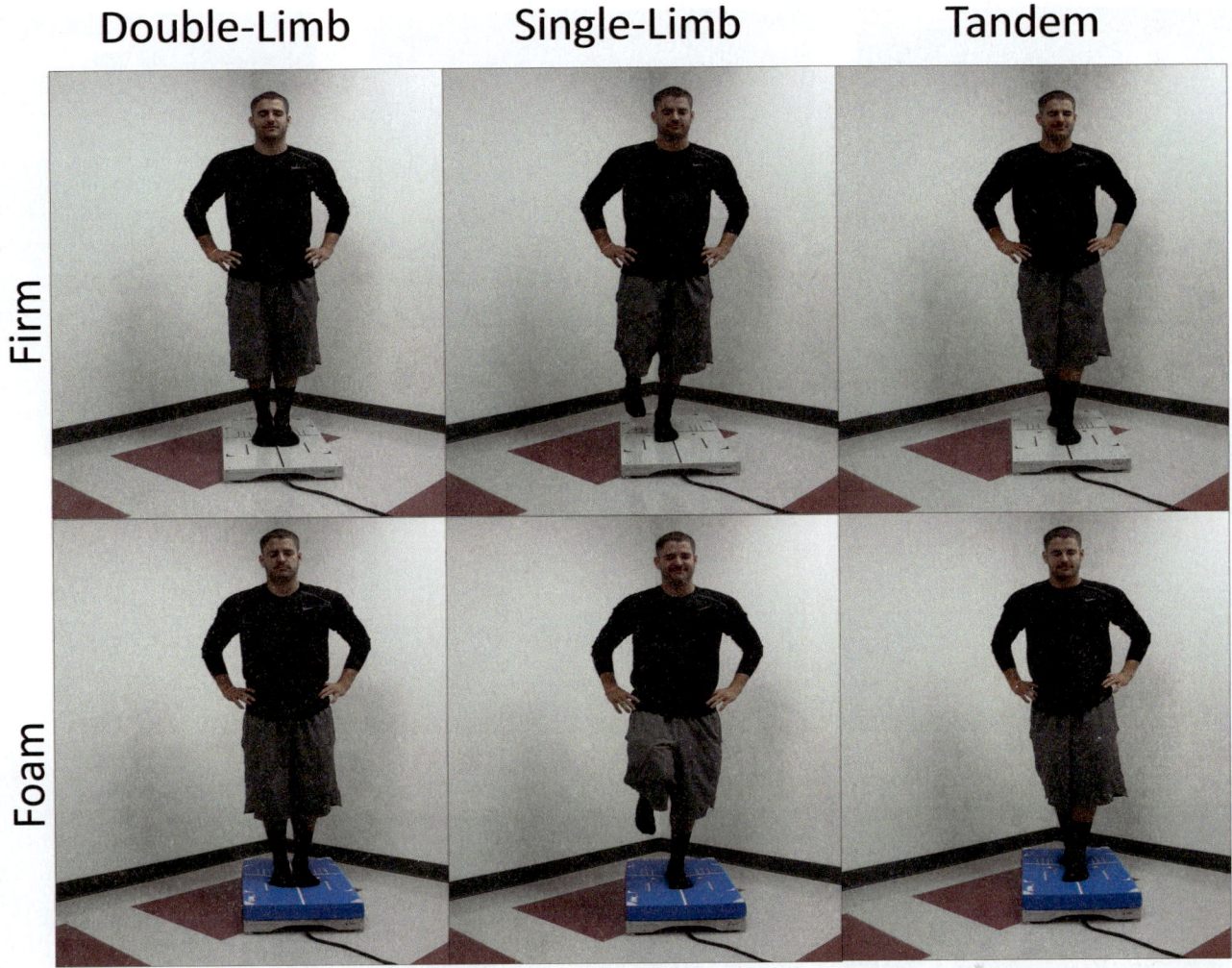

Figure 13.13 Clinical photographs demonstrating the Balance Error Scoring System.

Courtesy of Andrea Cripps.

cascade characterized by an increased energy demand in the presence of decreased cerebral blood flow.[2,3] Generally, following concussion, patients may appear dazed, "not quite right," or uncoordinated. The mechanism of injury may also have been observed. On inspection, the patients may be slow to follow commands or have trouble with normal activities. In more severe presentations of concussion, patients may present with nystagmus or other visual disturbances. These observations are red flags that more severe TBI may have occurred and further and immediate follow-up is needed. Additionally, a thorough neurologic evaluation that includes assessment of cranial nerves, dermatomes, and myotomes is necessary. In most cases, these examinations will be normal; however, they are important to help make a referral decision or a decision to initiate an emergency response, as they may be a sign of deterioration or of a more severe injury, such as intracranial hemorrhage.

Although the brain cannot be palpated, palpation of the scalp and areas of impact is important for differential diagnosis and assessment of vital signs, including blood pressure, and is also an important part of the concussion evaluation process. The special tests for concussion evaluation are focused on providing a multimodal assessment of concussion given that there is currently no gold standard diagnostic or evaluation tool.

> **Evidence for Tests**
>
> - Early studies on the multimodal assessment paradigm provide data that support the use of symptoms, cognitive assessment, and balance assessment.
> - When these are used in combination, the sensitivity to concussion is more than 90%; when used alone, sensitivity is below 65%.[18]

The battery of tests for concussion typically include use of the items included in the SCAT-5.[10] The SCAT-5 also includes a GCS, which may be used

598 Chapter 13 Head and Face

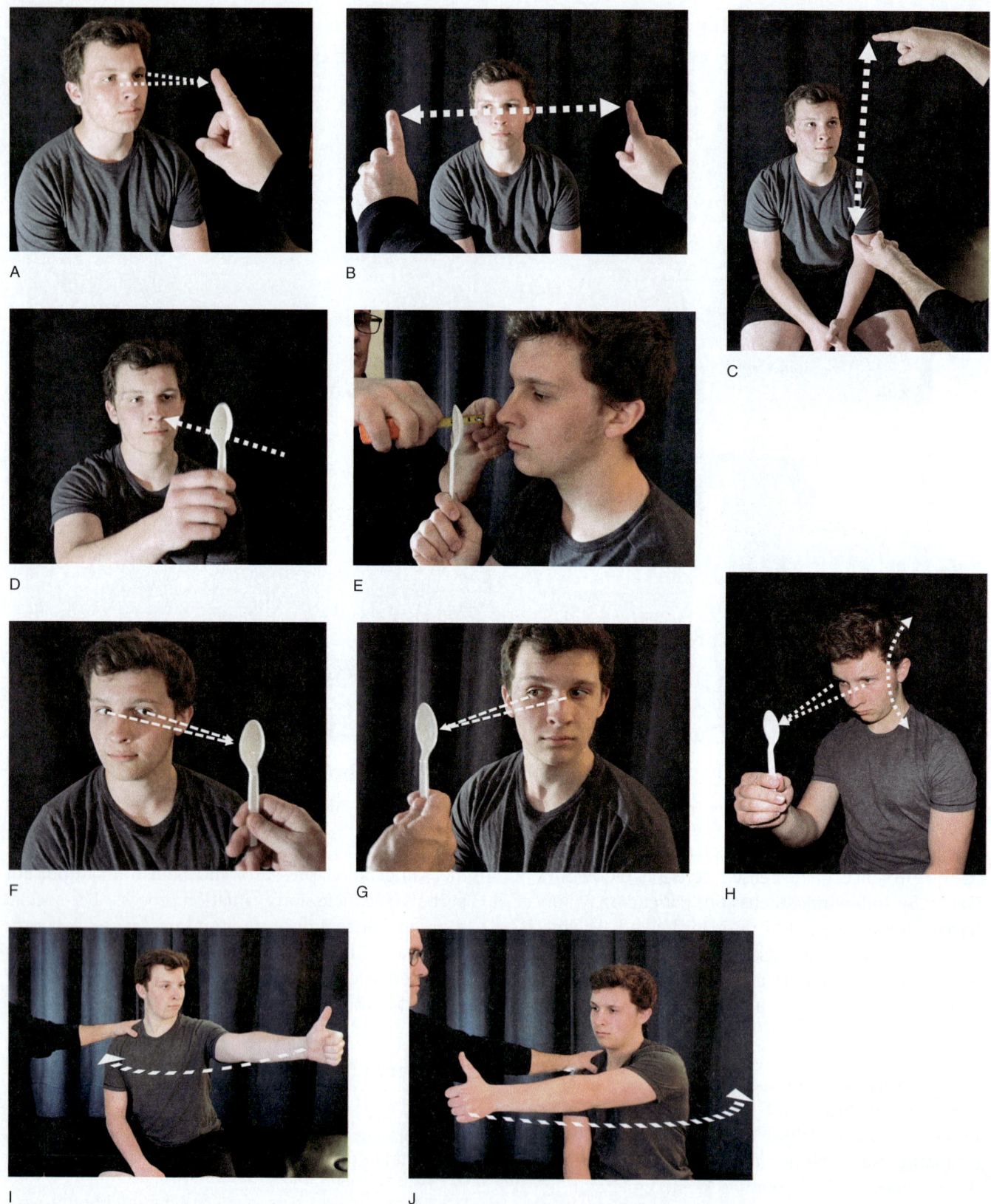

Figure 13.14 Clinical photographs demonstrating the vestibular-ocular motor screening. **A.** Smooth pursuits. **B.** Horizontal saccades. **C.** Vertical saccades. **D.** Convergence (part 1). **E.** Convergence (part 2). **F.** Horizontal vestibulo-ocular reflex (part 1). **G.** Horizontal vestibulo-ocular reflex (part 2). **H.** Vertical vestibulo-ocular reflex. **I.** Visual motion sensitivity (part 1). **J.** Visual motion sensitivity (part 2).

Courtesy of Andrea Cripps and Matt Kutz.

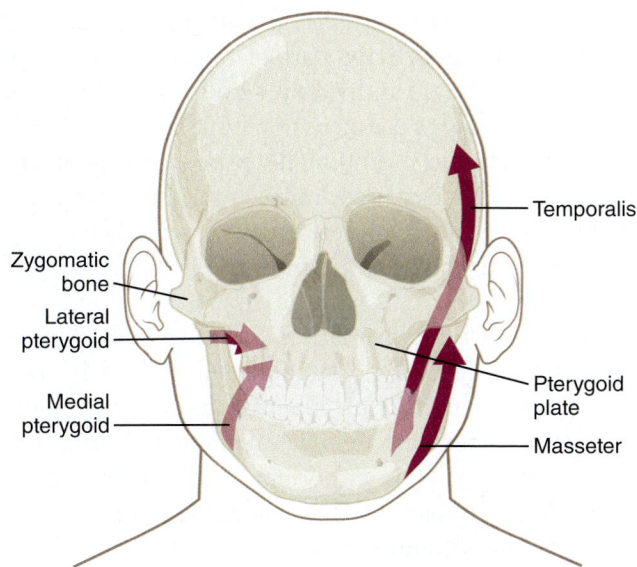

Figure 13.15 Drawing of the temporomandibular joint deviations.
© Jones & Bartlett Learning

as part of the primary survey as well as a postconcussion symptom scale, the SAC, the BESS, and the tandem gait task. Additional screening and tests to be considered are those that measure neurocognitive performance (eg, computerized neurocognitive tests)[19] and those that screen for visual-vestibular issues (eg, VOMS[13,20] and the King-Devick test).[21,22] As discussed previously, symptom assessment is key because those with increased initial symptom burden may have a delayed recovery.[8,9] Additionally, serial assessment of symptoms may help drive treatment and management decisions.

Regarding cognitive tasks, the SAC, an assessment of mental status, is most sensitive in the first 48 hours, when the deficits are often greatest.[11,12] For more expansive cognitive tests, such as traditional paper and pencil tests or computerized tests, patients often present with deficits concerning slower reaction time and memory issues beyond that initial acute window.[23,24]

Assessment of motor performance via a balance assessment, such as the BESS, or a tandem gait task provides clinicians with data concerning movement, coordination, and postural control, which are typically affected in some way following concussion. Deficits in these clinical measures of balance resolve on average in 3 to 5 days;[11] however, improvements in more functional measures that include both cognition and balance tasks together may take longer.[25] The results of these tests can help drive active management strategies, potential restrictions that may be needed on activity, and overall clinical decision making concerning return to school and sport. Recent data support that many active management strategies, such as symptom-limited activity once the patient has been stabilized, subsymptom–threshold aerobic exercise, and targeted rehabilitation paradigms (such as those treating visual-vestibular, attention, or cervicogenic issues), may be effective at improving outcomes from concussion.[26]

Although concussion cannot be detected using current clinical imaging techniques, other injuries, such as skull fracture or intracranial hemorrhage, can be ruled out using imaging techniques.[10] Sufficient

Table 13.6 Concussion Quick Tips

Pathology	Description	Presentation (HIPS)	Special Tests/Imaging	Differential Diagnosis	5-Min Sideline Assessment Tips
Concussion	Traumatic brain injury that results in diffuse presentation of symptoms following a blow to the head or body that transmits forces through the brain	Acute presentation. Primary survey important to rule out other conditions. MOI: Blow to the head or body. Transient presentation of neurologic dysfunction. Common symptoms include headache, confusion, and dizziness. Cognitive and motor dysfunction often present	Cognitive tests. Motor tests (balance, gait, etc). Imaging if red flags (routine imaging not recommended for concussion)	Dehydration. MOI can help rule out other conditions	SCAT-5 and VOMS can be useful

MOI, mechanism of injury; HIPS, history, inspection, palpation, special tests; SCAT-5, Sport Concussion Assessment Tool-5; VOMS, Vestibular-Ocular Motor Screening.

documentation is essential in the evaluation and management of concussion. This documentation should extend beyond noting the evaluation and management strategies to ensure the notes represent a clinical timeline from injury to recovery. These notes should be tailored around the evaluation format but also inclusive of the patient's short- and long-term goals.

An additional consideration following concussion is the functional aspects of return to learning and return to sports activity.[10] Although there is less consensus around a return-to-learning progression, there are guidance documents available, and a plan considering this guidance is essential in the evaluation and management of concussion.[27] Many patients with concussion are also students, and including this type of progression and assessment concerning school and learning-based activities is essential to ensuring proper care and management.

The return-to-sport progression is also a key part of the concussion evaluation, as this incorporates assessment of the level of exertion an individual can tolerate and be progressed through as he or she moves toward return to activity/sport. The most recent of these return-to-sport guidelines was published as part of the consensus statement on concussion in sport from the 5th International Conference on Concussion in Sport from 2016 (**Table 13.7**). This type of progression moves from initial removal from physical activity and progresses to low levels of exertion, resistance training, and sport-specific activity to eventual full return to sports activity. Part of this exertional progression is that no individual should return to play on the same day of a concussion or at any point while still symptomatic. Additionally, prior to fully returning to sports activity, clearance from an appropriate and trained medical professional is essential.[10]

Last, many signs and symptoms of concussion are present in individuals without concussion[28] and may overlap with other conditions, such as dehydration or migraine headache.[29] A thorough clinical history, including a potential mechanism and a multimodal assessment, can help delineate concussion amid the other concerns. It is important to consider that an individual may have a concussion in the presence of other conditions and issues.

Quick Tips for Evaluation of Concussion

- The primary survey is key in determining whether a life-threatening situation is occurring.
- If concussion is suspected, best practice is no return to play on the same day.
- Sideline evaluation tools can include the SCAT-5 components of symptoms, SAC, and BESS.
- When in doubt, the patient should not return to activity until a complete assessment can be completed to determine diagnosis.
- Patient must be cleared by a trained healthcare professional prior to return to sport.

Table 13.7 Fifth International Concussion in Sport Group: Return-to-Sport Guidelines

Rehabilitation Stage	Functional Exercise at Each Stage of Rehabilitation	Objective of Each Stage
1. Symptom-limited activity	Daily activities that do not provoke symptoms.	Gradual reintroduction of work/school activities.
2. Light aerobic exercise	Walking or stationary cycling at slow to medium pace. No resistance training.	Increase heart rate.
3. Sport-specific exercise	Skating drills in ice hockey, running drills in soccer. No head-impact activities.	Add movement.
4. Noncontact training drills	Progression to more complex training drills (eg, passing drills in football and ice hockey). May start progressive resistance training.	Exercise, coordination, and increased thinking.
5. Full-contact practice	Following medical clearance, participate in normal training activities.	Restore confidence and assessment functional skills by coaching staff.
6. Return to play	Normal game play.	

Modified from McCrory P, Meeuwisse W, Dvořák J, et al: Consensus statement on concussion in sport: the 5th international conference on concussion in sport held in Berlin, October 2016. *Br J Sports Med* 2017;51:838-847.

Skull Fracture

Skull fractures are often classified as linear, depressed, or comminuted and may occur in various locations and severities (**Figure 13.16**). Because of the forces that result in a skull fracture, there is always concern for TBI. Key history questions include queries about mechanism of injury, previous history of head trauma, and symptoms present. Although most skull fractures have an acute presentation, it is possible for a nondisplaced skull fracture to present after the time of injury. Key observation and inspection points include any appearance of deformity, hematoma, or lacerations as well as signs of additional head trauma, such as lack of coordination or loss of consciousness. Over time, ecchymosis may move to behind the ear (Battle sign) or around the eyes. Check for any leakage of CSF, as this would suggest, more severe brain injury (**Figure 13.17**). Palpation may reveal deformity

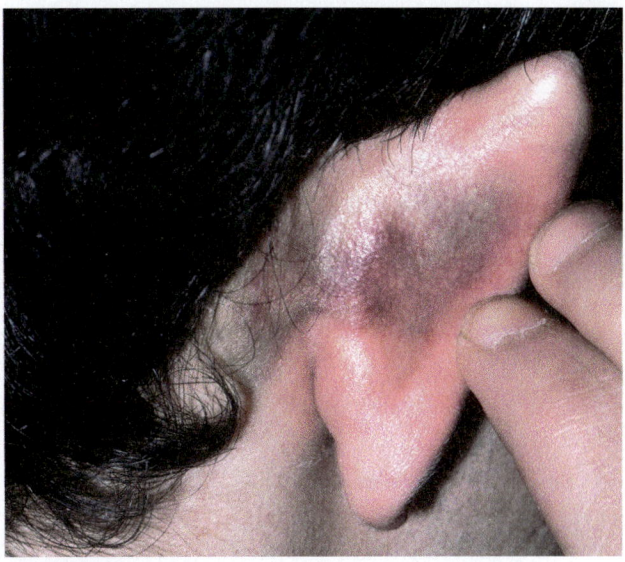

Figure 13.17 Photograph showing the Battle sign.
© Jones & Bartlett Learning

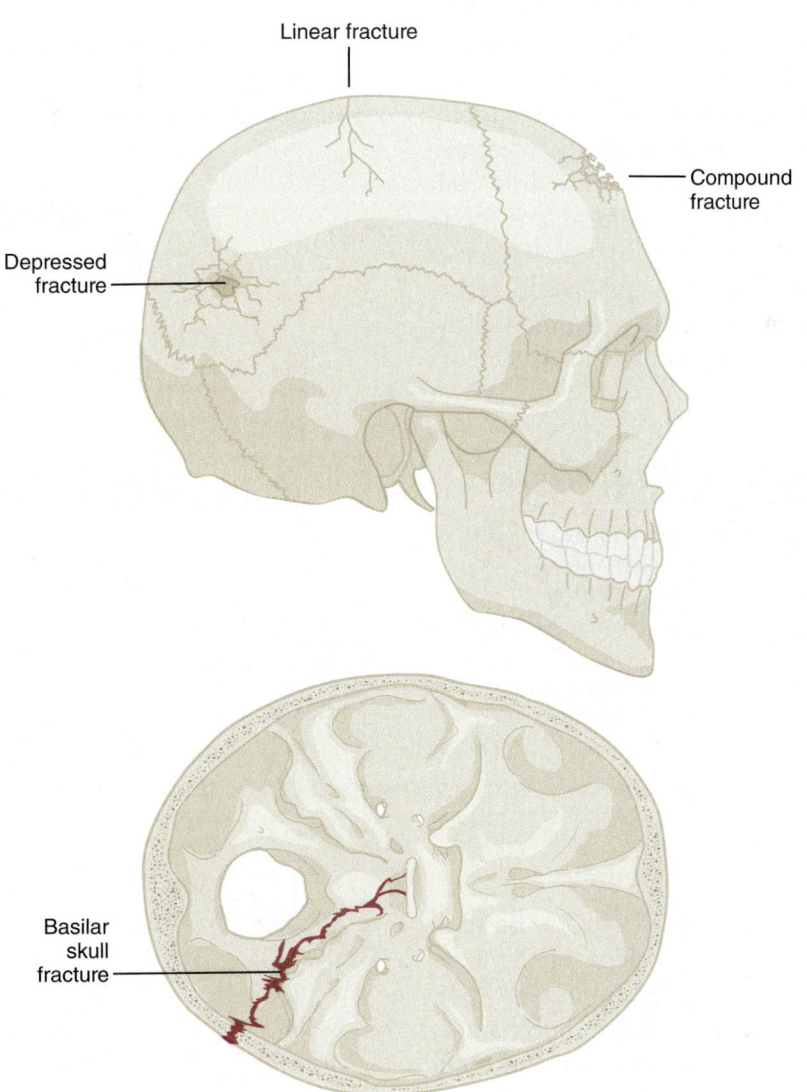

Figure 13.16 Drawings showing skull fractures.
© Jones & Bartlett Learning

Table 13.8 Skull Fracture Quick Tips

Pathology	Description	Presentation (HIPS)	Special Tests/Imaging	Differential Diagnosis	5-Min Sideline Assessment Tips
Skull fracture	Break fracture in the skull bones; often described as linear, depressed, or comminuted	Usually acute presentation May result in deformity, but not always Inspect for cerebrospinal fluid, discoloration, and deformity	Radiographs, CT, and/or MRI may be needed in many cases	Traumatic brain injury Facial contusion	Battle sign and raccoon eyes can be key May need immediate referral

HIPS, history, inspection, palpation, special tests.

if the fracture is depressed or comminuted. There may be pain at and around the site of the fracture on palpation.

Skull fractures are injuries that require immediate referral; if the fracture is depressed or comminuted, it is considered a medical emergency because of the likelihood of brain tissue involvement. Radiography, MRI, and CT may be used to evaluate the presence, severity, and location of skull fractures and to evaluate any additional trauma to the head and brain (**Table 13.8**). Any patient evaluated for a skull fracture should also be evaluated for concussion and severe TBI. Careful documentation should occur around the injury, specific to initial evaluation and management.

> **Quick Tips for Evaluation of Skull Fractures**
>
> - The primary survey is key in determining whether a life-threatening situation is occurring.
> - Any signs of a depressed or comminuted skull fracture should result in activation of the emergency action plan.
> - Evaluate for changing levels of consciousness.
> - Evaluate for TBI in any patient suspected of a skull fracture.

Nasal Fracture

A nasal fracture is a fracture of one or both of the nasal bones that form the bridge of the nose (**Figure 13.18**). Key history considerations are previous history of nasal fracture and the mechanism of injury, as these may affect presentation and other evaluation considerations. Deformity and epistaxis are commonly observed immediately following a nasal fracture; however, not all nasal fractures result in either presentation. Palpation may reveal deformity or crepitus in the area of the nasal bone and cartilage that may be affected. The palpation of this area will often result in reports of pain. There are no true special tests to evaluate a nasal fracture, but radiographs are often used to confirm fracture and rule out other structural involvement (**Table 13.9**).

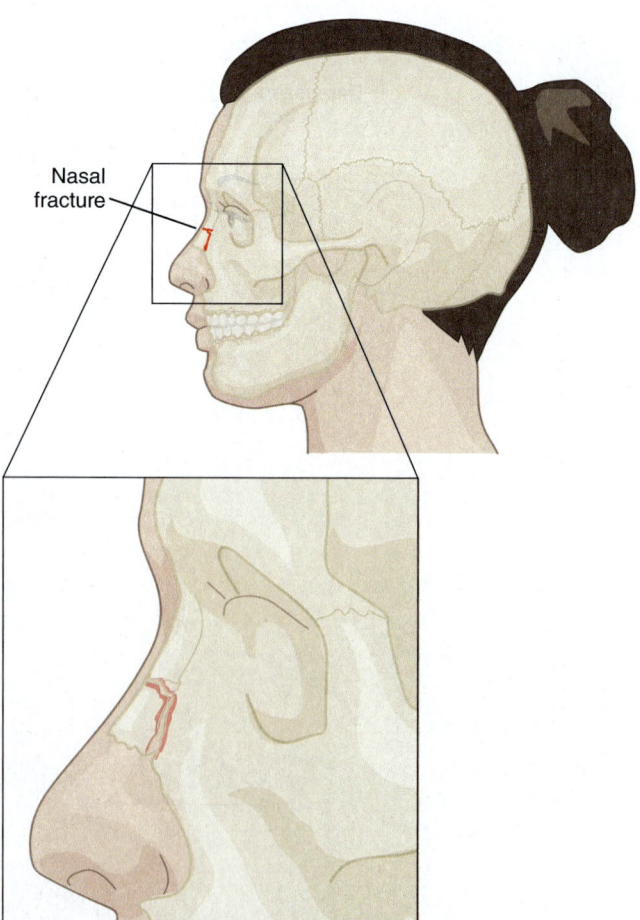

Figure 13.18 Drawing showing a nasal fracture.

© Jones & Bartlett Learning

Table 13.9 Nasal Fracture Quick Tips

Pathology	Description	Presentation (HIPS)	Special Tests/ Imaging	Differential Diagnosis	5-Min Sideline Assessment Tips
Nasal fracture	Fracture of the nasal bone; can be displaced or nondisplaced	Usually acute following blow to face May observe deformity Epistaxis often occurs	Radiographs often used to confirm the fracture	Facial fractures Traumatic brain injury	Consider other possible injuries Palpation and observation are key to sideline evaluation Consider sideline concussion assessment

HIPS, history, inspection, palpation, special tests.

Issues related to nasal fractures include the patient's pain and deformity in addition to possible airway complications if the fracture occludes or otherwise affects the nasal passages. Clinicians should be mindful of documenting the mechanism of injury and presentation so that resolution and improvements can be tracked over time. Differential diagnoses include other facial fractures and concussion. Individuals with a nasal fracture should also be evaluated for a concussion given overlap in mechanisms that can cause both injuries. Important consideration should also be given to other facial structures and eye involvement.

> **Quick Tips for Evaluation of Nasal Fractures**
>
> - Observe for deformity and epistaxis.
> - Sideline concussion assessment may be warranted.
> - Consider other facial structure and eye involvement.

Facial Laceration

Facial lacerations (**Figure 13.19**) are common in many sports and can result from an object or person coming in contact with the patient. Because many of the mechanisms that may lead to a facial laceration are shared by concussion and other injuries of the skull and face, it is important to gather a thorough history of the mechanism of injury and other complaints; in addition, the patient should be asked about any known history of bleeding or healing disorders (**Table 13.10**). Knowledge of the patient's sport and activities is also important, given the need to understand how the facial laceration may affect participation or use of equipment. Observations around a facial or head laceration include looking for signs of other injury, swelling, bleeding, size of the laceration, and any evidence of hematoma. It is typical with a facial or head laceration to see bleeding, bruising, and potentially a hematoma, especially for head lacerations. The size and depth of the laceration should be noted, as stitches or other wound closure measures may be necessary. If the patient has a concomitant injury, such as concussion, additional signs may be observed. Palpation around the area may reveal pain; there may also be palpable swelling.

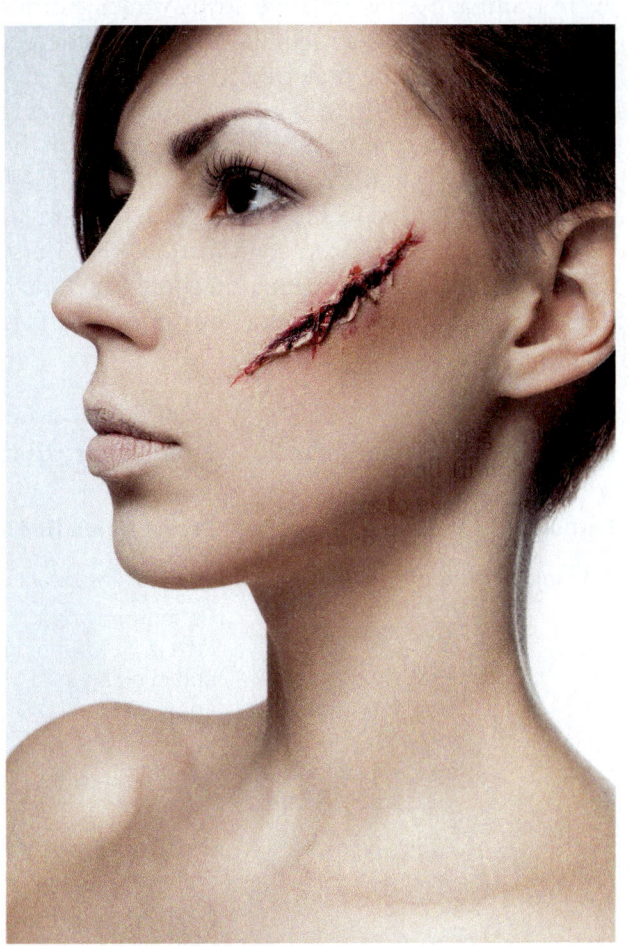

Figure 13.19 Photograph of a facial laceration.
© Vira/Shutterstock

Table 13.10 Facial Laceration Quick Tips

Pathology	Description	Presentation (HIPS)	Special Tests/Imaging	Differential Diagnosis	5-Min Sideline Assessment Tips
Facial laceration	Split in the skin in the facial/head region	Typically acute Split in skin present Inspect for hematoma	No special test, but may consider other conditions	Concussion Head/face fractures	Observe for size of laceration and bleeding Considerations for sterile adhesive strips versus sutures for closing

HIPS, history, inspection, palpation, special tests.

The evaluation may provide guidance in timing of referral in cases where the laceration is large or deep or in a location on the face that may lead to a noticeable scar. Additionally, the size of a hematoma with a head laceration may suggest additional testing and evaluation, as large and boggy hematomas have been associated with intracranial hemorrhage.[30] There are no specific special tests associated with evaluation of facial and head lacerations. Imaging may be ordered if other injuries are suggested via the evaluation process or to rule out additional and severe trauma. Sterile adhesive strips versus sutures for closure of the laceration should be considered. In general, sutures are preferred if bleeding does not stop with pressure, there is concern about scarring or cosmetic issues, muscle or fat is exposed, or the laceration is large and gaping. Differential diagnoses may include concussion and head or face fracture, as these injuries may occur in combination with a face or head laceration. Documentation should include a thorough history and an evaluation process to rule out other potential injuries.

> **Quick Tips for Evaluation of Facial Lacerations**
>
> - Observe for hematoma and other bleeding.
> - Sideline concussion assessment may be warranted.
> - Consider other facial or head bony involvement (eg, fracture).

TMJ Injury

Because the TMJ is the only freely moveable joint of the skull, TMJ injuries are a common facial injury. These injuries often occur from impact to the mandible (acute) or from grinding teeth (chronic). The injury can be either bony/joint or muscular in nature. It is important to consider how the injury occurred and when the pain first started (Table 13.11). Additionally, it is important to note what exacerbates the pain, including activities, such as mastication/chewing, talking over a period of time, or other activities that place pressure on the joint. Asking about activities, medications, or

Table 13.11 Temporomandibular Joint Injury Quick Tips

Pathology	Description	Presentation (HIPS)	Special Tests/Imaging	Differential Diagnosis	5-Min Sideline Assessment Tips
TMJ injury	Injury to the TMJ region may result from a variety of factors The injury may be primarily bone, muscular, articular, or a combination	Acute or insidious Patient may report lock jaw or popping and clicking in TMJ area In severe cases, swelling may be present Palpation over TMJ and surrounding muscles may be tender	Lateral deviation on opening and closing mouth Bite malocclusion MRI Ultrasonography	Concussion Facial contusion	Observe for deviations on opening and closing of mouth Feel for crepitus/popping and clicking on opening mouth In severe cases, observe for deformity and malocclusion

HIPS, history, inspection, palpation, special tests; TMJ, temporomandibular joint.

actions that improve the pain is also important. In many instances, there is not much to note on initial visual inspection of the TMJ. In more severe or traumatic injuries to the joint, there may be swelling or discoloration. The patient may have observable pain as he or she opens and closes the mouth when talking or chewing. Inspection should include postural observations of the cervical spine. Palpating over the TMJ externally and internally (Figure 13.12) will often be painful, and crepitus may be felt. There may also be soreness in the muscles surrounding the joint and additional muscles in the face and neck.

There are some tests specific to the TMJ that can provide additional clinical information. These tests are considered functional in nature. On average, the mouth can open to the size of two knuckles; however, with TMJ injury, the jaw may not be able to open and close in a smooth fashion. There may be lateral deviation to either side, or the bite may be maloccluded.[31] Deviations are observed using the lateral incisors as the reference point. When asking the patient to complete range of motion at the TMJ, observe for distance and quality. A C-shaped deviation represents hypomobility to the side of the deviation; an S-shaped deviation indicates a muscular problem with the muscles surrounding the TMJ. For muscular testing, the lateral pterygoids are tested for mouth opening, and the masseter, temporalis, and medial pterygoids are tested for mouth closing. MRI is one of the most commonly used imaging techniques for the TMJ; however, CT and ultrasonography can also be used to identify the various structures that may be injured.

Implications following TMJ diagnosis may include referral needs based on mechanism of injury and deficits. Additionally, any patient with dislocation or malocclusion should not be allowed to return to play until the issue is resolved. Differential diagnoses may include additional facial fracture or muscle injury. Documentation of the onset of pain, as well as progression of dysfunction, is important so that additional management strategies may be implemented and appropriate referrals may be given over the course of treatment.

Quick Tips for Evaluation for TMJ Injury

- Observe for mechanism of injury.
- Observe for obvious swelling, deformity, or malocclusion.
- Consider other facial or head bony involvement (eg, fracture).
- An injury that results in malocclusion, dislocation, or suspected fracture warrants removal from the game and referral.
- A dislocated TMJ may need to be immobilized.

Subdural and Epidural Hematomas

Subdural hematoma is the most common catastrophic sport-related traumatic brain injury.[32] (Although not as common, epidural hematomas, another type of intracranial hemorrhage, can also occur.) Subdural hematomas are caused from a bleed that typically occurs in a vein, leading to a slower bleed than an epidural hematoma; bleeding can be from an artery as well, however. A subdural bleed occurs below the dura mater and above the subarachnoid mater (**Figure 13.20**); an epidural bleed occurs above the dura mater.

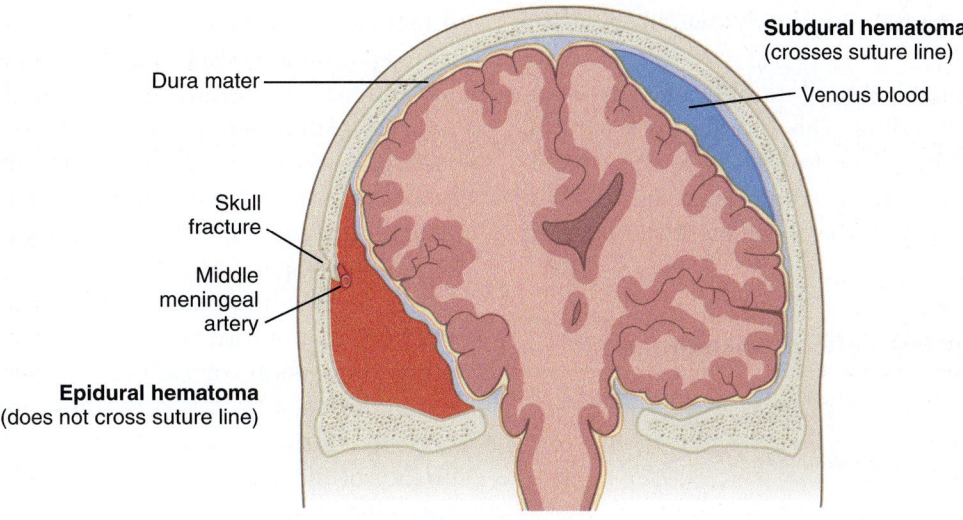

Figure 13.20 Drawing of a subdural hematoma.

Table 13.12 Subdural and Epidural Hematoma Quick Tips

Pathology	Description	Presentation (HIPS)	Special Tests/ Imaging	Differential Diagnosis	5-Min Sideline Assessment Tips
Subdural and epidural hematomas	Intracranial bleeds resulting from head trauma	Typically acute. Inspect for signs of concussion and traumatic brain injury. Patient may be disoriented or have lucid window prior to deterioration	MRI CT Skull radiograph	Concussion Cerebral contusion	Primary survey important. If suspected, activate emergency medical services

HIPS, history, inspection, palpation, special tests.

Key historical factors and questions to consider for intracranial bleeds include previous history of head injury, mechanism of injury, and general feelings of worsening along with other patient-reported symptoms. Because subdural hematomas are often venous bleeds, the deterioration may occur slowly over time, whereas epidural hematomas typically result in deterioration that occurs more quickly. In many cases, individuals have a short, lucid interval (10 to 15 minutes) followed by rapid deterioration. Individuals with a subdural or epidural hematoma may appear dazed and confused and present with signs of concussion. Palpation may not reveal anything, but palpation at the injury site is warranted to rule out skull fracture or other external head trauma. Neurologic assessment will often be abnormal with these injuries, and cranial nerve assessment may indicate involvement. Imaging is often ordered if one of these bleeds is suspected. This may include CT or MRI of the head. Functionally, patients may present with loss of consciousness and/or reduced mental status with lower GCS scores (**Table 13.12**).

There are many clinical implications concerning intracranial bleeding. This bleeding is a medical emergency and should be treated as soon as possible. Failure to treat this bleeding can result in death or permanent brain damage. Differential diagnosis primarily includes concussion. Careful documentation of mechanism of injury, initial evaluation, and all management actions is essential.

Postconcussion Syndrome/ Persistent Postconcussion Symptoms

Persistent postconcussion symptoms are defined as symptoms continuing beyond the typical window for concussion recovery and have been defined in a number of ways. One widely accepted definition used in the literature is that a patient has symptoms caused by the injury for at least 1 month.[33] This persistent symptom presence is frustrating for both the patient and clinician. Key history questions include queries about previous concussion history, time since concussion, and strategies used to reduce symptoms and stressors in the recovery process. Additionally, observation and inspection should assess vital signs and any noticeable effects on demeanor and coordination. There is no special test for postconcussion syndrome; however, the evaluative approach for concussion should be directly applied to these patients. Additionally, the BCTT, as described previously, may be useful in determining exercise tolerance and progression in these patients. Medical imaging cannot identify postconcussion syndrome. Functionally, patients may present in a manner similar to those with concussion but may exhibit more neurobehavioral-oriented symptoms, such as irritability, depression, or sadness. Implications include psychological effects of persistent symptoms and the need to consider potential interventions to improve quality of life. Referral to a concussion specialist or specialist with expertise specific to the patient's deficit may also be warranted. Documentation of any

---

Quick Tips for Evaluation of Hematoma

- Observe for altered consciousness, confusion, and deterioration.
- If suspected, activate emergency medical services.
- Continue to check vital signs.

Table 13.13 Postconcussion Syndrome Quick Tips

Pathology	Description	Presentation (HIPS)	Special Tests/Imaging	Differential Diagnosis	5-Min Sideline Assessment Tips
Postconcussion syndrome	Symptoms persisting beyond the typical window for concussion recovery (typically at least 1 month or more)	Full symptom and history assessment; Concussion assessment process over time	Cognitive and motor tests; Imaging may be necessary if intracranial bleed suspected	Psychiatric conditions; Initial concussion	Full concussion evaluation; Serial assessments important; Consider the many factors that may be influencing recovery

HIPS, history, inspection, palpation, special tests.

activities that improve or worsen symptoms is key to helping determine a progression of activity that may aid in recovery (**Table 13.13**).

Orbital Blowout Fracture

An orbital blowout fracture occurs when one of the walls of the orbit is fractured, but the rim remains intact. The most common mechanism is a direct blow to the orbit region. Key history questions include queries about previous injury to the head and face as well as location of pain and any complaints concerning vision and eye movement. Previous injury may affect the way things look on evaluation. If visual complaints are present, it is important to further evaluate for the primary cause, as these fractures can affect eye muscle function. Inferior orbit fractures are the most common, whereas lateral blowout fractures are the least common.

Observation and inspection may include enophthalmos (protruding eyes), diplopia, orbital emphysema, and malar region numbness due to potential inferior orbital nerve injury. Additional observations may include inability to track an object upward due to inferior rectus nerve involvement (**Figure 13.21**). Both radiography and CT are used in the evaluation of these fractures. A complete visual assessment is warranted to evaluate potential nerve and/or muscle involvement. Documentation of direct location of pain and specifically any eye involvement is key to determining management strategies (**Table 13.14**).

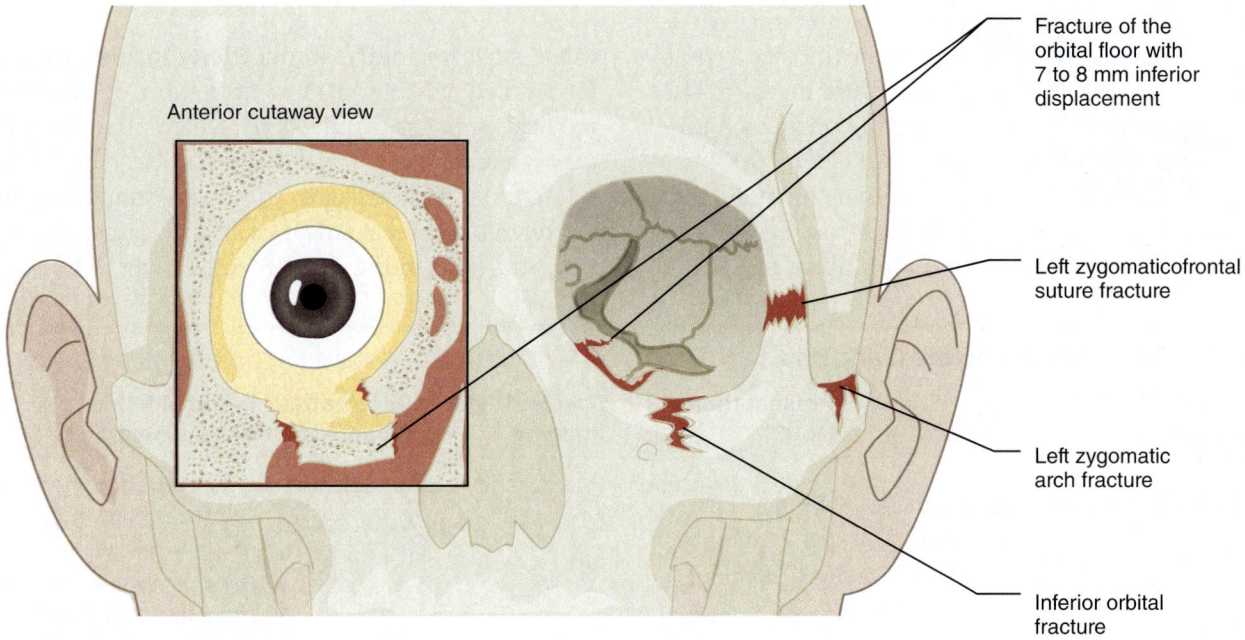

Figure 13.21 Drawing of an orbital fracture.
© Jones & Bartlett Learning

Table 13.14 Orbital Blowout Fracture Quick Tips

Pathology	Description	Presentation (HIPS)	Special Tests/ Imaging	Differential Diagnosis	5-Min Sideline Assessment Tips
Orbital blowout fracture	Wall of the orbit is fractured, but the rim remains intact	Acute presentation Deformity may be present Inability to look up if inferior rectus nerve is involved	Radiography CT	Facial fracture	Observe for deformity Inspect and test eye tracking/movement

HIPS, history, inspection, palpation, special tests.

Quick Tips for Evaluation of Orbital Blowout Fracture

- Observe for altered consciousness, confusion, and deterioration to suggest other injuries.
- Potential deformation.
- Eye tracking is a must to ensure eyes are moving smoothly and tracking objects appropriately.
- Patient should not return to sport the same day of an orbital fracture.

LeFort Fractures

LeFort fractures (**Figure 13.22**) are fractures of the midface. They occur in three different locations indicated numerically by 1, 2, 3 (or I, II, III). These fractures do not usually occur during sports participation, but more commonly occur with high-impact forces, such as motor vehicle collision. Classification of these fractures identifies the bony segments involved. LeFort fractures are very severe fractures that separate the upper teeth from the rest of the face. These fractures may result in sinus fluid running from the nose. Key historical considerations are previous injury and mechanism of injury that resulted in the fractures. Observations and inspection may include gross deformity and potential discoloration as well as signs of other injuries given the amount of force needed to

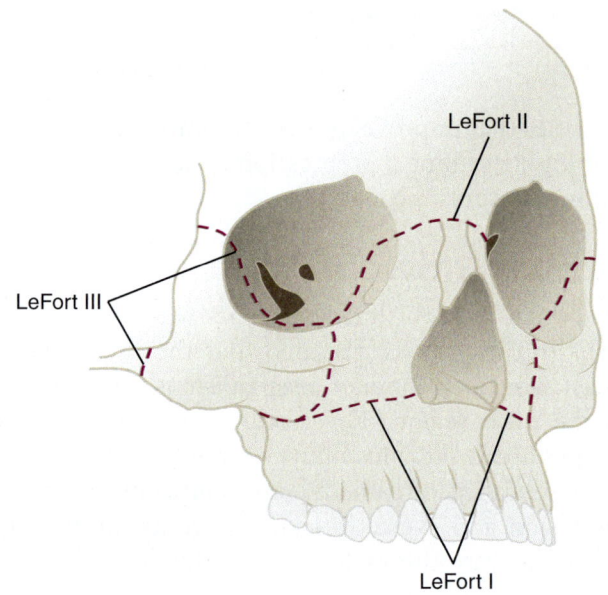

Figure 13.22 Drawing showing LeFort fracture.
© Jones & Bartlett Learning

cause such an injury. Implications include the need for immediate referral and activation of emergency medical services as needed. Differential diagnoses may include other facial fractures, concussion, and intracranial hemorrhages. Clinicians should carefully document the mechanism of injury, associated injuries, and steps in the care process (**Table 13.15**).

Table 13.15 LeFort Fracture Quick Tips

Pathology	Description	Presentation (HIPS)	Special Tests/ Imaging	Differential Diagnosis	5-Min Sideline Assessment Tips
LeFort fractures	Severe fractures that separate the upper teeth from the rest of the face	Acute presentation (usually not as a result of sports participation) Gross deformity	Radiography CT MRI	Concussion Other facial fractures	If suspected immediate referral/emergency medical services Gross force resulting in these fractures likely results in other injuries

HIPS, history, inspection, palpation, special tests.

Quick Tips for Evaluation of LeFort Fractures

- Primary survey due to severity of injury.
- Observe for deformity and any discoloration.
- Activation of emergency medical services.

Tooth Fractures and Luxations

Dental injuries are not uncommon in sport. Two of the most common are tooth fractures and luxations. These injuries may range in severity from a slightly chipped tooth to one that is fully avulsed. Key historical considerations include length of time since injury, mechanism of injury, and previous history of dental issues or trauma. These factors may influence decision making around timing and type of care needed. Tooth fractures result in parts of the tooth fracturing off the main tooth. Luxations occur when the tooth separates at the gomphosis.

Tooth fractures are classified into four types, three of which are shown in **Figure 13.23**. Type IV involves full separation of the top of the tooth, which, like type III, involves the dentin and the pulp cavity. As such, type III and IV fractures are more painful. Luxations refer to the tooth's root being avulsed from the socket, either outwardly or back toward the joint. As such, luxations include an intruded tooth, an extruded tooth, and a full tooth avulsion. Implications of a fracture or luxation are the need to seek dental care immediately to ensure the health of the tooth. Every effort should be made to find an outwardly avulsed tooth because replacement of the tooth is often possible. Differential diagnoses may include other facial fractures and concussion, as these injuries often occur with significant force directly to the mouth. Careful attention should be devoted to documenting the immediate response and care process for the injury (**Table 13.16**).

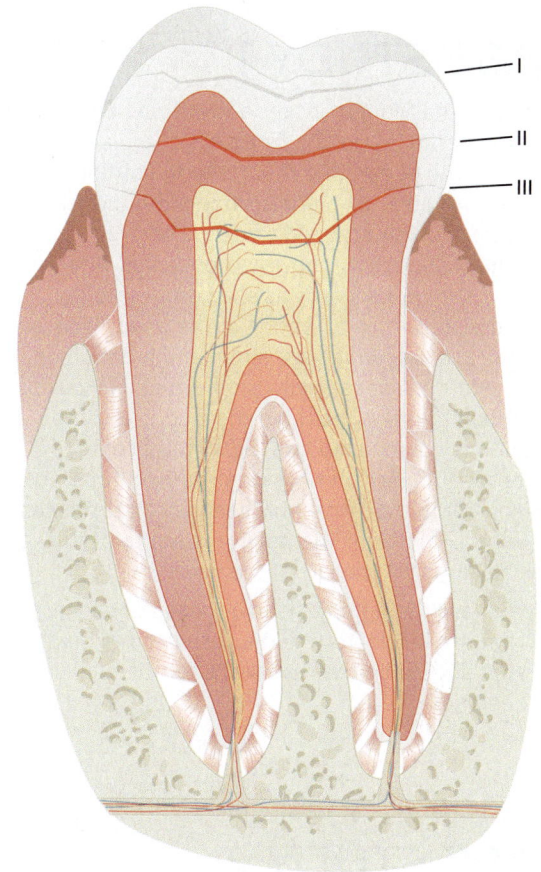

Figure 13.23 Drawing of tooth fracture classifications I, II, and III.

© Jones & Bartlett Learning

Quick Tips for Evaluation of Tooth Fractures

- Primary survey due to severity of injury.
- Observe for deformity and any discoloration.
- Make every effort to find a tooth that has been outwardly avulsed, because 90% of avulsed teeth can be replaced in children.
- Rinse found tooth and store it in a biocompatible storage environment.

Table 13.16 Tooth Fracture Quick Tips

Pathology	Description	Presentation (HIPS)	Special Tests/ Imaging	Differential Diagnosis	5-Min Sideline Assessment Tips
Tooth fractures	Fracture of the tooth	Acute presentation. Inspect for portion of tooth fractured/location of tooth affected	No specific special tests. Radiograph	Tooth luxation. Concussion. Other facial fractures	Observation is key. Immediate referral results in best outcomes

HIPS, history, inspection, palpation, special tests.

CASE STUDY 1

A 20-year-old female soccer athlete was elbowed in the head while going up for a header in her conference championship game last night. She said she "saw stars," had a headache, and felt dizzy immediately afterward but kept playing in the game. She reports to the athletic training clinic and states that she has started to feel a lot worse. She reports vomiting just before coming into the clinic. She has a history of three previous concussions and has received a diagnosis of generalized anxiety disorder.

Initial inspection shows no observed abnormalities; swelling; discoloration; or deformities on her head, face, or neck. She walks slowly as she comes into the clinic, and overall her demeanor appears fatigued. No abnormalities are suggested from palpation of the head, face, and neck. General neurologic evaluation of the cranial nerves suggests all cranial nerves are intact and functioning. However, the patient was dizzy on balance screening. Dermatome and myotome assessments are normal. No vascular compromise is noted.

Special testing included the BESS, a computerized neurocognitive test, and a visual-vestibular screening. The patient has balance deficits (BESS total score of 35). All neurocognitive testing outcomes are well below her baseline scores (particularly of note was reaction time and processing speed). She could not complete the visual-vestibular screen (VOMS) because she began to feel nauseated and dizzy at the beginning of the screening. Throughout the evaluation, it is clear the patient is not tolerating the testing activities or other stress well and that she is declining clinically over the course of the visit.

1. What are the differential diagnoses of concern in this case?
2. What are key factors in the patient's history that may be affecting the current presentation?
3. What should be the next steps for the clinician? What clues in the evaluation details lead to your decision for these next steps?

CASE STUDY 2

A 14-year-old male basketball player reports to you immediately after being hit on the right jaw by the elbow of an opponent during a game. The patient is not wearing a mouthguard. He cannot fully close his mouth when he first presents for evaluation and states his pain is worse on the right side. He also states he has a bad headache, his ear feels strange, and he feels a little dizzy. The patient eventually is able to close his mouth but states it still hurts. Inspection reveals that the patient is noticeably in pain and his skin is red where he was hit on the face.

The patient has limited depression of the mandible (opening of the mouth), and he feels a clunk at the restricted end range of motion. A noticeable C curve to the right side is observed as the patient opens his mouth. As he opens and closes his mouth, you can feel and hear a clicking/clunking noise on the right side.

1. What are the differential diagnoses of concern in this case?
2. What are the key anatomic structures that may be affected and why?
3. Should the patient be allowed to return to play that game? Why or why not?

ONE-IN-A-MILLION CASE STUDY

A 14-year-old male quarterback of a football team took a hit to the head on a sack during the first half. The player has a history of concussion and often takes risky plays leading with his head. After the play, he stumbled to get up but told his teammates he was OK and went back in for the next play. He continued to play in the game. During the latter part of the second half, he was sacked again but not noticeably hard. He again stumbled to get up, and, while walking back to the huddle, he went down on one knee and grabbed his head. His teammates walked over to check on him. While his teammates were talking with him, he fell to the ground and lost consciousness. His teammates began to try to move him to wake him up, but he would not respond.

1. What are key concerns for this patient?
2. What could have been done differently to potentially prevent negative outcomes for the patient?
3. What immediate next steps should be taken for this patient?
4. What are the differential diagnoses of concern?

WRAP-UP

Critical Thinking Questions

1. What is the purpose of the structure of the bones of the cranium and face?
2. Why does grinding one's teeth at night contribute to TMJ dysfunction?
3. Why are orbital fractures a cause of concern for normal eye function?
4. How should a full tooth avulsion be handled when at an away game with limited resources?
5. What are the red flags that may signal a more severe TBI or intracranial bleed? What steps should be taken if any of these red flags are found on evaluation?
6. When should a patient retire from contact/collision sports due to concussion?
   a. What are key factors to consider in this decision?
7. Is there any single component in the concussion evaluation process that is more important than another? Why or why not?

Pearls and Pitfalls

- There are 14 facial bones and 8 cranial bones.
- The TMJ is the only moveable joint of the skull.
- The cerebrum and the cerebellum make up most of the brain tissue.
- Key history points of consideration in evaluation of traumatic brain injury/concussion are family or personal history of psychological conditions, headache disorders, traumatic brain injury, learning disabilities, and attention deficit hyperactivity disorder.
- Key history for the face is previous history of facial trauma and any remaining deformities or considerations.
- Observe for any changes in mental status and consciousness, confusion, or deterioration with any injury to the head or face.
- For facial injuries, observe for any deformity or discoloration.
- A multimodal assessment paradigm, including the overall clinical interview and symptom, cognitive, and balance assessments, is the current recommended best practice.
- Imaging is useful for the head and face to evaluate for or rule out fractures or more severe injuries; however, this modality is not currently able to diagnose concussion.
- Serial assessment is key for concussion and other TBIs to ensure tracking of recovery and to inform management strategies.
- There should be no same-day return to play for a player with a concussion, and clearance from a trained healthcare provider is necessary prior to return to play.
- Patients with suspected skull fracture should also be evaluated for TBI.
- For almost all head and face injuries, other injuries should be considered, as the mechanisms that result in head and face injuries may also cause a variety of other issues.

References

1. Mueller FO: Catastrophic head injuries in high school and collegiate sports. *J Athl Train* 2001;36(3):312-315.
2. Giza CC, Hovda DA: The neurometabolic cascade of concussion. *J Athl Train* 2001;36(3):228-235.
3. Giza CC, Hovda DA: The new neurometabolic cascade of concussion. *Neurosurgery* 2014;75(Suppl 4):S24-33.
4. Meng L, Hou W, Chui J, Han R, Gelb AW: Cardiac output and cerebral blood flow: the integrated regulation of brain perfusion in adult humans. *Anesthesiology* 2015;123(5):1198-1208.
5. Iverson GL, Atkins JE, Zafonte R, Berkner PD: Concussion history in adolescent athletes with attention-deficit hyperactivity disorder. *J Neurotrauma* 2016;33(23):2077-2080.
6. Terry DP, Huebschmann NA, Maxwell BA, et al: Preinjury migraine history as a risk factor for prolonged return to school and sports following concussion. *J Neurotrauma* 2018.
7. Bahrami N, Sharma D, Rosenthal S, et al: Subconcussive head impact exposure and white matter tract changes over a single season of youth football. *Radiology* 2016;281(3):919-926.
8. Casson IR, Sethi NK, Meehan WP III: Early symptom burden predicts recovery after sport-related concussion. *Neurology* 2015;85(1):110-111.
9. Meehan WP III, O'Brien MJ, Geminiani E, Mannix R: Initial symptom burden predicts duration of symptoms after concussion. *J Sci Med Sport* 2016;19(9):722-725.
10. McCrory P, Meeuwisse WH, Dvorak J, et al: 5th International Conference on Concussion in Sport (Berlin). *Br J Sports Med* 2017;51(11):837.
11. McCrea M, Guskiewicz KM, Marshall SW, et al: Acute effects and recovery time following concussion in collegiate

football players: the NCAA Concussion Study. *JAMA* 2003;290(19):2556-2563.
12. McCrea M, Kelly JP, Randolph C, et al: Standardized assessment of concussion (SAC): on-site mental status evaluation of the athlete. *J Head Trauma Rehabil* 1998;13(2):27-35.
13. Mucha A, Collins MW, Elbin RJ, et al: A brief vestibular/ocular motor screening (VOMS) assessment to evaluate concussions: preliminary findings. *Am J Sports Med* 2014;42(10):2479-2486.
14. Leddy J, Hinds A, Sirica D, Willer B: The role of controlled exercise in concussion management. *PM R* 2016;8(3 Suppl):S91-S100.
15. Hinds A, Leddy J, Freitas M, Czuczman N, Willer B: The effect of exertion on heart rate and rating of perceived exertion in acutely concussed individuals. *J Neurol Neurophysiol* 2016;7(4).
16. Leddy JJ, Willer B: Use of graded exercise testing in concussion and return-to-activity management. *Curr Sports Med Rep* 2013;12(6):370-376.
17. Bryan MA, Rowhani-Rahbar A, Comstock RD, Rivara F, Seattle Sports Concussion Research Collaborative: Sports- and recreation-related concussions in US youth. *Pediatrics* 2016;138(1):e20154635.
18. Broglio SP, Macciocchi SN, Ferrara MS: Sensitivity of the concussion assessment battery. *Neurosurgery* 2007;60(6):1050-1057; discussion 1057-1058.
19. Alsalaheen B, Stockdale K, Pechumer D, Broglio SP, Marchetti GF: A comparative meta-analysis of the effects of concussion on a computerized neurocognitive test and self-reported symptoms. *J Athl Train* 2017;52(9):834-846.
20. Kontos AP, Sufrinko A, Elbin RJ, Puskar A, Collins MW: Reliability and associated risk factors for performance on the Vestibular/Ocular Motor Screening (VOMS) tool in healthy collegiate athletes. *Am J Sports Med* 2016;44(6):1400-1406.
21. Moran RN, Covassin T: King-Devick test normative reference values and internal consistency in youth football and soccer athletes. *Scand J Med Sci Sports* 2018;28(12):2682-2690.
22. Dickson TJ, Waddington G, Terwiel FA, Elkington L: The King-Devick test is not sensitive to self-reported history of concussion but is affected by English language skill. *J Sci Med Sport* 2019;22(Suppl 1):S34-S38.
23. Norris JN, Carr W, Herzig T, Labrie DW, Sams R: ANAM4 TBI reaction time-based tests have prognostic utility for acute concussion. *Mil Med* 2013;178(7):767-774.
24. Eckner JT, Kutcher JS, Broglio SP, Richardson JK: Effect of sport-related concussion on clinically measured simple reaction time. *Br J Sports Med* 2014;48(2):112-118.
25. Howell DR, Brilliant A, Berkstresser B, Wang F, Fraser J, Meehan WP III: The association between dual-task gait after concussion and prolonged symptom duration. *J Neurotrauma* 2017;34(23):3288-3294.
26. Schneider KJ, Leddy JJ, Guskiewicz KM, et al: Rest and treatment/rehabilitation following sport-related concussion: a systematic review. *Br J Sports Med* 2017;51(12):930-934.
27. Baker JG, Rieger BP, McAvoy K, et al: Principles for return to learn after concussion. *Int J Clin Pract* 2014;68(11):1286-1288.
28. Asken BM, Snyder AR, Clugston JR, Gaynor LS, Sullan MJ, Bauer RM: Concussion-like symptom reporting in non-concussed collegiate athletes. *Arch Clin Neuropsychol* 2017;32(8):963-971.
29. Register-Mihalik JK, Mihalik JP, Guskiewicz KM: Association between previous concussion history and symptom endorsement during preseason baseline testing in high school and collegiate athletes. *Sports Health* 2009;1(1):61-65.
30. Kuppermann N, Holmes JF, Dayan PS, et al: Identification of children at very low risk of clinically-important brain injuries after head trauma: a prospective cohort study. *Lancet* 2009;374(9696):1160-1170.
31. Vallerand AH, Russin MM, Vallerand WP: Taking the bite out of TMJ syndrome. *Am J Nurs* 1989;89(5):688-690.
32. Kucera KL, Yau RK, Register-Mihalik J, et al: Traumatic brain and spinal cord fatalities among high school and college football players - United States, 2005-2014. *MMWR Morb Mortal Wkly Rep* 2017;65(52):1465-1469.
33. Zemek R, Barrowman N, Freedman SB, et al: Clinical risk score for persistent postconcussion symptoms among children with acute concussion in the ED. *JAMA* 2016;315(10):1014-1025.

Appendix 13.A

Sport Concussion Assessment Tool-5

SCAT5 — SPORT CONCUSSION ASSESSMENT TOOL — 5TH EDITION
DEVELOPED BY THE CONCUSSION IN SPORT GROUP
FOR USE BY MEDICAL PROFESSIONALS ONLY

supported by

 FIFA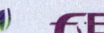

Patient details

Name: _____
DOB: _____
Address: _____
ID number: _____
Examiner: _____
Date of Injury: _____ Time: _____

WHAT IS THE SCAT5?

The SCAT5 is a standardized tool for evaluating concussions designed for use by physicians and licensed healthcare professionals[1]. The SCAT5 cannot be performed correctly in less than 10 minutes.

If you are not a physician or licensed healthcare professional, please use the Concussion Recognition Tool 5 (CRT5). The SCAT5 is to be used for evaluating athletes aged 13 years and older. For children aged 12 years or younger, please use the Child SCAT5.

Preseason SCAT5 baseline testing can be useful for interpreting post-injury test scores, but is not required for that purpose. Detailed instructions for use of the SCAT5 are provided on page 7. Please read through these instructions carefully before testing the athlete. Brief verbal instructions for each test are given in italics. The only equipment required for the tester is a watch or timer.

This tool may be freely copied in its current form for distribution to individuals, teams, groups and organizations. It should not be altered in any way, re-branded or sold for commercial gain. Any revision, translation or reproduction in a digital form requires specific approval by the Concussion in Sport Group.

Recognise and Remove

A head impact by either a direct blow or indirect transmission of force can be associated with a serious and potentially fatal brain injury. If there are significant concerns, including any of the red flags listed in Box 1, then activation of emergency procedures and urgent transport to the nearest hospital should be arranged.

Key points

- Any athlete with suspected concussion should be REMOVED FROM PLAY, medically assessed and monitored for deterioration. No athlete diagnosed with concussion should be returned to play on the day of injury.
- If an athlete is suspected of having a concussion and medical personnel are not immediately available, the athlete should be referred to a medical facility for urgent assessment.
- Athletes with suspected concussion should not drink alcohol, use recreational drugs and should not drive a motor vehicle until cleared to do so by a medical professional.
- Concussion signs and symptoms evolve over time and it is important to consider repeat evaluation in the assessment of concussion.
- The diagnosis of a concussion is a clinical judgment, made by a medical professional. The SCAT5 should NOT be used by itself to make, or exclude, the diagnosis of concussion. An athlete may have a concussion even if their SCAT5 is "normal".

Remember:

- The basic principles of first aid (danger, response, airway, breathing, circulation) should be followed.
- Do not attempt to move the athlete (other than that required for airway management) unless trained to do so.
- Assessment for a spinal cord injury is a critical part of the initial on-field assessment.
- Do not remove a helmet or any other equipment unless trained to do so safely.

© Concussion in Sport Group 2017
Echemendia RJ, et al. Br J Sports Med 2017;51:851–858. doi:10.1136/bjsports-2017-097506SCAT5

Appendix 13.A Sport Concussion Assessment Tool-5

Name:
DOB:
Address:
ID number:
Examiner:
Date:

IMMEDIATE OR ON-FIELD ASSESSMENT

The following elements should be assessed for all athletes who are suspected of having a concussion prior to proceeding to the neurocognitive assessment and ideally should be done on-field after the first first aid / emergency care priorities are completed.

If any of the "Red Flags" or observable signs are noted after a direct or indirect blow to the head, the athlete should be immediately and safely removed from participation and evaluated by a physician or licensed healthcare professional.

Consideration of transportation to a medical facility should be at the discretion of the physician or licensed healthcare professional.

The GCS is important as a standard measure for all patients and can be done serially if necessary in the event of deterioration in conscious state. The Maddocks questions and cervical spine exam are critical steps of the immediate assessment; however, these do not need to be done serially.

STEP 1: RED FLAGS

RED FLAGS:
- Neck pain or tenderness
- Double vision
- Weakness or tingling/burning in arms or legs
- Severe or increasing headache
- Seizure or convulsion
- Loss of consciousness
- Deteriorating conscious state
- Vomiting
- Increasingly restless, agitated or combative

STEP 2: OBSERVABLE SIGNS

Witnessed ☐   Observed on Video ☐

Lying motionless on the playing surface	Y	N
Balance / gait difficulties / motor incoordination: stumbling, slow / laboured movements	Y	N
Disorientation or confusion, or an inability to respond appropriately to questions	Y	N
Blank or vacant look	Y	N
Facial injury after head trauma	Y	N

STEP 3: MEMORY ASSESSMENT MADDOCKS QUESTIONS[2]

"I am going to ask you a few questions, please listen carefully and give your best effort. First, tell me what happened?"

Mark Y for correct answer / N for incorrect

What venue are we at today?	Y	N
Which half is it now?	Y	N
Who scored last in this match?	Y	N
What team did you play last week / game?	Y	N
Did your team win the last game?	Y	N

Note: Appropriate sport-specific questions may be substituted.

STEP 4: EXAMINATION GLASGOW COMA SCALE (GCS)[3]

Time of assessment			
Date of assessment			
Best eye response (E)			
No eye opening	1	1	1
Eye opening in response to pain	2	2	2
Eye opening to speech	3	3	3
Eyes opening spontaneously	4	4	4
Best verbal response (V)			
No verbal response	1	1	1
Incomprehensible sounds	2	2	2
Inappropriate words	3	3	3
Confused	4	4	4
Oriented	5	5	5
Best motor response (M)			
No motor response	1	1	1
Extension to pain	2	2	2
Abnormal flexion to pain	3	3	3
Flexion / Withdrawal to pain	4	4	4
Localizes to pain	5	5	5
Obeys commands	6	6	6
Glasgow Coma score (E + V + M)			

CERVICAL SPINE ASSESSMENT

Does the athlete report that their neck is pain free at rest?	Y	N
If there is NO neck pain at rest, does the athlete have a full range of ACTIVE pain free movement?	Y	N
Is the limb strength and sensation normal?	Y	N

In a patient who is not lucid or fully conscious, a cervical spine injury should be assumed until proven otherwise.

© Concussion in Sport Group 2017

Echemendia RJ, et al. Br J Sports Med 2017;**51**:851–858. doi:10.1136/bjsports-2017-097506SCAT5

OFFICE OR OFF-FIELD ASSESSMENT

Please note that the neurocognitive assessment should be done in a distraction-free environment with the athlete in a resting state.

STEP 1: ATHLETE BACKGROUND

Sport / team / school: _____

Date / time of injury: _____

Years of education completed: _____

Age: _____

Gender: M / F / Other

Dominant hand: left / neither / right

How many diagnosed concussions has the athlete had in the past?: _____

When was the most recent concussion?: _____

How long was the recovery (time to being cleared to play) from the most recent concussion?: _____ (days)

Has the athlete ever been:

Hospitalized for a head injury?	Yes	No
Diagnosed / treated for headache disorder or migraines?	Yes	No
Diagnosed with a learning disability / dyslexia?	Yes	No
Diagnosed with ADD / ADHD?	Yes	No
Diagnosed with depression, anxiety or other psychiatric disorder?	Yes	No

Current medications? If yes, please list:

_____
_____
_____
_____
_____

Name: _____
DOB: _____
Address: _____
ID number: _____
Examiner: _____
Date: _____

STEP 2: SYMPTOM EVALUATION

The athlete should be given the symptom form and asked to read this instruction paragraph out loud then complete the symptom scale. For the baseline assessment, the athlete should rate his/her symptoms based on how he/she typically feels and for the post injury assessment the athlete should rate their symptoms at this point in time.

Please Check: ☐ Baseline ☐ Post-Injury

Please hand the form to the athlete

	none	mild		moderate		severe	
Headache	0	1	2	3	4	5	6
"Pressure in head"	0	1	2	3	4	5	6
Neck Pain	0	1	2	3	4	5	6
Nausea or vomiting	0	1	2	3	4	5	6
Dizziness	0	1	2	3	4	5	6
Blurred vision	0	1	2	3	4	5	6
Balance problems	0	1	2	3	4	5	6
Sensitivity to light	0	1	2	3	4	5	6
Sensitivity to noise	0	1	2	3	4	5	6
Feeling slowed down	0	1	2	3	4	5	6
Feeling like "in a fog"	0	1	2	3	4	5	6
"Don't feel right"	0	1	2	3	4	5	6
Difficulty concentrating	0	1	2	3	4	5	6
Difficulty remembering	0	1	2	3	4	5	6
Fatigue or low energy	0	1	2	3	4	5	6
Confusion	0	1	2	3	4	5	6
Drowsiness	0	1	2	3	4	5	6
More emotional	0	1	2	3	4	5	6
Irritability	0	1	2	3	4	5	6
Sadness	0	1	2	3	4	5	6
Nervous or Anxious	0	1	2	3	4	5	6
Trouble falling asleep (if applicable)	0	1	2	3	4	5	6

Total number of symptoms:	of 22
Symptom severity score:	of 132
Do your symptoms get worse with physical activity?	Y N
Do your symptoms get worse with mental activity?	Y N
If 100% is feeling perfectly normal, what percent of normal do you feel?	

If not 100%, why?

_____
_____
_____

Please hand form back to examiner

© Concussion in Sport Group 2017

Appendix 13.A Sport Concussion Assessment Tool-5

3

STEP 3: COGNITIVE SCREENING
Standardised Assessment of Concussion (SAC)[4]

Name: _____
DOB: _____
Address: _____
ID number: _____
Examiner: _____
Date: _____

ORIENTATION

What month is it?	0	1
What is the date today?	0	1
What is the day of the week?	0	1
What year is it?	0	1
What time is it right now? (within 1 hour)	0	1
Orientation score		of 5

IMMEDIATE MEMORY

The Immediate Memory component can be completed using the traditional 5-word per trial list or optionally using 10-words per trial to minimise any ceiling effect. All 3 trials must be administered irrespective of the number correct on the first trial. Administer at the rate of one word per second.

Please choose EITHER the 5 or 10 word list groups and circle the specific word list chosen for this test.

I am going to test your memory. I will read you a list of words and when I am done, repeat back as many words as you can remember, in any order. For Trials 2 & 3: I am going to repeat the same list again. Repeat back as many words as you can remember in any order, even if you said the word before.

List	Alternate 5 word lists					Score (of 5) Trial 1	Trial 2	Trial 3
A	Finger	Penny	Blanket	Lemon	Insect			
B	Candle	Paper	Sugar	Sandwich	Wagon			
C	Baby	Monkey	Perfume	Sunset	Iron			
D	Elbow	Apple	Carpet	Saddle	Bubble			
E	Jacket	Arrow	Pepper	Cotton	Movie			
F	Dollar	Honey	Mirror	Saddle	Anchor			
					Immediate Memory Score			of 15
					Time that last trial was completed			

List	Alternate 10 word lists					Score (of 10) Trial 1	Trial 2	Trial 3
G	Finger	Penny	Blanket	Lemon	Insect			
	Candle	Paper	Sugar	Sandwich	Wagon			
H	Baby	Monkey	Perfume	Sunset	Iron			
	Elbow	Apple	Carpet	Saddle	Bubble			
I	Jacket	Arrow	Pepper	Cotton	Movie			
	Dollar	Honey	Mirror	Saddle	Anchor			
					Immediate Memory Score			of 30
					Time that last trial was completed			

CONCENTRATION

DIGITS BACKWARDS

Please circle the Digit list chosen (A, B, C, D, E, F). Administer at the rate of one digit per second reading DOWN the selected column.

I am going to read a string of numbers and when I am done, you repeat them back to me in reverse order of how I read them to you. For example, if I say 7-1-9, you would say 9-1-7.

Concentration Number Lists (circle one)					
List A	List B	List C			
4-9-3	5-2-6	1-4-2	Y	N	0
6-2-9	4-1-5	6-5-8	Y	N	1
3-8-1-4	1-7-9-5	6-8-3-1	Y	N	0
3-2-7-9	4-9-6-8	3-4-8-1	Y	N	1
6-2-9-7-1	4-8-5-2-7	4-9-1-5-3	Y	N	0
1-5-2-8-6	6-1-8-4-3	6-8-2-5-1	Y	N	1
7-1-8-4-6-2	8-3-1-9-6-4	3-7-6-5-1-9	Y	N	0
5-3-9-1-4-8	7-2-4-8-5-6	9-2-6-5-1-4	Y	N	1
List D	List E	List F			
7-8-2	3-8-2	2-7-1	Y	N	0
9-2-6	5-1-8	4-7-9	Y	N	1
4-1-8-3	2-7-9-3	1-6-8-3	Y	N	0
9-7-2-3	2-1-6-9	3-9-2-4	Y	N	1
1-7-9-2-6	4-1-8-6-9	2-4-7-5-8	Y	N	0
4-1-7-5-2	9-4-1-7-5	8-3-9-6-4	Y	N	1
2-6-4-8-1-7	6-9-7-3-8-2	5-8-6-2-4-9	Y	N	0
8-4-1-9-3-5	4-2-7-9-3-8	3-1-7-8-2-6	Y	N	1
Digits Score:					of 4

MONTHS IN REVERSE ORDER

Now tell me the months of the year in reverse order. Start with the last month and go backward. So you'll say December, November. Go ahead.

Dec - Nov - Oct - Sept - Aug - Jul - Jun - May - Apr - Mar - Feb - Jan	0 1
Months Score	of 1
Concentration Total Score (Digits + Months)	of 5

© Concussion in Sport Group 2017

Echemendia RJ, et al. Br J Sports Med 2017;**51**:851–858. doi:10.1136/bjsports-2017-097506SCAT5

Sport Concussion Assessment Tool-5

Name: _____
DOB: _____
Address: _____
ID number: _____
Examiner: _____
Date: _____

STEP 4: NEUROLOGICAL SCREEN

See the instruction sheet (page 7) for details of test administration and scoring of the tests.

Can the patient read aloud (e.g. symptom checklist) and follow instructions without difficulty?	Y	N
Does the patient have a full range of pain-free PASSIVE cervical spine movement?	Y	N
Without moving their head or neck, can the patient look side-to-side and up-and-down without double vision?	Y	N
Can the patient perform the finger nose coordination test normally?	Y	N
Can the patient perform tandem gait normally?	Y	N

BALANCE EXAMINATION
Modified Balance Error Scoring System (mBESS) testing[5]

Which foot was tested (i.e. which is the non-dominant foot)   ☐ Left   ☐ Right

Testing surface (hard floor, field, etc.) _____
Footwear (shoes, barefoot, braces, tape, etc.) _____

Condition	Errors
Double leg stance	of 10
Single leg stance (non-dominant foot)	of 10
Tandem stance (non-dominant foot at the back)	of 10
Total Errors	of 30

STEP 5: DELAYED RECALL:

The delayed recall should be performed after 5 minutes have elapsed since the end of the Immediate Recall section. Score 1 pt. for each correct response.

Do you remember that list of words I read a few times earlier? Tell me as many words from the list as you can remember in any order.

Time Started _____

Please record each word correctly recalled. Total score equals number of words recalled.

_____
_____
_____

Total number of words recalled accurately: ___ of 5   or   ___ of 10

STEP 6: DECISION

Domain	Date & time of assessment:		
Symptom number (of 22)			
Symptom severity score (of 132)			
Orientation (of 5)			
Immediate memory	of 15 of 30	of 15 of 30	of 15 of 30
Concentration (of 5)			
Neuro exam	Normal Abnormal	Normal Abnormal	Normal Abnormal
Balance errors (of 30)			
Delayed Recall	of 5 of 10	of 5 of 10	of 5 of 10

Date and time of injury: _____

If the athlete is known to you prior to their injury, are they different from their usual self?
☐ Yes ☐ No ☐ Unsure ☐ Not Applicable
(If different, describe why in the clinical notes section)

Concussion Diagnosed?
☐ Yes ☐ No ☐ Unsure ☐ Not Applicable

If re-testing, has the athlete improved?
☐ Yes ☐ No ☐ Unsure ☐ Not Applicable

I am a physician or licensed healthcare professional and I have personally administered or supervised the administration of this SCAT5.

Signature: _____
Name: _____
Title: _____
Registration number (if applicable): _____
Date: _____

SCORING ON THE SCAT5 SHOULD NOT BE USED AS A STAND-ALONE METHOD TO DIAGNOSE CONCUSSION, MEASURE RECOVERY OR MAKE DECISIONS ABOUT AN ATHLETE'S READINESS TO RETURN TO COMPETITION AFTER CONCUSSION.

© Concussion in Sport Group 2017

Echemendia RJ, et al. Br J Sports Med 2017;**51**:851–858. doi:10.1136/bjsports-2017-097506SCAT5

Appendix 13.A Sport Concussion Assessment Tool-5

CLINICAL NOTES:

Name: _____
DOB: _____
Address: _____
ID number: _____
Examiner: _____
Date: _____

CONCUSSION INJURY ADVICE

(To be given to the person monitoring the concussed athlete)

This patient has received an injury to the head. A careful medical examination has been carried out and no sign of any serious complications has been found. Recovery time is variable across individuals and the patient will need monitoring for a further period by a responsible adult. Your treating physician will provide guidance as to this timeframe.

If you notice any change in behaviour, vomiting, worsening headache, double vision or excessive drowsiness, please telephone your doctor or the nearest hospital emergency department immediately.

Other important points:

Initial rest: Limit physical activity to routine daily activities (avoid exercise, training, sports) and limit activities such as school, work, and screen time to a level that does not worsen symptoms.

1) Avoid alcohol

2) Avoid prescription or non-prescription drugs without medical supervision. Specifically:

   a) Avoid sleeping tablets

   b) Do not use aspirin, anti-inflammatory medication or stronger pain medications such as narcotics

3) Do not drive until cleared by a healthcare professional.

4) Return to play/sport requires clearance by a healthcare professional.

Clinic phone number: _____

Patient's name: _____

Date / time of injury: _____

Date / time of medical review: _____

Healthcare Provider: _____

© Concussion in Sport Group 2017

Contact details or stamp

Sport Concussion Assessment Tool-5

INSTRUCTIONS

Words in *Italics* throughout the SCAT5 are the instructions given to the athlete by the clinician

Symptom Scale

The time frame for symptoms should be based on the type of test being administered. At baseline it is advantageous to assess how an athlete "typically" feels whereas during the acute/post-acute stage it is best to ask how the athlete feels at the time of testing.

The symptom scale should be completed by the athlete, not by the examiner. In situations where the symptom scale is being completed after exercise, it should be done in a resting state, generally by approximating his/her resting heart rate.

For total number of symptoms, maximum possible is 22 except immediately post injury, if sleep item is omitted, which then creates a maximum of 21.

For Symptom severity score, add all scores in table, maximum possible is 22 x 6 = 132, except immediately post injury if sleep item is omitted, which then creates a maximum of 21x6=126.

Immediate Memory

The Immediate Memory component can be completed using the traditional 5-word per trial list or, optionally, using 10-words per trial. The literature suggests that the Immediate Memory has a notable ceiling effect when a 5-word list is used. In settings where this ceiling is prominent, the examiner may wish to make the task more difficult by incorporating two 5–word groups for a total of 10 words per trial. In this case, the maximum score per trial is 10 with a total trial maximum of 30.

Choose one of the word lists (either 5 or 10). Then perform 3 trials of immediate memory using this list.

Complete all 3 trials regardless of score on previous trials.

"I am going to test your memory. I will read you a list of words and when I am done, repeat back as many words as you can remember, in any order." The words must be read at a rate of one word per second.

Trials 2 & 3 MUST be completed regardless of score on trial 1 & 2.

Trials 2 & 3:

"I am going to repeat the same list again. Repeat back as many words as you can remember in any order, even if you said the word before."

Score 1 pt. for each correct response. Total score equals sum across all 3 trials. Do NOT inform the athlete that delayed recall will be tested.

Concentration

Digits backward

Choose one column of digits from lists A, B, C, D, E or F and administer those digits as follows:

Say: *"I am going to read a string of numbers and when I am done, you repeat them back to me in reverse order of how I read them to you. For example, if I say 7-1-9, you would say 9-1-7."*

Begin with first 3 digit string.

If correct, circle "Y" for correct and go to next string length. If incorrect, circle "N" for the first string length and read trial 2 in the same string length. One point possible for each string length. Stop after incorrect on both trials (2 N's) in a string length. The digits should be read at the rate of one per second.

Months in reverse order

"Now tell me the months of the year in reverse order. Start with the last month and go backward. So you'll say December, November ... Go ahead"

1 pt. for entire sequence correct

Delayed Recall

The delayed recall should be performed after 5 minutes have elapsed since the end of the Immediate Recall section.

"Do you remember that list of words I read a few times earlier? Tell me as many words from the list as you can remember in any order."

Score 1 pt. for each correct response

Modified Balance Error Scoring System (mBESS)[5] testing

This balance testing is based on a modified version of the Balance Error Scoring System (BESS)[5]. A timing device is required for this testing.

Each of 20-second trial/stance is scored by counting the number of errors. The examiner will begin counting errors only after the athlete has assumed the proper start position. The modified BESS is calculated by adding one error point for each error during the three 20-second tests. The maximum number of errors for any single condition is 10. If the athlete commits multiple errors simultaneously, only one error is recorded but the athlete should quickly return to the testing position, and counting should resume once the athlete is set. Athletes that are unable to maintain the testing procedure for a minimum of five seconds at the start are assigned the highest possible score, ten, for that testing condition.

OPTION: For further assessment, the same 3 stances can be performed on a surface of medium density foam (e.g., approximately 50cm x 40cm x 6cm).

Balance testing – types of errors

1. Hands lifted off iliac crest
2. Opening eyes
3. Step, stumble, or fall
4. Moving hip into > 30 degrees abduction
5. Lifting forefoot or heel
6. Remaining out of test position > 5 sec

"I am now going to test your balance. Please take your shoes off (if applicable), roll up your pant legs above ankle (if applicable), and remove any ankle taping (if applicable). This test will consist of three twenty second tests with different stances."

(a) Double leg stance:

"The first stance is standing with your feet together with your hands on your hips and with your eyes closed. You should try to maintain stability in that position for 20 seconds. I will be counting the number of times you move out of this position. I will start timing when you are set and have closed your eyes."

(b) Single leg stance:

"If you were to kick a ball, which foot would you use? [This will be the dominant foot] Now stand on your non-dominant foot. The dominant leg should be held in approximately 30 degrees of hip flexion and 45 degrees of knee flexion. Again, you should try to maintain stability for 20 seconds with your hands on your hips and your eyes closed. I will be counting the number of times you move out of this position. If you stumble out of this position, open your eyes and return to the start position and continue balancing. I will start timing when you are set and have closed your eyes."

(c) Tandem stance:

"Now stand heel-to-toe with your non-dominant foot in back. Your weight should be evenly distributed across both feet. Again, you should try to maintain stability for 20 seconds with your hands on your hips and your eyes closed. I will be counting the number of times you move out of this position. If you stumble out of this position, open your eyes and return to the start position and continue balancing. I will start timing when you are set and have closed your eyes."

Tandem Gait

Participants are instructed to stand with their feet together behind a starting line (the test is best done with footwear removed). Then, they walk in a forward direction as quickly and as accurately as possible along a 38mm wide (sports tape), 3 metre line with an alternate foot heel-to-toe gait ensuring that they approximate their heel and toe on each step. Once they cross the end of the 3m line, they turn 180 degrees and return to the starting point using the same gait. Athletes fail the test if they step off the line, have a separation between their heel and toe, or if they touch or grab the examiner or an object.

Finger to Nose

"I am going to test your coordination now. Please sit comfortably on the chair with your eyes open and your arm (either right or left) outstretched (shoulder flexed to 90 degrees and elbow and fingers extended), pointing in front of you. When I give a start signal, I would like you to perform five successive finger to nose repetitions using your index finger to touch the tip of the nose, and then return to the starting position, as quickly and as accurately as possible."

References

1. McCrory et al. Consensus Statement On Concussion In Sport – The 5th International Conference On Concussion In Sport Held In Berlin, October 2016. British Journal of Sports Medicine 2017 (available at www.bjsm.bmj.com)

2. Maddocks, DL; Dicker, GD; Saling, MM. The assessment of orientation following concussion in athletes. Clinical Journal of Sport Medicine 1995; 5: 32-33

3. Jennett, B., Bond, M. Assessment of outcome after severe brain damage: a practical scale. Lancet 1975; i: 480-484

4. McCrea M. Standardized mental status testing of acute concussion. Clinical Journal of Sport Medicine. 2001; 11: 176-181

5. Guskiewicz KM. Assessment of postural stability following sport-related concussion. Current Sports Medicine Reports. 2003; 2: 24-30

CONCUSSION INFORMATION

Any athlete suspected of having a concussion should be removed from play and seek medical evaluation.

Signs to watch for

Problems could arise over the first 24-48 hours. The athlete should not be left alone and must go to a hospital at once if they experience:

- Worsening headache
- Drowsiness or inability to be awakened
- Inability to recognize people or places
- Repeated vomiting
- Unusual behaviour or confusion or irritable
- Seizures (arms and legs jerk uncontrollably)
- Weakness or numbness in arms or legs
- Unsteadiness on their feet.
- Slurred speech

Consult your physician or licensed healthcare professional after a suspected concussion. Remember, it is better to be safe.

Rest & Rehabilitation

After a concussion, the athlete should have physical rest and relative cognitive rest for a few days to allow their symptoms to improve. In most cases, after no more than a few days of rest, the athlete should gradually increase their daily activity level as long as their symptoms do not worsen. Once the athlete is able to complete their usual daily activities without concussion-related symptoms, the second step of the return to play/sport progression can be started. The athlete should not return to play/sport until their concussion-related symptoms have resolved and the athlete has successfully returned to full school/learning activities.

When returning to play/sport, the athlete should follow a stepwise, **medically managed exercise progression, with increasing amounts of exercise.** For example:

Graduated Return to Sport Strategy

Exercise step	Functional exercise at each step	Goal of each step
1. Symptom-limited activity	Daily activities that do not provoke symptoms.	Gradual reintroduction of work/school activities.
2. Light aerobic exercise	Walking or stationary cycling at slow to medium pace. No resistance training.	Increase heart rate.
3. Sport-specific exercise	Running or skating drills. No head impact activities.	Add movement.
4. Non-contact training drills	Harder training drills, e.g., passing drills. May start progressive resistance training.	Exercise, coordination, and increased thinking.
5. Full contact practice	Following medical clearance, participate in normal training activities.	Restore confidence and assess functional skills by coaching staff.
6. Return to play/sport	Normal game play.	

In this example, it would be typical to have 24 hours (or longer) for each step of the progression. If any symptoms worsen while exercising, the athlete should go back to the previous step. Resistance training should be added only in the later stages (Stage 3 or 4 at the earliest).

Written clearance should be provided by a healthcare professional before return to play/sport as directed by local laws and regulations.

Graduated Return to School Strategy

Concussion may affect the ability to learn at school. The athlete may need to miss a few days of school after a concussion. When going back to school, some athletes may need to go back gradually and may need to have some changes made to their schedule so that concussion symptoms do not get worse. If a particular activity makes symptoms worse, then the athlete should stop that activity and rest until symptoms get better. To make sure that the athlete can get back to school without problems, it is important that the healthcare provider, parents, caregivers and teachers talk to each other so that everyone knows what the plan is for the athlete to go back to school.

Note: If mental activity does not cause any symptoms, the athlete may be able to skip step 2 and return to school part-time before doing school activities at home first.

Mental Activity	Activity at each step	Goal of each step
1. Daily activities that do not give the athlete symptoms	Typical activities that the athlete does during the day as long as they do not increase symptoms (e.g. reading, texting, screen time). Start with 5-15 minutes at a time and gradually build up.	Gradual return to typical activities.
2. School activities	Homework, reading or other cognitive activities outside of the classroom.	Increase tolerance to cognitive work.
3. Return to school part-time	Gradual introduction of schoolwork. May need to start with a partial school day or with increased breaks during the day.	Increase academic activities.
4. Return to school full-time	Gradually progress school activities until a full day can be tolerated.	Return to full academic activities and catch up on missed work.

If the athlete continues to have symptoms with mental activity, some other accomodations that can help with return to school may include:

- Starting school later, only going for half days, or going only to certain classes
- More time to finish assignments/tests
- Quiet room to finish assignments/tests
- Not going to noisy areas like the cafeteria, assembly halls, sporting events, music class, shop class, etc.
- Taking lots of breaks during class, homework, tests
- No more than one exam/day
- Shorter assignments
- Repetition/memory cues
- Use of a student helper/tutor
- Reassurance from teachers that the child will be supported while getting better

The athlete should not go back to sports until they are back to school/learning, without symptoms getting significantly worse and no longer needing any changes to their schedule.

© Concussion in Sport Group 2017

Index

Note: Page numbers followed by *f* and *t* indicate figures and tables, respectively

A

Abdomen and thorax
  cardiorespiratory assessment, 484–486
  clinical deductions, 415–416
  history of
    breathing evaluation, 415t–416t
    family medical history, 414
    general medical history, 414
    mechanism of injury, 414–416
    medication and drug use, 414
    onset of injury/illness, 415, 416
    past medical history, 414
  injury conditions to, 441–476
  muscles used for breathing, 440–441, 441t
  neurologic assessment, 484
  observation
    anatomic inspection, 418–419, 418f
    functional inspection, 417
  orthopaedic special tests (*see* Orthopaedic special tests)
  palpation
    articulations and ligamentous support, 421, 422
    muscles of the vertebral column, 424–425
    skeletal anatomy, 419–421, 419f, 420f
  PAR-Q, 477
  radiographic view, 483–484
  skin assessment, 486
  soft-tissue anatomy, 421t–422t
  special tests, 477–487
  vascular assessment, 487
Abdominal observation, 493, 495
Abnormal breathing patterns, 486t
Abnormal breath sounds, 493t
Accessory lateral collateral ligament, 277–278
ACL. *See* Anterior cruciate ligament
Acromioclavicular (AC) joint, 341, 342, 363t
  clinical diagnosis, 366
  functional assessment/outcome measures, 366
  history, 364–365
  inspection, 365
  palpation, 365
  Rockwood classification, 363–364, 364f
  special tests, 365, 365f, 366f
  sprain, 363–364
Active range of motion (AROM), 21, 22
Adhesive capsulitis, shoulder, 384–385, 384t, 385f
Adson test, 488
Allen test, 226, 227, 488
Anatomic snuffbox, palpation of, 229, 266t
Anterior cruciate ligament (ACL), 128–129
  anterior drawer test, 142, 142f
  differential diagnoses, 143
  evaluation, 141
  Lachman test, 141–142, 142f
  magnetic resonance imaging, 142, 143f
  mechanism of, 141
  pivot shift, 142
  radiography, 142, 142f
  rehabilitation, 143, 143t–144t
  treatment, 143
Anterior superior iliac spine (ASIS), 164
Aorta
  blood supply of heart, 422–423
  deep palpation of, 424, 424t, 423f
Appendicitis, 476t
  iliopsoas muscle test for, 496t
  obturator muscle test for, 497
  rebound sign for, 494, 496t
AROM. *See* Active range of motion
Athletes, sudden cardiac death syndrome in, 463–465
Athletic heart syndrome, 468
Axillary nerve, shoulder, 387, 387f
Axonotmesis, 11, 12

B

Babinski reflex, 26
Balance Error Scoring System (BESS), 596–597
Barrel chest, 417, 418f
Bennett fracture, 251–252, 251f, 251t
Bilateral comparison, 20
Blood pressure, 484–485
Blood supply to the heart
  aorta, 422–424
  inferior vena cava, 423
  renal arteries, 423
  renal veins, 424
  superior vena cava, 423
Brachial plexus neuropraxia, 563, 563t
Breathing, muscles used for, 440, 441
Bronchial circulation, 422
Brudzinski reflex, 26
Buffalo Concussion Treadmill Test (BCTT), 596

C

Carotid pulse, 487
Carpal bones of wrist and hand, 216
Carpometacarpal (CMC) joint, 216, 217
Central slip injury, 258–262, 259t, 259f, 260f, 261f
Cerebrospinal fluid (CSF), 582
Cervical spine
  history, 522
  inspection, 528
  palpation, 528–529, 529f
  range of motion, 530, 533
Clavicular fractures, 381–383
Cobb method, 482–484, 484f
Colles fracture, 233
Commotio cordis, 467t
Compression test for rib fracture, 487
Compressive force, 10
Computed tomography, 224
Costochondral joints, 421
Costochondral separation and dislocation, 452t
Costoclavicular syndrome tests for thoracic outlet syndrome, 489t
Costotransverse joints, 421
Costovertebral joints, 421
CSF. *See* Cerebrospinal fluid
Cubital tunnel syndrome, 307–308, 307t

621

Cyriax method, 358
Cyriax release test for thoracic outlet syndrome, 489t

D

de Quervain tenosynovitis, 230–233, 230t, 231f, 232f, 233t
Dermatome
    anatomic drawing, 25f
    testing, 478–480, 480t
Disk herniation, 455t
Distal biceps rupture, elbow, 298–300, 299f, 299t, 300f
Distal humerus, elbow, 274, 274f
Distal radioulnar joint, 217
Distal radius fractures, 233–236, 233t, 234f, 235f
Dorsal proximal interphalangeal joint dislocations, 258, 258t, 258f

E

Extensor carpi ulnaris synergy test, 246, 247
Extensor carpi ulnaris tendon injury, 245–247, 245t, 245f, 246f, 247f
Edema, 20
Elbow
    articulations and ligamentous support
        accessory lateral collateral ligament, 277–278
        annular ligament, 278
        elbow joint capsule, 276, 276f
        humeroradial joint, 276
        humeroulnar joint, 276
        lateral ligament complex, 277, 277f
        lateral ulnar collateral ligament, 277
        proximal radioulnar joint, 276
        radial collateral ligament, 277
        ulnar collateral ligament, 276–277, 277f
    bones of
        distal humerus, 274, 274f
        fracture/dislocation, 305–307, 306f
        proximal radius, 275, 275f
        proximal ulna, 275, 275f
    distal biceps rupture, 298–300, 299f, 299t, 300f
    evaluation, 289–294
        inspection, 292
        muscle strength, 311t–312t
        palpation, 292, 293t–294t
        patient history, 290
    lateral epicondylalgia, 294
        history, 295
        inspection, 295–296, 296f
        location, 295
        outcome measures, 295
        palpation, 296
        special tests findings, 296–297
    ligamentous-based pathology
        posterolateral rotatory instability, 303, 303f, 304t, 304f, 305
        ulnar collateral ligament injury, 300–303, 301t
    medial epicondylalgia, 297–298, 297t
    magnetic resonance imaging, 289
    myotomal testing, 313, 315t–316t
    neurologic-based pathology
        cubital tunnel syndrome, 307–308, 307t
        olecranon bursitis, 308–309, 309t
    neurologic testing, 312, 313t
    orthopaedic special tests, 316, 317t–328t
    radiology, 288–289, 288f
    range of motion, 309–311, 310t
    sensory testing, 312, 314f
    soft-tissue anatomy
        manual muscle testing, 278
        neurologic anatomy, 278, 285–286
        origin and insertion, 278–284, 279t–284t
        vascular anatomy, 286–288
    vascular assessment, 313–314, 316f
Elbow joint capsule, 276, 276f
Electromyography (EMG) analysis, 172, 173
Elson test, 261, 268
Epidural hematoma, 605–606
Evidence-based practice
    clinical evaluation of, 29–30
    diagnostic gold standard test, 32–34, 33t
    evaluation process, 31
    flow chart, 31f
    likelihood ratio, 35–37, 36t, 37t, 38f
    Potts maneuver, 31t
    reliability, 32
    sensitivity and specificity, 35t
    validity, 32
Examination process
    HIPS framework, 18t, 21f
    history, 18–19
    inspection, 19–20
    on-field and emergency evaluations, 26–28
    palpation, 19–20
    record-keeping format, 26, 27t
    special tests
        functional tests, 21
        ligamentous stress test, 23–24
        neurologic testing, 25–26
        range of motion and end feel, 21–23
Exhalation collapse, 449t
Extensor carpi ulnaris synergy test, 246
Extensor carpi ulnaris tendon injury, 245
Extensor tendon anatomy, 257
Extrinsic wrist
    and finger extensors, 219t–220t
    and finger flexors, 220t

F

Facet joints of spine, 422
False-negative ligamentous test, 24
False-positive ligamentous test, 24
Fibular collateral ligament, 129
Finger
    extensor hood of, 219f
    radiographs of, 223f
    range of motion, 225
Finger extensors, 219t–220t
Finger flexors, 220t
Finger joint injuries
    central slip injury, 258–262, 259t, 259f, 260f, 261f
    dorsal proximal interphalangeal joint joint dislocations and volar plate avulsion fractures, 258, 258t, 258f
    proximal interphalangeal joint fracture dislocations, 258, 259t
Finger tendon injuries, 262–266, 262f, 263t, 263f
Finkelstein test, 232, 266t
Flexion-adduction-internal rotation test, 191, 192t
Flexor digitorum brevis muscle, 68
Flexor digitorum longus, 68
Flexor tendon anatomy, 257, 260
Foot and ankle
    Achilles tendinosis, 107, 108t
    Achilles tendon rupture, 107–109, 109t, 110t
    anterior drawer test, 116t
    avulsion fracture, 111–113, 112f, 113t
    bones of
        forefoot joint, 60
        hindfoot joint, 62
        midfoot, 61–62, 61f, 62f
        phalanges and metatarsal, 58
        sesamoid bone, 58–59, 58f
        shank, 62–63
        talocrural joint, 62
        tarsal bone, 59, 59f
        tarsometatarsal joint, 60–61
        tibia and fibula, 59
        transverse tarsal joint, 62
    bump/percussion test, 121t
    calcaneal apophysitis, 112, 113
    case study, 122–124

common pathologies, 100, 100t
cotton test, 118t
dorsiflexion compression test, 119t
dorsiflexion eversion test, 120t
evaluation of
    activity changes, 87
    bilateral comparison, 93
    deformities present, 88
    foot type, 88, 89f, 89t
    hematomas, 90, 90f, 91t
    history of, injury, 87–88
    inspection, 88
    location of, pain, 87
    mechanism of injury, 87
    open- and closed-chain kinematics, 98
    palpation, 93, 94t–97t
    pes cavus, 93, 93f
    pes planus, 92–93, 93f
    phases of, gait, 98–99, 98f
    range of motion, 99–100, 99t
    skin abnormalities, 88–90
    toe deformities types, 90, 91
    valgus and varus alignment, 90, 92t, 92f
    weight-bearing status, 88
Feiss line, 115t
forced dorsiflexion test, 118t
growth plate fracture, 109
Jones fracture, 109, 111f, 112t
Kleiger test, 118t
lateral ankle sprain, 102–105, 103f, 104t, 105t
medial ankle sprain, 104, 106t, 107t
metatarsalgia, 100
musculotendinous anatomy
    intrinsic *vs.* extrinsic muscles, 69t–81t
    lower leg compartments, 68, 82t
navicular drop, 115t
neurologic anatomy, 68, 82, 83
neuroma, 100–101, 100f
plantar fascia, 101–103, 102f, 102t, 103t
radiology and imaging
    magnetic resonance image, 86
    Ottawa Ankle Rules, 86, 114
    radiograph, 84–86
soft-tissue anatomy, 63, 64f, 65f, 66t–67t
squeeze test, 119t
stress fracture, 113–114, 114t, 115t–121t
subtalar glides, 117t
syndesmotic sprain, 105, 107t
talar tilt test, 116t
Thompson test, 120t
tibia and fibular ankle fracture, 113
Tinel sign, 120t
tuning fork test, 121t
turf toe, 101, 101t
vascular anatomy, 83–86, 84f–86f, 86t
Frozen shoulder, 384–385, 384t, 385f
Functional testing, 21
Funnel chest, 417f

G

Gallbladder conditions, 474t
Ganglion cyst, 231
Gastroesophageal reflux disease, 475t
Glasgow Coma Scale (GCS), 590
Glenohumeral impingement
    arthrokinematics, 366
    glenohumeral joint testing, 371
    history, 367, 368f
    inspection, 368, 369f
    internal impingement, 366, 367f
    muscle-related special tests, 369–371
    palpation, 368–369
    primary impingement, 366
    subacromial space impingement, 371–372
Glenohumeral (GH) joint, 340–341
    clinical diagnosis, 363
    complications, 360
    functional assessment/outcome measures, 362–363
    history, 360–361
    incidence, 360
    inspection, 361
    palpation, 361
    special tests, 361–362
Gomphosis joint, 581–582
Goniometer, 21, 22, 23f

H

Hand. *See* wrist and hand
Hawkins-Kennedy test, 371, 372f
Head and face, 610
    articulations, 580–582, 580t–582t
    common skull views, 588, 588f–589f
    concussions, 596–597, 599–600, 613–620
    epidural hematoma, 605–606
    facial laceration, 603–604, 603f, 604t
    Glasgow Coma Scale, 590
    history, 590–591
    inspection, 591–595
    LeFort fractures, 608, 608f, 608t
    ligamentous support, 580–582
    luxations, 609
    magnetic resonance images, 589, 590f
    muscular anatomy, 582, 583t–587t
    nasal fracture, 602–603, 602f, 603t
    neurologic anatomy, 582, 588f
    orbital blowout fracture, 607–608, 607f, 607t
    palpation
        bones, 595, 596f
        soft tissue, 595
    postconcussion syndrome, 606–607, 607t
    skeletal anatomy, 579–580, 580f, 580t
    skull fractures, 601–602, 601f, 602t
    special tests, 595–598
    subdural hematoma, 605–606, 605f, 606t
    temporomandibular joint injury, 604–605, 604t
    tooth fractures, 609, 609f, 609t
    vascular anatomy, 582, 588f
Heart
    blood flow pathway to, 422, 423f
    blood supply, 422–424
    contusion, 469t
    pulse, 484
    rate, 484
Hematuria, 493–494, 496
Hip and thigh
    common hip pathologies, 191, 199
    electromyographic analysis, 172, 173
    FABER test, 192t, 206
    FADDIR test, 191, 192t
    FAIR test, 191, 192t
    hip pointer, 203
    history of, 184–185
    intra-articular pathology, 200–201
    muscle injuries, 199–200
    muscular anatomy, 168–180
    neurologic anatomy
        Achilles reflex, 181, 182f
        map of, dermatome, 179, 182f
        nerves of, 179, 180t
    neurologic assessment, 191
    Ober test, 192t, 202
    observation and inspection
        angle of, leg, 186
        approximation test, 194t
        coxa vara, 185, 186
        Ely test, 196t
        external/internal rotation, 186–188
        Gaenslen test, 196t, 206
        gapping test, 194t
        Gillet test, 195t, 205
        hip abduction, 189, 190f
        hip flexion, 186, 187f, 189f
        hip scoring test, 196t
        ipsilateral prone kinetic test, 193t, 205
        leg length discrepancy, 197t
        pelvic obliquity assessment, 185
        Prone knee bending test, 195t
        resisted hip rotation, 190f
        sacroiliac rocking test, 194t
        straight leg raise test, 195t, 198t

Hip and thigh (cont.)
    Thomas test, 186, 187f
    Trendelenburg test, 190f, 193t
    Weber-Barstow maneuver, 197t
  pediatric hip disease, 204–205
  piriformis syndrome, 202–203, 202f, 203t
  radiology and imaging
    AP radiographs, 183, 184, 207
    hip dysplasia, 183, 184f
    magnetic resonance arthrography, 184, 184f, 207
  sacroiliac joint pathology, 205–206
  skeletal anatomy
    acetabular labrum, 164, 166f
    angles of inclination, 166, 168
    anteversion and retroversion, 166, 168f
    bony fusion of, pelvis, 163, 164f
    femoral head, 166, 167f
    femur, 166, 167f
    sciatic foramen, 164, 165f
    triangular labrum, 164, 166
  snapping hip syndrome, 201–202, 201f, 201t, 202f
  soft-tissue anatomy
    Y-shaped iliofemoral ligament, 166–169
  vascular anatomy, 182, 183
HIPS framework, 18t, 21f
Hook of hamate fracture, 248–250
Hook of hamate pull test, 249, 267
Humeral fractures, shoulder, 383–384, 383f, 383t
Hyperabduction test for thoracic outlet syndrome, 490
Hyperventilation, 462t

I

Iliopsoas muscle test, appendicitis, 496t
Iliotibial (IT) band syndrome, 152–153
Inhalation
  expansion for, 442t–448t
Injury
  mechanism of, 414–416
  muscle, 458
  onset of, 415
  splenic, 472t–473t
  to lungs, 459t–461t
  to thorax and abdomen, 441–448
  types of
    bone injury, 12f
    bone spur, 13f
    ligament and capsular sprain, 11
    muscle and tendon strain, 11
    nerve injury, 11–12, 12f
    Salter-Harris classification, 12–13, 13t, 13f
    wounds, 13–14

Intercarpal joints, 217
Interphalangeal joints, 217
Intersection syndrome, 230–233, 230t, 231f, 232f, 233t

J

Jersey finger, 262–264, 262f, 263t, 263f
Jeune syndrome, 417

K

Kidney contusion/laceration, 470t
Knee joint
  anterior cruciate ligament injury
    anterior drawer test, 142, 142f
    differential diagnoses, 143
    evaluation, 141
    Lachman test, 141–142, 142f
    magnetic resonance imaging, 142, 143f
    mechanism of, 141
    pivot shift, 142
    radiography, 142, 142f
    rehabilitation, 143, 143t–144t
    treatment, 143
  inspection, 138–139, 139f
  iliotibial band syndrome
    differential diagnoses, 152
    evaluation, 152
    imaging, 152
    special tests, 152–153, 152f–153f
    treatment, 152–153
  lateral collateral ligament and posterolateral corner injury
    dial test, 147–148, 148f
    differential diagnoses, 148
    evaluation, 147
    imaging, 147–148
    peroneal nerve assessment, 147
    treatment, 148–149
    varus stress test, 147–148, 148f
  magnetic resonance imaging, 136–137
  manual muscle testing, 130, 140
  medial collateral ligament injury
    differential diagnosis, 146
    evaluation, 145–146
    imaging, 146
    overview, 145–146, 146t
    rehabilitation, 147
    treatment, 147
    valgus stress test, 146, 146f
  medial meniscus, 130
  meniscus tear
    Apley compression/distraction, 149–150
    differential diagnoses, 150

    evaluation, 149
    imaging, 150, 151f
    McMurray test, 149–150, 150f
    overview, 149
    rehabilitation, 151, 151f
    squat test, 149, 151
    Thessaly test, 149–150, 150f
    treatment, 151
  muscular anatomy, 130, 131t–134t, 135f
  neurologic anatomy
    motor testing, 130, 135t
    patellar tendon reflex, 130
    sensory testing, 130, 135t, 136f
  neurologic testing, 131–134, 140
  palpation, 140, 140f
  patellar instability
    differential diagnoses, 155
    evaluation, 154–155
    imaging, 155
    J sign, 155
    lateral patellar apprehension, 155, 155f
    rehabilitation, 155–156
    treatment, 155
  patellar tendinitis
    differential diagnoses, 156
    evaluation, 156
    imaging, 156
    overview, 156, 156t
    special tests, 156
    treatment, 156
  posterior cruciate ligament injury
    differential diagnosis, 145
    evaluation, 144
    imaging, 145, 145f
    overview, 143–144, 144t
    posterior drawer, 144
    posterior sag sign, 144–145, 145f
    rehabilitation, 145
    treatment, 145
  patellofemoral pain syndrome
    Clarke test, 153–154
    differential diagnoses, 154
    evaluation, 153
    imaging, 154
    pathologies, 153
    Q-angle assessment, 153–154, 154f
    treatment, 154
  special tests, 156, 157t–159t
  vascular anatomy, 130, 135–136
  vascular assessment, 141
Korotkoff sounds, 485
Kyphosis, 417

L

Labral tears, shoulder, 377–379, 378f, 378t, 379f

Index

Lateral collateral ligament (LCL) injury, 129
    dial test, 147–148, 148f
    differential diagnoses, 148
    evaluation, 147
    imaging, 147–148
    peroneal nerve assessment, 147
    treatment, 148–149
    varus stress test, 147–148, 148f
Lateral epicondylalgia, elbow, 294, 294t, 295f–296f, 297
Lateral ligament complex, 277, 277f
Lateral ulnar collateral ligament, 277
LeFort fractures, 608
Ligamentous anatomy, 63, 64f, 65f, 66t–67t
Ligamentous stress test, 23–24
Lister tubercle, 216
Liver contusion, 471t
Lumbar spine
    history, 522
    inspection, 528, 529f
    palpation, 530–532
    range of motion, 533
Lungs
    auscultations of, 488, 490, 492t
    blood supply of, 422
    injuries to, 459t–461t
    percussion of, 493, 494t
Lunotriquetral shear test, 240, 267

M

Magnetic resonance arthrography, 184
Magnetic resonance imaging, 222, 244
Mallet finger, 264–266, 264t, 264f, 265f, 266f, 266t–268t
Manual muscle testing, 24t, 24f
Mechanism of injury (MOI), 10, 18, 87
Medial collateral ligament (MCL) injury, 129
    differential diagnosis, 146
    evaluation, 145–146
    imaging, 146
    overview, 145–146, 146t
    rehabilitation, 147
    treatment, 147
    valgus stress test, 146, 146f
Medial epicondylalgia, elbow, 297–298
Medial patellofemoral ligament, 154–155
Median nerve, elbow, 285–286
Medication and drug use, 414
Meniscus tear
    Apley compression/distraction, 149–150
    differential diagnoses, 150
    evaluation, 149
    imaging, 150, 151f
    McMurray test, 149–150
    overview, 149
    rehabilitation, 151, 151f

squat test, 149, 151
Thessaly test, 149–150, 150f
treatment, 151
Metacarpal fractures, 252–253, 253t, 253f, 254f
Metacarpophalangeal joint, 216, 217f
Morley sign for thoracic outlet syndrome, 490
Motor testing, nerve root myotomes, 222
Multidirectional instability, 9
Murphy sign, 494, 496t
Musculoskeletal injuries
    advantages and disadvantages, 41, 42t
    computed tomography, 46–47, 47f
    diagnostic ultrasonography, 50–51, 51f
    factors, 41, 42t
    magnetic resonance imaging, 48–50
    nerve conduction study/electromyography, 51–53
    patient positioning, 42, 43f
    radiography, 44–46
    scintigraphy, 50, 50f
Musculotendinous anatomy, intrinsic vs. extrinsic muscle, 69t–73t
Myotomes, neuromuscular motion, 26t
Myotome testing, 480, 481t

N

Nasal fracture, 602–603
Neer impingement test, 371
Nerve conduction study, 51–53
Nerve root injury
    peripheral nerve damage, 561–563
    signs of, 560
    structural integrity of, 560
Neurapraxia, 11, 12
Neurologic anatomy
    Achilles reflex, 181, 182
    body map, 83, 83f
    map of, dermatome, 179, 182
Neurologic screening, 478t–479t
Neurologic testing, 25–26
Neurotmesis, 11, 12

O

Obturator muscle test, appendicitis, 497t
Olecranon bursitis, 308–309, 309t
Oppenheim reflex, 26
Orbital blowout fracture, 607–608
Orthopaedic special tests
    abdominal observations, 493, 495t
    auscultations of lungs, 488, 490, 492
    compression test for rib fracture, 487
    mobility of first rib, 487
    Murphy sign, 494, 496
    percussion of lungs, 493, 494

rebound sign for appendicitis, 494, 496t
    for thoracic outlet syndrome, 488
    urine test for hematuria, 493, 496t
Osteokinematic assessment
    thoracic spine flexion and extension, 477f
    thoracic spine rotation, 477, 478f
Oswestry Disability Index, 572–573
Oswestry Low Back Pain Disability Questionnaire, 572–573

P

PAR-Q. See Physical Activity Readiness Questionnaire
Passive range of motion, 21, 23
Patellar instability
    differential diagnoses, 155
    evaluation, 154–155
    imaging, 155
    J sign, 155
    lateral patellar apprehension, 155, 155f
    medial patellofemoral ligament, 154–155, 155t
    rehabilitation, 155–156
    treatment, 155
Patellar tendinitis
    differential diagnoses, 156
    evaluation, 156
    imaging, 156
    overview, 156, 156t
    special tests, 156
    treatment, 156
Patellofemoral pain syndrome
    Clarke test, 153–154
    differential diagnoses, 154
    evaluation, 153
    imaging, 154
    pathologies, 153
    Q-angle assessment, 153–154, 154f
    treatment, 154
Pectoralis major rupture, 390–392, 391f
Percussion of lungs, 493, 494
Pericardial tamponade, 466t
Perilunate fracture dislocation, 236
Peripheral nerve pathology, shoulder, 385–387, 385t, 386f
Persistent postconcussion symptoms, 606–607
Phalanges and metacarpals of wrist and hand, 216
Physical Activity Readiness Questionnaire (PAR-Q), 477
Piano key test, 244, 267
Pigeon chest, 417f
PIP. See Proximal interphalangeal joint (PIP)
Proximal interphalangeal joint fracture-dislocations, 257–259

Pleural cavity, 420f
Poland syndrome, 417
Postconcussion syndrome, 606–607
Posterior cruciate ligament injury, 129
    differential diagnosis, 145
    evaluation, 144
    imaging, 145, 145f
    overview, 143–144, 144t
    posterior drawer, 144
    posterior sag sign, 144–145, 145f
    rehabilitation, 145
    treatment, 145
Posterior superior iliac spine (PSIS), 164
Posterolateral corner (PLC) injury
    dial test, 147–148
    differential diagnoses, 148
    evaluation, 147
    imaging, 147–148
    peroneal nerve assessment, 147
    treatment, 148–149
    varus stress test, 147–148
Posterolateral rotatory instability, elbow, 303, 303f, 304t, 304f, 305
Proximal radioulnar joint, 276
Proximal radius, 275, 275f
Proximal ulna, 275, 275f
Pulmonary circulation, 422

R

Radial collateral ligament, 277
Radial nerve, 285, 286f
Range of motion (ROM), 5, 22t
    active, 480–481, 481t, 482f
    knee, 139
    methods to assess spinal, 483f
    passive, 481–482
    spine
        cervical, 530, 533
        lumbar spine, 533
    for thoracic spine, 480–482
Rebound sign, appendicitis, 494, 496t
Reflex testing, 477–478, 478t
Resisted range of motion, 21, 23
Reverse Bankart lesion testing, 378–379
Rib contusion, 449t
Rib fractures, 450t–451t, 487t
Ribs and thorax
    depression, 449t
    elevation, 442t–448t
Rib tip syndrome, 453t
Rigidity, abdominal postures, 27, 27f
Rockwood classification, 364, 364f
Roland-Morris Disability Questionnaire, 577
Rolando fracture, 251–252, 251f, 251t
Roos test for thoracic outlet syndrome, 491
Rotator cuff strain/tear, 372t
    history, 372–373
    inspection, 373
    palpation, 373
    special tests, 373
    supraspinatus, 372, 373f

S

Salter-Harris classification, 12–13, 13t, 13f
Scaphoid bone, blood supply of, 228
Scaphoid fracture, 227–229, 227t, 228f, 229f
Scaphoid tubercle, 216, 266t
Scapholunate ligament, 216
Scapular dyskinesis, shoulder, 380–381
Scheuermann kyphosis, 556–558
Scoliosis, 417, 484t
Sensory testing of nerve root dermatomes, 222
Shoulder
    acromioclavicular joint sprains, 363t
        clinical diagnosis, 366
        functional assessment/outcome measures, 366
        history, 364–365
        inspection, 365
        palpation, 365
        Rockwood classification, 363–364, 364f
        special tests, 365, 365f, 366f
    adhesive capsulitis, 384–385, 384t, 385f
    articulations and ligamentous support
        acromioclavicular joint, 341, 342f
        glenohumeral joint, 340, 340f, 341f
        sternoclavicular joint, 341–342, 342f
    clavicular fractures, 381–383
    evaluation
        inspection, 358
        palpation, 359
        pathology, 392, 393t–407t
        patient history, 356–358
        range of motion assessment, 358, 359t
        special tests, 360
    glenohumeral impingement, 366–372
    glenohumeral joint dislocation/subluxation, 360–363
    humeral fractures, 383–384, 383f, 383t
    labral tears, 377–379, 378f, 378t, 379f
    long head of biceps brachii strain/tear/impingement, 375–377, 376t, 377f
    peripheral nerve pathology, 385–387, 385t, 386f
    radiology and imaging, 355, 355f, 356f
    rotator cuff strain/tear, 372–373, 372t, 373f
    scapular dyskinesis, 380–381
    skeletal anatomy, 338, 339f–340f
    soft-tissue anatomy, 342–355, 343f–353f, 354f, 355f
    subscapularis muscle pathology, 374–375
Skeletal anatomy
    angles of, inclination, 166, 168f
    anteversion and retroversion, 166, 168f
    bony fusion of, pelvis, 163, 164f
Skin coloring evaluation, 486f, 487t
Skin temperature, 486
Skull fractures, 601–602
scapholunate and lunotriquetral ligament injury, 236–240, 236t, 237f, 238f, 239f, 240f
Smith fracture, 233–234
Spinal cord
    peripheral nerve damage, 561–563
    signs of, 560
    structural integrity of, 560
Spine, 564–566
    articulations
        cervical segment, 506
        intervertebral disks, 506–507, 507f
        spinal ligamentous support, 507–508, 507f–508f
    dislocation and subluxation, 556–557
    facet joint pathology, 554, 556t
    hyperextension, 521
    hyperflexion, 521
    imaging, 521, 521f
    inspection
        anterior anatomic view, 524, 524f
        cervical spine, 528
        ipsilateral rib cage, 525, 526f
        lumbar spine, 528
        mobility vs. stability, 522
        posterior view, 524–525, 525f
        postural assessment, 523, 523f
        scoliosis, 525–526, 525f–526f
        thoracic spine, 528–529
        upper and lower cross syndrome, 527–528, 527f–528f
    mobility and structural integrity, 504
    muscle strains, 521, 557–558
    muscular anatomy, 508–510, 509f, 510f
    neurologic anatomy, 513–514
    neurologic testing, 533–552
    occupational postures, 521–522

Index

palpation
    cervical spine, 528–529
    lumbar spine, 530–532
    thoracic spine, 529–530
patient-specific functional scale, 576
Roland-Morris Disability
    Questionnaire, 577
range of motion
    cervical, 530, 533
    lumbar spine, 533
Scheuermann kyphosis, 556–558
skeletal anatomy, 504–506, 504f–506f
spinal body fracture, 537, 553–554
spinal cord and nerve root injury
    peripheral nerve damage,
        561–563
    signs of, 560
    structural integrity of, 560
spinal stabilizing system, 510–511
spondylolisthesis, 553–555
spondylolysis, 553–555
vascular anatomy, 514, 515t–520t
vertebral disk injuries, 558–560, 559f
Spinous process, 420–421, 421f
Splenic injury, 472t–473t
Spondylolisthesis, 553–555
Spondylolysis, 553–555
Sport Concussion Assessment Tool-5
    (SCAT-5), 590, 596, 613–620
Sport-specific functional testing, 21
Standardized Assessment of Concussion, 596
Sternocostal joints, 421
Sternum fracture, 454t
Subdural hematoma, 605–606
Sudden cardiac death syndrome,
    463t–465t
Superior labrum anterior to posterior, 30
Supraclavicular pressure test for thoracic
    outlet syndrome, 491
Supraspinatus, rotator cuff strain/tear,
    372, 373f
Swan-neck deformity, 266f

T

Taxonomy of injury pathology
    acute injury, 10
    anatomic plane, 5, 8f
    anatomic position, 4–5, 6f
    chronic injury, 10
    common anatomic movements, 5–8,
        6t–8t
    disablement model framework, 8, 9f
    evaluation process, 5–8
    forces of, 10, 10f
    functional limitation, 9
    medical prefixes and suffixes, 4t–5t

physical maturity, 9
types of
    bone injury, 12, 12f
    bone spur, 13f
    ligament and capsular sprain, 11
    muscle and tendon strain, 11
    nerve injury, 11–12, 12f
    Salter-Harris classification, 12–13,
        13t, 13f
    wounds, 13–14
Temporomandibular joint, 581
    deviations, 596, 599
    injury, 604–605, 604t
TFCC. See Triangular Fibrocartilage
    Complex Injury (TFCC)
Thoracic outlet syndrome (TOS),
    456t–457t, 488
    Adson test for, 488t
    Allen test for, 488t
    costoclavicular syndrome tests for, 489t
    Cyriax release test for, 489t
    hyperabduction test for, 490t
    Morley sign for, 490t
    Roos test for, 491t
    supraclavicular pressure test for, 491t
    Tinel sign for, 491t
    Wright test for, 492t
Thumb ulnar collateral ligament injuries
    anatomy of, 255
    conditions causing ulnar-side wrist
        pain, 254–257, 254t, 255f,
        256f
    grading system for, 256
    stress testing of, 255, 256
    treatment of, 256
Tinel sign for thoracic outlet syndrome,
    491
Tinel test, 249
TOS. See Thoracic outlet syndrome
    (TOS)
Traumatic brain injury, 595
Triangular fibrocartilage complex (TFCC)
    injury, 242

U

Ulna fovea sign, 267
Ulnar collateral ligament, 254, 276–277
    pathology, elbow
        activities, 300, 301f
        history, 301–302
        inspections, 302
        outcome measures, 301
        palpation, 302
        special tests findings, 302, 303f
        stress test, 268
Ulnar grind test, 243, 267
Ulnar styloid, 216
Urine test for hematuria, 493–494, 496t

V

Vascular anatomy, myotome and reflex
    test, 83, 84
    obturator artery, 182, 183
    wrist and hand, 218–219
Vertebral column extension, 431t–434t
Vertebral column flexion, 426t–430t
Vertebral column lateral flexion,
    436t–439t
Vertebral column, muscles of, 424–440,
    424f–425f, 425t
Vertebral column rotation, 435t
Vertebral column stabilization, 440t
Vestibular-Ocular Motor Screening
    (VOMS), 596, 598
Volar plate avulsion fractures, 258, 258f

W

Watson scaphoid shift test, 238, 267
Wright test for thoracic outlet syndrome,
    492
Wrist and hand
    bones of, 215, 217
    case studies, 268–270
    clinical anatomy, 215–219, 218f,
        219f, 219t–221t
    compartments of, 231
    conditions of hand and fingers,
        251–257
        Bennett fracture and Rolando
            fracture, 251–252, 251f, 251t
        metacarpal fractures, 252–253,
            253t, 253f, 254f
        thumb ulnar collateral ligament
            injuries, 254–257, 254t, 255f,
            256f
    evaluation of, 224–226, 224t, 225t
        history, 224–225
        inspection, 225, 225t
        palpation, 225–226
        special tests, 226, 226f, 227f
    finger injuries, 257–266
    joints of, 217
    muscles and tendons of, 218, 219
    muscular anatomy, 217, 218f, 219f,
        219t–221t
    neurologic anatomy, 218, 222f, 222t
    radial-side wrist pain, 227–240
        de Quervain tenosynovitis and
            intersection syndrome,
            230–233, 230t, 231f, 232f, 233t
        distal radius fractures, 233–236,
            233t, 234f, 235f
        scaphoid fracture, 227–229, 227t,
            228f, 229f

Wrist and hand (*cont.*)
    scapholunate and lunotriquetral ligament injury, 236–240, 236*t*, 237*f*, 238*f*, 239*f*, 240*f*
    radiology and imaging, 219–224, 223*f*
        computed tomography, 224
        magnetic resonance imaging, 222
        radiography, 219, 221–223, 223*f*
        ultrasonography, 224
    special tests for, 266*t*–268*t*
    ulnar-side wrist pain, 240–250
        extensor carpi ulnaris tendon injury, 245–247, 245*t*, 245*f*, 246*f*, 247*f*
        hook of hamate fracture, 247–250, 248*t*, 248*f*, 249*f*, 250*f*
        triangular fibrocartilage complex injury, 240–245, 241*t*, 241*f*, 242*f*, 243*f*, 244*f*
    vascular anatomy, 218–219, 222*f*
Wrist arthroscopy, 238